Examination of Orthopedic & Athletic Injuries

FOURTH EDITION

Chad Starkey, PhD, AT, FNATA
Professor
Division of Athletic Training
School of Applied Health Sciences and Wellness
College of Health Sciences and Professions
Ohio University
Athens, OH

Sara D. Brown, MS, LAT, ATC
Clinical Associate Professor
Director, Programs in Athletic Training
Boston University
College of Health and Rehabilitation Sciences: Sargent College
Department of Physical Therapy and Athletic Training
Boston, MA

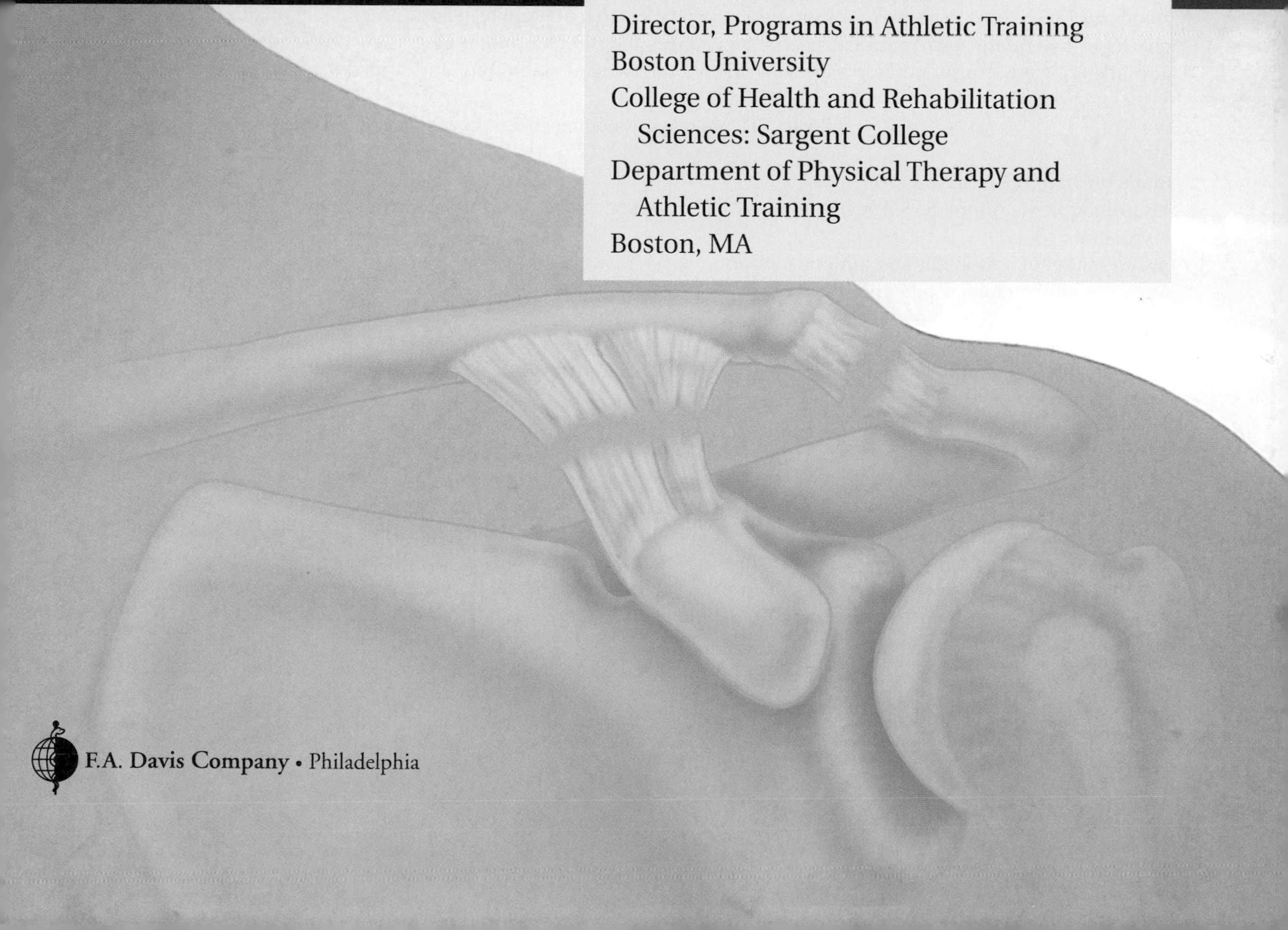

F.A. Davis Company • Philadelphia

F. A. Davis Company
1915 Arch Street
Philadelphia, PA 19103
www.fadavis.com

Printed in the United States of America

Last digit indicates print number: 10 9 8 7 6 5 4 3 2 1

Publisher: Quincy McDonald
Manager of Content Development: George W. Lang
Developmental Editor: Joanna E. Cain and Pamela Speh
Art and Design Manager: Carolyn O'Brien

As new scientific information becomes available through basic and clinical research, recommended treatments and drug therapies undergo changes. The author(s) and publisher have done everything possible to make this book accurate, up to date, and in accord with accepted standards at the time of publication. The author(s), editors, and publisher are not responsible for errors or omissions or for consequences from application of the book, and make no warranty, expressed or implied, in regard to the contents of the book. Any practice described in this book should be applied by the reader in accordance with professional standards of care used in regard to the unique circumstances that may apply in each situation. The reader is advised always to check product information (package inserts) for changes and new information regarding dose and contraindications before administering any drug. Caution is especially urged when using new or infrequently ordered drugs.

Library of Congress Cataloging-in-Publication Data

Starkey, Chad, 1959- , author.
Examination of orthopedic & athletic injuries / Chad Starkey, Sara D. Brown. — Fourth edition.
p. ; cm.
Examination of orthopedic and athletic injuries
Includes bibliographical references and index.
ISBN 978-0-8036-3918-8 — ISBN 0-8036-3918-X
I. Brown, Sara D., author. II. Title. III. Title: Examination of orthopedic and athletic injuries.
[DNLM: 1. Athletic Injuries—diagnosis. 2. Orthopedic Procedures—methods. QT 261]
RD97
617.1'027—dc23
2014041993

Whenever I put my foot in my mouth and
you begin to doubt
That it's you that I'm dreaming about
Do I have to draw you a diagram?

Chad Starkey, PhD, AT, FNATA

To my colleagues at Boston University, for your relentless curiosity, commitment to improvement, and willingness to laugh every day.

Sara D. Brown, MS, LAT, ATC

Preface

The continued evolution of health care necessitates careful changes in how we think about and approach the examination and diagnostic process for patients with orthopedic conditions. In this edition, we emphasize a patient-centered examination process using the World Health Organization's International Classification of Functioning, Disability, and Health disablement model. This model reminds us to look for connections between what the patient can and cannot do and the involved body structures and functions.

We continue to highlight the practical integration of evidence into practice. Updated information regarding the clinical usefulness of selective tissue tests and other examination techniques is presented in the associated boxes using a standardized format. Most notable, perhaps, is how little continues to be known about the validity and reliability of some of the commonly used techniques. We have added multiple new techniques that have promising or established diagnostic value. The values we present are dynamic and are not intended to supplant current systematic reviews or meta-analyses.

The values used to represent the range of scores for inter- and intrarater reliability, sensitivity, specificity, and positive and negative likelihood ratios were obtained from the references cited in the Appendix. Ranges for metrics that had 12 or more data points were calculated using the 95% confidence interval, while those having 5 to 11 data points were calculated using the interquartile range. For those tests having two to four data points, the low value, high value, and median value were reported. Instructors and students are encouraged to regularly scan the literature for the most recent information.

Integration of outcome measures into daily practice is becoming the expectation for high-quality health care. Outcome measures provide a standard approach to understanding the patient's current status, the impact of a condition on the patient's life, and the extent to which an intervention is helping the patient. This text emphasizes the incorporation of outcome measures into the examination process and connects these outcomes to a brief description of the interventions used. A new opener for each section describes commonly used patient-rated outcome measures and region-specific functional assessments, and clinician-rated outcome measures are incorporated into each chapter.

Some chapters have been reorganized, with the cervical and thoracic spine now bundled together to reflect clinical reality. The chapter on environmental conditions has been removed since this content is not typically included in courses relating to orthopedic examination. The relevant content on thoracic, abdominal, and cardiopulmonary pathologies, a stand-alone chapter in the third edition, has been redistributed to the specific systems.

The content is now organized into five discrete sections. **Section I** presents the foundations of the examination process. Chapter 1 describes the clinical examination process used, and Chapter 2 presents the on-field processes used throughout the text. Chapter 3 introduces the elements of diagnostic evidence and describes the measures commonly used for assessing outcomes (which are then presented in the relevant Section Openers). Chapter 4 gets the messy vernacular used to describe pathology out of the way and presents the examination findings of common musculoskeletal disorders (e.g., sprains, inflammatory conditions, fractures). Chapter 5 describes diagnostic imaging techniques that are often the gold standard used to confirm the clinical diagnosis. Chapters 6 (Assessment of Posture) and 7 (Evaluation of Gait) emphasize general alignment and function that can contribute to a patient's status.

Section II contains those chapters that describe the examination of the lower extremity. Although the content is presented in separate chapters, the actual clinical examination will most likely require the examination of the surrounding body parts. **Section III** presents the examination of the torso. Lumbar and sacral examination is presented in Chapter 13, while Chapter 14 covers the cervical and thoracic spine and the thorax. The upper extremity, shoulder and upper arm, elbow, wrist, hand, and fingers are covered in **Section IV**. The text concludes with **Section V**, involving injuries to the eye (Chapter 18), face (Chapter 19), and the brain and skull (Chapter 20).

The most visually striking change is the new full-color format, designed to provide still greater clarity of the pathologies and diagnostic techniques described in this text. We encourage both instructors and students to contact us with questions or comments. Chad's e-mail address is scalenes@gmail.com, and Sara's is sara@bu.edu. We also invite students and instructors to visit us on Facebook at facebook.com/EOAI4.

Contributors

Monique Mokha, PhD, ATC, LAT
Associate Professor
Division of Math, Science, and Technology
Farquhar College of Arts and Sciences
Nova Southeastern University
Fort Lauderdale-Davie, FL

Brady L. Tripp PhD, ATC
Clinical Associate Professor
Director of Graduate Athletic Training
Dept. Applied Physiology and Kinesiology
College of Health and Human Performance
University of Florida
Gainesville, FL

Reviewers

John W. Burns, MS, ATC, LAT
Program Director, Athletic Training Education
Kinesiology
Washburn University
Topeka, KS

Erin M. Jordan, MS, ATC
Clinical Instructor
Health and Kinesiology
Georgia Southern University
Statesboro, GA

Joanne Klossner, PhD, LAT, ATC
Clinical Assistant Professor
Kinesiology
Indiana University
Bloomington, IN

Heather Schuyler, MA, AT, MT, KTP
Assistant Professor
Athletic Training Education Program/ESPE
Adrian College
Adrian, MI

Bret A. Wood, MEd, LAT, ATC
Lecturer, Clinical Coordinator
Department of Kinesiology
University of North Carolina at Charlotte
Charlotte, NC

Acknowledgments

Sometimes, the actual writing seems simple when compared with the behind-the-scenes effort to produce a textbook. We thank the following people for their editorial and production assistance: Quincy McDonald, publisher; Joanna E. Cain and Pamela Speh, developmental editors of Auctorial Pursuits, Inc., and Athens' number one fan, photographer Jason Torres.

Monique Mokha, PhD, ATC, LAT was kind enough to again pen the Evaluation of Gait chapter, taking difficult laboratory concepts and contextualizing them in an easy-to-understand clinical format. Brady Tripp, PhD, ATC, LAT once again answered the call to assist us with the shoulder chapter, providing his expertise in scapular function and evaluation.

We would like to thank the many Ohio University and Boston University students and clinicians who volunteered their time to serve as models for the third and fourth editions. While the list of people involved in this process is too lengthy to include, we do need to recognize Frank Baker, Mary Wilson Connolly (YTB), Erica Dodge, Malcolm Ford, Nicole Ries, Nick Pfeifer, Dallin Tavoian, Taryn Pennington, Kristen Wells, and Amy Wyke for their time and effort. Many thanks are extended to Jessica Bennett for her organization in the scheduling and implementation of the (massive) photo shoot and surviving Chad's grumpiness prior to the shoot. We also recognize our colleagues at Coolidge Corner Imaging and Boston Medical Center, especially Dr. Akira Murakami, who provided images of injuries and their patients who sustained them.

Contents

Minimal Detectable Change: Variable based on the patient's condition

Minimally Clinically Important Difference: Variable based on the patient's condition

PROMIS®

Developed by the National Institutes of Health (NIH), the Patient Reported Outcomes Measurement Information System (PROMIS®) uses multiple instruments to assess domains of physical, mental, and social well-being. These instruments are available online at www.nihpromis.org.

Minimal Detectable Change: Variable based on the patient's condition and the instrument used

Minimally Clinically Important Difference: Variable based on the patient's condition and the instrument used

Global Rating of Change (GROC)

The patient responds to one question asked the same way during each administration: "With respect to <condition>, how would you describe yourself now compared with <sometime in the past>?" The patient marks a number on the 11-point scale:

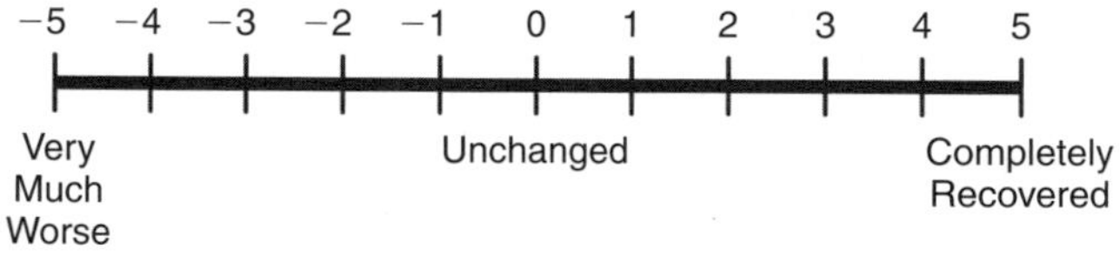

Minimal Detectable Change: 0.45 point

Minimally Clinically Important Change: 2[3]

Disablement in the Physically Active Scale

Specifically designed for use with active patients, for this scale, the patient responds to 16 questions in four domains: impairments, functional limitations, disability, and overall quality of life. Scores range from 0 to 64, with higher scores representing increased perceived disablement.[4]

Minimal Clinically Important Difference (in athletic patients with acute injuries): 9 points[5]

REFERENCES

1. Michener, LA: Patient- and clinician-rated outcome measures for clinical decision making in rehabilitation. *J Sport Rehabil*, 20:37, 2011.
2. Valovich McLeod, TC, and Register-Mihalik, JK: Clinical outcomes assessment for the management of sport-related concussion. *J Sport Rehabil*, 20:46, 2011.
3. Kamper, SK, Maher, CG, and Mackay, G: Global rating of change scales: a review of strengths and weaknesses and considerations for design. *J Man Manip Ther*, 17:163, 2009.
4. Vela, LI, and Denegar, C: Transient disablement in the physically active with musculoskeletal injuries, part 1: a descriptive model. *J Athl Train*, 45:615, 2010.
5. Vela, LI, and Denegar, C: The disablement in the Physically Active Scale, part II: the psychometric properties of an outcomes scale for musculoskeletal injuries. *J Athl Train*, 45:630, 2010.

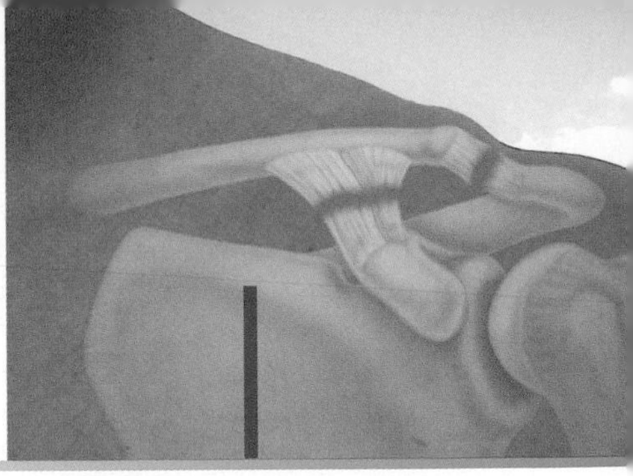

CHAPTER 1

Examination Process

Structure governs function. In the human body, anatomy is the structure, and physiology and biomechanics are the functions. To perform a competent orthopedic examination, a basic knowledge of the specific structure and function of the body part must be matched with an understanding of how these parts work together to produce normal movement (biomechanics). When injury occurs, **pathomechanics**, such as limping, may result. Conversely, an abnormal movement pattern, particularly one that is repeated thousands of times, such as a shortened stride length when running, can result in injury. The examination process consists of connecting the findings of dysfunctional anatomy, physiology, or biomechanics with the unique circumstances of the individual and correlating those findings to disruption in the patient's function.

The examination process is repeated throughout all phases of recovery. The effectiveness of the treatment and rehabilitation protocol, and subsequent modification, is based on the ongoing reexamination of the patient's functional status. Regardless of whether the examination is an initial **triage** of the injury or a reevaluation of an existing condition, a systematic and methodical evaluation model leads to efficiency, consistency, and accuracy in the evaluation process.

Some findings obtained during an examination will trigger referral to a physician for medical diagnosis and management. The examination process should always attempt to rule in or rule out these conditions. Much of the exclusionary process is intuitive: a patient who is talking is obviously breathing. Findings such as bone angulation associated with an obvious fracture may become evident during the secondary survey. Other findings such as localized numbness may become apparent later in the clinical examination. If the patient's **disposition** is not clear, err on the side of caution and refer the patient for further medical examination.

Differential Diagnosis

The differential diagnosis includes all those possible diagnoses that have not been excluded by the examination findings. As the examination continues, many pathologies are quickly excluded. For example, the patient who is walking does not have a femur fracture (ruling out a potential diagnosis). In the case of a patient with an acute ankle injury, the initial differential diagnosis must include the possibility of a fracture that must be ruled in or out during the examination process.

Following the examination, the differential diagnosis often contains more than one possible **pathology**. If arriving at a definitive diagnosis is necessary for treatment, additional testing, such as diagnostic imaging and obtaining laboratory values, is used to further narrow the differential diagnosis. In some cases, identification of the specific involved structure is not necessary (or even possible) for effective intervention. Many individuals with low back pain, for example, are diagnosed with "nonspecific low back pain."

Systematic Examination Technique

This chapter describes the examination model used in this text, one of many that are used. A comprehensive examination model must incorporate (1) the justifiable inclusion or exclusion of each step, (2) adaptability to the specific needs of the situation, and (3) the ability to rule in or rule out the possible differential diagnoses.

The examination should gather **objective data** to better organize, interpret, and monitor a patient's progress and

Triage The process of determining the priority of treatment

Disposition The immediate and long-term management of an injury or illness

Pathology A condition produced by an injury or disease

Objective data Finite measures that are readily reproducible regardless of the individual collecting the information develop treatment priorities. Baseline measurements such as pain scales obtained during the initial examination are recorded and referenced during subsequent reexaminations to document the patient's progress and identify the need for changes in the patient's treatment and rehabilitation protocol. The initial report serves as the baseline when planning the treatment and rehabilitation program.

The findings of the initial and follow-up examinations and any subsequent referrals must be documented in the patient's medical record. Besides serving a legal purpose, medical records have an important practical purpose. By using clear, concise terminology and objective findings, the medical record serves as a method of communicating the patient's current medical disposition to all who read it.

The Examination Model

For the purpose of explanation, the examination model is divided into multiple components, each with a defined objective. Each component, as well as the steps within each one, is presented sequentially, with one task completed before another is begun. Once the basic concepts are mastered, the examination sequence and content vary based on the findings obtained, and more experienced clinicians will combine tasks such as inspecting the injured area while conducting the history. Sometimes, too, findings during the examination dictate that components be omitted entirely. For example, when a long bone fracture is suspected, range of motion (ROM) of the adjacent joints should be excluded.

The goals of the examination process are to obtain a clinical diagnosis and to obtain sufficient information to determine a treatment plan that will improve the patient's quality of life. The need to consider the entire patient (and not just the injured body part) is captured in the World Health Organization's International Classification of Functioning, Disability, and Health (commonly abbreviated ICF).

The **ICF model** provides a broader framework for the examination process, encouraging the clinician to consider the patient beyond the immediate examination findings. The principles associated with the ICF model are applied in this text (Box 1-1). For example, identifying activity limitations by observing the patient performing the problematic tasks provides the foundation for the remainder of the examination. The clinical puzzle is to discover the underlying impairments to body structures and function that cause the activity limitations and result in participation restrictions.

Although the physical aspect of the examination is important, this model accounts for all aspects of a condition

Box 1-1
International Classification of Functioning, Disability, and Health

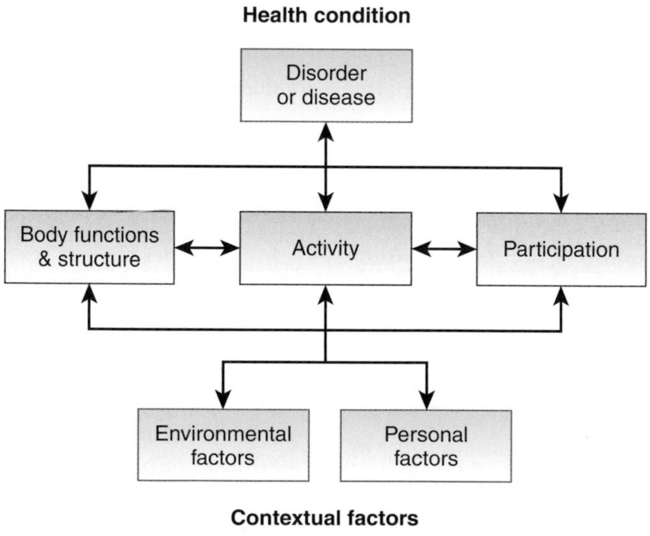

Traditional diagnostic models focus on the patient's pathology and tend to neglect the impact of the injury or illness on the person's ability to function on a personal and societal level. The International Classification of Functioning, Disability, and Health, or ICF, presents a conceptual framework demonstrating that impairments, or identified problems with body structures (anatomical parts) and functions (physiological functions), are inextricably connected to a person's activity and participation levels. Activities are those tasks or activities that are meaningful to the individual, and participation describes a person's involvement in life situations. Activity limitations and participation restrictions describe the extent to which the condition impacts a person individually and on the societal level. The model expands to provide individual context for each patient in the form of environmental and personal factors. Environmental factors are the physical and social environments in which the person lives. Personal factors describe the influence of a person's age, coping habits, social background, education, and experiences on the injury or illness experience.

Box 1-1
International Classification of Functioning, Disability, and Health—cont'd

While the examination process in this text focuses on the identification of impairments and activity limitations, doing this without understanding the resulting participation restriction leads to ineffective treatment. Likewise, not all impairments result in activity limitations. For example, a patient may have decreased ROM in a joint without impacting the ability to perform daily activities. In this example, a treatment approach that focuses on impairment-level treatment (increasing the ROM) will have limited impact on the patient's quality of life.

The following illustrates the primary components of the ICF model using a sprained knee ligament as the health condition:

	Definition	Examples of Assessment Techniques	Measurement/Finding
Health Condition	Interruption or interference of normal bodily processes or structures	Imaging Lab work	Ligament disruption
Body Structures and Functions	Structural, physiological, mental, or emotional impairments	History Pain questionnaires Instrumented testing Joint play Manual muscle tests Stress tests Selective tissue tests	Increased laxity with firm end-feel Pain at rest = 3.0/10 Pain at worst = 7.5/10
Activity Limitation	Restriction or lack of ability to perform a simple task that has meaning for the patient How the impairment(s) impacts the patient's ability to perform a task	Observation during a functional task such as walking or reaching that is necessary and/or important for the patient	Inability to go up stairs
Participation Restriction	An inability or limitation to perform in life situations	Question the patient regarding life impact. Which desired activities is the patient unable to do?	Unable to participate in football practice (but only if patient wants to participate in football)

that might influence recovery. For example, patients have a wide range of pain tolerance, apprehension, fear, and desire to return to activity. Each of these components will impact treatment and recovery, further illustrating the need to consider the patient's unique values and circumstances in the examination process.

Regional Interdependence

The concept of regional interdependence can be illustrated by walking without bending your knee. The resulting gait requires functional (movement) adaptations at the foot, ankle, hip, and lumbar spine. When prolonged aberrant motion occurs at one joint, potentially injurious stresses may be applied to the proximal and distal segments along the kinematic chain.

Historically, orthopedic diagnosis and the subsequent interventions have been derived using the biomedical model that focuses on the underlying pathology. The concept of regional interdependence recognizes that impairments in body regions other than the symptomatic one can contribute to the patient's complaints (see Chapter 6, p. 146).[1]

The Role of The Uninjured Paired Structure

The uninjured (opposite) body part provides an immediate reference point for comparison with the injured segment. In the case of an injured extremity, the patient may use the uninjured limb to demonstrate the mechanism of injury (MOI) or the movements that produce pain (Table 1-1). A portion of the history-taking process should be used to identify prior injury of the uninjured limb that could influence the bilateral comparison.

Although the role and importance of the uninjured body part are clear, where it fits into the evaluation process is not. One strategy is to perform each task on the uninjured body part before involving the injured side. The rationale for this technique is that the patient's apprehension will decrease if the evaluation is performed first on the uninjured side. The other school of thought suggests

Table 1-1 Role of the Noninjured Limb in the Examination Process

Segment	Relevance
History	**Past medical history:** Establishes preinjury health baseline and identifies conditions that can influence the current problem **History of present condition:** Replicates the mechanism of injury, primary complaint(s), activity limitations, and participation restrictions
Functional Assessment	Provides information regarding how the condition impacts the patient's ability to perform relevant tasks; may be influenced by arm dominance
Inspection	Provides a reference for symmetry, alignment, and color of the superficial tissues
Palpation	Provides a reference for symmetry of bones, alignment, tissue temperature, tissue density, or other deformity as well as the presence of increased tenderness
Joint and Muscle Function Assessment	Provides a reference to identify impairments relating to available ROM, strength, and pain with movement
Joint Stability Tests	Provides a reference for end-feel, hypermobility or hypomobility, and pain
Selective Tissue Tests	Provides a reference for pathology of individual ligaments, joint capsules, and musculotendinous units, as well as the body's organs
Neurological Test	Provides a reference for sensory, reflex, and motor function
Vascular Screening	Provides a reference for blood circulation to and from the involved extremity

that testing the uninvolved limb first may increase the patient's apprehension and cause **muscle guarding**. This text assumes that the noninjured body part will be evaluated first; however, the urgency of some acute injuries, such as joint dislocations, makes comparison with the noninjured limb irrelevant.

Clinical Assessment

The term "assessment" describes the broad array of techniques used to obtain information regarding the patient's condition and the impact of the condition on the patient's life, including physical activity. Compared with acute evaluations, clinical assessments are performed in a relatively controlled environment. In the clinical setting, the clinician has luxuries that are not available at an athletic venue, including evaluation tools (e.g., tape measures, goniometers), medical records, and, perhaps most importantly, time.

An injury evaluation normally includes physical contact between the patient and the clinician. At times, the physical contact may involve areas of the patient's body—such as the pelvic region or the chest in female patients—that call for the utmost in discretion. Regardless of the area of physical contact or the sex of the patient and clinician, the patient must always give informed consent for the clinician to perform the evaluation. Patients who are younger than 18 years old or who have a cognitive impairment that would preclude an informed consent must have their needs represented by a guardian if at all possible. A patient suffering a medical emergency may not be able to give consent for treatment. In this case, a clinician's duty to provide emergency medical care overrides obtaining consent.

History

The most informative portion of an examination is the patient's history. Identifying the MOI, appreciating the influence of any underlying medical conditions, and understanding the impact of the condition on the patient's life are examples of information obtained in this component. This process involves asking relevant questions, active listening, and note-taking.[2] Although "History" is identified as a discrete step in the diagnostic process, circumstances later in the examination may necessitate that the history be revisited, either to obtain more information or to confirm other findings.

The remainder of the examination refines the information derived from the history. The history provides information about the structures involved, the extent of the tissue damage, and the resulting activity limitations and participation restrictions. When examining acute conditions, identifying the MOI is vital to understanding the forces placed on certain structures. For chronic conditions, a determination of changes in training routines, equipment, or posture will help narrow the diagnostic possibilities and directly influence the intervention strategy.[2]

Obtaining a medical history relies on the ability to communicate with the patient. The quality, depth, and breadth

Muscle guarding Voluntarily or involuntarily assuming a posture to protect an injured body area, often through muscular spasm

Examination Map: Overview of the key elements of the examination model used throughout this text.

PAST MEDICAL HISTORY

Establish general information
- age, activities, occupation, limb dominance

Establish prior history of injury to area
- When (in years, months, days)?
- Number of episodes?
- Seen by physician or other healthcare provider?
- Immobilization? If so, how long?
- Surgery? Type?
- Limitation in activity? Duration?
- Residual complaints? (Full recovery?)
- Is this a similar injury? How is it different?

Establish general health status (medications, mental status, chronic or acute diseases, etc.)

HISTORY OF THE PRESENT CONDITION

Establish chief complaint
- What is the patient's level of function? What are the participation restrictions?
- What is the primary problem and resulting activity limitations with regard to activities of daily living (ADLs) and/or sport?
- What is the duration of the current problem?
- Mechanism of injury?
- Self-initiated treatment (ice, rest, continue to participate) and its effectiveness

Establish pain information
- Pain location, type, and pattern: does it change?
- What increases and decreases pain?
- Pattern relative to sport-specific demands

Establish changes in demands of activity and/or occupation
- Changes in activity?
- New activity pattern?
- New equipment?
- ADLs?

Other relevant information
- Pain/other symptoms anywhere else?
- Altered sensation?
- Crepitus, locking, or catching?

FUNCTIONAL ASSESSMENT

What functional limitations does the patient demonstrate?

What impairments cause the functional limitations?

Which are most problematic?

INSPECTION*

Obvious deformity

Swelling and discoloration

General posture

Scars, open wounds, cuts, or abrasions

PALPATION*

Areas of point tenderness

Change in tissue density (scarring, spasm, swelling, calcification)

Deformity

Temperature change

Texture

JOINT AND MUSCLE FUNCTION ASSESSMENT*

Active range of motion
- Evaluate for ease of movement, pain, available ranges (quantified via goniometry)

Manual muscle tests
- Evaluate for pain and weakness

Passive range of motion
- Evaluate for difference from active ROM, pain, end-feel, available range (quantified via goniometry)

JOINT STABILITY TESTS*

Stress testing
- Evaluate for increased pain and/or increased or decreased laxity relative to opposite side

Joint play
- Evaluate for increased pain and/or increased or decreased mobility relative to opposite side

SELECTIVE TISSUE TESTS*

Provocation testing
- Stress increases pain/symptoms and/or indicates instability

Alleviation testing
- Application of force decreases pain or symptoms

NEUROLOGICAL ASSESSMENT*

Sensory
- Assess spinal nerve root and peripheral nerve sensory function

Motor
- Determine spinal nerve root and peripheral motor nerve function

Reflex
- Assess spinal level reflex function

VASCULAR ASSESSMENT*

Capillary refill
- Assess for adequate perfusion

Distal pulses

Assess for adequate blood supply

DIFFERENTIAL DIAGNOSIS

Include all diagnoses that have not been excluded by the differential diagnosis process.

Ideally, the clinical diagnosis is obtained by ruling out all of the potential differential diagnoses.

DISPOSITION

rognosis
- Predict probable short- and long-term outcome of the intervention

Intervention
- Identify treatment goals (such as return to activity) based on identified impairments, activity limitations, and participation restrictions

*Compare bilaterally

of information gained from the patient's responses will correspond to the clinician's communication skills. Sociocultural differences between the clinician and patient may create an unrecognized communication barrier that can negatively influence the rest of the evaluation. An awareness of these differences can facilitate communication and improve patient care (Box 1-2).

Open-ended inquiries are useful during the history-taking process because they encourage the patient to describe the nature of the complaint in detail. Asking questions that can be answered "yes" or "no" limits the amount of information that can be deduced from the patient's response. Consider the different responses to, "Does your shoulder hurt when you raise your arm?" versus, "Tell me about what makes

Box 1-2
Culturally Competent Care

The information gained during a patient examination must be pertinent and accurate to arrive at the proper clinical diagnosis. The environmental factors described in the ICF model capture the influence of culture on an individual's response to an injury or illness. Miscommunication or misinterpretation often can occur because of differing cultural conventions between the clinician and the patient, possibly leading to an incorrect diagnosis, inappropriate care, or patient noncompliance.[3,4] To minimize this risk, clinicians should learn to:

- Involve patients in their own health care
- Understand cultural groups' attitudes, beliefs, and values as related to issues of health and illness
- Use cultural resources and knowledge to address health care problems
- Develop care plans that are holistic and include patients' cultural needs

"Culture" is the values, beliefs, and practices shared by a group and influences an individual's health beliefs, practices, and behaviors. Evaluating patients within a cultural context helps the clinician gain accurate information. It also conveys concern about the patient as a person, not as a body part or injury (e.g., "my ACL patient"). Therefore, using patient-first language, that is, addressing the patient rather than the condition is more appropriate (e.g., "my patient who has an ACL injury").

Remember that culture is present, operating, and influencing the interchange in every evaluation (whether the interaction is between members of different cultures or within the same culture). The following are some cultural aspects that must be considered during the evaluation process.

History

Clear communication between the clinician and patient is critical for taking an accurate history. Whether you are using verbal and/or nonverbal communication skills, it is important to understand the cultural context in which the exchange is occurring.

- Convey respect: Patients, particularly adult patients, are addressed formally (Miss, Mr., Mrs., Ms.) unless otherwise directed to do so by the patient.
- Language: Barriers can exist when English is spoken as a second language or if the patient does not speak English. Likewise, barriers can exist even when speaking the same language or dialect. Some communication interventions include:
  - Determine the level of English fluency.
  - Obtain the services of an interpreter, if needed.
  - Recognize that dialects are acceptable.
  - Avoid stereotyping because of language and speech patterns.
  - Clarify slang terms.
  - Use jargon-free language.
  - Use pictures, models, or materials written in the patient's language.
  - Speak more slowly, not more loudly.
  - Ask about one symptom at a time.

To ensure that the patient understands your instructions, have him or her paraphrase what you said. If you are working in a setting where other languages are spoken, consider learning the languages of the patient or obtain the services of an interpreter. If an interpreter is used, speak to, and make eye contact with, the patient, not the interpreter.

- **Verbal versus nonverbal communication:** The actions of the clinician can be just as important as what is said (or not said). If patients have difficulty understanding what you are saying, they will increase their reliance on secondary forms of communication such as body language and facial expressions. Likewise, the clinician should be familiar with assessing patients' body language from a cultural perspective, including level of eye contact and use of silence.
- **Narrative sequence:** Clinicians often ask history questions and expect answers in a chronological order. However, not all patients describe the history chronologically. Some relay what happened episodically, indicating those "episodes" or "stories" deemed important to the injury. Allow patients to respond to the question in the sequence that is comfortable for them. Taking notes will help organize the pertinent information.
- **Religious considerations:** Some religions prohibit or limit the amount of medical intervention that can occur. In organized sports, obtaining cultural information, including religious considerations, as part of the preparticipation medical examination history potentially minimizes the risk of providing unwanted or prohibited care. For example, if an acute injury situation arises where the patient is unconscious, knowledge about the patient's preferences will assist the clinician in providing care that is consistent with those preferences.
- **Family considerations:** Including immediate and extended family in the decision-making process is often important. Family members can assist with therapeutic regimens, thereby improving compliance.
- **Use of complementary and alternative medicine (CAM); traditional and folk medicines or practices:** Ask patients if they are using home remedies, traditional medicines or practices, herbal supplements, or other healthcare practices not considered a part of conventional medicine. As a clinician, you want to work cooperatively with patients, understanding and respecting their healthcare practices in order to provide the best possible care. In addition, some alternative medicines or treatments may negatively interact with mainstream medical care.

Box 1-2
Culturally Competent Care—cont'd

Inspection

When inspecting your patient, remember that differences in skin pigmentation and conditions must be considered.

- **Skin assessment (coloration and discoloration):** Skin pigmentation varies between and within cultural groups. Use enough lighting to differentiate changes in skin tone. When inspecting dark-pigmented skin for pallor, cyanosis, and jaundice, check the mucous membranes, lips, nail beds, palms of hands, and soles of feet to determine the problem.
- **Skin conditions:** Be aware that keloids, scars that form at the site of a wound and grow beyond its boundaries, are most common in African American and Asian patients. Ascertain whether the patient is prone to keloids, particularly if surgery is indicated. There may be steps the physician can take to minimize the scarring.

Issues Regarding Physical Contact

When palpating the patient, care must be taken to touch in a manner that is culturally appropriate.

- **Religious considerations:** Permission must be granted before touching any patient. In some cultures and religions, the act of physically being touched or exposing body areas may carry with it certain moral and ethical issues.
- **Gender considerations:** The standard for the "appropriateness" of touching can be influenced by the gender of the patient and the clinician. Some patients may not feel comfortable being examined by an individual of the opposite gender. If a clinician is of the opposite gender of the patient, the process should be observed by a third party (e.g., another clinician, coach, parent/guardian, or family member).

Not all individuals in a given ethnic or racial group behave the same way. The levels of acculturation and socioeconomic status are just two factors that influence healthcare beliefs and practices. Therefore, use this information as a guide during the evaluation process.

your shoulder hurt." Occasionally, however, when time is critical, such as the immediate examination of an acute, potentially **catastrophic** injury, closed-ended questions are necessary; for example, "Can you move your fingers?" (see Chapter 2).

Past Medical History

For nonacute examinations, patients or their parents are usually asked to complete medical history forms that detail baseline information such as any underlying health conditions, prior injuries, factors that might predispose them to injury, and the course of the current condition. Increasingly, clinicians are asking patients to complete questionnaires that quantify the extent and nature of the impact of a condition on a patient's life. These questionnaires provide valuable baseline information and can be repeated to determine the effectiveness of any intervention. Commonly used outcome measures are described in each Section Opener. When used over a large population, outcome measures help to identify optimal interventions.[5]

The past medical history portion of the examination includes the items below. Information such as operative reports or documentation from other providers should be reviewed.

- **Previous history:** Is there is a history of injury to this region on either side? If so, ask the patient to describe and compare this injury with the previous injury. Was the onset similar? Do the present **symptoms** duplicate the previous symptoms? Asking about injury to the entire extremity is important because injury to one structure, even though not currently symptomatic, can impact forces imposed on the adjacent, currently injured structure.

  A history of injury to the body area, prior medical conditions, and **congenital** conditions can predispose the person to further injury or influence the evaluation findings. If the injury appears to be a chronic condition or if previous injury to this body part has occurred, determine the prior medical intervention. Understanding how similar prior injuries were managed and their subsequent outcome provides a baseline reference for future diagnostic procedures and rehabilitation planning.
  - When did this episode occur? Has it reoccurred since the initial onset?
  - Who evaluated and treated this injury previously?
  - What diagnosis was made?
  - What diagnostic tests were performed? (e.g., radiographs, magnetic resonance imaging [MRI], blood work)
  - What was the course of treatment and rehabilitation?
  - Was surgery performed or medication prescribed?
  - Did the previous treatment plan change the symptoms?
  - Was there a successful return to the desired level of activity?

Catastrophic An injury that causes permanent disability or death

Symptom A condition not visually apparent to the examiner, indicating the existence of a disease or injury; symptoms usually obtained during the history-taking process

Congenital A condition existing at or before birth

- **General medical health:** What is the patient's general health status and what, if any, **comorbidities** are present? Athletes are often assumed to be in prime physical health. Unfortunately, this is not always correct. Prior physical examinations, including preparticipation and annual physical examinations, may reveal congenital abnormalities or diseases that could affect the evaluation and treatment of the injury.

The use of medications and other medical treatments now allows individuals to compete with conditions that once would have excluded them from competition. Conditions such as **cystic fibrosis**, asthma, **human immunodeficiency virus** (HIV), spastic colitis, **Crohn disease**, renal disease, hypertension, and undescended testicles may not preclude strenuous physical activity. A prudent examination involves questions regarding the existence of any underlying medical conditions and review of any existing medical records.

The **signs** and symptoms of certain tumors and other systemic pathologies may masquerade as overuse injuries, strains, sprains, and other inflammatory conditions.[6,7] For example, testicular cancer may clinically appear to be a chronic adductor injury. Patients who present with apparent musculoskeletal injuries, but are lacking a relevant history to explain the symptoms or have symptoms that fail to resolve within a typical time frame, must be promptly referred to a physician (Table 1-2). Many of these referral alerts may be first recognized during the acute (on-field) examination (see Chapter 2).

- **Relevant illnesses and lab work:** Chronic systemic illnesses or laboratory findings that can affect injury management and influence the healing process should be noted at the time of examination. For example, people with diabetes often have associated sensory and vascular deficits that delay healing and alter pain perception.
- **Medications:** What prescription or over-the-counter medications, supplements, and/or herbal remedies is the individual taking? Certain medications impede tissue healing and may interact with any medications used to treat the current condition (Table 1-3).
- **Smoking:** Cigarette smoking is associated with a decreased tolerance for exercise, an increased risk for low back pain and musculoskeletal disorders, and an increased risk for cardiovascular disease. In addition, smoking is associated with delayed fracture and wound healing.[14]
- **Family medical history:** Some conditions have a hereditary component, such as osteochondral defects, anterior cruciate ligament tears, or foot abnormalities. A family history of cardiac abnormalities and cardiac-related **sudden death** are strong predictors for **hypertrophic cardiomyopathy**, myocardial infarction, and other heart-related conditions.[15-17] The strongest indicator of an athlete's predisposition to sudden death is a family history of cardiovascular-related sudden death. The preparticipation examination's medical history questionnaire must identify any family history of cardiac-related sudden death and any such history warrants full examination by a cardiologist.

Table 1-2 Referral Alerts

Finding	Possible Active Pathology or Condition
Chest pain	Congestive heart failure
Dizziness	Myocardial infarction
Shortness of breath	Splenic rupture
Unexplained pain in the left arm	
Unexplained swelling of the ankles/legs	
Unexplained weight gain	
Unexplained weight loss	Cancer
Moles or other acute skin growths	
Slow-to-heal skin lesions	
Blood in the stool	
Unremitting night pain	
Blood in the urine	Kidney stones
Pain in the flank following the course of the ureter	Kidney/bladder infections
Low back pain associated with the above	
Loss of balance/coordination	Neurological involvement
Loss of consciousness	
Bilateral hyperreflexia	
Acute hyporeflexia	
Inability to produce voluntary muscle contractions	
Unexplained general muscular weakness	
Bowel or bladder dysfunction	
Fever, chills, and/or night sweats	Systemic disease or infection
Insidious joint or bone pain	Ankylosing spondylitis (spine)
	Rheumatoid arthritis
	Lyme disease
	Osteomyelitis
	Osteosarcoma
	Septic arthritis
	Gout
Amenorrhea	Pregnancy
Severe dysmenorrhea	Ectopic pregnancy

Comorbidities Disorder(s) unrelated to the condition for which the patient seeks assistance

Sign An observable condition that indicates the existence of a disease or injury

Sudden death Unexpected and instantaneous death occurring within 1 hour of the onset of symptoms; most often used to describe death caused secondary to cardiac failure

Table 1-3 Potential Medication Effects on Musculoskeletal Healing

Medication (or medication family)	Generic Name (trade name) Example	Potential Negative Effect
Beta-blockers	Metoprolol (Lopressor®) Propranolol (Inderal®) Atenolol (Tenormin®)	Decreased tolerance to exercise coupled with reduced perceived exertion
Corticosteroid	Methylprednisolone (Medrol®) Dexamethasone (Decadron®)	Prolonged use: Muscle weakness, loss of muscle mass, tendon rupture, osteoporosis, aseptic necrosis of femoral and humeral heads, spontaneous fractures[8]
Cox-2 Inhibitor	Celecoxib (Celebrex®)	Possible inhibition of soft tissue and bone healing[9]
Nonsteroidal Anti-Inflammatory Drugs (NSAIDs)	Ibuprofen (Motrin®) Diclofenac (Voltaren®)	The effect of NSAIDs on bone healing is unclear. Some studies indicate a delay,[10-12] but a systematic review indicated that there was no detrimental effect on bone healing.[13]
Salicylate	Aspirin	Prolonged bleeding times
Anticoagulant	Warfarin (Coumadin®)	Prolonged bleeding times

History of the Present Condition

The following information should be obtained during the history-taking process:

- **Mechanism of the injury:** How did the injury occur? The description of the MOI helps to identify the involved structures and the forces placed on them (see Chapter 4). Was the trauma caused by a single traumatic force (macrotrauma), or was it the accumulation of repeated forces (microtrauma), resulting in an **insidious** onset of the symptoms? For example, "I got hit on the outside of my knee" describes a mechanism that produces compressive forces laterally and tensile forces medially.

  For athletic injuries, practice and game videos can be used to help identify the MOI. These films may allow the medical team to actually view the mechanism and circumstances surrounding the injury.
- **Relevant sounds or sensations at the time of injury:** What sensations were experienced? Did the patient or bystanders hear any sounds, such as a "pop" that could be associated with a tearing ligament or a "crack" associated with bone fracturing? Determining the relationship between true physical dysfunction and the reported sensations is useful. For example, true "giving way" or instability would involve the subluxation of a joint (see Chapter 4). The physical sensation of a joint's giving way, but without true joint subluxation, indicates pain inhibition or weakness of the surrounding muscles.
- **Onset and duration of symptoms:** When did this problem begin? With acute macrotrauma, the signs and symptoms tend to present themselves immediately. The signs and symptoms associated with chronic or insidious microtrauma, such as **overuse syndromes**, tend to progressively worsen with time and continued stresses. In the early stages, patients with overuse syndromes complain of pain associated with fatigue and after activity. As the condition progresses, pain is also described at the onset of activity and then progresses to pain of a constant nature.
- **Pain:** Because of changes in physiology following an injury, acute injuries often have a localized "stinging" type pain. A few hours later, the pain becomes more diffuse and may be described as "burning" or "aching." Valuable outcome measures to gauge a patient's progress, the location, type, and severity of pain should be quantified and documented whenever possible (Box 1-3).
  - **Location of pain:** Ask the patient to point to the area of pain. In many cases, the location of the pain correlates with the damaged tissue. Conversely, the patient may be experiencing referred or radicular pain in a region without tissue damage. Often, following an acute injury, the patient is able to use one finger to isolate the area of pain and is more likely to isolate the involved structure or structures. As time passes following the injury, pain becomes more diffuse, and the patient tends to identify the painful area by sweeping the hand over a general area.
  - **Referred pain:** Referred pain, or pain at a site other than the actual location of trauma, can mislead the patient and the clinician as to the actual location of the pathology. Resulting when the central nervous system (CNS) misinterprets the location and source of the painful stimulus, referred pain patterns can indicate internal injury, such as when damage to the spleen results in left shoulder pain (Fig. 1-1). Musculoskeletal injury can also cause

Insidious Of gradual onset; with respect to symptoms of an injury or disease having no apparent cause

Overuse syndrome Injury caused by accumulated microtraumatic stress placed on a structure or body area

Box 1-3
Pain Rating Scales

Visual Analog Scale (VAS)

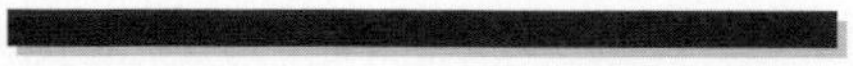

Using a 10-cm line, the patient is asked to mark the point that represents the current intensity of pain. The VAS value is then calculated by measuring the distance in centimeters from the right edge of the line.

Numeric Rating Scale (NRS)

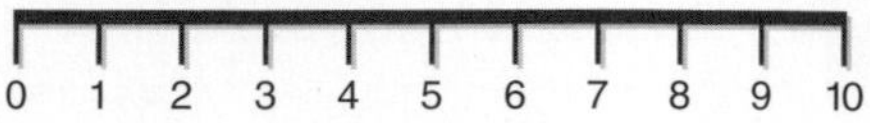

The patient is asked to circle the number from 0 (no pain) to 10 (worst pain imaginable) that best describes the current level of pain. Only whole numbers are used with this scale.

The VAS and NRS are common outcome measures that are used to quantify the amount of pain that a patient is experiencing over time. They are also useful for measuring pain before and after treatment.

McGill Pain Questionnaire

A. Where is your pain?

Using the drawing on the right, please mark the area(s) where you feel pain. Mark an "E" if the source of the pain is external or "I" if it is internal.. If the source of the pain is both internal, please mark "B".

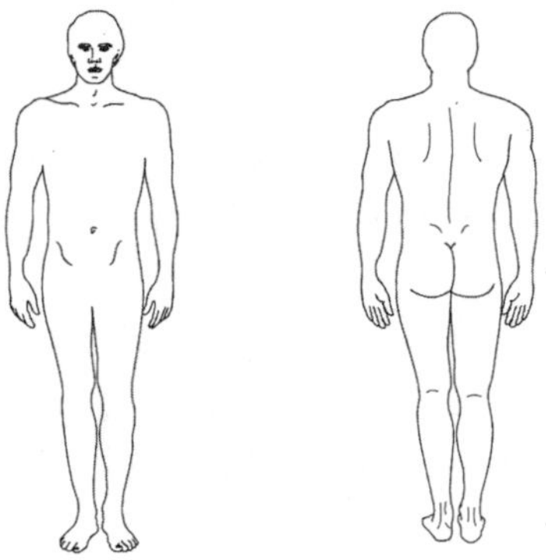

B. Pain rating index

Many different words can be used to describe pain. From the list below, please circle those words that best describe the pain you are currently experiencing. Use only one word from each category. You do not need to mark a word in every – **Only mark those words that most accurately describe your pain.**

1. Flickering Quivering Pulsing Throbbing Beating Pounding	2. Jumping Flashing Shooting	3. Pricking Boring Drilling Stabbing	4. Sharp Cutting Lacerating	5. Pinching Pressing Gnawing Cramping Crushing
6. Tugging Pulling Wrenching	7. Hot Burning Scalding Searing	8. Tingling Itchy Smarting Stinging	9. Dull Sore Hurting Aching Heavy	10. Tender Taut Rasping
11. Tiring Exhausting	12. Sickening Suffocating	13. Fearful Fightful Terrifying	14. Punishing Grueling Cruel Vicious Killing	15. Wretched Blinding
16. Annoying Troublesome Miserable Intense Unbearable	17. Spreading Radiating Penetrating Piercing	18. Tight Numb Drawing Squeezing Tearing	19. Cool Cold Freezing	20. Nagging Nauseating Agonizing Dreadful Torturing

Pain assessment instruments such as the McGill Pain Questionnaire are often used for patients who have complex pain problems. In Part A, the patient identifies the area(s) of pain and whether the pain is deep or superficial. Part B provides descriptors that the patient uses to determine the intensity and nature of the pain. A visual analog or numeric rating scale is often included as a part of the outcome measure.

Figures from Starkey, C. *Therapeutic Modalities* (ed 4). Philadelphia: FA Davis, 2013, pp. 49-50.

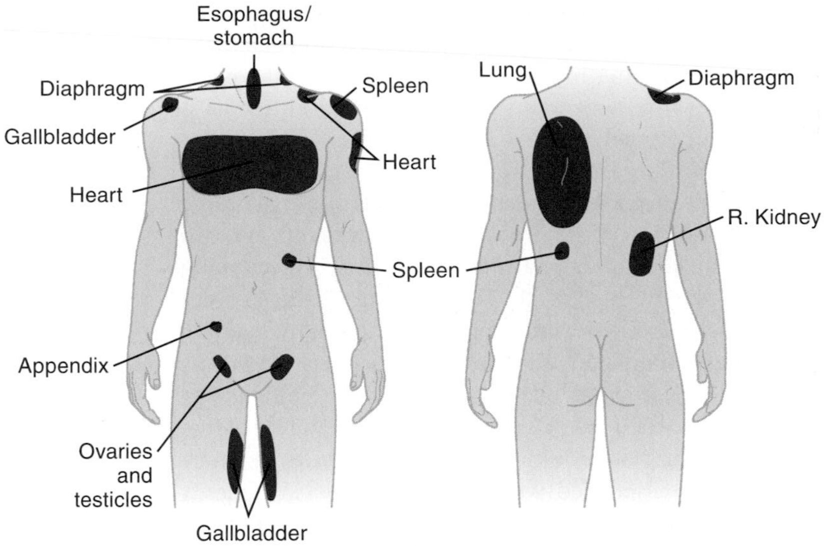

FIGURE 1-1 ■ Referred pain patterns from the viscera. Pain from the internal organs tends to radiate along the corresponding somatic sensory fibers.

referred pain, such as when rotator cuff involvement refers pain to the insertion of the deltoid muscle.

- **Radicular pain:** Radicular symptoms can result when a nerve root or peripheral nerve is compressed or otherwise damaged. Radicular pain occurs along relatively common distributions of innervation (dermatomes) and is discussed further in the appropriate chapters of this text.
- **Type of pain:** When injured, different tissues may respond by producing different types of pain. Pain associated with fractures is often described as "sharp" due to the rich innervation of the periosteum. Nerve pathology can be described as "electricity," "lightning," or "pins and needles" extending from **proximal** to **distal** (or, on rare occasions, distal to proximal) in the extremity. Sharp, localized "stinging" pain is common immediately following acute injury; with time, the pain will transition to an "aching" or "throbbing" sensation.
- **Daily pain patterns:** When during the course of the day is the pain worse? Better? What is the pattern during activity? Does the location vary throughout the day? Pain that is worse in the morning and eases as the day progresses may be associated with **tissue creep** that occurs when tissues are shortened during the night (see Chapter 4). The opposite pattern, better in the morning and worse later in the day, can be associated with muscular fatigue or prolonged compressive forces, as in the case of a herniated disc.
- **Provocation and alleviation patterns:** What activities or positions relieve and worsen the pattern? The patient's description of a position that provokes the pain may direct the sequence of the examination and also helps identify what tissues may be stretched or compressed. For example, a patient may describe the activity limitation of increased shoulder pain with overhead movement, a provoking movement that can be replicated during the ROM portion and selective tissue testing portion of the examination. Patients with a cervical disc problem may describe certain positions that decrease pain, such as lateral bending, illustrating an alleviation pattern.

- **Other symptoms:** Does the patient describe other symptoms, such as weakness or **paresthesia**? Does the limb "give out"? Does the patient complain that the extremity feels "cold," indicating possible arterial involvement, or "heavy," indicating possible venous or lymphatic involvement? Questioning the patient about the onset of symptoms such as **effusion** may help identify the involved structure.
- **Treatment to date:** Has the patient attempted any self-treatment or sought help from anyone else for this condition? A complete description of medications, alternative therapies, first aid procedures, and any other interventions such as prescription or over-the-counter foot orthotics is necessary to understand the full scope of the condition.
- **Affective traits:** Does the patient have any influences that would impede or exaggerate the desire to return

---

Proximal Toward the midline of the body; the opposite of distal

Distal Away from the midline of the body, moving toward the periphery; the opposite of proximal

Tissue creep The gradual and progressive deformation of tissues to adapt to postural changes including immobilization or pathomechanics

Paresthesia The sensation of numbness or tingling, often described as a "pins and needles" sensation, caused by compression of or a lesion to a peripheral nerve

Effusion The accumulation of excess fluid within a joint space or joint cavity to activity? Patients may understate the magnitude of their symptoms if an injury may prevent them from participating. Sometimes patients may overstate—or exaggerate—their symptoms either as a reason for poor performance or for possible financial gain.

Depression is frequently associated with chronic pain, such as with nonspecific low back pain, and can negatively impact treatment outcomes.[18] Questioning the patient specifically about recent feelings of depression and a decline in interest or pleasure in doing things can help identify those with depressive tendencies.[19] Fear-avoidance behaviors, where patients opt not to participate in a given activity due to fear of further injury or re-injury, and emotional distress may also be associated with poor outcomes in patients with chronic musculoskeletal conditions; however, treatment plans tailored to the individual may equalize outcomes.[20]

- **Resulting activity limitations and participation restrictions:** What is the patient unable to accomplish and what activities are restricted? As described in Box 1-1, the concept of connecting identified impairments with activity limitations and resulting participation restrictions is key to developing an effective intervention strategy that works for the individual. For example, a runner who experiences pain at mile 20 may not have a disability if his goals can be met with runs of 10 miles.

At the conclusion of the initial history-taking process, a clear picture of the events causing the injury; predisposing conditions that may have led to its occurrence; and the activities, motions, and postures that increase or decrease the symptoms should be formed. The impact of the injury on the patient's life should be known. The remainder of the examination is used to further investigate the findings obtained during the history-taking process. Expand on the history during the remainder of the examination, backtracking or asking further questions as you follow leads to fully ascertain all the facts regarding the patient's condition.

Physical Examination

Next in the process is the physical examination, during which the clinician continues to pare down the differential diagnosis, determine a clinical diagnosis, and identify activity limitations and underlying impairments.

Blood, synovial fluid, saliva, and other bodily fluids can potentially transmit bloodborne pathogens such as the **hepatitis B virus** (HBV) and HIV. All bodily fluids must be treated as though they contain these viruses. The treatment of acute injuries that involve bleeding, postsurgical wounds, and the handling of soiled dressings, instruments, or other blood- or fluid-soiled objects must be managed as if contaminated.

Functional Assessment

Ask the patient to perform those functional tasks that are performed regularly and/or were identified as problematic during the history-taking portion of the clinical examination. The patient might describe problems with tasks during ADLs, such as reaching or walking or during more complex tasks such as throwing a baseball. Consider the underlying impairment that could lead to the activity limitations. For example, painful or limited knee flexion can cause a compensatory hip hike to sufficiently shorten the limb while climbing stairs. The results of the functional assessment form the framework for the remaining physical examination, where the impairments are identified and measured.

Standardized, reproducible functional tests are designed to assess how the body parts work together to produce functional activity (e.g., reaching, one leg hop for distance, ROM, strength, and balance). These assessments are then expanded to replicate the activity to be performed by the patient under the precise demands faced during real-life situations (e.g., running, jumping, stair climbing, stacking boxes on a pallet). Specific functional tests, which can also serve as outcome measures, are described in the Section openers. By assessing a patient's functional status throughout the course of a condition, the relative effectiveness of an intervention can be determined.

Inspection

The inspection is a continual process that begins as soon as the patient enters the facility. Bilateral comparison of paired body parts such as the extremities or eyes must be performed when applicable, noting and exploring any deviation from the expected mirror image of the **contralateral** side.

Inspect the injured body part and compare the results with the opposite structure for:

- **Deformity:** Visual deviations from normal can be subtle, **gross**, or somewhere in between. Some fractures and joint dislocations result in gross deformity, with angulation or clear disruption of normal joint contour. Signs of joint displacement or bony fracture warrant ruling out any other significant trauma, appropriate splinting, and the immediate referral to a physician. This process is explained further in Chapter 2.

  Careful bilateral inspection may reveal differences in otherwise healthy-looking body parts (Fig. 1-2).
- **Swelling:** Any enlargement of a body part can be subtle or dramatic and occur rapidly or over time. The onset, look, and feel of a swollen body part can help identify

Contralateral Pertaining to the opposite side of the body or the opposite extremity

Gross Visible or apparent to the unaided eye

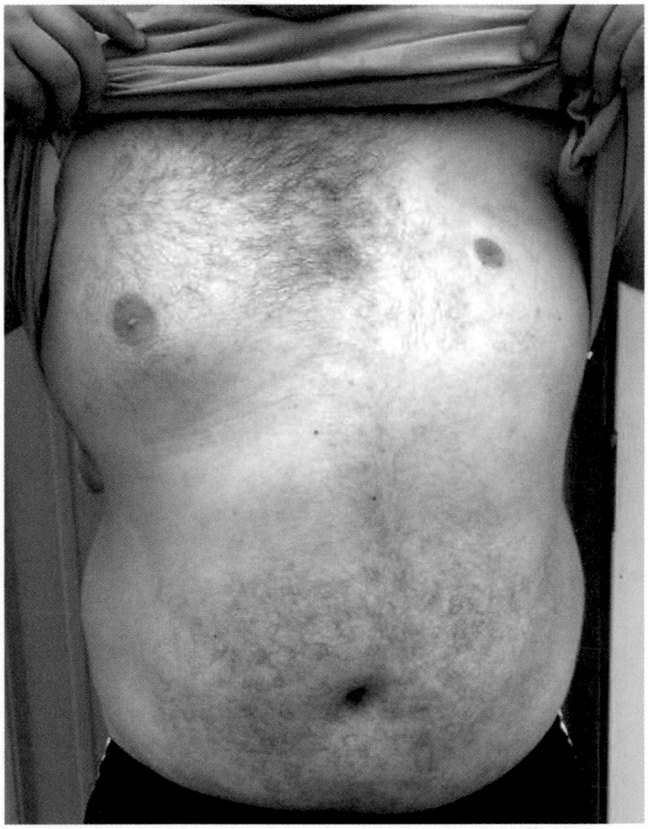

FIGURE 1-2 ■ What's wrong with this picture? (The answer is given in the legend of Fig. 1-3.) The patient has decreased scapular control. There is no history of trauma to the body area. Carefully observe this picture to determine the cause of the lack of scapular control.

the nature of injury. Increased girth (volume) across the joint line relative to the opposite limb suggests the presence of swelling. Increased girth across muscle mass is indicative of hypertrophy or edema; decreased girth across muscle mass is indicative of atrophy.

For example, an acute joint effusion resulting from a **hemarthrosis** is typically readily apparent. Joint swelling that forms over a number of hours or days is most likely the result of excess synovial fluid production. **Edema** resulting from a tibial stress fracture can be slight and localized. The amount of swelling can be measured in a quantifiable manner using girth measurements (Selective Tissue Tests 1-1) or volumetric measurements (Fig. 1-3). Girth measurements require less equipment and demonstrate high interrater reliability, and results closely represent the results of volumetric measurements.[21-23]

*** Practical Evidence**

When used to determine muscle volume, most body-composition methods, including girth measurements, tend to be more accurate on males than females because of the overlying adipose tissue layer in females.[24] Intrarater and interrater reliability of girth measurement are significantly improved when landmarks are consistently identified and used.

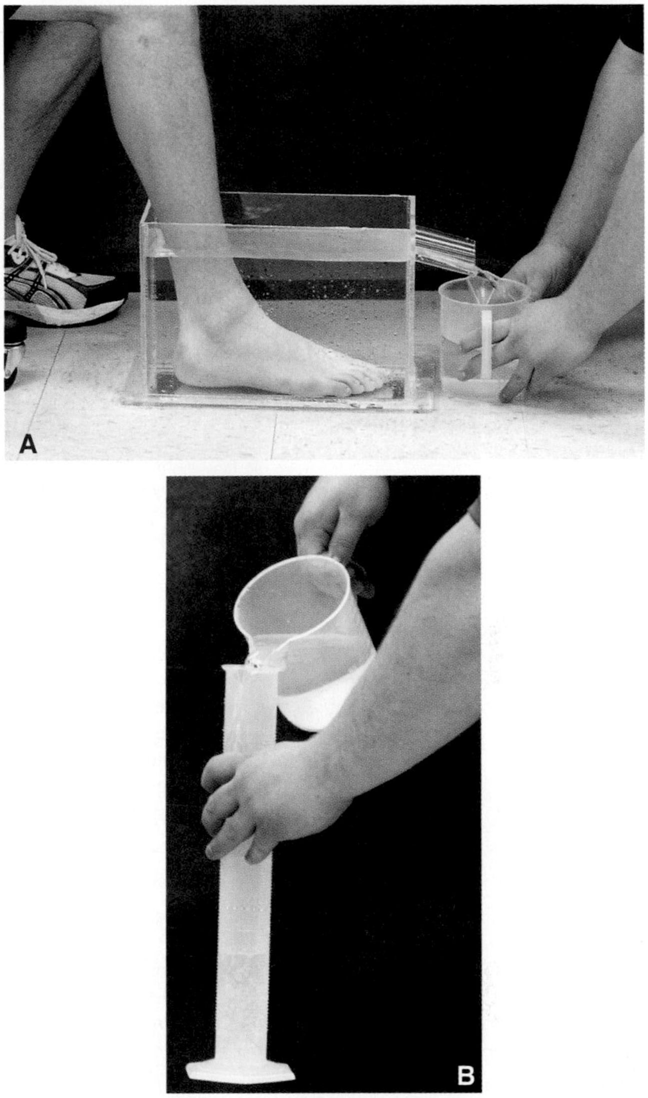

FIGURE 1-3 ■ Volumetric Measurement. (A) The tank is filled with water up to the specified level and the limb is gently immersed. (B) The overflow water is collected and poured into a calibrated beaker to determine the mass (volume) of the limb. This measurement is obtained by either reading a graduate cylinder or, more accurately, by weighing the water expelled. Volumetric measurement of limb volume is most commonly used as a research tool, but can provide important clinical information. Answer to Figure 1-2: The patient is missing his left pectoralis minor muscle.

- **Skin:** Does the area show redness that may be associated with inflammation? Is **ecchymosis** present, indicating a contusion or other **soft tissue** disruption? Is the ecchymosis located at or distal to the injured structure? Ecchymosis located distal to the site of injury indicates pooling of the blood secondary to the effects of gravity. Are there any open wounds that warrant referral or first aid? Are there signs of

---

Hemarthrosis Bleeding into a joint cavity

Edema The collection of fluids in the intercellular spaces

Ecchymosis A blue or purple area of skin caused by blood escaping into the extravascular spaces under the skin

Selective Tissue Test 1-1
Ankle Girth Measurement

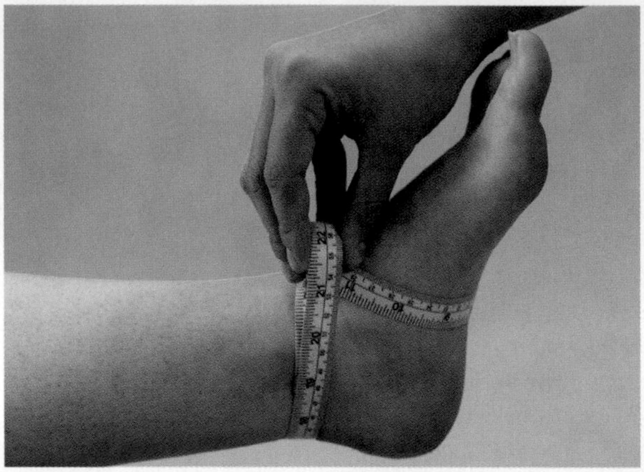

Girth measurements provide a quantifiable and reproducible measure of a limb's volume.

Patient Position	Supine
Position of Examiner	Standing to access the body part
Evaluative Procedure	Do not use a measuring tape made of cloth. (They tend to stretch and fade.) To measure ankle girth, use a figure-8 technique with the patient's ankle in 20° of plantarflexion. Position the zero point of the tape measure at the anterior edge of the medial or lateral malleolus. Circle the tape medially around the foot to the fifth metatarsal and then continue around the medial malleolus to return to the start point. **1.** Pull the tape snugly and read the circumference in centimeters or inches. **2.** Take three measurements and record the average. **3.** Repeat these steps for the uninjured limb.
Positive Test	A significant difference in the girth (volume) between the two ankles
Implications	The minimal clinically important difference is approximately 1 cm.[23]
Evidence	

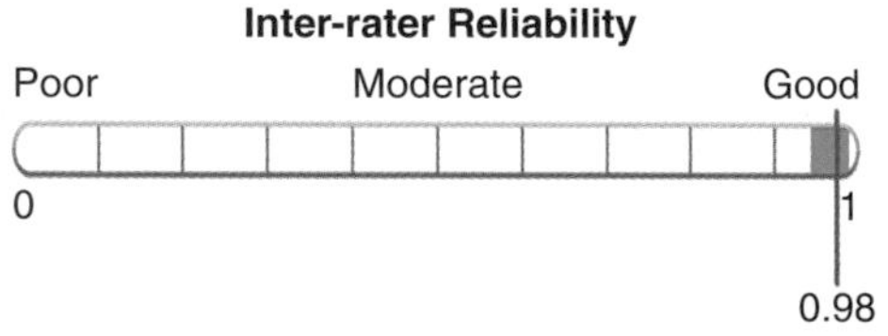

previous trauma or surgical scars that have not been explained in the history? Dark-skinned individuals are at an increased risk of hypertrophic scarring (excessive scar formation that does not grow beyond the wound boundaries) or keloids (irregularly shaped scars that exceeds the boundaries of the original wound).[25]

- **Infection:** Does the body area show signs of infection (e.g., redness, swelling, pus, red streaks, swollen **lymph nodes**)? Infections can occur in both open and closed wounds. Red streaks that follow the lymphatic system necessitate immediate physician referral.

Palpation

Palpation, the process of touching and feeling the tissues, allows the examiner to detect tissue damage or change by comparing the findings of one body part with those of the opposite one. It also helps to identify areas of point tenderness. Palpation is performed bilaterally and in a specific

Lymph nodes Nodules located in the cervical, axillary, and inguinal regions, producing white blood cells and filtering bacteria from the bloodstream. Lymph nodes become enlarged secondary to an infection.

sequence, beginning with structures away from the site of pain and progressively moving toward the potentially damaged tissues. Thus, different potential sources of pain can be ruled out, and possible involved secondary structures can be identified. While assessing pulse and sensation technically involves palpation, these assessments are typically classified with other parts of the examination.

One method of sequencing is to palpate the bones and ligaments first, then palpate the muscles and tendons, and then, finally, locate any other areas such as pulses. The second form of sequencing is to palpate all structures (e.g., bones, muscles, ligaments) farthest from the suspected injury and then palpate progressively toward the injured site. Regardless of the palpation strategy used, a thorough knowledge of topical anatomy is crucial to ensure that the connection is made between the location of the finding and the associated structure. Some examination models delay the palpation process until the end of the evaluation because this is often the most painful aspect of the evaluation. Excess pain with palpation can produce apprehension, causing the patient to guard the area and thus altering the remainder of the evaluation.

During the palpation, make note of the following potential findings:

- **Point tenderness:** Begin with gentle and progressively increasing pressure, visualizing the structures that lie beneath your fingers. Certain areas of the body (e.g., the anatomical snuff box in the wrist, orbital rim, costochondral joints) are normally tender. To be a meaningful finding, palpation should elicit increased tenderness of the structure relative to the surrounding structures and the same structure on the opposite side of the body.
- **Trigger points:** A trigger point is a hypersensitive area located in a muscle belly that, when irritated as during palpation, refers pain to another body area. Trigger points feel like small nodules within the tissue. The cause-and-effect relationship between the symptoms and the patient's pathology should be determined.
- **Change in tissue density:** Determine any differences in the density or "feel" of the tissues, possibly indicating muscle spasm, hemorrhage, edema, scarring, heterotropic ossification, or other conditions (Table 1-4).

Table 1-4 Possible Causes of Changes in Tissue Density

Tissue Feel	Possible Cause
Spongy, boggy over a joint	Synovitis
Thickened, warm	Blood accumulation, infection
Dense thickening	Scar tissue formation
Dense/viscous	Pitting edema
Increased muscle tone	Muscle spasm, muscle hypertrophy
Hard	Bone or bony outgrowth (exostosis)

- **Crepitus:** Note a crunching or crackling sensed with the rubbing of tissues. Termed *crepitus*, this may indicate a fracture when felt over bone or inflammation when felt over a tendon, bursa, or joint capsule. **Crepitus** is sometimes audible such as when bony fracture sites grind against each other or when air enters the tissues after an orbital fracture or pneumothorax.
- **Tissue temperature:** Feel for an altered temperature of the injured area relative to the surrounding sites. An increased temperature is typical during an active inflammatory process such as one that occurs following an acute injury or in the presence of infection. A decreased temperature is associated with vascular insufficiency.

Joint and Muscle Function Assessment

The results of active and passive ROM assessments and manual muscle testing help quantify impairments that contribute to functional changes. As with all evaluation tools, bilateral comparison is used, and, when possible, results are compared against established **normative data**. The examination includes assessment of all available motions at the involved joint and the joints proximal and distal to the affected area. Pain and/or dysfunction proximal or distal to the involved structure can change the stress on that tissue and must be addressed for full recovery.

Common terminology such as *flexion, extension, abduction*, and *adduction* describes most joint motions. Some joint motions, such as ankle inversion, are unique to specific joints. These specific motions are discussed in the individual chapters.

The evaluation of active and passive ROM may be made by gross observation or, more precisely, objectively measured with the use of a goniometer or inclinometer (GON 1-1). The patient's age and gender influence ROM. In the high school and college-aged population, women have a greater ROM in all planes than do men. Age-related ROM decreases in women are generally small, with a notable exception of progressively decreasing glenohumeral external rotation.[26]

Active Range of Motion

Joint movement occurs through physiological and accessory motions. Active range of motion (AROM), joint motion produced by the patient contracting the muscles, assesses physiological motion and osteokinematics. AROM is evaluated first unless it is **contraindicated** by immature fracture sites or recently repaired soft tissues. Accessory motions, or arthrokinematics, are those patterns that must occur for normal osteokinematic motion but are not under voluntary control. For example, to flex the glenohumeral

Normative data Normal ranges of data collected for comparison during the evaluation of an athlete. On many measures, athletes have norms different from the general population.

Contraindication (contraindicated) Procedure that may prove harmful given the patient's current condition

Goniometry 1-1
Goniometer Use Guidelines

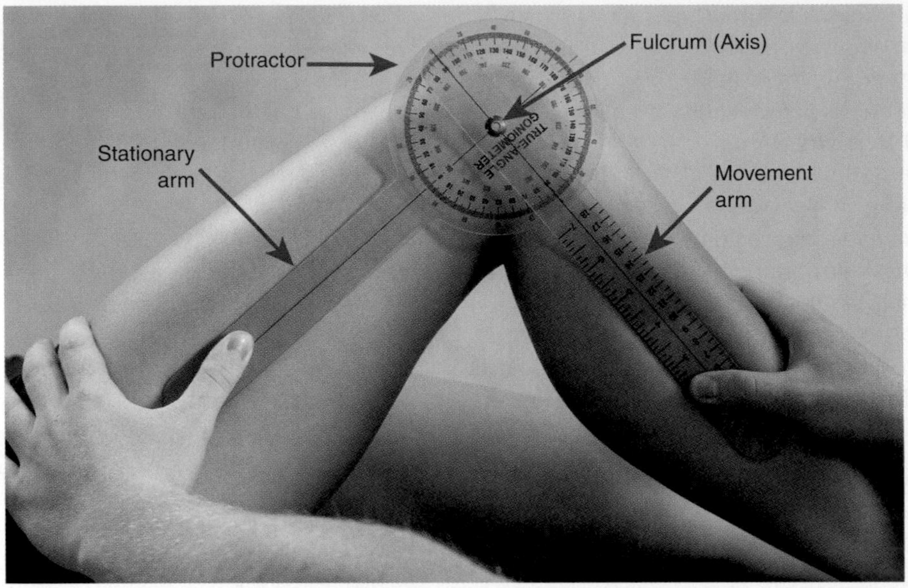

With proper training and practice, goniometers can yield accurate and quantifiable measures of a patient's active and passive ROM. Each joint has different landmarks for the fulcrum, stationary arm, and movement arm. ROM may also be measured using inclinometers or electronic goniometers and also via smartphone apps.[27]

Goniometer Segments	*Protractor:* Measures the arc of motion in degrees. Full-circle goniometers have a 360° protractor; half-circle goniometers have a 180° protractor. *Fulcrum:* The center of the axis of rotation of the goniometer *Stationary arm:* The portion of the goniometer that extends from, and is part of, the protractor *Movement arm:* The portion of the goniometer that moves independently from the protractor around an arc formed by the fulcrum
Procedure	**1.** Take the joint through the motion passively, assessing the end-feel and estimating ROM. **2.** Select a goniometer of the appropriate size and shape for the joint being tested. **3.** Position the joint in its starting position. **4.** Identify the center of the joint's axis of motion. **5.** Locate the proximal and distal landmarks that align with the joint's axis of motion. **6.** Align the fulcrum of the goniometer over the joint axis. **7.** Align the stationary arm along the proximal body segment and the movement arm along the distal segment. **8.** Read and record the starting values from the goniometer. **9.** Move the distal joint segment through its ROM. **10.** Reapply the goniometer as described in Steps 5 and 6. **11.** Read and record the ending values from the goniometer.
Recording Results	There are several different methods and documentation forms for recording goniometric data. Most systems use the neutral position as "0" and document the amount of motion from this point. For example, 10° of knee extension and 120° of knee flexion would be recorded as: **10°–0°–120°** In a case where the patient is unable to obtain the starting ("0") position, zero is the first number cited or is omitted. For example, a limitation in the ROM, lacking 10° of knee extension, would be recorded as: **0°–10°–120°** or **10°–120°** Do not use negative numbers.

joint (osteokinematics), the humeral head must slide inferiorly (arthrokinematics). Accessory motions are assessed using joint play (p. 22).

First evaluating the AROM determines the patient's willingness and ability to move the body part through any or all of the ROM. An unwillingness to move the extremity could signify extreme pain, neurological deficit, or possible **malingering**.

While the joint is actively moved through all the possible motions in the cardinal planes, observe the ease with which the movement is made and the total ROM obtained (Fig. 1-4). Also note any compensation or abnormal movement in the surrounding structures. The patient may verbally or nonverbally describe a **painful arc** within the ROM, representing compression, impingement, or abrasion of the underlying tissues.

Manual Muscle Testing

Manual muscle testing (MMT) is used to assess for strength and provocation of pain by relatively isolating muscles or groups of muscles. True isolation of a muscle, where no other muscles are active, is not possible to achieve clinically, but EMG analysis can assess the positions in which muscles are most active. These positions are used for MMT.

Resisted range of motion (RROM), alternatively, assesses gross strength of an entire muscle group throughout a cardinal plane of motion. Often, movements assessed during manual muscle testing are the same as those assessed with RROM. For example, strength of the quadriceps is assessed using knee extension. While RROM is used to assess the strength of muscle groups throughout the full ROM within the cardinal planes, its usefulness is relegated to determining a general weakness. Any evoked pain cannot be attributed to muscle because other tissues are stressed. MMTs are described throughout this text.

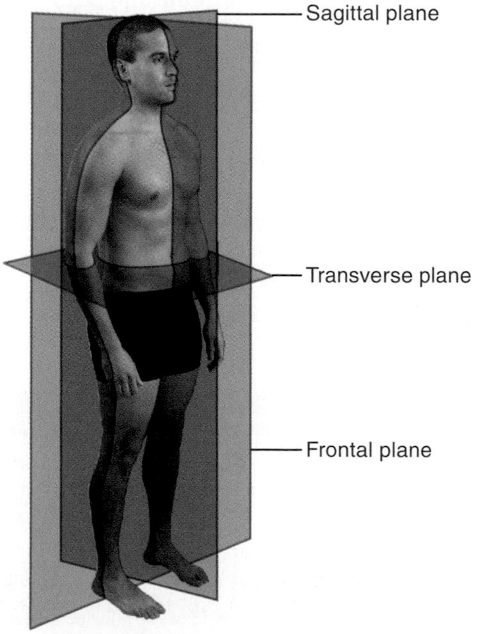

FIGURE 1-4 ■ The cardinal planes of the body. The sagittal plane divides the body into left and right sides. The transverse plane bisects the body into superior and inferior or proximal or distal segments. The frontal (coronal) plane divides the body into anterior and posterior segments. Movement in the frontal plane occurs around an anterior–posterior axis; movement in the sagittal plane occurs around a medial–lateral axis; movement in the transverse plane occurs around a vertical axis.

* Practical Evidence

Because of the relative lack of testosterone, girls are typically weaker than boys from the age of 9 and beyond.[28] Strength normally increases with age until 20 to 30 years. In the fifth or sixth decade of life, the rate of muscle strength decay increases.[29]

Isometric MMT performed in the midrange of the joint's ROM, also known as a **break test**, better differentiates between muscle pathology and injury of noncontractile tissues such as ligaments. Noncontractile tissues are less likely to be taut in a joint's midrange. Instrumented testing such as a handheld dynamometer allows the muscle force being generated to be quantitatively assessed.

The ability to perform AROM serves as the foundation for grading manual muscle tests. The ability to perform pain-free AROM against gravity would receive a minimum score of "Fair" or "3/5" as gravity is providing resistance to the motion. If the patient were unable to achieve a grade of Fair, the position would be changed to reduce the effects of gravity. If the patient is able to achieve a grade of Fair, then resistance is progressively added to determine the final grade. With the exception of identifying neurological involvement, the use of these grading scales to quantify strength in athletes and others involved in strenuous physical activity is rarely beneficial (Fig. 1-5). Multiple repetitions of a single test may be needed before weakness is apparent, particularly when the patient notes that symptoms are present only when fatigue is a contributing factor.

Manual muscle tests (MMTs) are useful in determining the strength of muscles and muscle groups when administered by highly trained personnel, but they are prone to low interrater and intrarater reliability measures, especially for grades 4 and 5 (Manual Muscle Test 1-1).[30] Procedural consistency using standardized positions, hand placements, and instructions to the patient is important for maximum reliability and validity during MMTs.

During manual resistance, the limb is stabilized proximally to prevent other motions from compensating for weakness of the involved muscle. Resistance is provided distally on the bone to which the muscle or muscle group attaches, not distal to a second joint. **Compensation** occurs when postural changes are used to substitute for a loss of motion or weakness, such as using shoulder girdle elevation to compensate for a loss of glenohumeral abduction. Compensation may also occur through muscular **substitution**, especially by more proximal muscle groups, as the patient attempts to overcome weaknesses of the muscle being

---

Malingering Faking or exaggerating the symptoms of an injury or illness

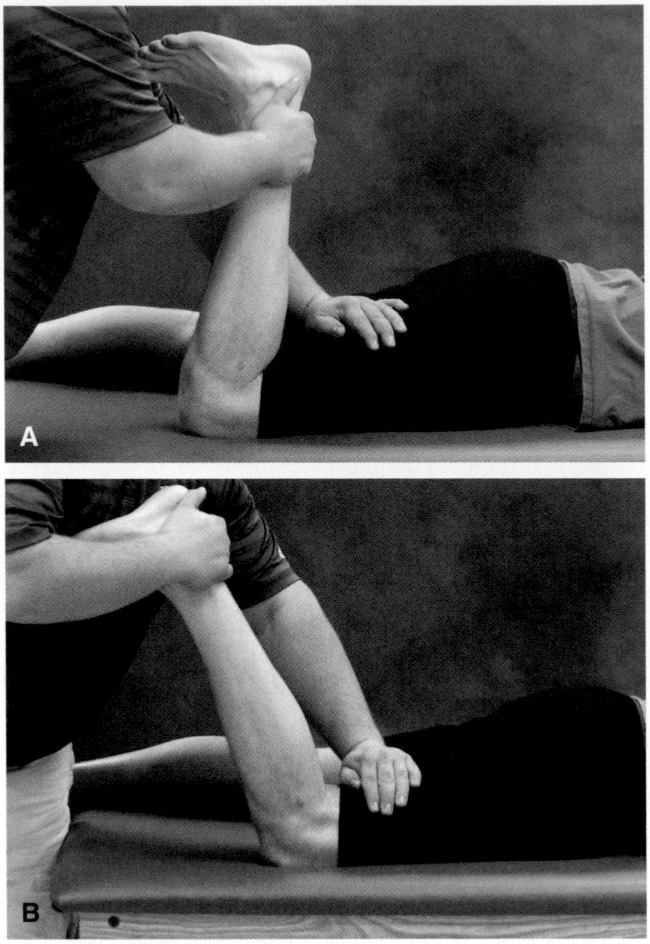

FIGURE 1-5 ■ Manual muscle test of the hamstring muscle group. (A) When the knee is flexed beyond 90° in the prone position gravity assists the motion of the hamstrings. (B) If the knee is flexed less than 90° the hamstring muscles must work to overcome both gravity and the examiner's manual resistance.

tested by recruiting other muscles (e.g., upper trapezius recruitment during shoulder abduction to compensate for a torn supraspinatus tendon). When the patient uses compensatory motions, the amount of resistance used against the contraction should be reduced and the patient's MMT grade reduced accordingly.

✱ Practical Evidence

The clinical relevance (and interrater reliability) of manual muscle testing are improved when muscle strength is described as "normal" or "not normal" rather than ordinal grading systems such as 0 to 5.[31]

Passive Range of Motion

After muscle function is assessed, passive range of motion (PROM), where the clinician moves the joint through the ROM, is evaluated for the quantity of available movement as compared with AROM and changes in the pain pattern. **Overpressure** should be applied at the end of the ROM to identify the **end-feel** that indicates which type of structures are stressed at the terminal ROM. The different end-feels as established by the Cyriax method are listed in Table 1-5.[32] Certain movements have particular normal end-feels (e.g., elbow extension should have a hard or bony end-feel). Knowledge of these end-feels is necessary to identify pathological limits to ROM (Table 1-6).

A capsular pattern is the characteristic loss of motion caused by shortening or adhesions of the joint capsule. Each synovial joint has a unique capsular pattern. Full joint motion cannot occur if the capsular fibers are shortened. Noncapsular patterns occur when nonjoint capsular structures are involved. The capsular patterns for the major joints of the body are described in the relevant chapters of this text.

Useful information can be obtained by comparing the range of movement obtained for AROM with that obtained for PROM. Typically, PROM is greater than AROM. When AROM and PROM are equal and both fall short of the expected ROM, capsular adhesions or joint tightness may be restricting the motion. AROM that is less than PROM signifies a muscular weakness or a lesion within the active **contractile tissue** that is causing pain and inhibiting motion. Although data exist describing normal ROM, this information may not be helpful in determining whether a functionally sufficient amount of range is available for the

Contractile tissue Muscle tissue

Table 1-5 Physiological (Normal) End-Feels to PROM

End-Feels	Structure	Example
Soft	Soft tissue approximation	Knee flexion (contact between soft tissue of the posterior leg and posterior thigh)
Firm	Muscular stretch	Hip flexion with the knee extended (passive elastic tension of hamstring muscles)
	Capsular stretch	Extension of the metacarpophalangeal joints of the fingers (tension in the palmar capsule)
	Ligamentous stretch	Forearm supination (tension in the palmar radioulnar ligament of the inferior radioulnar joint, interosseous membrane, oblique cord)
Hard	Bone contacting bone	Elbow extension (contact between the olecranon process of the ulna and the olecranon fossa of the humerus)

From: Norkin, CC, and White, DJ: *Measurement of Joint Motion: A Guide to Goniometry* (ed 4). Philadelphia: FA Davis, 2009.

Manual Muscle Test 1-1
Muscle Testing Guidelines

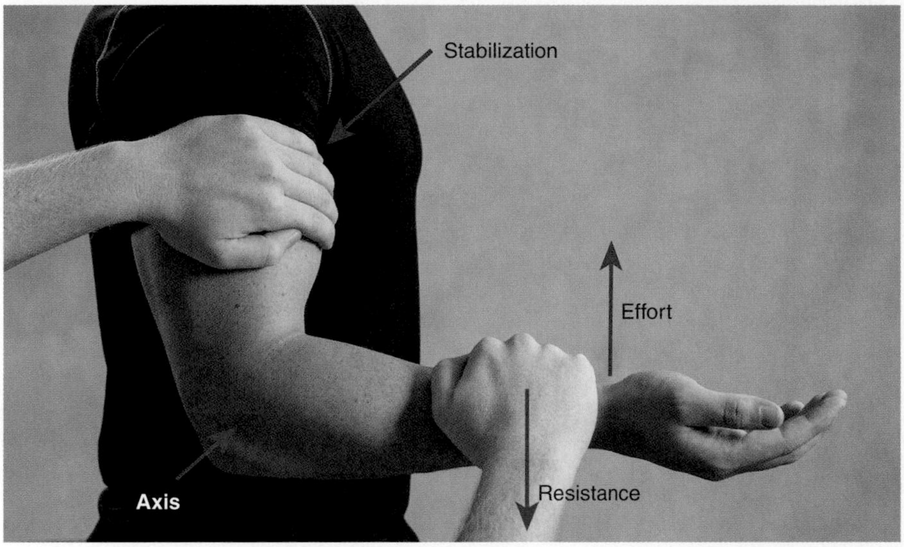

These procedures are used when attempting to isolate an individual muscle or muscle group (manual muscle test). Specific techniques are described in the appropriate chapters throughout this text.

Patient Position	Position the patient so that the muscle(s) tested must work against gravity.
Position of Examiner	As needed to stabilize proximal to the joint being tested and provide resistance distal to the joint
Evaluative Procedure	**1.** Provide stabilization proximal to the joint to isolate the joint to the motion/muscle(s) being tested. Do not apply resistance at this point. **2.** Instruct the patient to perform the requested motion, such as elbow flexion with the forearm supinated. **3.** If the patient is able to complete the ROM against gravity, a starting grade of "Fair" or "3" is assigned. **4.** Position the joint in the mid-ROM and apply resistance. Instruct the patient, "Don't let me move you." Gradually increase the resistance. **5.** Apply resistance as far away as possible from the target joint without crossing the distal joint. **6.** Ensure that the muscles distal to the joint being tested are relaxed. **7.** If the patient is unable to complete the ROM against gravity, reposition the body part to a gravity-eliminated position and request that the patient attempt to perform AROM again.
Positive Test	Weakness and/or pain compared with the contralateral side
Implications	A numerical or verbal grade is assigned as follows: *Normal (5/5)* The patient can resist against maximal pressure. The examiner is unable to overcome the patient's resistance. *Good (4/5)* The patient can resist against moderate pressure. *Fair (3/5)* The patient can move the body part against gravity through the full ROM. *Poor (2/5)* The patient can move the body part in a gravity-minimized position through the full ROM. *Trace (1/5)* The patient cannot produce movement, but a muscle contraction is palpable. *Zero (0/5)* No contraction is felt.

AROM = active range of motion; ROM = range of motion

Table 1-6 Pathological (Abnormal) End-Feels to PROM

End-Feels	Description	Example
Soft	Occurs sooner or later in the ROM than is usual or occurs in a joint that normally has a firm or hard end-feel; feels boggy	Soft tissue edema Synovitis
Firm	Occurs sooner or later in the ROM than is usual or occurs in a joint that normally has a soft or hard end-feel	Increased muscular tone, capsular, muscular, ligamentous shortening Osteoarthritis
Hard	Occurs sooner or later in the ROM than is usual or occurs in a joint that normally has a soft or firm end-feel; feels like a bony block	Loose bodies in joint Heterotopic ossification Fracture
Spasm	Joint motion is stopped by involuntary or voluntary muscle contraction.	Inflammation Muscle tear Joint instability
Empty	Has no real end-feel because end of ROM is never reached owing to pain; no resistance felt except for patient's protective muscle splinting or muscle spasm	Acute joint inflammation Bursitis Abscess Fracture Psychogenic origin

From: Norkin, CC, and White, DJ: *Measurement of Joint Motion: A Guide to Goniometry* (ed 4). Philadelphia: FA Davis, 2009.

individual. For example, consider a gymnast who must have 0 to 140 degrees of hip flexion (as opposed to the normal value of 0 to 120 degrees) in order to execute a move. Even if the patient is able to complete full AROM, PROM should be performed with emphasis on the quality of the end-feel.

✱ Practical Evidence

The consistency of the findings between multiple clinicians (interrater reliability) for lower extremity PROM is poor. Much of the difference is accounted for by the wide variation of situations in which PROM is assessed.[33]

Joint Stability Tests

Joint stability is provided by contractile and noncontractile tissue, including ligaments and the joint capsule. The contribution of these noncontractile tissues to joint stability is assessed by stress testing and joint play. Stress testing isolates specific ligaments and/or portions of the joint capsule, while joint play assesses accessory motions, those motions that are essential for normal physiological movement.

Joints may be either **hypermobile** (having more laxity than the norm) or **hypomobile** (having mobility that is considered below the normal limits). Joints must have an appropriate amount of accessory motion for proper motion to occur. However, some adaptations may occur normally as the result of repeated activity. Athletes may demonstrate expected mobility patterns in some joints. For instance, baseball pitchers tend to have an increased amount of glenohumeral external rotation and a decreased amount of internal rotation than the rest of the population.

Testing involves the application of a specific stress to a noncontractile tissue to assess its laxity. However, a distinction must be made between laxity and instability. Laxity is a clinical sign, and instability is the symptom. Laxity describes the amount of "give" within a joint's supportive tissue (Fig. 1-6). A person may have congenital laxity throughout all joints as determined by generalized measures. One indicator is the ability to pull the thumb to the forearm (Fig. 1-7). Instability is a joint's inability to function under the stresses encountered during functional activities. The amount of joint laxity does not always correlate with the degree of joint instability.[34] The case of laxity in the absence of reported instability illustrates an identified impairment without an activity limitation.

To limit the potential splinting effects of patient apprehension, joint stability tests should first be performed on the injured limb and then the uninjured extremity.[35]

Stress Testing

Ligamentous stress testing is used to identify the presence of joint laxity. Sprains are graded on a three-degree scale that is based on the amount that the joint opens and the quality of the **endpoint** relative to the opposite uninvolved, uninjured joint (Table 1-7).

End point The quality and quantity at the end of motion for any stress applied to a tissue

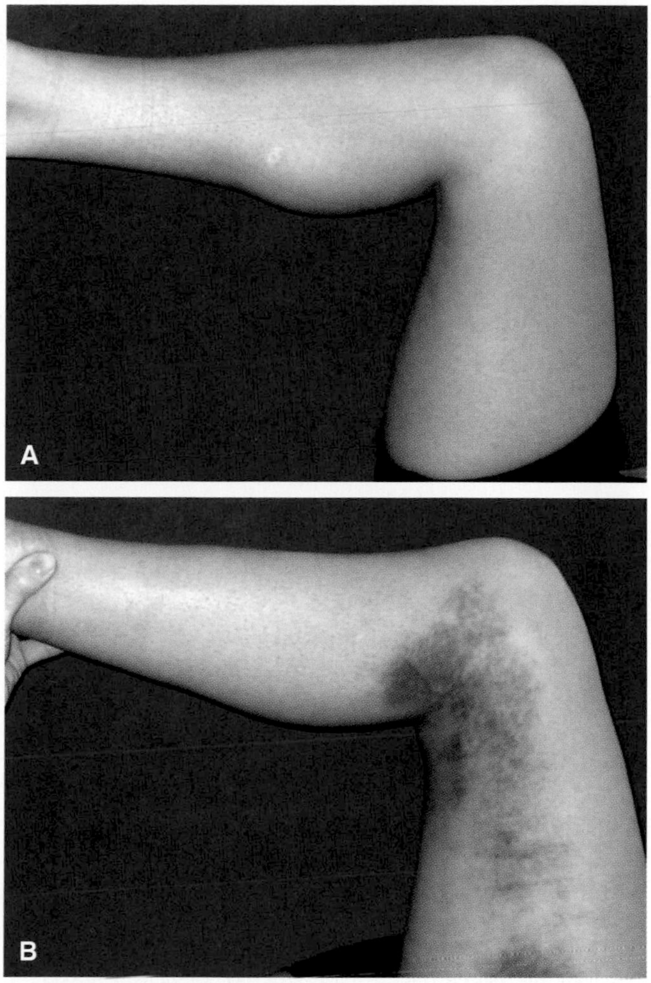

FIGURE 1-6 ■ Clinical laxity. As demonstrated by the Godfrey Test, the posterior cruciate ligament (PCL) supports the tibia when the patient is lying supine with the hip and knee flexed to 90 degrees (A). The ankle is supported by the examiner. (B) When the posterior cruciate ligament is torn, the proximal tibia sags inferiorly (see Chapter 10).

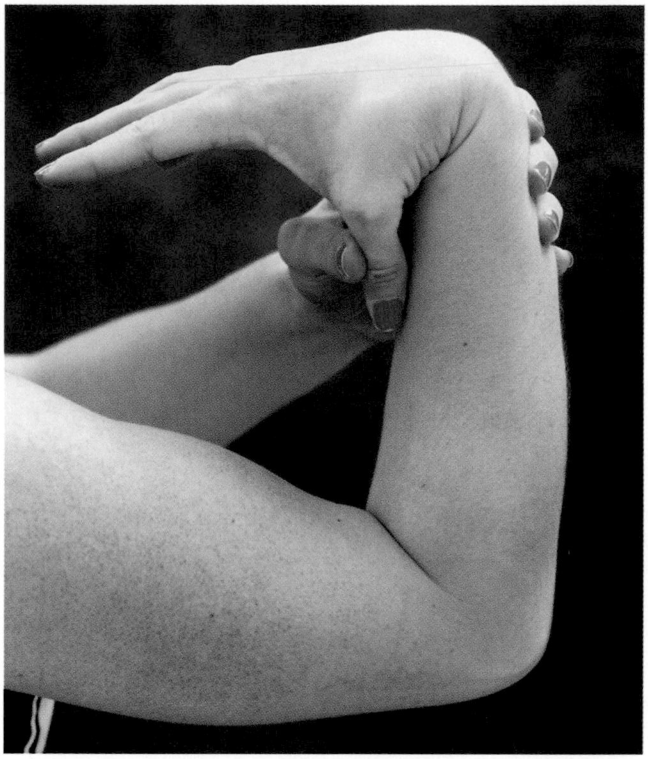

FIGURE 1-7 ■ Determining systemic laxity (hypermobility). Some patients may be naturally lax in all joints. A simple test to determine laxity is to have the patient attempt to pull the thumb to the forearm.

Table 1-7 Grading System for Ligamentous Laxity

Grade	Ligamentous End-Feel	Damage
I	Firm (normal)	Slight stretching of the ligament with little, if any, tearing of the fibers. Pain is present, but the degree of laxity roughly compares with that of the opposite extremity.
II	Soft	Partial tearing of the fibers. There is increased play of the joint surfaces upon one another or the joint line "opens up" significantly when compared with the opposite side.
III	Empty	Complete tearing of the ligament. The motion is excessive and becomes restricted by secondary restraints, such as tendons.

Joint Play

Normal observable ROM cannot be achieved without sufficient accessory (arthrokinematic) motion. These accessory motions occur via rolling, spinning, or gliding of the joint surfaces and are assessed using joint play. The concave–convex rule identifies the direction of accessory motions based on the shape of the joint surfaces (Fig. 1-8).

Joint play is assessed with the patient relaxed and the joint in the loose-packed, or resting, position to minimize the influence of bony congruency. A gliding or distracting stress is then applied and the relative amount of movement assessed and compared bilaterally. The findings of joint play assessment can be rated as normal; hypermobile, such as following injury to a ligament; or hypomobile, such as following a period of immobilization. A seven-point scale is typically used, with a score of 3 indicating normal mobility:

0 = **ankylosed**
1 = considerably decreased
2 = slightly decreased
3 = normal
4 = slightly increased
5 = considerably increased
6 = dramatically increased; pathological

Ankylosed Fusion of a joint as the result of pathology or surgical design

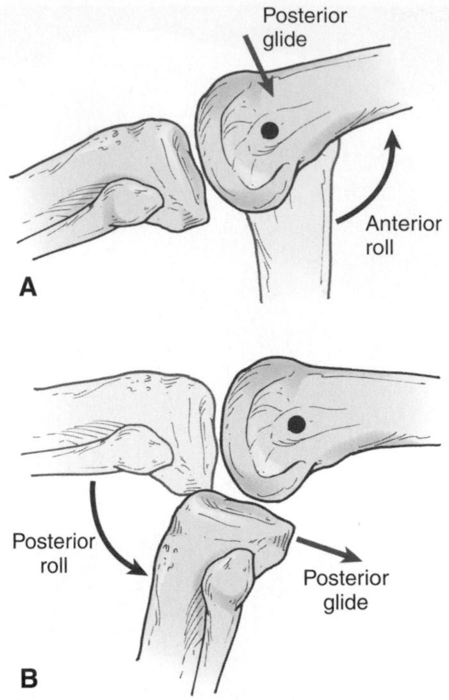

FIGURE 1-8 ■ The convex–concave rule. (A) Moving convex joint surface rolls and glides in opposite directions to offset natural translation. (B) A moving concave joint surface rolls and slides in the same direction.

All stress tests are evaluated bilaterally and, whenever possible, compared with baseline measures. The proper joint angle must be obtained to isolate specific tissues within the joint. Performing joint mobility tests with the joint in the incorrect position can yield false results.

Selective Tissue Tests

Selective tissue tests involve specific stresses or procedures applied to specific tissues or functions. Therefore, these tests are unique to each structure, joint, body part, or system. Examples of selective tissue tests include the impingement test in the shoulder or the Thessaly test for a meniscal tear. Like all examination techniques, some selective tissue tests are more helpful to the diagnostic process than others. The concepts introduced in Chapter 3 are used to determine whether tests should be included in the examination. Increasingly, positive or negative findings of clusters of selective tissue tests are being examined to improve diagnostic accuracy.[36]

Unlike stress testing, selective tissue tests are typically not graded based on the magnitude of the findings (e.g., grade 1, grade 2, grade 3), but rather are evaluated as being "positive" or "negative" relative to the opposite side. Selective tissue tests are further classified as provocation (causing pain or instability) or alleviation (reducing pain or other symptoms) tests.

Neurological Screening

Neurological assessments involve an upper and lower quarter screen of sensation, motor function, and deep tendon reflexes. Neurological tests are used to identify nerve root impingement, peripheral nerve damage or entrapment, central nervous system (CNS) trauma, or disease. Any neurological signs must be determined so that proper management techniques may be performed. Lower quarter screens are presented in Neurological Screening 1-1, and upper quarter screens are presented in Neurological Screening 1-2. Interrater reliability in identifying patterns associated with nerve root or peripheral nerve involvement is good between experienced examiners.

During the clinical evaluation of orthopedic injuries, neurological examination is indicated when the patient complains of numbness, paresthesia, muscular weakness, or pain of unexplained origin or when the patient has sustained a cervical or lumbar spine injury.

Sensory Testing

Each spinal nerve root innervates a discrete area of skin. These areas, known as dermatomes, have central autogenous zones that are supplied by only one nerve root, with the peripheral areas being supplied by other nerve roots. When standing upright, the dermatomes appear to have a random pattern (Fig. 1-9). However, when the body is placed in the quadruped position, the order becomes clear (Fig. 1-10).

When a single nerve root is compressed or otherwise inhibited, the skin in the autogenous zone will have reduced sensory function (paresthetic or anesthetic). The remaining portion of the dermatome may have altered sensory function.

*** Practical Evidence**

Having the patient indicate areas of pain or unusual sensation on a drawing of the human body and then mapping the results to dermatome charts is reliable in identifying pain of neurological origin.[37]

Sensory testing involves a bilateral comparison of light touch discrimination, using a light stroke within the central autogenous zone of the dermatome to avoid overlap of multiple nerve roots and more accurately identify the breadth of the involved area. The stroke should be felt to an equal extent on each side. Sensory tests using sharp and dull discrimination and two-point discrimination may also be used to assess sensation in a more quantified manner (Fig. 1-11).[38] Different types of sensory tests are used to differentiate between the types of nerves involved. All sensory testing begins with a thorough explanation of the test to the patient; however, actual testing should be conducted with the patient's eyes closed or head averted to avoid visual influence. The technique should first be tried on an area of normal sensation so that the patient has an accurate understanding of expected sensations.[39]

Motor Testing

Manual muscle tests using the procedures described in Manual Muscle Test 1-1 are used to assess the motor nerves that are innervating the extremities (see Neurological

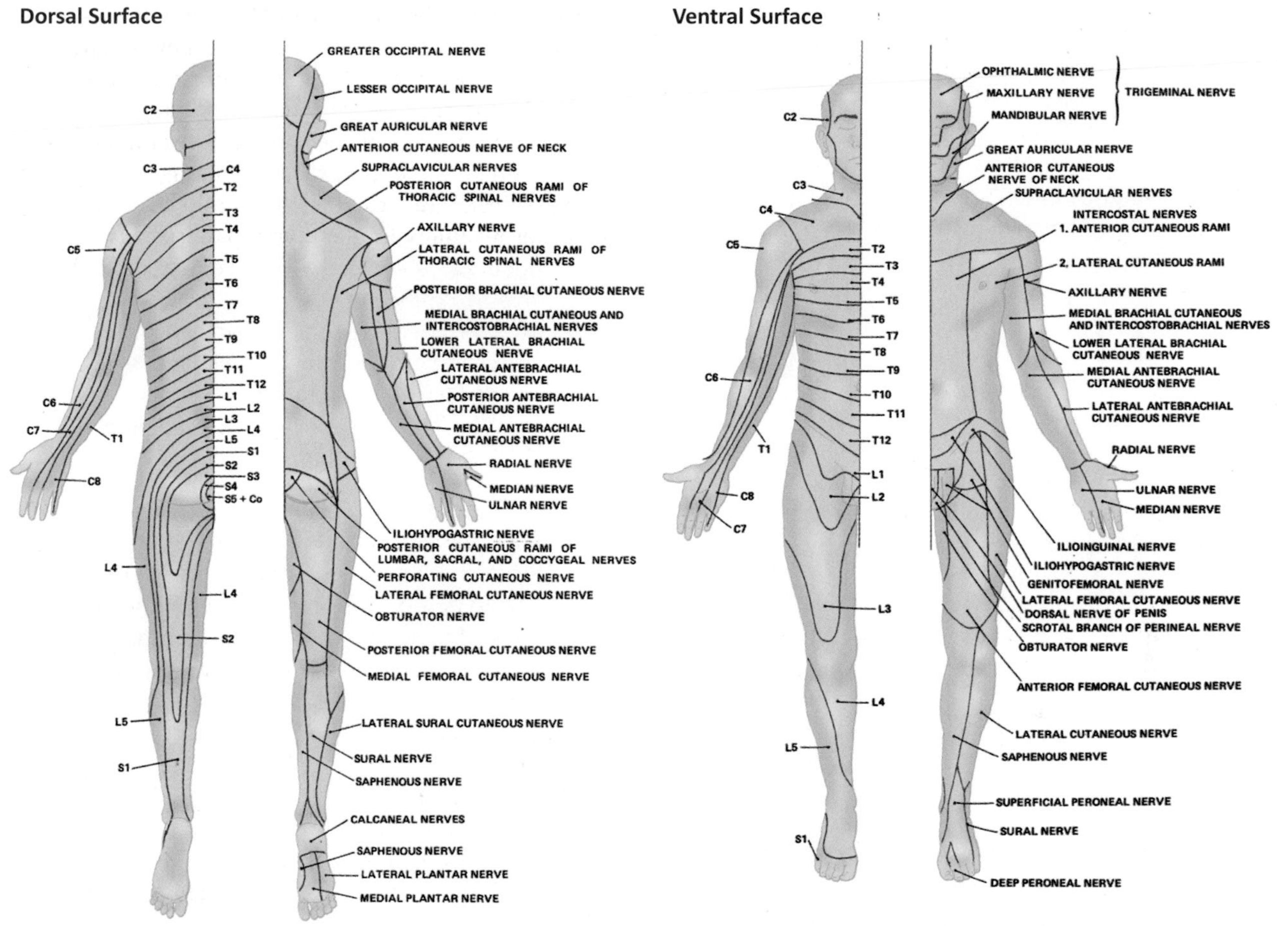

FIGURE 1-9 ■ Cutaneous innervation of the front and back of the body. Dermatomes are on the left and peripheral nerves are on the right. These charts describe the area of skin receiving sensory input from each of the nerve roots. Note that there are many different dermatome references.

Screenings 1-1 and 1-2). Although innervation of all muscles tends to overlap, some muscles are more pure than others with regard to their innervation and are initially tested. If weakness is detected in a neurological motor test screen that is innervated by a specific nerve root, identify another muscle that shares that innervation and perform a manual muscle test. If only one muscle is weak, pathology to the muscle or the peripheral nerve supplying it (if different from the second muscle) should be suspected. If both muscles are weak, then the nerve root or peripheral nerve supplying the muscles is implicated.

Reflex Testing

Deep tendon reflexes (DTRs), myotatic reflexes, provide information about the integrity of the cervical and lumbar nerve roots and their afferent (from the periphery to the CNS) and efferent (from the CNS to the periphery) pathways. The impact of the reflex hammer on the muscle tendon stretches the tendon, stimulating Golgi tendon organs and muscle spindles. These receptors send a signal to the spinal cord indicating that the muscle is being stretched. In turn, the spinal cord sends a motor impulse to the muscle instructing it to fire and therefore take the stretch off of the muscle.[39]

Reflex testing is limited because not all nerve roots have an associated DTR. A standard scale for grading DTRs is used (Table 1-8). Differences in reflexes on the left and right sides are more significant than hyper- or hyporeflexia occurring on both sides (if a spinal cord or brain pathology is not suspected). Because of natural variability, the results of reflex testing should be interpreted in light of other examination findings.[40] Increased response to a reflex test indicates an **upper motor neuron lesion**, while decreased responses could signify a **lower motor neuron lesion**.

Upper motor neuron lesion A lesion proximal to the anterior horn of the spinal cord that results in paralysis and loss of voluntary movement, spasticity, sensory loss, and pathological reflexes

Lower motor neuron lesion A lesion of the anterior horn of the spinal cord, nerve roots, or peripheral nerves resulting in decreased reflexes, flaccid paralysis, and atrophy

Neurological Screening 1-1
Lower Quarter Neurological Screen

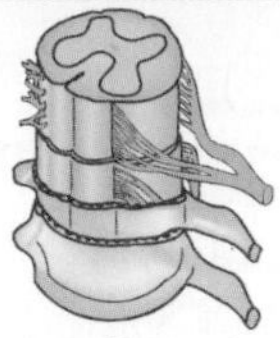 Nerve Root Level	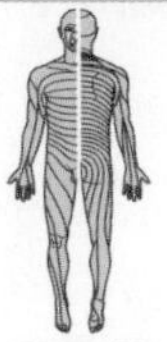 Sensory Testing	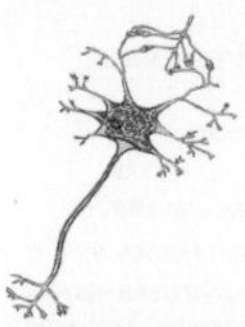 Motor Testing	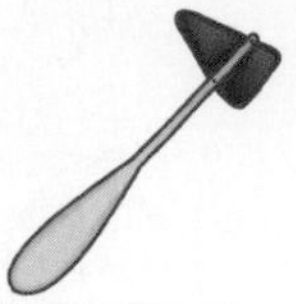 Reflex Testing
L1	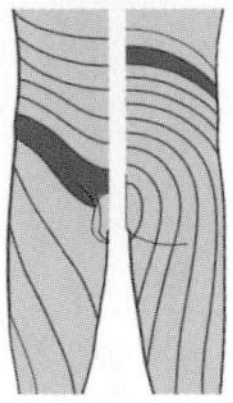 Femoral cutaneous n.	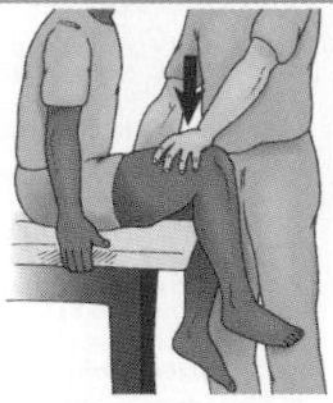 Lumbar plexus	 None
L2	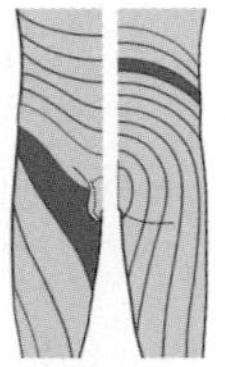 Femoral cutaneous n.	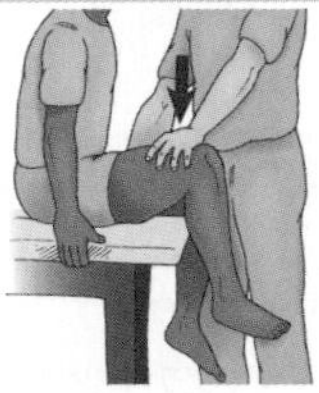 Lumbar plexus	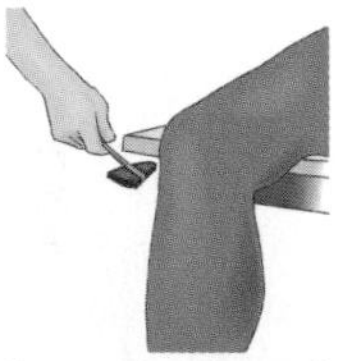 Femoral n. (partial)
L3	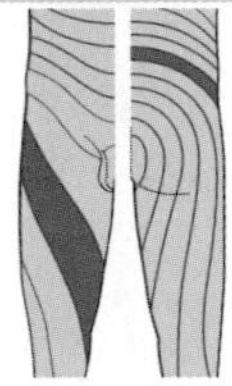 Femoral cutaneous n.	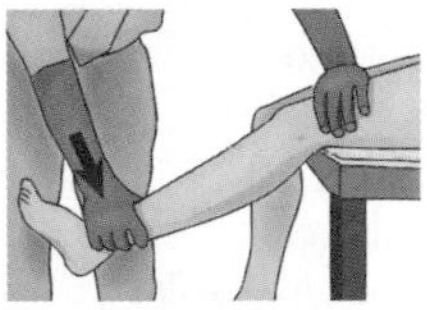 Femoral n.	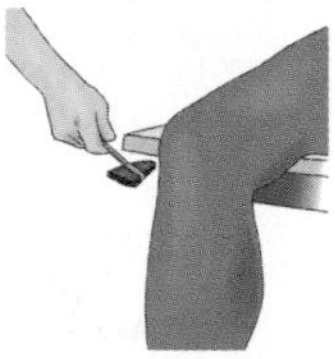 Femoral n. (partial)
L4	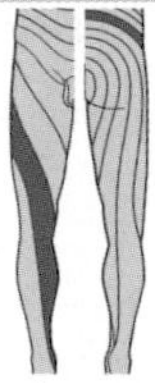 Saphenous n.	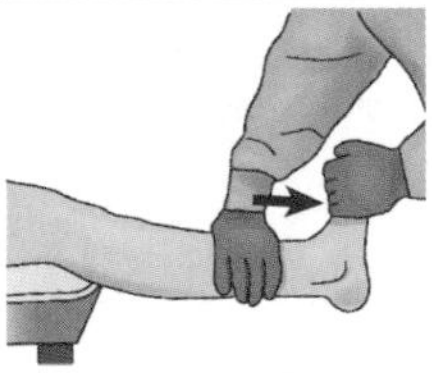 Deep peroneal n.	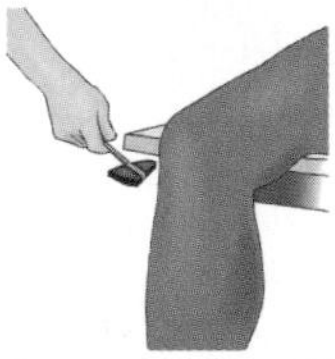 Femoral n. (partial)
L5	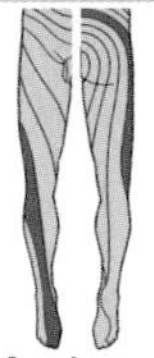 Superficial peroneal n.	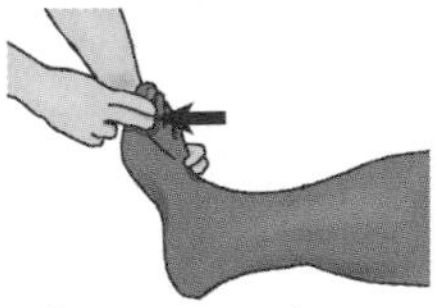 Deep peroneal n.	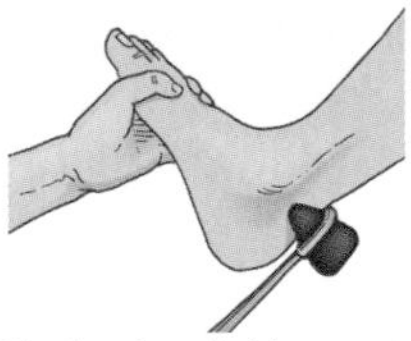 Tibial n. (medial hamstring or tibialis posterior)
S1	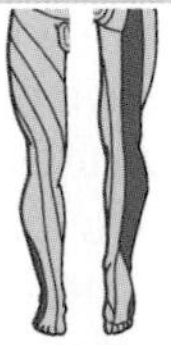 Posterior femoral cutaneous n. and sural n.	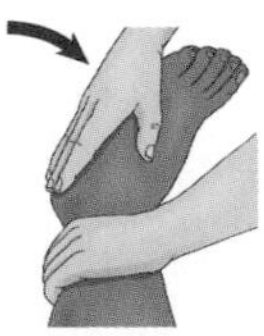 Superficial peroneal n.	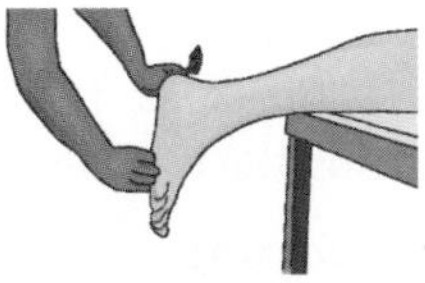 Tibial n. (Achilles)
S2	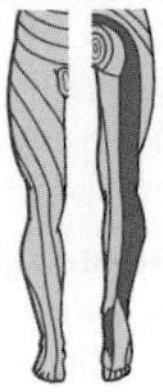 Posterior femoral cutaneous n.	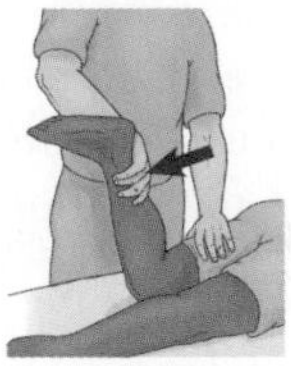 Tibial n. and common peroneal n.	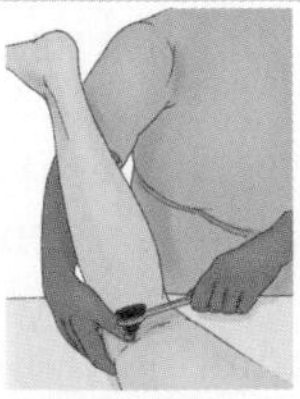 Tibial n. (lateral hamstring)

Neurological Screening 1-2

Upper Quarter Neurologic Screen

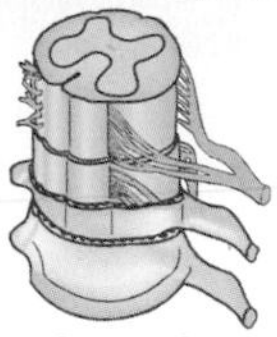 Nerve Root Level	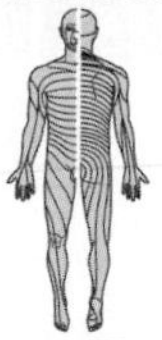 Sensory Testing	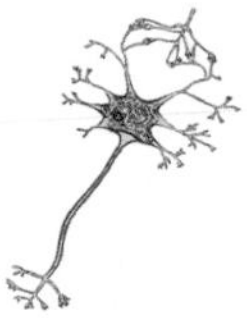 Motor Testing	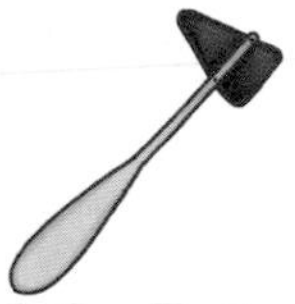 Reflex Testing
C4	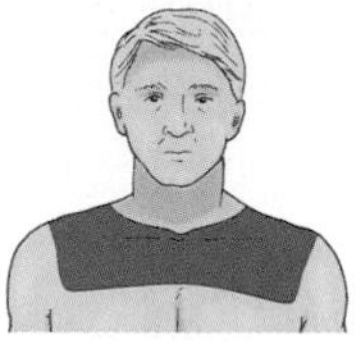 Supraclavicular n.	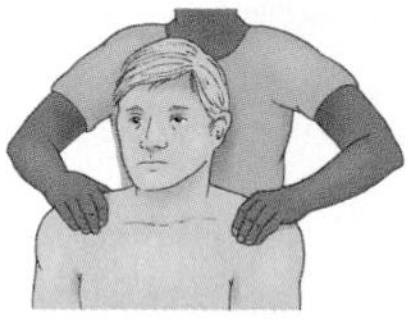 Shoulder shrug Dorsal scapular n.	None
C5	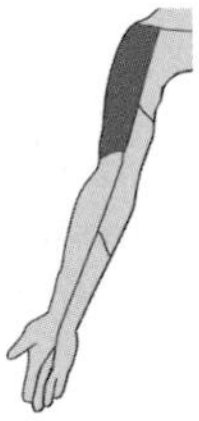 Proximal lateral brachial	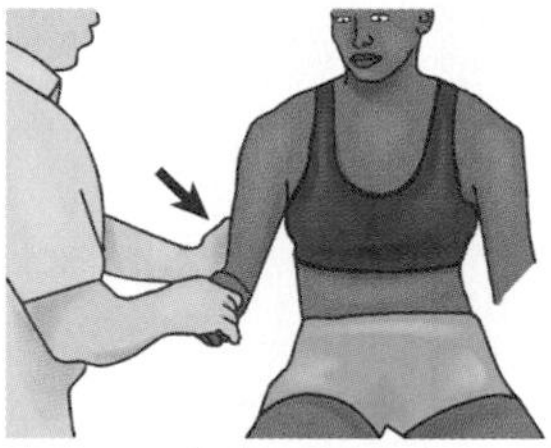 Axillary n.	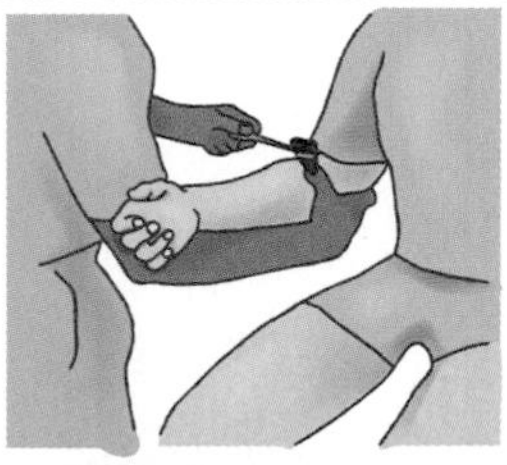 Musculocutaneous n.
C6	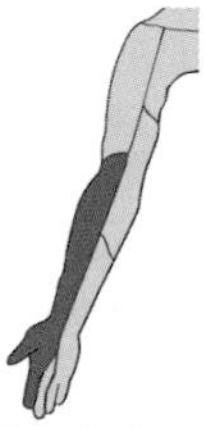 Lateral antebrachial Cutaneous n.	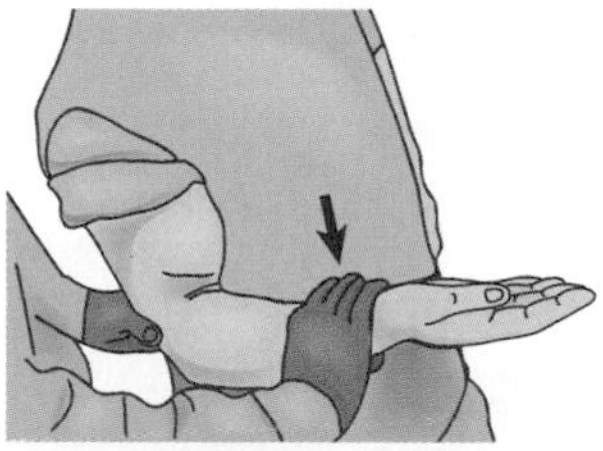 Musculocutaneous n. (C5 & C6)	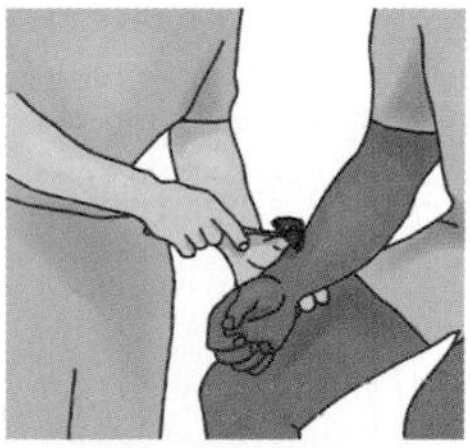 Musculocutaneous n.
C7	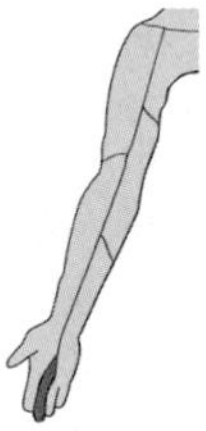 Radial n.	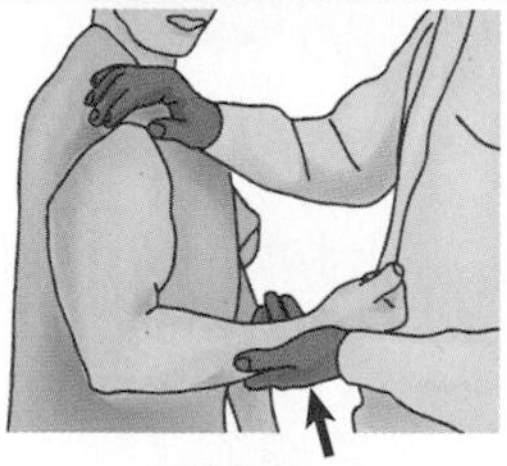 Radial n.	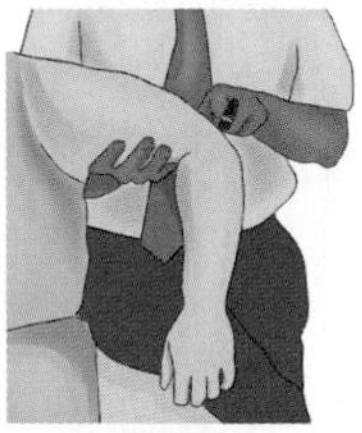 Radial n.
C8	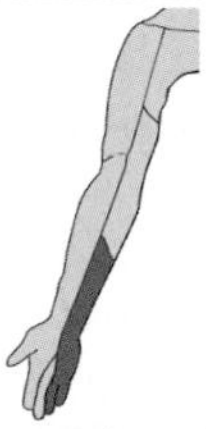 Ulnar n. (mixed)	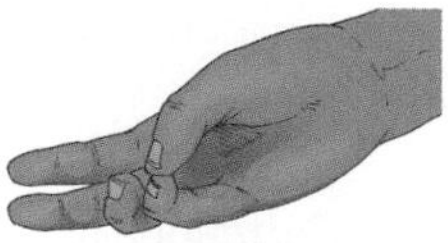 Median n.	None
T1	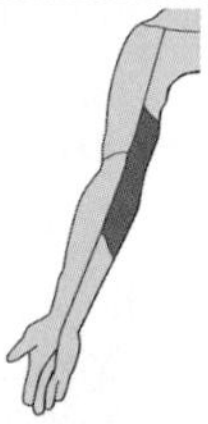 Med. brachial cutaneous n.	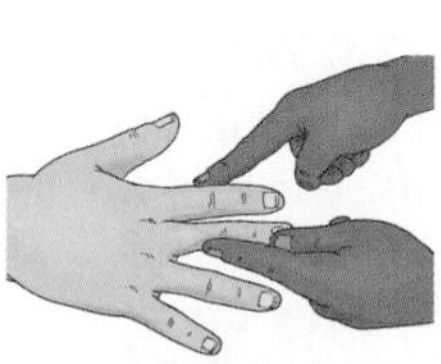 Med. brachial cutaneous n.	None

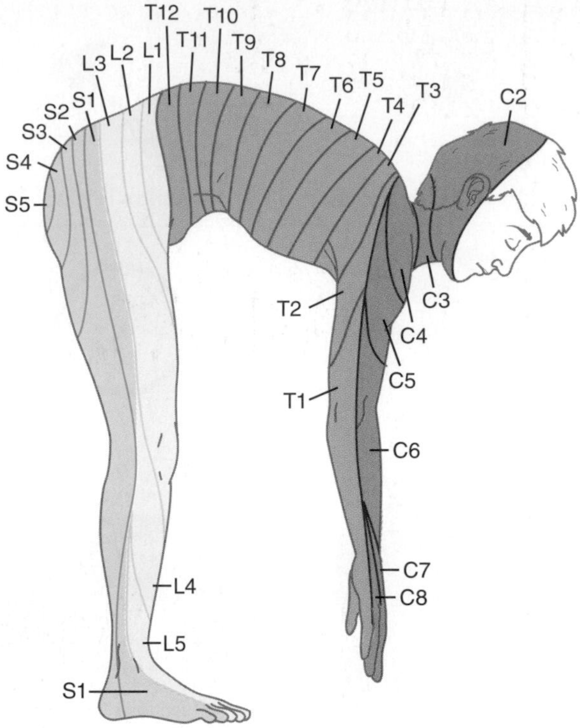

FIGURE 1-10 ■ When the body is placed in the quadruped position the sequence and position of the dermatomes become orderly, starting with C2 (there is no C1 dermatome) at the skull and progressing to S5 at the "tail."

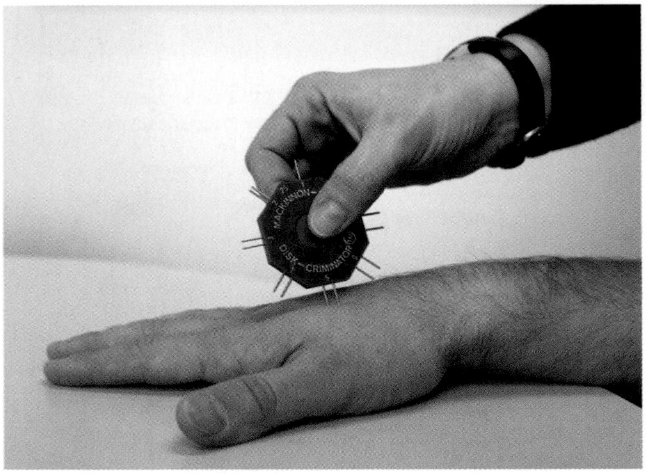

FIGURE 1-11 ■ Two-point discrimination test. This examination procedure is used to determine the amount of sensory loss. Normal results are that the patient can distinguish points that are at most 4 to 5 mm apart.

DTRs are assessed with the target muscle/tendon on slight stretch and relaxed. The patient should be instructed to look away from the target site. The tendon should be struck briskly by the reflex hammer and the reaction noted. The reflex should be elicited multiple times, with any change in response noted. In some patients, eliciting a reflexive response is difficult. For these individuals, the technique of having the patient contract a muscle away from the target area, the **Jendrassik maneuver**, may be helpful (Fig. 1-12).[41]

All of the reflexes in the extremity being tested should be assessed and compared with the same reflex in the opposite extremity. For example, in a patient who exhibits poor muscle tone, a reflex that is elicited with reinforcement might be assessed as abnormal. However, further assessment would reveal that all of the remaining reflexes are also grade 1. Therefore, this is the baseline assessment naturally found in this individual.

Table 1-8 Deep Tendon Reflex Grading

Grade	Response
0	No reflex elicited
1+	Hyporeflexia: Reflex elicited with reinforcement (precontracting the muscle)
2+	Normal response
3+	Hyperreflexia (brisk)
4+	Hyperactive with **clonus**

Nerve root–specific reflex tests are presented in Reflex Testing 1-1 through 1-8.

Vascular Screening

Clinical examination of the vascular system provides a gross assessment of the blood flow to and from the extremities. Decreased arterial blood flow can produce pain by depriving the tissues of oxygen; inhibition or failure of the vascular return network can produce pain secondary to edema (Table 1-9).[42] Symptoms often worsen during and following activity. It is often useful to have the patient repeat the motions and/or positions that provoke the symptoms.[42]

Adequate arterial supply to the extremity is grossly determined by establishing the presence of a pulse. Lower extremity pulses are assessed at the femoral, posterior tibial, and dorsal pedal arteries. In the upper extremity, the brachial, radial, and ulnar arteries are frequently used. The carotid artery (supplying the brain) is used to determine a systemic pulse.

The capillary refill in the nail beds of the toes and fingers can provide some clinical evidence as to the status of the cardiovascular and respiratory systems (Selective Tissue Test 1-2). If blood and/or oxygen supply to the extremities is diminished, the nail beds often become cyanotic. Capillary refill should be assessed in digits that have a unique blood supply.

Unexplained vascular symptoms such as discoloration (cyanosis or pallor), swelling, or lack of capillary refill can be indicative of other cardiovascular or metabolic conditions such as diabetes. The insidious onset of vascular symptoms warrants referral for further medical examination.[42]

Review of Systems

The focus of this text is an assessment of the musculoskeletal system. All systems should be reviewed in the examination process. Even if the exam is for a nonmusculoskeletal

---

Clonus Neuromuscular activity in the skeletal muscle marked by rapidly alternating involuntary contraction followed by relaxation

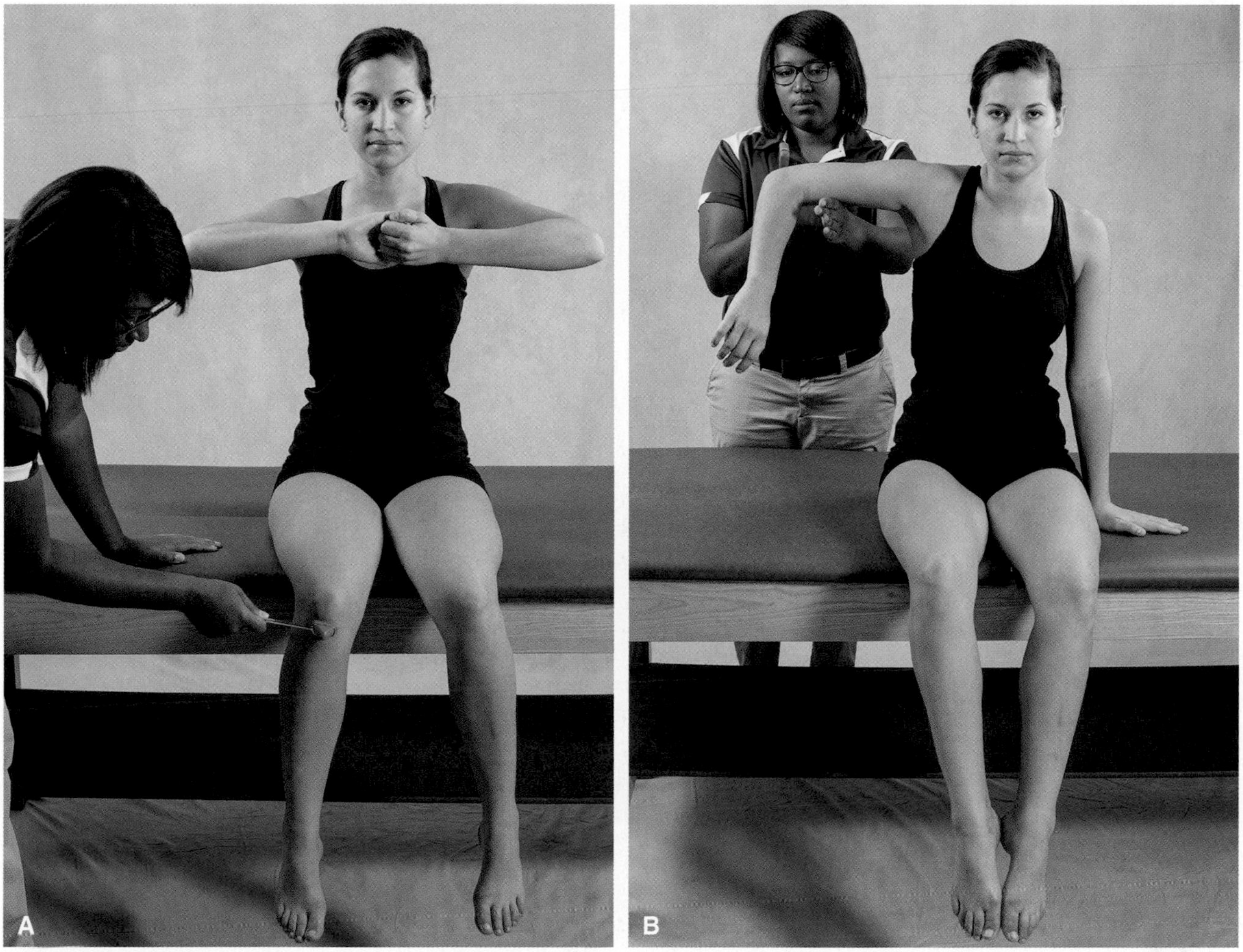

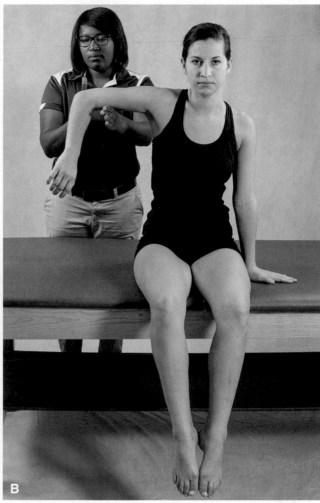

FIGURE 1-12 ■ The Jendrassik maneuvers. (A) To facilitate muscle function during lower extremity reflex testing, have the patient attempt to pull the hands apart as shown. (B) Muscle facilitation during upper extremity reflex testing. The patient presses the medial aspects of the feet against each other.

Table 1-9 Signs of Vascular Inhibition in the Extremities

Arterial Deficiency	Venous Inhibition
Decreased pulse	Edema in the distal extremity
Decreased capillary refill	Noticeable "pitting" after removing the socks
Cyanotic color	Dark discoloration

condition, such as an illness, a routine assessment of blood pressure or resting pulse may detect an underlying condition that warrants further examination. In the case of urgent conditions, the vital signs acquired during the review of systems should be recorded and repeated periodically to identify decline or improvement.

Cardiopulmonary System

Blood pressure, heart rate, oxygenation, and auscultation are the components of assessing the cardiopulmonary system. When assessing patients in acute stress, certain cardiopulmonary findings are characteristic of shock, a condition that warrants referral (Table 1-10). The vascular screen presented on page 28 is used to assess distal circulation following orthopedic injury. The review of the cardiovascular system is used to identify systemic involvement.

Table 1-10 Signs and Symptoms of Shock

Rapid, weak pulse
Decreased blood pressure
Rapid, shallow breathing
Excessive thirst
Nausea and vomiting
Pale, bluish skin
Restlessness or irritability
Drowsiness or loss of consciousness

Text continued on page 34

Reflex Testing 1-1
C5 Nerve Root Reflex

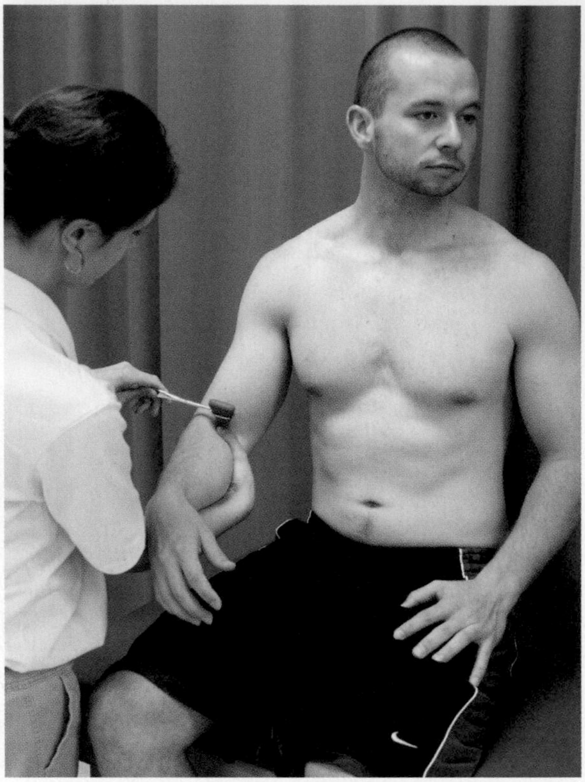

Muscle	Biceps brachii
Patient Position	Seated looking away from the tested side
Position of Examiner	Standing to the side of the patient, cradling the forearm with the thumb placed over the tendon
Evaluative Procedure	The thumb is tapped with the reflex hammer.
Innervation	Musculocutaneous nerve
Nerve Root	C5, C6

Reflex Testing 1-2
C6 Nerve Root Reflex

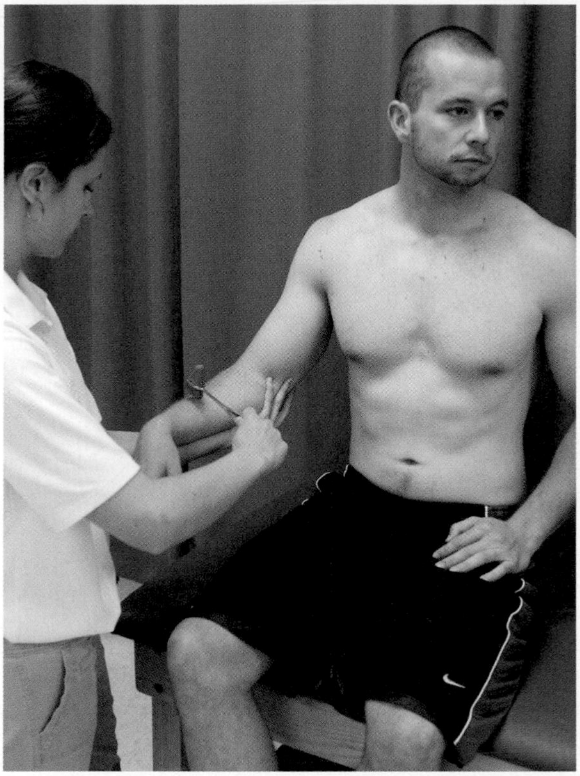

Muscle	Brachioradialis
Patient Position	Seated looking away from the tested side The elbow is passively flexed to between 60° and 90°.
Position of Examiner	Cradling the patient's arm
Evaluative Procedure	The distal portion of the brachioradialis tendon is tapped with the reflex hammer. The proximal tendon may also be used.
Innervation	Radial nerve
Nerve Roots	C5, C6

Reflex Testing 1-3
C7 Nerve Root Reflex

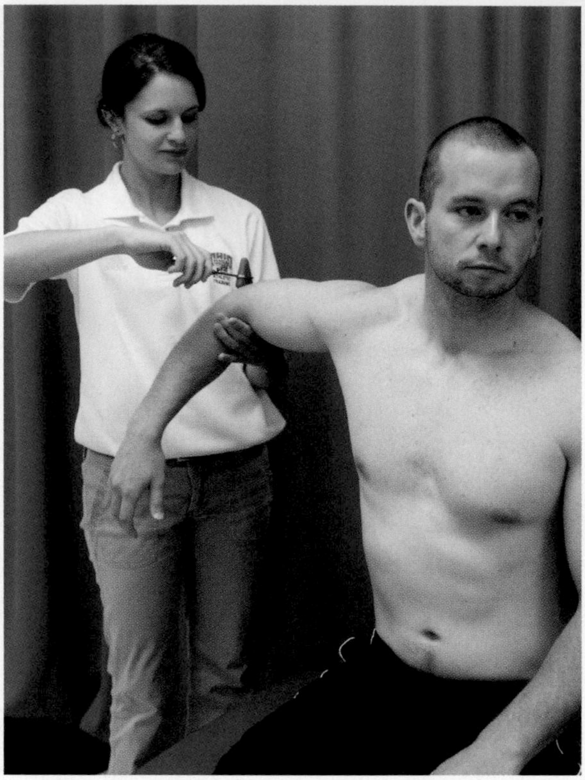

Muscle	Triceps brachii
Patient Position	Seated looking away from the tested side
Position of Examiner	Supporting the patient's shoulder abducted to 90° and the elbow flexed to 90°
Evaluative Procedure	The distal triceps brachii tendon is tapped with the reflex hammer.
Innervation	Radial nerve
Nerve Roots	(C6), C7, C8

Reflex Testing 1-4
L4 Nerve Root Reflex

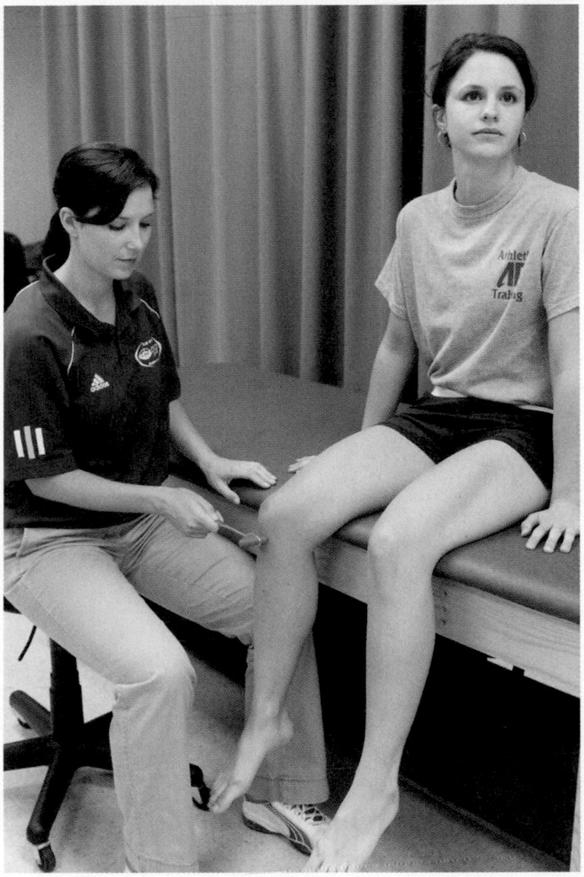

Muscle	Patellar tendon (quadriceps femoris)
Patient Position	Sitting with the knees flexed over the end of the table looking away from the tested side
Position of Examiner	Standing or seated to the side of the patient
Evaluative Procedure	The patellar tendon is tapped with the reflex hammer.
Innervation	Femoral nerve
Nerve Roots	(L2), L3, L4

Reflex Testing 1-5
L5 Nerve Root Reflex (Tibialis Posterior)

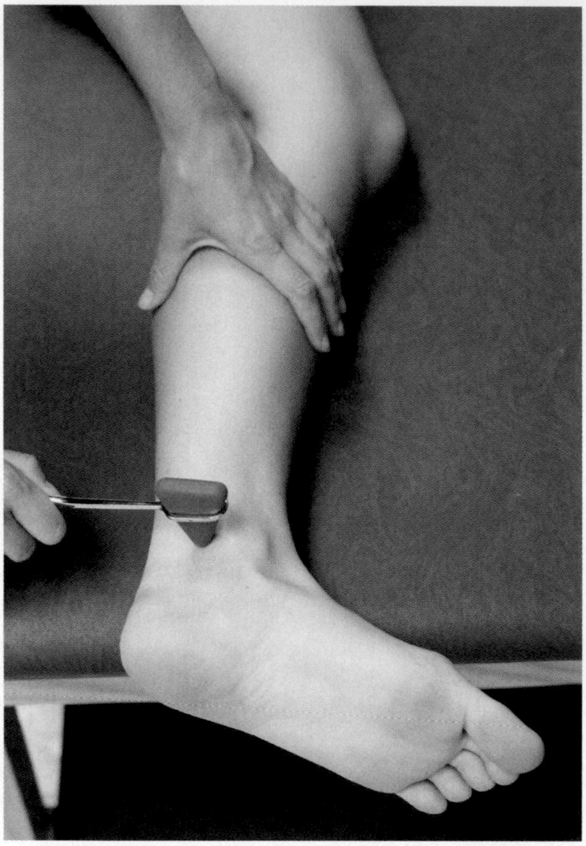

Muscle	Tibialis posterior
Patient Position	Side-lying on test side The test foot is off the edge of the table.
Position of Examiner	Standing or seated to the side of the patient
Evaluative Procedure	The tibialis posterior tendon is tapped with the reflex hammer posteriorly and just proximal to the medial malleolus.
Innervation	Tibial nerve
Nerve Roots	L5, (L4, S1)

Heart Rate

The heart rate is determined by palpating the carotid, radial, femoral, or brachial pulse (Selective Tissue Test 1-3). An athlete's resting heart rate typically ranges from 60 to 100 beats per minute (bpm). Highly conditioned athletes have lower heart rates. Older or recreational athletes have heart rates at the higher end of the scale. When assessing the heart rate of an athlete who has just stopped exercising, an increased heart rate caused by the demands of exercise should be considered.

Palpable pulses should have a consistent rhythm with a smooth, quick upstroke, consistent summit, and a gradual downstroke. An abnormal rate or irregular rhythm could be indicative of an arrhythmia, stimulant use, or anxiety. A rapidly rising, large-amplitude pulse (water-hammer pulse) suggests hypertrophic cardiomyopathy, or aortic or mitral valve regurgitation; a slowly rising, small-amplitude pulse suggests aortic stenosis or heart failure.[17]

Simultaneous palpation of the radial and femoral pulses can identify narrowing (coarctation) of the aorta. A delay of

Reflex Testing 1-6
L5 Nerve Root Reflex (Medial hamstrings)

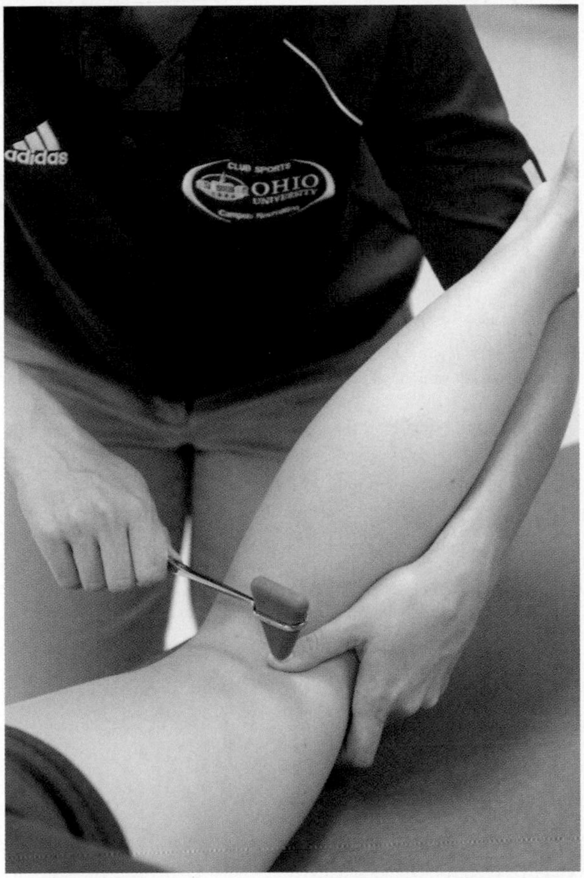

Muscle	Medial hamstrings
Patient Position	Prone with the knee slightly flexed looking away from the tested side
Position of Examiner	Standing or seated to the side of the patient The thumb or finger is placed over the semitendinosus tendon immediately superior to the medial joint line.
Evaluative Procedure	The finger is tapped with the reflex hammer.
Innervation	Tibial nerve
Nerve Roots	L5, S1, (S2)

the femoral pulse relative to the radial pulse warrants further cardiovascular examination.[17]

Blood Pressure

A measurement of the pressure exerted by the blood on the arterial walls, blood pressure is affected by a decrease in blood volume (severe bleeding or dehydration), a decreased capacity of the vessels, shock, or a decreased ability of the heart to pump blood (cardiac arrest or fibrillation). Decreased blood pressure indicates a decreased ability to deliver blood, with its nutrients and oxygen, to the organs of the body. Organs are highly susceptible to **anoxia** and can be severely damaged secondary to a decrease in blood pressure.

High blood pressure, or hypertension, is commonly seen in the general population. A dangerous precursor to cardiovascular problems, high blood pressure can exert extreme

anoxia Without oxygen

Reflex Testing 1-7
S1 Nerve Root Reflex

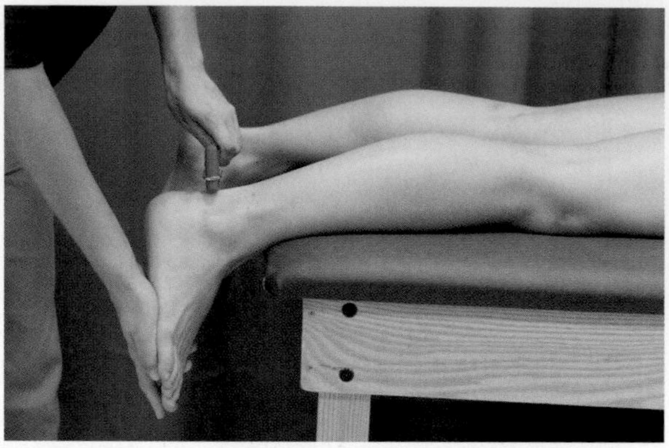

Muscle	Achilles tendon (triceps surae muscle group)
Patient Position	Prone with the feet off the edge of the table
Position of Examiner	Seated or standing next to the patient, supporting the foot in its neutral position
Evaluative Procedure	The Achilles tendon is tapped with a reflex hammer.
Innervation	Tibial
Nerve Roots	S1, S2

pressure on the blood vessels, particularly in the smaller vasculature of the brain. Excessive pressure causes these vessels to rupture, resulting in a **cerebrovascular** accident (CVA) or stroke.[43] The presence of high blood pressure warrants referral to a physician for further evaluation (Selective Tissue Test 1-4).

*** Practical Evidence**

Manual sphygmomanometers are associated with less error than digital sphygmomanometers and should be used when a high level of accuracy is needed, such as in patients with known hypertension or arrhythmias or those who have experienced trauma.[46]

Heart Auscultation

Auscultation of the heart should be performed with the patient sitting or standing (Selective Tissue Test 1-5).[47] Normally, the heart makes "lub" and "dub" sounds as the valves close. The "lub" (or S_1) represents the closing of the mitral and tricuspid valves—between the atria and the ventricles—as the ventricles begin to contract to push blood out through the aorta and pulmonary artery. The "dub" (or S_2) occurs as the aortic and pulmonary valves close as the ventricles finish pushing out the blood and begin to relax.[48] Any reflux of blood through a faulty or leaking valve causes a decrease in the heart's ability to efficiently deliver the needed metabolites to the tissues of the body and alters the characteristic heart sounds (Table 1-11).

*** Practical Evidence**

Athletes with a murmur that becomes louder when squatting should be referred for evaluation for hypertrophic cardiomyopathy, a potentially fatal condition.[15,17]

Respiratory System

Intense exercise dramatically changes the respiratory rate and pattern. In the event of abnormal changes, the individual will be anxious and may have trouble speaking. Any **sputum** that may be produced as the person coughs should be checked for the presence of blood. Pink or bloody sputum indicates internal bleeding requiring emergency treatment.

Breath Sounds

Auscultate breath sounds over all the lobes of each lung, noting the pitch, intensity, quality, and duration of inspirations and exhalations (Selective Tissue Test 1-6).[49] Inhalation typically reveals a dry, smooth, unobstructed sound that is equal throughout each lobe. The absence of breath sounds may indicate a collapsed lung associated with a pneumothorax. Pneumonia or other buildup of fluid within the lungs may produce rhonchi, a localized moist-sounding movement of air.[50]

Respiratory Flow

Peak flow meters (spirometers) assist in diagnosing and monitoring asthma by determining the peak expiratory

cerebrovascular Relating to the brain and its blood vessels

Reflex Testing 1-8
S2 Nerve Root Reflex

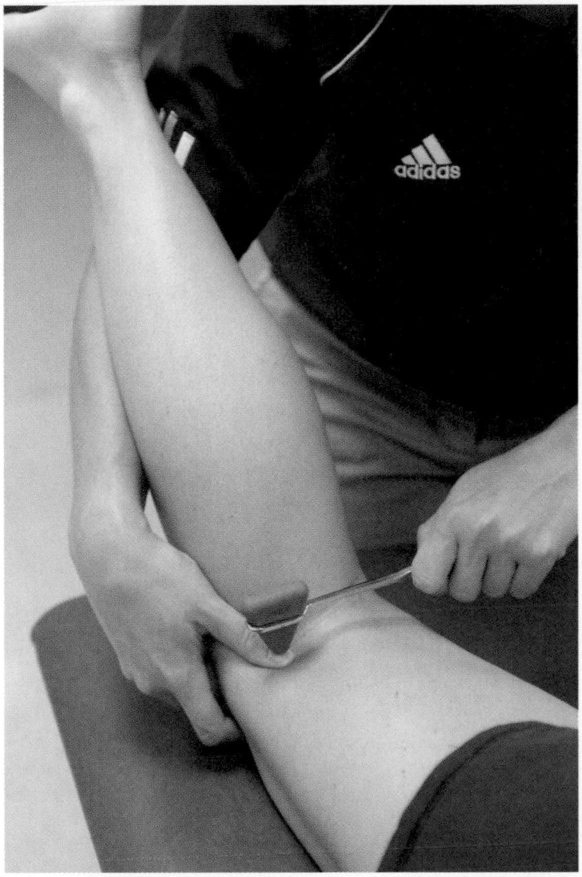

Muscle	Biceps femoris
Patient Position	Prone with the knee flexed to approximately 20°
Position of Examiner	Standing next to the patient The thumb is placed over the biceps femoris tendon just proximal to the joint line.
Evaluative Procedure	The thumb is tapped with a reflex hammer.
Innervation	Tibial, common peroneal
Nerve Roots	L5, S1, S2, (S3)

Table 1-11 Examples of Heart Sounds

Sound	Status	Possible Interpretation
"Lub"	Normal systole	Closure of the mitral and tricuspid valves
"Dub"	Normal diastole	Closure of the aortic and pulmonary valves
Soft, blowing "lub"	Abnormal systole	Associated with anemia or other changes in blood constituents
Loud, booming "lub"	Abnormal systole	Aneurysm Incomplete closure of the valves; blood heard regurgitating backward
Sloshing "dub"	Abnormal diastole	Friction sound Abnormal inflammation of the heart's pericardial lining; pericarditis

Selective Tissue Test 1-2
Capillary Refill Testing

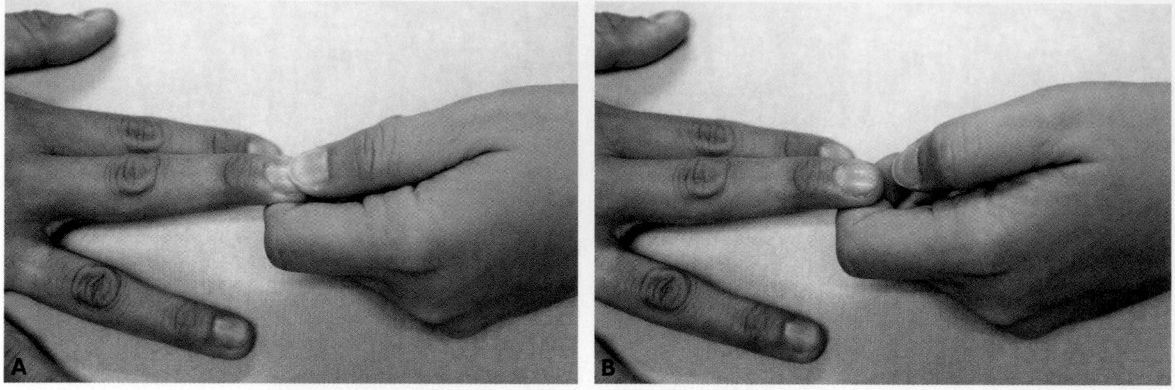

The capillary refill test provides gross information on the quality and quantity of blood flow to the extremities.

Patient Position	*Fingers:* Sitting or lying supine. The extremity is placed in a gravity-neutral position (horizontal). *Toes:* Lying supine
Position of Examiner	In front of or beside the patient
Evaluative Procedure	Observe the color of the nail bed. **(A)** Squeeze the fingernail so that the nail bed turns white or a lighter shade and hold for 5 seconds. **(B)** Release the pressure and note the speed of the refill as indicated by the baseline color returning to the nail bed. Repeat using the other fingers or toes and then perform on the opposite extremity.
Positive Test	Markedly slow or absent return of the nail's natural color
Implications	*Unilateral:* Occlusion of an artery or arteriole supplying the finger *Bilateral:* Possible systemic cardiovascular compromise or disease
Evidence	Absent or inconclusive in the literature

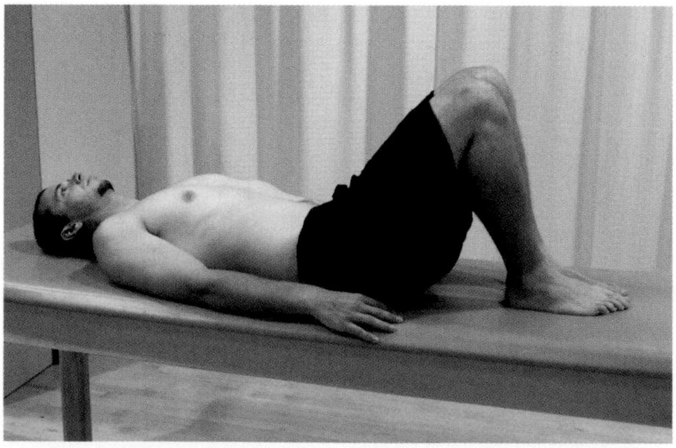

FIGURE 1-13 ■ Positioning of the patient during palpation of the abdomen. The hook-lying position relaxes the abdominal muscles, easing palpation of the underlying structures.

flow rate (PEFR). The PEFR represents the maximum velocity of air that can be forced from the lungs after taking a deep breath.[52] This is directly affected by changes in the airways such as those found with increases or decreases in secretion buildup or bronchospasm.

Gastrointestinal System

Assessment of the gastrointestinal system generally occurs following trauma to the thorax or if the patient reports symptoms that suggest gastrointestinal involvement.

Auscultation of the Abdomen

Perform auscultation, listening to sounds with a stethoscope, to help establish the presence of internal injury (Selective Tissue Test 1-7). The abdomen typically makes an occasional "gurgling" sound as **peristalsis** occurs. After injury, the peristaltic mechanism may be inhibited or may sympathetically shut down. In either case, the bowel sounds are absent. The exact placement of the stethoscope over specific portions of the bowel is not crucial because these sounds resound throughout the cavity. Auscultate the abdomen before palpating it. Manipulation of the abdomen during palpation may falsely produce normal bowel sounds.

Selective Tissue Test 1-3
Determination of Heart Rate Using the Radial Pulse

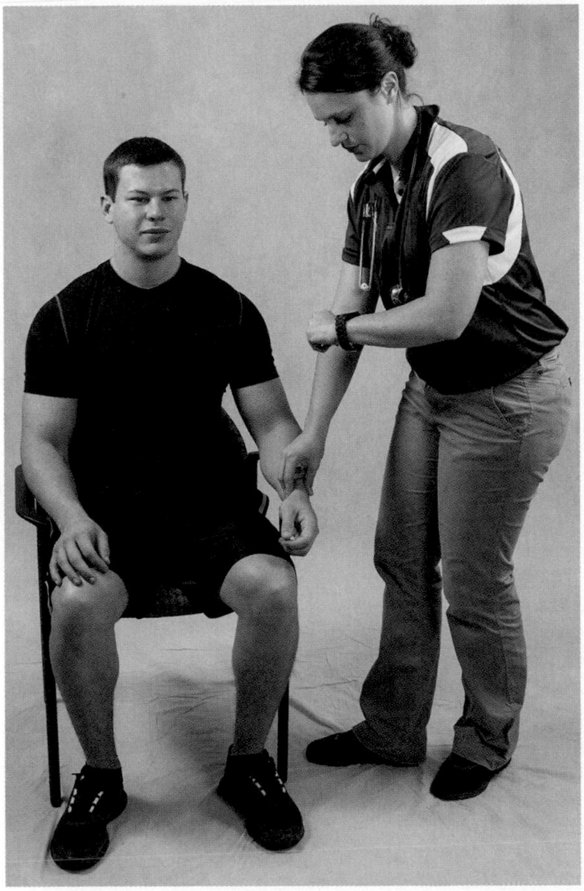

The radial artery, palpated just proximal to the thumb on the palmar side of the radial aspect of the wrist, is used to determine the frequency, quality, and rhythm of the pulse.

Patient Position	Seated
Position of Examiner	Use the index and middle fingers to locate the radial pulse.
Evaluative Procedure	Count the number of pulses in a 15-second interval and multiply that number by 4 to determine the number of beats per minute. The examiner also attempts to determine the quality of the pulse: strong (bounding) or weak.
Positive Test	Heart rate outside of expected values or values that deviate from any baseline values Bounding or irregular pulse
Implications	The quality and quantity of the heart rate established: Normal (general population): 60–100 bpm Well-trained athletes: 40–60 bpm Tachycardia: Greater than 100 bpm Bradycardia: Less than 60 bpm
Comments	The baseline heart rate should be recorded and rechecked at regular intervals. Note the rhythm of the beats for symmetry and strength.
Evidence	Absent or inconclusive in the literature

Selective Tissue Test 1-4
Blood Pressure Assessment

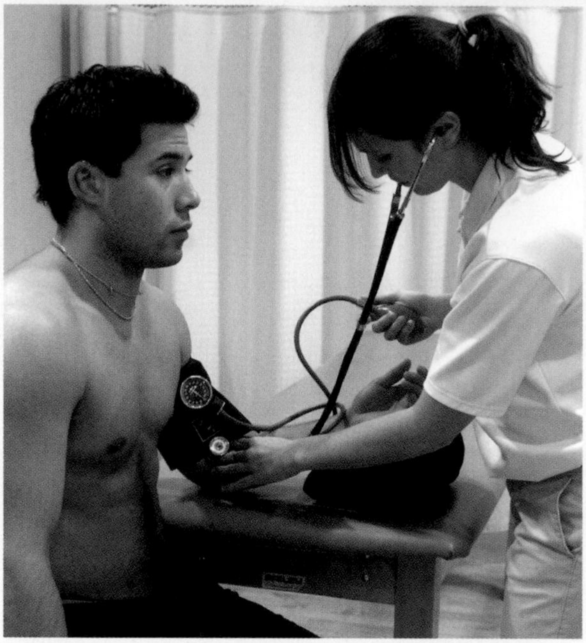

Blood pressure assessment at the brachial artery. Based on the findings of the systolic and diastolic pressures, the patient's blood pressure is categorized as hypertensive, prehypertensive, normal, or hypotensive.

Patient Position	If possible, the patient should be seated; support the arm so that the middle section of the upper arm is at heart level.
Position of Examiner	In front of or beside the patient in a position to read the gauge on the BP cuff
Evaluative Procedure	The sphygmomanometer (cuff) is secured over the upper arm, with the lower edge of the bladder approximately 1 inch above the antecubital fossa. Many cuffs have an arrow that must be aligned with the brachial artery. The stethoscope is placed over the brachial artery. The cuff is inflated to 180 to 200 mm Hg. The air is slowly released from the cuff at a rate of 2 mm per second until the initial beat is heard.[44] While reading the gauge, note the point at which the first pulse sound, the systolic pressure, is heard. Continuing to slowly release the air from the cuff (approximately 2 mm Hg per second), note the value at which the last pulse, the diastolic value, is heard. Record to the nearest 2 mm Hg.
Positive Test	*Hypertension:* Systolic pressure greater than 140 mm Hg Diastolic pressure greater than 90 mm Hg *Prehypertension:* Systolic pressure 120–139 mm Hg Diastolic pressure 80–89 mm Hg *Normal:* Systolic pressure 90–119 mm Hg Diastolic pressure 60–79 mm Hg *Hypotension:* Systolic pressure less than 90 mm Hg Diastolic pressure less than 60 mm Hg
Implications	Low BP may indicate shock or internal hemorrhage. High BP indicates hypertension.

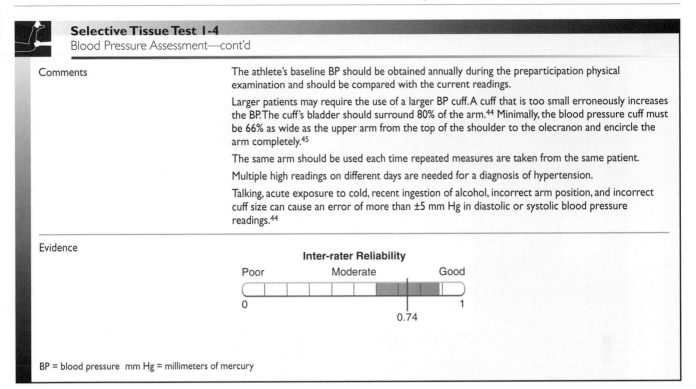

Selective Tissue Test 1-4
Blood Pressure Assessment—cont'd

Comments	The athlete's baseline BP should be obtained annually during the preparticipation physical examination and should be compared with the current readings. Larger patients may require the use of a larger BP cuff. A cuff that is too small erroneously increases the BP. The cuff's bladder should surround 80% of the arm.[44] Minimally, the blood pressure cuff must be 66% as wide as the upper arm from the top of the shoulder to the olecranon and encircle the arm completely.[45] The same arm should be used each time repeated measures are taken from the same patient. Multiple high readings on different days are needed for a diagnosis of hypertension. Talking, acute exposure to cold, recent ingestion of alcohol, incorrect arm position, and incorrect cuff size can cause an error of more than ±5 mm Hg in diastolic or systolic blood pressure readings.[44]
Evidence	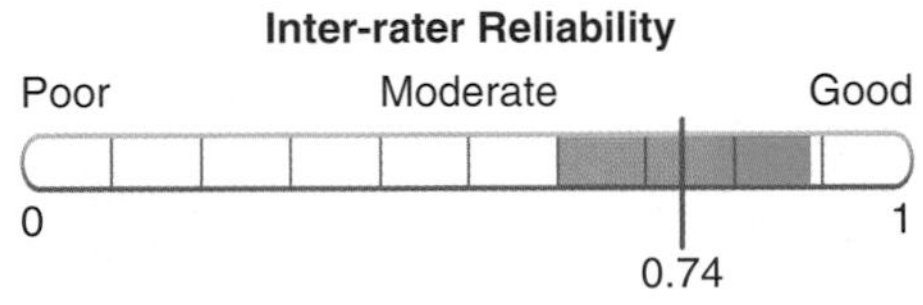

BP = blood pressure mm Hg = millimeters of mercury

Abdominal Palpation

To palpate the abdomen, place the patient in the hook-lying position (Fig. 1-13). During palpation of the four abdominal quadrants, note for areas of pain, increased tissue density, rigidity, and rebound tenderness (pain experienced when pressure is released, suggesting inflammation of the peritoneum) (Selective Tissue Test 1-8). Findings are correlated with the structures within the associated abdominal quadrant:

Quadrant Segment (Relative to the Patient)

	Right	Left
Upper	Liver (cholecystitis or liver laceration) Gallbladder (Pain in the absence of trauma suggests gallbladder disease.)	Spleen (Rigidity under the lower ribs suggests trauma to the spleen.)
Lower	Appendix (Rebound tenderness suggests appendicitis.) Colon (Colitis or diverticulitis may cause pain.) Pelvic inflammation results in diffuse pain.	Colon (Colitis or diverticulitis may cause pain.) Pelvic inflammation results in diffuse pain.

Genitourinary System

Consider genitourinary involvement if the patient describes acute trauma to the mid- or lower thorax or describes abdominal pain or symptoms with urination or intercourse. Kidney stones and urinary tract infections are both associated with low back pain. A central disc protrusion that compresses the spinal cord or cauda equina may result in loss of bowel and/or bladder control.

Urinalysis

If a patient report spainful urination or **hematuria** or has sustained trauma to the midthoracic region, obtain a urine sample, if possible, and note its appearance. Hematuria may indicate significant injury to the kidneys and warrants immediate referral to a physician. Any patient suspected of having an internal injury must be instructed to observe the color of the urine upon the next voiding. Immediately after the injury, blood may not be visible to the unaided eye but can be detected using a microscope or chemically with specially formulated strips dipped into the urine (Selective Tissue Test 1-9). Note that hematuria may normally be present after certain athletic events such as long-distance running or when an athlete is menstruating.

Excessive protein (proteinuria) or evidence of a urinary tract infection (elevated blood, protein, and nitrite or leukocyte esterase levels) may also be detected using a dipstick. The dipstick is far more useful at ruling out urine abnormalities rather than ruling them in.[53]

The Role of Evidence in the Examination Process

With more than 100 orthopedic tests available for the knee alone, it quickly becomes clear that not all of them can be performed during the examination of each patient. Using the results of the history and functional assessment conducted early in the process helps whittle

Selective Tissue Test 1-5
Heart Auscultation

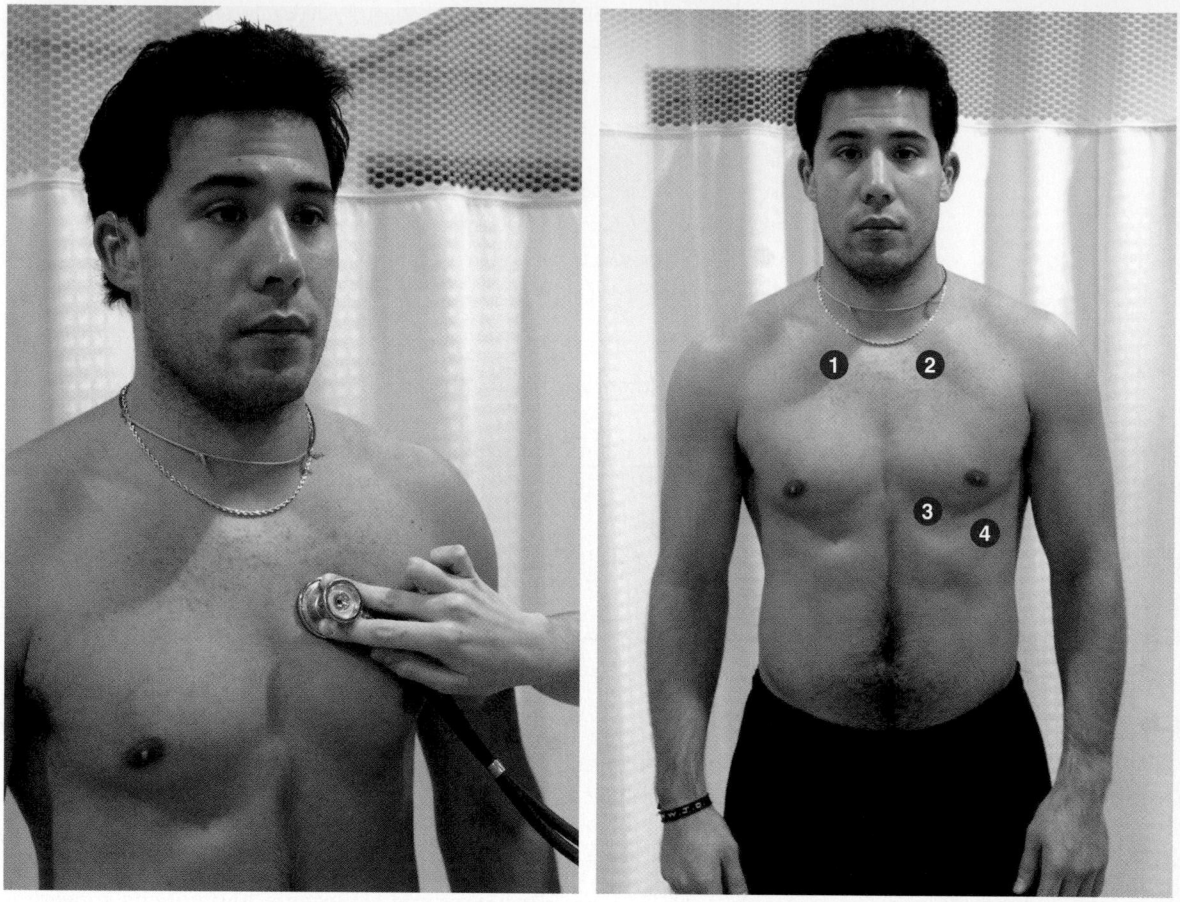

Heart auscultation identifies the presence or absence of abnormal heart sounds.

Patient Position	Sitting and/or standing
Position of Examiner	Stand facing the patient's right side
Evaluative Procedure	Listen at four locations: **1.** Right sternal border between ribs 2 and 3: Aortic area **2.** Left sternal border between ribs 2 and 3: Pulmonary area **3.** Left sternal border between ribs 5 and 6: Tricuspid area **4.** Left midclavicle line between ribs 5 and 6: Mitral area
Positive Test	Any deviation from typical "lub" and "dub" warrants referral to a physician. For examples, see Table 15-5.
Implications	A range of cardiac conditions
Comments	Do not auscultate over clothing.
Evidence	Absent or inconclusive in the literature

Selective Tissue Test 1-6
Lung Auscultation

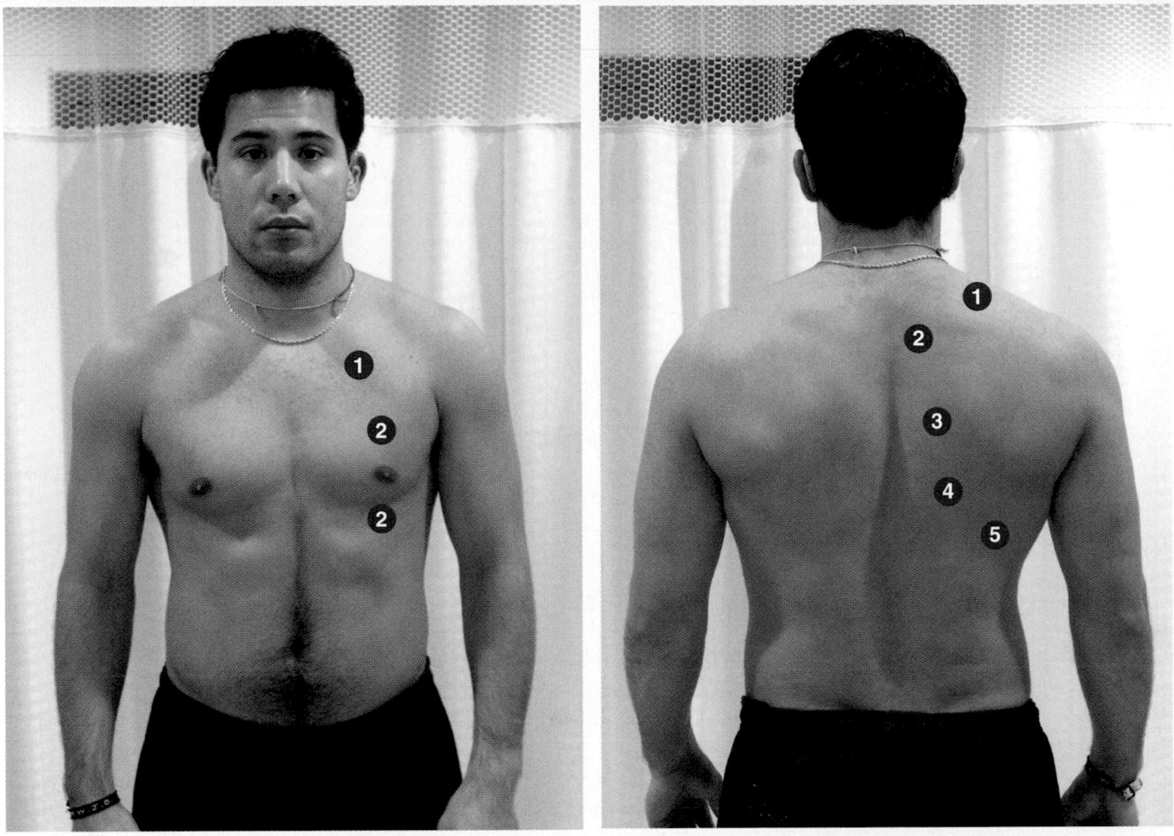

Lung sounds are obtained from the anterior and posterior thorax to determine the quality and quantity of respirations, noting for abnormal sounds.

Patient Position	Sitting
Position of Examiner	Standing beside the patient, ideally with the ability to move behind
Evaluative Procedure	Instruct the patient to breathe slowly and deeply through the mouth. Listen left and then right at each level. *Anterior:* **1.** Midclavicle line just below the clavicle **2.** Above and below the nipple line under breast tissue if present *Posterior:* Five spots on each side, taking care to not listen over the scapula **1.** Above the spine of scapula **2.** At the level of scapula spine **3.** Midscapula **4.** Distal scapula **5.** Below the inferior angle
Positive Test	Absence of sound: Collapsed lung Hyperresonance: Fluid in lung Crackles: Representing small airways "popping open" Wheeze: Narrowed airway (high pitch) Rhonchi: Secretions in larger airway (lower pitch); gurgling[51]
Comments	Do not auscultate over clothing.
Evidence	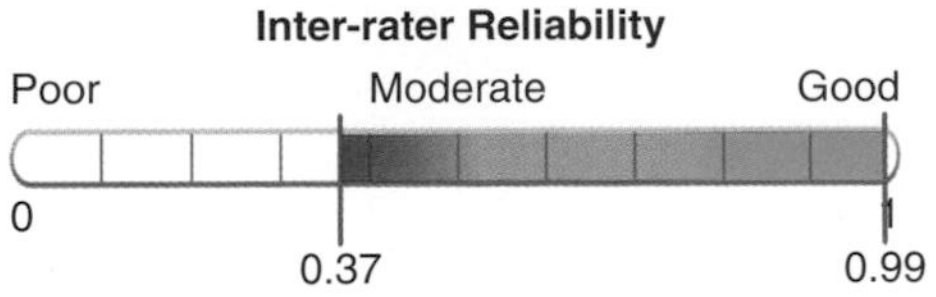

Selective Tissue Test 1-7
Abdomen Auscultation

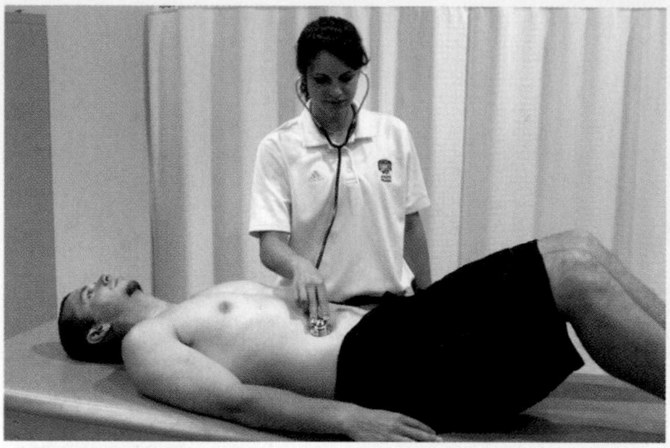

Auscultation of the abdomen. The integrity of the abdomen, the hollow organs, lungs, and descending blood vessels can be assessed through listening to the bowel sounds. Although the abdomen typically makes a gurgling sound, abdominal trauma reduces or eliminates this noise.

Patient Position	Supine; hook lying
Position of Examiner	Standing at the side of the patient
Evaluative Procedure	Examine the patient with an empty bladder if possible. Bowel sounds: Place diaphragm of stethoscope gently over the lower-right quadrant for 30 seconds. Medium-pitched gurgles every 5–10 seconds are normal. If these are absent, listen in all other quadrants. Listen for bruits (the sound of turbulent air rushing past an obstruction) at the top border of the right and left upper quadrants and the lower border of the right and left lower quadrants.
Positive Test	Bowel sounds that are high pitched or tinkle indicate possible partial obstruction or early complete bowel obstruction. Absent sounds indicate bowel paralysis possibly secondary to complete obstruction or **peritonitis**. To be sure that bowel sounds are truly absent, listen for 5 minutes. Bruits at the top border of the upper quadrant indicate renal artery stenosis.
Implications	Bowel obstruction, peritonitis, internal injury
Comments	Auscultate before palpation. Palpation can stimulate the bowel and give a false impression.
Evidence	Absent or inconclusive in the literature

Selective Tissue Test 1-8
Abdominal Percussion

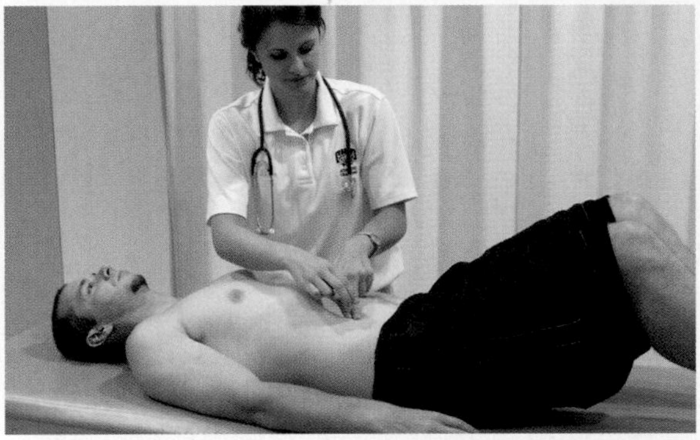

The abdominal quadrants are percussed by a quick tap of the fingertips lying gently on the abdomen. The resulting sound provides context to the density of the underlying tissues. Solid (or fluid-filled) areas produce a dull thud; hollow areas yield a more resonant sound.

Patient Position	Hook lying
Position of Examiner	Standing to the patient's side The examiner lightly places one hand palm down over the area to be assessed. The index and middle fingers of the opposite hand tap the DIP joints of the hand placed over the patient's abdomen.
Evaluative Procedure	The fingertips of the top hand quickly strike the middle phalanges of the bottom hand in a tapping motion. The sound of the echo within the abdomen is noted. Areas over solid organs have a dull thump associated with them. Hollow organs make a crisper, more **resonant** sound.
Positive Test	A hard, solid-sounding echo over areas that should normally sound hollow
Implications	Internal bleeding filling the abdominal cavity
Evidence	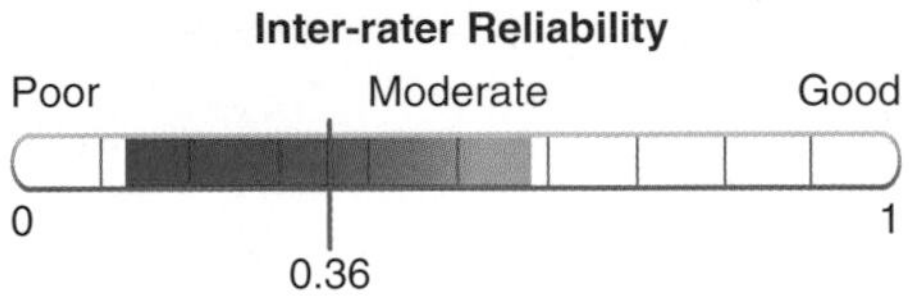

DIP = distal interphalangeal

Selective Tissue Test 1-9

"Clean Catch" Dipstick Urinalysis

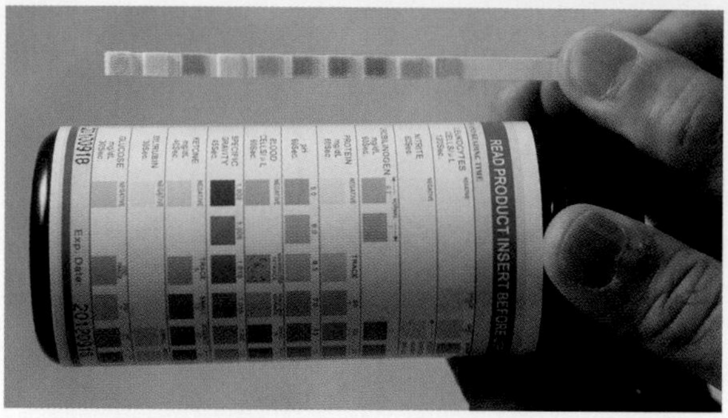

Dipstick urinalysis provides information regarding the patient's health and relative hydration level.

Evaluative Procedure

The external urethra and surrounding area is cleansed using soap and water and then rinsed.

To clear the urethra, the initial flow of urine is into a toilet bowl or "dirty" collection container.

One to 2 oz. of urine is then collected in a clean specimen cup.

The dipstick is then immersed into the specimen cup.

Follow the manufacturer's recommendations for immersion and interpretation times.

Test Results

The colors produced on the dipstick are matched to the values provided by the manufacturer.

Implications

Element	Normal	Interpretation
Specific Gravity:	1.006–1.030	Low reading: Diabetes mellitus, excessive hydration, renal failure High reading: Dehydration; heart or renal failure
pH:	4.6–8.0	Low reading: Chronic obstructive pulmonary disease, diabetic ketoacidosis High reading: Renal failure, urinary tract infection
Glucose, glucose dehydrogenase:	<0.5	Diabetes mellitus, stress
Ketones:	0	Anorexia, poor nutrition, alcoholism, diabetes mellitus
Protein:	-8	Congestive heart failure, polycystic kidney disease
Hemoglobin:	Trace	Urinary tract infection, kidney disease or trauma
RBC:	0	Kidney disease or trauma, kidney stones, bladder infection, urinary tract infection

Comments

The above interpretations are partial lists. High or low readings should be interpreted by a physician.

Factors such as diet and the level of exercise can alter the urinalysis readings.

Evidence

Hematuria

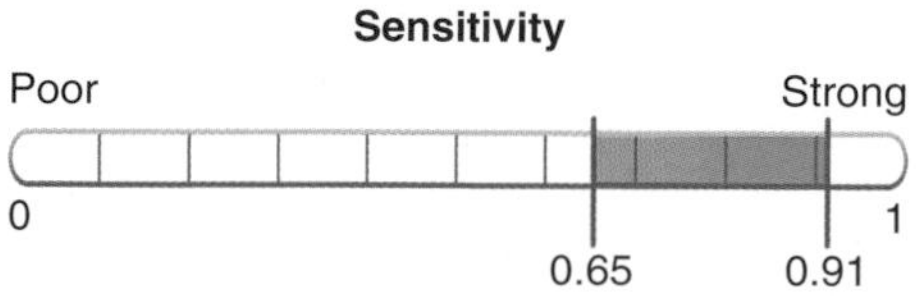

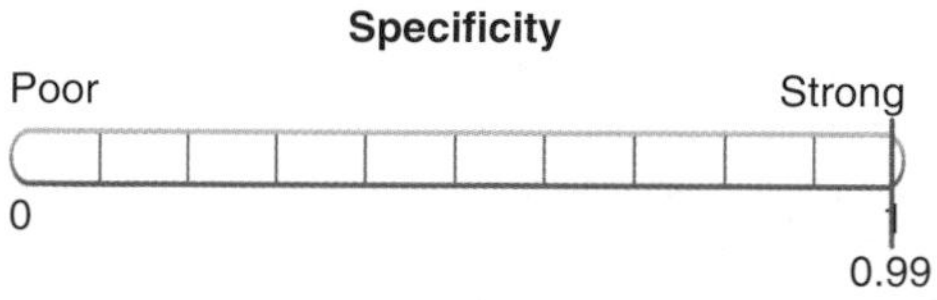

LR+: 65–91

LR−: 0.09–0.35

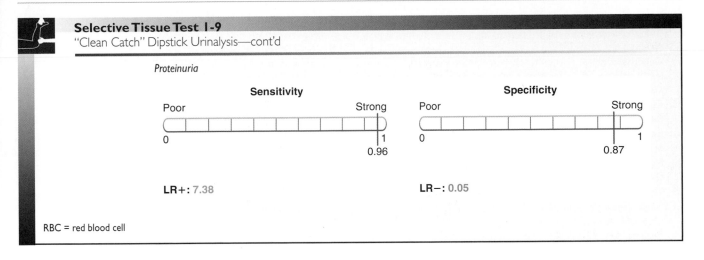

Selective Tissue Test 1-9
"Clean Catch" Dipstick Urinalysis—cont'd

Proteinuria

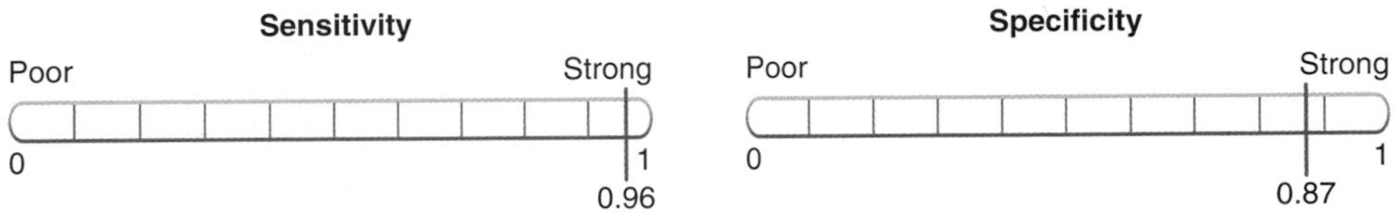

LR+: 7.38

LR−: 0.05

RBC = red blood cell

down or modify the orthopedic tests to be included. If the patient is complaining of a condition with a gradual onset, examination techniques to help identify an acute fracture can be omitted.

Applying the best evidence allows us to pare the list still further. Incorporating tests and measures that change the probability (or likelihood) of a certain diagnosis and eliminating those that do not help include or exclude diagnoses makes the examination still more refined, accurate, and efficient. When clinical prediction rules, such as the Ottawa Ankle Rules, exist, they should be followed whenever possible. The role of evidence in the clinical examination process is described in Chapter 3.

REFERENCES

1. Wainner, RS, et al: Regional interdependence: a musculoskeletal examination model whose time has come. *J Orthop Sports Phys Ther*, 37:658, 2007.
2. Spanjer, J, et al: Disability assessment interview: the role of detailed information on function in addition to medical history-taking. *J Rehabil Med*, 41:267, 2009.
3. McHenry, DM: A growing challenge: patient education in a diverse America. *J Nurses Staff Dev*, 23:83, 2007.
4. Spector, RE: *Cultural Diversity in Health and Illness*, ed 6. Stamford, CT: Appleton & Lange, 2003.
5. Bakhsh, H, et al: Assessment of the validity, reliability, responsiveness and bias of three commonly used patient-reported outcome measures in carpal tunnel syndrome. *Ortop Traumatol Rehabil*, 14:335, 2012.
6. Muscolo, DL, et al: Tumors about the knee misdiagnosed as athletic injuries. *J Bone Joint Surg*, 85(A):1209, 2003.
7. Jennings, F, Lambert, E, and Fredericson, M: Rheumatic diseases presenting as sports-related injuries. *Sports Med*, 38:917, 2008.
8. Roach, S: Hormones and related drugs. In *Pharmacology for Health Professionals*. Baltimore, MD: Lippincott Williams & Wilkins, 2005, pp 355-356.
9. Abdul-Hadi, O, et al: Nonsteroidal anti-inflammatory drugs in orthopaedics. *J Bone Jt Surg*, 91(A):2020, 2009.
10. Cohen, DB, et al: Indomethacin and celecoxib impair rotator cuff tendon-to-bone healing. *Am J Sports Med*, 34:352, 2006.
11. Pountos, I, Georgouli, T, and Giannoudis, PV: Do nonsteroidal anti-inflammatory drugs affect bone healing? A critical analysis. *ScientificWorld Journal*. 2012:606404, 2012.
12. Warden, SJ, et al: Low-intensity pulsed ultrasound accelerates and a nonsteroidal anti-inflammatory drug delays knee ligament healing. *Am J Sports Med*, 34:1094, 2006.
13. Kurmis, AP, et al: The effect of nonsteroidal anti-inflammatory drug administration on acute phase fracture healing: a review. *J Bone Jt Surg*, 94(A):815, 2012.
14. Warner, DO: Perioperative abstinence from cigarettes: physiologic and clinical consequences. *Anesthesiology*, 104:356, 2006.
15. Sen-Chowdhry, S, and McKenna, WJ: Sudden cardiac death in the young: a strategy for prevention by targeted evaluation. *Cardiology*, 105:196, 2006.
16. Leski, M: Sudden cardiac death in athletes. *South Med J*, 97:861, 2004.
17. Giese, EA, et al: The athletic preparticipation evaluation: cardiovascular assessment. *Am Fam Physician*, 75:1008, 2007.
18. George, SZ, et al: Depressive symptoms, anatomical region, and clinical outcomes for patients seeking outpatient physical therapy for musculoskeletal pain. *Phys Ther*, 91:358, 2011.
19. Haggman, S, Maher, CG, and Refshauge, KM: Screening for symptoms of depression by physical therapists managing low back pain. *Phys Ther*, 84:1157, 2004.
20. George, SZ, and Stryker, SE. Fear-avoidance beliefs and clinical outcomes for patients seeking outpatient physical therapy for musculoskeletal pain conditions. *J Orthop Sports Phys Ther*, 41:249, 2011.
21. Mawdsley, RH, Hoy, DK, and Erwin, PM: Criterion-related validity of the figure-of-eight method of measuring ankle edema. *J Orthop Sports Phys Ther*, 30:149, 2000.
22. Peterson, EJ, et al: Reliability of water volumetry and the figure of eight method on subjects with ankle joint swelling. *J Orthop Sports Phys Ther*, 29:609, 1999.
23. Rohner-Spengler, M, Mannion, AF, and Babst, R: Reliability and minimal detectable change for the figure-of-eight-20 method of measurement of ankle edema. *J Orthop Sports Phys Ther*, 37:199, 2007.
24. Daniel, JA, Sizer, PS, and Latman, NS: Evaluation of body composition methods for accuracy. *Biomed Instrum Technol*, 39:397, 2005.
25. Gerd, G, et al: Hypertrophic scarring and keloids: pathomechanisms and current and emerging treatment strategies. *Mol Med*, 17:113, 2011.
26. Macedo, LG, and Magee, DJ. Effects of age on passive range of motion of selected peripheral joints in healthy adult females. *Physiother Theory Pract*, 25:145, 2009.
27. Ockendon M, and Gilbert RE: Validation of a novel smartphone accelerometer-based knee program. *J Knee Surg*, 25:341, 2012.

28. Round, JM, et al: Hormonal factors in the development of differences in strength between boys and girls during adolescence: a longitudinal study. *Ann Hum Biol*, 26:49, 1999.
29. Goodpaster, BH, et al: The loss of skeletal muscle strength, mass, and quality in older adults: the health, aging and body composition study. *J Gerontol A Biol Sci Med Sci*, 61:1059, 2006.
30. Cuthbert, SC, and Goodheart, GJ: On the reliability and validity of manual muscle testing: a literature review. *Chiropr Osteopath*, 15:4, 2007.
31. Jepsen, JR, et al: Manual strength testing in 14 upper limb muscles: a study of inter-rater reliability. *Acta Orthop Scand*, 75:442, 2004.
32. Norkin, CC, and White, DJ: *Measurement of Joint Motion: A Guide to Goniometry*, ed 4. Philadelphia, PA: FA Davis, 2009, p 9.
33. van Trijffel E, et al: Inter-rater reliability for measurements of passive physiological movements in the lower extremity joints is generally low: a systematic review. *J Physiother*, 56:223, 2010.
34. Ageberg, E, et al: Balance in single-limb stance in patients with anterior cruciate ligament injury: relation to knee laxity, proprioception, muscle strength, and subjective function. *Am J Sports Med*, 33:1527, 2005.
35. Smith, CC: Evaluating the painful knee: a hands-on approach to acute ligamentous and mensical injuries. *Adv Stud Med*, 4:362, 2004.
36. Hegedus, EJ, et al: Which physical examination tests provide clinicians with the most value when examining the shoulder? Update of a systematic review with meta-analysis of individual tests. *Br J Sports Med*, 46:964, 2012.
37. Bertilson, B, et al: Pain drawing in the assessment of neurogenic pain and dysfunction in the neck/shoulder region: inter-examiner reliability and concordance with clinical examination. *Pain Med*, 8:134, 2007.
38. Dehghani, M, et al: Diagnostic accuracy of preoperative clinical examination in upper limb injuries. *J Emerg Trauma Shock*, 4:461, 2011.
39. Reese, NB: Techniques of the sensory examination. In *Muscle and Sensory Testing*, ed 2. St. Louis, MO: Elsevier Saunders, 2005, p 522.
40. Dick, JPR: The deep tendon and the abdominal reflexes. *J Neurol Neurosurg Psychiatry*, 74:150, 2003.
41. Delwaide, PJ, and Toulouse, P: The Jendrassik maneuver: quantitative analysis of reflex reinforcement by remote involuntary muscle contraction. In: Desmedt, JE, et al. *Motor Control Mechanisms in Health and Disease*. New York, NY: Raven Press, 1983, pp 661-669.
42. Perlowski, AA, and Jaff, MR: Vascular disorders in athletes. *Vasc Med*, 15:469, 2010.
43. Edmonds, ZV, et al: The reliability of vital sign measurements. *Ann Emerg Med*, 39:233, 2002.
44. McAlister, FA, and Straus, SE: Measurement of blood pressure: an evidence based review. *BMJ*, 322:908, 2001.
45. Kaplan, NM, Deveraux, RB, and Miller, HS: Task force 4: systemic hypertension. *J Am Coll Cardiol*, 24:885, 1994.
46. Young, E: A systematic review of variability and reliability of manual and automated blood pressure readings. *J Clin Nurs*, 20:602, 2011.
47. Barrett, MJ, Ayub, B, and Martinez, MW: Cardiac auscultation in sports medicine: strategies to improve clinical care. *Curr Sports Med Rep*, 11:78, 2012.
48. Karnath, B, and Thornton, W: Auscultation of the heart. *Hosp Physician*, 39, 2002.
49. Yen, K, et al: Interexaminer reliability in physical examination of pediatric patients with abdominal pain. *Arch Pediatr Adolesc Med*, 159:373, 2005.
50. Brooks, D, and Thomas, J: Interrater reliability of auscultation of breath sounds among physical therapists. *Phys Ther*, 75:1082, 1995.
51. Karnath, G, and Boyars, MC: Pulmonary auscultation. *Hosp Physician*, 22, 2002.
52. Aaron, SD, Dales, RE, and Cardinal, P: How accurate is spirometry at predicting restrictive pulmonary impairment? *Chest*, 115:869, 1999.
53. Simerville, JA, Maxted, WC, and Pahira, JJ: Urinalysis: a comprehensive review. *Am Fam Physician*, 71:1153, 2005.

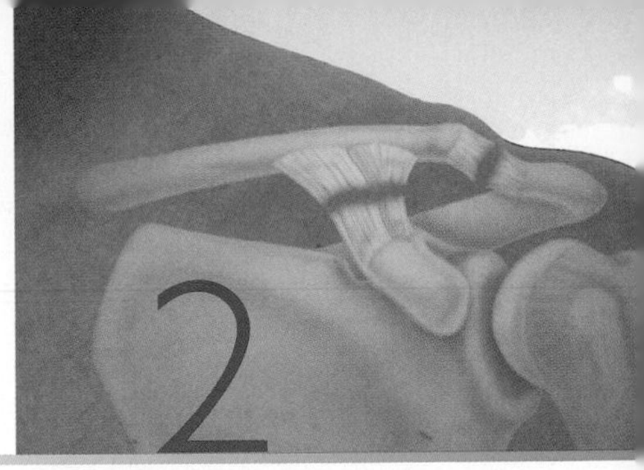

CHAPTER 2

Examination and Management of Acute Conditions

The circumstances surrounding an acute orthopedic injury influences the nature and duration of the initial examination. Consider the ambulatory evaluation, characterized by the patient coming to you for care on the sidelines. In many cases, this examination process mimics that described in Chapter 1. As used in this text, an acute examination is one that occurs immediately following the onset of the injury, often on the court or field. The acute examination initially focuses on determining the absence of severe injury, progresses through a series of examination techniques designed first to identify gross pathology, establishes the patient's ability and willingness to move and bear weight, and finally, if indicated, ends with a decision regarding return to play.

This chapter focuses on the immediate management of orthopedic pathology. Other possible **emergent** conditions, such as **anaphylaxis**, myocardial infarctions, and other medical conditions, that may require emergency interventions are not covered.

The first goal of the immediate examination is to determine if the condition requires emergency management to save the patient's life or extremity. In order of their importance, the immediate examination must rule out:

- Inhibition of the cardiovascular and respiratory systems (i.e., whether or not the person is breathing and has a pulse)
- Life-threatening trauma to the head or spinal column
- Profuse bleeding
- Fractures
- Joint dislocation
- Peripheral nerve injury
- Other soft tissue trauma

Based on the findings of this triage, the immediate disposition of the patient must be determined. The acute management of the injury, the safest method of removing the athlete from the field, and the urgency of referral for further medical care are the focus of the decision-making process.

On-field examinations are best performed with two responders. In cases of head or spine trauma, one individual is responsible for stabilizing the cervical spine, while the other performs the needed examination techniques. For noncatastrophic conditions, one responder conducts the examination while the other communicates with and calms the athlete and controls the surrounding scene (Fig. 2-1). In all cases, the responders should ensure that play has stopped (or has been moved in the event of a practice-related injury)

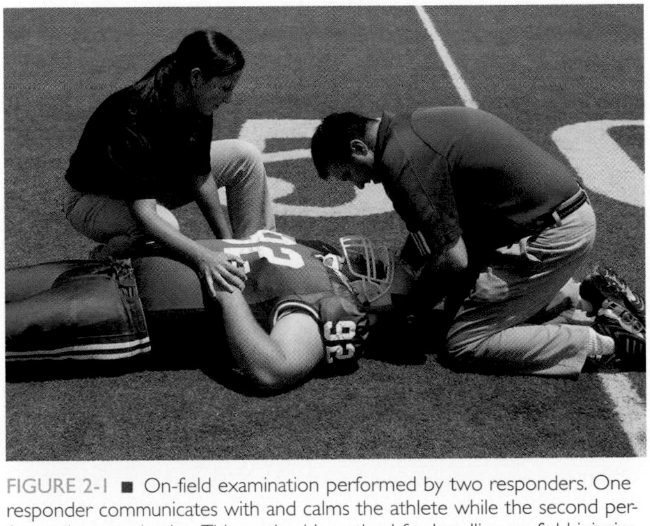

FIGURE 2-1 ■ On-field examination performed by two responders. One responder communicates with and calms the athlete while the second performs the examination. This method is optimal for handling on-field injuries, especially in emergency situations.

Emergent In need of prompt care; emergency

Anaphylaxis A severe, potentially life-threatening allergic reaction so that the responders and the victim are protected from further sports-related activity.

When one responder is responsible for the on-field injury examination, a clear communication and examination protocol is needed so that relatively untrained people can assist (Fig. 2-2). The coaching staff and other personnel should receive regular training in cardiopulmonary resuscitation (CPR), including use of an automated external defibrillator (AED), and be prepared to provide assistance in the event of a catastrophic injury.

Practical Evidence

Early defibrillation using an AED saves lives. Early defibrillation is the single most important intervention in improving survival following sudden cardiac arrest (SCA). For every minute that defibrillation is delayed, the chance of surviving SCA declines by 10%.[1,2]

Emergency Planning

The planning of event medical coverage must account for the worst-case scenario: catastrophic conditions to athletes, spectators, and others at the venue. Each institution should have a written **emergency action plan (EAP)** that identifies the personnel, equipment, lines of communication, and standard procedures should a potentially catastrophic event occur.[3] When visiting an away site, communicate with the host institution to determine the EAP for that venue.

An on-field communication plan must be established for managing on-field injuries. Pre-established hand signals or walkie-talkies allow the individuals on the field to communicate with sideline personnel. This makes it easy to quickly relay the need for emergency equipment, the team physician, other emergency personnel, and a transport squad on the field.

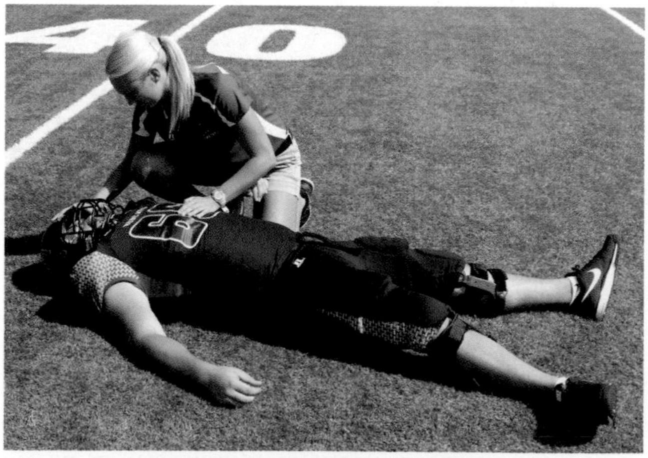

FIGURE 2-2 ■ One examiner responding to an on-field injury. This method requires that the individual perform the evaluation, communicate with the athlete, and, if necessary, summon emergency personnel.

Sport-Specific Rules

Each sport at each level of competition has rules governing the on-field management of injuries during sanctioned competition. In most cases, the official must summon assistance to the playing area, and, in some sports such as wrestling, the examination must be completed and the disposition of the athlete determined within a limited period of time. Once that time ends, the athlete is disqualified from competition regardless of ability to continue based on a medical evaluation.

Clinicians must stay current with concussion management guidelines as they frequently change. In 2008, the Consensus Statement on Concussion in Sport at the International Conference on Concussion in Sport in Zurich recommended that a concussed athlete shall not return to competition on the day of the injury (see Chapter 20).[4] These guidelines form the basis for most athletic leagues and state-based concussion regulation.

Table 2-1 provides a general summary of sport-specific rules as they pertain to medical examination and care. These rules vary by governing organization, state, and venue. The medical staff is responsible for knowing the rules governing medical assistance. Before each contest, meet with the officials and other emergency personnel to clarify rules as they pertain to injury examination and protective equipment.

Critical Findings

During the examination of an acute injury, a finding may be so profound that no other information need be collected; management procedures are implemented, and the athlete is immediately transported to an appropriate medical facility. Such findings include acute neurological symptoms (indicative of cervical spine or head pathology), signs of cardiovascular distress, bone angulations or deformity (associated with fractures or joint dislocations), gross joint instability, and vascular deficits. When the severity of the condition is uncertain, always err on the side of caution and refer the athlete for further medical attention.

If the initial examination cannot rule out a catastrophic condition, management of the condition becomes the first priority (Table 2-2). In addition to activating the EAP, injury-management strategies must be implemented.

The On-Field Examination

When examining an on-field injury, obtaining a precise clinical diagnosis and identifying the functional limitations are less important than determining the extent of the injury and how to safely transport the athlete. Immediately after the injury, the examination focuses on determining if—and how—to splint the body part, how to remove the athlete from the playing area, and whether the athlete should be transported to the sidelines, to a

Table 2-1 Rules Affecting Examination During Athletic Competition

Sport	Rule(s)
Baseball	Hard casts must be properly padded. Players are permitted to wear only one elbow pad that does not exceed 10 inches in length.[5] No player may wear a nonstandard elbow protection pad, or any pad designed to protect the upper or lower arm, unless the player has an existing elbow or other arm injury and the team carries with it the following documentation: (a) A letter identifying the player and describing both the nature of the injury and the proposed elbow protection pad; (b) A physician's report diagnosing the injury; and 26 Rule 1 / The Game, Playing Field and Equipment; (c) A physician's determination of the length of time the protective pad will be necessary.[5[pp 25-26]]
Basketball	An injured player must temporarily leave the contest if the athletic trainer or other staff member comes onto the court requiring a stoppage in play.[6] Pliable (flexible or easily bent) material, covered on all exterior sides and edges with no less than 1/2-inch thickness of a slow-rebounding foam, may be used to immobilize and protect an injury. Equipment deemed dangerous to others by the officiating crew is prohibited.[6] Pre-event approval of protective equipment is required.
Field Hockey	Protective equipment that increases the size of the goalkeeper is not allowed.[7]
Football	No equipment that would endanger others, such as that made of metal, is allowed. Hard equipment must be covered with thick foam padding; functional/preventative knee braces must be covered or worn under clothing.[8] After an injury timeout, the injured player must leave for at least one down.[8]
Ice Hockey	When there is a stoppage of play because of an injury to a player other than the goalkeeper, the injured player must leave the ice until the completion of the ensuing faceoff. Use of pads or protectors made of metal or any hard substance that could cause injury is prohibited.[9]
Soccer	Athletic trainers or other staff may not enter the field unless instructed by an official. Casts, knee braces, and other hard braces must be properly padded.[10]
Softball	Casts, braces, splints, and/or prostheses may be worn provided they are well padded and not distracting.[11]
Tennis	Time-limited medical and bleeding timeouts may be used to treat the athlete.[12]
Wrestling	Medical personnel may leave the restricted zone only during an injury timeout. Two injury timeouts may be given for a cumulative maximum of 90 seconds for the entire match. A third nonbleeding injury will end the match. Bleeding timeouts do not count as an injury timeout, but the number of timeouts and the length of time allowed to treat the wound are left to the official's discretion. If a contestant is rendered unconscious or shows signs of a concussion or spinal injury, that wrestler shall not be permitted to continue in the match or return to competition without approval of the team physician or the team physician's designee according to each institution's concussion management plan. Student athletes diagnosed with a concussion shall not return to activity (or competition) for the remainder of that day. No more than two attendants may be allowed on the mat during these timeouts.[13]
All Sports	Athletes who have an open wound must be removed from competition until the bleeding is controlled and the wound appropriately covered. Uniforms that are saturated with blood must be changed. NCAA sports are bound by a uniform concussion policy: www.NCAA.org/health-safety.

Refer to current national governing agencies and individual conference rules regarding competitor safety.

sports medicine facility, or directly to the hospital. The examination must first rule out life- or limb-threatening conditions (including head and spinal cord trauma), followed by assessment for fractures/dislocations, peripheral nerve pathology, joint instability, and muscle trauma.

Because the purpose of the on-field examination differs from that of a clinical examination, the model used will also differ. Part of the inspection process begins before a history is taken, and only gross measures of joint range of motion (ROM), muscle function, and joint stability are assessed. Selective tissue tests are usually not performed at this point. In the event of possible vertebral fracture or dislocation, or spinal cord or nerve root trauma, neurological testing will assume increased importance, as will vascular screening if a fracture or dislocation of a major joint is present.

Table 2-2 Findings that Warrant Immediate Physician Referral

Segment	Findings
History	Reports of the inability to feel or move one or more limbs (confirm with neurological screen)
	Reports of significant chest pain
	Reports of difficulty breathing (e.g., anaphylaxis, pneumothorax)
Inspection	Obvious fracture
	Obvious joint dislocation
	Loss of consciousness
	Cyanosis
	Unequal chest expansion
Palpation	Disruption in the contour of bone, indicating a fracture or joint dislocation
	Malalignment of joint structures
Joint and Muscle Function Assessment	Inability of the muscle to produce torque secondary to spinal cord or peripheral nerve injury
Joint Stability Tests	Gross joint instability
Neurological Tests	Sensory dysfunction
	Motor dysfunction
	Pathological changes in reflex
	Inability to maintain balance, loss of coordination, and other signs and symptoms of brain injury
Vascular Screening	Diminished or absent pulse
	Pooling of venous blood, suggesting inhibition of venous return

Another difference between clinical and on-field acute examinations is the less-than-ideal conditions in which the acute examination is conducted. The luxury of an examination table is replaced by the challenge of examining an athlete who is **prone** on the ground or sitting awkwardly on a bench. The examination may also be complicated by protective equipment and environmental conditions.

The best way to acclimate yourself to performing an on-field examination is to practice these skills with a person lying on the ground wearing football equipment or on the ice while wearing hockey equipment. The mechanics of the ROM, stress, and selective tissue tests described in this text are more difficult to perform while kneeling. Other athletic venues, such as swimming pools and gymnastics pits, also present challenges to those conducting acute examinations.

Prone Lying face down

Equipment Considerations

Athletic equipment can hinder many components of the on-field examination. In most cases, clothing is not removed to conduct the on-field examination, but protective equipment such as ankle or knee braces can impede the immediate examination and must be removed or loosened to permit a complete evaluation. Methods to remove protective equipment safely are discussed in the on-field management sections in the applicable chapters of this text. Helmets, face masks, and shoulder pads present a unique challenge to the on-field examination of suspected cervical spine trauma (see Chapter 20).

✱ Practical Evidence

Football face mask removal using a cordless screwdriver is easier than using tools that cut through the straps and results in less head movement.[14]

Primary Survey

The acute examination begins with the primary survey (Fig. 2-3). As you approach the athlete, observe for signs of movement. An athlete who is moving normally, holding an injured body part, or writhing in pain indicates consciousness, a functioning central nervous system (CNS), and cardiovascular function. Far more critical are athletes who show no signs of movement or who are seizing, indicating possible CNS trauma. All unconscious individuals should be managed as if they are suffering from cervical spine trauma (see Chapter 20), with the emergency action plan immediately activated. When multiple providers are present, a prone, unconscious athlete with a pulse and who is breathing should be rolled to the supine position to facilitate the possible use of CPR or AED. An athlete who is not breathing or who does not have a pulse should be immediately rolled to the supine position.

Stabilize the head and cervical spine, unless this is clearly not indicated by the mechanism of injury (Fig. 2-4). Establish the level of consciousness by speaking to the athlete. Do not use "smelling salts" (e.g., ammonia capsules) in an attempt to determine the athlete's level of consciousness or to revive the athlete.

Pulses

For unconscious athletes, determine if a normal pulse is present. If no pulse is present, bare the chest, begin chest compressions and prepare to use an AED. Abnormal pulses are classified by the heart's rate and rhythm:

Type	Characteristics	Implication
Accelerated	Pulse >150 beats per minute (bpm) (>170 bpm usually has fatal results).	Pressure on the base of the brain; shock
Bounding	Pulse that quickly reaches a higher intensity than normal, then quickly disappears	Ventricular systole and reduced peripheral pressure

Deficit	Pulse in which the number of beats counted at the radial pulse is less than that counted over the heart itself	Cardiac arrhythmia
High Tension	Pulse in which the force of the beat is increased; an increased amount of pressure is required to inhibit the radial pulse.	Cerebral trauma
Low Tension	Short, fast, faint pulse having a rapid decline	Heart failure; shock

Airway

The conscious athlete may show signs of **apnea** or **dyspnea**, in which case an obstructed airway should be suspected. Possible causes of obstructed airways on the playing field include mouthpieces, dislodged teeth, and swelling of the esophagus secondary to anaphylaxis. If the airway is blocked, clear it using the Heimlich maneuver (sharp, rapid abdominal thrusts) or, if that fails, manually removing the obstacle.

Respiratory Rate and Pattern

At rest, normal respiration ranges from 12 to 20 breaths per minute, with well-conditioned athletes falling on the lower end of the range. Abnormal breathing patterns and the possible causes of their onset include:

- **Rapid, shallow breaths:** Rib fracture; internal injury; shock
- **Deep, quick breaths:** Pulmonary obstruction; asthma
- **Noisy, raspy breaths:** Airway obstruction

Apnea The temporary cessation of breathing

Dyspnea Air hunger marked by labored or difficult breathing; may be either a normal occurrence after exertion or an abnormal occurrence indicating cardiac or respiratory distress

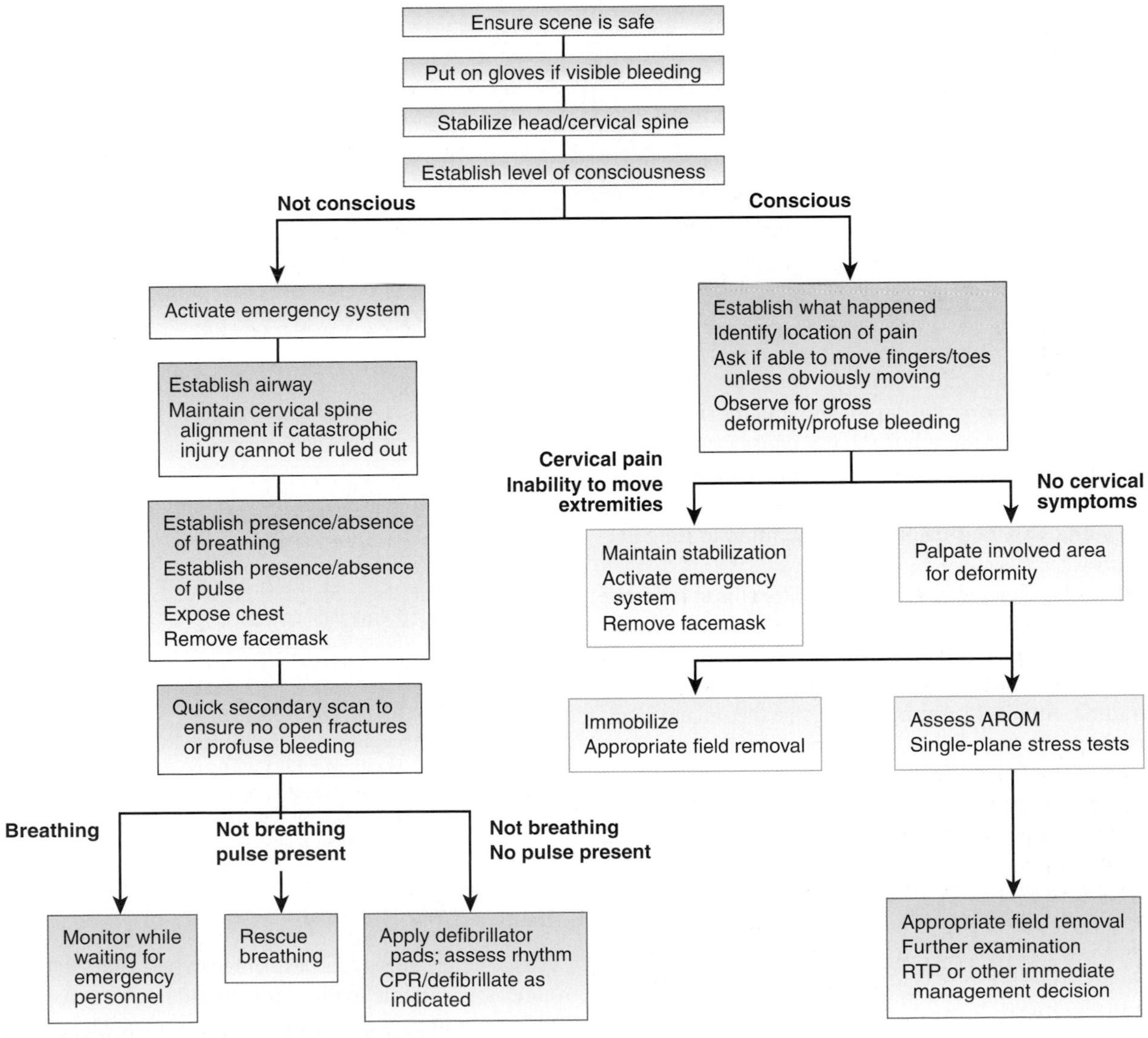

FIGURE 2-3 ■ Schematic representation of the on-field decision-making process.

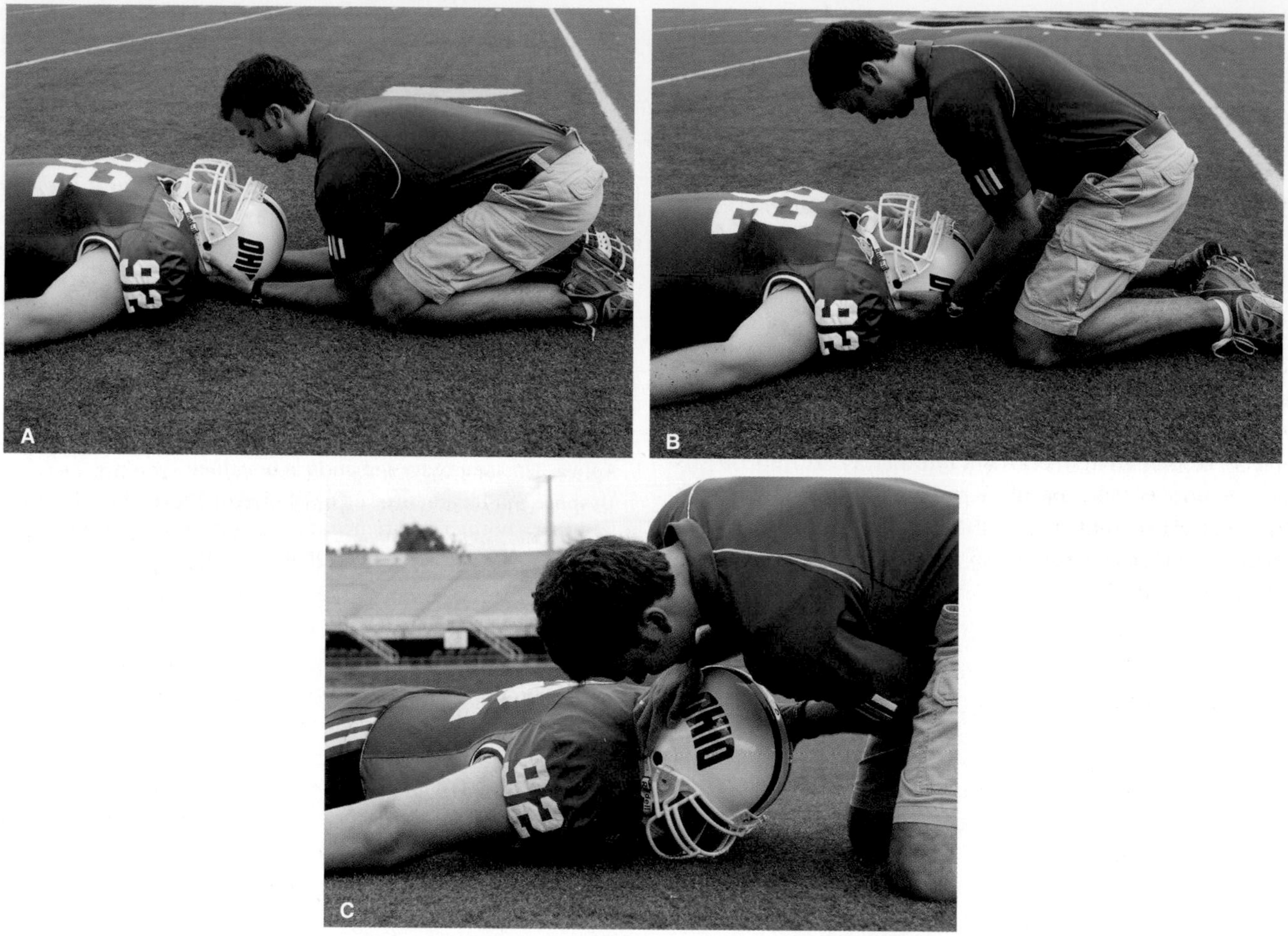

FIGURE 2-4 ■ Different cervical spine stabilization techniques. (A, B) In-line stabilization and (C) prior to rolling the athlete supine.

Note the respiration rate, depth, and quality. Difficulty in breathing, or stridor, may have many causes that include asthma, allergies, cardiac contusion, injury to the ribs or costal cartilage, lung trauma (e.g., pneumothorax, hemothorax, or pulmonary contusion), or other injury to the internal organs.

Observe the chest wall movement. The ribs should rise and fall in a symmetrical pattern with each breath; any deviation in this pattern could be the result of fractured ribs or a pneumothorax. **Subcutaneous emphysema** may indicate lung trauma. Atypical prominence of the secondary inspiration muscles (e.g., scalenes, sternomastoid) indicates that the patient is having difficulty breathing.

Abnormal breathing patterns are further classified based on the tempo and relationship between inspirations and exhalations:

Type	Characteristics	Implications
Apneustic	Prolonged inspirations unrelieved by attempts to exhale	Trauma to the pons
Biot's	Periods of apnea followed by hyperapnea	Increased intracranial pressure
Cheyne-Stokes	Periods of apnea followed by breaths of increasing depth and frequency	Frontal lobe or brain stem trauma
Slow	Respiration consisting of fewer than 12 breaths per minute	CNS disruption
Thoracic	Respiration in which the diaphragm is inactive and breathing occurs only through expansion of the chest; normal abdominal movement is absent	Disruption of the phrenic nerve or its nerve roots

Subcutaneous emphysema Air trapped beneath the skin.

Secondary Survey

A secondary survey is performed when the athlete is unconscious, unable to move (or should not be moved), or unable to communicate with the responder. The purpose of the secondary survey is to identify other serious conditions that require immediate management or that will change how emergency care is implemented. For example, CPR cannot effectively be administered when there is bleeding from a large artery because chest compressions will cause more bleeding.

Observe and palpate the other body areas, noting for the presence of any bleeding, gross deformity, or other signs of trauma to other parts of the body. In cases in which the injury is apparent, such as an obvious fracture or dislocation, the history of the injury often becomes irrelevant. In these cases, rule out the possibility of head and/or spinal trauma, calm the athlete, and perform a secondary screen to rule out injury to other body areas while initiating appropriate management of the condition. When appropriate, treat for shock.

The results of the primary and secondary survey are used to make the next clinical decision. Options at this point are: (1) activate the EAP and provide emergency intervention such as controlling bleeding and/or administering CPR or AED, or (2) continue with the examination process.

On-Field History

Once the presence of the athlete's airway and circulation has been established, the history-taking process continues. If the athlete is unconscious or disoriented, as much information as possible is obtained from those who witnessed the episode. The history portion of the on-field evaluation is relatively brief compared with that associated with the clinical evaluation and tends to focus on the immediate events. The information to be identified includes:

- **Location of the pain:** Identify the site of pain as closely as possible. Although the athlete may be holding a particular area, do not assume that this is the only site of trauma because multiple injuries may have occurred. Ask the question, "Do you have pain anywhere else?"
- **Peripheral symptoms:** Question the athlete about the presence of pain or altered sensation that radiates into the distal extremities, suggesting spinal cord, nerve root, or peripheral nerve trauma.
- **Mechanism of the injury:** Identify the force that caused the injury (e.g., contact vs. noncontact injuries).
- **Associated sounds and symptoms:** Note any reports of a "snap" or "pop" at the time of injury, which may indicate either a fracture or a torn ligament or tendon.
- **History of injury:** Identify any relevant history of injury that may have been exacerbated by the current trauma or may influence the physical findings during the current evaluation.

On-Field Inspection

The observation process begins as soon as the athlete is in the responder's sight. As described in the Primary Survey section, observe for signs of movement and determine the level of consciousness first. Once it has been determined that the athlete has a pulse and is breathing, note the following:

- **Position of the athlete:** Is the athlete prone, **supine**, or side-lying? Is a body part in an awkward position? Is any gross deformity evident? Athletes experiencing cardiac episodes will most likely be clutching their chest and possibly bending over in pain. Patients in respiratory distress characteristically bend over with their hands on their knees. This closed chain position allows the secondary muscles of respiration (sternocleidomastoid and pectoral muscles) to aid breathing. In labored breathing, these muscles may be observed to be contracting forcefully. The athlete may recruit the secondary muscles of respiration by sitting with the elbows on the knees and the head hanging between the legs.
- **Inspection of the injured area:** This process is an abbreviated version of the steps presented in the Clinical Evaluation section, specifically observing for signs of a fracture (such as long-bone angulation), joint dislocation (gross deformity), or edema.
- **Vomiting:** Observe the patient for and question about any vomiting after injury. Blood in the vomitus may also signify injury to the stomach, esophagus, pulmonary trauma, or chronic conditions such as ulcers.
- **Skin color:** The color of the athlete's skin is normally flushed because of exercise. Cardiopulmonary distress results in pale or ashen skin. First appearing in the lips, the discoloration progresses to cyanosis as the skin's tissues are deprived of oxygen. An unexpected change in skin tone or color from that which is normally associated with exercise should be a "red flag" for the examiner.
- **Sweating:** Anyone suffering from cardiac problems may perspire profusely. However, the athlete involved in vigorous physical activity normally exhibits perspiration as a result of the activity. In the absence of physical activity, complaints of chest pain and profuse sweating are classic symptoms of cardiac distress. Absence of sweating during exercise can suggest heat-related illness.

On-Field Palpation

Two major areas to palpate are the bony structures and soft tissues. Findings of possible fractures, joint dislocations, or neurovascular pathology warrant terminating the evaluation and transporting the athlete to a medical facility.

Palpation of Bony Structures

- **Bony alignment:** Palpate the length of the injured bone to identify any discontinuity. Although fractures of long bones are often accompanied by gross deformity, those of smaller bones may present no outward signs but are exquisitely tender during palpation.

Supine Lying face up

- **Crepitus:** Note any crepitus, associated with fractures, swelling, inflammation, or air entering the subcutaneous tissues.
- **Joint alignment:** If the injury involves a joint, palpate along the joint line to determine whether the joint is aligned normally.

Palpation of Soft Tissues

- **Swelling:** Swelling immediately after the injury is often associated with a major disruption of the tissues. Trauma to bursae tend to swell disproportionately to the severity of the injury. Tissues that have a rich blood supply, such as those in the face, may present with a rapid formation of localized edema.
- **Painful areas:** Areas that are painful when palpated can indicate trauma to underlying tissue. Associate the painful area to both the underlying structure or, in the case of neurological conditions, the associated nerve pathway.
- **Deficit in the muscles or tendons:** Severe tearing of a muscle or tendon can result in a palpable defect. There is a "golden period" immediately after an injury that allows for defects to be palpated. After this period, edema and muscle spasm mask any underlying defect.

On-Field Joint and Muscle Function Assessment

While evaluating acute injuries on the field, ROM and functional testing provide information about the athlete's ability and willingness to move the involved extremity. Active range of motion (AROM) is the most important test to perform while the athlete is still on the field, as this demonstrates willingness to move and an intact contractile structure. If the injury involves the lower extremity, expand functional testing to include the ability to bear weight.

Do not perform an on-field assessment of joint function when a fracture, dislocation, or muscle or tendon rupture is suspected. An approach to assessing the limb's function in a progressive manner includes:

- **Active range of motion:** The athlete is asked to move the limb through the ROM, while the quality and quantity of movement are noted.
- **Strength assessment:** If ROM test results are normal, break pressure can be used to determine the involved muscle group's ability to sustain a forceful contraction. Similar to passive range of motion (PROM), the more specific manual muscle tests are delayed until a more detailed examination is performed.
- **Passive range of motion:** The decision to include PROM assessment is made on a case-by-case basis and is frequently delayed until the clinical evaluation. The degree of muscular and/or ligamentous damage and capsular disruption is assessed by placing the tissues on stretch. Do not perform PROM evaluations on the field if the athlete is unable to actively move the joint.
- **Weight-bearing status (lower extremity injuries):** If the athlete is able to complete the ROM tests, the athlete can be permitted to walk off the field, with assistance if necessary. If the athlete is unable to perform these tests or signs and symptoms of a potential fracture or dislocation exist, the athlete is removed from the field in a non–weight-bearing manner.

On-Field Joint Stability Tests

The purpose of on-field stress testing is to gain an immediate impression of the integrity of the capsule and ligaments involved in the injury before muscle guarding or swelling masks the degree of laxity. Often, on-field stress testing involves only single-plane tests that are compared with the opposite side. Because these evaluations are performed on the playing surface, stress testing is often conducted in less-than-ideal conditions.

On-Field Neurological Testing

Neurological testing becomes particularly important in the on-field evaluation of the athlete with a suspected head or spine injury. A thorough evaluation can ensure the proper management of these potentially catastrophic injuries. When responding to acute neurological injuries, tests for cervical nerve root and cranial nerve involvement are needed (see Chapters 14 and 20).

Fractures or dislocations can impinge or lacerate peripheral nerves. Assessing motor function distal to the site of injury is indicated if it can be done without moving the involved bone or joint. For example, the athlete might be asked to move his or her fingers in the presence of an anterior glenohumeral joint dislocation. An assessment of distal sensation should also be included.

On-Field Vascular Assessment

After the dislocation of a major joint or the fracture of a large bone, the integrity of the distal vascular structures must also be determined. As with nerves, bony displacement may impinge on or lacerate the arteries and veins supplying the distal portion of the extremity. An athlete with damaged arteries may still present with an intact distal pulse, so further diagnostic testing is indicated after joint dislocation and reduction. Capillary refill should be assessed, and formation of edema distal to the injured area, possibly signifying blockage of the venous return system, should be noted.[15] The specific processes for identifying these deficits are described in the appropriate chapters of this text.

*** Practical Evidence**

Identifying a distal pulse after knee dislocation does not rule out vascular damage. Following a dislocation, angiography is recommended even with normal pulse and a well-perfused limb. Angiography is not recommended if vascular injury is obvious (diminished pulse, signs of ischemia) because any delay in surgery worsens the patient's outcome.[16]

Immediate Management

Upon completion of the on-field examination, a determination must be made regarding how to manage the athlete. Possible conclusions are:

- **No splinting is needed:** The athlete walks off under his or her own power.
- **No splinting is needed:** The athlete is assisted off the field.
- **No splinting is needed:** The athlete is transported directly to the hospital.
- **Splinting is needed:** The athlete walks off the field (upper extremity injury).
- **Splinting is needed:** The athlete is assisted off the field (lower extremity injury).
- **Splinting is needed:** The athlete is transported directly to the hospital.

The decision-making model will change according to physician availability and institutional protocol. Refer to Chapter 20 regarding the on-field management of head and spine injuries. On-field management strategies for upper and lower extremity injuries are presented in the corresponding chapters.

Splinting

Most fractures, dislocations, and significant joint sprains will need to be immobilized before removing the athlete from the field. A variety of splints are available for use, but vacuum splints are arguably the most widely used. The basic principles of immobilization are the same regardless of the type of splint used (Box 2-1).

Transportation

A decision must be made regarding how and when to transport the athlete from the playing area in the safest manner possible. If a fracture, dislocation, gross joint instability, or other significant musculoskeletal trauma is suspected, the involved body part must be splinted as described in the previous section before moving the athlete.

Based on the severity and type of injury being managed, one of several methods may be used to remove the athlete from the field (Fig. 2-5). In the case of most upper extremity injuries, immobilize the body part and walk the athlete off the field. In cases of lower extremity injuries in which the athlete is unable to bear weight or upright posturing is contraindicated, several types of stretchers may be used; avoid carrying the athlete if possible. Suspected injury to the spine requires the use of a spine board and rigid cervical collar.

Injured athletes who are lying on the field should first be moved to a sitting position, where they are again monitored for dizziness and light-headedness. If sitting is achieved without a problem, the athlete is assisted to a standing position. Finally, give instructions regarding the extent of weight bearing. If non–weight bearing on the injured limb, provide two human "crutches" of similar size.

Box 2-1
Principles of Splinting and Immobilization

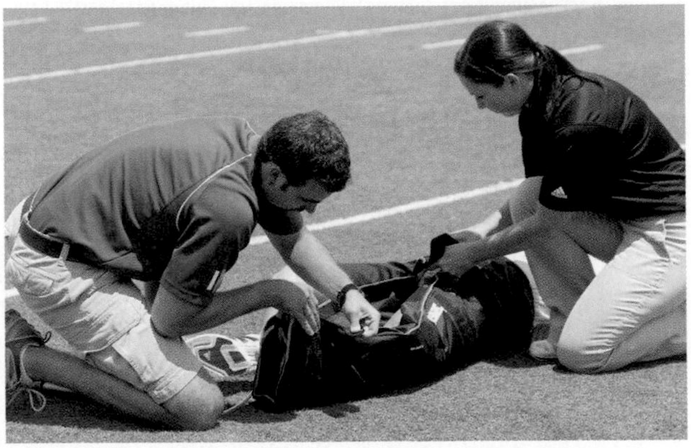
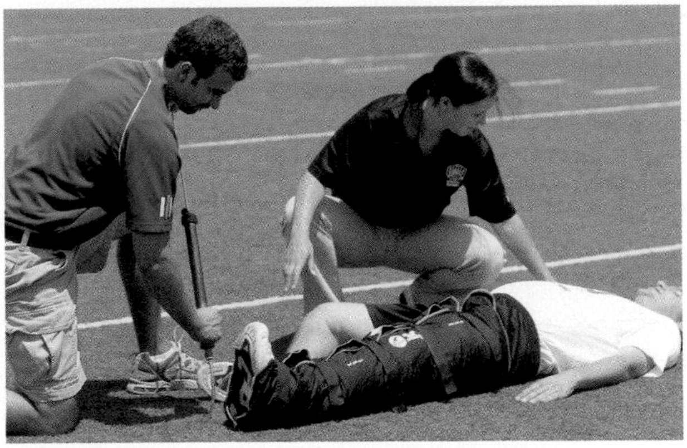

In most sports medicine settings, commercial splints will be used to immobilize the body part, although upper extremity injuries can often be splinted against the torso. Regardless of the type of splint used, the splinting technique should limit motion of the involved joint and/or bone in three dimensions.

1. Unless otherwise directed by a physician, splint the extremity in the position in which it was found.
2. Establish a baseline level of sensation and skin temperature so that any changes can be noted.
3. Immobilize the joint(s) proximal and distal to the injured site.
4. Edema will most likely form soon after the injury. The splint should allow for edema and be regularly readjusted to account for swelling.[17]
5. To allow capillary refill to be checked, leave the fingers or toes uncovered when possible. Regularly assess capillary refill.
6. After immobilization, periodically question the athlete about increased pain, diminished or altered sensation, and changes in skin temperature.

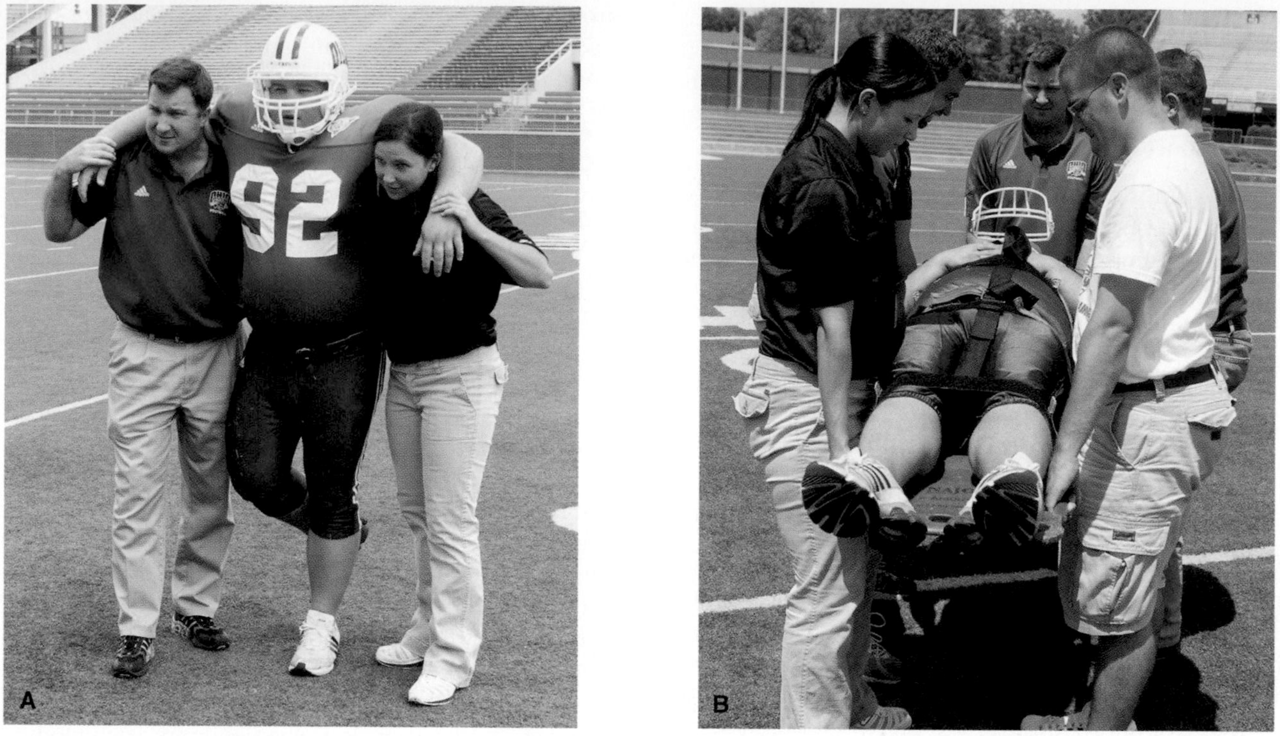

FIGURE 2-5 ■ Various athlete extraction techniques. (A) Assisted walking; and (B) full spine board.

Disposition

After removing the athlete from the field, a more detailed examination can be performed. The goals of this examination are to obtain enough information to determine a clinical diagnosis, make a return-to-play decision, and decide on an immediate plan of care. The plan of care could include immediate referral for more advanced medical care, immediate treatment such as cold and compression, and/or home instructions for continued monitoring.

Return-to-Play Decision Making

Following the acute examination, there will be instances in which the athlete obviously cannot continue to participate and other cases where the trauma was obviously minor and the athlete's ability to play is evident. The challenging decision is a case that lies in between these two extremes. A physician may need to be consulted when making the return-to-play decision.

The return-to-play decision should be based on the relative risk of reinjury and on the athlete's functional ability. The athlete's age and level of competition also factor into the decision-making process. Younger individuals are generally managed more conservatively than older athletes; for example, an injury that would not disqualify a professional athlete often disqualifies a child from participating in a recreational league.

This decision is often made in an environment that is not conducive to obtaining objective measures (e.g., the sidelines). The final determination is based on the assessment of function:

- **Strength and range of motion:** The athlete's strength and ROM should be approximately equal bilaterally and sufficient to protect both the injured area—and the athlete in general—from further injury.
- **Pain:** The athlete should report tolerable pain during exertional activities that does not result in noticeable change in function or worsen the condition.
- **Proprioception:** The athlete's involved extremity should demonstrate proprioceptive ability sufficient to protect the body part from further injury.
- **Functional activity progression:** Gradually increase the demands of the activity by introducing progressively more challenging tasks. For example, for a soccer player with a lower-extremity injury, the functional progression would include demonstrating the ability to walk, jog, run straight ahead, change direction when jogging, and then change direction at high speed. Sport-specific skills such as dribbling are added once the athlete can complete this progression.

REFERENCES

1. Marenco, JP, et al: Improving survival from sudden cardiac arrest: the role of the automated external defibrillator. *JAMA*, 285:1193, 2001.
2. Zipes, DP, et al: ACC/AHA/ESC 2006 guidelines for management of patients with ventricular arrhythmias and the prevention of sudden cardiac death—executive summary. A report of the American College of Cardiology/American Heart Association Task Force and the European Society of Cardiology Committee for Practice Guidelines. *J Am Coll Cardiol*, 48:1064, 2006.
3. Andersen, JC, et al: National Athletic Trainers' Association position statement: emergency planning in athletics. *J Athl Train*, 37:99, 2002.
4. McCrory, P, et al. Consensus statement on consussion in sport. The 4th International Conference on Concussion in Sport held in Zurich, November 2012. *Clin J Sport Med.* 23:90, 2013.
5. Paronto, J: *2011 & 2012 NCAA Baseball Rules*. Indianapolis, IN: The National Collegiate Athletic Association, 2010. Retrieved from http://www.ncaapublications.com/productdownloads/BA12.pdf (Accessed January 18, 2013).
6. Hyland, A, and Williamson, D: *2012 & 2013 NCAA Men's and Women's Basketball Rules and Interpretations*. Indianapolis, IN: The National Collegiate Athletic Association, 2011. Retrieved from http://www.ncaapublications.com/productdownloads/BR13.pdf (Accessed January 18, 2013).
7. The International Hockey Federation: *Rules of Hockey-Including Explanations*. Lausanne, Switzerland: The International Hockey Federation, 2006.
8. Redding, R: *Football 2011 and 2012 Rules and Interpretations*. Indianapolis, IN: The National Collegiate Athletic Association, 2011. Retrieved from http://www.ncaapublications.com/productdownloads/FR12.pdf (Accessed January 18, 2013).
9. Piotrowski, S: *2010-12 NCAA Men's and Women's Ice Hockey Rules and Interpretations*. Indianapolis, IN: The National Collegiate Athletic Association, 2011. Retrieved from http://www.ncaapublications.com/productdownloads/IH12.pdf (Accessed January 18, 2013).
10. Andres, K: *2004 Men's and Women's Soccer Rules*. Indianapolis, IN: The National Collegiate Athletic Association, 2004.
11. Abrahamson, D: *2011 2012 and 2013 NCAA Softball Rules and Interpretations*. Indianapolis, IN: The National Collegiate Athletic Association, 2011. Retrieved from http://www.ncaapublications.com/DownloadPublication.aspx?download=SR13.pdf (Accessed January 18, 2013).
12. United States Tennis Association: USTA Regulations: Part 3, Section W, 2005. Retrieved from http://www.usta.com/Active/Rules/1122_USTA_Regulations/ (Accessed January 18, 2013).
13. Bubb, RG: *Wrestling 2011-12 and 2012-13 Rules and Interpretations*. Indianapolis, IN : The National Collegiate Athletic Association, 2011. Retrieved from http://www.ncaapublications.com/productdownloads/WR13.pdf (Accessed May 29, 2014).
14. Jenkins, HL, et al: Removal tools are faster and produce less force and torque on the helmet than cutting tools during face-mask retraction. *J Athl Train*, 37:236, 2002.
15. Miranda, FE, et al: Confirmation of the safety and accuracy of physical examination in the evaluation of knee dislocation for injury of the popliteal artery: a prospective study. *J Traum Inj Infect Crit Care*, 52:247, 2002.
16. Barnes, CJ, Pietrobon, R, and Higgins, LD: Does the pulse examination in patients with traumatic knee dislocation predict a surgical arterial injury? A meta-analysis. *J Trauma*, 53:1109, 2002.
17. Spain, D: Casting acute fractures. Part 1—Commonly asked questions. *Aust Fam Physician*, 29:853, 2000.

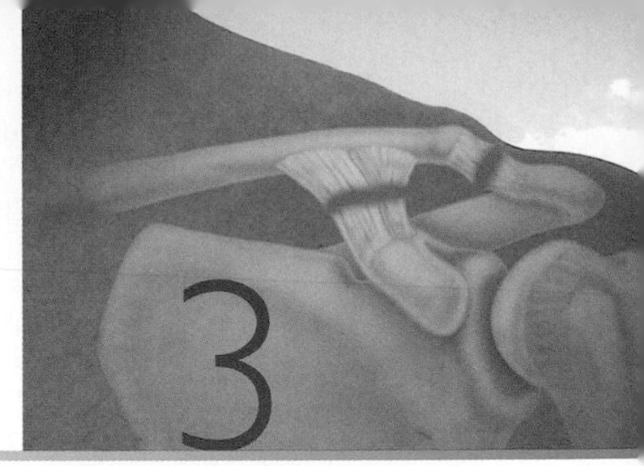

CHAPTER 3

Evidence-Based Practice in the Diagnostic Process

Evidence-based practice (EBP) in health care is an old concept with a new name, with the principles embedded in everyday life. EBP is the integration of current, best research results, clinical expertise, and the unique circumstances and values of the patient.[1] These components are used in everyday life. Consider helping a friend buy a new computer. First, you would **research** the various brands and models that are on the market; some are better than others. For a few more dollars, you may be able to purchase a computer with more features, but are they worth it? During this process, you would call on the second element, your **personal experience and expertise**. What brands have worked well in the past? Finally, you must consider the **circumstances and values** of your friend. Is cost or portability more significant? Failure to recognize these personal needs and values could lead to inaccurate results (unless you guessed correctly). If your friend simply must have a portable computer, no amount of research will make a desktop computer a good choice.

*** Practical Evidence**

Evidence-based practice, a foundation of **best practice**, is the incorporation of three elements into the decision-making process of patient care: (1) best available research, (2) clinical expertise, and (3) the circumstances and values of the individual patient. These concepts are intertwined with the patient examination, the clinical diagnosis, and subsequent intervention plan.[2]

EBP came into focus as the result of rising medical costs, including surgery and other interventions that are paid for by insurance companies. As a result of the costs associated with these techniques, insurance companies began to question their **efficacy**. Research indicated that some techniques did not provide significant improvement in patient outcomes. Other procedures required prolonged follow-up care or repeat surgeries, provided no additional benefit to the patient, or were less efficient and more expensive than other techniques.[3] To receive payment, insurance companies began to require that the procedures being billed actually helped patients improve in a timely, efficient manner. Thus began the modern movement toward evidence-based practice.

Applying EBP to patient care assists in making informed decisions about the most effective approaches to maximize the outcome for the client/patient. Each disease or injury is associated with multiple prevention strategies, diagnostic approaches, and intervention strategies. EBP provides a framework to determine if one strategy is better than another, if both strategies are similar, or if one is just simply wrong.

EBP is a process rather than a technique.[4] Information—evidence—is gathered from unbiased sources such as peer-reviewed journals that address the clinical problem. Some types (levels) of information are more compelling than others (Box 3-1). For example, a **meta-analysis** collectively examines a body of research on a specific topic. Combined with **randomized clinical trials**, these types of research provide the strongest arguments for the inclusion or exclusion of a particular technique for a specified population. The weakest level of evidence, although not always "bad" or unusable, is often the most prevalent and from the most surprising source: expert opinion (including textbooks).

Best practice Methods or procedures that through research and experience have demonstrated the optimal, most expedient results

Efficacy The ability of a protocol to produce the intended effects

Meta-analysis A research technique that combines the results of multiple studies that have similar research hypotheses

Randomized clinical trial A study in which subjects are randomly assigned to a control group or a treatment group

Box 3-1
Puzzlin' Evidence

Not all evidence is created equally. The data and methods used to derive conclusions are varied, some stemming from well-constructed research designs and others that do not pass muster with the scientific community. Certainly, the findings of double-blind, randomized control studies are (or should be) more meaningful than an advertisement claiming that "4 out of 5 doctors recommend..."

The Centre for Evidence-Based Medicine has developed criteria to evaluate the quality of research. Termed "Levels of Evidence," it describes a hierarchy of the different sources of data from which clinical decisions are made. Accurate and generalizable studies are more useful in making clinical decisions.[5] Those at the top of the hierarchy carry more weight than the ones ranked lower:

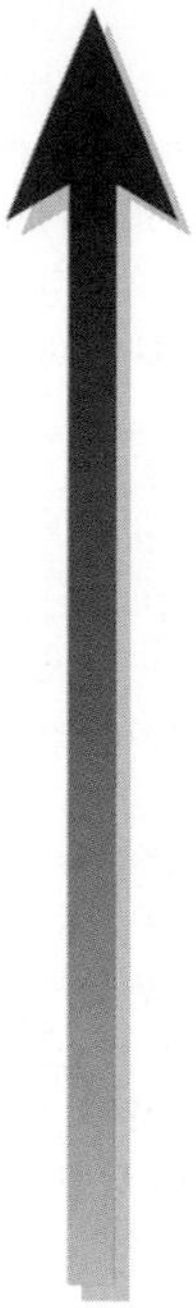

Meta-analysis: Technique that combines the results of similar high-quality research studies and draws a conclusion based on statistical results.

Systematic review: A literature review that critiques and synthesizes high-quality research relating to a specific, focused question.

Randomized clinical trials: A research technique in which subjects are randomly assigned to an experimental or control group. The experimental group receives the treatment. The control group does not. The results for each group are statistically compared to identify any differences.

Cohort studies: Two groups, one that receives the treatment and one that does not, are studied forward over time to determine the impact of the treatment.

Case-control studies: Similar to cohort studies, but groups are studied from a historical perspective (backwards in time). Differences between groups of patients with the specified condition (the case group) and without the specified condition (the control group) are identified.

Case series: A report on a series of patients with a particular condition; no control group is used.

Expert opinion: An opinion based on general principles, animal or human-based laboratory research, physiology, and clinical experience.

Often two sources may be contradictory regarding the usefulness of clinical techniques. In this case, it is important to factor in the strength of the source (based on the hierarchy above) and the weight of the recommendations. The recommendations derived from a randomized clinical trial must be given more consideration than those from a case report.

Much of what we learn, practice, and teach has either not been critically analyzed or is still used despite the fact that the evidence does not support its inclusion in the diagnostic process.

Your clinical expertise and the input from others also contribute to obtaining the best outcome for your patient. Quality published research on the clinical signs and symptoms, examination techniques, and management of many conditions may simply not exist. In other cases, the research may not be applicable to your patient.[6] For example, research on the diagnosis of shoulder conditions in the elderly may not be applicable to the diagnosis of shoulder conditions in the younger population. This is compounded by limited research on relatively rare conditions and new clinical diagnostic techniques. In these instances, your clinical judgment, based on your knowledge of anatomy, biomechanics, examination techniques, and past experiences, serves as the best available evidence.

The process from the initial diagnosis through management and rehabilitation must be **patient-centered**, accounting for the patient's circumstances, values, and long-term goals. A patient who has no desire to return to competitive athletics after an injury would be managed much differently than a patient who does. A patient with an anterior cruciate ligament (ACL) injury and a comorbidity of diabetes would be managed differently than a patient without diabetes. At times, the patient's family should be involved in the decision-making process to ensure agreement and compliance with the recommended course of care. Failure to personalize care, regardless of the research findings for the condition being managed, may alienate the patient and detract from the final outcome. Refer to Box 1-2, Culturally Competent Care, for more information about interpersonal aspects of the examination process.

Evidence-based practice serves as the foundation for best healthcare practice. Adopting this approach provides a systematic method for structuring the clinical diagnostic approach and determining management strategies. This chapter details the components of EBP only as it relates to clinical diagnostic techniques and describes how these components are incorporated into the remainder of this text. Many excellent resources describe the process of researching and interpreting the literature and present a broader picture of the evidence-based process.

The Role of Evidence-Based Practice in Orthopedic Examination and Diagnosis

Hundreds, if not thousands, of orthopedic examination techniques are described in the literature. Which ones are best suited for which patient? Does every known orthopedic test need to be performed on each patient? EBP principles are used as a framework to improve the precision and efficiency of the diagnostic process. Let us assume that there are 50 selective tissue tests for the glenohumeral joint. Even if time allowed, do all of the 50 tests need to be performed for each patient complaining of shoulder pain you examine? Identifying the tests that are most appropriate and accurate for the activity limitations identified during the functional screening and symptoms obtained during the history-taking process reduces the number of procedures that must be performed. When we weigh the evidence of how useful these tests are in identifying pathology, we could potentially pare their number down to three or four (Fig. 3-1).

Understanding the principles that assess the relative usefulness of the examination features is needed to interpret and incorporate research findings. The diagnostic accuracy of many common clinical tests is yet to be determined. Although this is far from ideal, the absence of evidence does not mean that the procedure should not be used. Conversely, some clinical tests have been studied and identified as not reliable and/or not accurate in identifying the condition. These techniques should no longer be used because of their potential to influence clinical decisions inaccurately.

Fundamentals of Interpreting Research

EBP requires thoughtful interpretation and integration of published research. This section introduces the EBP concepts used throughout this text by describing the basic interpretation and clinical application of research findings. We will use a hypothetical example to illustrate these points. For our example, we will walk through the process of determining the usefulness of the McManus test, a new (and fictitious) stress test that is intended to identify damage to the ACL (Fig. 3-2). To determine if we should include the McManus test as a part of our ACL examination procedure, we must consult the literature to determine the test's reliability and its ability to rule in or rule out ACL sprains.

Reliability

Before the **diagnostic accuracy** of a test can be established, its reliability—how often the same results are obtained—must be determined.[7] A test cannot be diagnostically useful without acceptable reliability. Clinically, there are two types of reliability: intrarater reliability and interrater reliability.

Intrarater (intraexaminer) reliability describes the extent to which the same examiner obtains the same results on the same patient. If the same examiner performs the McManus test on the same patient multiple times, how consistently will the same result (positive or negative) be obtained?

Interrater (interexaminer) reliability describes the extent to which different examiners obtain the same results for the same patient. If different examiners perform the McManus test on the same patient multiple times, how consistently will they obtain the same findings?

Depending on the type of test, statisticians report reliability using the kappa coefficient (κ) or intraclass correlation coefficient (ICC) (Box 3-2). Clinically, however, the most important aspect of these statistical measures is the interpretation of their relative usefulness. Remember that

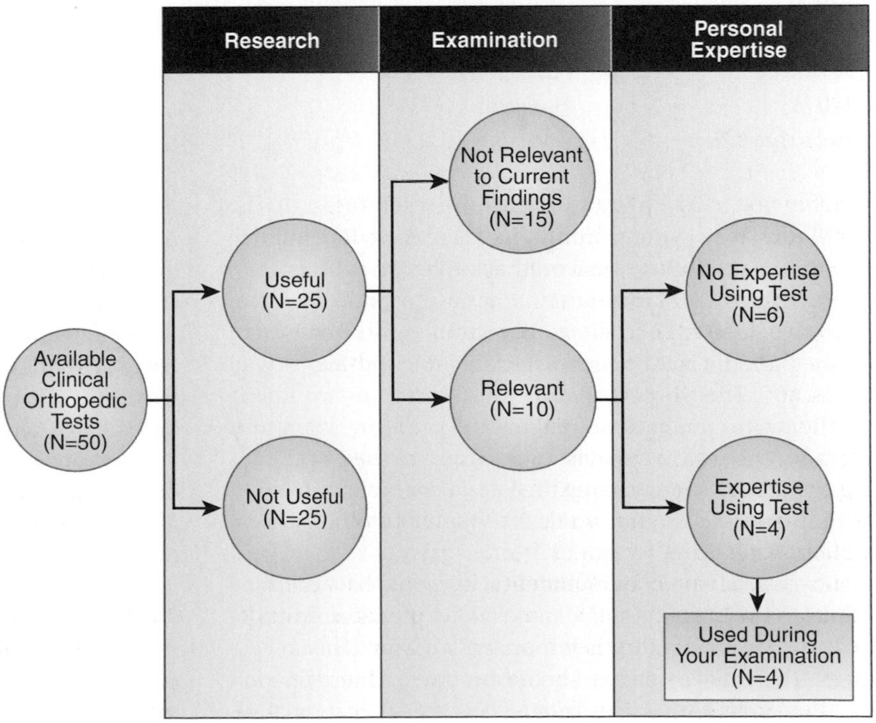

FIGURE 3-1 ■ Paring down the number of clinical tests to use in an examination. Consider a pool of 50 orthopedic diagnostic tests for a particular body area. After researching the various tests (hopefully found in one or two journal articles), we find that 25 of them are clinically useful and 25 are not. Based on the patient's history and clinical signs and symptoms, 15 are not needed for the differential diagnosis, leaving 10 in the pool. Of these 10, there are 6 procedures that you are not versed in. Assuming that the remaining 4 tests are accurate (which we deduced from the research phase), we can be more certain that we will reach a correct diagnosis by including these 4 tests in our overall examination of this patient.

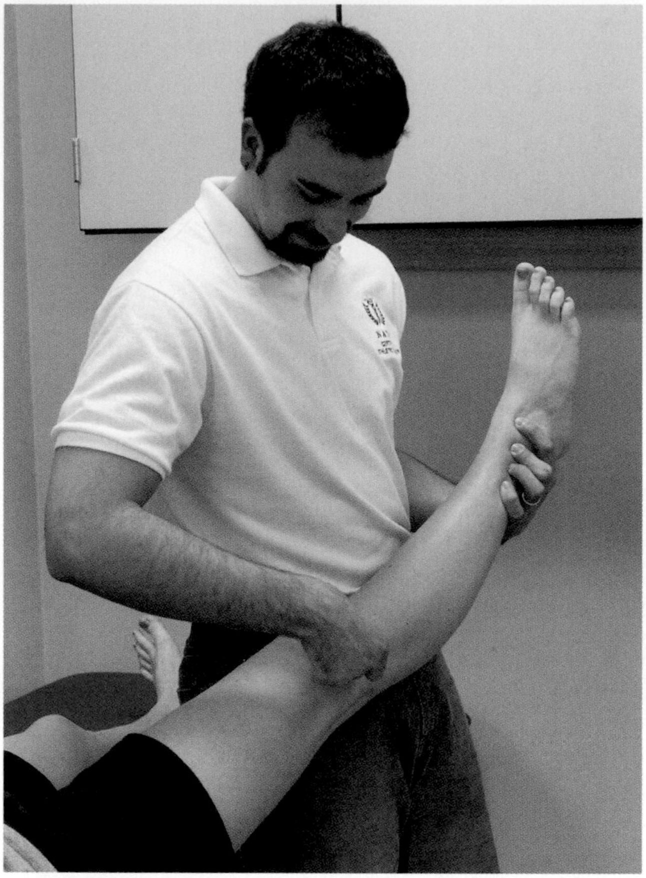

FIGURE 3-2 ■ The McManus test, a fictitious test used to identify ACL pathology as an illustration of EBP concepts.

the closer the reliability measure is to 1.0, the better it is, and the closer to 0.0, the less reliable it is:

If the reliability measure is . . .	. . . then the clinical usefulness falls within this range
Less than 0.5	Poor
0.5–0.75	Moderate
Greater than 0.75	Good

The first step in establishing the usefulness of the McManus test is determining its reliability. To establish **intrarater reliability**, we would ask the same clinician to perform the McManus test on multiple patients on at least two different occasions. The sample would consist of some patients who were ACL-deficient and some who were not. The clinician would not know (or would be "blinded" to) the patient's history or condition when performing the test. We would then compare the examiner's result for consistency using the kappa coefficient. To what extent does the examiner reach the same finding on each patient each time?

To establish **interrater reliability**, we would have multiple clinicians perform the McManus test on the same group of patients. Again, blinding is important. We would then measure the extent of agreement in the examiners' determination of positive and negative results. Fortunately, the McManus test performed well, yielding an interrater reliability of 0.76 and an intrarater reliability of 0.86.

Box 3-2
Measures of Reliability

When a statistician determines the percentage agreement of positive or negative findings for procedures that produce a "yes/no" or "true/false" result (nominal data), the **kappa coefficient** is used. This statistic accounts for differences attributed to chance alone. When one outcome is far more common than the other (for example, almost everyone will have a negative result), agreement needs be extremely high for an acceptable kappa coefficient. Most STTs yield this type of result, meaning that it is either positive or negative, rather than graded on a scale (such as seen with ligamentous tests). Reliability between two or more repeated interval measurements (e.g., temperature) or ratio measurements (e.g., range of motion [ROM]) are expressed using an **intraclass correlation coefficient**.

The closer the reliability measures (k or ICC) are to 1.0, the more reliable are the findings; the closer to 0.0, the more unreliable they are. The diagnostic accuracy of a test is suspect in the presence of low reliability.[8]

Reliability is influenced by factors such as consistency in performing a skill, how the results are interpreted, the experience and training of the examiner, and the equipment used.

* Practical Evidence

When a task is correctly repeated multiple times by a trained practitioner using the same technique and the same scale is applied to interpret the results, intrarater reliability improves.

Diagnostic Accuracy

After determining that the McManus test is reliable, the test is then assessed for its diagnostic accuracy. How often do the results correctly identify whether or not the pathology is present?

To assess diagnostic accuracy, we first identify a population of individuals on whom to perform the test. In this example, our population would be individuals presenting to us with knee pain. We know that a certain number of these individuals have sustained an ACL injury (the **prevalence** of a condition) and are trying to determine how effective our test is at correctly categorizing those people who have an ACL tear and those who do not.

Prevalence, the extent to which a condition is present in a specific population, is an important consideration for diagnostic statistics. The prevalence of any condition can change based on the group being studied. For example, prevalence of ACL sprains for everyone in the United States would be much different than the prevalence in a population that reports to an orthopedic clinic because of acute knee pain. In your group of friends, there is a chance (probability) that one or more has an ACL-deficient knee. In an orthopedic clinic, the chance of finding someone who has ACL pathology is much greater simply because of the types of patients seen at the facility. Prevalence information is helpful to establish the **pretest probability** that a condition exists in a given population.

✻ Practical Evidence

Simply because of random chance, changes in the prevalence of a condition affect the ability to identify the pathology. If 1 in 100 patients has a torn ACL, then there is a 1% chance of simply guessing (or pulling out of a hat the name of) the person who is injured, and a 99% chance that you can correctly identify people who have intact ACLs. If 50 in 100 patients have a torn ACL, there is a 50% chance of randomly identifying those with ACL deficiency.

Diagnostic Gold Standard

To determine accuracy, our test results are compared with a **diagnostic gold standard** (also known as the reference standard). Gold standards have the highest diagnostic accuracy but are generally more expensive, less accessible, slower, invasive, and/or require additional personnel as compared with the clinical test. **Arthroscopy** is the gold standard for diagnosing ACL tears.[9,10] The clinical results of the McManus test will be compared with those obtained during arthroscopy.

The clinical diagnostic results are compared with the gold standard via a table consisting of two columns and two rows (a 2 × 2 contingency table). One of four outcomes can occur:

	Gold Standard	
	Positive	Negative
Clinical test positive	True Positive (TP)	False Positive (FP)
Clinical test negative	False Negative (FN)	True Negative (TN)

- **True positive:** The clinical test and the gold standard are both positive, and the condition is correctly identified. The McManus test and arthroscopy both indicate ACL pathology.
- **False positive:** The clinical test incorrectly identifies a condition as present when, in fact, there is no pathology. The McManus test indicates ACL pathology, but the ACL is shown to be intact during arthroscopy.
- **True negative:** The clinical test and the gold standard are both negative. The absence of the pathology is correctly identified. The McManus test indicates no ACL pathology, and the ACL is shown to be intact during arthroscopy.
- **False negative:** The clinical procedure identifies a condition as not present when, in fact, it is present. The McManus test indicates no ACL pathology, but the arthroscopy shows the ACL as torn.

The best diagnostic accuracy is achieved with a high rate of true positives and true negatives. Following a trial involving 40 patients with knee pain, the results of the McManus test are classified as positive or negative and are grouped by arthroscopic findings of the intactness of the ACL. In this case, the comparison of the McManus test with the reference standard of arthroscopy results in the 2 × 2 table below:

	Arthroscopy	
	Arthroscopy Positive for ACL Pathology	Arthroscopy Negative for ACL Pathology
McManus test positive	17 (TP)	3 (FP)
McManus test negative	6 (FN)	14 (TN)

FN = False Negative; FP = False Positive; TN = True Negative; TP = True Positive

Diagnostic Predictive Value

The **accuracy** of a test is determined by comparing the number of correctly classified patients (true positives + true negatives) to the total number of patients examined. A test that is 100% accurate correctly classifies every single patient; however, this level of accuracy is highly unlikely. Relying on accuracy to determine a test's usefulness can be deceptive because it is impacted by the prevalence of a condition.[7]

Research on the usefulness of diagnostic techniques may report the **positive predictive value** (PPV) and **negative predictive value** (NPV). By comparing the true positive rate to the overall positive rate (or true positive/true positive + false positive), PPVs depict how often a positive finding is correct. Conversely, NPVs identify how often a negative finding is correct (true negative/true negative + false negative).

Although useful, predictive values are less valuable than likelihood ratios because a low prevalence of a condition in a given population deflates the PPV and inflates the NPV. In other words, when the number of those who will test negative is large simply because of the low prevalence, the true positives will be much more difficult to find without including more false positives in the process.[11] Failing to consider prevalence rates when comparing predictive values from two different studies can lead to false conclusions. Because of the wide spectrum of prevalence rates and the resulting difficulty in making comparisons, predictive values are not reported in this text. See Box 3-3 for a further description of the influence of prevalence on predictive values.

Sensitivity and Specificity

Sensitivity and specificity describe how often the technique identifies the true positive and true negative

Pretest probability The likelihood that a specific condition is present before the diagnostic test results are known

Arthroscopy A minimally invasive procedure in which a tube-like instrument is inserted through the skin to visualize and repair underlying tissues

Box 3-3
Relationship Between Prevalence and Predictive Value

Prevalence is the number of people affected by a condition. Depending on the group of people studied, the prevalence of a condition will change. Because of the differences in the physical demands of the sport, it is more likely that more cases of patellar tendinopathy would be identified in a group of 100 professional basketball players (say 25 out of 100) than in a group of 100 golfers (say 5 out of 100).

Prevalence affects the positive and negative predictive values. In our example of basketball players and golfers, random chance gives us a greater probability of finding a basketball player with patellar tendinopathy than a golfer. Differences in the prevalence of a condition make comparison of PPVs and NPVs between two different studies problematic.

The tables below illustrate the effect of two different prevalences on the PPV and NPV for the McManus test. Group I assumes that the prevalence of ACL pathology in the entire adult population of the United States is 0.02%, or 20 out of every 100,000 individuals. Because the number of those without the pathology is so overwhelmingly high, it makes sense that the NPV will be very high: almost everyone is already negative. Because so few individuals have the pathology, the rate of false positives will also be high, and the PPV will be decreased.

The prevalence of ACL pathology changes in a sports medicine facility (Group II). First, our target population is those exclusively complaining of acute knee pain. In this population, a much higher proportion will have sustained damage to the ACL. Let us assume a prevalence of 20%, or 20,000 out of 100,000 patients, have injured their ACL. Now, we can expect a slightly lower NPV and a largely increased PPV. There are fewer false positives simply because there are more people with ACL trauma.

Using the 2 × 2 tables below, compare the PPVs and NPVs for Groups I and II. Although the rate of detection for the McManus test is the same, the predictive values change based on the prevalence of ACL trauma in the two groups. The increased proportion of ACL-deficient people most significantly affects the PPV. When examining the predictive values, the population used must be considered before making a determination of a test's usefulness.

Group I Prevalence = 20/100,000 (0.02%)

	Arthroscopy		
	Positive ACL Pathology	Negative ACL Pathology	Predictive Value
McManus test positive	15	18,000	PPV = 15/18,015 = 0.08
McManus test negative	5	82,000	NPV = 82,000/82,005 = 99.99

Group II Prevalence = 20,000/100,000 (20.0%)

	Arthroscopy		
	Positive ACL Pathology	Negative ACL Pathology	Predictive Value
McManus test positive	15,000	14,400	PPV = 15,000/29,400 = 51.02
McManus test negative	5000	65,600	NPV = 65,600/70,600 = 92.92

PPV = positive predictive value; NPV = negative predictive value

results. **Sensitivity** describes the test's ability to detect those patients who actually have the disorder relative to the gold standard.[11] Also known as the *true positive rate,* sensitivity describes the proportion of positive results a technique identifies relative to the actual number of positives. Sensitivity is calculated as true positives/(true positives + false negatives).[12] Compared with arthroscopy, the McManus test correctly identified 17 out of 23 individuals who have ACL pathology, yielding a sensitivity of 0.74.

	Arthroscopy	
	Arthroscopy Positive for ACL Pathology	Arthroscopy Negative for ACL Pathology
McManus test positive	17 (TP)	3 (FP)
McManus test negative	6 (FN)	14 (TN)

Sensitivity = TP/(TP+FN)
= 17/(17 + 6)
= 0.74

TP = True Positive; FP = False Positive; TN = True Negative; FN = False Negative

Tests with high sensitivity accurately identify all or most patients with a given condition. The sensitivity value alone, however, can be misleading. While all true positives are likely to be identified, the number of false positives obtained along the way can also be high. To gain a better understanding of a test's overall usefulness, specificity must also be considered.

Specificity, the *true negative rate*, describes the test's ability to detect patients who do not have the disorder. The specificity of a diagnostic technique identifies the proportion of true negatives the technique detects compared with the actual number of negatives in a given population. Specificity is calculated as true negatives/(true negatives + false positives).[12] With a specificity of 0.82, the McManus test correctly identified those without ACL damage by yielding a negative result 82% of the time.

	Arthroscopy	
	Arthroscopy Positive for ACL Pathology	Arthroscopy Negative for ACL Pathology
McManus test positive	17 (TP)	3 (FP)
McManus test negative	6 (FN)	14 (TN)
	Sensitivity = TP/(TP+FN) = 17/(17 + 6) = 0.74	Specificity = TN/(TN + FP) = 14/(14 + 3) = 0.82

TP = True Positive; FP = False Positive; TN = True Negative; FN = False Negative

A high sensitivity tells us that, in most cases, this test will identify someone with an ACL sprain. Because of this, negative tests results strongly rule out the presence of an ACL tear. **SnNout** is a useful reminder: In tests with a high sensitivity (Sn), a negative finding (N) effectively rules *out* the condition. Alternatively, a high specificity, where most of those without the condition are identified, makes positive results more convincing. The reminder **SpPin** is used: In tests with a high specificity (Sp), a positive finding (P) convincingly rules *in* the condition.[8]

The meaningfulness of sensitivity and specificity values changes relative to the condition being studied. When the failure to identify some conditions could produce catastrophic results, a high sensitivity is required and can come at the expense of specificity. Using our SnNout acronym, we would need to use a test with a high sensitivity in which a negative result is truly negative. For example, when examining a "high-stakes" orthopedic condition such as a cervical spine fracture or joint dislocation, the test with the highest sensitivity is used first to identify all potentially positive cases.

*** Practical Evidence**

Failure to detect arterial insufficiency could result in the loss of the distal extremity. Because palpation of a distal pulse (e.g., the dorsalis pedis pulse) is not highly sensitive in detecting damage to the proximal artery, a more definitive (sensitive) technique such as Doppler ultrasound should be used to determine if there is arterial damage.[13]

As with sensitivity, using only the specificity values is misleading in determining the usefulness of a diagnostic test. Detecting all of the true negatives may also be at the expense of misclassifying those who actually do have the condition as false negatives. Sensitivity and specificity determine how well a test detects true positives and true negatives. Yet, taken individually, these measures may not be sufficiently useful. Unless both the sensitivity and specificity values are high, determining the procedure's clinical usefulness is difficult (and often inconclusive). To avoid these pitfalls, sensitivity and specificity values are considered together and are expressed as likelihood ratios (LRs).

Likelihood Ratios

Likelihood ratios provide information on how positive and negative findings on a particular test determine a test's diagnostic usefulness. Likelihood ratios incorporate a test's sensitivity and specificity and are not influenced by the prevalence of a condition (see Box 3-3).

Likelihood ratios explain the shift in the pretest probability that a patient has a condition after a test result is obtained. Pretest probabilities are population specific and derived from prevalence data from regional or national databases, practice databases, published research findings, or clinical experience.[7] Often, pretest probabilities must be estimated based on clinical experience because specific data are not available.

An LR that is near or at 1 indicates that there is little to no shift in the pretest probability that a condition is present after the results—either positive or negative—of the test are considered. An LR that is greater than 1 increases the probability that the condition exists, and an LR of less than 1 decreases the probability that the condition exists.[2] Consideration of LR results can lead to one of three clinical decision options:[8]

- The posttest probability is so high that there is acceptable certainty that the pathology is present.
- The shift in posttest probability is inconclusive. A stronger test or tests, if available, are needed to rule in or rule out the pathology.
- The posttest probability is so low that there is acceptable certainty that the pathology is not present. Other diagnoses must be considered.

Following a positive or negative test result, how sure are we that the patient has the condition in question? A positive LR describes the shift in the pretest probability that the condition is present based on a positive test result. A negative LR describes the change in the pretest probability that a condition exists based on a negative test result.

Positive Likelihood Ratio

The positive likelihood ratio (LR+) expresses the change in our confidence that a condition is present when the test is positive. The higher the LR+, the more a positive test enhances the probability that the pathology is present.

The LR+ is calculated as:

$$\text{sensitivity}/(1 - \text{specificity})$$

Using our sensitivity and specificity information for the McManus test presented earlier, the LR+ can be calculated:

	Arthroscopy	
	Arthroscopy Positive for ACL Pathology	Arthroscopy Negative for ACL Pathology
McManus test positive	17 (TP)	3 (FP)
McManus test negative	6 (FN)	14 (TN)
	Sensitivity = 0.74	Specificity = 0.82

LR+ = Sensitivity / (1 − specificity)
= 0.74 /(1 − 0.82)
= 4.11

Positive likelihood ratios cannot be calculated for those tests that have a specificity of 1.0 since a division by 0 error occurs.

TP = True Positive; FP = False Positive; TN = True Negative; FN = False Negative

A positive result using the McManus test is about four times more likely to be seen in a patient with our target condition.

Negative Likelihood Ratio

The negative likelihood ratio (LR−) expresses the probability that the pathology is still present even though the test was negative. How convincing is a negative test in diminishing the likelihood that the patient has the pathology? The closer the LR− is to 1, the less significant is the change in pretest probability. The lower the LR− is, the lower is the probability that the condition exists.
The LR−is calculated as:

(1 − sensitivity)/specificity

A high sensitivity (or true positive rate), will deflate the LR−. A negative McManus test would not convincingly rule out the possibility of an ACL tear because there is only a small shift in the pretest probability.

	Arthroscopy	
	Arthroscopy Positive for ACL Pathology	Arthroscopy Negative for ACL Pathology
McManus test positive	17 (TP)	3 (FP)
McManus test negative	6 (FN)	14 (TN)
	Sensitivity = 0.74	Specificity = 0.82

LR+ = 4.11
LR− = (1 − Sensitivity)/ Specificity
= (1 − 0.74)/0.82
= 0.32

Negative likelihood ratios cannot be calculated for tests having a specificity of 0.

TP = True Positive; FP = False Positive; TN = True Negative; FN = False Negative

Interpreting Likelihood Ratios

Likelihood ratios tell us the extent to which the outcome of our test changes the probability that the patient has the suspected condition. This change in probability can be interpreted using an LR nomogram (Fig. 3-3) or general guidelines. The general guidelines for interpretation of LRs are presented in Table 3-1.[14,15]

To use the nomogram, the pretest probability that the patient has the condition must be known or estimated. Remember that the pretest probabilities are based on a specific group of people (e.g., athletes, construction workers, the elderly) and are derived from the results of ongoing research.[7] Often, pretest probabilities must be estimated based on clinical experience because specific data are not available.

If the pretest probability that a specific pathology exists is already high, then only a test having a large LR+ will help confirm the diagnosis. If the pretest probability that a specific pathology exists is low, then only a test with a very small LR− will lower that probability even more.

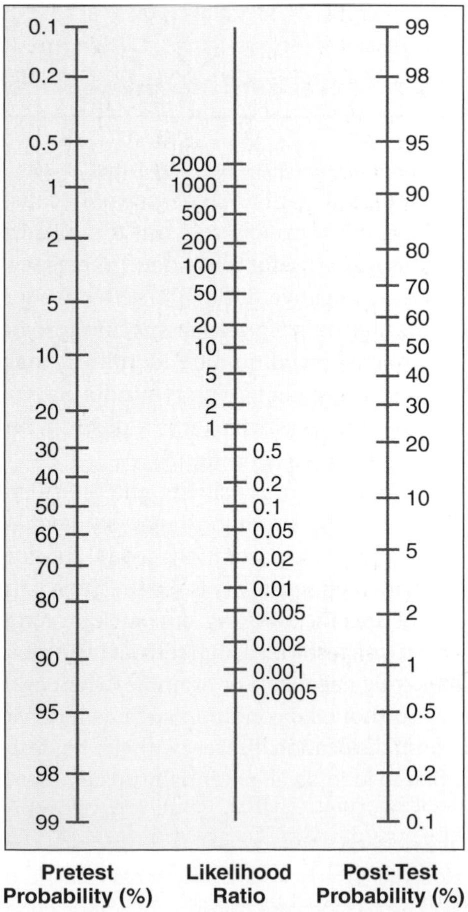

FIGURE 3-3 ■ Nomogram. The pretest probability is identified on the left side of the nomogram, the positive or negative likelihood ratio is plotted on the middle column, and a line connecting the two points is continued through the third column. The intersection in the third column indicates the change in probability that the condition exists given the results of the test.

Table 3-1 Interpretation of Likelihood Ratios

Positive Likelihood Ratio	Negative Likelihood Ratio	Shift in Probability Condition Is Present
>10	<0.1	Large, often conclusive
5–10	0.1–0.2	Moderate but usually important
2–5	0.2–0.5	Small, sometimes important
1–2	>0.5	Very small, usually unimportant

Tests with LR+ or LR− values that approach 1.0 have little clinical usefulness and can be omitted from the clinical diagnostic procedure.

Ample data exist on knee injuries and the incidence of injury to the ACL. In a recent study of knee injury in high school athletes, 25% of those with an acute knee injury sustained damaged to their ACL.[16] Risk factors or reported history also help in generating a pretest probability hypothesis. For example, girls who play basketball or soccer are two to three times more likely to sustain an ACL injury as compared with their male counterparts, and around 5% of females who play soccer and basketball year round will sustain an ACL injury.[16,17] Athletes between 15 and 25 years of age sustain more than 50% of all ACL injuries.[18] The majority of noncontact ACL injuries occur from planting and pivoting.[19]

Using our example, consider a 17-year-old woman who comes in seeking evaluation for an acute knee injury that occurred yesterday while she was playing basketball. Our initial differential diagnosis includes about a 25% probability that she has sustained injury to her ACL. In this case, the McManus test is positive, and we know its LR+ is 4.11. Using a nomogram to plot our results, we find that the posttest probability that she has injured her ACL is approximately 50% (Fig. 3-4). Had we obtained a negative result with the McManus test, the posttest probability that she has injured her ACL would be between 5% and 10%, using the test's LR− of 0.32. Using the interpretation guidelines, we have obtained a small but potentially useful shift in probability that she has injured her ACL.

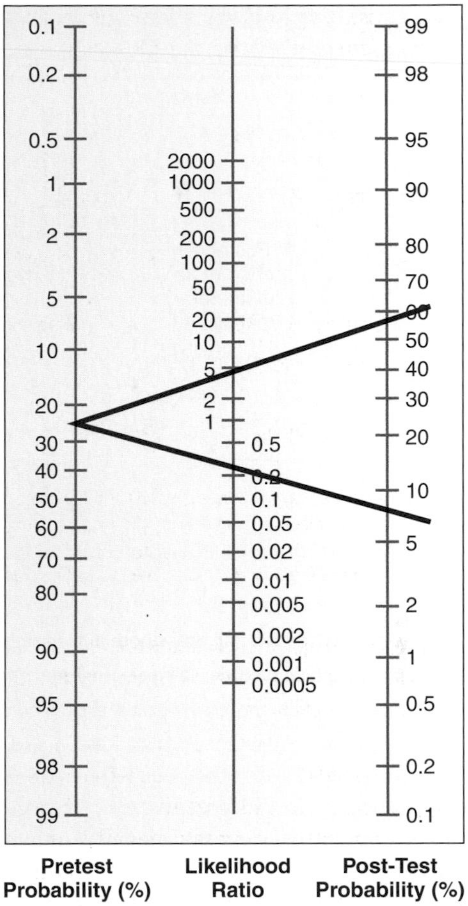

FIGURE 3-4 ■ Nomogram for the McManus test. These lines show the changes in pretest probability of a patient having an ACL sprain with a positive or negative McManus test result. Use the nomogram in Figure 3-2 to plot the changes in posttest probability for a condition that has a low pretest probability that is diagnosed using a test with a high LR+.

Clinical Decision Rules

Clinical decision rules (CDRs), also known as clinical prediction rules, are developed in response to a clinical problem that, when applied correctly, improve the consistency and efficiency of clinical practice.[20, 21] CDRs are developed around the findings of **predictor variables** that determine the presence or absence of an **outcome variable**. As used in this text, the outcome variable is the presence or absence of a condition or the need for further testing such as radiographs. The predictor variables are categorical in nature and should represent all possible outcomes (e.g., Pain "Yes" or "No"). The initial list of predictor variables is then pared down to at least three that, if present, are indicative of the outcome.[21]

Data from this collection of validated, reliable items are analyzed to identify the items that contribute most to making an accurate clinical decision, providing the basis of the CDR. These rules must then be tested in various groups to ensure that they should, in fact, be included. Finally, the impact of the CDR on cost, patient satisfaction, and/or outcome is evaluated.[20,22]

For example, the Ottawa Ankle Rules were developed to reduce unnecessary radiographs for patients presenting to emergency rooms after traumatic foot and ankle injuries (Box 3-4; also see Chapter 9). Using only the clinical findings of the ability to bear weight and areas of point tenderness, this simple diagnostic protocol results in fewer radiographs, lower costs, decreased time in the emergency room, increased patient satisfaction, and (most importantly) no undetected fractures (100% sensitivity).[23,24]

Box 3-4
Ottawa Ankle Rules

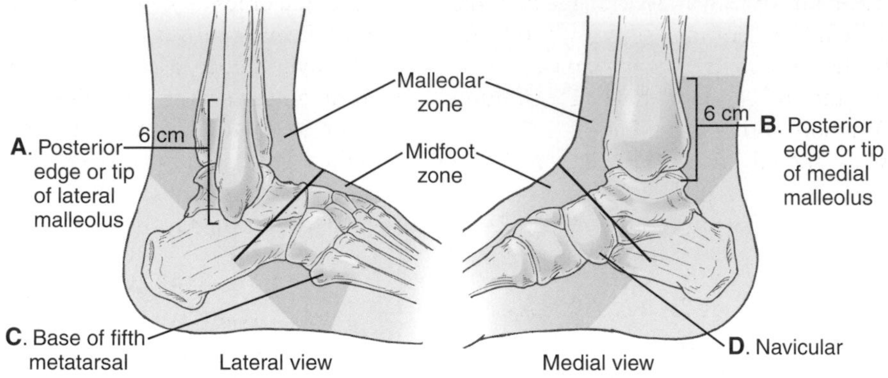

Description

The Ottawa Ankle Rules provide evaluative criteria to identify when the patient should be referred for radiography.

Criteria for Radiographic Referral

The patient's inability to walk four steps both immediately after the injury and at the time of examination.

Ankle radiographs should be ordered if pain is elicited during palpation of zone A or B.

Foot radiographs should be ordered if pain is elicited during palpation of zone C or D.

The clinical application of the Ottawa Ankle Rules is discussed in Chapter 9.

Common diagnostic CDRs include those used for the diagnosis of deep vein thrombosis, mild traumatic brain injuries, cervical spine injuries, ankle fractures, and knee fractures.[24,25]

Clinical Practice Guidelines

Intended to help healthcare providers and patients make informed decisions, clinical practice guidelines (CPGs) are recommendations that guide the care of patients with specific conditions. Starting with a clinical question, a CPG is based on a systematic review of published evidence and evaluation of those findings by experts. The end product is a set of recommendations that involves both evidence and value judgments regarding the patient's course of care for a given condition.[8] The National Guideline Clearinghouse is an indexed repository for CPGs and provides a mechanism for locating guidelines that meet specific inclusion criteria.

Outcome Measures

Historically, the diagnostic process and subsequent interventions have primarily focused on the pathology (a disease-oriented approach) rather than addressing those factors that are meaningful to the patient (a patient-oriented approach). Clinician-based measures primarily assess impairments at the body structure and function level (see Box 1-1).[26,27] Patient-based measures are self-evaluations of activity limitations and participation restrictions (Table 3-2).[28]

Table 3-2 Clinician- and Patient-Based Outcome Measures

Measure	Description
Clinician-based outcomes	Measures used to assess the results of interventions from the clinician's perspective; can include objective measures of strength, ROM, edema, etc. or clinician-report instruments.
Patient-based outcomes	Measures used to assess concerns important to the patient that often relate to symptoms, functional ability, or health-related quality of life. **Condition-specific measures:** Specific to a joint (e.g., Foot and Ankle Disability Index) or body area (e.g., Lower Extremity Functional Scale). These scales use multiple questions to assess the patient's level of function and may also include clinician-based measures. **Generic measures:** Global Rating of Change: A single question to determine improvement over time

Functional assessment tools are patient-centered instruments that focus on the impact of the pathology on their daily lives.

Patient-oriented evidence that matters (POEM) identifies the effect that an injury has on the patient's health status and health-related quality of life (HRQOL). While the clinical examination is used to identify impairments, the effect of the condition on the patient's physical, psychological, and social needs must be considered. For example, a 10-degree improvement in knee ROM may be measurable and significant to the clinician but may still result in functional limitations for the patient. The patient's past experiences, expectations, and perceptions have a profound influence on pain, function, and quality of life.[26]

Each outcome scale should have values that assist in determining improvement in the patient's condition. Depending on how well the instrument has been validated, the following measures may be available for interpreting scores:[26]

- **Minimum Detectable Change (MDC):** The smallest clinically significant difference in the scores of two administrations of the instrument; useful in determining the efficacy of an intervention
- **Minimal Clinically Important Difference (MCID):** A measure of responsiveness, the MCID identifies the smallest change that is important or beneficial to the patient.

The most important and meaningful of these measures, the MCID, is still being developed for many instruments. As a result, there are many MCIDs that have a large amount of variability, and others are volatile (meaning that a single study could create a significant shift in the MCID).[29]

Incorporating Evidence-Based Practice into Clinical Diagnosis

A clinical diagnostic technique is useful—and should be included in the examination process—if it meaningfully assists in identifying the presence (or absence) of the pathology. Many of the clinical techniques are used more because of tradition than science, with a positive or negative finding adding little to the diagnostic picture. Other techniques have been examined only by the individual(s) who developed the procedure, adding a bias to the outcome (who would publish a paper declaring "I developed this test, but it does not work"?). Lastly, a large percentage of the orthopedic clinical techniques used have not been the subject of rigorous study.

To be determined as useful, a clinical technique must be reliable, and it must increase or decrease the probability that the condition is present. If a procedure has low intra- or interrater reliability, then the usefulness is limited because the technique is not accurately reproducible, and the findings will vary from attempt to attempt (intrarater reliability) or from clinician to clinician (interrater reliability). To be clinically useful, a procedure must demonstrate moderate (>0.5) to good (>0.75) reliability. Of course, the closer the reliability is to 1.0, the more comfortable we are with the reproducibility of the results.

Likelihood ratios combine the influences of sensitivity and specificity to determine the impact that a positive or negative test finding has on the probability that a given condition exists. A positive test result must have a minimum LR+ value of 2.0 (small) to add significantly to the pretest probability that the condition is present. A LR− value of 0.2 or less meaningfully lowers the probability that the condition is present.

Our hypothetical McManus test passed the first criterion of intra- and interrater reliability, yielding 0.76 interrater reliability and 0.86 intrarater reliability values. This means that the test is reproducible, and we can accept the findings of the same person over time and the results of two different clinicians. The LRs, although not as strong as we would like, did generate a meaningful shift in posttest probability. The McManus test has a 4.11 LR+, meaning that a positive finding increases the chance that ACL damage is present. The LR− value of 0.32 means that a negative test finding decreases the chance that the ACL has been torn.

Given that other tests, such as the Lachman's or pivot-shift test, have higher LR+ and lower LR− values, it is unlikely that the McManus test will significantly contribute to making a clinical diagnosis. As such, we should use the Lachman's and/or pivot-shift test rather than the McManus test. We can efficiently examine a knee for ACL pathology and accurately conclude that the ACL is torn without performing the McManus test. Likewise, because the Lachman's test has a higher LR+ value >10, if it was positive, there would be no need to perform other orthopedic tests such as the pivot-shift or McManus to confirm the presence of an ACL tear.

Adopting an evidence-based approach to patient care requires a commitment to asking well-formed clinical questions and seeking answers from contemporary resources. As is the nature of research, much of the EBP information presented in this text will change with time. The reader is advised to supplement the information provided in this text with that found in current peer-reviewed journals.

Use of Evidence in This Text

Developing an evidence-based approach will increase efficiency, improve outcomes, and provide a thoughtful, individualized strategy for examination and diagnosis of those with orthopedic conditions. Throughout this text, we have incorporated the best evidence as it is currently available. While we used an orthopedic STT as an example in this chapter, the principles of EBP apply to all components of the examination process.

*** Practical Evidence**

Remaining current with *all* the literature is impossible. Use clinical questions that relate to your patient as the foundation for evidence-based practice. When faced with a clinical challenge, refer to the current literature on that topic and incorporate he published findings into your decision-making process.

We report relevant diagnostic information in a consistent format throughout this text (Fig. 3-5). This provides you with a quick summary of the relative usefulness of a

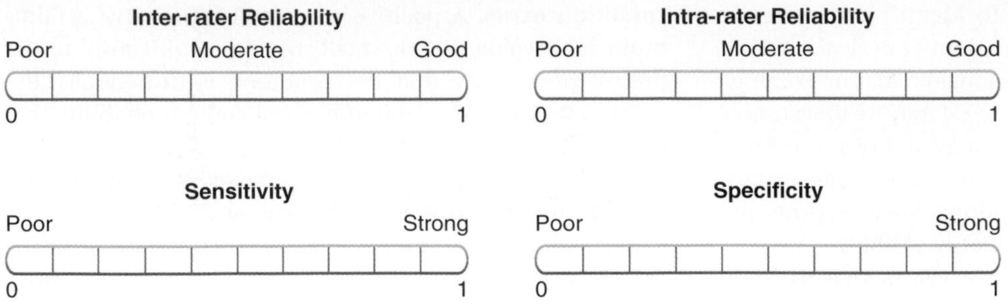

FIGURE 3-5 ■ Presentation of reliability, sensitivity, and specificity values used in this text. Likelihood ratios will be presented numerically.

positive or negative test in arriving at a diagnosis. Likelihood ratios were calculated from available specificity and sensitivity data when not provided. When specificity equals 1 (indicating that all of those without the condition were correctly identified), we did not calculate the LR+ because the denominator will be 0. In this case, you can assume that a positive finding generates a large shift in the posttest probability that the condition exists.[7]

REFERENCES

1. Fetters, L, Tilson, J: *Evidence-Based Physical Therapy*. Philadelphia, PA: FA Davis Company, 2012.
2. Fritz, JM, Wainner, RS: Examining diagnostic tests: an evidence-based perspective. *Phys Ther*, 81:1546, 2001.
3. Bourne, RB, Maloney, WJ, Wright, JG: An AOA critical issue: the outcome of the outcomes movement. *J Bone Joint Surg Am*, 86-A:633, 2004.
4. Steves, R, Hootman, JM: Evidence-based medicine: what is it and how does it apply to athletic training? *J Athl Train*, 39:83, 2004.
5. Daly, J, et al: A hierarchy of evidence for assessing qualitative health research. *J Clin Epidemiol*, 60:43, 2007.
6. Cook, DJ, Levy, MM: Evidence-based medicine: a tool for enhancing critical care practice. *Crit Care Clin*, 14:353, 1998.
7. Cleland, J: *Orthopedic Clinical Examination: An Evidence-Based Approach for Physical Therapists*. Carlstadt, NJ: Icon Learning Systems, 2005.
8. Straus, SE, et al: *Evidence-Based Medicine: How to Practice and Teach It* (ed 4). Philadelphia, PA: Elsevier Churchill Livingstone, 2011.
9. Scholten, RJ, et al: Accuracy of physical diagnostic tests for assessing ruptures of the anterior cruciate ligament: a meta-analysis. *J Fam Pract*, 52:689, 2003.
10. Moore, SL: Imaging the anterior cruciate ligament. *Orthop Clin North Am*. 33:663, 2002.
11. Loong, T-W: Understanding sensitivity and specificity with the right side of the brain. *BMJ*, 327:716, 2003.
12. Gatsonis, C, Paliwal, P: Meta-analysis of diagnostic and screening test accuracy evaluations: methodologic primer. *AJR Am J Roentgenol*, 187:271, 2006.
13. Barnes, CJ, Pietrobon, R, Higgins, LD: Does the pulse examination in patients with traumatic knee dislocation predict a surgical arterial injury? A meta-analysis. *J Trauma*, 53:1109, 2002.
14. Denegar, CR, Fraser, M: How useful are physical examination procedures? Understanding and applying likelihood ratios. *J Athl Train*, 41:201, 2006.
15. Jaeschke, R, Guyatt, JH, Sacket, DL: User's guide to the medical literature, III: how to use an article about a diagnostic test. B: What are the results and how will they help me in caring for my patients? The Evidence-Based Medicine Working Group. *JAMA*, 271:703, 1994.
16. Swenson, DM, et al: Epidemiology of knee injuries among US high school athletes, 2005/06-2010/11. *Med Sci Sports Exerc*, e-pub, 2012.
17. Prodromos, CC, et al. A meta-analysis of the incidence of anterior cruciate ligament tears as a function of gender, sport, and a knee injury-reduction regimen. *Arthroscopy*, 23:11320, 2007.
18. Griffin, LA, et al: Understanding and preventing noncontact anterior cruciate ligament injuries: a review of the Hunt Valley II meeting, January 2005. *Am J Sports Med*, 34:1512, 2006.
19. Shultz, SJ, et al: ACL Research Retreat V: an update on ACL injury risk and prevention, March 25–27, 2010, Greensboro, NC. *J Athl Train*, 45:499, 2010.
20. Toll, DB, et al: Validation, updating, and impact of clinical prediction rules: a review. *J Clin Epidemiol*, 61:1085, 2008.
21. Shapiro, SE: Guidelines for developing and testing clinical decision rules. *West J Nurs Res*, 28:244, 2006.
22. Childs, JD, Cleland, JA: Development and application of clinical prediction rules to improve decision making in physical therapist practice. *Phys Ther*, 86:122, 2006.
23. Stiell, IG, et al: A study to develop clinical decision rules for the use of radiography in acute ankle injuries. *Ann Emerg Med*, 21:384, 1992.
24. Nugent, PJ: Ottawa Ankle Rules accurately assess injuries and reduce reliance on radiographs. *J Fam Pract*, 53:785, 2004.
25. Perry, JJ, Stiell, IG: Impact of clinical decision rules on clinical care of traumatic injuries to the foot and ankle, knee, cervical spine, and head. *Injury*, 37:1157, 2006.
26. Snyder, AR, et al: Using disablement models and clinical outcomes assessment to enable evidence-based athletic training practice, part I: disablement models. *J Athl Train*, 43:428, 2008.
27. Snyder, AR, et al: Using disablement models and clinical outcomes assessment to enable evidence-based athletic training practice, part II: clinical outcomes assessment. *J Athl Train*, 43:437, 2008.
28. Michner, LA: Patient- and clinician-rated outcome measures for clinical decision making in rehabilitation. *J Sport Rehabil*, 20:37, 2011.
29. Cook, CE: Clinimetrics Corner: the minimal clinically important change score (MCID): a necessary pretense. *J Man Manip Ther*, 16:E82, 2008.

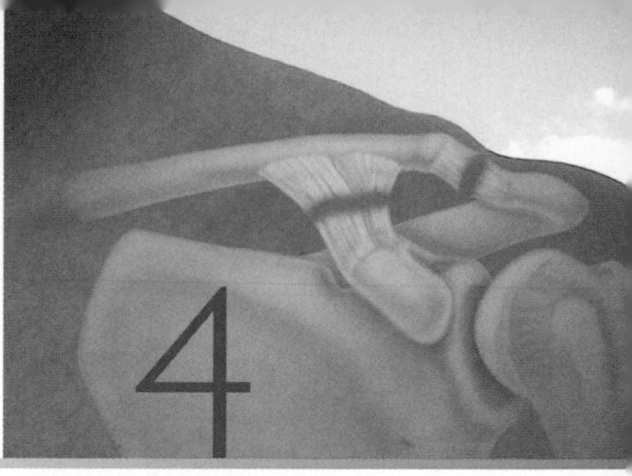

CHAPTER 4

Injury Pathology Nomenclature

A standard approach to describing the body and its conditions is essential for communication among healthcare providers and insurers. Use of standardized terminology is increasingly important with the expanded use of electronic medical records that follow the patient among providers. The use of standardized language improves the validity and reliability of outcome measures and interpreting evidence as it applies to the diagnosis and management of the pathology.

Interestingly, even terminology changes as more and more is known about the body. For example, until recently "tendinitis" was used to describe most nonacute tendon pathologies. We now know that many tendon conditions are not inflammatory in nature, as the "itis" suffix implies. Instead, tendon pathology often results from degenerative changes, and the term "tendinosis" is more appropriate. It is easy to see how the nomenclature might influence the treatment. A patient with an "itis" might effectively be treated with agents designed to reduce inflammation. Treatment of a patient with an "osis" would likely take a different path. In addition to a common labeling approach, a common understanding of how different tissues respond to different types of stress is critical to understanding how various mechanisms result in injury.

Tissue Response to Stress

The tissues that form the human body react to the forces—stress—placed on them in a meaningful and predictable manner, as described by the **Physical Stress Theory** (Fig. 4-1).[1] The term "stress" is broad and encompassing enough to describe physical forces applied to the body as well as psychological, social, and emotional factors. This chapter focuses on the physical forces applied to human tissues, but one should recognize that social stresses are an important factor in determining the patient's level of disability. Emotional stresses will affect both the patient's reaction to the injury and also the perception of pain. In addition, stress can affect the body systemically, such as cardiovascular and muscular enhancements when running, or regionally, such as when performing a one-armed biceps curl.

Some stress is needed for soft tissue and bone to maintain homeostasis (maintenance level). This level of activity varies from person to person, but, as long as the stressors applied to the body stay within this range, no physiological changes occur. When the relative level of applied stress falls below the maintenance level, the tissues **atrophy**. This can be seen after long-term immobilization of an arm or leg: when the cast or brace is removed, the girth of the muscles of the immobilized portion of the limb is significantly less than the healthy limb.

Hypertrophy occurs when the duration and magnitude of the stress applied to the body are progressively increased at a rate that allows the tissues to accommodate their cellular structure and composition to meet the imposed demands.[1] Examples of the beneficial changes in this stage include increased muscle girth and increased bone mineral density and strength. If the body cannot adapt to these forces, tissue **injury** or **cell death** occurs.[1]

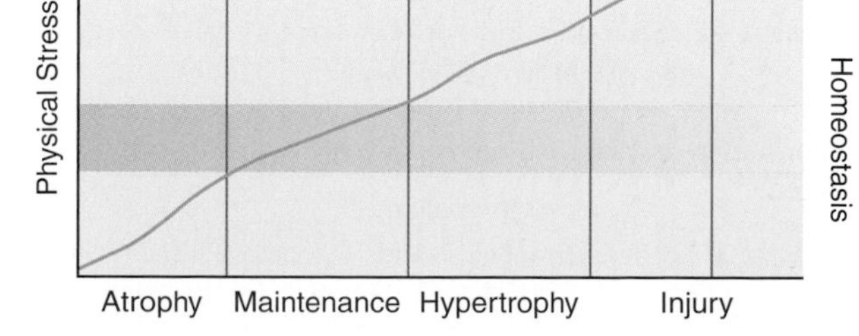

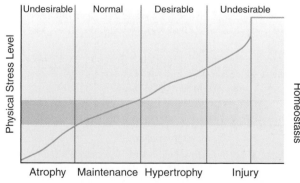

FIGURE 4-1 ■ Physical Stress Theory. The body and specific tissues respond in a predictable manner to stresses placed upon them.

Stress–Strain Relationships

Stress–strain curves (Fig. 4-2) describe the amount of tensile load specific tissues can tolerate before damage results. During the early stages of tension development, called the **toe region**, the tissue slack is being taken up, and there is relatively little change in strength. When no more slack remains, elongation continues, and stiffness increases. At some point, maximum stiffness occurs, and any further stress results in tissue failure. Tissue stiffness increases with aging, a predisposing factor in many soft tissue injuries.

Mechanisms of Injury

Identifying the mechanism of injury is one of the goals of the history-taking process. In response to questions, the patient tends to describe what happened: "I fell with my arm outstretched and landed on my hand" or "It started hurting when I started running outside." **Macrotrauma** occurs when a single force exceeds the tissue's failure point. **Microtrauma** occurs when the body receives repeated submaximal forces over time, and the tissue is unable to adapt.

The most common forms of acute musculoskeletal trauma are the result of tensile, compression, shear, or torsion forces (Fig. 4-3). Certain parts of the body have unique descriptors of the forces leading to injury. For example, whiplash describes a rapid flexion–extension injury to the cervical spine.

Tensile Forces

A tensile force exerts a longitudinal "tearing" stress on the structure, such as a weight suspended by a rope. Tissues, especially muscles and tendons, are better able to adapt and accommodate to tensile forces when they are gradually applied than those that are received abruptly (see Stress–Strain Relationships.

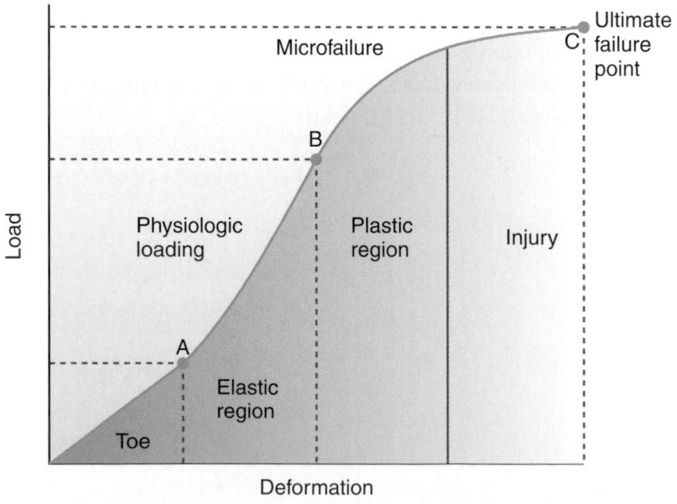

FIGURE 4-2 ■ Load-deformation curve for a connective tissue tested in tension. Initially, the crimp straightens with little force (toe region). Then, collagen fibers are stretched as the elastic region begins at A. After the elastic region ends (B), further force application causes a residual change in tissue structure (plastic region). Continuation of load may case the tissue to rupture at its ultimate failure point (C).

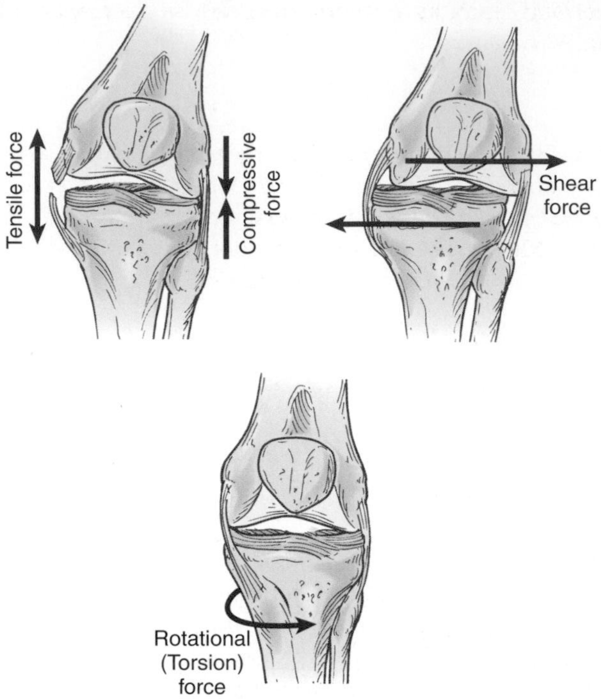

FIGURE 4-3 ■ Forces placed on a joint. Tensile forces "tear" the structure by stretching the tissue. Compressive forces place opposing forces on the structure. Note that tensile forces and compressive forces may occur on opposite sides of the joint. Shear forces place a stress perpendicular to the tissues. Rotational forces (torsion) place an angular stress on the tissues.

Muscle tissue (including tendons), ligaments, and fascia are most prone to injury as the result of tensile forces. Motion that stretches these structures beyond their normal limits and exceeds the tissues' tensile strength results in tearing of the structure. In ligaments, tensile forces are caused by an overstretching of the structure, such as a valgus force stressing the medial collateral ligament of the knee. In muscles and tendons, tensile injury occurs when the joint's normal range is exceeded. A muscle that crosses two joints, for example, the rectus femoris, is more apt to be injured as the result of overstretching than a one-joint muscle such as the vastus lateralis. More commonly, musculotendinous strains are the result of **dynamic overload** where the muscle is contracting eccentrically while an opposing force attempts to elongate the muscle. For instance, tears of the hamstring group often occur while the muscle is eccentrically contracting to slow knee extension during running.

Compression Forces

Compression forces result when stresses are applied at each end of a structure. Compressive injuries can result from an acute mechanism, such as a distal radius fracture after falling on an outstretched arm, or from chronic overload, such as vertebral disc failure from repetitive forces in diving.

Shear Forces

Shear forces occur perpendicularly across the long axis of a structure. When a shear force of sufficient magnitude is applied across a bone, a transverse fracture may occur (see p. 97). When a shear force of sufficient magnitude is applied across a joint, dislocation is imminent.

Torsion Forces

Torsion forces occur with twisting, such as when the foot is fixed and the knee rotates during a change of direction. Torsion forces are magnified by shoes that fix the foot more firmly to the ground and may result in fractures and sprains.

Direct Blow

The term describes exactly what occurs: a blow directly to the body part. Resulting in contusions, fractures, and possibly dislocations, direct blows are easily described by the patient.

Soft Tissue Pathology

Soft tissue pathology, the most common form of orthopedic injury, includes damage to the muscles and their tendons, skin, joint capsules, ligaments, nerves, and bursae. These injuries hinder motion at one or more joints, decrease the ability of the muscle to produce force, create joint instability, make volitional control difficult or impossible, or mechanically limit the amount of motion available.

Musculotendinous Injuries

Muscle injury can be related to overexertion (functional injury) or direct injury to the tissue (structural muscle injury). Injuries to a muscle belly or tendon adversely affect the muscle's ability to generate and sustain tension within the muscle because of mechanical insufficiency or pain. If the **musculotendinous unit** has been mechanically altered through partial or complete tears, the muscle can no longer produce the forces required to perform simple movements or meet the demands required by athletic or work activity. Partial muscle or tendon tears cause decreased force production secondary to pain elicited during the contraction. Complete tears of the unit result in the muscle's mechanical inability to produce force.

Muscle Injury

Terminology describing muscle injury has been reexamined to fully capture the breadth of conditions affecting this tissue (Table 4-1).[2] Functional muscle injuries cause pain and impact movement but do not have identifiable structural changes. Structural injuries involve actual damage to the muscle fibers. While the term "strain" is frequently used to describe these injuries, the term "muscle tear" better reflects the structural damage.

Functional muscle injuries are caused by overexertion or neurological input. Overexertion can result in fatigue-induced muscle disorder with the primary symptoms of "aching" and "tightness." Delayed onset muscle soreness (DOMS) is the latent development of pain following unaccustomed activity, usually including decelerating movements and **eccentric muscle contraction**. DOMS is characterized by pain during activity and at rest, muscle stiffness, and altered movement patterns.

Muscle pain of neurological origin can stem from the spine (e.g., nerve root compression) or from dysfunctional

Musculotendinous unit The group formed by a muscle and its tendons

Eccentric muscle contraction A contraction in which the elongation of the muscle is voluntarily controlled, such as when lowering a weight

Table 4-1 Comprehensive Muscle Injury Classification: Type-specific Definitions and Clinical Presentations

Type	Classification	Symptoms	Clinical Signs
Exertional			
1A	Fatigue-induced disorder	Increase in the longitudinal muscle tone as the result of overexertion, change of playing surface, or activity patterns	Diffuse, dull pain; "tight muscles" reported
1B	Delayed-onset muscle soreness (DOMS)	Generalized muscle pain following exercise, especially those involving eccentric contractions	Acute inflammation-related pain; pain at rest that persists hours to days following activity
Neuromuscular			
2A	Spine-related neuromuscular muscle disorder	Increase in longitudinal muscle tone as the result of structural spinal or lumbopelvic disorders	Increased muscle tension that increases with activity and decreases at rest. Pain may increase with muscle stretching or the application of pressure.
2B	Muscle-related neuromuscular muscle disorder	Spindle-shaped area of increased muscle tone as the result of dysfunctional neuromuscular control (e.g., reciprocal inhibition)	Aching with progressive muscle tension (spasm)

Continued

Table 4-1 Comprehensive Muscle Injury Classification: Type-specific Definitions and Clinical Presentations—cont'd

Type	Classification	Symptoms	Clinical Signs
Muscle Tension Related			
3A	Minor partial muscle tear	Tearing of less than one muscle fascicle/bundle	The patient may report a "snap" followed by a sharp, stabbing pain.
3B	Moderate partial muscle tear	Tear diameter is greater than one muscle fascicle/bundle.	The patient reports a "snap" at the time of injury, with a noticeable sensation of tearing. Muscle function will be limited.
4	(Sub)total muscle tear/tendinous avulsion	Tear involving the complete—or near complete—diameter of the muscle or tendon, frequently located at the musculotendinous junction	Noticeable tearing. The patient experiences a definite snap followed by immediate disability of the muscle.
Direct Blow			
Contusion	Direct injury	Trauma caused by blunt trauma leading to hematoma	Dull pain that may increase with time (proportional to the increased size of the hematoma)

Adapted from: Mueller-Wohlfahrt, H, et al: Terminology and classification of muscle injuries in sport: The Munich consensus statement. *Br J Sports Med*, 47:342, 2013.

local neuromuscular control mechanisms. Spine-related muscle disorders are characterized by increased tone and "aching," and the underlying source must be identified and managed. Muscle-related neuromuscular disorders are characterized by cramp-like pain, aching, and localized increased tone. These symptoms may be relieved by stretching.

Structural muscle injuries involve an acute episode and often result from a sudden forced lengthening. Often occurring at the weaker musculotendinous junction, muscle tears are further classified as minor partial, moderate partial, and total, depending on the amount of involved tissue. Patients will often describe a "snap" following by a sharp localized pain at the time of injury. Moderate and total tears result in palpable defects, ecchymosis, and edema that may extravasate distally (Fig. 4-4). Functionally, patients will compensate to avoid activating or elongating the involved muscle. Total tears may not result in a complete loss of joint function due to compensation by secondary movers (Examination Findings 4-1).

The same mechanism that produces a tear in a skeletally mature individual may result in an avulsion of the muscle's origin or insertion in skeletally immature individuals. Radiographs and magnetic resonance imaging (MRI) are used to rule out apophyseal avulsions.

Muscle Injury Intervention Strategies

Muscle injury that occurs as the result of exertion is often managed symptomatically using thermal modalities. Light to moderate exercise and stretching assist in reducing symptoms and restoring muscle function. The interventions for neuromuscular-related conditions focus on resolving the underlying neurological condition (e.g., nerve impingement, disc herniation). Type 3A and 3B muscle tears are initially managed using cryotherapy and stretching as tolerated. Rehabilitation focuses on strengthening both the involved muscle(s) and the **antagonist** muscle group with the goal of restoring appropriate muscle balance. Type 4 muscle tears (ruptures) often require surgical correction.

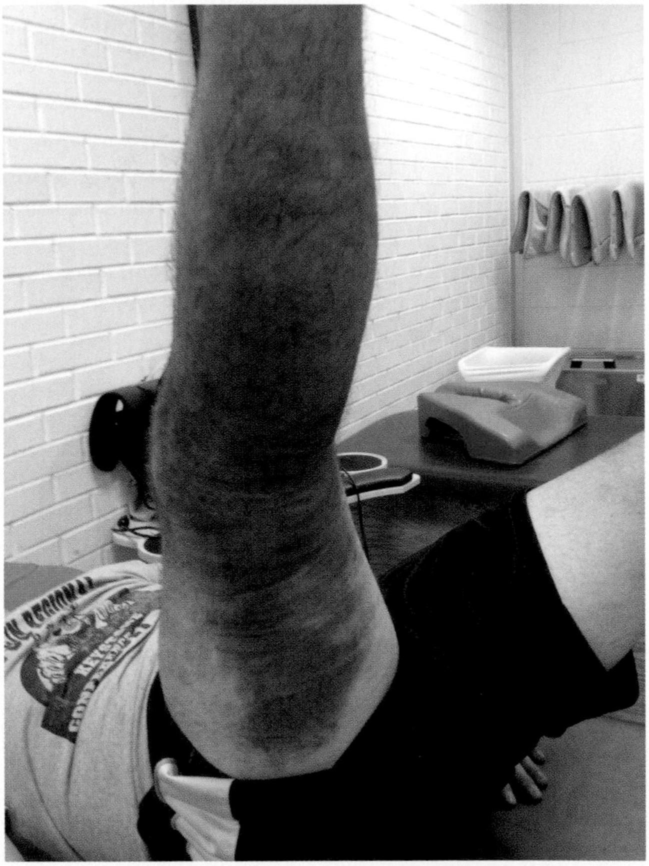

FIGURE 4-4 ■ Ecchymosis associated with a muscular strain and concurrent ligament damage. Gravity causes blood that has seeped into the tissues to drift distally.

Antagonist Muscle that produces a motion that is opposite of another muscle (e.g., the antagonistic motion of extension is flexion)

Examination Findings 4-1
Muscle Tears

Examination Segment	Clinical Findings
History of Current Condition	*Onset:* Acute *Pain characteristics:* Pain is initially located at the site of the injury, which tends to be at or near the junction between the muscle belly and tendon. After a few days, pain becomes more diffuse and difficult to localize. The distal musculotendinous junction is most often involved. *Mechanism:* Tears usually result from a single episode of overload of the muscle as the result of an eccentric contraction. *Risk factors:* Imbalance in the strength of the agonist/antagonist muscle groups; History of injury to the involved muscle; Muscle tightness and improper warm-up before activity.
Functional Assessment	Compensatory movement patterns will be observed in motions requiring control or strength from the involved muscles.
Inspection	Ecchymosis may be evident in cases of moderate or total muscle tears. Gravity causes the blood to pool distal to the site of trauma. Swelling may be present over or distal to the involved area. In severe acute cases or in a chronic condition, a defect may be visible in the muscle or tendon.
Palpation	Point tenderness and increased tissue density associated with spasm exist over the site of the injury, with the degree of pain increasing with the severity of the injury. A defect may be palpable at the injury site.
Joint and Muscle Function Assessment	*AROM:* Pain is elicited at the injury site. In the case of moderate or total tears, the patient may be unable to complete the movement. *MMT:* Muscle strength is reduced. Pain increases as the amount of resistance is increased. Total tears result in total a loss of function of the involved muscle. *PROM:* Pain is elicited at the injury site during passive motion in the direction opposite that of the muscle, placing it on stretch.
Joint Stability Tests	*Stress tests:* Stress tests of the ligaments crossing the joint(s) serviced by the muscle should be performed. Tears may occur as the body attempts to protect against ligament injury. *Joint play:* Rule out hypermobility.
Selective Tissue Tests	As indicated to rule out underlying pathology
Neurological Screening	Use to rule out nerve entrapment that clinically appears as a strain. Tearing of muscle may also damage peripheral nerves.
Vascular Screening	Within normal limits
Imaging Techniques	MRI can be used to identify tears and the resulting edema in the muscle and/or tendon. Diagnostic ultrasound
Differential Diagnosis	Tendinopathy, underlying joint instability, stress fracture, nerve entrapment, avulsion fracture
Comments	Tears occur more frequently in muscles that span two joints than they do in one-joint muscles. In the presence of a complete muscle tear (rupture), trauma to the associated joint structures should be ruled out. AROM does not rule out a complete tear of the muscle belly or rupture of the tendon. Secondary movers may still produce active motion.

AROM = active range of motion; MMT = manual muscle test; PROM = passive range of motion

Examination Findings 4-10
Exostosis

Examination Segment	Clinical Findings
History of Current Condition	*Onset:* Insidious *Pain characteristics:* Exostosis involving the extremities most often results in localized pain. Spinal exostosis can result in pain radiating along the distribution of affected nerve roots. *Mechanism:* Exostosis is the result of repeated stress placed on a bone or the bony insertion of a tendon. It may also result from repeated compressive forces. *Risk factors:* Previous trauma to the area, osteoarthritis, instability
Functional Assessment	The patient demonstrates avoidance of movements that add tensile stress or compress the exostosis.
Inspection	Deformity may be noted over the site of pain.
Palpation	Point tenderness is present. A large bony outgrowth may be palpable.
Joint and Muscle Function Assessment	*AROM:* Limited secondary to pain and/or bony block *MMT:* Dependent on joint position *PROM:* Equal to AROM
Joint Stability Tests	*Stress tests:* May be present with underlying instability *Joint play:* May be restricted in the direction of exostosis
Selective Tissue Tests	Not applicable
Neurological Screening	Within normal limits
Vascular Screening	Within normal limits
Imaging Techniques	Radiograph
Differential Diagnosis	Tumor, apophysitis (e.g., Osgood-Schlatter disease)

AROM = active range of motion; MMT = manual muscle test; PROM = passive range of motion

Stress Fractures

A stress fracture is classified as a fatigue fracture or insufficiency fracture. **Fatigue fractures** occur when normal bone is subjected to abnormally high, repeated submaximal stresses and is linked to sudden changes in the frequency, intensity, or duration of activity beyond which the bone is accustomed. **Insufficiency fractures** occur when abnormally weak bones are subjected to normal forces.[22]

Although stress fractures most commonly occur in the lower extremities, this condition can be found in any bone that absorbs repetitive stress.[23,24] Stress fractures present as a complex injury because of their nondescript initial findings and their tendency to mimic the signs and symptoms of soft tissue injuries (Table 4-3).[25] Stress fractures occur when the bone's osteoclastic activity outweighs **osteoblastic** activity, causing a weakened area along the line of stress. If the external stress is not reduced (e.g., the patient continues running), the bone eventually fails.

The history reveals a chronic condition caused by repetitive stresses to the involved area. There may have been a recent change in the patient's workout routine, including changes in equipment, playing surfaces, frequency, duration, or intensity. Because of the related reduction in levels of estrogen and progesterone, **amenorrheic** women may be predisposed to developing stress fractures. With specific palpation, an area of exact tenderness can be discerned along any bony surface. Compression of long bones may result in increased pain (Examination Findings 4-11).

Osteoblasts (osteoblastic) Cells responsible for the formation of new bone

Amenorrheic (amenorrhea) The absence of menstruation

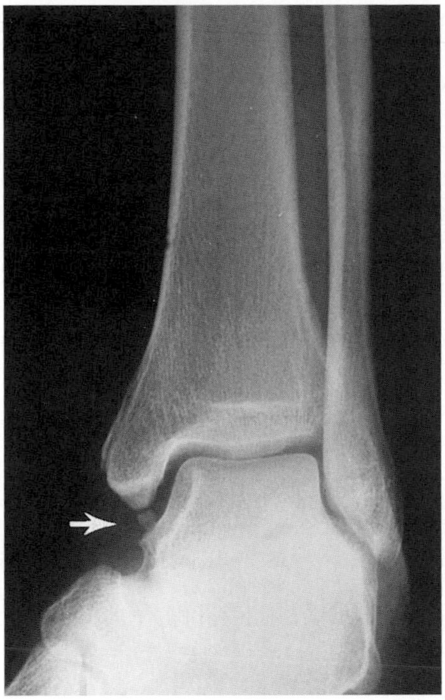

FIGURE 4-15 ■ Radiograph (anterior view of the left ankle) of an avulsion fracture of the attachment of the deltoid ligament (arrow).

✱ Practical Evidence

MRI and bone scans are the preferred modalities for diagnosing stress fractures. By comparison, tuning forks and therapeutic ultrasound (with a positive result of pain with application) lack diagnostic accuracy.[26]

Neurological and Vascular Pathologies

Trauma to the nerves, arteries, and veins is often a consequence of joint dislocation, bony displacement, concussive forces, or compartment syndromes (see Box 4-1). If untreated, vascular disruption can lead to the loss of the affected body part. Neurological inhibition can lead to the loss of function in the involved part.

Peripheral Nerve Injury

Entrapment injuries to the peripheral nerves are common at the ankle, elbow, wrist, and cervical spine. Peripheral nerves located more distally from the spinal column have a greater probability of regeneration than a lesion that occurs more proximal to the central nervous system.

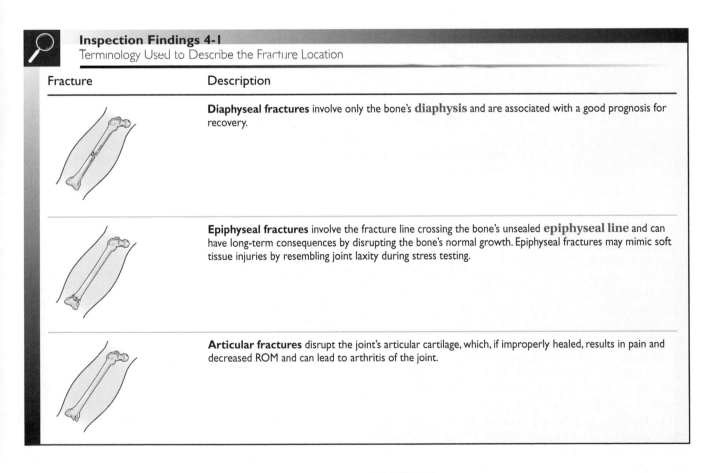

Inspection Findings 4-1
Terminology Used to Describe the Fracture Location

Fracture	Description
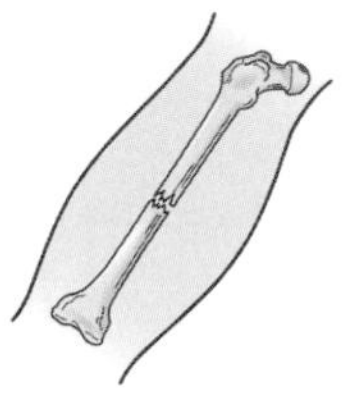	**Diaphyseal fractures** involve only the bone's **diaphysis** and are associated with a good prognosis for recovery.
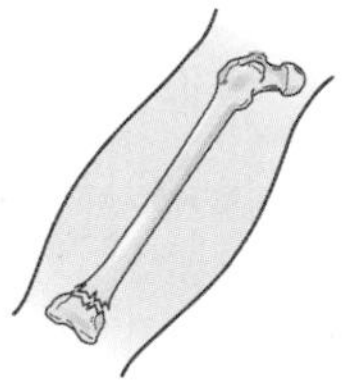	**Epiphyseal fractures** involve the fracture line crossing the bone's unsealed **epiphyseal line** and can have long-term consequences by disrupting the bone's normal growth. Epiphyseal fractures may mimic soft tissue injuries by resembling joint laxity during stress testing.
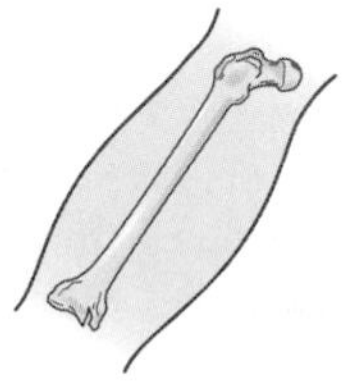	**Articular fractures** disrupt the joint's articular cartilage, which, if improperly healed, results in pain and decreased ROM and can lead to arthritis of the joint.

Diaphysis The shaft of a long bone

Epiphyseal line The area of growth found between the diaphysis and epiphysis in immature long bones

Table 4-3 Classification of Stress Fractures

Grade	Imaging Findings
1	Incidental "stress reaction" found on imaging; patient may be asymptomatic
2	Patient describes pain as a part of the history of the condition; pain elicited during palpation; stress reaction (bone fatigue found on imaging)
3	Nondisplaced fracture line on imaging
4	Fracture displacement $\geq$ 2 mm identified on imaging
5	Nonunion fracture identified on imaging

In some cases, nonneurological tissue or swelling entraps the nerve, causing dysfunction in the form of paresthesia and muscular weakness. This condition is most commonly seen at the ulnar tunnel, pronator teres muscle, carpal tunnel, and tarsal tunnel. In each case, the complaints are of specific pain patterns and paresthesia. With careful manual muscle testing, muscle weakness may be elicited. Although these syndromes may be suspected on evaluation, they are confirmed via electrodiagnostic testing.

Stretch injuries to peripheral nerves may be divided into three categories based on the pathology and the prognosis for recovery. **Neurapraxia** is the mildest form of peripheral nerve stretch injury. The nerve, **epineurium**, and **myelin sheath** are stretched but remain intact. Symptoms are usually transient and include burning, pain, numbness, and temporary weakness on clinical evaluation.

Axonotmesis involves a disruption of the axon and the myelin sheath, but the epineurium remains intact. The

Neurapraxia A stretch injury to a nerve resulting in transient symptoms of paresthesia and weakness

Epineurium Connective tissue containing blood vessels surrounding the trunk of a nerve, binding it together

Myelin sheath A fatty-based lining of the axon of myelinated nerve fibers

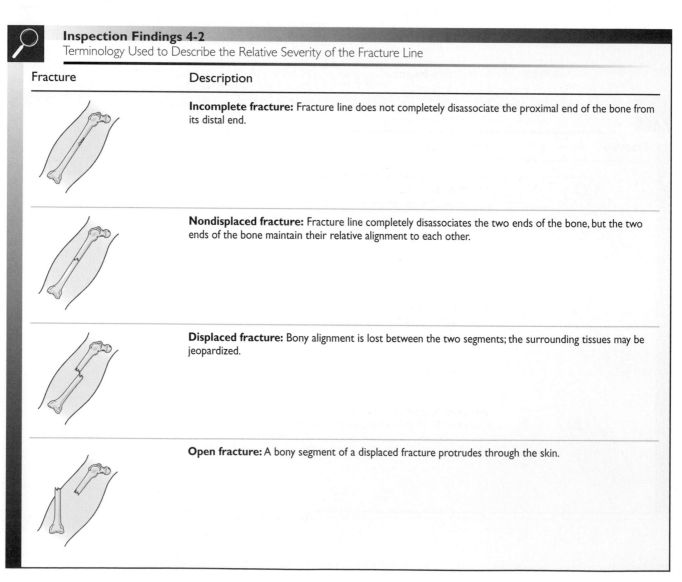

Inspection Findings 4-2

Terminology Used to Describe the Relative Severity of the Fracture Line

Fracture	Description
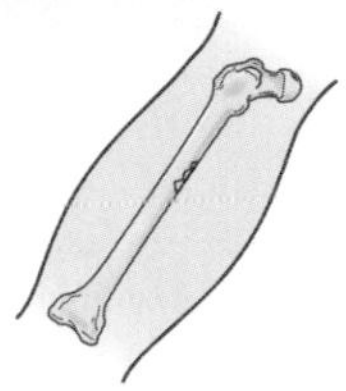	**Incomplete fracture:** Fracture line does not completely disassociate the proximal end of the bone from its distal end.
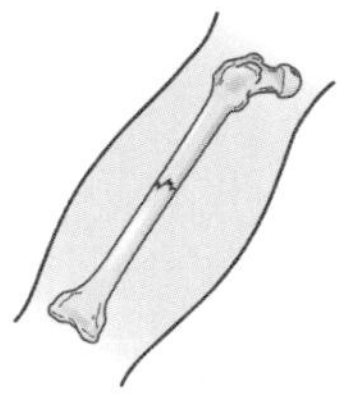	**Nondisplaced fracture:** Fracture line completely disassociates the two ends of the bone, but the two ends of the bone maintain their relative alignment to each other.
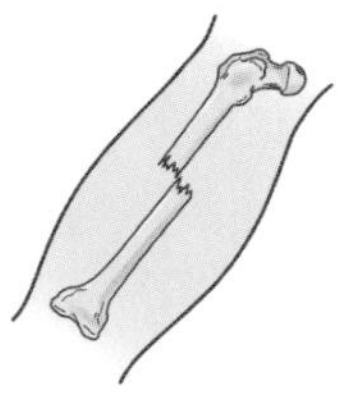	**Displaced fracture:** Bony alignment is lost between the two segments; the surrounding tissues may be jeopardized.
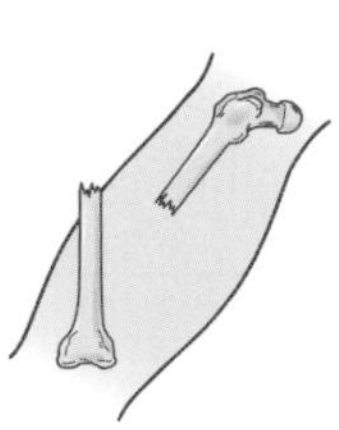	**Open fracture:** A bony segment of a displaced fracture protrudes through the skin.

Inspection Findings 4-3
Terminology Used to Describe the Fracture Line

Fracture	Description
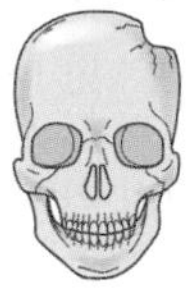	**Depressed fracture:** Results from direct trauma to flat bones, causing the bone to fracture and depress
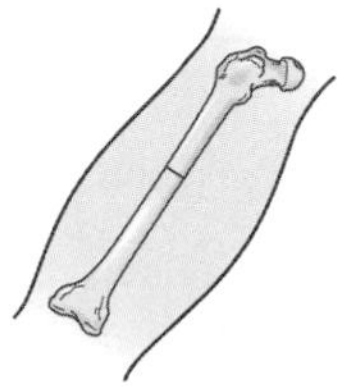	**Transverse fracture:** Caused by a direct blow, shear force, or tensile force being applied to the shaft of a long bone and results in a fracture line that crosses the bone's long axis
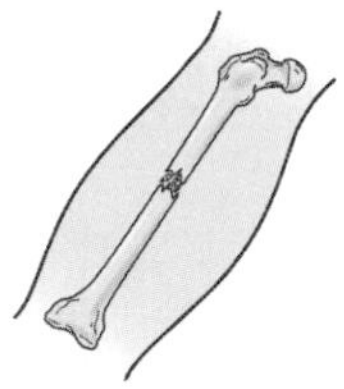	**Comminuted fracture:** Result of extremely high-velocity impact forces that cause the bone to shatter into multiple pieces. This type of fracture often requires surgical correction.
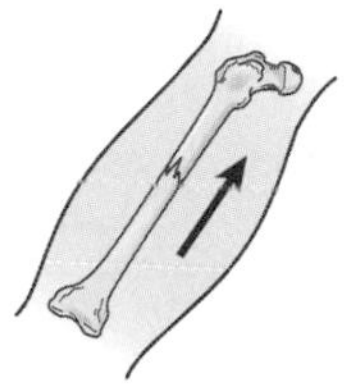	**Compacted fracture:** Results from compressive forces applied through the long axis of the bone. One end of a fractured segment is driven into the opposite piece of the fracture, leading to a shortening of the involved bone.
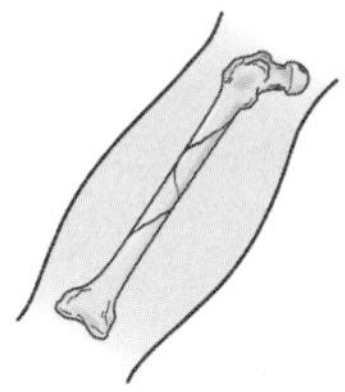	**Spiral fracture:** The result of a rotational force placed on the shaft of a long bone, such as twisting the tibia while the foot remains fixated. The fracture line assumes a three-dimensional S-shape along the length of the bone.
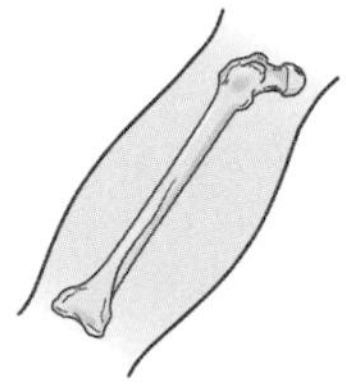	**Longitudinal fracture:** Most commonly occurs as the result of a fall and has a fracture line that runs parallel to the bone's long axis
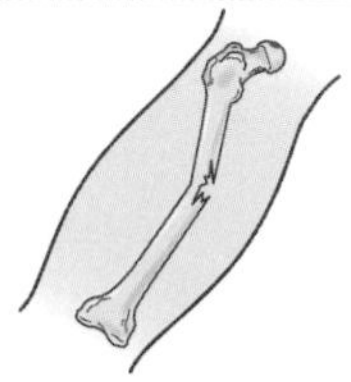	**Greenstick fracture:** Generally specific to the pediatric and adolescent population, this involves a displaced fracture on one side of the bone and a compacted fracture on the opposite side. The name is derived from an analogy to an immature tree branch that has been snapped.

Examination Findings 4-11
Stress Fractures

Examination Segment	Clinical Findings
History of Current Condition	*Onset:* Insidious The patient cannot report a single traumatic event causing the pain. *Pain characteristics:* Pain tends to localize to the involved bone. *Other symptoms:* Not applicable *Mechanism:* Cumulative microtrauma causes stress fractures or underlying bony deficiency. *Risk factors:* Overtraining, poor conditioning, amenorrhea, low energy availability, and improper training techniques may be noted.
Functional Assessment	The patient can often function normally during low-load, short-duration activity; symptoms increase as activity and duration increase, eventually leading to disability.
Inspection	Usually no bony abnormality is noted. Soft tissue swelling may be present.
Palpation	Point tenderness exists over the fracture site.
Joint and Muscle Function Assessment	*AROM:* All motions are generally within normal limits. *MMT:* Pain is increased if tension is added at the fracture site. *PROM:* Unremarkable
Joint Stability Tests	*Stress tests:* Unremarkable *Joint play:* Unremarkable
Selective Tissue Tests	Long bone compression test
Neurological Screening	Within normal limits
Vascular Screening	Within normal limits
Imaging Techniques	Bone scans, MRI
Differential Diagnosis	Tumor, tendinopathy, compartment syndrome, periostitis
Comments	For repetitive stress fractures, seek the underlying cause.

AROM = active range of motion; MMT = manual muscle test; MRI = magnetic resonance imaging; PROM = passive range of motion

signs and symptoms are the same as for neurapraxia, but those associated with axonotmesis have a longer duration. Because the axon undergoes **Wallerian degeneration**, the return of normal innervation is unpredictable, and sustained weakness may be experienced.

Neurotmesis, a complete disruption of the nerve, is the most severe form of peripheral nerve injury. The prognosis for the return of normal innervation is poor. This injury occurs under extremely high forces and usually entails concurrent injury to bones, ligaments, and tendons. Many times, a nerve **graft** or tendon transfer is required to return function to the extremity. These procedures meet with limited success and are not conducive to the return to competitive athletics.

Complex Regional Pain Syndrome

Complex regional pain syndrome (CRPS), previously known as reflex sympathetic **dystrophy** (RSD), is characterized by continuing pain that is out of proportion to the instigating injury. CRPS often develops following injury or a condition that requires immobilization. The pain is regional and not isolated to a specific dermatome. Other common findings include **vasomotor** disturbances (e.g., side-to-side temperature differences, skin color changes), edema, decreased motor function, and **trophic** changes.[27] With Type I CRPS, there is no measureable nerve damage. Type II CRPS involves nerve involvement that is detectable through electrodiagnostic testing. The classification of CRPS-NOS (not otherwise specified) is used for patients who partially meet diagnostic criteria and for whom no more compelling diagnosis is available.[27]

Signs and symptoms of CRPS may include:

- Pain that is disproportionately increased relative to the severity of the injury
- Superficial hypersensitive areas (e.g., pain when clothing touches the skin)
- Edema
- Decreased motor function, leading to dystrophy
- Muscle spasm
- Dermatologic alterations, including the integrity of the skin, skin temperature changes, hair loss, and changes in the nailbed
- Vasomotor instability: **Raynaud disease**, **vasoconstriction**, **vasodilation**, **hyperhydrosis**
- Skeletal changes, including osteoporosis

Complex Regional Pain Syndrome Intervention Strategies

The prognosis for patients with CRPS is extremely variable, but early intervention appears to improve the probability of a favorable outcome, making early recognition and referral a priority. Intervention is focused on restoration of function and generally includes modalities, therapeutic exercise, medications, and psychotherapy. In unyielding cases, surgical dissection of the nerve may be required to prevent the pain causing nerve transmission.[27]

REFERENCES

1. Mueller, MJ, and Maluf, KS: Tissue adaptation to physical stress: a proposed "Physical Stress Theory" to guide physical therapist practice, education, and research. *Phys Ther*, 82:383, 2002.
2. Mueller-Wohlfahrt, H, et al: Terminology and classification of muscle injuries in sport: the Munich consensus statement. *Br J Sports Med*, 47:342, 2013.
3. Maffulli, N: Basic science and clinical aspects of Achilles tendinopathy. *Sports Med Arthrosc*, 17:190, 2009.
4. Asplund, CA, and Best, TM: Achilles tendon disorders. *BMJ*, 346:f1262, 2013.
5. Sharma, P, and Maffulli, N: Tendon injury and tendinopathy: healing and r epair. *J Bone Joint Surg Am*, 87:187, 2005.
6. Wilson, JJ, and Best, TM: Common overuse tendon problems: a review and recommendations for treatment. *Am Fam Physician*, 72:811, 2005.
7. Kijowski, R, De Smet, A, and Mukharjee, R: Magnetic resonance imaging findings in patients with peroneal tendinopathy and peroneal tenosynovitis. *Skelet Radiol*, 36:105, 2007.
8. It's bursitis, but which type? *Emerg Med*, 21:71, 1989.
9. Kary, JM: Diagnosis and management of quadriceps strains and contusions. *Curr Rev Musculoskelet Med*, 3:26, 2010.
10. Pape, HC, et al: Current concepts in the development of heterotopic ossification. *J Bone Joint Surg*, 86-B:783, 2004.
11. Thacker, SB, et al: The impact of stretching on sports injury risk: a systematic review of the literature. *Med Sci Sport Exer*, 36:371, 2004.
12. Jackson, WM, et al: Cytokine expression in muscle following traumatic injury. *J Orthop Res*, 29:1613, 2011.
13. Aronen, JG, et al: Quadriceps contusions: clinical results of immediate immobilization in 120 degrees of knee flexion. *Clin J Sport Med*, 16:383, 2006.
14. Drakos, MC, et al: Injury in the National Basketball Association: a 17-year overview. *Sports Health*, 2:284, 2010.
15. Mithoefer, K, et al: Current concepts for rehabilitation and return to sport after knee articular cartilage repair in the athlete. *J Orthop Sports Phys Ther*, 42:254, 2012.
16. Pascual-Garrido, C, McNickle, AG, and Cole, BJ: Surgical treatment options for osteochondritis dissecans of the knee. *Sports Health*, 1:326, 2009.
17. Chan, KKW, and Chan, LWY: A qualitative study on patients with knee osteoarthritis to evaluate the influence of different pain patterns on patients' quality of life and to find out patients' interpretation and coping strategies for the disease. *Rheumatol Rep*, 3:9, 2011.

Wallerian degeneration Degeneration of a nerve's axon that has been severed from the body of the nerve

Neurotmesis Complete loss of nerve function with little apparent anatomic damage to the nerve itself

Graft An organ or tissue used for transplantation. An allograft is a donor tissue transplanted from the same species. An autograft tissue is transplanted from within the same individual.

Dystrophy The progressive deterioration of tissue

Vasomotor Pertaining to nerves controlling the muscles within the walls of blood vessels

Trophic Pertaining to efferent nerves controlling the nourishment of the area they innervate

Raynaud disease A reaction to cold consisting of bouts of pallor and cyanosis, causing exaggerated vasomotor responses

Vasoconstriction A decrease in a vessel's diameter

Vasodilation An increase in a vessel's diameter

Hyperhydrosis Excessive or profuse sweating

18. Jouben, LM, Steele, RJ, and Bono, JV: Orthopaedic manifestations of Lyme disease. *Orthop Rev*, 23:395, 1994.
19. Marzan, KAB, and Shaham, B: Early juvenile idiopathic arthritis. *Rheum Dis Clin N Am*, 38:355, 2012.
20. McKinnis, LN: Radiologic evaluation of fracture. In McKinnis, LN: *Fundamentals of Musculoskeletal Imaging*, ed 2. Philadelphia, PA: FA Davis, 2005, p 94.
21. Starkey, C: The injury response process. In Starkey, C: *Therapeutic Modalities*, ed 4. Philadelphia, PA: FA Davis, 2013.
22. Ha, YJ, et al: Osteoporotic calcaneal stress fractures mistaken for aggravation of rheumatoid arthritis. *Arthritis Rheum*, 2013 [epub ahead of print].
23. Miller, TL, Harris, JD, and Kaeding, CC: Stress fractures of the ribs and upper extremities: causation, evaluation, and management. *Sports Med*, 43:665, 2013.
24. Hutchinson, PH, et al: Complete and incomplete femoral stress fractures in the adolescent athlete. *Orthopedics*, 31:604, 2008.
25. Kaeding, CC, and Miller, T: The comprehensive description of stress fractures: a new classification system. *J Bone Joint Surg*, 95:1214, 2013.
26. Schneiders, AG, et al: The ability of clinical tests to diagnose stress fractures: a systematic review and meta-analysis. *J Orthop Sports Phys Ther*, 42:760, 2012.
27. Harden, RN, et al: Complex regional pain syndrome: Practical diagnostic and treatment guidelines, ed 4. *Pain Med*, 14:180, 2013.

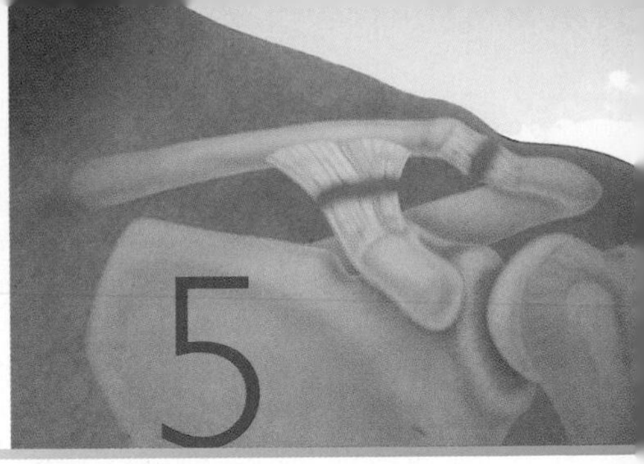

CHAPTER 5

Musculoskeletal Diagnostic Techniques

Multiple laboratory-based neuromuscular diagnostic techniques are referenced throughout this text. Although typically ordered and interpreted by physicians, knowledge of when these techniques are indicated, what conditions they identify, and basic interpretation techniques are valuable clinical skills. Table 5-1 presents an overview of the techniques discussed in this chapter and their most common uses.

Imaging Techniques

Radiographs, magnetic resonance images (MRIs), computed tomography (CT), bone scans, and diagnostic ultrasounds are collectively referred to as **diagnostic imaging**. They are obtained by exposing the body to electromagnetic energy, or in the case of diagnostic ultrasound, acoustical

Table 5-1 Selected Diagnostic Techniques and Their Use

Technique	Best Use
Radiography	**Standard:** Bone lesions, joint surfaces, and joint spaces **Arthrogram:** Capsular tissue tears and articular cartilage lesions **Angiogram:** Blood vessels **Myelogram:** Pathologies within the spinal canal
Computed Tomography (CT)	Bony or articular cartilage lesions and some soft tissue lesions Quantify detailed bony lesions (e.g., size and location) Identify tendinous and ligamentous injuries in varying joint positions **Angiography:** Artery and/or vein pathologies, including stenosis, aneurysms, and thrombi (clots)
Magnetic Resonance Imaging (MRI)	Visualize soft tissue structures, especially ligamentous and meniscal injuries **Magnetic resonance arthrography (MRA):** Used to image blood vessels **Functional magnetic resonance imaging (fMRI):** Assesses metabolic activity associated with brain function
Nuclear Medicine	**Bone scan:** Identifies increased metabolic activity but may yield false-positive findings, especially in endurance athletes **Positron emission tomography (PET):** Creates a three-dimensional image of physiological function in the body **Single photon emission computed tomography (SPECT):** Produces three-dimensional images of internal structures
Ultrasonic Imaging	Detects joint and soft tissue disorders; used to guide injections
Electromyography	Evaluates muscle physiology at rest and with activity Identifies pathology of muscle secondary to nerve supply dysfunction or change in the muscle itself Used in conjunction with a nerve conduction study
Nerve Conduction Study	Assesses function of motor and sensory nerves to detect nerve pathology, including axonal degeneration and neurotmesis

energy, and determining how much of that energy is absorbed by the body, is reflected, or passes through the tissues. Most imaging techniques use a source (generator) that transmits the energy to the body and a collector that captures energy that has not been absorbed or scattered. From this, two- or three-dimensional images are constructed.

To obtain the clearest images of the involved structure(s), the diagnostic energy must strike the body from a specific direction and angle. Energy may pass from the anterior through the posterior tissues (anteroposterior [AP]), posterior to anterior (posteroanterior [PA]) or from a left or right lateral projection. The patient and generator may be aligned so that the energy strikes the body at a right angle, or images may be obtained using an oblique or acute angle (Fig. 5-1).

Cost, accuracy, risk to the patient, the patient's tolerance, skill of the operator, and availability are factors in

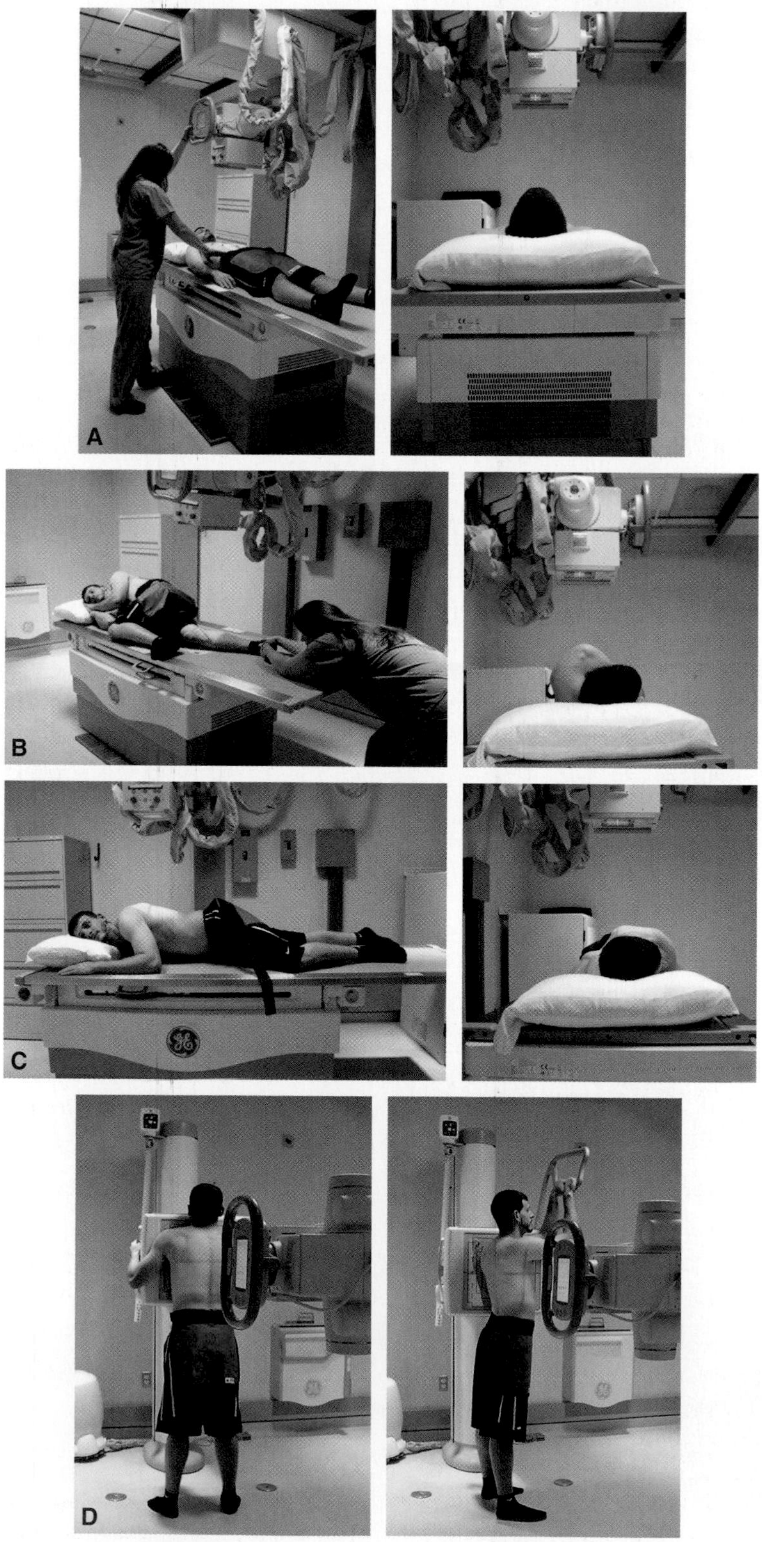

FIGURE 5-1 ■ Patient positioning for common radiographic imaging series. Position for (A) anterior to posterior view, (B) lateral view, (C) oblique view, and (D) chest view. Images courtesy of Nicole Ries.

determining which diagnostic technique is used. Because of its low cost and availability, radiography is a frequent first step to determine if there is bony pathology. For some suspected pathologies, other imaging techniques are quickly ordered in the presence of a negative radiograph and persistent symptoms.

Radiography

Radiographs are the most common imaging technique used in the diagnosis of orthopedic injuries. Discovered in 1895, x-rays made it possible for the first time to view the internal structures without invasive techniques.[1] Before this, the only method of viewing the internal structures was to actually cut the individual open. Note that "x-ray" describes the form of electromagnetic energy that is used; radiography describes the process of acquiring images (Fig. 5-2).

Although radiographs have limited utility beyond identification of fractures, because of their relatively low cost they are often obtained before MRI or CT scans. However, they are not sensitive in acutely identifying some forms of acute fractures, such as those involving the scaphoid and acute stress fractures. [2,3] Because of its improved sensitivity and lack of radiation exposure, MRI is replacing scintigraphy (bone scan) as the imaging of choice in detecting stress fractures early in the pathological process.[4]

Radiographic examination uses **ionizing radiation** to penetrate the body. Depending on the density of the underlying tissues, the radiation is absorbed or dispersed in varying degrees. High-density tissues such as bone absorb more radiation and are therefore more difficult to penetrate than less-dense tissue. The exposure to radiation leaves an imprint on special x-ray film (radiographic plate), producing the familiar radiographic image. Overexposure to ionizing radiation is hazardous, and care must be taken to protect the reproductive organs by using a lead apron.

Patient Information
Radiograph

Patient Preparation	The patient should wear clothes that are easy to put on and remove because the part to be imaged needs to be exposed.
Duration of Procedure	Radiograph: 5–10 minutes Arthrogram: 45–60 minutes
Procedure	Patients are positioned to expose the involved body part to the x-ray beam. Patients must remain still while the picture is taken. Generally, multiple views are taken. Arthrogram: A local anesthetic injection precedes the injection of the contrast medium. After a waiting period, radiographs are obtained.
Comments	Patients who are—or who suspect that they may be—pregnant should inform the technician. When possible, a lead shield is placed over the reproductive organs to protect them from radiation exposure. Stress radiographs determine the effects of stress on a joint. These require special positioning using either weights or manual stress applied by the technician. Patients undergoing arthrography should inform the technician of any allergies to medication.[6] Joint discomfort is common for 24–48 hours following arthrogram.

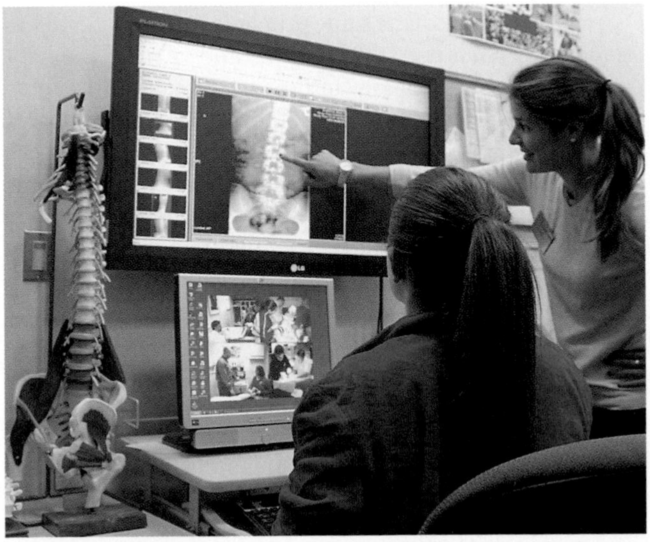

FIGURE 5-2 ■ Interpretation of radiographs is performed using the ABCS method: Alignment, Bones, Cartilage, and Soft tissue.

The interpretation of radiographic images can be based on the ABCS method:[5]

A—Alignment: Observe for the normal continuity of the bones and joint surfaces and the alignment of one bone with another.

B—Bones: Bones should have normal density patterns, presenting with uniform color throughout the bone as compared bilaterally. Cortical bone appears brighter; cancellous bone is darker. Areas of decreased density appear as darkened areas within the bone. Fractures and abnormal bony outgrowths such as exostoses can also be visualized.

Ionizing radiation Electromagnetic energy that causes the release of an atom's protons, electrons, or neutrons. Ionizing radiation is potentially hazardous to human tissue.

C—Cartilage: Although cartilage itself does not produce a radiographic image, the cartilage and ligamentous structures are inspected for what does not appear. The joint spaces should be smooth and uniform.

S—Soft tissue: Although soft tissue cannot be imaged, swelling within the confines of the soft tissue or between the soft tissue and the bones can be determined. In addition, the outline of soft tissues and even pockets of edema within soft tissue can be identified with adjusted exposure techniques.

Each body area has a standard series of radiographic views that are obtained to rule in or rule out a diagnosis (Table 5-2). The views ordered may be expanded based on the differential diagnosis, the patient's symptoms, or findings of earlier imaging series.

Assessment of a joint's ligamentous integrity often requires the use of imaging techniques, during which stress is applied to a joint to measure the amount of laxity—a stress radiograph (Fig. 5-3). This requires application of a force that stretches the ligament during the x-ray exposure, allowing for the measurement of excessive motion, determining a third-degree ligament injury, or ascertaining the amount of overall joint laxity.

Other forms of radiographic screening involve the use of radio-opaque dyes that are absorbed by the tissues, allowing visualization by radiographic examination. Collectively known as **contrast imaging**, arthrograms, myelograms, and angiograms have various applications to specific body systems. With the availability of MRI techniques, these types of studies are less frequently used in the diagnosis of orthopedic injuries.

Table 5-2 Routine Radiologic Series by Body Area

Body Area	Views
Foot	AP, lateral, oblique
Ankle	AP, AP mortise, lateral, oblique
Knee	AP, lateral, intercondylar fossa
Patellofemoral	AP, lateral, merchant
Hip	AP, lateral
Lumbar Spine	AP, lateral, oblique (right and left)
Thoracic Spine	AP, lateral
Cervical Spine	AP, lateral, oblique (right and left), open mouth
Shoulder	AP (internally rotated), AP (externally rotated), axillary
Elbow	AP, lateral, oblique (internal and external)
Wrist, Hand, and Fingers	PA, lateral, oblique

AP = anteroposterior; PA = posteroanterior

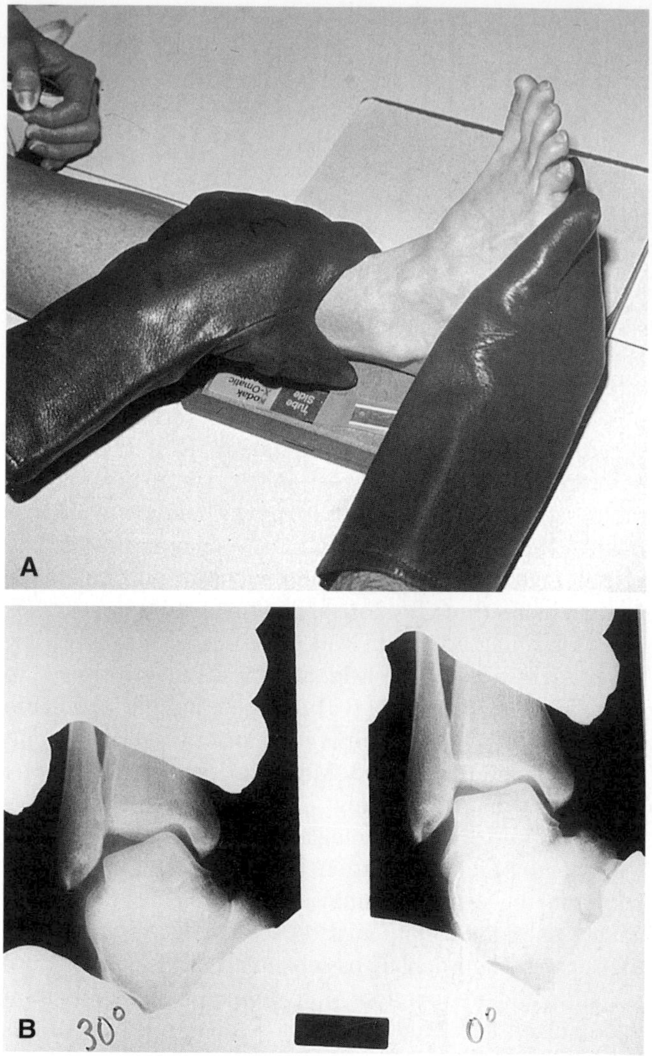

FIGURE 5-3 ■ Stress radiograph for inversion of the ankle. (A) Setup of the stress radiograph. (B) Resulting images.

Computed Tomography Scan

CT scan uses many of the same principles and technology as radiography but is used to determine and quantify the presence of a specific pathology rather than as a general screening tool. In the case of CT scans, the x-ray source and x-ray detectors rotate around the body (Fig. 5-4). Instead of the images being produced on film, a computer determines the density of the underlying tissues based on the absorption of x-rays by the body, allowing for more precision in viewing soft tissue. This information is then used to create a two-dimensional image, or slice, or a three-dimensional image of the body.[1] These slices can be obtained at varying positions and thicknesses, allowing physicians to study the area and its surrounding anatomical relationships (Fig. 5-5).

In traditional CT imaging, the x-ray source rotates 360 degrees around the body to obtain one slice. In spiral, or helical, CT, the x-ray source scans in a continuous arc around the body (Fig. 5-6). The speed and number of slices

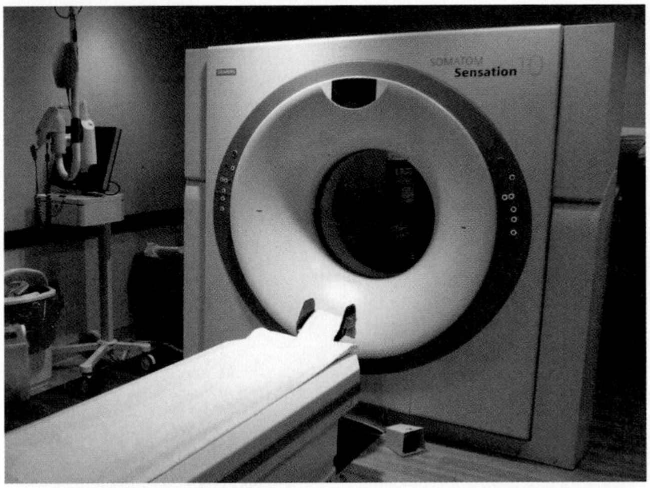

FIGURE 5-4 ■ CT scan device. Image courtesy of Shields MRI.

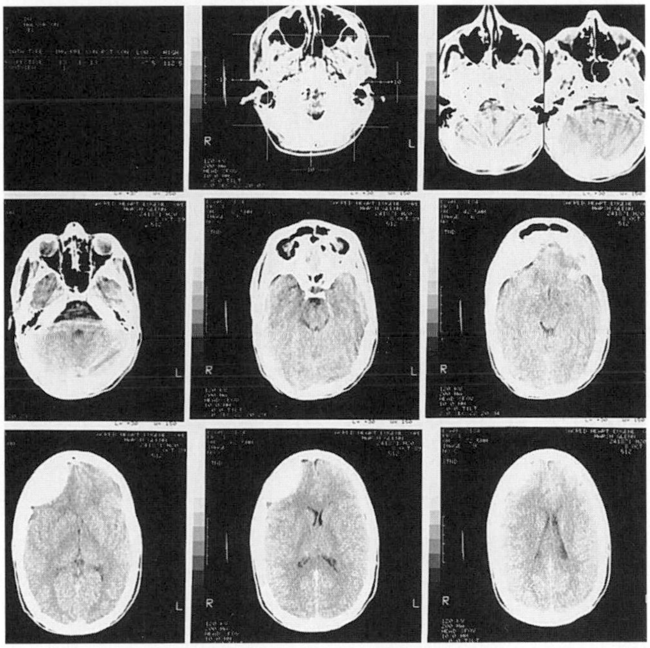

FIGURE 5-5 ■ CT scan of a cranium.

acquired depends on the number of detectors. Spiral CT has improved accuracy, requires less radiation exposure, and has a faster acquisition time than traditional CT.

Practical Evidence

Because of a small increased risk of future cancer secondary to radiation exposure, CT scans for children are used only when other forms of imaging are inadequate.[7]

Optimal visualization of certain tissues requires injection or swallowing of a contrast medium prior to the scan. CT angiography, which involves use of a contrast medium injected into a vein, is often used to visualize blood vessels. SPECT merges multiple two-dimensional images obtained from different angles and assembles them to form a three-dimensional image.

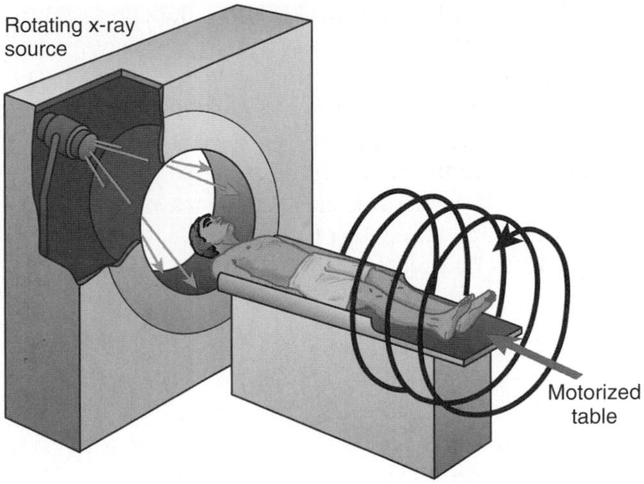

FIGURE 5-6 ■ Spiral (helical) CT scan. The patient table moves through the generator as the x-ray source rotates around the body, allowing the scan to be performed in a continuous arc.

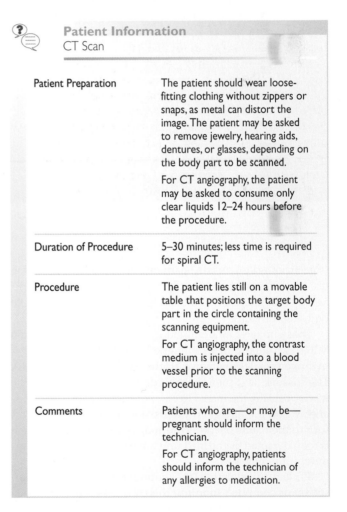

Patient Information
CT Scan

Patient Preparation	The patient should wear loose-fitting clothing without zippers or snaps, as metal can distort the image. The patient may be asked to remove jewelry, hearing aids, dentures, or glasses, depending on the body part to be scanned. For CT angiography, the patient may be asked to consume only clear liquids 12–24 hours before the procedure.
Duration of Procedure	5–30 minutes; less time is required for spiral CT.
Procedure	The patient lies still on a movable table that positions the target body part in the circle containing the scanning equipment. For CT angiography, the contrast medium is injected into a blood vessel prior to the scanning procedure.
Comments	Patients who are—or may be—pregnant should inform the technician. For CT angiography, patients should inform the technician of any allergies to medication.

Magnetic Resonance Imaging

MRI acquires a detailed picture of the body's soft tissues (Fig. 5-7). Similar to a CT scan, MRI is generally used to identify specific pathology or visualize a soft tissue structure

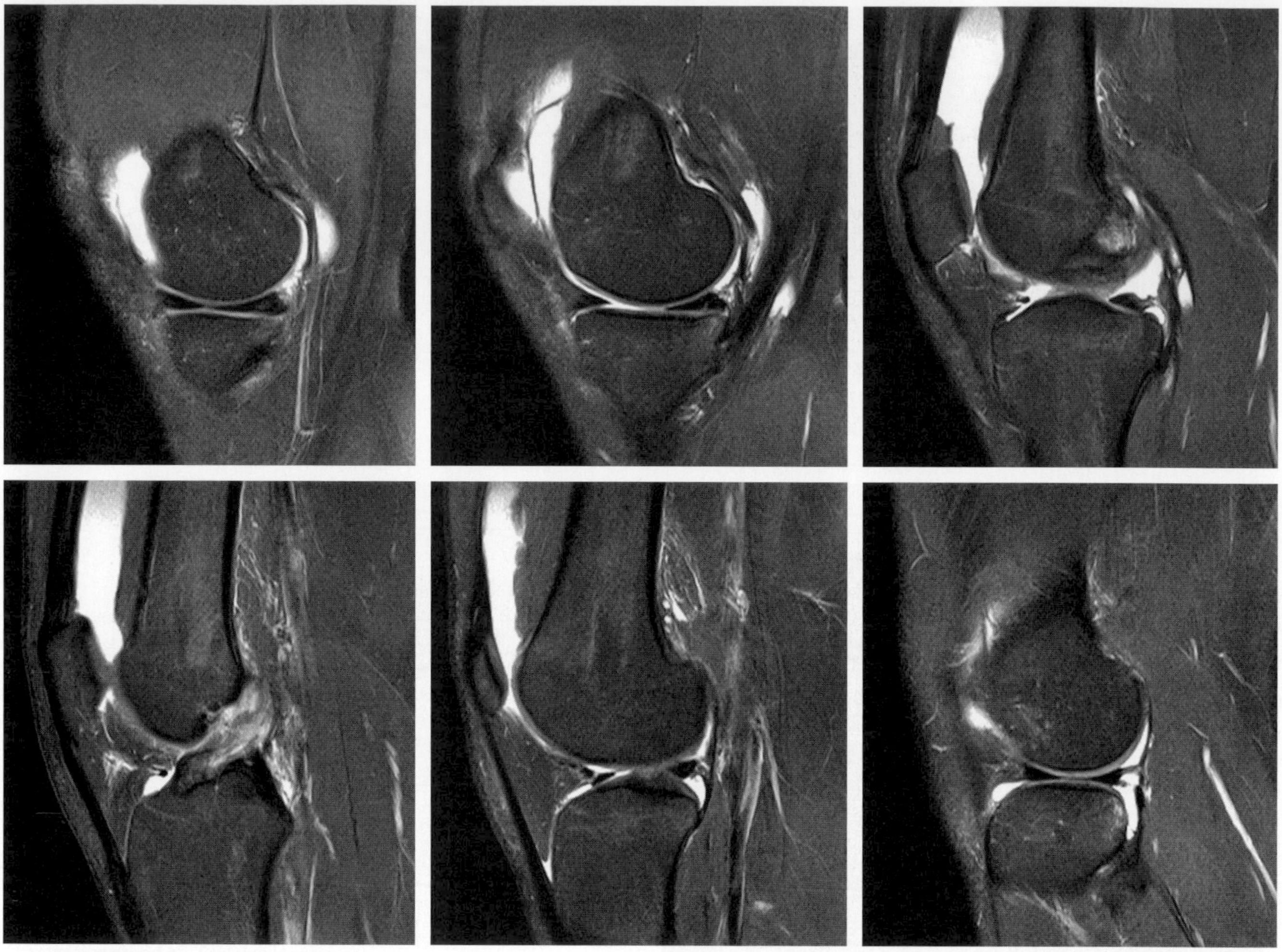

FIGURE 5-7 ■ MRI image showing sagittal slices through the knee with an ACL tear (lower left image) and meniscal lesion (lower middle image).

(e.g., an anterior cruciate ligament sprain) rather than being used as a general screening tool. Compared with other imaging techniques, MRI offers superior visualization of the body's soft tissues.

These images are obtained by placing the patient in an MRI tube that produces a magnetic field, causing the body's hydrogen nuclei to align with the magnetic axis (Fig. 5-8). The tissues are then bombarded with electromagnetic waves, causing the nuclei to resonate as they absorb the energy. When the energy to the tissues ceases, the nuclei return to their state of equilibrium by releasing energy, which is then detected by the MRI unit and transformed by a computer into images.[1]

Similar to adjusting the contrast on your television screen or computer monitor, the contrast of the MR image can be "weighted" to better identify specific types of tissues (Box 5-1). Contrast imaging media may be introduced into the tissues to delineate the structures further.

Unlike the ionizing radiation associated with radiographs and CT scans, the energy used during the MRI process produces no known potentially harmful effects. The only known limitations to the administration of this procedure lie with individuals who suffer from claustrophobia (who are fearful of entering the imaging tube) or those who have some types of implanted metal. MRI can often be safely used even if the patient has implanted metal such as surgical staples, pins, plates, and screws, as long as it has been in place for longer than 4 to 6 weeks. The open MRI eliminates or reduces

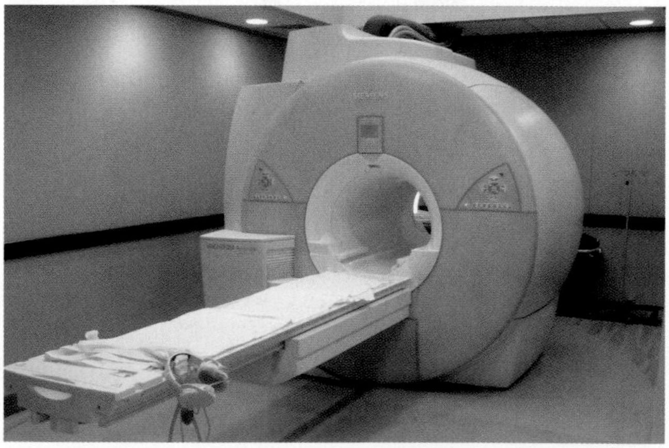

FIGURE 5-8 ■ MRI unit. Courtesy of Shields MRI.

Box 5-1

Relative Signal Intensities of Selected Structures in Musculoskeletal Magnetic Resonance Imaging

	Sequence		
Structure	T1-Weighted	Proton Density	T2-Weighted
	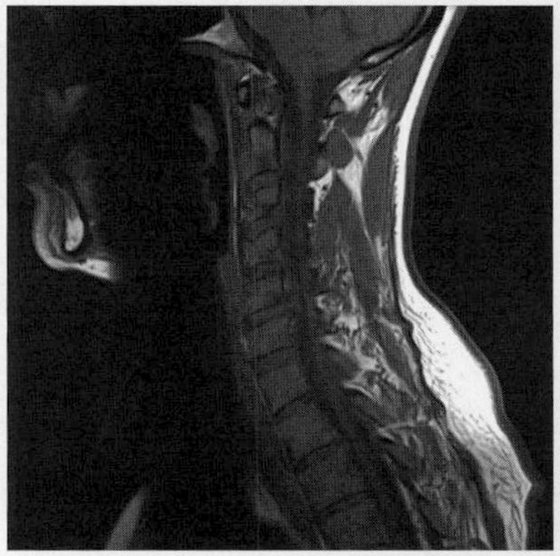	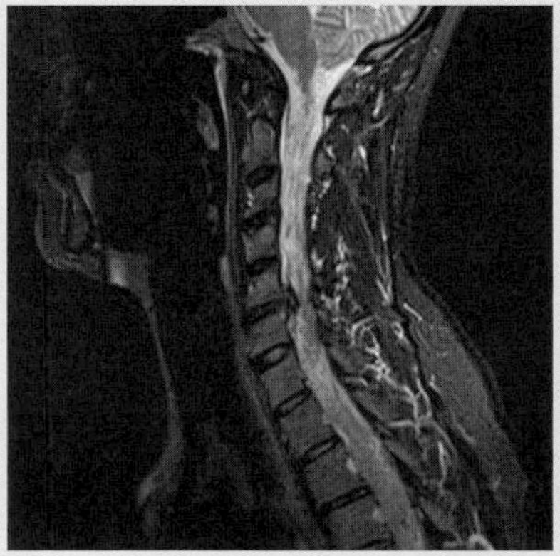	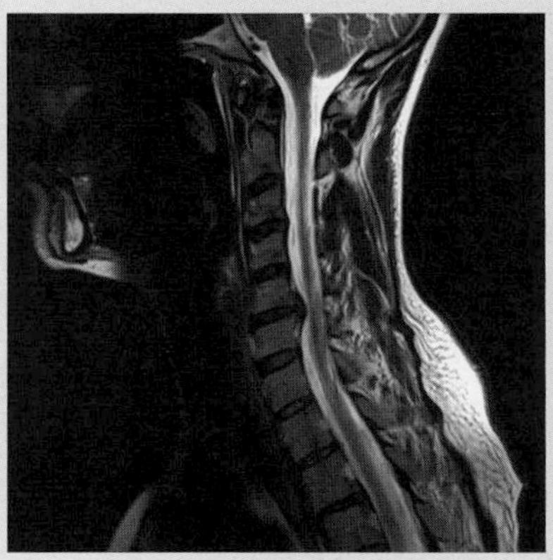
Fat[a]	Bright	Bright	Intermediate
Fluid[b]	Dark	Intermediate	Bright
Fibrocartilage[c]	Dark	Dark	Dark
Ligaments, Tendon[d]	Dark	Dark	Dark
Muscle	Intermediate	Intermediate	Dark
Bone Marrow	Bright	Intermediate	Dark
Nerve	Intermediate	Intermediate	Intermediate

[a] Includes bone marrow.
[b] Includes edema, most tears, and most cysts.
[c] Includes labrum, menisci, triangular fibrocartilage.
[d] Signal may be increased because of artifacts.

Patient Information
MRI

Patient Preparation	The patient should wear loose-fitting, comfortable clothes without zippers or snaps. The facility may provide hospital scrubs or a gown. Remove all jewelry and glasses, including any body piercings, before the procedure.
Duration of Procedure	15–45 minutes
Procedure	Patients lie on a sliding table for positioning inside the MRI tube. Patients are asked to remain still inside the tube while the images are being taken. The MR generator produces loud, clanging noises. Many imaging centers provide earplugs or headphones for music and to allow the MR technologist to communicate with the patient during the procedure.
Comments	Patients who are claustrophobic may have increased anxiety within the enclosed tube of the MRI. A mild sedative can be administered, or, if available, an open MRI can be used. Patients who have pacemakers, implanted metal (such as pins, plates, screws), or the possibility of pregnancy should inform the technician. While tooth fillings and braces are not a contraindication, their presence should be noted for accurate tuning of the MRI. Some tattoos and permanent eyeliner contain metal. If contrast medium is needed, it will be administered during the procedure. The patient should alert the technician to any medication allergies.

claustrophobia by minimizing the immersion in the imaging tube and reducing the level of magnetism required to produce images.

Functional MRIs (fMRIs) are used to detect metabolic changes in the brain. fMRIs are useful in tracking changes in brain activity following stroke, traumatic brain injury, or tumor.

Magnetic resonance angiography (MRA) uses MRI to study blood vessels, and its relative lack of invasiveness makes it preferable to a catheter study. Contrast material is sometimes injected into the bloodstream to better visualize the vessels (Fig. 5-9).

MRI images are referenced from the frontal, sagittal, and transverse planes. They are read using a legend that numbers the slices as they progress through the body part. Each image can be referenced back to the legend image to determine

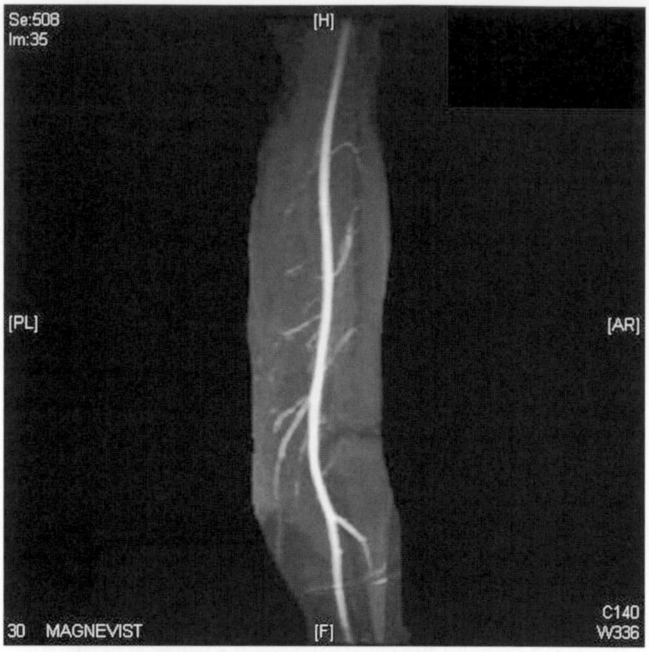

FIGURE 5-9 ■ Magnetic resonance angiography.

where the slice is located. Sprains or other connective tissue damage involving loss of tissue continuity, fluid accumulation, or nerve entrapment are common pathologies that can be discovered via MRI (Fig. 5-10).

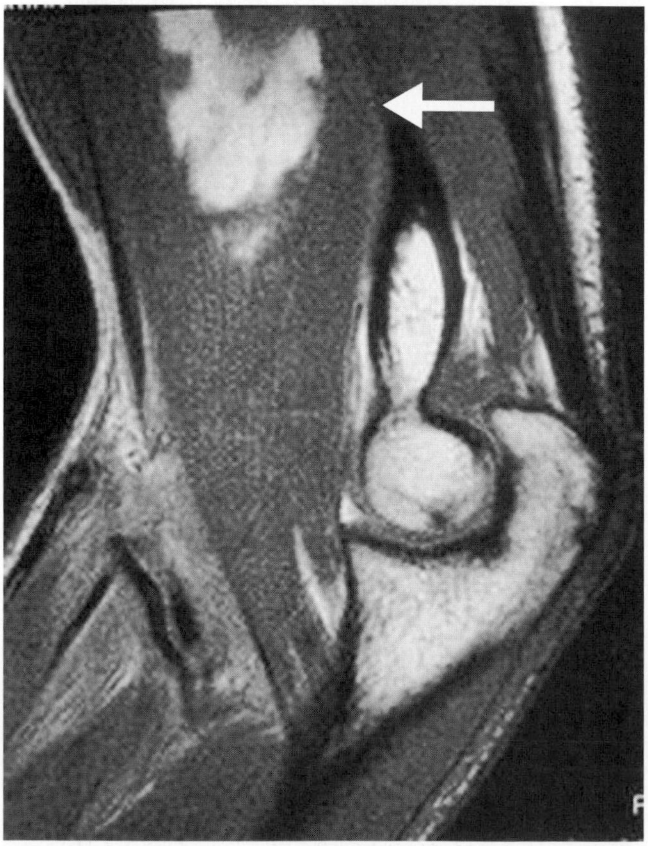

FIGURE 5-10 ■ MRI of a soft tissue injury. The arrow is indicating a hematoma in the right brachialis muscle (medial view).

Bone Scan

Bone scans are a form of nuclear medicine used to detect bony abnormalities that are not normally visible on a standard radiograph. The patient receives an injection of a **radionuclide**, technetium-99m (Tc-99m), a **tracer element** that is absorbed by areas of bone undergoing excessive remodeling, or hotspots. These areas appear as darkened spots on the image and must be correlated with clinical signs and symptoms (Fig. 5-11). Bone scans can identify common pathologies, including degenerative disease, bone tumors, and stress fractures of the long bones and the vertebrae.[8]

Patient Information
Bone Scan

Patient Preparation	The patient should wear comfortable clothing.
Duration of Procedure	This depends on the type of scan and the time it takes for radioactive tracer to reach the target tissue. The imaging procedure itself takes 20–45 minutes.
Procedure	The radioactive agent is delivered into a vein. After waiting the prescribed period, the patient is asked to lie still on a table while the detector obtains and records the data.
Comments	Patients who are—or may be—pregnant should inform the technician. Patients should inform the technician of any allergies to medications.

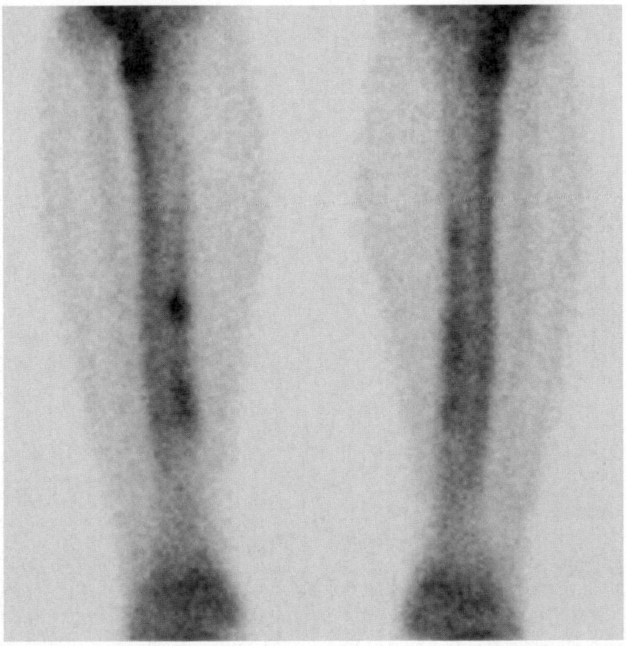

FIGURE 5-11 ■ Bone scan of the lower extremity. The darkened areas indicate "hot spots" of high uptake of the tracer element. Image courtesy of Akira Murakami, MD. Boston Medical Center.

Diagnostic Ultrasound

Defects in soft tissue structures, primarily superficial muscle, the Achilles tendon, patellar tendon, and the rotator cuff tendons, can be identified using diagnostic ultrasound (sonograms). Some internal organs, the testes, breasts, and a fetus can also be viewed using sonograms. Diagnostic ultrasound uses sound waves having a frequency between 1 and 15 **megahertz** (MHz) depending on the depth and type of tissues being imaged.

The frequency of the ultrasonic energy used is inversely proportional to the depth of the target tissue. Superficial structures such as muscle and tendon require energy with a higher frequency, normally in the range of 7 to 15 MHz. Imaging of deep internal organs requires energy with a lower frequency.

A piezoelectric transducer delivers a brief pulse of ultrasonic energy into the tissues, then "listens" for a return echo. A computer interprets the strength of the returning sound wave and converts this information to display the type and depth of each structure (Fig. 5-12). The resulting image presents the tissues in cross section. Advanced units can generate color and three-dimensional images of the tissues and also assess for blood flow.

Sonograms are relatively inexpensive, easy to obtain, and risk-free to the patient, but the quality of the resulting image is significantly influenced by the skill of the operator. Accessibility and portability of the imaging devices is also an advantage. In some cases, the quality of images obtained from obese patients may be degraded as the result of scattering of the ultrasonic energy as it passes through dense

Patient Information
Diagnostic Ultrasound

Patient Preparation	The body part to be examined must be exposed. The patient should wear clothing that is easy to remove and put on.
Duration of Procedure	15–45 minutes
Procedure	The patient lies on a table. Gel, a coupling medium, is applied to the skin over the target, and the technician runs the transducer head over the target area, capturing specific images on the computer.
Comments	Diagnostic ultrasound should not be confused with therapeutic ultrasound.

Radionuclide An atom undergoing disintegration, emitting electromagnetic radiation

Tracer element A substance that is introduced into the tissues to follow or trace an otherwise unidentifiable substance or event

Megahertz One million cycles per second

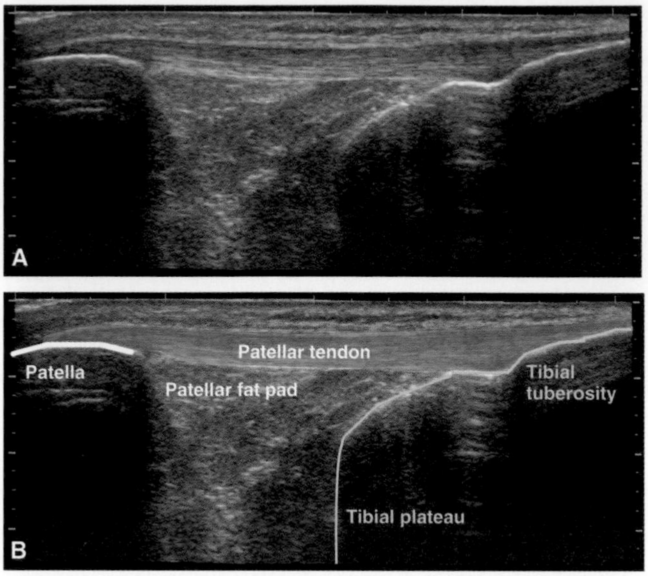

FIGURE 5-12 ■ Ultrasonic image of the patellar tendon. (A) Raw view. (B) View identifying specific structures.

pockets of adipose tissue. An equal level of skill is required to interpret the resulting image.

Nerve Conduction Study/Electromyography

Nerve conduction studies (NCS) and electromyography (EMG) are diagnostic techniques used to detect pathology in peripheral nerves and the muscles they innervate. The techniques are performed by a trained health practitioner, often a neurologist or **physiatrist**. Peripheral nerve entrapments (such as carpal tunnel syndrome and tarsal tunnel syndrome), neurotmesis, nerve root injury, or muscle diseases such as **muscular dystrophy** and **myasthenia gravis** can be detected via NCS/EMG.

A motor NCS is used to examine motor peripheral nerve function and detect pathology along its path. In this procedure, the peripheral nerve is stimulated with an electrical current, and activity from a muscle innervated by the nerve is identified and recorded. Two primary measurements are obtained: (1) **latency**, the time it takes for the impulse to travel to the target muscle and (2) **amplitude**, the magnitude of the nerve's response (Fig. 5-13). Comparing the amplitude of the muscle's electrical activity with the initial current strength provides a measure of the nerve's health. By stimulating different points along a peripheral nerve, NCS can detect the location of entrapments and isolate the location of specific pathology. An NCS is usually conducted in conjunction with an EMG study.

An EMG study is an invasive procedure that involves inserting a thin detecting needle electrode into the muscle. The initial electrical activity with insertion of the electrode, which follows a characteristic pattern in a healthy muscle, is noted. The electrical activity of the resting muscle is then assessed. In normal muscle, the muscle should be electrically inactive. Spontaneous activity, or depolarizations, at rest could be indicative of muscle pathology. Finally, the patient is then asked to contract the muscle. The shape, size, and frequency of motor unit action potentials are noted.

Physiatrist A physician who specializes in physical medicine and rehabilitation

Muscular dystrophy An inherited disease of the muscles causing progressive atrophy and weakness

Myasthenia gravis A disease caused by a malfunction of the body's immune system, interrupting communication with motor nerves and causing weakness and fatigue

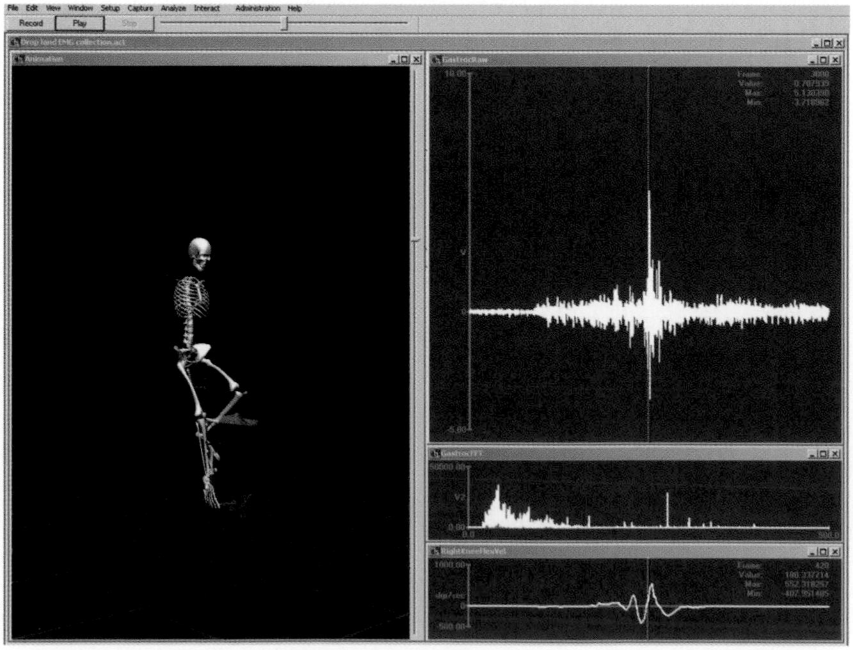

FIGURE 5-13 ■ EMG of a muscle contraction with 3D representation of movement.

Patient Information

Nerve Conduction Study/Electromyography

Patient Preparation	The body part to be examined will need to be exposed. The patient should wear clothing that is easy to remove and put on.
Duration of Procedure	30 minutes to 2 hours, depending on the extent of the examination
Procedure	**NCS:** The patient lies on a table. Electrodes are placed on the skin at various points along the course of the peripheral nerve. An electrical current is applied, which may be perceived as a small shock. **EMG:** Small, thin needle electrodes are placed in the target muscle. The patient is first asked to relax the muscle and then to contract it. The procedure is repeated in each muscle of interest.
Comments	Patients who are taking anticoagulant medications such as warfarin should inform the person conducting the test. Some patients complain of muscle soreness after the EMG procedure.

REFERENCES

1. D'Orsi, CJ: Radiology and magnetic resonance imaging. In Greene, HL, Glassock, RJ, and Kelley, MA: *Introduction to Clinical Medicine*. Philadelphia, PA: BC Decker, 1991, p 91.
2. Chakravarty, D, Sloan, J, and Brenchley, J: Risk reduction through skeletal scintigraphy as a screening tool in suspected scaphoid fracture: a literature review. *Emerg Med J*, 19:507, 2002.
3. Chakravarty, D, Sloan, J, and Brenchley, J: Risk reduction through skeletal scintigraphy as a screening tool in suspected scaphoid fracture: a literature review. *Emerg Med J*, 19:507, 2002.
4. Gaeta, M, et al: CT and MR imaging findings in athletes with early tibial stress injuries: comparison with bone scintigraphy findings and emphasis on cortical abnormalities. *Radiology*, 235:553, 2005.
5. Schuerger, SR: Introduction to critical review of roentgengrams. *Phys Ther*, 68:1114, 1988.
6. Schopp, JG, et al: Allergic reactions to iodinated contrast media: premedication considerations for patients at risk. *Emerg Radiol*, 2013. [Epub ahead of print].
7. Pearce, MS, et al: Radiation exposure from CT scans in childhood and subsequent risk of leukaemia and brain tumours: a retrospective cohort study. *Lancet*, 380:499, 2012.
8. Patton, DO, and Doherty, PN: Nuclear medicine studies. In Greene, HL, Glassock, RJ, and Kelley, MA: *Introduction to Clinical Medicine*. Philadelphia, PA: BC Decker, 1991, p 81.

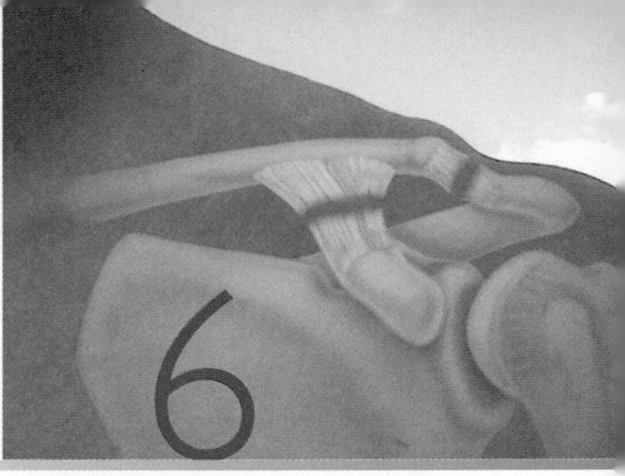

CHAPTER 6

Assessment of Posture

The term *posture* is used to describe the position of the body at a given point in time. Ideal posture is characterized by specific landmarks being aligned with the force of gravity, minimizing energy expenditure and maximizing function.[1] Proper posture requires the least amount of muscular effort, resulting in reduced stress on the joints and surrounding structures. Faulty posture produces an increased amount of muscular activity and places increased stress on the joints and surrounding soft tissues, resulting in impairments.[2] Conversely, impairments can result in faulty posture. Clinically, it is difficult to determine if the faulty posture is the result of muscle imbalances, caused by overuse of certain muscles during the **activities of daily living** (ADLs), or if these imbalances are the result of faulty posture. Poor posture in and of itself usually does not prompt people to seek medical attention.

Postural assessment is used to identify postural deviations that may be contributing to the patient's pain or abnormal movement patterns. The postural examination begins with the patient in a standing or sitting position but can progress to include the dynamic postures of walking and running (see Chapter 7).[3] Static positions assessed in a health-care facility may not replicate the postures that the patient normally assumes during athletic, school, home, or work activities.

This chapter describes the relationship between common postural deviations and the resulting clinical examination findings. The cause-and-effect relationship between faulty posture, common compensatory motions, and associated musculoskeletal dysfunctions is also discussed.

Clinical Anatomy

Before understanding how deviations in one region of the body affect another region, a review of basic anatomical and biomechanical concepts is needed. The musculoskeletal system is designed to function in a mechanically and physiologically efficient manner to use the least possible amount of energy. The change in position of one joint results in a predictable change in position of the other interrelated joints.[4] When a postural deviation or skeletal malalignment occurs, other joints in the kinetic chain undergo compensatory motions or postures to allow the body to continue to function as efficiently as possible. For example, a forward shoulder posture can result from tightness of the pectoralis minor. This, in turn, changes the functional positions of the scapula and may predispose the patient to chronic shoulder pain.[5]

The Kinetic Chain

The musculoskeletal system is a series of kinetic chains in which different joints are directly or indirectly linked to each other (Fig. 6-1). In a kinetic chain, movement occurring at one joint causes motion at an adjacent joint, creating a "chain reaction" of movements up or down the associated kinetic chain. Kinetic chains are classified as **open chain** (non–weight-bearing) or **closed chain** (weight-bearing). Because the definitions of open and closed kinetic chain motions become blurred, the terms "weight-bearing" and "non–weight-bearing" are often used instead. The lower extremity-pelvis-lumbar complex functions primarily in a closed kinetic chain; the upper extremity, scapulothoracic, and cervical spine function primarily in an open kinetic chain.[6]

A closed kinetic chain is formed when the distal segment meets sufficient resistance or is fixated, such as the weight-bearing limb during walking or the upper extremity during push-ups or weight lifting. Because of the interdependency of each joint within a closed chain, the associated joints undergo predictable changes in position in response to a change in position of another joint along the chain. This can be demonstrated by standing up and

---

Activities of daily living (ADLs) The skills and motions required for the day-to-day activities of life

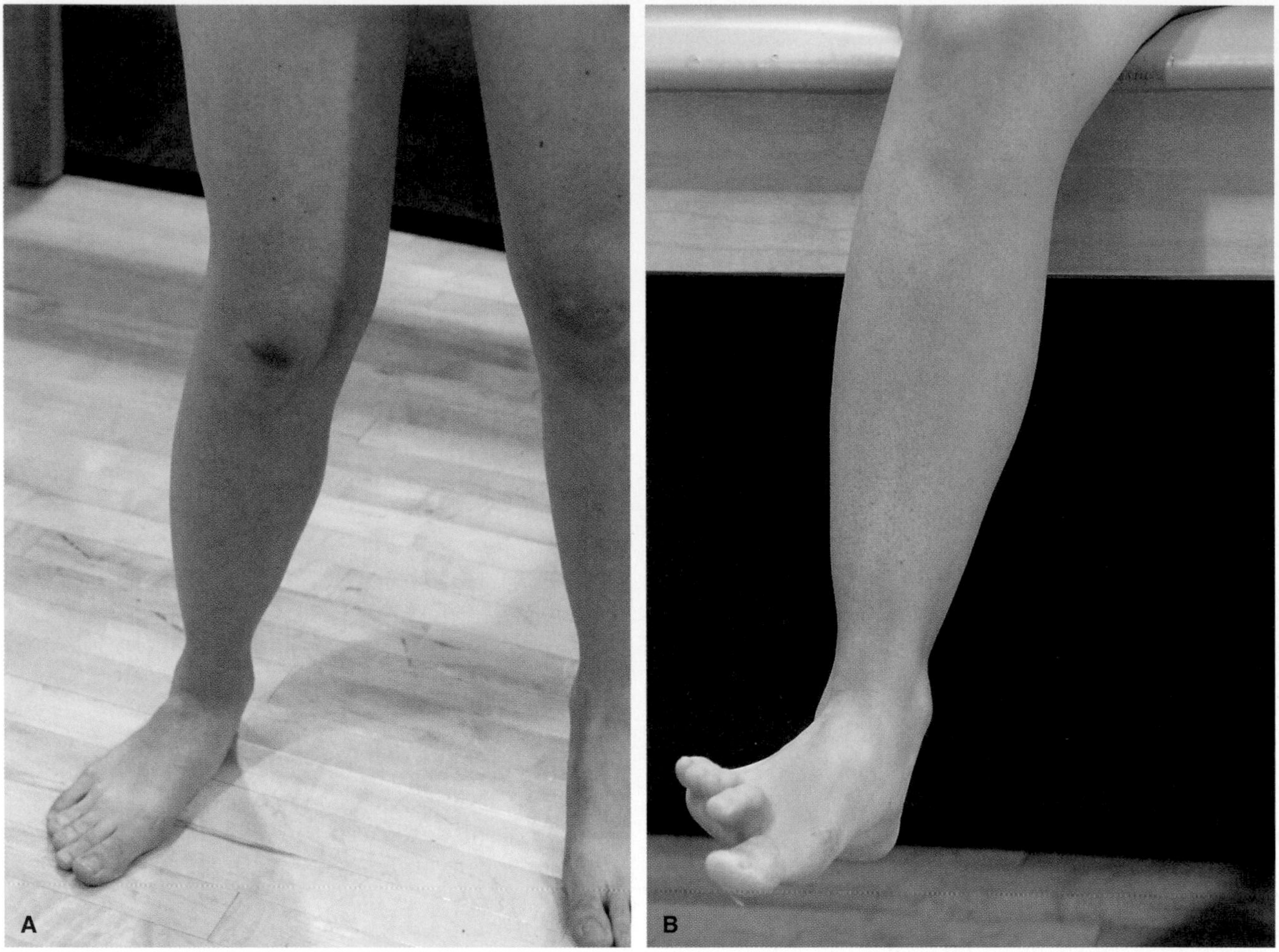

FIGURE 6-1 ■ (A) Weight-bearing and (B) Non–weight-bearing examples of kinetic chains in the musculoskeletal system.

"rolling" the foot inward. When maximum pronation is reached, the ankle naturally dorsiflexes, the tibia internally rotates, the knee flexes, and the hip internally rotates and flexes (see Fig. 6-1A). In an open kinetic chain, the distal portion of the chain (the distal extremity) moves freely in space. When the inward rolling of the foot used in the closed kinetic chain is repeated with the foot non–weight-bearing, only the foot pronates, and motion does not occur at the joints proximal to the foot and ankle (see Fig. 6-1B).

Kinetic chains are the underlying principle in determining the cause of postural deviations. Soft tissue dysfunction or bony anomaly occurring in one part of the kinetic chain can affect the proximal or distal joints and soft tissues along the chain, causing a specific postural deviation (Table 6-1).[7] The body attempts to compensate for these deviations to maintain efficient movement. An example of this compensatory strategy involves a structural condition of the foot called **forefoot varus**. If the body were unable to compensate for the abnormal position of the forefoot, a person would walk on the outside of the foot, not a very functional or efficient motion. To maximize propulsion and reduce the effect on gait, the foot compensates for forefoot varus by excessively pronating at the subtalar joint (STJ) and midtarsal joints to reach a foot-flat position (Fig. 6-2).

Table 6-1 Examples of Compensatory Strategies of the Body

Skeletal Malalignment	Subtalar Joint	Tibiofemoral Joint	Hip Joint	Pelvis and Lumbar Spine
Forefoot or Rearfoot Varus	Excessive and/or prolonged pronation	Flexion Internal tibial rotation	Flexion Internal femoral rotation	Anterior rotation and excessive lumbar extension
Forefoot Valgus	Early supination	Extension External tibial rotation	Extension External femoral rotation	Posterior rotation and excessive flexion

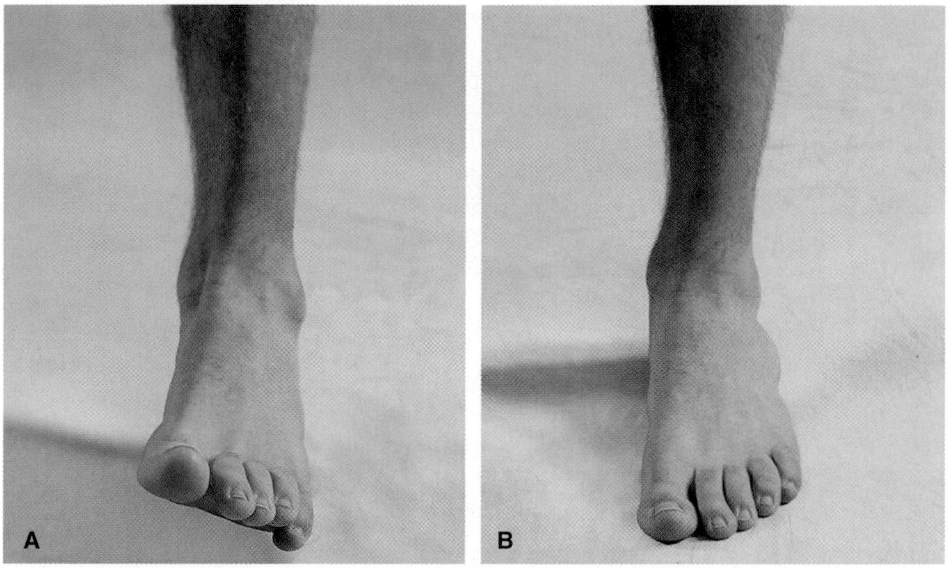

FIGURE 6-2 ■ (A) Uncompensated (STJ neutral) and (B) Compensated forefoot varus.

Adhesive capsulitis is another example of a soft tissue pathology that can alter the kinetic chain. In adhesive capsulitis, the **arthrokinematic** motions of the glenohumeral (GH) joint are decreased, prohibiting normal humeral elevation. Because the scapulothoracic articulation is included in the upper extremity kinetic chain, it compensates for the hypomobility of the GH joint by allowing excessive upward scapular rotation to permit functional humeral elevation (Fig. 6-3). When compensatory movement patterns or postures occur over a prolonged period, they become "learned," and the body interprets them as being correct.[8]

Arthrokinematic Action and reaction of articular surfaces as a joint travels through its range of motion

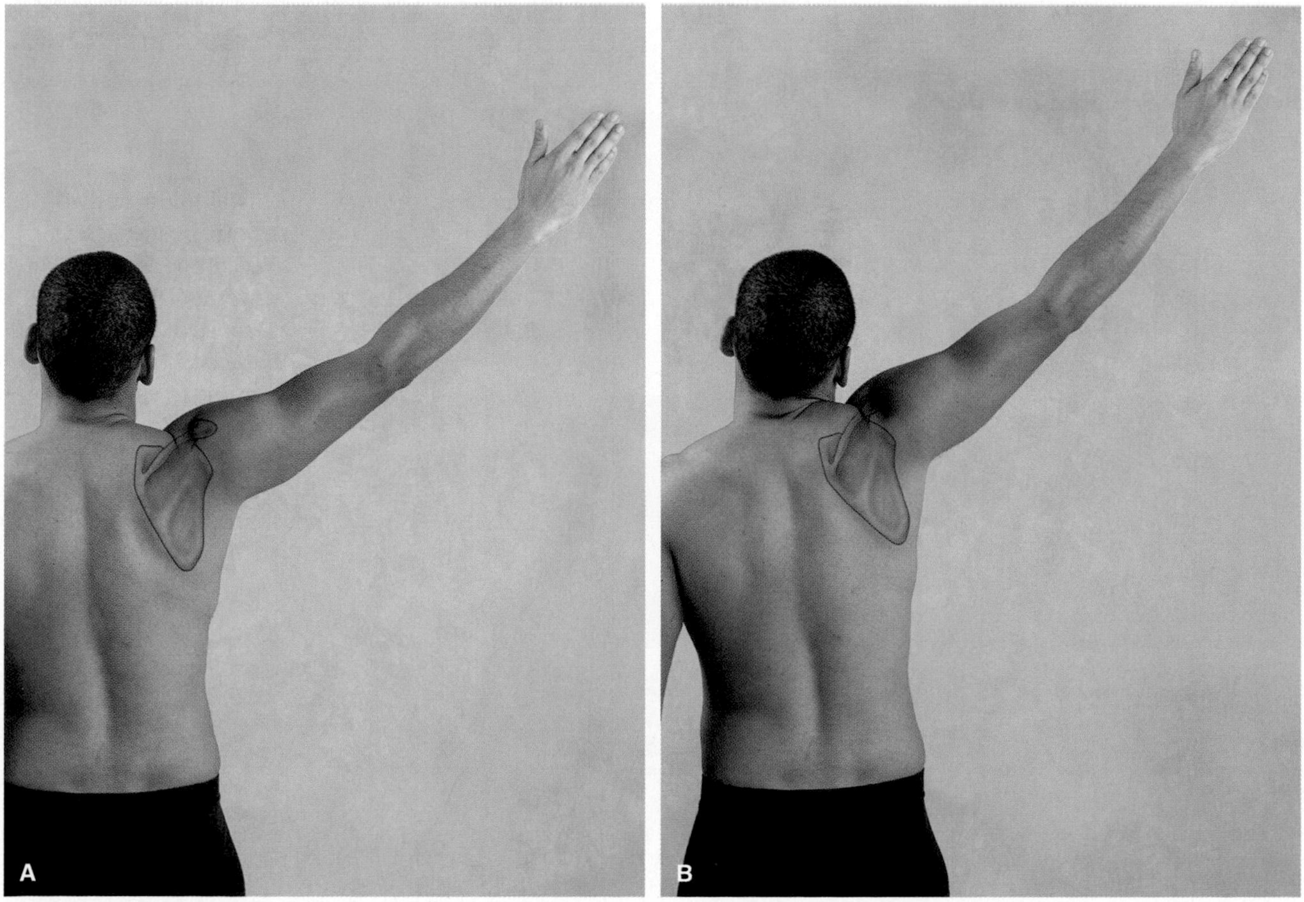

FIGURE 6-3 ■ (A) Normal scapulohumeral elevation. (B) Scapulohumeral elevation compensated with increased upper trapezius activity.

Not all compensatory postures are detrimental. Some allow the body to function more efficiently, with less discomfort, or both. Such is the case for someone with **stenosis** in the lumbar spine. The individual assumes a flexed posture in the lumbar spine (decreased lumbar **lordosis**) to increase the otherwise narrowed space in the vertebral canal caused by stenosis. All the findings obtained during a postural evaluation must be interpreted before attempting to correct a compensatory postural deviation.

Muscular Function

Muscle contractions produce joint motion and provide dynamic **joint stability**. To perform these tasks properly, the muscles must have an optimal length–tension relationship. Muscles that are functionally too short or too long can produce adverse stress on the joints, work inefficiently, or create the need for compensatory motions during activity (Table 6-2). Different abnormal postures provide clues as to which muscles might be problematically shortened or lengthened. For example, increased lordosis is commonly associated with lengthened abdominal muscles. A passive insufficiency is created, making the abdominals less capable of working effectively.

Muscular Length–Tension Relationships

The **muscular length–tension relationship** describes the effect of muscle length and the amount of tension (force) produced. The tension-developing capacity of a muscle occurs within the **sarcomere** unit at the cross-bridges formed between **actin** and **myosin** myofilaments. The optimal relationship between length and tension is the **resting position**, the joint position where the muscle can generate the greatest amount of tension with the least amount of effort. At this length, the cross-bridges between actin and myosin filaments within the sarcomere are at their most efficient position.

If a muscle is shortened or lengthened, the interaction of the cross-bridges between actin and myosin filaments is reduced because there is either too much or too little overlap, resulting in a decreased ability to produce force (Fig. 6-4). **Active insufficiency** occurs when a muscle is shortened and the actin and myosin myofilaments overlap to the point where maximum tension cannot be produced. Changes in leverage and passive restraint from the antagonists also contribute to active insufficiency.[9] **Passive insufficiency** occurs when the length limits of a musculotendinous unit are reached and further movement results in passive joint movement or a restriction of joint movement. Passive insufficiency usually occurs in muscles that cross multiple joints. For example, when the fingers are actively flexed, the long finger extensors are stretched to the limit and wrist flexion is restricted. If the hip is flexed, the hamstrings may limit knee extension.[9]

Agonist and Antagonist Relationships

A muscle that contracts to perform the primary movement of a joint is termed the **agonist muscle**. The **antagonist**

Table 6-2 Muscle Length and the Ability to Function

Muscle Length	Ability to Provide Mobility	Ability to Provide Stability
Normal	Efficient	Efficient
Shortened	Inefficient	Efficient
Elongated	Efficient	Inefficient

Stenosis (spinal) A narrowing of the vertebral foramen through which the spinal cord or spinal nerve root pass

Lordosis Anterior curvature of the spine

Joint stability The integrity of a joint when it is placed under a functional load

Sarcomere A portion of striated muscle fiber lying between two membranes

Actin A contractile muscle protein

Myosin A contractile muscle protein

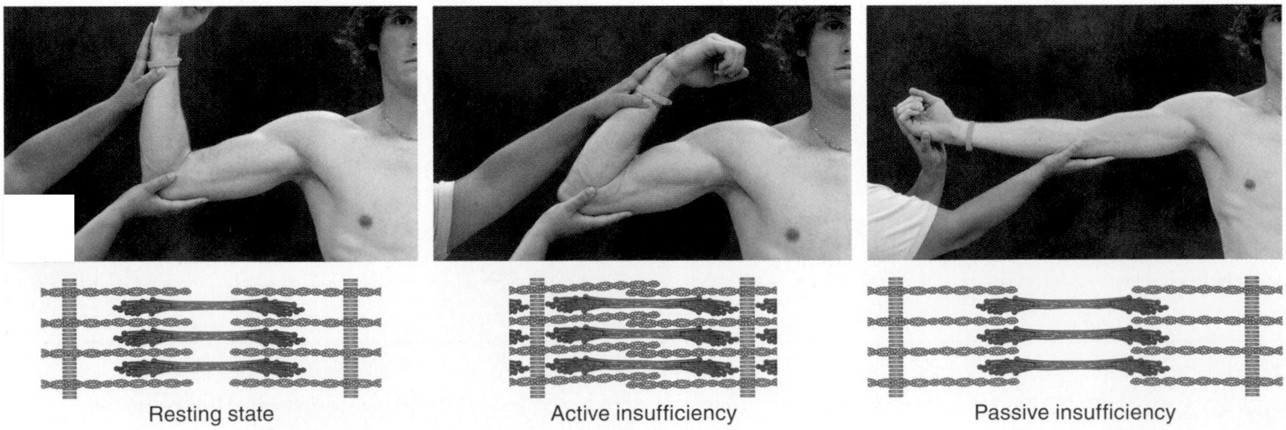

FIGURE 6-4 ■ Relationship of actin and myosin cross bridges. When the muscle is in its resting state, there is full communication between the actin and myosin, allowing for a strong contraction. Active insufficiency is created when the muscle has maximally shortened to its fullest point and the filaments can no longer slide. When the muscle is fully elongated, passive insufficiency, there is decreased communication between the actin and myosin, decreasing the strength the muscle can generate.

muscle performs the opposite movement of the agonist muscle and must reflexively relax to allow the agonist's motion to occur. This reflexive response is termed **reciprocal inhibition**. The biceps brachii and triceps brachii muscles are examples of agonist and antagonist muscles. During elbow flexion, the biceps brachii is the agonist performing the action of elbow flexion. The antagonist is the triceps brachii because it performs the opposite motion of elbow extension. The triceps brachii must reflexively relax and elongate while the biceps brachii contracts to allow normal, smooth elbow flexion. If an antagonist muscle did not receive an inhibitory impulse to relax, but instead received an excitatory stimulus of the same magnitude as the agonist, the joint would not move because both sets of muscles would be equally contracting. This concurrent contraction of the agonist and antagonist muscles, **co-contraction**, is a key feature of dynamic joint stability. The smooth, deliberate movements of the body during normal ADLs are allowed to occur because of this excitatory/inhibitory reflex loop between the agonist and antagonist muscle groups.

Muscle Imbalances

Length–tension relationships and agonist versus antagonist muscles allow us to better understand the implications of muscle imbalance. Muscle imbalances occur due to muscle weakness or spasm, asymmetrical strength relationships, changed muscle length–tension relationships, or aberrant nerve input. Table 6-3 lists some of the common causes of muscle imbalances.

Different muscle types exhibit different patterns of activity. Skeletal muscles are classified as either postural (also referred to as tonic) or phasic (Table 6-4). Postural muscles primarily function to support the body against the forces of gravity. They are composed of a higher percentage of slow-twitch muscle fibers, are slower to fatigue, and do not respond as quickly when activated.[9] Postural muscles have a greater tendency to become overactivated and shortened in response to stresses or pain (Fig. 6-5). **Trigger points** are hypersensitive contraction knots that are painful to pressure and common sources of pain in postural muscles.[10]

Phasic muscles are primarily responsible for movement of the body. With a higher proportion of fast-twitch muscle fibers than postural muscles, phasic muscles contract more quickly and generate a greater amount of force. Phasic muscles tend to rapidly fatigue because of the higher percentage of fast-twitch fibers. Muscle tears and tendinopathies are common soft tissue dysfunctions seen in phasic muscles.

When a muscle becomes overactivated and shortened and its antagonist is weakened, the muscular balance around the joint changes. The overactivated muscle influences the manner in which the underlying joint (or joints) move and alter the compressive or tensile forced placed on the joint. Muscle imbalances expend more energy and create inefficient and stressful movement patterns and postures for the body.[6,10]

When an impairment resulting from a muscle imbalance is problematic, the intervention must first restore normal joint kinematics by emphasizing elongation of the shortened, overactivated muscle group before strengthening the inhibited and weakened group.

Table 6-3 Causes of Muscle Imbalances

Cause	Result
Nerve Pathology	Paralysis, muscle weakness, or muscle spindle inhibition
Pain	Inhibition or muscle spasm
Joint Effusion	Reflexive inhibition of muscle
Poor Posture	Alteration in muscle length–tension relationship
Repetitive Activity of One Muscle Group	Adaptive shortening and increased recruitment

Noncontractile Soft Tissue Influences

Faulty posture and associated muscle imbalances can alter the joint position, causing increased stress on different portions of the joint capsule and surrounding ligaments. While areas of a joint capsule that are continually stressed may adapt by elongating, areas that are slack and not stressed (usually on the opposite side of the tensile forces) may undergo adaptive shortening. The shoulder provides an example of a common noncontractile soft tissue imbalance. A person who has acquired pronounced rounded, forward shoulders can experience adaptive shortening of the posterior portion of the GH capsule and

Trigger point A pathological condition characterized by a small, hypersensitive area located within muscles and fasciae

Table 6-4 Postural versus Phasic Muscles

Characteristic	Postural Muscles	Phasic Muscles
Function	Support body against forces of gravity	Movement of the body
Muscle Fiber Type	Higher percentage of slow-twitch fibers	Higher percentage of fast-twitch fibers
Response to Dysfunction	Become overactivated and tightened or shortened	Become inhibited and weakened
Common Soft Tissue Dysfunction	Prone to trigger points	Prone to tears and tendinopathies

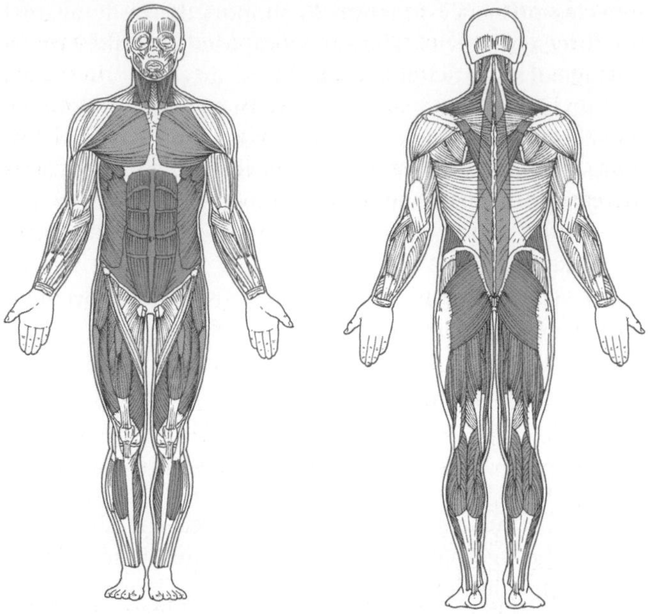

FIGURE 6-5 ■ Postural and phasic muscles. Blue = postural; Green = phasic.

Common Postural Muscles	Common Phasic Muscles
Sternocleidomastoid	Scalenes
Pectoralis major	Subscapularis
Upper trapezius	Lower trapezius
Levator scapula	Rhomboids
Quadratus lumborum	Serratus anterior
Iliopsoas	Rectus abdominis
Tensor fascia latae	Internal obliques
Rectus femoris	External obliques
Piriformis	Gluteus minimus
Hamstring group	Gluteus maximus
Short hip adductors	Gluteus medius
Gastrocnemius	Vastus medialis
Erector spinae	Vastus lateralis
Soleus	Tibialis anterior
Longissimus thoracic	Peroneals
Multifidus or rotatores	
Tibialis posterior	

elongation of the anterior portion of the GH capsule. To compensate for forward shoulder posture, the humeral head externally rotates to allow the hands to assume a more functional posture. This reduces normal stresses on the posterior capsule, which, in turn, adaptively shortens. This position is further exaggerated as the anterior chest muscles adaptively shorten to maintain the posture while the posterior muscles—the middle and lower trapezius and serratus anterior—elongate and become inefficient in maintaining dynamic stability of the scapula.

Clinical Examination of Posture

Posture plays both direct and indirect roles in the onset of overuse injuries. Overuse injuries are characterized by pain with an insidious onset, often brought on by repetitive tasks performed in specific postures.[10] When evaluating a musculoskeletal injury, general observation of posture must occur early in the examination process.

The clinical examination of posture is not an exact science. Although the use of radiographs, photographs, and computer analyses are the gold standards for determining skeletal postural deviations, clinical tools such as **plumb lines**, goniometers, flexible rulers, and inclinometers are more readily available and have demonstrated reliability (Fig. 6-6).[11] Whenever possible, use measurements to further quantify the malalignments causing postural deviations. Objective, quantifiable measurements can also assist in determining whether the current treatment plan is effective and the patient's posture is improving.

The use of inspection and palpation in the assessment of posture varies from that during the examination of specific body areas. Although inspection and palpation are described as separate entities in this chapter, in practice these two segments occur simultaneously, each validating or refuting the findings of the other. As posture is being observed, the clinician simultaneously palpates to determine specific positions of joints and structures.

Posture is commonly assessed in two positions: standing and sitting. In addition, assessment of posture in other static or dynamic positions that produce the patient's symptoms should also be performed, including postures assumed by the patient for prolonged periods during the day or during normal ADLs. In standing, ask the patient to assume a natural posture.

History

A thorough history assists in determining whether postural dysfunction is contributing to the patient's pathology and symptoms (Table 6-5). Repetitive tasks while maintaining a certain posture can lead to overuse injuries as well, so the

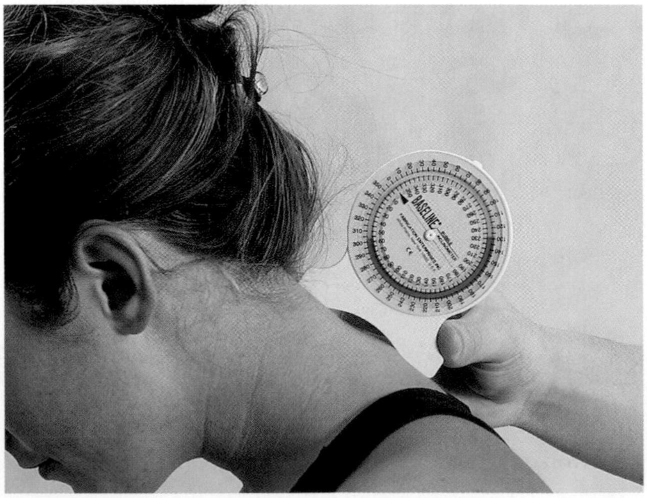

FIGURE 6-6 ■ An inclinometer can be used to the measure range of motion.

Plumb line A string and pendulum that hangs perpendicular to a surface

Table 6-5 Factors Influencing Posture

Factor	Example
Neurologic Pathology	Winging of the scapula secondary to inhibition of the long thoracic nerve
Muscle Imbalances	Increased pelvic angles secondary to weak abdominal muscles
Hypermobile Joints	Genu recurvatum
Hypomobile Joints	Flexion contracture
Decreased Muscle Extensibility	Decreased pelvic angles secondary to tightness of the hamstring muscles
Bony Abnormalities	Toe in or toe out posture secondary to internal or external tibial torsion
Leg-Length Discrepancies	Functional scoliosis
Pain	Antalgic posture (e.g., side bending cervical spine to decrease compression on a nerve root)
Lack of Postural Awareness	Acquired bad habits (e.g., slouching in chair)

history needs to identify any repetitive motions that are routinely performed.

If the patient describes an insidious onset and symptoms that gradually increase over time, a portion of the history-taking process should be devoted to investigating the person's day-to-day tasks and postures. In the absence of acute trauma, the patient's symptoms may be the result of posture and biomechanics. The following information should be obtained to determine whether posture is contributing to the current pathology.

*** Practical Evidence**

As the weight of a backpack increases, there is a proportional increase in the risk of onset of low back pain in college students and adolescents.[12,13]

Mechanism of Injury

Many overuse injuries associated with postural faults have an insidious onset with no specific cause of the pain. Other common responses pointing toward possible postural involvement in an injury include:

- Pain worsening as the day progresses
- Description of pain associated with specific posture
- Complaints of intermittent pain
- Vague or generalized pain descriptions
- Pain initially starting as an ache that has progressively worsened over time

Level and Intensity of Exercise

Is exercise performed on a regular or sporadic basis or not at all? Has the exercise routine changed in any way? A rapid change in exercise duration or intensity may make a previously benign postural fault problematic.

Type, Location, and Severity of Symptoms

Are the symptoms constant or intermittent? Are they worse during a certain time of the day (i.e., morning, afternoon, evening)? Many postural dysfunctions are worse, or produce more symptoms, in the evening after the individual has maintained the posture all day. Which positions or postures increase or decrease the symptoms? Some activities, such as gymnastics, regularly require unusual postures. If the symptom is primarily pain, then what type of pain is it: burning, sharp, aching, pulsating? Is the patient experiencing paresthesia? If so, is it constant or intermittent?

Side Dominance

Is the patient right- or left-side dominant? If one side is used for most, if not all, tasks, then bilateral imbalances are likely to occur, exposing the patient to overuse injuries.

Medical History

Has this problem occurred before? If so, was medical attention sought and what treatments were rendered? Are there any medical problems that should be identified? A general health questionnaire may be helpful to use before the evaluation to uncover any medical conditions.

Functional Assessment

Observation of posture during activities that increase symptoms or are repeated throughout the day forms the basis of functional assessment. Postural adaptations and/or compensations are associated with specific activities. For example, the resting scapular position is different in throwing athletes than in the population as a whole.

Activities of Daily Living

What is the patient's usual day like? Many people have repetitive daily schedules. Which types of activities does the patient perform and for what duration and frequency? To better understand the motions associated with specific pain-producing tasks, have the patient demonstrate specific motions as they are being described (Table 6-6).

Driving, Sitting, and Sleeping Postures

Has anything been changed in the person's daily routine over the past few months (Table 6-7)? Changes in a routine often provide information about the instigating factor. For example, a change in mattress could provoke or decrease symptoms.

*** Practical Evidence**

Replacing an older mattress with a medium-firm mattress is associated with decreased pain and disability for individuals with low back pain.[15]

Inspection

Ensure that the area used for postural assessment is private to protect the modesty of the patient and is at a comfortable temperature. When possible, males should wear only shorts that expose most of the legs. Females also wear shorts that expose most of their legs and a halter-type top that exposes the whole back. To allow observation of foot positions, shoes should not be worn. Do not alert the patient that posture is being assessed at this time.

Table 6-6 Examples of Daily Stresses and Their Possible Resulting Pathologies

Activity	Associated Tasks	Possible Postural Deviations	Possible Soft Tissue Dysfunctions	Corrections
Desk Job	Computer use: Is the station ergonomically correct? Is it a multiuse station?	FHP, FSP, general postural faults caused by muscle fatigue or poor postural sense throughout trunk and upper quadrant	Soft tissue syndromes of the cervical, thoracic, and shoulder regions, including, myofascial syndromes, muscle imbalances, thoracic outlet syndrome, carpal tunnel syndrome, or other nerve-entrapment syndromes throughout the upper extremity	1. Proper ergonomic design of workstation 2. Frequent breaks with performance of postural exercises and stretches 3. Maintenance of proper sitting posture at work 4. Periodic use of standing desk[14]
	Telephone use: How is the phone held? Is the phone cradled between the ear and shoulder? Is the same side used?	Prolonged cervical lateral flexion, shoulder elevation	Adaptive shortening of cervical lateral flexors, lengthening of contralateral muscles, myofascial syndromes in all the above areas mentioned, joint or nerve root related problems in the cervical spine caused by compression of one side (narrowing of intervertebral foramen and compression of the ipsilateral facet joints)	Use of a telephone headset to maintain the head in the neutral position and leave the hands free to perform other tasks with minimal strain
	What type of chair is used? Is it ergonomically correct?	Inadequate lumbar support: Leads to "slouched" posture and flexed lumbar, thoracic spine, FSP, and FHP Inadequate arm rests: Leads to increased upper extremity work causing fatigue of shoulder girdle muscles	Muscle imbalances throughout trunk, shoulder girdle region, upper extremities; myofascial syndromes; TOS at any of three entrapment sites (anterior or middle scalenes, first rib and clavicle, pectoralis minor and rib cage); other nerve-entrapment syndromes	1. Ergonomically correct chair with adequate lumbar support and arm rests at correct height 2. The chair placed correctly in front of the computer and not angled to perform computer work and other tasks at the same time 3. Frequent breaks from computer work to perform postural exercises or stretches 4. Maintenance of proper sitting posture at work
	Are bifocals worn? Are regular glasses worn and is the prescription up to date? Is there glare on the computer screen?	FHP, FSP from straining to read the screen	TMJ dysfunctions; myofascial syndromes; joint and nerve dysfunctions; muscle imbalances; headaches	1. Change of computer screen angle or height 2. Change of glasses as needed 3. Use of antiglare screens and shields; decrease in glare from overhead fluorescent lighting

Manual Labor	Frequency of bending, lifting, repetitive motions? (If possible, the patient should demonstrate the actual positions assumed and motions performed.)	Improper spinal flexion; decreased use of leg muscles or increased use of back muscles; flexed thoracic and cervical spine with increased stress of soft tissue structures of back; combined motions of lumbar spine flexion and rotation	Muscle imbalance; myofascial syndrome; muscle tears or ligamentous sprains; joint or disc pathology	1. Teach proper lifting technique: maintenance of neutral spine; flexing at hips; use of legs rather than back muscles; maintenance of cervical lordosis or thoracic kyphosis; use of pivoting with feet versus rotation of spine when turning 2. Perform extension exercises throughout day to counteract flexion 3. Use assistive devices to lift heavy objects; use more trips with less weight per trip; and use partner to lift heavy and bulky objects
	Repetitive overhead tasks?	Cervical spine in prolonged extension	Muscle imbalances; cervical spine facet joint or nerve compression; myofascial syndromes; with the presence of an FSP, patients are more prone to shoulder impingement syndromes	1. Frequent breaks from overhead activities 2. Use of stool or device to attempt to keep work at eye level
	Is any specific equipment used repetitively?	Repetitive motions with use of specific tool increasing stress on certain tissues	Muscle imbalances; tendinopathy; strains; nerve-entrapment syndromes	1. Stretching of muscles used during operation of tools 2. Ergonomically correct tools
Student	Is a backpack used? How heavy is the backpack?	FHP; FSP; flexed trunk and lumbar spine	Myofascial syndromes; TOS; facet or disc pathology; muscle imbalances	1. Use of both shoulder straps while wearing backpack to avoid carrying the weight over one shoulder 2. Limiting the weight of the backpack as much as possible
Athletics	Sports and position? Frequency, duration, and intensity of involvement?	Adaptation depends on position assumed (e.g., swimmers who emphasize the butterfly stroke develop increased thoracic kyphosis/cervical lordosis)	Myofascial syndrome; muscle tears or ligamentous sprains; muscle imbalances	1. Conditioning to prepare specific tissues for the rigors of the sport and position. Proper stretching before and after participation 2. Change in training regimen as necessary 3. Change of position 4. Increased awareness of stresses

FHP = forward head posture; FSP = forward shoulder posture; TMJ = temporomandibular joint; TOS = thoracic outlet syndrome

Table 6-7 Driving, Sitting, and Sleeping Postures

ADL	Posture	Possible Postural Deviations	Postural Correction
Driving	Inadequate lumbar support?	Flexion of lumbar spine and thoracic spine, FSP, and FHP	Use lumbar support cushion
	Reclined seat angle—hips flexed less than 90°?	Flexion of lumbar and thoracic spine; increased scapula protraction; excessive arm elevation to reach steering wheel; FSP; FHP	Adjust seat angle so hips are at 90° of flexion
	Seat distance too far from steering wheel and pedals?	Flexion of lumbar and thoracic spine; protraction of scapula; FSP; FHP; increased pelvis and leg activity to reach for pedals	Adjust seat distance so elbows and knees are flexed approximately 30°–45°; the hands should reach the steering wheel, and the thoracic spine and scapula should maintain contact with the seatback
	Frequency, length of time spent driving?	Muscle imbalances and overuse syndromes when incorrectly postured with prolonged sitting position	1. Use correct posture while driving 2. Take frequent rest stops and perform stretching exercises (e.g., trunk extension, hamstring stretches)
Sitting	Although some sitting postures are covered in Table 6-6, it is important to identify all different types of sitting postures assumed throughout the day	See Table 6-6 for description of postural deviations while sitting.	Use proper sitting posture that incorporates the following: body weight slightly anterior to ischial tuberosities; maintenance of normal lumbar lordosis; hips slightly higher than knees; feet flat on floor; shoulders maintained in a "back and down" position (retracted and depressed); arms supported at the proper height to maintain good shoulder position; head retracted and in a neutral position Postures may vary from the above description; the key is to understand what correct posture entails for that individual and to work from that position, changing various amounts of each movement to find a more "correct or functional" position for each individual
Sleeping	Mattress support (firm or soft)? Recent change in mattress?	A soft mattress may not provide adequate support; firm mattresses may be too rigid to conform to the natural curves of the body.	Change mattress according to desired support. Replace old mattress.
	Number of pillows used? Type of pillow used?	Using too many pillows places the head and neck in excessive lateral flexion toward the opposite side during sleeping; may cause prolonged compression and distraction at the neck on the weight-bearing side	Use an adequate number (and size) of pillows to maintain the head in the neutral position while sleeping.
	Sleep posture?	Different positions place abnormal stresses on the soft tissues or may perpetuate postural changes.	Use positions that are not at the extremes of motion (i.e., too much flexion or extension); use pillows between the legs when side-lying

ADL = activity of daily living; FHP = forward head posture; FSP = forward shoulder posture

Patients who are aware that posture is being assessed will become conscious about their posture and may stand more erect than usual.

Use a systematic approach when assessing posture to avoid overlooking a specific region. The evaluation process may start at the foot and work superiorly or vice versa. This chapter describes posture starting at the feet and working superiorly. Whenever comparing bilaterally for symmetry, place your eyes at the same level as the region you are observing.

Overall Impression

The first component of a postural assessment is the determination of the patient's general body type: ectomorph, mesomorph, or endomorph (Inspection Findings 6-1). A person's body type is largely inherited and can influence the types of activity in which he or she may engage. For example, an ectomorph is more apt to be a distance runner than an endomorph. The body mass index (BMI) describes the person's relative mass based on height and weight (Box 6-1).

Inspection Findings 6-1
Classifications of Body Types

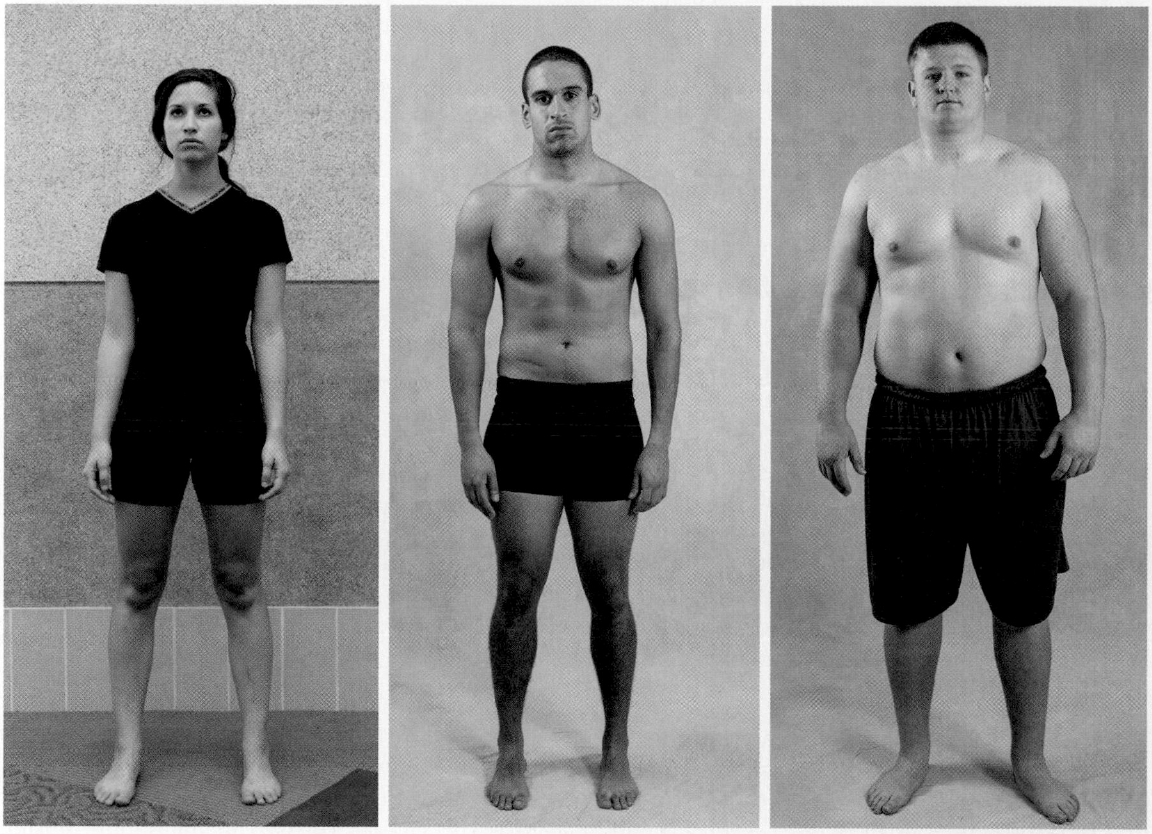

	Ectomorph	Mesomorph	Endomorph
Description	Slender, thin build; relatively low body mass index	Medium, athletic build, relatively average body mass index	Stocky build; relatively high body mass index
Joint Shape	Small, flat joint surfaces	Medium-sized joint surfaces	Large, concave-convex joint surfaces
Muscle Mass	Minimal muscle bulk, thin muscles	Medium muscle build	Thick muscle mass
Joint Mobility	Increased	Within normal limits	Decreased
Joint Stability	Decreased	Within normal limits	Increased

Box 6-1
Body Mass Index

Historically, the medical determination of obesity was made based on the percentage of body fat or total body weight. Depending on the measure being used, obesity is used to describe a person who is 20% to 30% over the average weight based on gender, age, and height. Body mass index (BMI) is an indirect estimation of the percentage of body fat. The BMI, based on height and weight, is calculated by:

(Weight [lbs.] × (705)/(height [in.] × (height [in.])
or
Weight (kg)/(height [m]×(height [m])

A BMI of 27.0 is the most commonly used threshold to define obesity. The National Center for Health Statistics proposes the following classification scheme for adult BMI. Note that there are specific BMI ranges for children and teenagers:[16i]

Underweight: <18.5

Normal: 18.5–24.9

Overweight: 25.0–29.9

Class I obesity: 30.0–34.9

Class II obesity: 35.0–39.9

Class III obesity: ≥40.0

BMI does not accurately describe the amount of body fat for certain groups of people, especially athletes.[17] For example, a 6-foot-tall (1.83 m) muscular basketball player who weighs 200 pounds (90.7 kg) would have a BMI of 27.1 (90.7 kg/[1.83 m × 1.83 m]). This individual would fall into the preobese classification, even though he or she may have a low percentage of body fat. Therefore, obesity should be determined on a case-by-case basis, taking the individual's sex, height, weight, age, BMI, percentage of body fat, and level of activity into consideration.

Views of Postural Inspection

Posture is inspected from all views or planes with the body in a natural stance: lateral (sagittal plane), anterior (frontal plane), and posterior (frontal plane). A plumb line may be used to assist in identifying postural deviations. When using a plumb line, align the patient using the feet as the permanent landmark. Position the plumb line slightly anterior to the lateral malleolus from the lateral view and equidistant from both feet from the anterior and posterior views. Inspection Findings 6-2 presents ideal posture in each of the three planes. Deviation from ideal posture forms the basis for identifying the possible underlying impairments.

Leg-Length Discrepancy

A leg-length discrepancy (LLD) can contribute to lower limb and back pathology.[18] Hip osteoarthritis and lower extremity stress fractures are more frequent on the longer limb.[19] The amount of LLD that results in pathology is debatable. In general, those who develop LLD early in life tolerate more difference, while those who are athletic, stand on their feet frequently, or develop LLD later in life tolerate less difference.[19]

The two categories of LLDs are structural (true) and functional (apparent) (Table 6-8).[18] Although the most accurate methods for determining unequal leg lengths are by radiograph and CT evaluation, several methods can be used clinically.[18]

LLD can be determined using indirect methods, including premeasured blocks to level the pelvis (Selective Tissue Test 6-1) or measuring the distance between established landmarks using a tape measure (Selective Tissue Test 6-2). In addition to using the more functional position of standing, the block method has improved reliability and validity when compared with the tape measure method.[18,19] If a functional leg-length discrepancy is suspected, further assessment of soft tissue lengths and joint range of motion (ROM) must be used to determine the source (or consequence) of the difference.[20, 21]

An actual difference in lengths of the femurs or tibias can be grossly assessed in the supine position with the feet placed flat and in equal positions on the examining table with the knees flexed to 90 degrees. Observing the height of the knees from the anterior view will determine whether one tibia is longer than the other. Observing the length of the

Table 6-8 Leg-Length Differences

Category Type	Description	Possible Causes
Functional or Apparent Leg Length	Leg-length difference that is attributed to something other than the length of the tibia and/or femur	Tightness of muscle or joint structures or muscular weakness in the lower extremity or spine; examples include knee hyperextension, scoliosis, or pelvic muscle imbalances.
Structural or True Leg Length	An actual difference in the length of the femur or the tibia of one leg compared with the other	Possibly from disruption in the growth plate of one of the long bones or a congenital anomaly

Inspection Findings 6-2
Assessment of Ideal Posture

Lateral	Anterior	Posterior
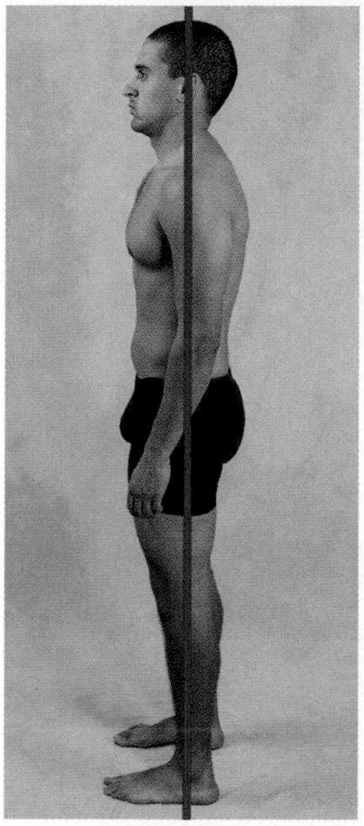	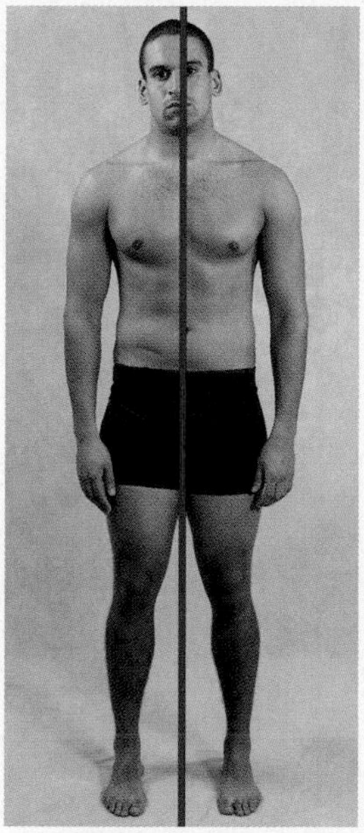	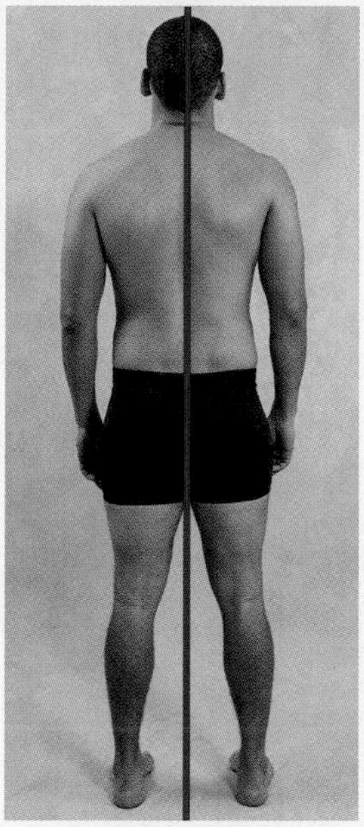
Alignment relative to plumb line:	Alignment relative to plumb line:	Alignment relative to plumb line:
Lower extremity • Lateral malleolus: Slightly posterior • The tibia should be parallel to the plumb line, and the foot should be at a 90° angle to the tibia • Lateral femoral epicondyle: Slightly anterior • Greater trochanter: Plumb line bisects	• Feet: Evenly spaced from plumb line • Tibial crests: Slight external rotation • Knees: Evenly spaced from plumb line • Patella: Facing anteriorly • Consistent angulation from joint to joint • The lateral malleoli, fibular head, and iliac crests should be bilaterally equal.	• Feet evenly spaced from plumb line • Feet in slight lateral rotation: Lateral two toes are visible • Knees evenly spaced from plumb line • Consistent angulation from joint to joint
Torso • Midthoracic region: Plumb line bisects	• Umbilicus: Plumb line bisects, although abdominal surgical procedures may alter the alignment. • Sternum: Plumb line bisects • Jugular notch: Plumb line bisects	• Median sacral crests: Plumb line bisects • Spinous processes: Plumb line bisects • Paraspinals musculature bilaterally symmetrical
Shoulder • Acromion process: Plumb line bisects	• Acromion processes: Evenly spaced from plumb line • Shoulder heights equal or dominant side slightly lower • Deltoid, anterior chest musculature bilaterally symmetrical and defined	• Scapular borders: Evenly spaced from plumb line • Acromion processes: Evenly spaced from plumb line • Deltoid, posterior musculature bilaterally symmetrical • Shoulder heights equal or dominant side slightly lower
Head and Neck • Cervical bodies: Plumb line bisects • Auditory meatus: Plumb line bisects	• Head: Plumb line bisects • Nasal bridge: Plumb line bisects • Frontal bone: Plumb line bisects	• Cervical spinous processes: Plumb line bisects • Occipital protuberance: Plumb line bisects

Selective Tissue Tests 6-1
Measured Block Method of Determining Leg-Length Discrepancy

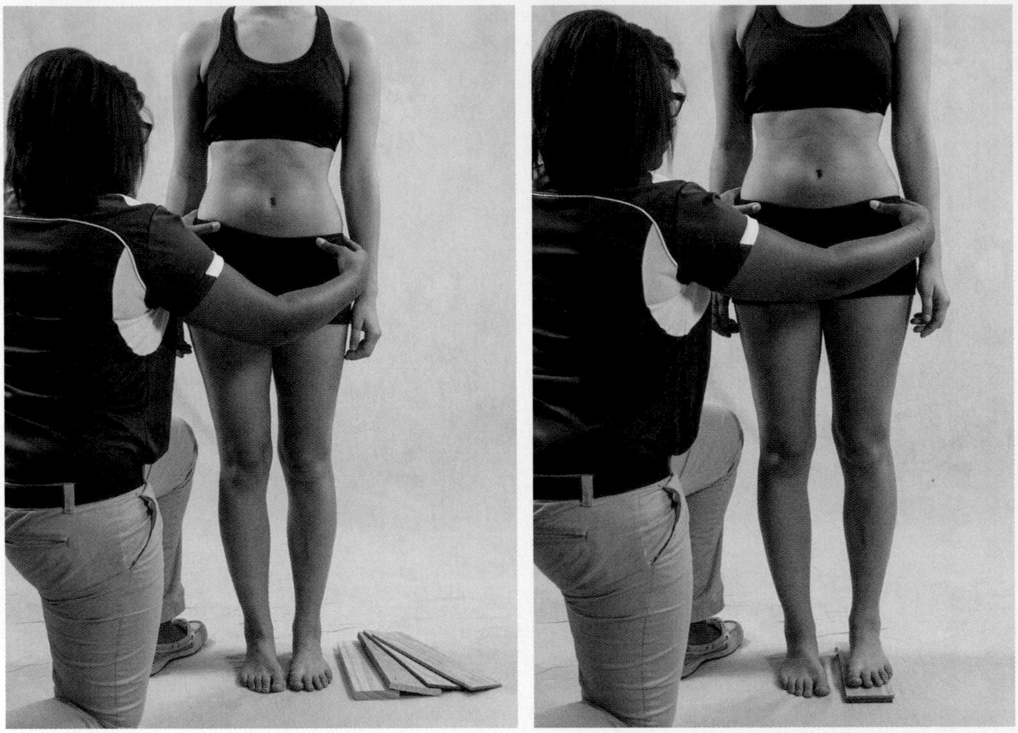

The block method of determining a leg-length difference. Blocks of a known thickness are placed under the shorter extremity.

Patient Position	Standing on a firm surface with the feet shoulder-width apart and the weight evenly distributed
Position of Examiner	Standing in front of the patient
Evaluative Procedure	The starting levels of the iliac crests are noted. If heights are determined to be unequal, blocks of known height (measured in millimeters) are placed under the shorter leg until the iliac crests are of equal height. The leg-length difference is calculated by adding the heights of the individual blocks.
Positive Test	A leg-length difference of 10–20 mm is frequently cited as the level at which gait is affected.[18] Patients who acquire the LLD at an early age may tolerate more difference. Patients who are athletic or must stand for much of the day may tolerate less.[19,21]
Comments	When the iliac crests are level, palpate the heights of the anterior superior iliac spine (ASIS). If these are not an equal height, then the patient has asymmetrical innominate bones.
Evidence	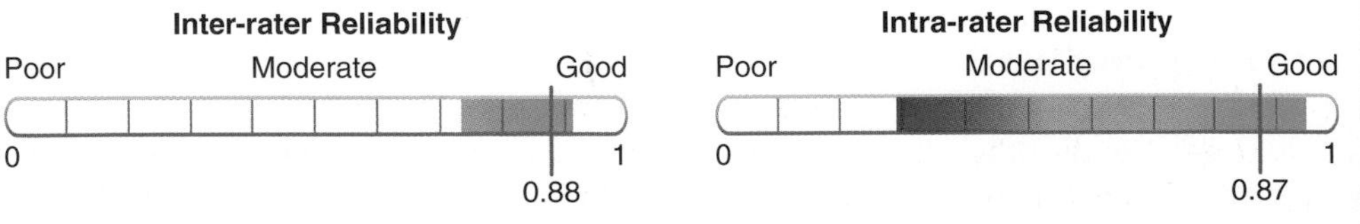

ASIS = anterior superior iliac spine; LLD = leg-length discrepancy

Selective Tissue Tests 6-2
Tape Measure Method of Detecting Leg Length Discrepancy

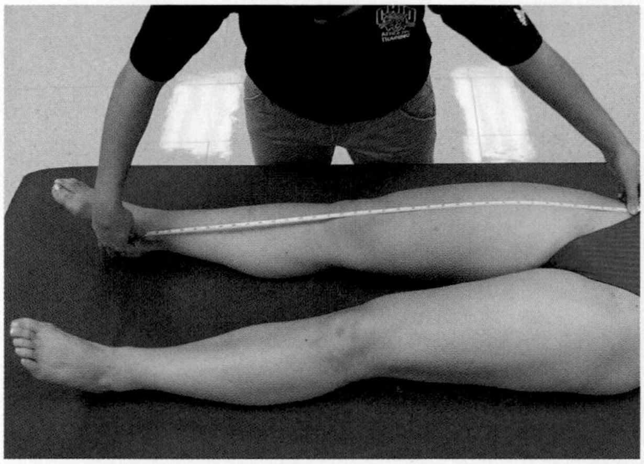
True Leg-Length Discrepancy

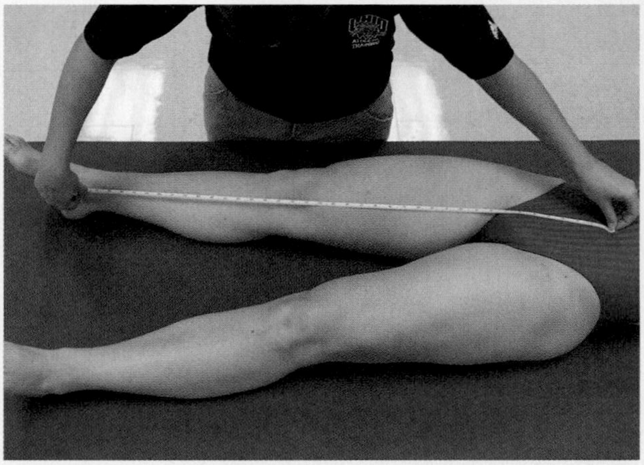
Apparent Leg-Length Discrepancy

Patient Position	Supine
Position of Examiner	Standing to the side of the patient
Evaluative Procedure	*True LLD:* Measure the distance from the ASIS to the distal tip of the medial malleolus. Do this bilaterally. *Apparent LLD:* Measure the distance from the umbilicus to the distal tip of the medial malleolus. Do this bilaterally.
Positive Test	A true leg-length difference of 10–20 mm is frequently cited as the level at which gait is affected.[18] Patients who acquire the LLD at an early age may tolerate more difference. Patients who are athletic or must stand for much of the day may tolerate less.[19,21]
Comments	A side-to-side difference in the measurements from the bony landmarks indicates a true (structural) LLD. A side-to-side difference in the measurements from the umbilicus indicates a functional leg-length discrepancy. Some clinicians use the tip of the lateral malleolus as the distal reference.
Evidence	

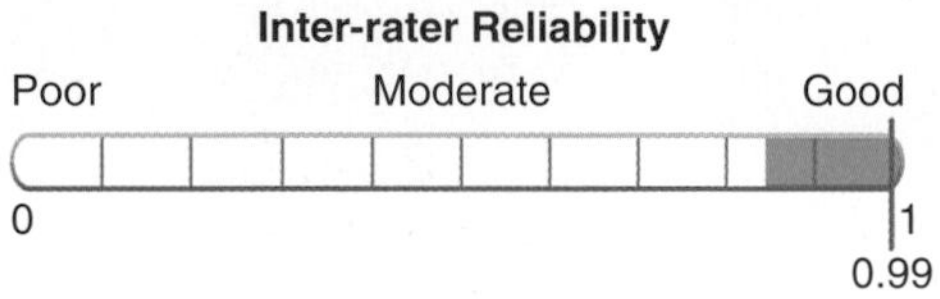

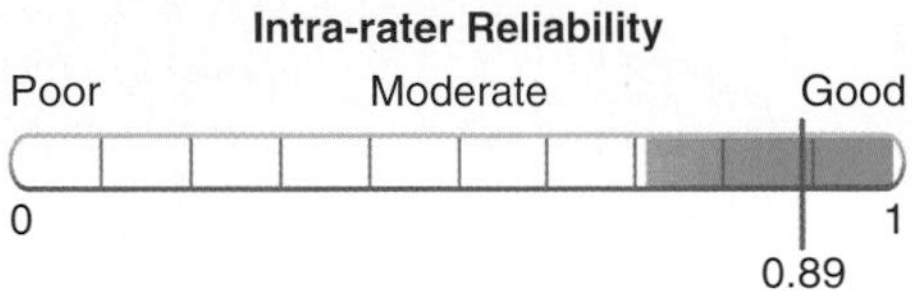

ASIS = anterior superior iliac spine; LLD = leg-length discrepancy

knees from the lateral view can be used to determine if one femur is longer than the other but does not rule out apparent leg-length discrepancies caused by the shape and position of the pelvis (Fig. 6-7). During weight bearing, the position of the feet can also provide evidence of a functional compensation for LLD. The foot on the shorter leg supinates, and the foot on the longer leg pronates in an attempt to compensate for the discrepancy in length (Fig. 6-8).

Palpation

When assessing posture, accurate palpation of key landmarks assists in identifying various postural deviations.

Lateral Aspect

- **Pelvic position:** Palpate the ASIS and posterior superior iliac spine (PSIS) on the same side. Because palpation of bony landmarks in this region is unreliable to start, the ability to detect asymmetry is questionable.[22] Furthermore, side-to-side asymmetry is common in asymptomatic individuals[23] and does not appear to be associated with low back pain.[24]

Anterior Aspect

- **Patellar position:** Before palpating for patellar position, ensure that the patient is standing comfortably with the feet symmetrically rotated and in an equal stance.

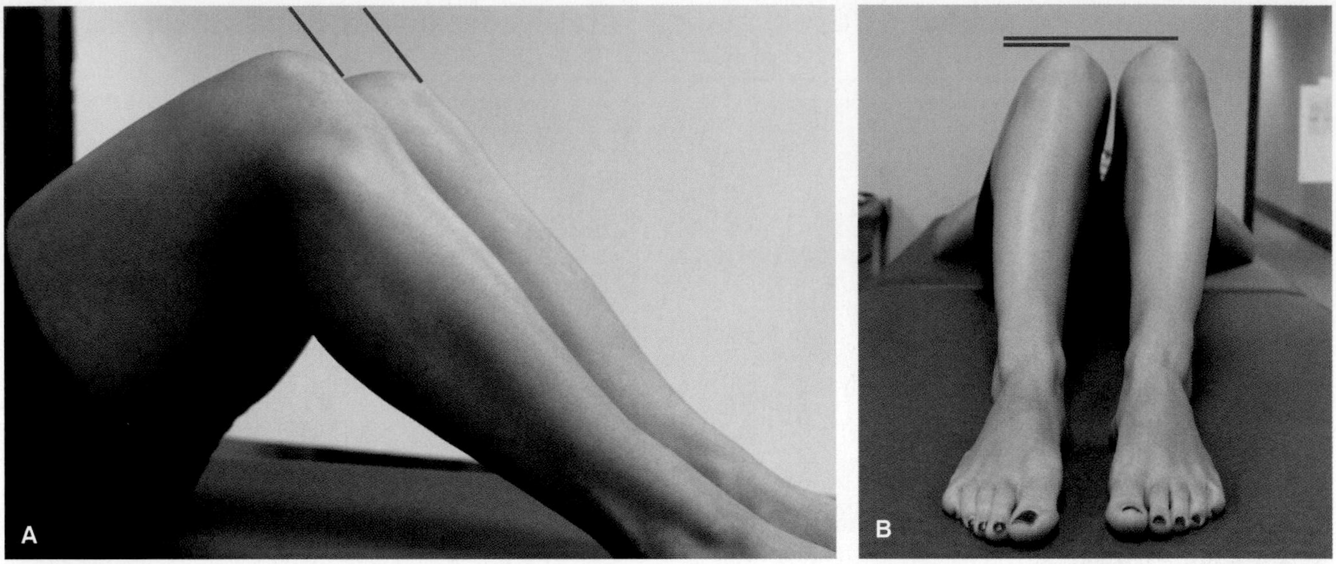

FIGURE 6-7 ■ Clinical discrimination between femoral and tibial leg length differences. (A) When viewing the patient from the lateral side, an increased anterior position of one knee indicates a discrepancy in the lengths of the femurs. (B) When viewing the knees from the front, a difference in height indicates a discrepancy in the lengths of the tibias.

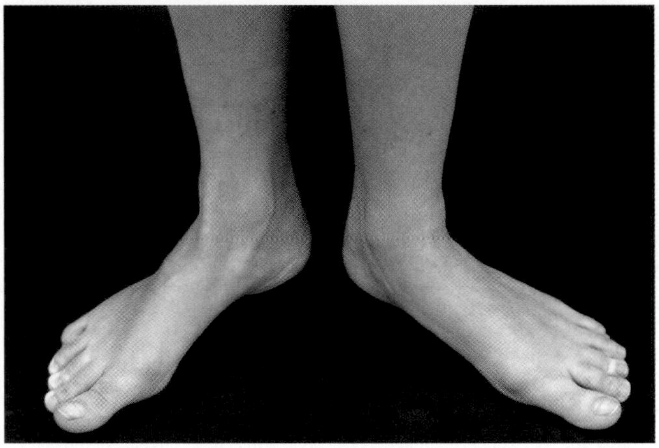

FIGURE 6-8 ■ Foot posture associated with leg length difference. The foot on the long-leg side (the patient's left foot) is pronated while the foot on the short-leg side is supinated.

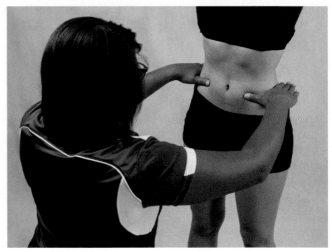

FIGURE 6-9 ■ Finding the heights of the iliac crests.

Patellar position is observed while the patient is standing, lying supine, long sitting, and during dynamic moment. To assist in determining patellar position, place the thumbs on the medial borders of the patellae and the index fingers on the lateral borders. Further information regarding patellar position is provided in Chapter 11.

- **Iliac crest heights:** Palpate the lateral portions of both ilia moving superiorly until reaching the most superior aspect of the iliac crests. Place the palmar aspects of the index and middle fingers on top of the iliac crests as if forming two "tabletops." When you have located the landmarks, determine if your hands are level and that the iliac crest heights are equal (Fig. 6-9). If one hand is higher than the other, then the iliac crests are unequal. Causes of unequal iliac crest height include true leg-length discrepancy or functional LLD resulting from soft-tissue changes or excessive or restricted joint motion.
- **ASIS heights:** Trace your thumbs down the anterior portion of both iliac crests until coming to the ASIS protuberance. Hook the thumbs on the most inferior ridges of the ASIS to ensure that the same aspect of the ASIS is being palpated on both sides. Determine if your thumbs are equal heights (Fig. 6-10).
- **Lateral malleolus and fibula head heights:** Bilaterally palpate the most prominent projections of the lateral malleolus to determine whether each is of equal height. Repeat this process for the fibular heads.
- **Shoulder heights:** Place the palmar aspect of the index and middle fingers on the superior surface of the

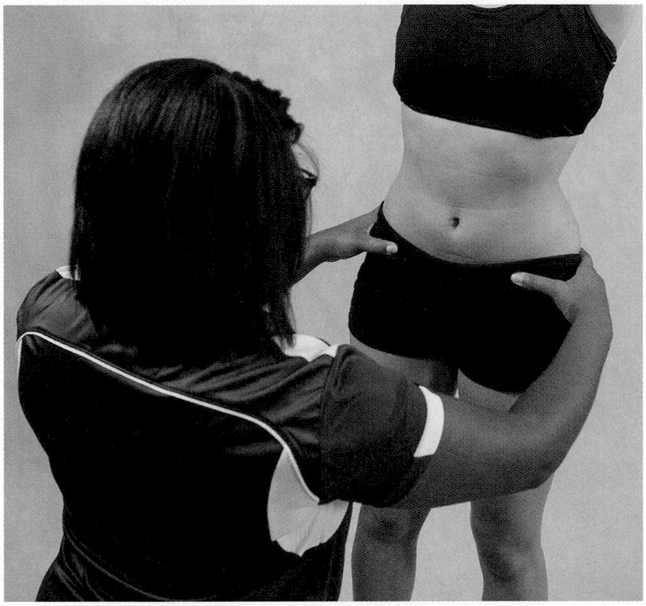

FIGURE 6-10 ■ Identifying the anterior superior iliac spine.

acromion processes. The fingers should sit flatly on both acromion processes and be parallel to the ground (Fig. 6.11).

Posterior Aspect

Many of the same landmarks used for the anterior view are also used in the posterior view. This section discusses only landmarks that are specific to the posterior view.

- **PSIS positions:** Keeping the index and middle fingers in the position for measuring iliac crest heights, angle the thumbs 45 degrees downward and medially. Palpate for the PSIS, a relatively large, round protuberance, and hook your thumbs under the inferior margins of the PSIS. Determine if your thumbs are at equal heights (Fig. 6-12).

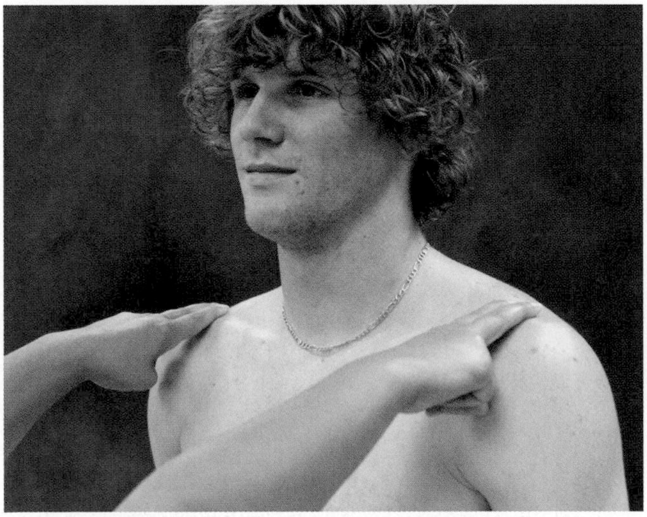

FIGURE 6-11 ■ Identifying the level of the shoulders.

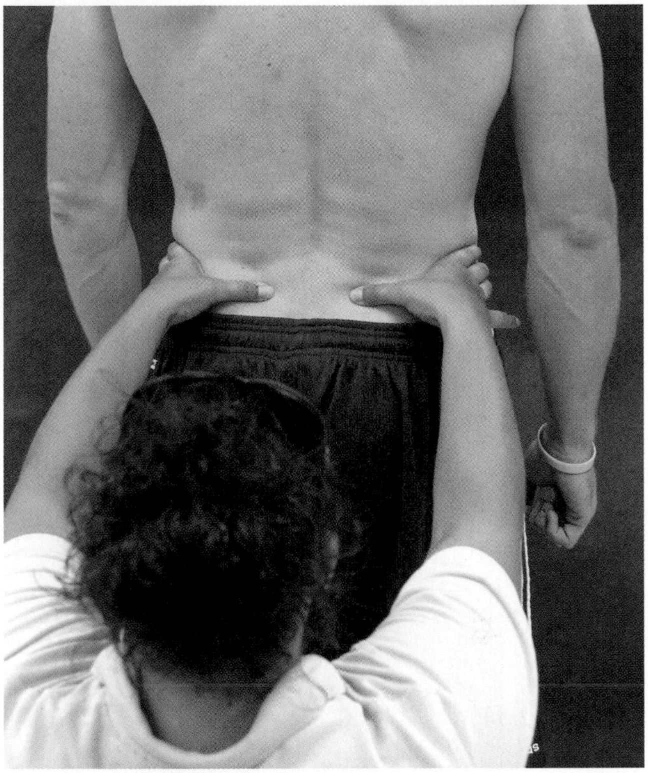

FIGURE 6-12 ■ Palpating the posterior superior iliac spines.

- **Spinal alignment:** Starting from the cervical vertebrae, trace your finger down each spinous process to the sacrum. A lateral deviation where more than one spinous process is not aligned vertically may reflect scoliosis. Refer to the section of this chapter on the spine for definitions of functional versus structural scoliosis.
- **Scapular position:** With the patient standing and relaxed, evaluate the scapula's resting position and note bilateral or unilateral elevation or depression, **protraction** or **retraction**, **rotation**, and **winging** (Box 6-2). Normally, the scapula on the dominant side is slightly more protracted than the nondominant shoulder. In normal posture, the scapula is angled 30 to 40 degrees relative to the frontal plane (the plane of the scapula) with the medial (vertebral) border parallel to the spine. The superior angle is located at about the level of the third or fourth thoracic vertebra, while the inferior angle is at the level of the seventh to ninth thoracic vertebra. The scapula should be anteriorly tilted around 10 degrees with the arms at the side.[25]

Protraction (scapular) Movement of the vertebral borders of the scapula away from the spinal column

Retraction (scapular) Movement of the scapular vertebral borders toward the spinal column

Rotation (scapular) Spin of the scapula in the frontal plane

Winging (scapular) The medial border of the scapula lifting away from the thorax

Box 6-2
Resting Scapular Postures

Vertical Scapular Position

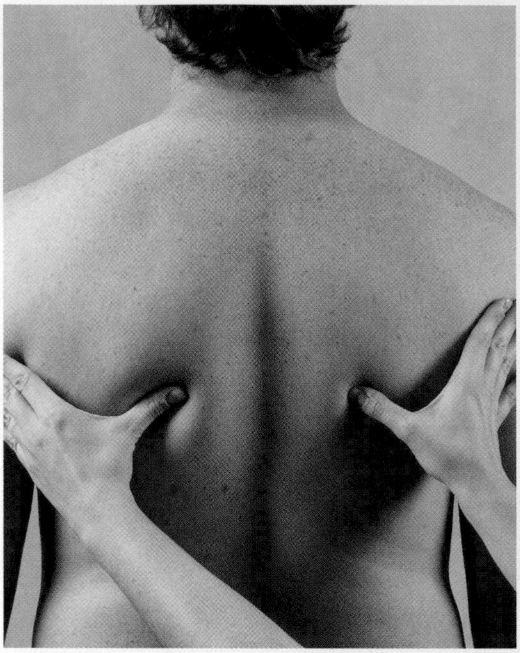

The vertical alignment of the scapulae is compared using the inferior angle as a landmark. The normal height correlates to thoracic vertebrae 7–9.[25]

Horizontal Scapular Position

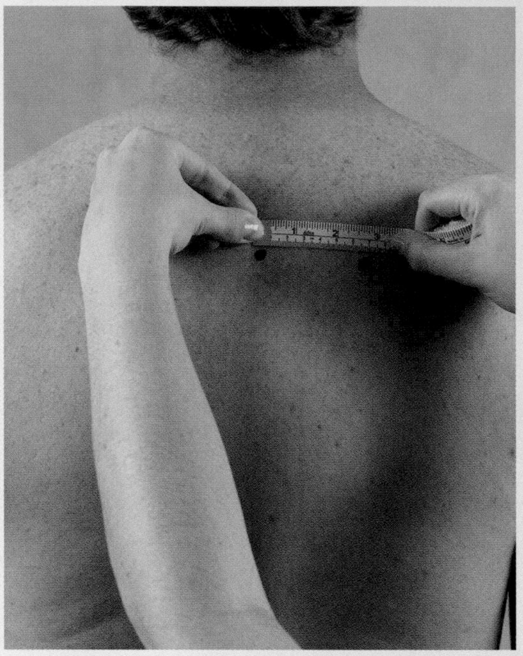

The distance from the T4 spinous process to the medial border of the scapula is measured with the patient standing. The measurement can be repeated with the patient actively retracting both scapulae. The normal resting value is approximately 6 cm.[25] An increased distance represents a protracted scapular position, a decreased distance, or a retracted scapula.

Scapular Rotation

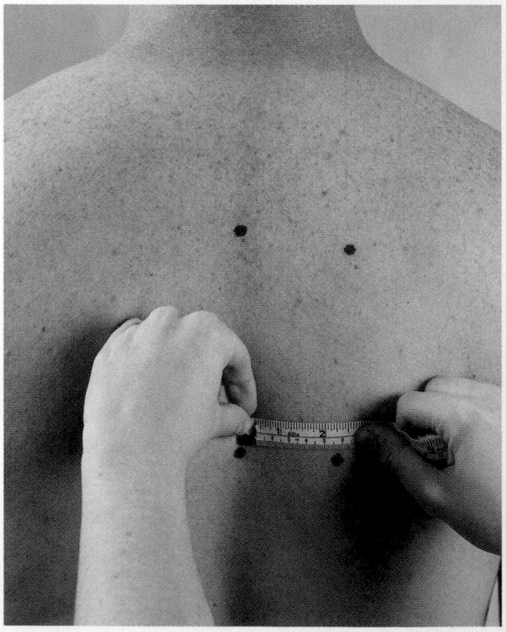

The distance from the T7 vertebra to the inferior angle of each scapula is measured. An increased distance indicates an upwardly rotated scapula.

Scapular Winging

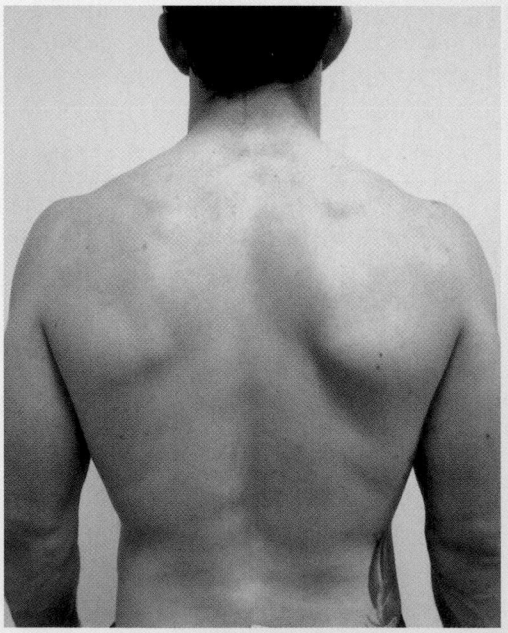

Protrusion of the medial border of the scapula

"Pseudowinging" is apparent when the inferior angle (not the entire medial border) is prominent and is associated with increased anterior tipping of the scapula.

Muscle-Length Assessment

Muscle-length assessment objectively measures whether specific muscles are shortened or elongated, contributing to postural abnormality. Abnormal stresses can occur if a muscle crossing a specific joint is shortened because the necessary ROM required for normal function may be lacking. If a muscle crossing a specific joint is abnormally elongated, the joint may be affected by the lack of stability required for efficient movement. Consider a patient with low back pain who has increased anterior pelvic tilt. The next task is to identify the underlying impairments and whether or not these contribute to activity limitations. The anterior tilt may be caused by a tight rectus femoris or iliopsoas muscles with lengthened hamstrings, but this assumption must be confirmed using, objective, measurable tests. As with all aspects of a clinical examination, muscle-length assessment should use standard measures to be as objective as possible.

Before assessing the length of a muscle, rule out any bony or soft tissue restrictions that could be involved in the joint or joints that the muscle crosses. Muscles that cross more than one joint (two-joint muscles) have a greater tendency to become shortened during normal ADLs than do muscles crossing only one joint. Specific, measurable tests are available for many of the **two-joint muscles** that commonly create postural problems as they become shortened in length. When assessing muscle length for most of the **one-joint muscles**, the normal ranges (measurements) for passive joint ROM are used. One-joint muscles are less likely to become shortened. A goniometer used to measure joint angles assists in the objectivity of muscle-length assessment.

Assessing for Shortness of the Lower Extremity Muscles

When muscle shortening occurs, various postural deviations may result. The specific procedures for assessing muscle length in selected lower extremity muscles are described in Muscle Length 6-1 through 6-3. The Ober test (see Selective Tissue Test 10-19) and the Thomas test (see Selective Tissue Test 12-3) are two additional tests for muscle length.

Assessing for Shortness of the Upper Extremity Muscles

When shortening occurs in upper extremity muscles, various postural deviations may result. The specific procedures for assessing muscle length in selected upper extremity muscles are described in Muscle Length 6-4 through 6-6.[26]

Common Postural Deviations

Many people have less-than-ideal posture. However, not all postural deviations cause pathology or result in symptoms. Clinicians must be able to identify normal posture, **asymptomatic** deviations, and postural deviations possibly causing soft tissue dysfunction and pain. When evaluating postural deviations, keep in mind that any potential muscle imbalances can either cause the poor posture or be a result of the poor posture. The next section discusses some common postural deviations observed for each joint.

Foot and Ankle

Pronated Foot

A pes planus foot, or a flattened medial longitudinal arch, is characteristic of excessively pronated subtalar and midtarsal joints. Excessive pronation is characterized by adduction and plantarflexion of the talus and eversion of the calcaneus when the foot is weight bearing (refer to Table 8-1 for a description of foot pronation and supination while weight bearing and non–weight bearing).

Two weight-bearing methods used to measure foot posture are the longitudinal arch angle and the navicular drop test (see Chapter 8, Selective Tissue Tests 8-1 and 8-4). The subtalar neutral position is commonly used to determine non–weight-bearing foot position. In this position, the clinician is observing for static foot positions such as forefoot or rearfoot varus, which contribute to compensatory prolonged or hyperpronation and the resulting compensations up the kinetic chain (Fig. 6-13).

Supinated Foot

Excessive weight-bearing supination is characterized by abduction and dorsiflexion of the talus and inversion of the calcaneus. A heightened medial longitudinal arch is also

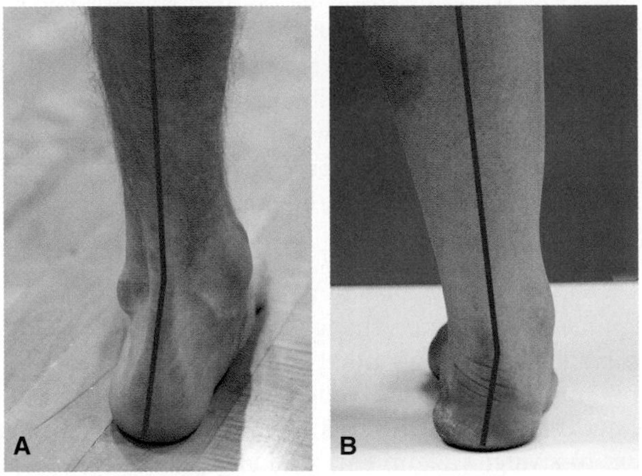

FIGURE 6-13 ■ Alignment of the calcaneus and tibia. (A) Calcaneal eversion (calcaneovalgus). (B) Calcaneal inversion (calcaneovarus).

Two-joint muscle A muscle that exerts its force across two different joints and whose strength depends on the position of those joints

One-joint muscle A muscle that exerts force across only one joint

Asymptomatic Without symptoms

commonly observed. Forefoot valgus in the subtalar neutral position during non–weight bearing can be a structural cause for excessive supination. A supinated or cavus foot has less shock-absorbing capacity, predisposing the foot to a number of stress-related conditions.

Foot Posture Index

The Foot Posture Index© (FPI) was designed to improve the reliability and validity of classification of foot postures as supinated, neutral, or pronated and may be useful in predicting injury predisposition (Fig. 6-14).[28-30] Using simple palpation and inspection metrics with the patient in a relaxed stance, the FPI uses a five-point Likert scale to assess six aspects of foot position:

1. Talonavicular congruence
2. Supra- and infralateral malleolar curvature
3. Calcaneal frontal plane position
4. Bulge in the region of the talonavicular joint
5. Height and congruence of the medial longitudinal arch
6. Abduction or adduction of the forefoot on the rear foot (too many toes sign)

Each feature is assigned a rating from –2 to +2. Negative values reflect more supinated positioning, and positive values reflect pronated positioning. The scores are added, and the composite score is used. In an adult population, the normal range is from +1 to +7, with an average of +4 (slightly pronated). Scores of less than or equal to –3 or greater than or equal to +10 are considered pathological.[31]

*** Practical Evidence**

A pronated foot type (FPI score of +7 to less than +10) is associated with less injury risk compared with a neutral foot type (FPI score of +1 to less than +7) in novice runners.[31] Children and older adults have more pronated feet than middle-aged adults. FPI scores create a U-shaped curve. In children, the FPI score is high, indicating a pronated foot. During early adulthood, the FPI score decreases, suggesting a more normal arch structure. Then, later in life, FPI scores increase.[31]

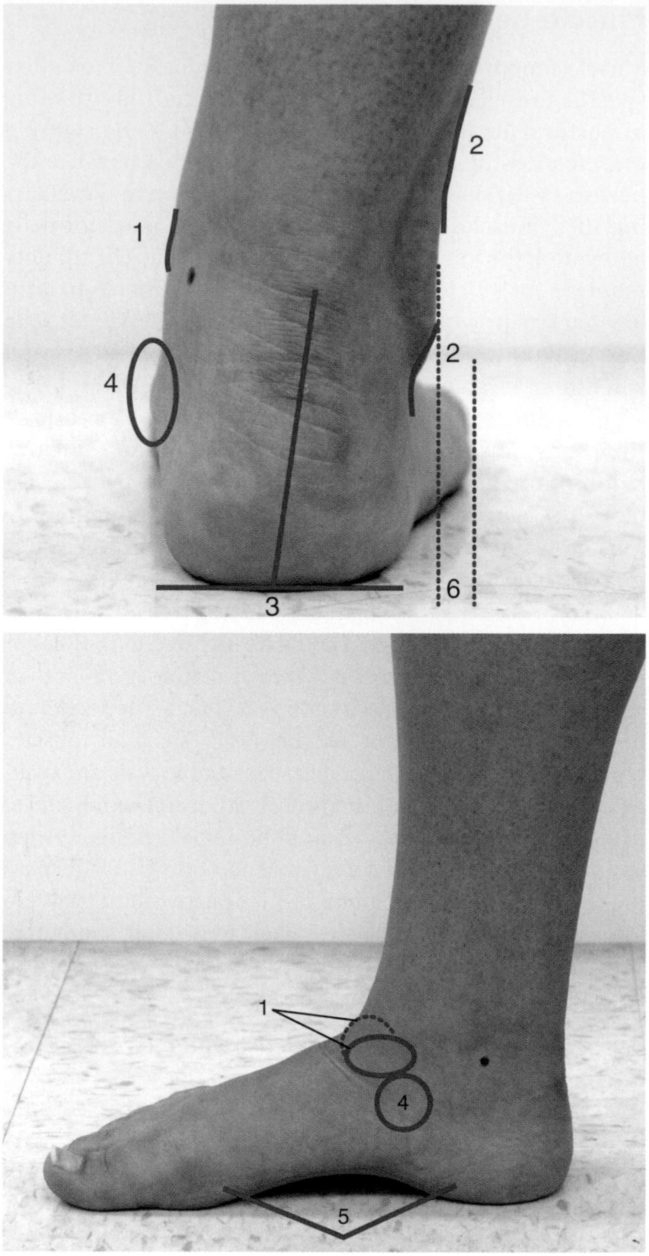

FIGURE 6-14 ■ Posterior view of a pronated foot as defined by the Foot Posture Index©. 1, talar navicular congruence; 2, inferior and superior lateral malleolar curves; 3, calcaneal frontal plane position; 4, bulging of the talonavicular joint; 5, height and congruence of the medial longitudinal arch; 6, forefoot abduction/adduction on the rearfoot.

The Knee

Alignment of the knee changes with age. Young children display a greater tibiofemoral angle than adults. The stressors introduced as the toddler transitions to walking change the knee from a varus alignment to a vertical alignment to a valgus alignment, gradually leading to a valgus alignment of less than 6 degrees by early adolescence.[32] See Inspection Findings 10-1 for more description of knee malalignments.

Genu Recurvatum

This postural deviation is noted when the knee's axis of motion is significantly posterior relative to the plumb line, the person has greater than 5 degrees of knee hyperextension as measured with a goniometer, or the hyperextension is asymmetrical. More pronounced in women, a person with genu recurvatum often stands with the knee(s) "locked" in an extreme extended position.[33] Genu recurvatum may be congenital or may be caused by pathology such as a combined tear of the anterior and posterior cruciate ligaments.

Genu Valgum

Genu valgum is a medial angulation of the femur and tibia occurring at the knee. Normally, a slight medial angulation

Muscle Length 6-1
Assessment of the Gastrocnemius

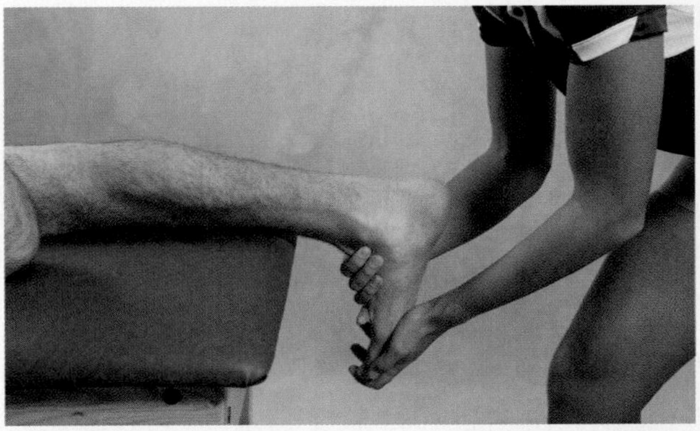

Patient Position	Prone with the foot off the edge of the table with the knee extended
Position of Examiner	One hand palpating the STJ The other hand grasping the foot
Evaluative Procedure	While maintaining the STJ in the neutral position, the ankle is taken into dorsiflexion. ROM can be measured goniometrically by placing the axis over the lateral malleolus, the distal arm aligned parallel to the bottom of the foot, and the proximal arm aligned with the fibula.
Positive Test	Less than 10° of dorsiflexion may affect normal walking gait; less than 15° of dorsiflexion may affect normal running gait.
Implications	Tightness of the gastrocnemius can create overuse pathology at the foot, ankle, and knee.
Possible Pathologies	Plantar fasciitis, Sever's disease, Achilles tendinopathy, calcaneal bursitis, patellofemoral pathology
Comments	The length of the soleus is assessed using dorsiflexion ROM with the knee flexed to at least 60°.
Evidence	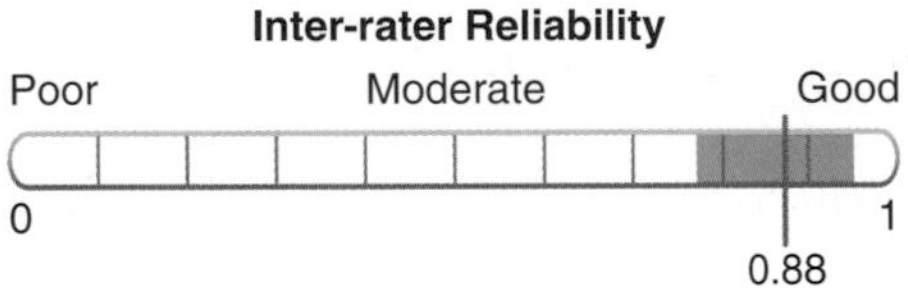

ROM = range of motion; STJ = subtalar joint

at the knee is present. However, with excessive genu valgum ("knock-kneed"), the knees are visibly closer together than the ankles during stance. Objectively measuring a person's Q angle determines whether excessive genu valgum is present (see Chapter 10).

Genu valgum occurs because of structural anomalies at the hip, contributing muscular weaknesses occurring at the hip, or secondary to excessively pronated feet. Genu valgum can lead to or result from a number of other different postural deviations in the lower extremity, such as, internal tibial rotation, medial patellar positioning, and internal femoral rotation.

Genu Varum

Genu varum ("bow-legged") is a lateral angulation of the femur and tibia occurring at the knee. The knees are farther apart than the ankles in standing. Genu varum occurs because of structural anomalies at the hip or from excessive supination of the feet. Other different postural deviations in the lower extremity can occur because of genu varum; these include external tibial rotation, lateral patellar positioning, and external femoral rotation. Participating in load-bearing sports during adolescence is associated with increased varus alignment, a predisposing factor to the later development of osteoarthritis.[34]

Muscle Length 6-2
Assessment of the Hamstring Group

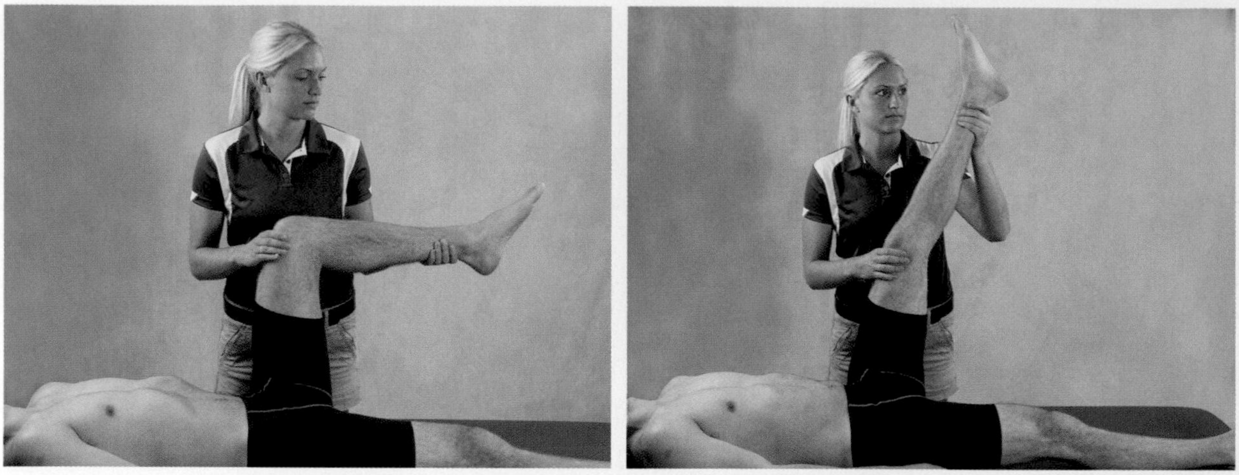

Patient Position	Supine
Position of Examiner	Standing at the side of the patient; the leg being assessed is placed in 90° of hip flexion and 90° of knee flexion (90/90 position)
Evaluative Procedure	The upper leg is stabilized in 90° of hip flexion, and the knee is extended.
Positive Test	Lacking more than 20° of full knee extension or asymmetry in movement
Implications	Tightness of the hamstrings may affect the knee, thigh, hip, and spine.
Possible Pathologies	Muscle tears, patellofemoral dysfunction, ischial tuberosity inflammation, low back dysfunction
Evidence	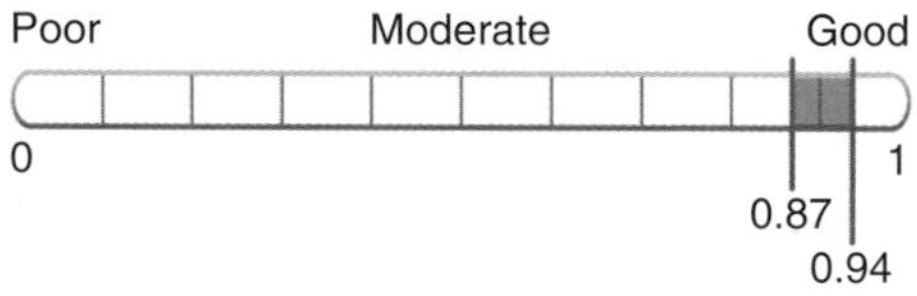

Spine and Pelvis

Hyperlordotic Posture

This postural deviation entails an increase in the lumbar lordosis without compensation in the thoracic or cervical spines (Inspection Findings 6-3). Increased lower lumbar lordosis (anterior convexity) may have been acquired secondary to adaptive shortening of the hip flexors, rotating the ilia anteriorly and pulling the lumbar spine anteriorly. A large anterior abdominal mass, including during pregnancy, obesity, poor postural awareness, ligamentous laxity, and muscle weakness may also increase lumbar lordosis.

Normally, there is an 8° to 10° angle between the ASIS and PSIS relative to horizontal. Anterior pelvic tilt is characterized by an angle greater than 10° between the ASIS and PSIS. Posterior pelvic tilt is marked by an angle less than 8° between the ASIS and PSIS.

Kypholordotic Posture

Kypholordotic posture is similar to hyperlordotic posture in that the patient has an increased lumbar lordosis; however, there is also a compensatory increase in thoracic **kyphosis** as an attempt to maintain the spine in a position of equilibrium (Inspection Findings 6-4). Kypholordotic posture increases the normal curvature in both the lumbar and thoracic spines. The lordosis cervical spine also increases, and a forward head posture (FHP) is assumed in an attempt to compensate for the other regions of the

Kyphosis Posterior curvature of the spine

Muscle Length 6-3
Assessment of the Rectus Femoris

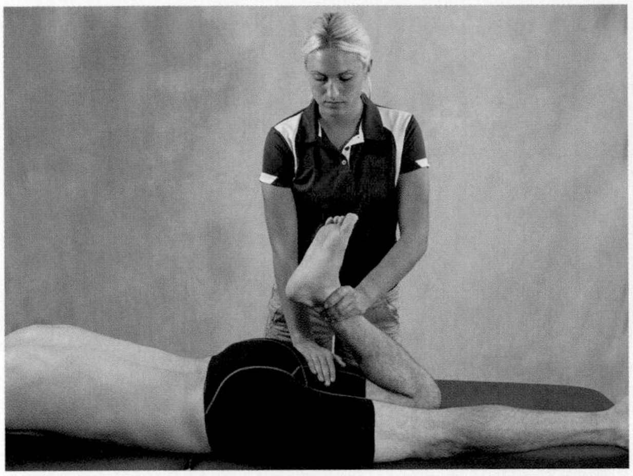

Patient Position	Prone
Position of Examiner	At the side of the patient
Evaluative Procedure	The knee is flexed. ROM can be measured using a goniometer with the axis placed over the lateral epicondyle, the distal arm aligned with the lateral malleolus, and the proximal arm aligned with the greater trochanter.
Positive Test	10° or greater difference as compared with the nonaffected side
Implications	Tightness of the quadriceps may affect the knee, thigh, hip, and spine.
Possible Pathologies	Muscle tears, patellofemoral dysfunction, low back dysfunction
Comments	This procedure is also known as Ely's test (see Chapter 13).
Evidence	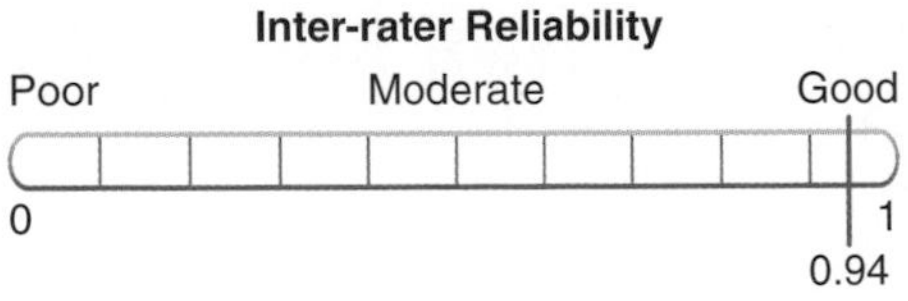

ROM = range of motion

spinal column. With this posture, adaptive changes in the lengths of the muscles can be observed throughout the entire trunk.

Swayback Posture
Swayback posture is marked by increased lumbar lordosis and thoracic kyphosis that cause the hips to extend. This creates a position of instability because the spinal column relies on ligaments rather than muscles for support (Inspection Findings 6-5). Swayback posture commonly is associated with an ectomorph or a lax ligamentous mesomorph body type. The joints are usually at the ends of their ranges, placing excessive strain on the surrounding ligamentous structures. In ideal posture, stability occurs because of a balance of static support from the ligamentous structures and dynamic support from surrounding muscles.

Flat Back Posture
An individual displaying a flat back posture has lost the normal "S"-shaped curvature of the spine in the sagittal plane (Inspection Findings 6-6). The thoracic and lumbar curvatures are decreased, and the spine is relatively straight. Often an associated FHP occurs to counteract the

Muscle Length 6-4
Assessment of the Shoulder Adductors

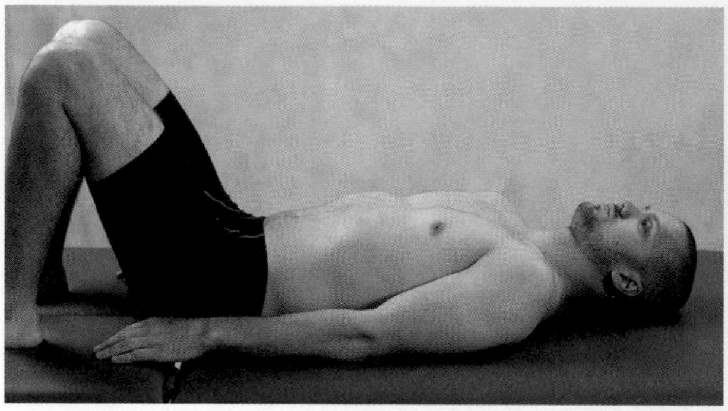

Starting Position

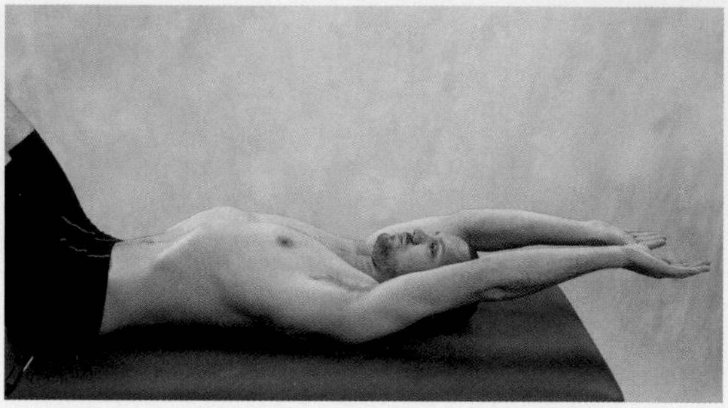

Ending Position

Patient Position	In the hook-lying position with the arms at the side
Position of Examiner	At the side of the patient
Evaluative Procedure	The patient flexes the shoulders above the head and attempts to place the arms on the table.
Positive Test	The patient cannot flex the arms above the head or the lumbar spine lifts off the table.
Implications	Shortness of the latissimus dorsi and teres major muscles
Evidence	Absent or inconclusive in the literature

Muscle Length 6-5
Assessment of the Pectoralis Major

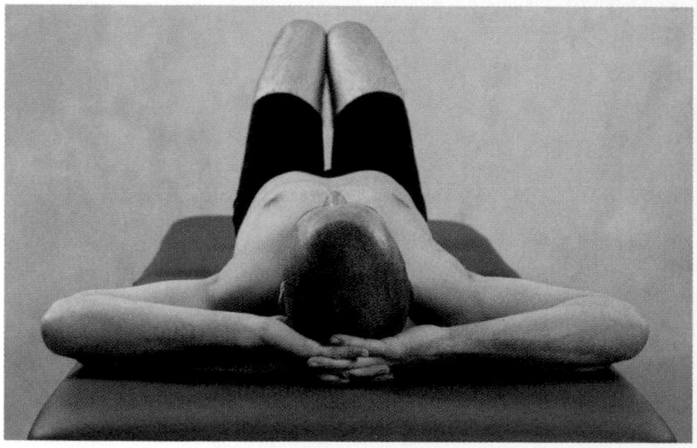

Normal Finding

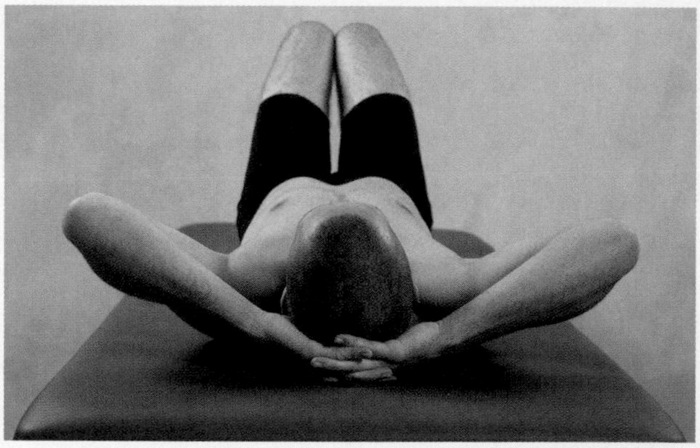

Positive Finding

Patient Position	In the hook-lying position with the arms abducted, externally rotated, with the elbows flexed and the hands locked behind the head
Position of Examiner	At the head of the patient
Evaluative Procedure	The patient attempts to position the elbows flat on the table.
Positive Test	The elbows do not rest on the table. To establish an objective baseline, measure (in centimeters) the distance from the posterior aspect of the acromion process to the tabletop.
Implications	Tight pectoralis major muscles may create rounded shoulders and subsequent FHP, although shortness of the pectoralis minor is most commonly implicated.
Evidence	Absent or inconclusive in the literature

FHP = forward head posture

Muscle Length 6-6
Assessment of the Pectoralis Minor

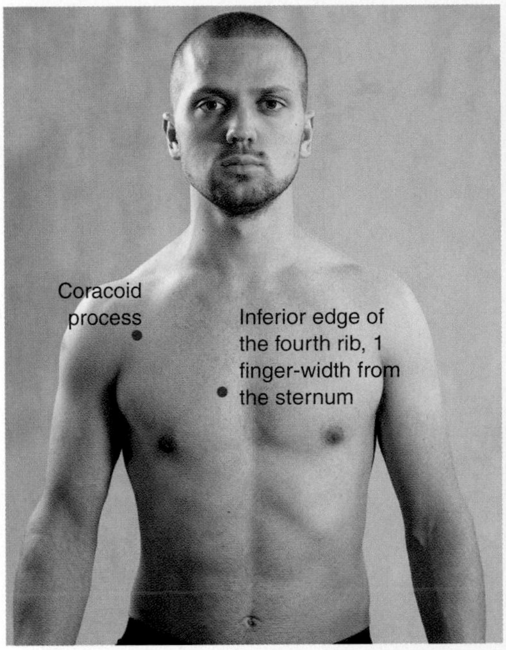

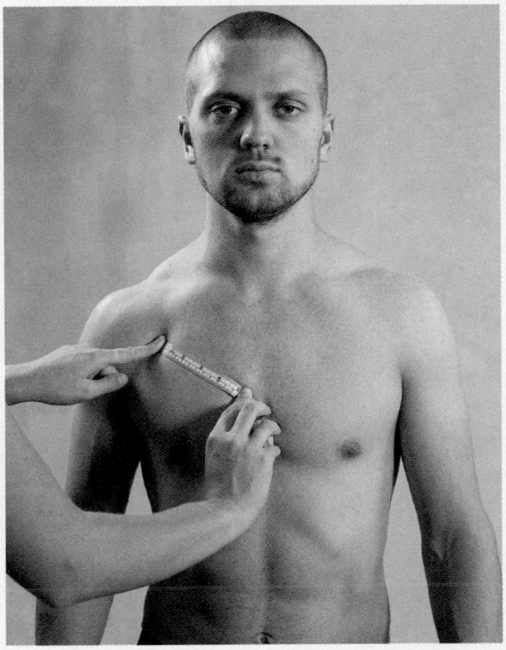

Patient Position	Seated or standing
Position of Examiner	At the side of the patient
Evaluative Procedure	Locate the coracoid process at its medial inferior border. Locate the 4th rib at its anterior inferior edge, 1 finger-width lateral to the sternum. Using a tape measure, measure the distance in centimeters between these two points.[26]
Positive Test	A side-to-side difference in length While normative values have not been established, a length of 14.1 cm has been considered normal, with a length of 8.1 cm considered pathological.[27]
Implications	Tight pectoralis minor muscles may create forward shoulder posture and contribute to FHP. Tight pectoralis minor muscles are associated with limited posterior tipping of the scapula and limited external rotation during elevation, both of which may contribute to the development of impingement.[26]
Evidence	ICC (compared with digitized measurement): 0.82-0.86[26]

FHP = forward head posture

Inspection Findings 6-3
Hyperlordotic Posture

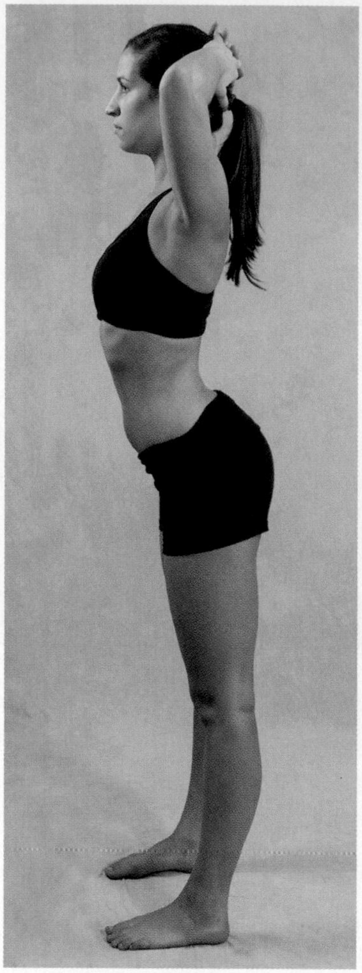

Observable Deviations	Increased lumbar lordosis Anterior pelvic tilt Hip assuming a slightly flexed position
Potential Causes	Tightened or shortened hip flexor muscles or back extensors Weakened or elongated hip extensors or abdominals Poor postural sense
Resulting Forces and Adaptations	Increased shear forces placed on lumbar vertebral bodies secondary to psoas tightness Increased compressive forces on lumbar facet joints Adaptive shortening of the posterior lumbar spine ligaments and the anterior hip ligaments Elongation of the anterior lumbar spine ligaments and the posterior hip ligaments Narrowing of the lumbar intervertebral foramen

Inspection Findings 6-4
Kypholordotic Posture

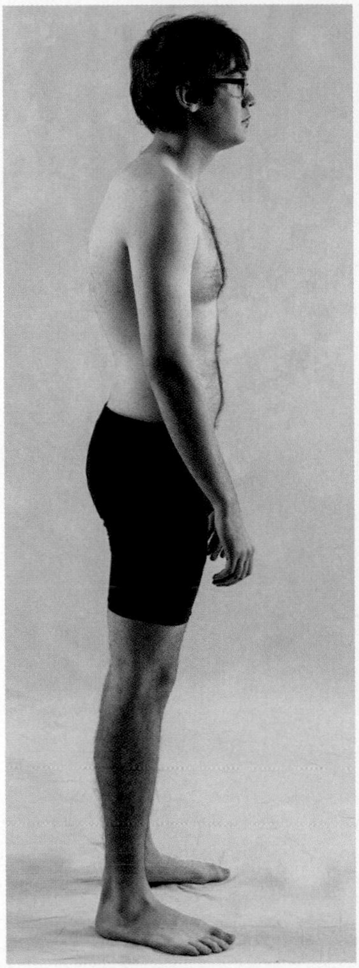

Observable Deviations	Anterior pelvic tilt Flexed hip joint Increased lumbar lordosis Increased thoracic kyphosis Commonly associated with FSP and FHP
Potential Causes	Poor postural sense Tightened or shortened hip flexors or back extensors Weakened or elongated hip extensors or trunk flexors
Resulting Forces and Adaptations	Adaptive shortening of anterior chest musculature Elongation of thoracic paraspinal musculature Increased tensile forces on ligamentous structures in posterior aspect of thoracic spine and anterior aspect of lumbar spine Increased compression of lumbar facet joints Increased compression of thoracic anterior vertebral bodies

FHP = forward head posture; FSP = forward shoulder posture

Inspection Findings 6-5
Swayback Posture

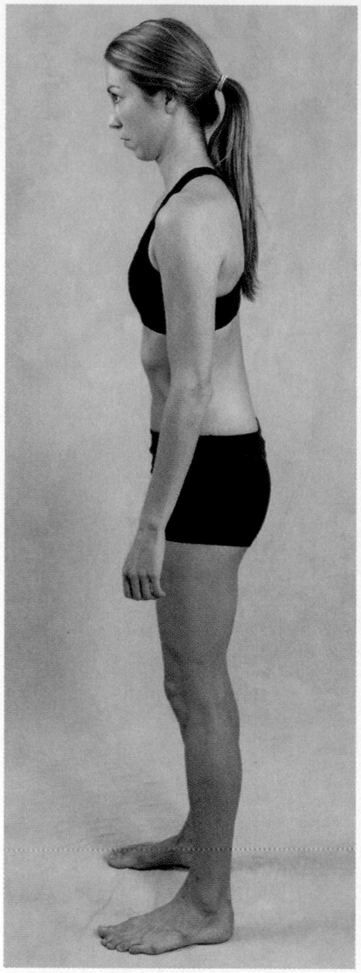

Observable Deviations	Genu recurvatum Extended hip joint Posterior pelvic tilt Anterior shift of the lumbosacral region Lumbar spine in neutral or minimal flexed position Increase in lower thoracic, thoracolumbar curvature (increase in lower thoracic kyphosis to cause posterior shift of trunk to compensate for anterior shift of L5/S1) Commonly associated with FSP and FHP
Potential Causes	Poor postural sense Tightened or shortened hip extensors Weakened or elongated hip flexors or lower abdominals Decreased general muscular strength
Resulting Forces and Adaptations	Elongation or increased tensile forces on the ligamentous structures at the anterior hip joint and posterior aspect of the lower thoracic spine Adaptively shortened or increased compressive forces on the posterior ligamentous structures at the hip joint and anterior aspect of the lower thoracic spine Increased tensile forces on the soft tissue structures of the posterior knee; compressive forces on anterior knee Increased shearing forces L5/S1

FHP = forward head posture; FSP = forward shoulder posture

Inspection Findings 6-6
Flat Back Posture

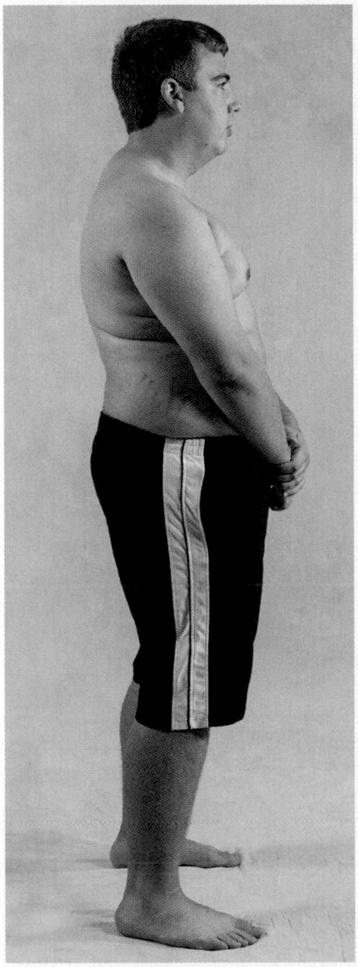

Observable Deviations	Extended hip joint Posterior pelvic tilt Decreased lumbar lordosis and lower thoracic kyphosis Increased upper thoracic kyphosis and cervical lordosis Commonly associated with FHP
Potential Causes	Shortened or tightened hip extensors, abdominal musculature Weakened/elongated hip flexors, back extensors Poor postural sense
Resulting Forces and Adaptations	Adaptive shortening of soft tissue and compressive forces in the posterior hip joint, anterior lumbar and lower thoracic regions, posterior upper thoracic and cervical regions, and upper chest region. Elongation of soft tissue and tensile forces on the anterior hip joint; posterior lumbar and lower thoracic regions, and anterior upper thoracic and cervical regions.

FHP = forward head posture

posterior displacement of the thoracic and lumbar spines. A decreased lumbar lordosis is associated with a posterior pelvic tilt.

Scoliosis

Scoliosis is a 3-dimensional deformity including torsion and lateral curvature of the spine and trunk (Inspection Findings 6-7). Scoliosis is named for the side of convexity and the region of the spine in which it is observed. There are two types of scoliosis: functional and structural. Functional scoliosis occurs because of extraspinal causes such as muscle imbalance, muscle guarding, or a limb-length discrepancy.[33] A structural scoliosis is caused by a defect or congenital bony anomaly of the vertebrae. A subcategory of structural scoliosis is **idiopathic** scoliosis. Idiopathic scoliosis affects up 2% to 3% of the population and females more often than males.[35] Idiopathic scoliosis is structural in nature but does not involve bony abnormalities of the vertebral body. Associated with "growth spurts," the exact cause of idiopathic scoliosis is multifactorial, with a genetic predisposition to the condition.[35] Only about 10% of those with idiopathic scoliosis have progressive deformities that require intervention such as therapeutic exercises or bracing.

To determine if a scoliosis is structural or functional, observe the patient's spine during erect posture and then while prone or in a forward flexed trunk posture (Adams forward bend test; see Selective Tissue Test 13-2). A structural scoliosis is present in both positions. In contrast, functional scoliosis is demonstrated only while the individual stands erect and disappears during spinal flexion. Patients with functional scoliosis must be further examined to determine the underlying cause. School screening for scoliosis in childhood is no longer recommended.[36] Referrals for school-detected scoliosis result in unnecessary radiographs and bracing, which has negative psychosocial consequences. The long-term consequences of most cases of untreated idiopathic scoliosis are minimal.[35]

Shoulder and Scapula

Forward Shoulder Posture

Forward shoulder posture (FSP) is characterized by the scapula resting in a protracted position (Inspection Findings 6-8). A shortened pectoralis minor and increased thoracic kyphosis are associated with this posture.[25,37] FSP often occurs concurrently with forward head posture.

When observed from the lateral view, FSP is associated with an anterior displacement of the acromion process in relation to the plumb line. Common causes of FSP include poor postural sense (i.e., a person assuming a "slouched" posture); adaptively shortened anterior chest muscles (particularly the pectoralis minor); associated elongation of the posterior interscapular muscles (lower and middle trapezius, rhomboids); and abnormal cervical and thoracic spine sagittal plane curvatures, altering the resting position of the scapula.[1,37]

*** Practical Evidence**

Functionally, FSP restricts scapular upward rotation, posterior tipping, and external rotation during elevation secondary to tightness of the pectoralis minor.[37] All of these mechanical changes decrease the subacromial space and predispose the patient to subacromial impingement.[37] In this case, interventions must emphasize restoring the proper length of the pectoralis minor.

Several consequences result from the presence of prolonged FSP. Biomechanical changes in the shoulder girdle can cause any number of the following soft tissue dysfunctions: degeneration of the acromioclavicular joint; bicipital or rotator cuff tendinopathy or impingement; muscular weakness; **myofascial** pain and trigger points; posterior capsular tightness; and abnormal scapulohumeral rhythm. They can be attributed to excessive and habitual flexion of the back.[38,39] Adaptive shortening of the pectoralis minor or the anterior and middle scalene muscles can compress the subclavian artery, vein, and medial cord of the brachial plexus, resulting in **thoracic outlet syndrome** (Chapter 14).[40] An FSP can also be associated with traction placed on the brachial plexus at the origin of the suprascapular and dorsal scapular nerves, causing associated pain and muscle weakness of the supraspinatus, infraspinatus, and rhomboids in which they innervate.[41]

Scapula Winging

Scapula winging, where the medial border projects posteriorly, can occur because of weakness of the periscapular muscles, especially the serratus anterior and middle and lower trapezius, and often occurs secondary to trauma to the long thoracic nerve. Winging is often more apparent with overhead movements. Scapula stabilization is essential for allowing normal arm mobility and biomechanics of the shoulder joint.

Head and Cervical Spine

Forward Head Posture

FHP, the anterior displacement of the head relative to the thorax, is a common postural deviation.[42] Observed from the lateral view, FHP is characterized by the external auditory meatus aligning anterior to the plumb line and anterior to the acromion process (Inspection Findings 6-9). This posture results in flexion of the lower cervical spine, flattening or flexion of the midcervical spine, and extension of the upper cervical spine (suboccipital region).

Causes of FHP include poor postural sense, use of bifocal lenses, muscle fatigue, FSP, and the need for glasses.[43] Several possible dysfunctions of the cervical spine, shoulder, temporomandibular joint, and general upper quadrant can occur as a result of FHP.[43,44] The head weighs approximately 13 lbs. Displacing this weight anteriorly on the cervical spine increases the amount of muscular activity in the posterior neck muscles and upper shoulder girdle muscles.[40]

Idiopathic Of unknown origin

Myofascial A muscle and its associated fascia

Inspection Findings 6-7
Scoliosis

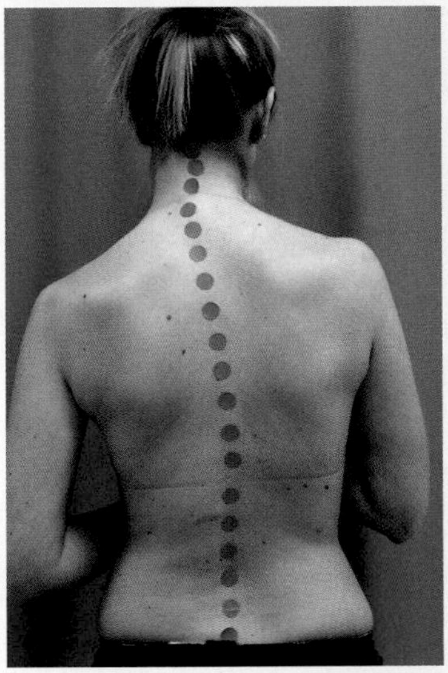

Left thoracic curve. Note the resulting asymmetrical scapular position.

Observable Deformity	Curvature of spine in frontal plane
Potential Causes	Structural scoliosis: Anomaly of vertebrae Functional scoliosis: Muscle imbalance, leg-length discrepancy
Resulting Forces and Adaptations	Compression of one facet joint; distraction of the opposite facet joint Shortened or tightened trunk muscles on concave side of the curvature Weakened or elongated trunk muscles on convex side of the curvature Decreased mobility of spine and chest cage Asymmetry in chest expansion with deep breathing Decreased pulmonary function (if excessive in thoracic region) Alteration of pattern of mechanical stresses on joint involved If caused by limb-length inequality: Degenerative changes in lumbar spine, hip, knee joints in longer limb Muscle overuse on longer limb caused by increased muscle activity Excessive pronation of longer limb with associated dysfunctions

FHP can also affect normal shoulder elevation. Elevation of the upper extremity requires cervical spine extension. If the middle and lower cervical spine remains in a flexed position, then full shoulder elevation cannot occur. Certain muscle imbalances also result when FHP occurs concurrently with FSP (Table 6-9). Normally, the external auditory meatus aligns with the acromion process of the shoulder. If the AC joint and external auditory meatus are in alignment, but both landmarks are forward of the plumb line, then both FSP and FHP are present.

Table 6-9 Combination of Forward Head Posture and Forward Shoulder Posture

Muscles That Become Overactivated and Tightened	Muscles That Become Inhibited and Weakened
Pectoralis minor	Lower trapezius
Pectoralis major	Middle trapezius
Upper trapezius	Serratus anterior
Upper rhomboids	
Levator scapulae	

Regional Interdependence

Because each body part is closely linked to corresponding body parts, it is difficult to determine whether poor postural habits cause impairments or whether the impairments were the cause and poor posture was the result (Table 6-10). It is more important to understand the relationship and importance of correcting these factors because it is impossible to determine which was the cause or the effect after the fact.

Inspection Findings 6-8
Forward Shoulder Posture

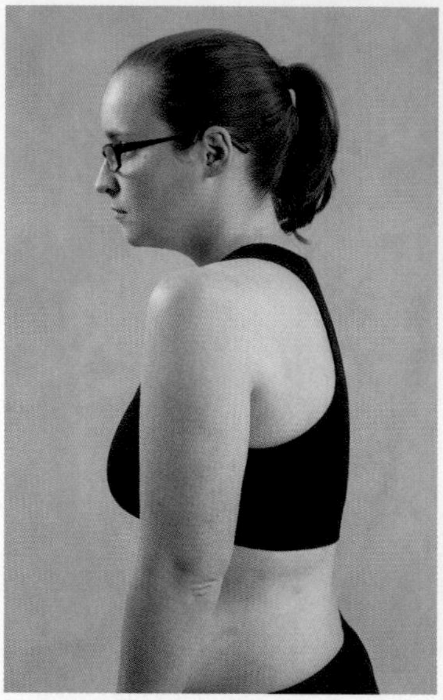

Observable Deformities	Humeral head anterior to line bisecting the body in the frontal plane Internal GH rotation Associated with FHP
Potential Causes	Shortened or overdeveloped anterior shoulder girdle muscles (primarily pectoralis minor) Weakened or elongated scapular stabilizing muscles (middle trapezius, rhomboid, lower trapezius) Poor postural awareness Abnormal cervical and thoracic spine sagittal plane alignments[37] Postural muscle fatigue Large breast development Repetitive occupational and sporting positions
Resulting Forces and Adaptations	Restricted scapular upward rotation, posterior tipping, and external rotation during elevation[37]

FHP = forward head posture; GH = glenohumeral

Postural assessment is an important part of the evaluation process. Recognizing postural faults that are contributing to activity limitations and participation restrictions and establishing a plan to work toward correcting or minimizing these faults is an essential role for a clinician. Most soft tissue dysfunctions that have a gradual, insidious onset have, at least, a minimal postural component. This postural component may result in or cause imbalances between agonist and antagonist muscle groups or **inert soft tissue** structures. Clinicians must learn to investigate and observe the entire body and the interrelationships between regions when evaluating a specific body part. Learning to look at the "whole picture" makes someone a more effective clinician and more successful in treating patients.

Documentation of Postural Assessment

Documentation of posture needs to be concise, yet as detailed as possible for the clinician to correlate possible postural impairments to the patient's functional limitations and disability. Table 6-11 presents a sample postural assessment that would be recorded in the impairment section of an initial evaluation. A sample of a standard postural assessment form is provided in Figure 6-15.

Inert soft tissue Noncontractile soft tissue, including the joint capsule and ligaments supporting the joint capsule

Inspection Findings 6-9
Forward Head Posture

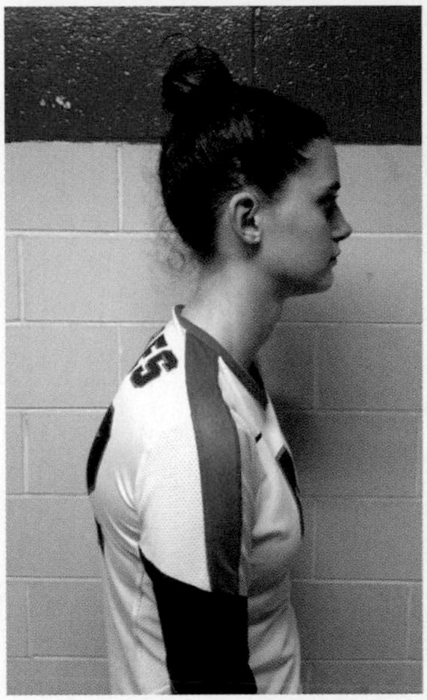

Observable Deformities	Flexed lower cervical spine Flattening or flexion of midcervical spine Extended upper cervical spine Associated with FSP
Potential Causes	Wearing of bifocals Poor eyesight and need for glasses Muscle fatigue and weakness Poor postural sense Compensatory mechanism for other postural deviations (occupational activities and ADLs)
Resulting Forces and Adaptations	Adaptively shortened suboccipital muscles (capital extensors), scalenes, upper trapezius, and levator scapulae Elongated and weakened anterior cervical flexors and scapular depressors Hypomobile upper cervical region with compensatory hypermobility of the midcervical spine Abnormal shoulder (GH joint) biomechanics; decrease in shoulder elevation Decreased cervical range of motion[42]

ADLs = activities of daily living; FSP = forward shoulder posture; GH = glenohumeral

Table 6-10 Regional Interdependence in Weight Bearing

Structure or Interconnecting Joints	Position of One Joint or Structure	Effect of Position of Other Joint or Structure
STJ and Tibia	STJ pronated	Tibia internally rotated
	STJ supinated	Tibia externally rotated
Tibia and Femur	Internal tibial rotation	Femur internally rotated
	External tibial rotation	Femur externally rotated
Tibiofemoral Joint and the Talocrural Joint	Knee joint flexed, decreasing the angle between the tibia and foot	Talocrural joint dorsiflexed
	Knee joint hyperextended, increasing the angle between the tibia and foot	Talocrural joint plantarflexed
Femur and Tibia	Femoral anteversion	Tibia internally rotated*
	Femoral retroversion	Tibia externally rotated*
Femur and Patella	Internal femoral rotation	Squinting patellae
	External femoral rotation	Frog-eye patellae
Pelvic Position and the Hip Joint	Pelvis in an anterior pelvic tilt, decreasing the angle between the pelvis and femur	Hip flexed
	Pelvis in a posterior pelvic tilt, increasing the angle between the pelvis and femur	Hip extended
Position of the Pelvis and the Lumbar Spine	Pelvis in an anterior pelvic tilt, flexing the sacrum (nutation) and extending the lumbar spine	Increased lumbar lordosis
	Pelvis in a posterior pelvic tilt, extending the sacrum (counternutation) and flexing the lumbar spine	Decreased lumbar lordosis

*A developmental compensation for femoral anteversion is tibia external rotation of the tibia to maintain the feet positioned straight ahead.
STJ = subtalar joint

Table 6-11 Documentation of Impairments Identified in a Full Postural Assessment

View	Characteristics
Anterior	Minimal pes planus bilateral feet
	Moderate bilateral squinting patellae
	Moderate bilateral genu valgum
	Minimal increase in right ASIS height
	Minimal bilateral internal rotation shoulder, right greater than left
Posterior	Minimal bilateral calcaneal valgum
	Moderate bilateral genu valgum
	Minimal decrease in right PSIS height
	Minimal bilateral protraction scapulae, right greater than left
Right Lateral	Minimal genu recurvatum
	Moderate anterior pelvic tilt, 20°
	Minimal increase in lumbar lordosis
	Minimal FHP
Left Lateral	Moderate genu recurvatum
	Moderate anterior pelvic tilt, 20°
	Minimal increase in lumbar lordosis
	Minimal FHP

ASIS = anterior superior iliac spine; FHP = forward head posture; PSIS = superior posterior iliac spine

The following are guidelines for documenting posture:

- Document the view that is being observed (i.e., anterior, posterior, right lateral, left lateral).
- Quantify each postural deficit using minimum, moderate, or severe and, whenever possible, objectively measure the deficits. When measuring the deficit, note the specific landmarks used, specific positions measured, or any specific techniques used to measure them. This will assist in reproducibility of the measurement.
- Document the side of the body where the deficit occurs. If it involves unequal heights, choose whether to document the higher or lower side and then be consistent with your documentation.
- To avoid medical transcription errors, do not use abbreviations.
- Document in an outline form (rather than paragraph form) to make the assessment easier to read and to identify specific regions quickly.
- Document only postural deficits in the assessment. Identify normal regions as within normal limits.
- Use an asterisk (*) to emphasize a significant finding by placing the * beside the deficit.
- When evaluating an upper quarter condition, include the pelvis, lumbar spine, and all joints proximal to the injury in the postural assessment.

Standard Postural Assessment Form

Name: ______________________

Clinician: ______________________

ANTERIOR VIEW

Alignment of plumb line with trunk: ______________________

Alignment of plumb line with head: ______________________

Calluses, bunions, blisters on feet: ______________________

Lower Extremity

Arch Position:	□ pes planus	□ pes cavus	□ neutral
Subtalar Joint:	□ pronated	□ supinated	□ neutral
Tibia Position:	□ medial rotation	□ lateral rotation	□ neutral
Patella Position	□ squinting	□ frog-eyed	□ neutral
Leg Position:	□ genu valgum	□ genu varum	□ neutral

Q-angle: □ left: □ right:

Muscle mass/girth comments: ______________________

Other comments: ______________________

____

Pelvis/Trunk

Iliac crest symmetry: ______________________

ASIS symmetry: ______________________

Abdominal muscle mass: ______________________

Chest Shape: □ pectus excavatum □ pectus recurvatum □ normal

Shoulder Girdle, Cervical Spine, and Head

Shoulder Position:	□ internally rotated	□ externally rotated	□ neutral
Shoulder Heights:	□ right elevated right	□ depressed	□ neutral
Head Position:	□ side bent	□ rotated	□ neutral

Pectoral muscle mass: ______________________

Upper trapezius muscle mass: ______________________

Painful area: ______________________

Date: ____________

POSTERIOR VIEW

Alignment of plumb line with trunk: ______________________

Alignment of plumb line with head: ______________________

Note calluses, blisters on heels: ______________________

Lower Extremity

Calcaneal Position:	□ genu valgum	□ genu varum	□ neutral
Leg Position:	□ genu valgum	□ genu varum	□ neutral

Muscle mass calves: ______________________

Muscle mass posterior thighs: ______________________

Pelvis/Trunk

Spinal Alignment: □ scoliosis □ neutral

Iliac crest symmetry: ______________________

PSIS symmetry: ______________________

Gluteal muscle mass: ______________________

Shoulder Girdle, Cervical Spine, and Head

Scapula Positions: ______________________

Elevation/depression: ______________________

Protraction/retraction: ______________________

Upward/downward Rotation: ______________________

Winging: ______________________

Periscapula muscle mass: ______________________

Upper trapezius muscle mass: ______________________

Shoulder height: ______________________

Head Position: □ side bent □ rotated □ neutral

Duration of symptoms (months): ________

LATERAL VIEW: RIGHT or LEFT (circle which):

Note alignment of following structures relative to plumb line:

Lat. Malleolus:	□ anterior	□ posterior	□ bisecting
Talocrural Joint:	□ plantarflexed	□ dorsiflexed	□ neutral
Lat. Femoral Epicondyle:	□ anterior	□ posterior	□ bisecting
Knee Position:	□ flexed	□ extended	□ neutral
Greater Trochanter:	□ anterior	□ posterior	□ bisecting
Mid-Thorax:	□ anterior	□ posterior	□ bisecting
Acromion Process:	□ anterior	□ posterior	□ bisecting
Cervical Vertebral Bodies:	□ anterior	□ posterior	□ bisecting
External Auditory Meatus:	□ anterior	□ posterior	□ bisecting
Pelvic Position:	□ ant. rotation	□ post. rotation	□ neutral
Shoulder Position:	□ forward	□ neutral	
Head Position:	□ forward	□ neutral	

Lumbar Spine Position: ______________________

Thoracic Spine Position: ______________________

Cervical Spine Position: ______________________

Shoulder/Head: ______________________

LATERAL VIEW: RIGHT or LEFT (circle which):

Note alignment of following structures relative to plumb line:

Lat. Malleolus:	□ anterior	□ posterior	□ bisecting
Talocrural Joint:	□ plantarflexed	□ dorsiflexed	□ neutral
Lat. Femoral Epicondyle:	□ anterior	□ posterior	□ bisecting
Knee Position:	□ flexed	□ extended	□ neutral
Greater Trochanter:	□ anterior	□ posterior	□ bisecting
Mid-Thorax:	□ anterior	□ posterior	□ bisecting
Acromion Process:	□ anterior	□ posterior	□ bisecting
Cervical Vertebral Bodies:	□ anterior	□ posterior	□ bisecting
External Auditory Meatus:	□ anterior	□ posterior	□ bisecting
Pelvic Position:	□ ant. rotation	□ post. rotation	□ neutral
Shoulder Position:	□ forward	□ neutral	
Head Position:	□ forward	□ neutral	

Lumbar Spine Position: ______________________

Thoracic Spine Position: ______________________

Cervical Spine Position: ______________________

Shoulder/Head: ______________________

FIGURE 6-15 ■ Standard postural assessment form

- When evaluating a lower quarter condition, include the lumbar spine, pelvis, and all joints distal to the painful site in the postural assessment.
- Include the entire body in the postural assessment of a patient with a spinal injury.

REFERENCES

1. Kendall, FP, et al: *Muscles: Testing and Function, with Posture and Pain*, ed 5. Baltimore, MD: Lippincott Williams & Wilkins, 2005.
2. Kisner, C, and Colby, LA: *Therapeutic Exercise: Foundations and Techniques*, ed 5. Philadelphia, PA: FA Davis, 2007.
3. Norkin, CC: Posture. In Levangie, PK, and Norkin, CC (eds): *Joint Structure and Function: A Comprehensive Analysis*, ed 5. Philadelphia, PA: FA Davis, 2011, pp 483-523.
4. Rieger-Krugh, C, and Keysor, JJ: Skeletal malalignments of the lower quarter: Correlated and compensatory motions and postures. *J Orthop Sports Phys Ther*, 23:164, 1996.
5. Ludwig, PM, Reynolds, JR: The association of scapular kinematics and glenohumeral joint pathologies. *J Orthop Sports Phys Ther*, 39:90, 2009.
6. Houglum, PA: Muscle Strength and Endurance. In *Therapeutic Exercise for Musculoskeletal Injuries*. Champaign, IL: Human Kinetics, 2010, pp 199-251.
7. Massie, DL, and Haddox, A: Influence of lower extremity biomechanics and muscle imbalances on the lumbar spine. *Athl Ther Today*, 4:46, 1999.
8. Whilt, SG, and Sahrmann, SA: A movement system approach to management of musculoskeletal pain. In Grant, R: *Clinics in Physical Therapy: Physical Therapy of the Cervical and Thoracic Spine*. New York, NY: Churchill Livingstone, 1994.
9. Chleboun G. Muscle Structure and Function. In Levangie, PK, and Norkin, CC (eds): *Joint Structure and Function: A Comprehensive Analysis*, ed 5. Philadelphia, PA: FA Davis, 2011, pp 483-523.
10. Houvet, P, and Obert, L: Upper limb cumulative trauma disorders for the orthopaedic surgeon. *Orthop Traumatol Surg Res*, 99S:S104, 2013.
11. Fortin, C, et al: Clinical methods for quantifying body segment posture: A literature review. *Disabil Rehabil*, 33:367, 2011.
12. Heuscher, Z, et al: The association of self-reported backpack use and backpack weight with low back pain among college students. *J Manipulative Physiol Ther*, 33:432, 2010.
13. Skaggs, DL, et al: Back pain and backpacks in school children. *J Pediatr Orthop*, 26:358, 2006.
14. Gilson, ND, et al: Does the use of standing 'hot' desks change sedentary work time in an open plan office? *Prev Med*, 54:65, 2012.
15. Jacobson, BH, Boolani, A, and Smith, DB: Changes in back pain, sleep quality, and perceived stress after introduction of new bedding systems. *J Chiropr Med*, 8:1, 2009.
16. Ehrman, JK: *ACSM's Resource Manual for Guidelines for Exercise Testing and Prescription*, ed 6. Philadelphia, PA: Lippincott Williams & Wilkins, 2010, pp 266-277.
17. Turocy, PS, et al: National Athletic Trainers' Association position statement: safe weight loss and maintenance practices in sport and exercise. *J Athl Train*, 46:322, 2011.
18. Sabharwal, S, and Kumar, A: Methods for assessing leg length discrepancy. *Clin Orthop Relat Res*, 466:2910, 2008.
19. Gurney, B: Leg length discrepancy. *Gait Posture*, 15:195, 2002.
20. Raczkowski, JW, Daniszewska, B, and Zolynski, K: Functional scoliosis caused by leg length discrepancy. *Arch Med Sci*, 6:393, 2010.
21. Defrin, R, et al: Conservative correction of leg-length discrepancies of 10 mm or less for the relief of chronic low back pain. *Arch Phys Med Rehabil*, 86:2075, 2005.
22. Stovall, BA, and Kumar, S: Anatomical landmark asymmetry assessment in the lumbar spine and pelvis: a review of reliability. *PMR*, 2:48, 2010.
23. Krawiec, CJ, et al: Static innominate asymmetry and leg length discrepancy in asymptomatic collegiate athletics. *Man Ther*, 8:207, 2003.
24. Levangie, PK: The association between static pelvic asymmetry and low back pain. *Spine*, 24:1234, 1999.
25. Struyf, F: Clinical assessment of the scapula: A review of the literature. *Br J Sports Med*, 2012. [Epub ahead of print].
26. Borstad, JD. Measurement of pectoralis minor muscle length: Validation and clinical application. *J Orthop Sports Phys Ther*, 38:169, 2008.
27. Borstad, JD, and Ludewig, PM: The effect of long versus short pectoralis minor resting length on scapular kinematics in healthy individuals. *J Orthop Sports Phys Ther*, 35:227, 2005.
28. Keenan, A, et al: The Foot Posture Index: Rasch analysis of a novel, foot-specific outcome measure. *Arch Phys Med Rehabil*, 88:88, 2007.
29. Redmond, AC, Crossbie, J, and Ouvrier, RA: Development and validation of a novel rating system for scoring standing foot posture: the Foot Posture Index. *Clin Biomech*, 21:89, 2006.
30. Redmond, A: The Foot Posture Index© . Easy quantification of standing foot posture. Six item version FPI-6. User's guide and manual. 2005. Retrieved from http://www.leeds.ac.uk/medicine/FASTER/z/pdf/FPI-manual-formatted-August-2005v2.pdf. (Accessed August 22, 2013).
31. Redmond, AC, Crane, YZ, and Menz, HB: Normative values for the Foot Posture Index. *J Foot Ankle Res*, 1:6, 2008.
32. Yates, B, and White, S: The incidence and risk factors in the development of medial tibial stress syndrome among naval recruits. *AJSM*, 32:772, 2004.
33. Medina McKeon, JM, and Hertel J: Sex differences and representative values for 6 lower extremity alignment measures. *J Athl Train*, 44:249, 2009.
34. Thijs, Y, et al: Is high-impact sports participation associated with bowlegs in adolescent boys? *Med Sci Sports Exerc*, 44:993, 2012.
35. Negrini, S, et al. 2011 SOSORT guidelines: orthopaedic and rehabilitation treatment of idiopathic scoliosis during growth. *Scoliosis*, 7:3, 2012.
36. U.S. Preventive Services Task Force: Screening for idiopathic scoliosis in adolescents: recommendation statement. *Am Fam Physician*, 71:1975, 2005.
37. Borstad, JD: Resting position variables at the shoulder: evidence to support a posture-impairment association. *Phys Ther*, 86:549, 2006.
38. Ayub, E: Posture and the upper quarter. In Donatelli, RA (ed): *Physical Therapy of the Shoulder*, ed 2. New York, NY: Churchill Livingstone, 1991.
39. Greenfield, B, et al: Posture in patients with shoulder overuse injuries and healthy individuals. *J Orthop Sports Phys Ther*, 21:287, 1995.
40. Langford, ML: Poor posture subjects a worker's body to muscle imbalance, nerve compression. *Occup Health Saf*, 63:38, 1994.
41. Howell, JW: Evaluation and management of thoracic outlet syndrome. In Donatelli, RA (ed): *Physical Therapy of the Shoulder*, ed 2. New York, NY: Churchill Livingstone, 1991.
42. De-la-Llave-Rincón, AI, et al: Increased forward head posture and restricted cervical range of motion in patients with carpal tunnel syndrome. *J Orthop Sports Phys Ther*, 39:658, 2009.
43. Garrett, TR, Youdas, JW, and Madison, TJ: Reliability of measuring forward head posture in a clinical setting. *J Orthop Sports Phys Ther*, 17:155, 1993.
44. Harrison, AL, Barry-Greb, T, and Wojtowicz, G: Clinical measurement of head and shoulder posture variables. *J Orthop Sports Phys Ther*, 23:353, 1996.

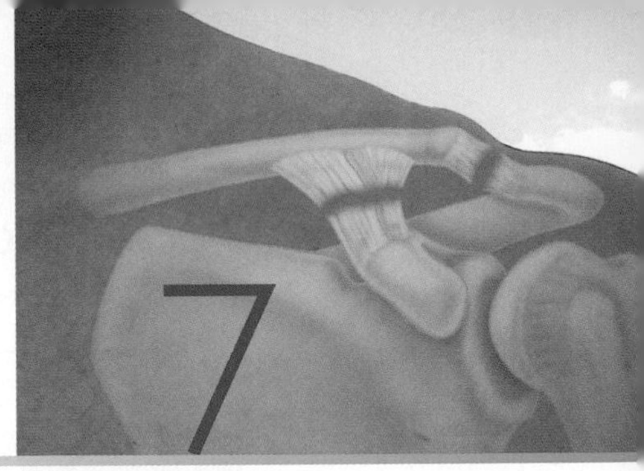

CHAPTER 7

Evaluation of Gait

Monique Mokha, PhD, ATC, LAT

Gait is the manner in which a person walks or runs. As a key component of the assessment of patient function, gait evaluation can provide diagnostic information about underlying conditions such as functional ankle instability, traumatic brain injury, and low back pain that disrupt these factors.

Observational Gait Analysis

Gait can be evaluated qualitatively or quantitatively. In settings where clinicians are professionally trained in gait analysis, these two techniques are combined to yield comprehensive results that serve as the basis for intervention planning. This chapter focuses on qualitative evaluation using observational gait analysis (OGA) (Box 7-1).

OGA is a functional evaluation of a person's walking or running style where gait deviations are identified from gross observation. Several tools have been developed to guide and organize an OGA such as Rancho Los Amigos Medical Center's *Observational Gait Analysis Handbook*[1] and the Rivermead Visual Gait Assessment (RVGA).[2] The patient is asked to walk and/or run with and without shoes on a treadmill or in a designated area. Although this is the most common[3] method of gait analysis, it has poor to moderate intrarater reliability.[4] Reliability improves with training, experience, by using recorded video that can replay and slow motion, and by using a specific observational tool (Fig. 7-1).

*** Practical Evidence**

Using a formal approach to an OGA recorded on a structured form improves reliability.[2]

OGA tools may be helpful to identify gross gait abnormalities such as those associated with neurological disorders (e.g., stroke, Parkinson's disease); however, these tools lack the sensitivity needed to document subtle gait deviations.

Box 7-1
Observational Gait Analysis

Using an OGA written tool, the presence or absence of the critical events in the gait cycle can be determined. When preparing for your analysis, refer to the following OGA guidelines:

1. Prepare the area and materials ahead of time.
2. Avoid clutter in the viewing background.
3. Have the patient wear clothing that does not restrict viewing of joints.
4. Ensure that the patient is at a self-selected walking pace; otherwise, gait will be altered.
5. Position yourself so you can view the individual segments (i.e., if you are observing for forefoot pronation and supination, then squat down so your eyes are in line with the patient's feet).
6. Observe the subject from multiple views (anterior, posterior, and both lateral views) but not from an oblique angle.
7. Look at the individual body parts first, then the whole body, then the individual parts again.
8. Conduct multiple observations or trials.
9. Conduct the analysis with the patient barefoot and wearing shoes.
10. Label all video files.

Observational Gait Analysis Model

STRENGTH (MMT and Functional)

	Quads	Hams	Hip IR	Hip ER	TA	TP	Peroneals	Gastroc	Core Squat
R	/5	/5	/5	/5	/5	/5	/5	/5	
L	/5	/5	/5	/5	/5	/5	/5	/5	

FLEXIBILITY

	RF (Kendall)	Iliopsoas (Thomas)	Hams (deg)	Gastroc (deg)	IT Band (Ober's)
R					
L					

NON–WEIGHT BEARING ALIGNMENT

	Rearfoot	Forefoot	Hallux	Toes	Med Long Arch	LLD	Callus location
R	□ valgus □ varus	□ valgus □ varus	□ valgus □ bunion	□ claw □ hammer	□ planus □ cavus		
L	□ valgus □ varus	□ valgus □ varus	□ valgus □ bunion	□ claw □ hammer	□ planus □ cavus		

FUNCTIONAL STANDING ALIGNMENT

Navicular Drop (mm)	Toe Raise*	SL Squat*	DBL Squat*
R L	R L	R L	

*assess and document stability and/or alignment changes during test

STANDING POSTURE & ALIGNMENT (FRONTAL PLANE)

Achilles	Toe In/Out	Knee (valgus/varus)	Popliteal Creases	Iliac Crests (level, rotation)	Shoulders (level)
□ valgus □ R □ L □ varus □ R □ L	□ in □ R □ L □ out □ R □ L □ WNL	□ valgus □ varum □ recurvatum □ WNL	□ level □ uneven	□ level □ R > L □ L > R	□ level □ R > L □ L > R

STANDING POSTURE & ALIGNMENT (SAGITTAL PLANE)

Knee (recurvatum)	Lumbar	Thoracic	Shoulders	Cervical
□ yes □ no	□ lordosis □ flat	□ kyphosis	□ rounded	□ excessive lordosis

FIGURE 7-1 ■ Sample observational gait analysis tool.

For example, a small amount of toeing out might qualify as "unremarkable" on the Los Ranchos Amigos or RVGA OGA instruments, yet, in an athletic patient performing repetitive, high-force movements, this could be a significant finding. Additionally, an OGA tool used for walking gait must be adapted to use with running. The differences between running and walking are discussed later in this chapter.

Gait changes can be caused by acute injury, chronic conditions, or improper biomechanics. The resulting gait deviations may have a subtle or dramatic presentation. Consider, for example, an athlete who limps off the basketball court after suffering an ankle sprain. Because of pain and/or instability, we observe that the athlete quickly pulls the foot off the ground (decreased stance time), takes short steps, and does not dorsiflex his ankle. This, in turn, alters the mechanics of the knee, the hip, and possibly the lumbar spine.

Theoretically, when acute trauma is resolved, normal gait should return. Chronic conditions (e.g., peroneal tendinopathy) or congenital abnormalities (e.g., tarsal coalition) can permanently alter gait. Consequently, altered stresses caused by improper biomechanics may lead to injury or pain along the kinetic chain. An analysis of running gait is critical in the athletic patient as improper biomechanics may amplify from walking to running. This analysis also yields more sport-specific information.

The results of the OGA are combined and compared with the results from the remainder of the clinical examination. The patient is examined to identify underlying impairments that might result in the abnormal gait patterns. For example, a limitation in dorsiflexion may cause an early heel raise. A meaningful OGA requires a keen eye, guided practice, a planned system of observation, and a detailed understanding of the components of walking and running gait.

Gait Terminology

Reliable OGA is rooted in well-defined standard terminology. The functional unit of gait is the **gait cycle**, or stride, consisting of two successive steps. We typically focus our analysis on a single gait cycle with the reasonable assumption that it will represent the patient's general gait. Spatial (space) and temporal (time) variables such as step length, step width, stride length, foot angle, cadence, velocity, and comfortable walking speed are measurable variables of the gait cycle that provide information of function. Boxes 7-2 and 7-3 present the definitions, expected findings (normative values), and the clinical significance of these variables.

Walking Gait Phases

There are two prerequisites for walking: (1) the person must periodically move the foot from one position of support to the next, and (2) the person must be able to produce sufficient **ground reaction forces** (GRFs) to support the body. Because walking gait is a cyclic function, each leg alternates between a supportive (stance) and a nonsupportive (swing) phase (Fig. 7-2). While one leg is in the stance phase, the

Box 7-2
Common Spatial Gait Terminology

	Definition	Significance	Adult Norm
Step Length 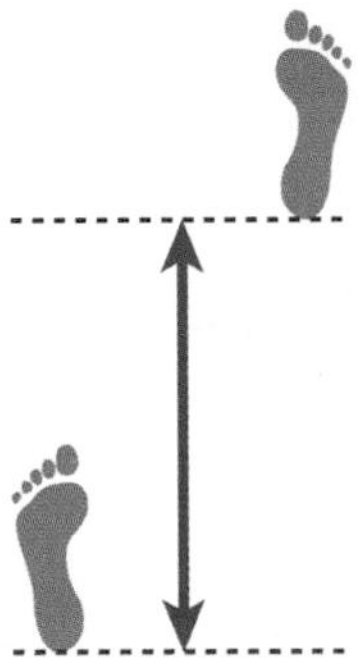	Linear distance between successive points of contact of contralateral feet	Should be symmetrical right to left; shortens in attempt to decrease contact time; shortens on one side with limb injury or pain; shortens bilaterally with injury (e.g., low back pain) or complex disorders such as multiple sclerosis; increases typically as velocity increases	75 ± 1.6 cm[5]
Step Width 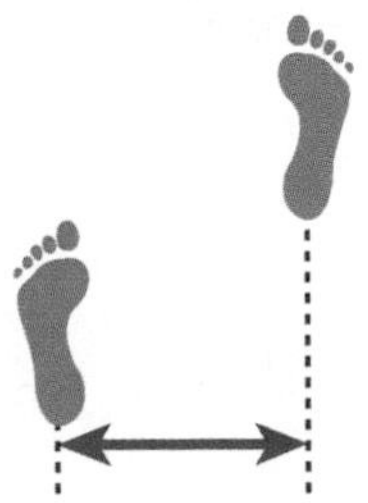	Mediolateral distance between successive points of contact of contralateral feet	A function of balance; if increased, suspect pathology (e.g., traumatic brain injury, tight hip abductors, inner ear infection); decreases typically as velocity increases and may even see a crossover	8.2 ± 0.8 cm[5]

Continued

Box 7-2
Common Spatial Gait Terminology—cont'd

	Definition	Significance	Adult Norm
Stride Length 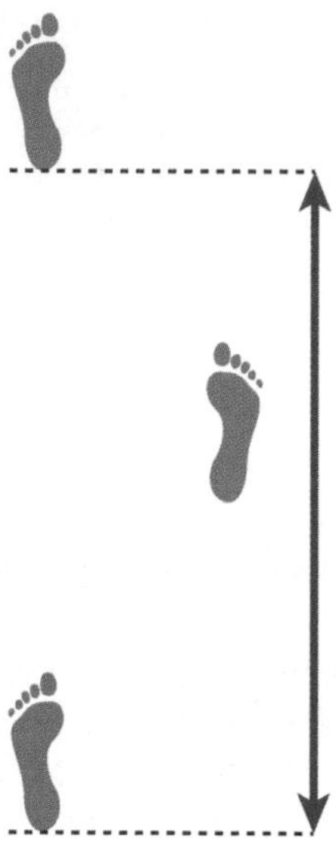	Linear distance between points of contact of ipsilateral foot; length of two sequential steps	See step length	150 ± 3.2 cm[5]
Foot Angle 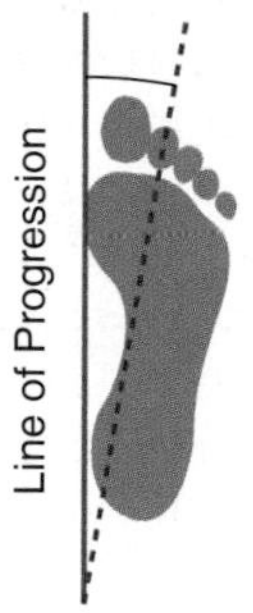	Angle of the foot (imaginary line from heel to second toe) relative to the line of progression	Negative value can indicate internal rotation (toeing in), and positive value can indicate external rotation (toeing out) of the lower extremity during stance	+10 degrees indicating slight external rotation is normal

Box 7-3
Common Temporal Gait Terminology

	Definition	Significance	Adult Norm
Cadence	Walking rate measured in the number of steps per minute	Slow <70 steps/min Fast >120 steps/min	107 ± 2.7 steps/min[5]
Velocity	Distance walked per unit time such as meters or centimeters per second	Overall predictor of functional disability	140 ± 4.8 cm/s[5]
Comfortable Walking Speed	"Free speed," or the speed selected by the patient that feels most natural	The speed that expends the least amount of energy; decreases with age	80 m/min
Stance Time	Amount of time spent in contact with surface by single limb	Increases at slower walking velocities; decreases with faster walking velocities; decreases on side with limb pain	~ 60% of total gait cycle

Box 7-3
Common Temporal Gait Terminology—cont'd

	Definition	Significance	Adult Norm
Swing Time	Amount of time spent not in contact with surface by single limb	Increases with faster velocities	~ 40% of total gait cycle
Double Support Time	Amount of time spent in contact with surface by both limbs simultaneously; occurs at two time intervals during stance phase: (1) when right limb makes initial contact and left limb is in preswing (2) when right limb is in preswing and left limb makes initial contact	Increases at slower walking velocities; decreases with faster walking velocities	Each double support occurrence constitutes ~ 10% total stance time (20% of total gait cycle)

other leg is in the swing phase. At two points in the gait cycle, midstance and terminal stance, the body is supported by a single limb. At two points in the gait cycle, initial contact and preswing, the body is supported by both limbs. Three basic functional tasks are accomplished in the gait cycle: weight acceptance, single-limb support, and limb advancement. These tasks are further broken down into the events that occur within the stance and swing phases below.

Efficient gait incorporates minimal upward and side-to-side motion of the body's **center of mass** (COM). The patient's COM travels along a smooth, sinusoidal up-and-down and side-to-side path. As the patient steps forward with a limb creating double support, the center of gravity (COG) lowers, and, as the patient brings the opposite limb forward creating single support, the COG rises. The COG's vertical rise and fall is approximately 5 cm. This pattern is also accompanied by slight lateral motion as a patient steps from right to left and vice versa as well as by horizontal plane rotation (Fig. 7-3). To lengthen a step, the pelvis rotates on the supporting femur, internally rotating the hip joint. At the same time, the swinging limb is rotated externally at the hip to keep the foot aligned with the direction of movement.

An efficient gait pattern requires the least amount of energy expenditure. Patients will choose a **comfortable walking speed** (CWS) that requires the least energy expenditure per unit of distance. CWS decreases with age, most likely as a result of decreased strength.[5]

The hip flexors, knee extensors, and ankle plantarflexors are the primary muscle groups contributing to energy generation in the sagittal plane during level surface walking.[6] Other muscle groups are also involved in producing successful walking and are discussed for each gait period.

Concentric muscle work, also called positive work, results in energy flow from the muscles to the segments to accelerate the body. Conversely, eccentric muscle work, also called negative work, results in energy flow from the segments to the muscles to decelerate the body. It is the

Center of mass The point inside or outside the body where the body is equally balanced or where gravitational pull is concentrated

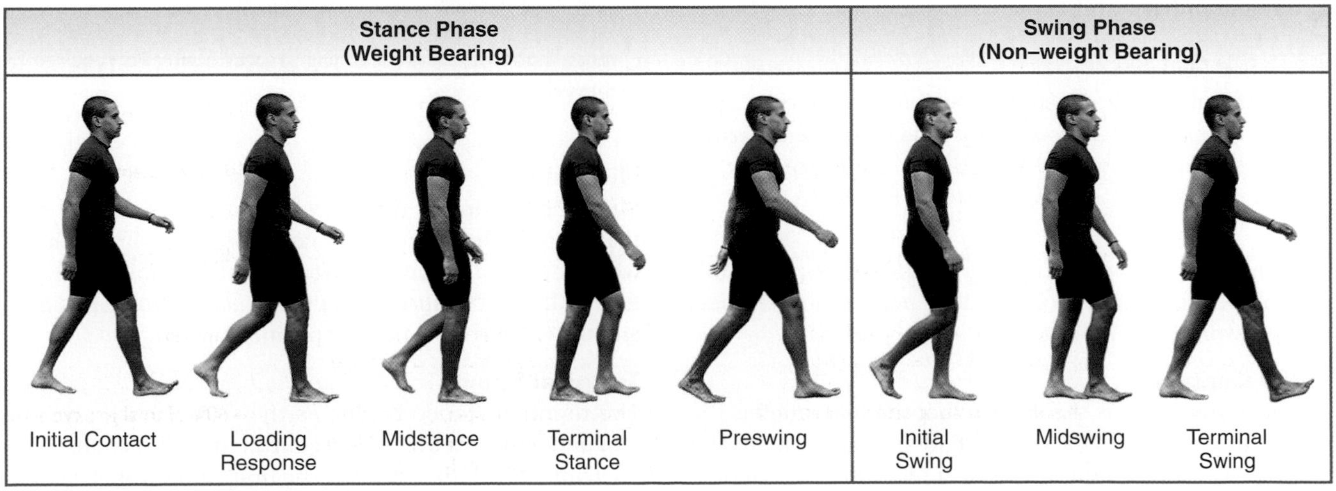

FIGURE 7-2 ■ Phases of the gait cycle.

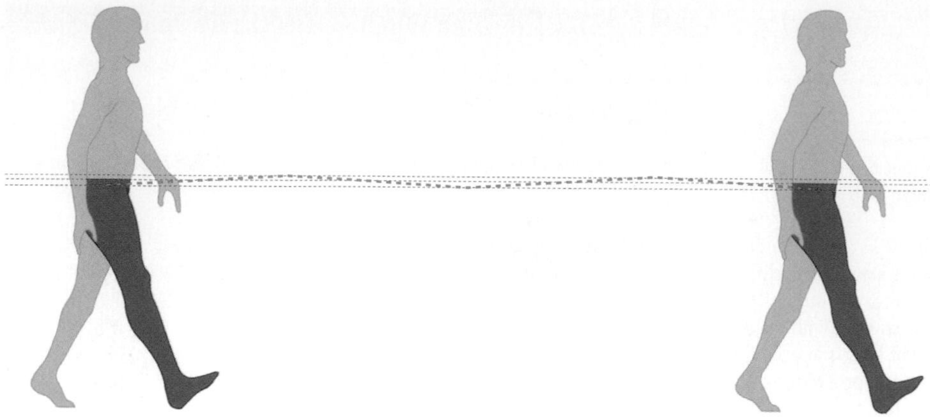

FIGURE 7-3 ■ Path of the center of mass during gait. The body's center of mass, typically located near the L5/S1 joint, moves approximately 2 cm in the frontal plane and 4 cm in the transverse plane during normal gait.

coordination between these energy sources that produces successful walking.

Stance Phase

The stance phase constitutes approximately 60% of the gait cycle and lasts about 600 ms. There are two periods of double-limb support (initial stance and preswing), beginning with initial contact of the foot on the surface and ending as the foot breaks the contact with the ground. This is the high-energy portion of the gait cycle where a closed kinetic chain is created between the foot and the surface, allowing forces from the lower extremity to be transferred to the ground and back, thereby moving the body forward.[7,8] GRFs are created during the stance phase. When measured using a force platform, the vertical, or impact, GRF is shaped somewhat like the letter "m." The first hump represents initial contact, and the second hump represents the push-off that occurs in preswing. Nearly 60% of the body's weight is loaded abruptly (less than 20 ms) onto the limb during the early stance phase, highlighting the importance of muscle strength and coordination in attenuating shock, preserving gait velocity, and maintaining stability.

*** Practical Evidence**

Increases in walking or running speed, downhill running, aging, and harder contact surfaces increase the magnitude of vertical GRFs.[9-11] Large vertical GRFs (>3 times the body weight) at initial contact can lead to injury.[12]

Five distinct periods occur during the stance phase: initial contact, loading response, midstance, terminal stance, and preswing (Box 7-4).

Initial Contact

Initial contact begins the instant that the foot touches the supporting surface. The foot is rigid as it approaches the surface, with the subtalar joint in supination and the tibia in external rotation. Initial contact should occur on the lateral aspect of the heel, then move forward toward the lateral edge of the foot through the loading response and midstance phases and finally diagonally toward the undersurface of the great toe at terminal stance. Although this pattern is similar among individuals, each person's pressure pattern is unique.[13]

During initial contact, both limbs are in contact with the ground at the same time. This is the first double-support period and represents approximately 10% of the total gait cycle. This is the point when the COM is at its lowest position.

Loading Response

The loading response occurs immediately after initial contact. During this period, the limb reacts to accepting the impact of the body weight. The body weight is then advanced onto the foot by midtarsal and subtalar joint pronation, coupled with internal tibial rotation. This period lasts until the opposite extremity has left the surface and double-limb support has ended.

*** Practical Evidence**

The ratio of pronation to tibial internal rotations varies from 2.5:1 during walking to 1.5:1 during running.[14] The tibialis posterior and triceps surae group provide eccentric control of these motions.[8] During running, greater control is required by these muscles.

Midstance

Midstance begins as the body weight moves directly over the support limb and stationary foot, and it concludes when the COM is directly over the foot. At this point, the foot is flat on the surface, the knee is in a stable position, and the COM is at its highest position.

Terminal Stance

The terminal stance begins as the COG passes over the foot and ends just before the contralateral limb makes initial contact with the ground. The body moves ahead of the supporting foot with the weight shift over the metatarsal

Box 7-4
Stance Phase

	Stance phase (60%)				
Gait period	Initial contact	Loading response	Midstance	Terminal stance	Preswing
	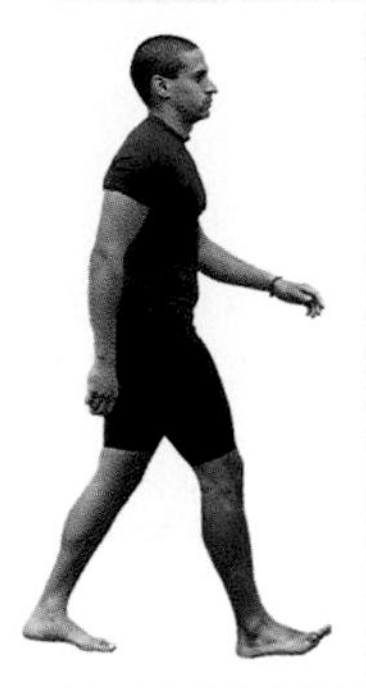	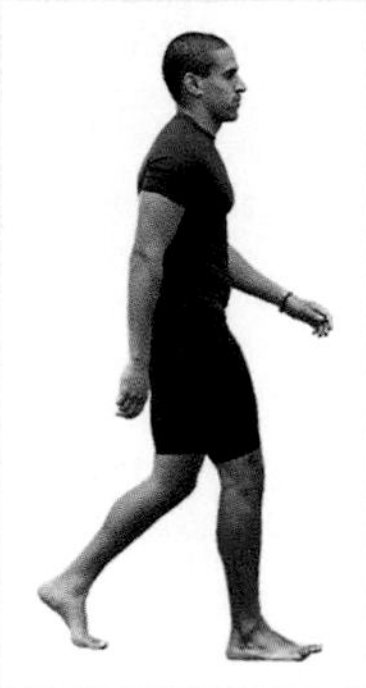	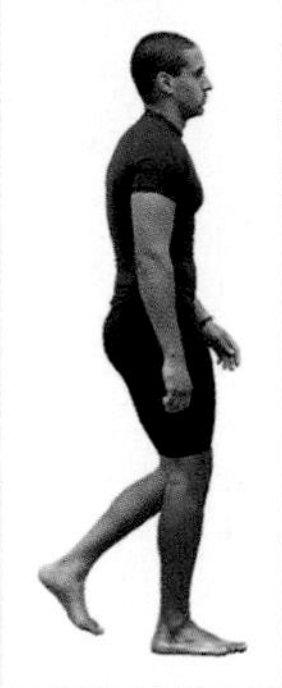	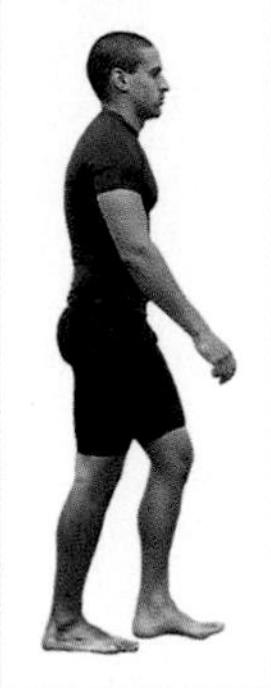	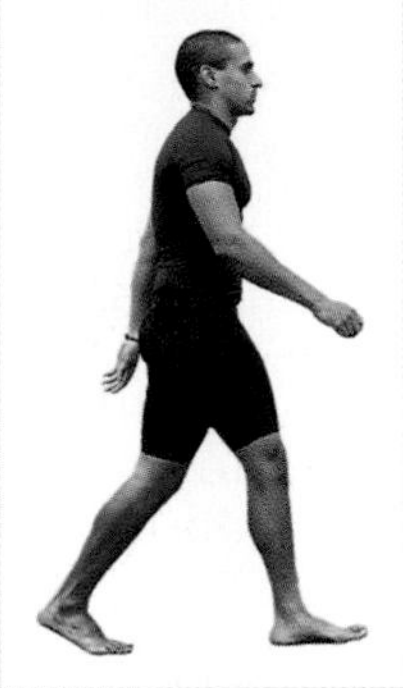
Limb support	Double-limb support		Single-limb support		Double-limb support
% total cycle	0%–2%	0%–10%	10%–30%	30%–50%	50%–60%
Critical event	Heel strike	Flat foot	Single-limb support	Heel off	Toe off
			Muscle activity		
Iliopsoas	Becomes active in terminal stance to eccentrically control rate of hip extension				
Gluteus maximus	Lower portion primarily contracts to control hip flexion; lower portion contracts to assist in control of drop of contralateral pelvis				
Gluteus medius and minimus	Contract to control drop of contralateral pelvis and hip internal rotation				
Hamstrings	Contract eccentrically at knee right at heel strike; contract at hip to control hip flexion				
Quadriceps	Initially contract eccentrically to control knee flexion at contact then concentrically at midstance to initiate knee extension				
Ankle dorsiflexors	Contract eccentrically to prevent foot from slapping on ground				
Ankle plantarflexors	Largely inactive until midstance when they contract eccentrically to limit dorsiflexion; concentric contraction begins at terminal stance to initiate plantarflexion				
Foot intrinsics	Contract to convert foot into rigid structure with weight bearing				
			Joint angles		
Hip angle	30° flexion; slight external rotation	30° flexion; femur reaches peak external rotation then begins internally rotating	25° flexion to 0°; femur internally rotates and slightly adducts	0°to 10° extension; femur continues to internally rotate and adduct	20° extension to 0°; femur reaches peak internal rotation then begins externally rotating with slight abduction
Knee angle	0° flexion; tibia externally rotates	20° flexion; tibia internally rotates and begins to externally rotate as knee extends	20° flexion to 0°; tibia externally rotates	5° flexion to 0°; tibia externally rotates	0°–40° flexion; tibia externally rotated

Continued

Box 7-4
Stance Phase—cont'd

	Joint angles				
Talocrural angle	Neutral or slightly plantarflexed moving in plantarflexion direction	Reaches maximum of 7° plantarflexion	Reaches maximum of 15° dorsiflexion as lower leg moves anteriorly over foot	5°–10° dorsiflexion moving toward plantarflexion	0°–20° plantarflexion
Subtalar angle	5° supination; quickly moves into pronation	10° pronation	5° pronation, supinating toward neutral	5° supination	10° supination

heads until the contralateral limb provides a new base of support. As the heel begins to rise, the gastrocnemius continues to contract to begin active plantarflexion. The subtalar joint begins supinating to create a rigid lever for propulsion. The plantar fascia also helps to create a solid structural platform needed for the pushing off in the preswing period.

Preswing

Preswing is the final period of the stance phase, the transitional period of double support during which the limb is rapidly unloaded from the ground and prepared to swing forward. This is the second of the two periods with double-limb support in a normal walking gait cycle. Preswing begins with the initial contact of the contralateral limb and ends with the toe-off of the stance limb. With the weight over the first metatarsophalangeal joint, the ankle plantarflexors act concentrically to generate force for pushing off. As metatarsophalangeal joint extension occurs, the plantar fascia tightens and pulls the calcaneus and metatarsal heads together. This heightens the medial longitudinal arch of the foot, thereby creating a rigid structural support, also known as the windlass effect (see Chapter 8, p. 178).

*** Practical Evidence**

Eccentric muscle activity in the lower extremity occurs primarily when the subtalar joint is pronating in order to provide joint control and shock absorption. Concentric muscle activity in the lower extremity occurs primarily when the subtalar joint is supinated in order to provide propulsion and acceleration.[8]

Swing Phase

The low-energy phase of the gait cycle occurs during the acceleration portion, or swing phase, and represents approximately 38% of the gait cycle.[7] The **swing phase** begins as soon as the toes leave the surface and ends when the limb next makes contact with the surface. The swing phase achieves foot clearance and advancing of the trailing limb and limb repositioning for subsequent initial contact. Gravity is working in favor of the pendulum swing of the limb by pulling the leg mass down toward the surface. The momentum gained at toe-off helps carry the leg through the swing phase, requiring considerably less energy than that expended in the stance phase.[8] Three distinct periods occur during the swing phase: initial swing, midswing, and terminal swing (Box 7-5).

Initial Swing

Initial swing begins at the point when the toes leave the ground, creating a propulsive force, and continues until the knee reaches its maximum range of flexion, approximately 60 degrees. The thigh is advanced, and the ankle dorsiflexes through concentric contraction to begin toe clearance. The ankle dorsiflexors remain active throughout the swing phases.

Midswing

During midswing, the knee extends from the point of maximum flexion to the point at which the tibia reaches a vertical position perpendicular to the ground. The thigh continues to advance, toe clearance is ensured, and the propulsion force continues to be developed.

Terminal Swing

The final period of the swing phase is the terminal swing, which occurs from the end of the midswing to the initial contact period of the stance phase. The momentum gained from toe-off assists in carrying the leg through in a pendulum-like motion. The trunk is erect, the thigh decelerates for heel contact, and the knee extends to create a step length for initial contact.

Running Gait Cycle

Running is a modification of walking but with two distinct differences: (1) presence of a **flight or float phase** during

Box 7-5
Swing Phase

	Swing phase (40%)		
Gait period	Initial swing	Midswing	Terminal swing
	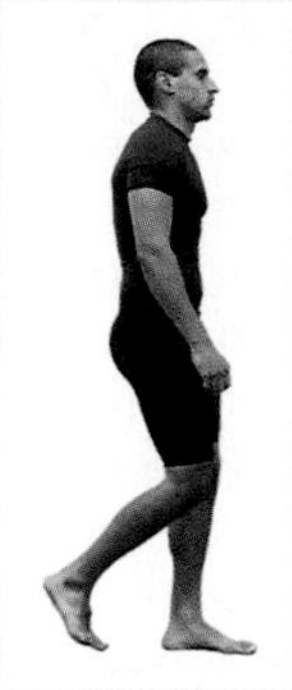	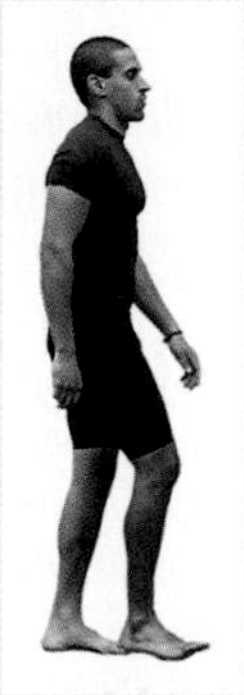	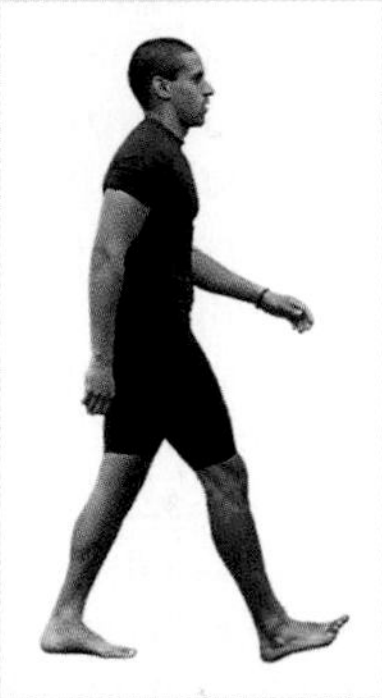
% total cycle	60%–73%	73%–87%	87%–100%
Critical event	Limb accelerates	Toe clearance	Limb decelerates
		Muscle activity	
Iliopsoas	Initially acts concentrically to flex hip and then becomes inactive as hip flexion continues from momentum		
Gluteus maximus	Largely inactive		
Gluteus medius and minimus	Largely inactive		
Hamstrings	Contract concentrically to initiate knee flexion (only at slower walking speeds)		
Quadriceps	Rectus femoris contracts to limit knee flexion, and then, just prior to initial contact, quadriceps group initiates activity to prepare for contact		
Ankle dorsiflexors	Contract concentrically to assist with toe clearance during swing phase		
Ankle plantarflexors	Largely inactive		
Foot intrinsics	Largely inactive		
		Joint angles	
Hip angle	0°–20° flexion; femur externally rotates to neutral	20°–30° flexion; femur externally rotates	30° flexion; femur externally rotates
Knee angle	30°–70° flexion; tibia internally rotates	30°–0° flexion; tibia externally rotates	0°; tibia externally rotates
Talocrural angle	Reaches maximum of 20° rapid dorsiflexion for toe clearance	Neutral	Neutral
Subtalar angle	Pronating	Neutral	5° supination

which neither foot is in contact with the supporting surface and (2) absence of a period of double-limb support. This means that the impacts per limb will be greater and occur over a shorter time. Various aspects of running, such as arm swing range of motion (ROM), stride length, cadence, and knee flexion ROM, change in proportion to the speed. Muscular force and speed of contraction requirements change, particularly with the eccentric contractions required to control pronation during the loading response and to initiate supination prior to preswing.[8] Less upward and downward motion of the total body also accompanies faster speeds.

During running, the stance phase accounts for approximately one-third of the cycle (depending on the speed of running).[15] Greater vertical GRFs are produced during running. Decreased stance phase time (250 ms versus 600 ms) and increased vertical GRFs (2.0 to 6.0 times the body weight versus 0.7 to 0.8 times the body weight) contribute to the greater number of injuries that occur during running versus walking (Fig. 7-4). In addition, runners classified as low arch runners tend to incur soft tissue injuries such as posterior tibial tendinopathy, while high arch runners are more likely to sustain bony injuries such as stress fractures.[16]

Because the critical features occur at a quicker rate, detecting subtle abnormalities with the naked eye can be difficult. Use of a video camera for stop-action playback along with a carefully developed observational gait analysis tool can assist in the viewing of events and subsequent diagnosis of technique. Further, evaluation of running on a treadmill is recommended so running velocity and observational distance remain constant.

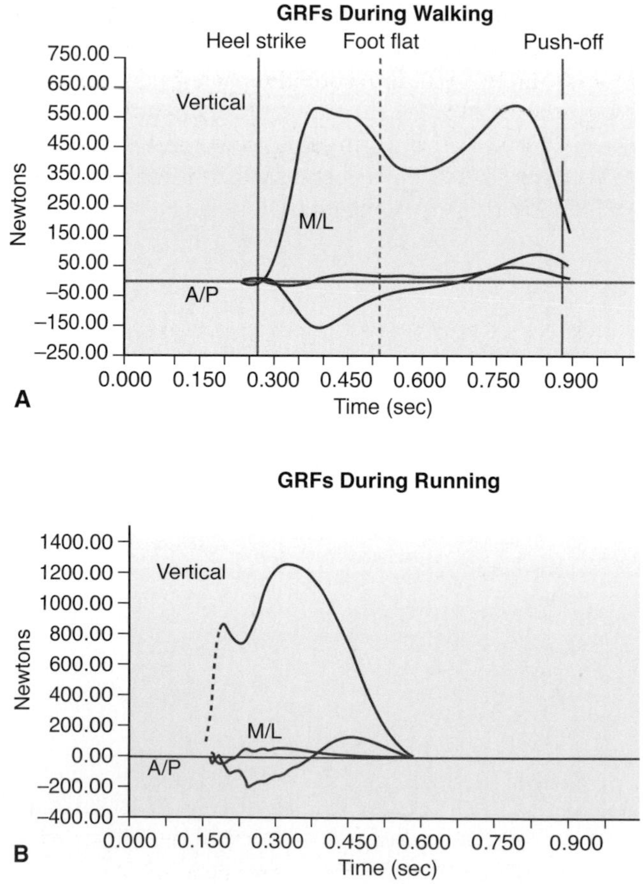

FIGURE 7-4 ■ Ground reaction forces. (A) During walking. (B) During running.

Stance Phase

The running gait cycle begins with the initial contact of the limb in the stance phase. The loading response and the midstance period occur more rapidly during running gait. The end of the stance phase is a significant biomechanical sequence necessary to generate quick, forceful forward propulsion. Time spent in stance diminishes as running speed increases. This results in increased velocity of ROM since the periods of the gait cycle need to occur within a shorter time as well as higher eccentric contractions of the muscles to control joint motion.

At initial contact, the hip is flexed to approximately 50 degrees. From this point, the hip moves toward extension during the remainder of the stance phase. The knee, flexed approximately 30 degrees at initial contact, reaches a maximum range of 50 degrees of flexion during the loading response and then moves into extension through the rest of the stance phase.[17] Full extension is not reached at push-off, and greater extension values are generally associated with faster running speeds.

The talocrural joint is dorsiflexed to a maximum range of 25 degrees at the point of initial contact. The subtalar joint is supinated at initial contact and then pronates to allow for adaptation to uneven surfaces and absorption of forces. In running, there is no plantarflexion after initial contact like there is in walking. This causes increased pronation and less supination.[8] The tibialis anterior acts eccentrically during walking to eccentrically control plantarflexion, but it contracts concentrically during running to stabilize the ankle and possibly accelerate the tibia over the foot.[8] At the same time, the gastrocnemius and soleus contract eccentrically to control the forward progression of the tibia. As the limb continues from midstance to preswing, the subtalar joint supinates to form a rigid lever for push-off. At push-off, hip and knee extension are needed to assist in thrusting the body as it progresses into flight. The hamstrings convert from stabilizing knee flexors to active hip extensors.

Swing Phase

The swing phase clears the non–weight-bearing limb over the ground and positions the foot to accept weight bearing. Because weight-bearing forces are not involved, the probability of injury during the swing phase is less than during the weight-bearing stance phase. Most injuries occurring during the swing phase of the running cycle involve the lower extremity muscles that decelerate and control the limb when running. The hamstring muscle group is often injured during the swing phase as it eccentrically contracts to slow knee extension.[18]

During the initial swing phase, the hip is in 10 degrees of extension. The hip then flexes during the remainder of the swing period, reaching approximately 50 to 55 degrees of flexion during the terminal swing period.

The knee moves through its greatest ROM during the swing phase, and the motion varies with the intensity of running (e.g., jog or sprint). While fully extended at initial swing, the knee can reach 125 degrees of flexion during midswing. Extreme knee flexion is characteristic of sprinters. By increasing the knee flexion angle, the radius of rotation is decreased, reducing the **moment of inertia**, thus making it easier to rotate the limb about the hip joint. In walking or distance running, in which less angular acceleration of the legs is required, knee flexion during the swing phase remains relatively small, and the leg's moment of inertia relative to the hip is increased. In terminal swing, the knee extends in preparation for initial contact.

Initially during the swing period, the talocrural joint is at 25 degrees of plantarflexion but proceeds rapidly to 20 degrees of dorsiflexion, where it remains until initial contact during the stance phase. Runners are classified as rearfoot, midfoot, or forefoot strikers, according to the portion of the foot first making contact with the ground.

Factors influencing GRF patterns include running speed, running style, ground surface,[19] and grade of incline.[20] The running shoes worn[21] and the use of orthotics may also affect GRF patterns. Overstriding can be counterproductive to producing speed because GRFs with larger retarding horizontal components are generated. Also, with longer strides, muscles crossing the knee absorb more of the shock that is transmitted upward through the musculoskeletal system, which may translate to additional stress being placed on the knees.[22]

Moment of inertia The amount of force needed to overcome a body's or body part's present state of rotatory motion

General Approach to Patient Evaluation

While there are common gait pattern pathologies, each patient has a unique set of functional limitations and physical examination findings.[23] The general approach to gait evaluation is similar to medical examinations and includes a history and physical examination prior to the gait assessment. This allows the clinician to determine the possible cause(s) of the gait pattern pathology.

History

A comprehensive gait evaluation begins with a thorough medical history. It is typically during the history taking that we are posed with the "chicken or the egg" paradox, meaning is a preexisting injury a contributor to dysfunctional gait or is a preexisting dysfunctional gait a contributor to a particular injury. An example of the first is the "limp" that occurs after an ankle sprain. An example of the second is the medial tibial stress syndrome that occurs in a runner who pronates excessively and has an abductory twist compensatory gait pattern (see Box 7-4). When the underlying diagnosis is known, certain gait patterns that are associated with the condition can be anticipated. Table 7-1 describes common impairments and the compensations produced during the stance phase; Table 7-2 presents common impairments and the compensations produced during the swing phase.

Table 7-1 Effects of Impairments During the Stance Phase of the Gait Cycle

	Compensation			
Impairment	Initial Contact	Loading Response	Midstance	Terminal Stance
Decreased Dorsiflexion	Increased subtalar pronation Forefoot abduction	Increased and prolonged midtarsal joint pronation		Decreased ability to toe-off Premature heel raise
Extrinsic Leg or Thigh Muscle Weakness	Variable foot/ground contact points	Increased subtalar joint pronation Increased tibial rotation	Impaired supination	Decreased ability to toe-off
Hip Rotator Muscle Weakness	Toe-in gait	Increased rotation of femur		
Rearfoot Varus	Increased subtalar pronation Increased medial leg or foot stresses	Excessive pronation		
Hypomobile First Ray	Altered midfoot and forefoot position	Instability in midtarsal joints and forefoot	Altered distribution of ground reaction forces	Decreased ability to toe-off Premature heel raise Reduced resupination

Continued

Table 7-1 Effects of Impairments During the Stance Phase of the Gait Cycle—cont'd

	Compensation			
Impairment	Initial Contact	Loading Response	Midstance	Terminal Stance
Plantarflexed First Ray	First ray contacts the ground	Decreased subtalar pronation	Early resupination Decreased ability to absorb shock	Increased force on first ray
Forefoot Varus		Increased and prolonged pronation	Delayed supination.	Incomplete resupination with decreased force at toe-off
Forefoot Valgus		Early supination Decreased ability to absorb shock	Decreased force at toe-off	
Tarsal Coalition	Decreased or absent subtalar joint motion			
Tibial Torsion	Increased compensatory subtalar joint pronation			
Femoral Anteversion	Toe-in gait Increased subtalar joint pronation secondary to internal rotation			
Leg-Length Discrepancy	Compensatory pronation of the longer leg with compensatory supination of the shorter leg			

Table 7-2 Effects of Impairments During the Swing Phase of the Gait Cycle

	Compensation		
Impairment	Initial Swing	Midswing	Terminal Swing
Hamstring Weakness		Decreased knee flexion leading to shortened step length	
Hip Flexor Weakness	Decreased hip flexion propulsion causing inability to achieve toe clearance; compensatory hip elevation occurs along with a shortened step length		
Hamstring Tear or Sciatic Nerve Pathology			Decreased knee extension and impaired ability to decelerate leg for contact
Leg-Length Discrepancy	Pelvic drop when short side in swing phase		
Hip External Rotator Tightness	Toeing out		

Physical Examination

Gait assessment is a component of the functional assessment portion of the clinical examination.[23] One approach is to identify the gait deviation(s) and then determine the underlying impairments through the physical examination. Findings such as tight hip flexors, weak hip abductors, or tight soleus may affect a patient's gait pattern. Structural abnormalities such as a leg-length discrepancy, genu varum, or pes cavus may also affect a patient's gait pattern as identified in the observational gait analysis findings.

Observational Gait Analysis Findings

Correlating the findings of the gait analysis with the activity limitations described by the patient and the impairments identified during the clinical examination completes the examination picture. This section presents common deviations and their associated pathologies.

Shortened Step Length

Pain or weakness anywhere along the kinetic chain will produce a shortened step length. Other causes include inadequate push-off by the ankle plantarflexors or pull-off by the hip flexors at the end of the stance phase, which will shorten the time during swing, bringing the leg back to the surface quicker (Fig. 7-5).[3]

Shortened Stance Time

Spending less time on one side contacting the ground is typically due to pain. This compensation helps the patient avoid load absorption for any length of time. It may be necessary to fit the patient for crutches or a protective brace to avoid gait asymmetry. Gait asymmetry can lead to injury and pain elsewhere due to the unequal distribution of the load.

Pelvic Drop

Hip drop that occurs when the opposite limb is weight bearing could be the result of either a leg-length discrepancy (the shorter side shows a dropped hip) or a weak gluteus medius muscle causing a short-leg or Trendelenburg gait, respectively (see Box 7-6). The cause of the pelvic drop should be identified during the physical examination.

Asymmetrical Arm Swing

Arm swing occurs primarily to counterbalance the activity of the hips and pelvis during walking and running. When an asymmetry is observed, consider what is being seen in the lower extremity unless the patient has an upper extremity injury. Leg-length discrepancies and spine deformities such as scoliosis can cause an asymmetrical arm swing. If motion is limited or exaggerated on one side of the pelvis or hip, then, most likely, arm swing motion will follow suit (Fig. 7-6).

Plantarflexed Ankle at Initial Contact

An ankle that remains plantarflexed can be the result of spasticity of the gastrocnemius-soleus complex or denervation of the tibialis anterior preventing active dorsiflexion ("drop foot"). A hamstring or knee injury will result in the patient assuming a plantarflexed position during gait, causing predominant weight bearing on the toes.[3] This is usually accompanied by a flexed knee to decrease tension on the hamstrings or to put the knee in a flexed position to accommodate swelling and decrease pain.

Flat Foot at Initial Contact

A flat-footed gait most likely indicates an ankle sprain or gastrocnemius or soleus tear. Usually, an absence of initial contact with the heel is observed. Patients often move the center of mass quickly over the foot, making contact with a flat foot instead. Plantarflexion at the ankle, the open-packed position, is avoided in the terminal stance and preswing phases as the limb is quickly brought into swing phase.

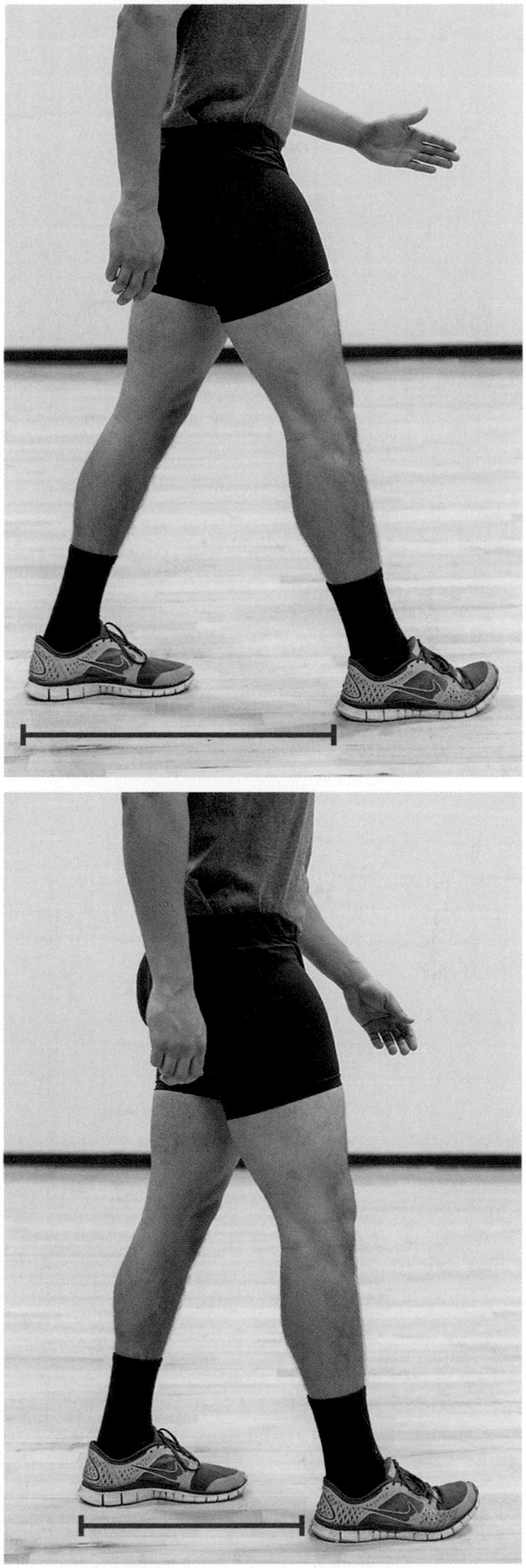

FIGURE 7-5 ■ Shortened step length.

Inadequate Ankle Plantarflexion at Push-Off

Insufficient plantarflexion at push-off is noted as a weak push-off and may be caused by inadequate strength from

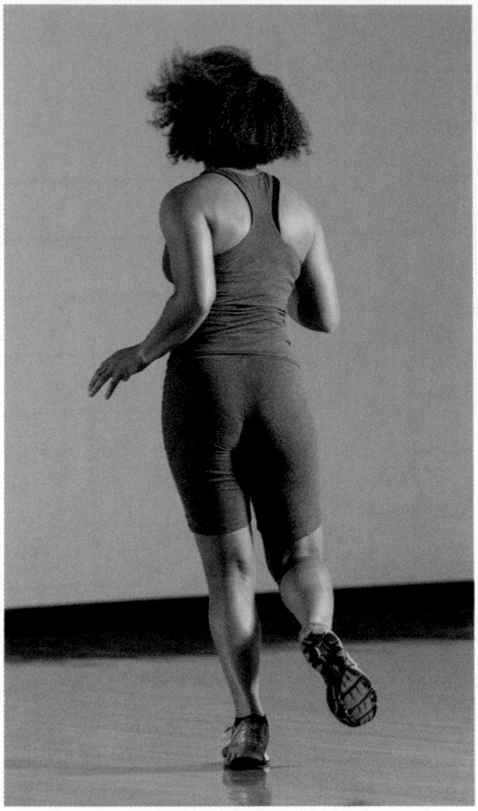

FIGURE 7-6 ■ Asymmetrical arm swing.

the triceps surae (tibial nerve pathology, atrophy), an acute ankle sprain with pain and swelling as limiting factors, or forefoot pathology where the patient is avoiding contact over the area.[3]

Excessive Knee Flexion at Initial Contact

Patients with a hamstring tear, tight hamstring, or spasm will avoid full extension to prevent lengthening of the affected muscle, which causes pain. Similarly, sciatic nerve pathology either from a herniated disk or piriformis syndrome will also prevent the knee from being extended at contact to avoid tension on the nerve and a consequent exacerbation of symptoms. Hip adductor tears may also result in a gait that shows a more flexed knee at contact in addition to an internally rotated hip. This is an attempt to keep the muscle in a shortened state in order to avoid pain.

Inadequate Knee Flexion Angle During Stance

To absorb shock, the knee flexes to about 20 degrees during stance. This flexion is controlled by the eccentric contraction of the quadriceps muscle. Thus, any pathology to this muscle may hinder its ability to control the knee flexion angle, leaving it in a more extended position. Joint pain can also limit the flexion angle.

Inadequate Knee Flexion During Swing

The knee is flexed 30 to 60 degrees in the swing phase during walking and more than 90 degrees during fast running speeds. Hamstring-related pathologies such as tears, spasms, or sciatica could limit the flexion used during swing.

Inadequate Hip Extension at Terminal Stance

The hip extends as the body has been propelled forward onto the swing leg in walking and into the air in running. Inadequate hip extension could be the result of a contracture of the hip flexor muscles.[3] The limited extensibility prevents the hip from achieving necessary extension.

Forward Trunk Angle

The trunk is relatively upright during walking and running. A forward trunk could indicate pathology such as a herniated disk, weak and painful hip flexors, or weak ankle plantarflexors.

Toe-In or Toe-Out Gait

The lower limb should move through the sagittal plane with minimal deviation. Toe-in or toe-out gait can be witnessed at either midstance or just after push-off. Most often, it is the result of malalignment, muscle weakness, or muscle inhibition further along the kinetic chain (tibial rotation, hip rotation, inhibited hip external rotators). Toe-in during midstance can place stress on the lower leg's lateral soft tissues (e.g., peroneus longus), contributing to pain and injury at that site. Toe-out during midstance places the foot in an overpronated position, causing stress on the foot's medial and plantar structures. Sometimes toe-out, when observed just after push-off, is the result of an excessively pronated foot during stance that has placed the limb in a more medial position (Fig. 7-7). The lower leg compensates by rotating externally, giving the toe-out appearance.

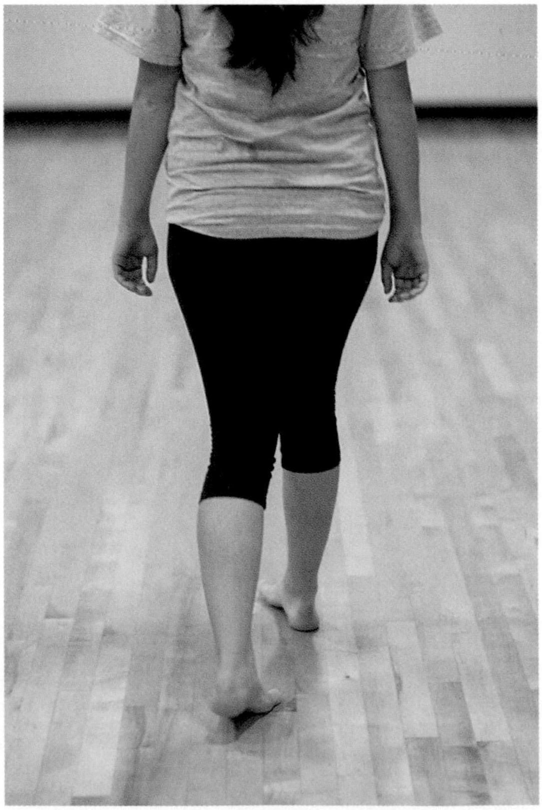

FIGURE 7-7 ■ Toe-in on left lower leg during walking.

Excessive Foot Pronation

Foot pronation is necessary during stance for shock absorption. Further, a pronated foot in a static position does not necessarily dictate faulty mechanics.[24] However, increased or prolonged pronation coupled with increased pressure on the medial aspect of the foot during running is associated with the development of lower leg pain.[25] Weak or inhibited hip abductors and external rotators may contribute to excessive pronation. Runners who make initial contact on the central heel versus lateral heel must move through their pronation at a quicker rate, thus not allowing the foot adequate shock absorption, which may increase the risk for lower extremity injury.[26]

*** Practical Evidence**

Pronating more than approximately 15.5 degrees during running has been linked with increased risk of lower extremity injury.[27]

Compensatory Gait Deviations

Compensatory gait deviations are atypical gait patterns that occur as a result of the patient accommodating for a deficit. For example, in the Trendelenburg gait, a patient has weakness or inhibition of the right gluteus medius muscle, and this can cause a lateral trunk lean during the stance phase on the right side and a hip drop on the left side. Another example is the abductory twist, which occurs when the heel rises at the end of the stance phase and the foot goes into a rapid abduction. This has also been called a "medial heel whip." It occurs when there is excessive pronation accompanied by femoral internal rotation and tibial external rotation or because of a rigid hallux hindering proper extension during push-off. Compensatory gait deviations often require more energy. Therefore, being able to identify and improve them may improve walking efficiency (Box 7-6).

Quantitative Gait Analysis

Quantitative gait analysis is the gold standard for assessing gait function.[23] It provides more precise information to develop the treatment plan. It includes measurement of three primary components: **kinematics**, kinetics, and muscle activity. Because it requires sophisticated equipment and expert personnel, clinicians may need to establish relationships with hospital or university gait or biomechanics laboratories. Box 7-7 provides more detail on the type of equipment used in quantitative gait analysis.

Kinematics The characteristics of movement related to time and space (e.g., range of motion, velocity, and acceleration); the effect of joint action

Box 7-6
Compensatory Gait Deviations

Gluteus Maximus Gait

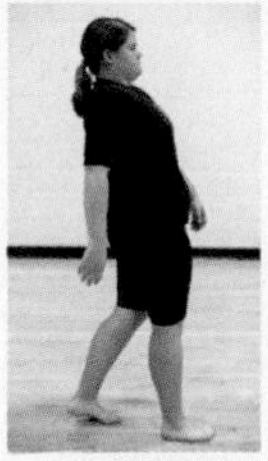

At initial contact, the thorax is thrust posteriorly to maintain hip extension during the stance phase, often causing a lurching of the trunk.

Cause: Weakness or paralysis of the gluteus maximus muscle

Stiff Knee or Hip Gait

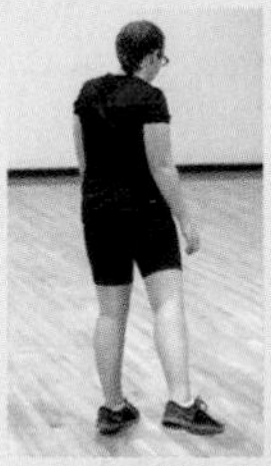

In the swing phase, the affected extremity is lifted higher than normal to compensate for knee or hip stiffness. To accomplish this, the uninvolved extremity demonstrates increased plantarflexion.

Cause: Knee pathologies such as meniscal or ligamentous tears or hip pathologies such as bursitis or muscle tears that result in decreased ROM

Continued

Box 7-6
Compensatory Gait Deviations—cont'd

Trendelenburg Gait (gluteus medius gait)

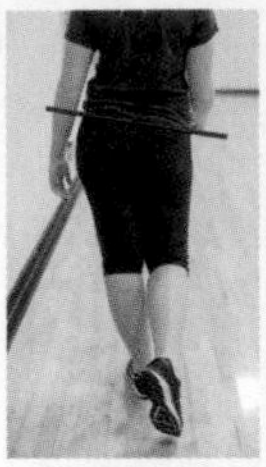

During the stance phase of the affected limb, the thorax lists toward the involved limb. This serves to maintain the COM and prevent a drop in the pelvis on the affected side.

Cause: Weakness of the gluteus medius muscle

Calcaneal Gait

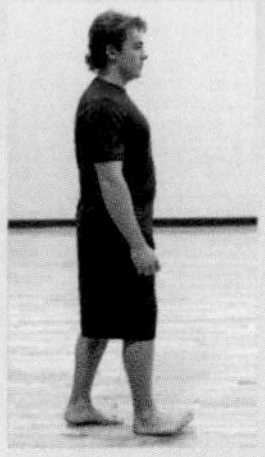

During the stance phase, increased dorsiflexion and knee flexion occur on the affected side, resulting in a decreased step length.

Cause: Paralysis or weakness of the plantarflexors or pain when weight bearing on the forefoot or toes caused by such conditions as blisters, hallux rigidus, sesamoiditis, or ankle sprains

Psoatic Limp

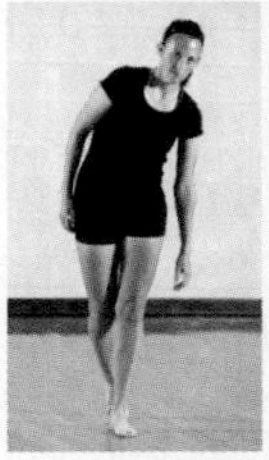

To compensate during the swing phase, lateral rotation and flexion of the trunk occurs with hip adduction. The trunk and pelvic movements are exaggerated.

Cause: Weakness or **reflex inhibition** of the psoas major muscle (i.e., the result of Legg-Calvé-Perthes disease)

Short Leg Gait

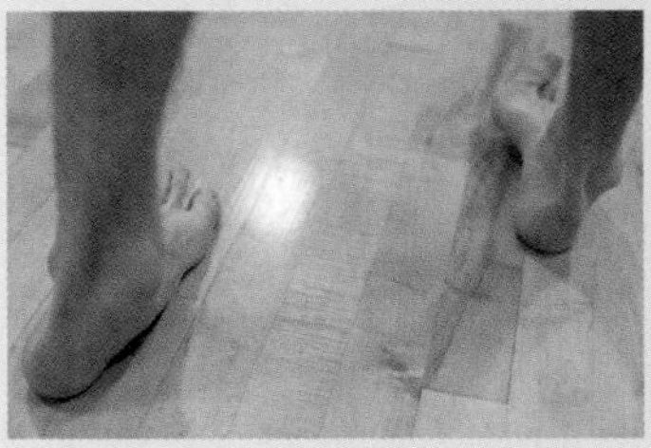

Increased pronation occurs in the subtalar joint of the long leg, accompanied by a shift of the trunk toward the longer extremity.

Cause: True (anatomical) leg-length discrepancy; the right (facing) leg is longer.

Steppage Gait (drop foot)

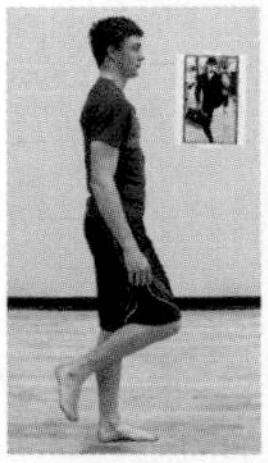

The foot slaps at initial contact, owing to drop foot. During the swing phase, the affected limb demonstrates increased hip and knee flexion to avoid toe dragging, producing a "high-step" pattern.

Cause: Weakness or paralysis of the dorsiflexors

Abductory Twist Gait

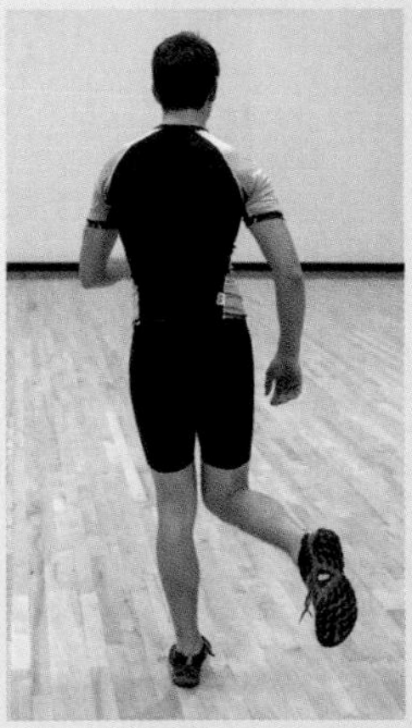

The foot abruptly abducts beginning at heel-off and then rotates into adduction through swing; it is often seen with excessive pronation.

Cause: Weak hip external rotators and abductors; contracture at 1st metatarsophalangeal joint

COM = center of mass; ROM = range of motion

Reflex inhibition A reflex arc prohibiting the contraction of a specific muscle or muscle group

Box 7-7
Quantitative Gait Analysis

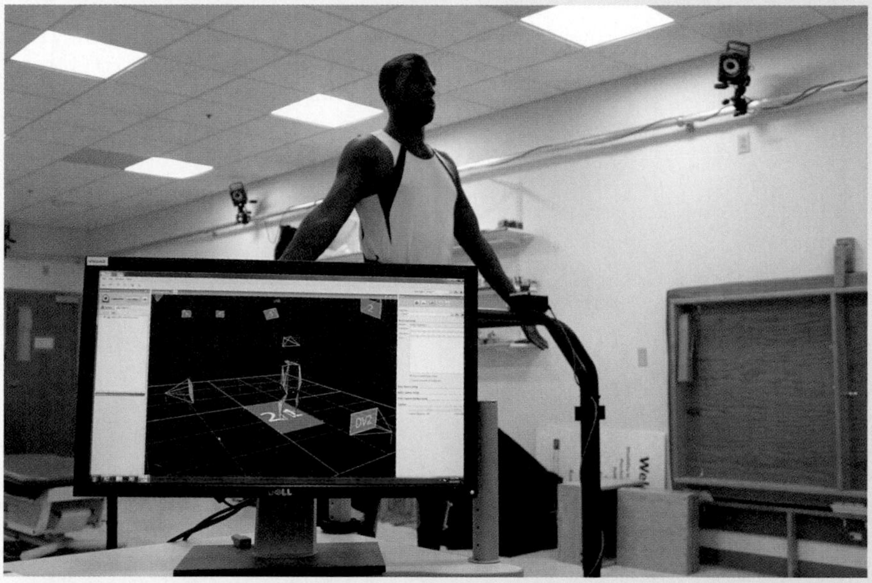

A quantitative gait analysis yields numerical results for the motion, force, and muscle activity characteristics during gait and may be conducted with simple tools such as a stopwatch and camcorder or with a motion measurement system that may also include instrumented walkways, force plates, pressure mats, and/or electromyography (EMG) capabilities. Other more sophisticated methods include the use of (1) electromechanical instruments such as imbedded pressure-sensitive switches in the patient's shoe or inserts or the same switches applied to the bottom of the foot and (2) optoelectronic techniques such as video capture.

Video capture requires the use of reference markers attached to the patient, careful calibration of the video space, a computerized digitizing process of the reference markers, and mathematical equations to yield the results. Motion measurement systems are usually housed in gait analysis laboratories. Angular kinematics, such as knee extension ROM or hip flexion velocity, are measured using electrogoniometry, accelerometry, or optoelectronic techniques. Electrogoniometers, available in uniaxial and multiaxial designs, attach to the body segments for a direct measure of angular displacement (ROM) of a joint. Accelerometers are similar. They are attached to the body segments of interest but directly measure segmental acceleration. Segmental velocities and displacements are then determined.

EMG techniques are used to measure the timing and amplitude of muscle activity and help to describe the motor performance underlying the kinematic and kinetic characteristics of gait. Surface EMG, which involves attaching electrodes directly to the skin over the muscles of interest, is more common in clinical gait analyses. Intramuscular EMG, in which needles are inserted through the skin and into the muscles of interest, is primarily used in gait research.

EMG, force, and pressure plates are typically integrated with a motion measurement system to enable simultaneous acquisition of kinematic, kinetic, and muscle activity information. These systems are also helpful in producing gait reports.

REFERENCES

1. Perry, J: Observational Gait Analysis, ed 4. Downey, CA: Ranchos Los Amigos Education Institute, 2001.
2. Lord, SE, Halligan, PW, and Wade, DT: Visual gait analysis: the development of a clinical assessment and scale. Clin Rehabil, 19:107, 1998.
3. Kirtley, C: Clinical Gait Analysis. London, UK: Elsevier, 2006.
4. Toro, B, Nesto, C, and Farren, P: A review of observational gait assessment in clinical practice. Physiother Theory Pract, 19:137, 2003.
5. Kang, HG, and Dingwell, JB: Separating the effects of age and gait speed on walking variability. Gait Posture, 27:572, 2008.
6. Teixeira-Salmela, L, et al: Effects of cadence on energy generation and absorption at lower extremity joints during gait. Clin Biomech, 23:769, 2008.
7. Root, ML, Orient, WP, and Weed, JH: Normal and abnormal function of the foot. Clinical Biomechanics, Vol. II. Los Angeles, CA: Clinical Biomechanics Corp, 1977.
8. Dugan, SA, and Bhat, KP: Biomechanics and analysis of running gait. Phys Med Rehabil Clin N Am, 16:621, 2005.
9. Bus, S: Ground reaction forces and kinematics in distance running in older-aged men. Med Sci Sports Exerc, 35:1167, 2003.
10. Dixon, S, Collop, A, and Batt, M: Surface effects on ground reaction forces and lower extremity kinematics in running. *Med Sci Sports Exerc*, 32:1919, 2000.
11. Gottschall, JS, and Kram, R: Ground reaction forces during downhill and uphill running. *J Biomech*, 38:445, 2005.
12. Hreljac, AA: Impact and overuse injuries in runners. *Med Sci Sports Exerc*, 36:845, 2004.
13. Donatelli, R: *The Biomechanics of the Foot and Ankle*, ed 2. Philadelphia, PA: FA Davis, 1996.
14. Powers, CM: The influence of altered lower-extremity kinematics on patellofemoral joint dysfunction: a theoretical perspective. *J Orthop Sports Phys Ther*, 33:639, 2003.
15. Enoka, R: *Neuromechanics of Human Movement*, ed 4. Champaign, IL: Human Kinetics, 2008.
16. Williams, DS, McClay, IS, and Hamill, J: Arch structure and injury patterns in runners. *Clin Biomech*, 16:341, 2001.

17. Hamill, J, and Knutzen KM: *Biomechanical Basis of Human Movement,* ed 2. Philadelphia, PA: Lippincott Williams & Wilkins, 2003.
18. Crossier, J: Factors associated with recurrent hamstring injuries. *Sports Med*, 34:681, 2004.
19. Stiles, V, et al: Biomechanical response to changes in natural turf during running and turning. *J Appl Biomech*, 27:63, 2007.
20. Gottschall, J, and Kram, R: Ground reaction forces during downhill and uphill running. *J Biomech*, 38:445, 2005.
21. Logan, S, et al: Ground reaction force differences between running shoes, racing flats, and distance spikes in runners. *J Sports Sci Med*, 9:147, 2010.
22. Derrick, TR, Hamill J, and Caldwell, GE: Energy absorption of impacts during running at various stride lengths. *Med Sci Sports Exerc*, 30:128, 1998.
23. Exell, TA, et al: Gait asymmetry: composite scores for mechanical analyses of sprint running. *J Biomech*, 45:1108, 2012.
24. Butler, RJ, Davis, IS, and Hamill, J: Interaction of arch type and footwear on running mechanics. *Am J Sports Med*, 34;1998, 2006.
25. Williams, DS, et al: Lower extremity kinematic and kinetic differences in runners with high and low arches. *J Appl Biomech*, 17:153, 2001.
26. Willems, TM, et al: A prospective study of gait related risk factors for exercise-related lower leg pain. *Gait Posture*, 23:91, 2006.
27. Willems, TM, et al: Gait-related risk factors for exercise-related lower-leg pain during shod running. *Med Sci Sports Exerc*, 39:330, 2007.

SECTION 2

Lower Extremity Examination

In addition to describing lower extremity patient-based outcomes, this section also incorporates clinician-rated outcome measures designed to objectively and reliably rate an athlete's function. Although these tests may be sensitive in some patients, subjective complaints of difficulty with pivoting, cutting, and twisting may be the most sensitive determination of the ability to function. These concerns should be captured using patient-rated outcome measures.

Patient-Reported Outcome Measures

The following scales represent a selection of the wide range of lower extremity scales that are used clinically. Many other scales are available to clinicians and researchers.

Lower Extremity Functional Scale (LEFS)

The LEFS comprises 20 questions relating to a patient's ability to participate in everyday tasks, and can be used with patients with unilateral or bilateral lower extremity conditions. The patient selects a number from 0 (Extreme Difficulty or Unable to Perform Activity) to 4 (No Difficulty). Scores range from 0 to 80, with higher scores reflecting less disability.[1]

Minimal Detectable Change: 9
Minimal Clinically Important Difference: 9

Knee Injury Osteoarthritis and Outcome Score (KOOS)

This patient-rated outcome measure is designed for use by patients with knee osteoarthritis or by patients who have injuries that are associated with the development of osteoarthritis such as ACL tears and meniscal lesions. The patient responds to 42 items in terms of symptoms and disability over the past week. A normalized score ranging from 0 to 100 is calculated for each of five subscales: Pain, Other Symptoms, Activities of Daily Living (ADLs), Sports and Recreation Function, and Knee-related Quality of Life. Lower scores indicate more symptoms and larger life impact. A pediatric version, used in those aged 9 to 12, is also available at: http://www.koos.nu/

Minimal Detectable Change (for patients with knee injury):
Pain subscale: 6–6.1
Symptoms subscale: 5–8.5
ADL subscale: 7–8
Sport/Recreation subscale: 6–12
Quality of Life subscale: 7
Minimal Clinically Important Difference: 8–10. However, this value likely changes based on patient population, intervention, and time since initial injury.[2]

Foot and Ankle Ability Measure (FAAM)

The patient-rated FAAM consists of 21 items relating to ADLs and an 8-item sports subscale. Patients with leg, foot, and/or ankle disorders respond to the items on a 5-point scale, with lower scores indicative of greater levels of disability.

Minimal Detectable Change: 5.7 points (ADLs); 12.3 points (sports subscale)
Minimal Clinically Important Difference: 8 points (ADLs); 9 points (sports subscale)[3]

International Knee Documentation Committee – Subjective Knee Form (IKDC)

Specific to knee injuries, the IKDC is considered a good general measure for all knee conditions.[4] The patient-reported IKDC includes 18 total items (7 for symptoms, 1 for sports participation, 9 for ADLs, and 1 for current knee function) with varying response types. Some items require a 5-point Likert scale, and others use an 11-point numerical rating scale. A final score from 0 to 100 is calculated, with higher scores associated with improved perceived function.

Minimal Detectable Change: 9 – 16 (depending on time between test administrations)
Minimal Clinically Important Difference: 12

Hip Outcome Score (HOS)

Developed specifically to assess outcomes following arthroscopic hip surgery, the HOS asks the patient to respond to 26 items regarding perceived function in ADLs (19 items; 7 scored) and sports (9 items). The five descriptors for each item range from 4 or "no difficulty at all," to 0 or "unable to do." Two subscores, adjusted to range from 0 to 100, are calculated: one for ADLs and one for sports. Higher scores represent better perceived function. Patients also report their current level of function as a percentage of ability prior to the hip condition.[5]

Minimal Detectable Change: 3 points
Minimal Clinically Important Difference: 9 points for ADL subscale; 6 points for sports subscale[6]

Functional Outcome Measures

These tests are contraindicated for patients who display gross joint laxity or muscle weakness.

Star Excursion Balance Test (SEBT)

The SEBT assesses dynamic postural control by requiring the patient to stand on one leg and then squat and reach to different points on the floor with the other leg. The distance reached in the anterior, posteromedial, and posterolateral directions is recorded. The SEBT challenges the patient's control in multiple planes of movement and can be used to both identify those at risk for lower extremity injury and as an assessment of progress following injury.[7]

Standardized procedures are important to test–retest reliability. Using three tape measures, position one anteriorly and the other two at 45-degree angles from the first. The patient stands on one leg in the middle of the testing grid. Maintaining this stance, the patient reaches with the nonstance limb as far as possible along one of the lines, lightly touching the line with the foot and returning to bilateral stance. Failure to maintain balance results in a nonscored trial. The patient should have four warm-up trials to become familiar with the process.[7]

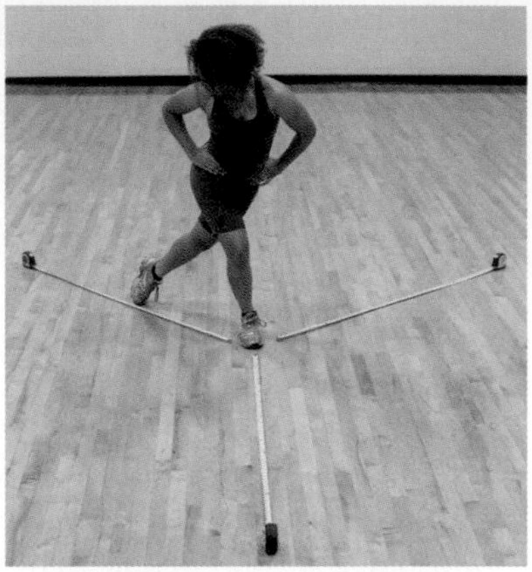

Star Excursion Balance Test

Side-to-side results are compared and deficits noted. For comparison among multiple individuals, results must be standardized to leg length and are expressed as a percentage.

Single-legged Hop Tests

Single-legged hop tests are functional assessments that assess an individual's dynamic stability. Using a single leg for a functional task helps identify unilateral deficits that may not be apparent doing two-legged activities.[8] Different assessments that have been used include a single hop for distance, a crossover hop for distance, a triple hop for distance, and the time to hop 6 meters.

A right-to-left comparison is made, with results reported using the hop limb symmetry index, a percentage calculated by dividing the longest distance hopped by the involved limb by the longest distance hopped by the uninvolved limb. Time is used instead of distance for the 6-meter timed hop. For the single-legged hop, a score of 88% or greater is associated with improved perceived function following ACL injury.[8]

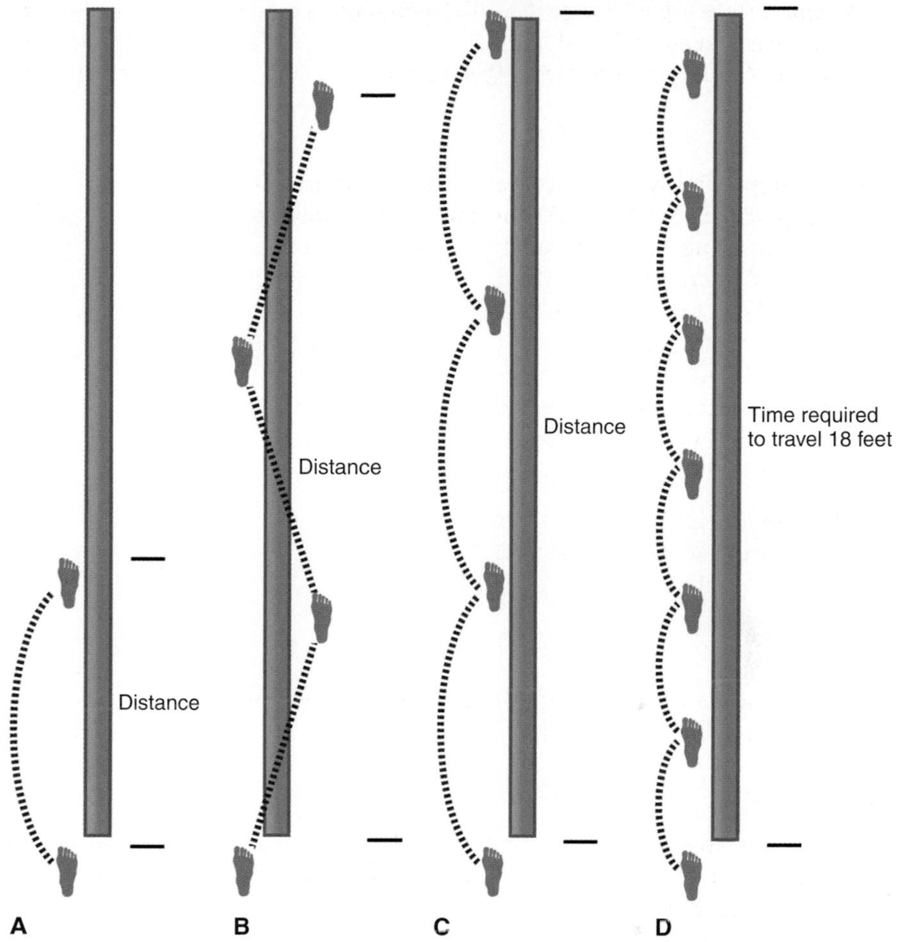

Single-legged Hop Tests

REFERENCES

1. Binkley, JM, et al: The Lower Extremity Functional Scale (LEFS): scale development, measurement properties, and clinical application. *Phys Ther*, 79:371, 1999.
2. Collins, NJ, et al: Measures of knee function: International Knee Documentation Committee (IKDC) Subjective Knee Evaluation Form, Knee Injury and Osteoarthritis Outcome Score (KOOS), Knee Injury and Osteoarthritis Outcome Score Physical Function Short Form (KOOS-PS), Knee Outcome Survey Activities of Daily Living Scale (KOS-ADL), Lysholm Knee Scoring Scale, Oxford Knee Score (OKS), Western Ontario and McMaster Universities Osteoarthritis Index (WOMAC), Activity Rating Scale (ARS), and Tegner Activity Score (TAS). *Arthritis Care Res*, 63(suppl 11):S208, 2011.
3. Martin, RL, et al: Evidence of validity for the Foot and Ankle Ability Measure (FAAM). *Foot Ankle Int*, 26:968, 2005.
4. Wang, D, et al: Patient-reported outcome measures for the knee. *J Knee Surg*, 23:137, 2010.
5. Tijssen, M, et al: Patient-Reported Outcome questionnaires for hip arthroscopy: a systematic review of the psychometric evidence. *BMC Musculoskelet Disord*, 12:117, 2011.
6. Martin, RL, and Philippon, MJ: Evidence of reliability and responsiveness for the hip outcome score. *Arthroscopy*, 24:676, 2008.
7. Gribble, PA, Hertel, J, and Plisky, P: Using the Star Excursion Balance Test to assess dynamic postural-control deficits and outcomes in lower extremity injury: a literature and systematic review. *J Athl Train*, 47:339, 2012.
8. Myer, GD, et al: Utilization of modified NFL combine testing to identify functional deficits in athletes following ACL reconstruction. *J Orthop Sports Phys Ther*, 41:377, 2011.

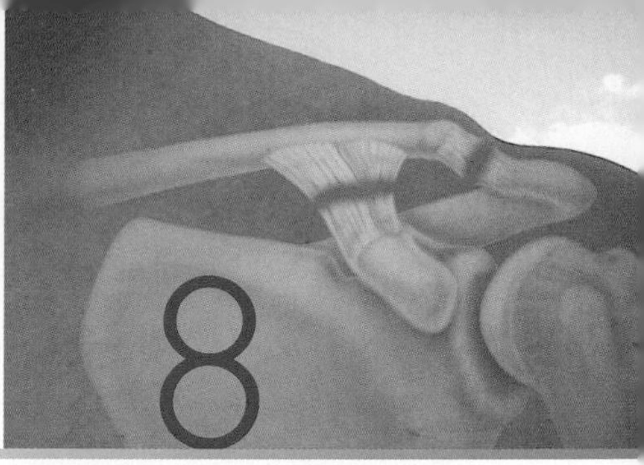

CHAPTER 8

Foot and Toe Pathologies

The demands placed on the foot and toes require a delicate balance between the need to provide a rigid platform and the ability to remold itself to adapt to uneven terrain. The foot acts as a rigid lever during the preswing phase of gait and as a shock absorber during the initial contact and loading response phases (Fig. 8-1). When running, the foot is required to absorb and dissipate about three times the person's body weight.[1]

Biomechanically, the functions of the foot, toes, and ankle are highly interrelated, as is the examination of these areas. This chapter describes the diagnostic techniques for the foot and toes. Chapter 9 covers the examination of the ankle and leg. Additionally, impairments and biomechanical abnormalities proximal to the foot and ankle may also influence the mechanics of the foot, a concept known as **regional interdependence**.[2] An examination of the foot and toes should also include the trunk, hip, and knee. The functional assessment frequently includes a gait analysis, described in Chapter 7.

Clinical Anatomy

The foot relies on intimate and precise relationships with the various surrounding structures. True one-on-one articulation between its bones is rare, tending to be limited to the joints of the toes. The majority of the remaining bones have multiple articulations with their contiguous structures. The muscles originating off the bones of the foot (intrinsic muscles) and the extrinsic muscles originating from the lower leg provide motion and support.

Zones of the Foot

Formed by 26 structural bones, the foot has three regions: the **rearfoot**, the **midfoot**, and the **forefoot** (Fig. 8-2). The **tarsals** consist of the calcaneus, talus, navicular, cuboid, and three cuneiforms. Articulating with the distal tarsals, each of the five **metatarsals** (MTs) leads to the proximal phalanges. Each toe consists of three **phalanges** (proximal,

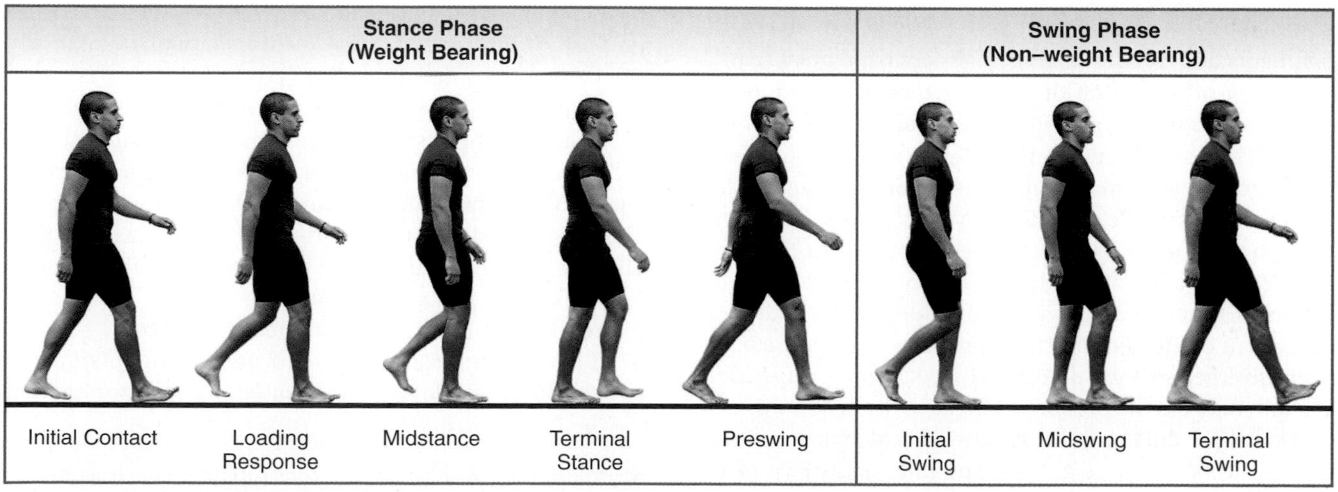

FIGURE 8-1 ■ Phases of gait for the right foot as defined by the Los Ranchos Medical Center system of gait analysis. This system, described in Chapter 7, divides the gait into weight-bearing and non–weight-bearing phases.

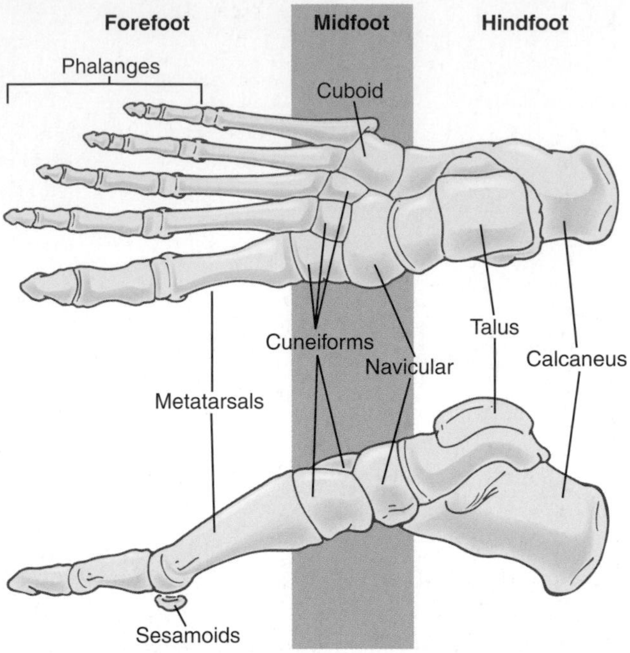

FIGURE 8-2 ■ Anatomical zones of the foot. The talus and calcaneus form the rearfoot; the 3 cuneiforms, the navicular, and the cuboid form the midfoot; and the 5 metatarsals, 14 phalanges, and 2 sesamoid bones form the forefoot.

middle, and distal), with the exception of the great toe, which has only two bones (proximal and distal). Two sesamoid bones are found in the flexor hallucis brevis tendon beneath the first **metatarsophalangeal (MTP) joint**.

Rearfoot

The rearfoot, formed by the calcaneus and talus, provides stability and shock absorption during the early stance phase of gait and serves as a lever arm for the Achilles tendon during plantarflexion. The calcaneus is the largest of the tarsal bones. Its most prominent feature is the posteriorly projecting **calcaneal tubercle**. The large size of this tubercle provides a mechanically powerful lever for increasing the muscular force produced by the **triceps surae muscle group** (the gastrocnemius and soleus). The large calcaneal body is the origin of insertion for many of the ligaments and muscles acting on the foot and ankle.

Arising off the anterior superior medial surface of the calcaneal body, the **sustentaculum tali** (*tali* is Latin for "shelf") helps support the talus (Fig. 8-3). On the inferior surface of the sustentaculum tali is a groove through which the tendon of the flexor hallucis longus passes. The lateral portion of the anterior calcaneus articulates with the cuboid. Projecting off the lateral side of the calcaneus, the **peroneal tubercle** assists in maintaining the stability and alignment of the peroneal tendons. Here, the peroneal tendons diverge, with the peroneus brevis running superior to the tubercle and the peroneus longus coursing inferior to it.

The distal tibia and fibula form an articular mortise in which the talus sits (Fig. 8-4). The inferior surface of the **talus** is marked by anterior, middle, and posterior ***facets*** that provide a weight-bearing surface with the calcaneus. The superior surface is marked with facets that articulate with the tibia.

The saddle-shaped talus is the interface between the foot and ankle. Its unique shape is necessitated by its five functional articulations: (1) superiorly with the distal end of the tibia, (2) medially with the medial malleolus, (3) laterally with the lateral malleolus, (4) inferiorly with the calcaneus, and (5) anteriorly with the navicular. There is no muscle attachment on the talus—the only axial skeletal bone to have this distinction.

Midfoot

Serving as the shock-absorbing segment of the foot, the midfoot is composed of the **navicular**, three cuneiforms, and the cuboid bones. The **keystone** of the medial longitudinal arch, the navicular, articulates anteriorly with the three cuneiforms, the cuboid laterally, and the talus posteriorly. The medial aspect of the navicular gives rise to the **navicular tuberosity**, the primary insertion for the tibialis posterior muscle. In some cases, the navicular tuberosity is detached, creating an **accessory navicular**.

The **cuboid** articulates with the third (lateral) cuneiform and navicular medially, the fourth and fifth MTs anteriorly, and the calcaneus posteriorly. A palpable **sulcus** is formed anterior to the cuboid tuberosity and posterior to the base of the fifth MT, where the peroneus longus begins its course along the foot's plantar surface.

Adding to the flexibility of the midfoot and forefoot, the three **cuneiforms** are identified by their relative position on the foot: medial (first), intermediate (second), and lateral (third). Each cuneiform articulates with the navicular posteriorly, the corresponding MT anteriorly, and its contiguous cuneiform medially and laterally. The lateral border of the third cuneiform also articulates with the medial aspect of the cuboid.

Forefoot and Toes

The forefoot and toes, formed by the 5 MTs and 14 phalanges, act as a lever during the preswing phase of gait. The MTs and phalanges are long bones, each having a proximal base, body, and distal head. The MTs are referenced numerically from first (medial) to fifth (lateral). Proximally, the bases of the first three MTs articulate with the corresponding cuneiform, except the second MT, which also articulates with the first cuneiform. The fourth and fifth MTs articulate with the cuboid. Each of the MT heads articulates with the proximal phalanx of the corresponding toe and loosely with the neighboring MT heads (see Fig. 8-3). Like the MT heads, the bases articulate with the contiguous MTs, but with a tighter fit. The toes are numerically referenced as 1 through 5 from medial to lateral.

At least three sesamoids are located on the plantar aspect of the great toe. Two are located in the flexor hallucis

Keystone The crown of an arch that supports the structures on either side of it

Sulcus A groove or depression within a bone

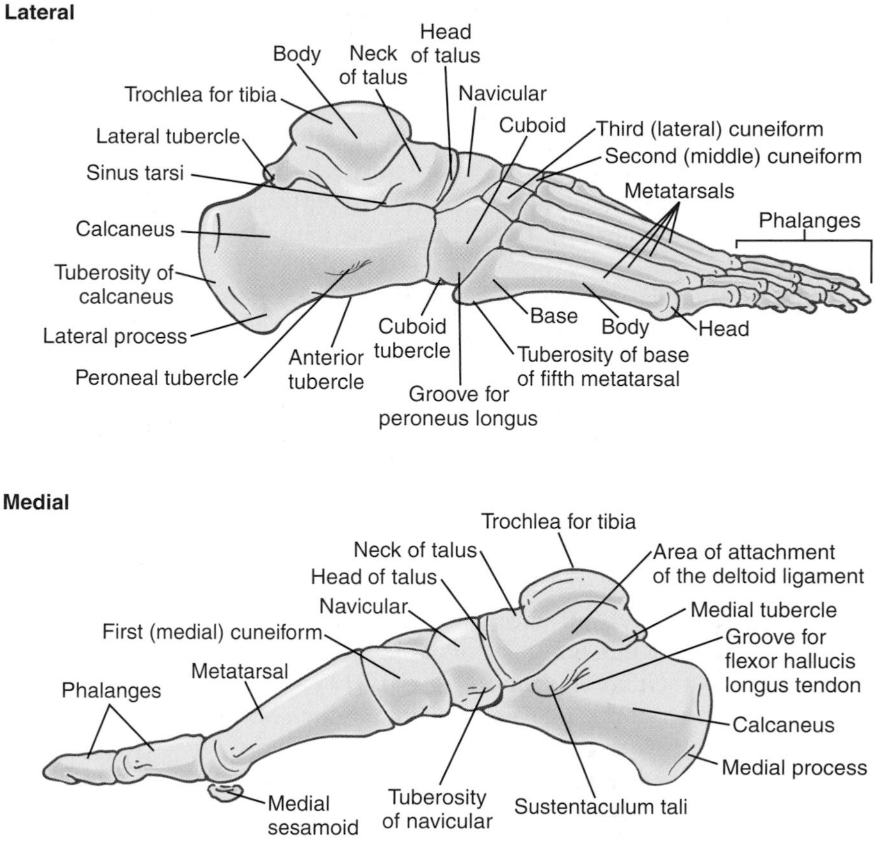

FIGURE 8-3 ■ Anatomy of the foot showing prominent bony landmarks.

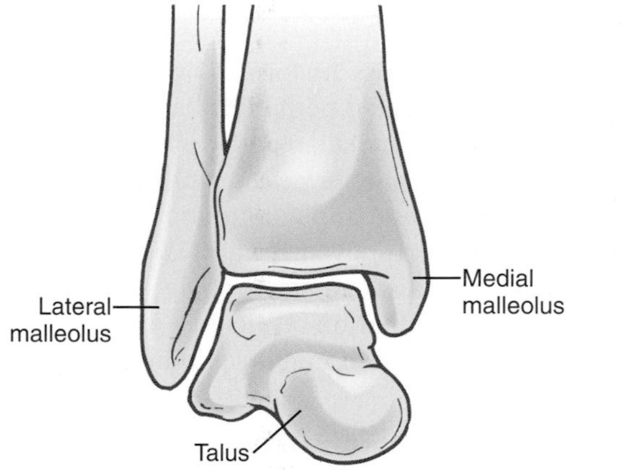

FIGURE 8-4 ■ The ankle mortise (anterior view). The articulation formed by the talus, tibia, and fibula. The subtalar joint is formed by the articulation between the inferior talus and the superior portion of the calcaneus."

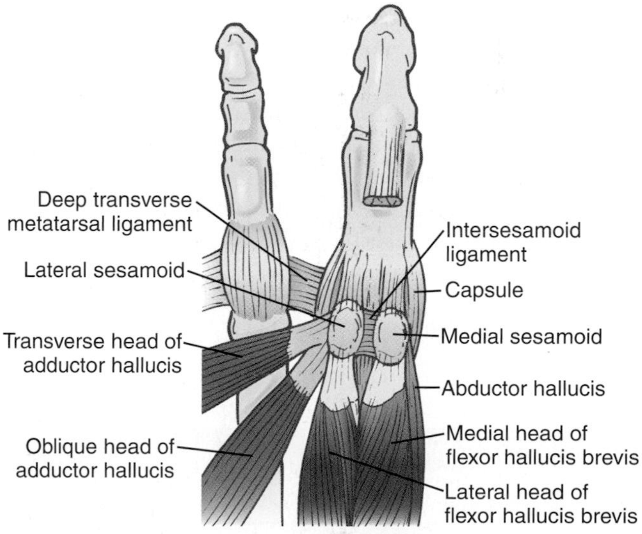

FIGURE 8-5 ■ Sesamoids overlying the first MTP joint.

brevis (FHB) tendon beneath the MTP joint, one medially and one laterally. A third sesamoid is often located on the plantar aspect of the interphalangeal joint. These sesamoids absorb and redirect weight-bearing forces, reduce friction, and protect the tendon.[3] Within the FHB tendon, the two sesamoids lie in separate grooves and are bound by the intersesamoid ligament (Fig. 8-5). The medial (tibial) sesamoid is usually larger than the lateral (fibular) sesamoid and is therefore more affected by weight bearing.[4]

Articulations and Ligamentous Support

The ligaments joining the tarsal bones of the foot are collectively grouped into three sets: (1) the thin **dorsal tarsal ligaments**, (2) the relatively thick **plantar tarsal ligaments**, and (3) the **interosseous** tarsal ligaments that stretch between contiguous bones and interrupt the synovial cavities. The specific names given to these ligaments typically reflect the bones they connect.

Subtalar Joint

Located at the junction between the inferior surface of the talus and the superior surface of the calcaneus, the subtalar (talocalcaneal) joint has three articular facets. The posterior articular surface is a concave facet on the talus. The anterior and middle articular surfaces are convex facets. A sulcus that allows for the attachment of an intra-articular ligament, the tarsal canal, obliquely crosses the talus and calcaneus.

Although often misused, the single-plane motion terms "inversion" and "eversion" do not accurately describe the joint biomechanics. The subtalar joint is a uniaxial joint with 1 degree of **freedom of movement**, pronation and supination, which occurs around an oblique axis and cuts through all three cardinal planes. Supination and pronation do not occur only at the subtalar joint. Rather, they are the composite motion of the talocrural joint, subtalar joint, midtarsal joints, and distal tibiofibular syndesmosis (see Chapter 9).[5]

Pronation of the foot and ankle influence proximal joint mechanics, causing internal tibial rotation, knee flexion, and hip internal rotation. Supination also changes proximal joint mechanics, resulting in external tibial rotation, knee extension, and hip external rotation.

Talar motions are identified by the direction in which the talar head moves. The bony motion that occurs during subtalar joint motion differs when the extremity is weight bearing and when it is non–weight bearing (Table 8-1). When non–weight bearing, the calcaneus moves on the talus. When the extremity is weight bearing, the talus moves on the calcaneus.

Because no muscles attach to the talus, the stability of the subtalar joint is derived from ligamentous and bony restraints. The **interosseous talocalcaneal ligament** lies in the tarsal canal. In addition to assisting in maintaining the alignment between the talus and calcaneus, this ligament serves as an axis for talar tilt and divides the subtalar joint into two articular cavities. A second intra-articular ligament, the **ligamentum cervicis**, lies laterally in the tarsal canal. Collateral support is gained from the lateral and medial (deltoid) ankle ligaments. A segment of the deltoid ligament, the **medial talocalcaneal ligament**, provides medial intrinsic support to the subtalar joint, and the **lateral talocalcaneal ligament** provides lateral support. Anterior glide of the talus on the calcaneus is partially restrained by the **posterior talocalcaneal ligament**.

Freedom of movement The number of cardinal planes in which a joint allows motion

Midfoot

The **talocalcaneonavicular (TCN) joint** and the **calcaneocuboid (CC) joint** represent the junction between the rearfoot and midfoot. The TCN joint is formed by the articulation between the talar head, the posterior aspect of the navicular, and the anterior border of the calcaneus and its sustentaculum tali. The **plantar calcaneonavicular ("spring") ligament** provides soft tissue support to the inferior portion of the joint capsule. Spanning the distance from the sustentaculum tali to the inferior surface of the posterior navicular and blending in with the deltoid ligament of the ankle, this ligament forms a "socket" for the talar head and supports the medial longitudinal arch.

Formed by the anterior border of the calcaneus and the posterior aspect of the cuboid, the CC joint is reinforced by the plantar and dorsal **calcaneocuboid ligaments**. Support is also gained from the **long plantar ligament** and **plantar fascia** (plantar aponeurosis) that attaches to the three primary weight-bearing points on the foot: medial tubercle of the calcaneus, head of the first metatarsal, and head of the fifth metatarsal.[6]

The **midtarsal joints** are formed by the articulations of the tarsal bones located perpendicular to the long axis of the foot—the talonavicular and calcaneocuboid joints. The midtarsal joints increase the range of motion (ROM) during pronation and supination and allow the forefoot to compensate for uneven terrain. With pronation, the axes of the midtarsal joints become parallel, allowing more mobility. Supination results in a less-parallel orientation of the axes at the midtarsal joints, resulting in increased stability.

Table 8-1 Summary of Non–Weight-Bearing and Weight-Bearing Pronation and Supination

	Component Movements of Subtalar Supination/Pronation	
Motion	Non–Weight Bearing	Weight Bearing
Supination	Calcaneal inversion (or varus)	Calcaneal inversion (or varus)
	Calcaneal adduction	Talar abduction (or lateral rotation)
	Calcaneal plantarflexion	Talar dorsiflexion
		Tibiofibular lateral rotation
Pronation	Calcaneal eversion (or valgus)	Calcaneal eversion (or valgus)
	Calcaneal abduction	Talar adduction (or medial rotation)
	Calcaneal dorsiflexion	Talar plantarflexion
		Tibiofibular medial rotation

Forefoot

The junction between the midfoot and forefoot is demarcated by the **tarsometatarsal joints** (Lisfranc joint). Here the five MTs form gliding articulations with the bones of the midfoot. Proximal and distal **intermetatarsal joints** are formed between the bases and heads of adjacent MTs. Permitting a slight amount of dorsal/plantar glide, the proximal joints between the second through fifth MTs are bound together by the plantar, dorsal, and interosseous ligaments. There are no proximal intermetatarsal ligaments between the first and second proximal metatarsals, resulting in increased mobility of the first **ray**.[7] The deep transverse ligament and the interosseous ligament support the distal joints.

A condyloid articulation between the MTs and the toes, the MTP joints allows flexion and extension, as well as limited degrees of abduction, adduction, and rotation of the toes. Synovial and fibrous joint capsules surround each MTP joint. The plantar portion of the capsule is reinforced by the plantar fascia and thickened portions of the capsule, the plantar ligament. The medial and lateral joint capsule is reinforced by **collateral ligaments**.

With the exception of the first toe (hallux), each toe has two **interphalangeal (IP) joints**: a proximal interphalangeal (PIP) joint and a distal interphalangeal (DIP) joint. The hallux has only one IP joint. These hinge joints allow only flexion and extension to occur. Similar to the MTP joints, each joint is reinforced by the plantar and dorsal joint capsule and collateral ligaments.

Muscles Acting on the Foot and Toes

The intrinsic foot muscles are those originating on the foot and directly influencing the motion of the foot and toes. The extrinsic foot muscles originate on the lower leg or the distal femur. In addition to producing motion at the foot and toes, the extrinsic foot muscles cause motion at the ankle. The gastrocnemius and plantaris also flex the knee.

Intrinsic Muscles of the Foot

The foot's intrinsic muscles originate and insert from the foot and are grouped into four layers (Table 8-2). The origins, insertions, actions, and innervations of the intrinsic muscles are presented in Table 8-3.

The **superficial layer** contains the primary abductor of the first toe, the abductor hallucis; the primary abductor of the fifth toe, the abductor digiti minimi; and the secondary flexor of the second through fifth toes, the flexor digitorum brevis (Fig. 8-6). The **middle layer** is formed by the quadratus plantae, a muscle that, when contracted, changes the angle of pull for the flexor digitorum longus and the lumbricals that flex the MTP joints and extend the IP joints. The tendons of the flexor hallucis longus and flexor digitorum longus also pass through this layer. The **deep layer** consists of the secondary flexors of the first and fifth toes, the flexor hallucis brevis and the adductor hallucis, and the flexor digiti minimi brevis. The **interosseous layer**, found beneath the deep layer, contains the plantar and dorsal interossei. The three plantar interossei adduct the lateral three toes, and the four dorsal interossei abduct the middle three toes (in relation to the second MT).

Table 8-2 Layers of the Foot's Intrinsic Muscles

Layer	Muscles
1st: Superficial Layer	Abductor hallucis Flexor digitorum brevis Abductor digiti minimi
2nd: Middle Layer	Tendon of flexor hallucis longus Tendons of flexor digitorum longus Quadratus plantae Lumbricals
3rd: Deep Layer	Flexor hallucis brevis Adductor hallucis Flexor digiti minimi brevis
4th: Interosseous Layer	Plantar interossei Dorsal interossei

Extrinsic Muscles Acting on the Foot

Arising from the leg compartments described in Chapter 9, the muscles that cross the talocrural and subtalar joints affect the position of the foot. The flexor hallucis longus assists in plantarflexion and adduction and supination of the foot and ankle. The flexor digitorum longus also plantarflexes the ankle while supinating the foot (Table 8-4). The long toe extensors, extensor hallucis longus (EHL) and extensor digitorum longus (EDL), assist in ankle dorsiflexion. Based on their lines of pull, the EHL also supinates the foot, and the EDL slightly contributes to pronation (Table 8-5).

Arches of the Foot

Serving primarily as shock absorbers to buffer and dissipate the **ground reaction forces**, the three arches of the foot increase its flexibility. Normal arches are more prominent in the non–weight-bearing position than in the weight-bearing position. When non–weight bearing, the medial longitudinal arch is the most noticeable; the lateral longitudinal arch and the transverse arch are less distinct. With weight bearing, the arches flatten as the foot contacts the ground at multiple points.

Medial Longitudinal Arch

Five bones form the prominent medial longitudinal arch: the calcaneus, talus, navicular, first cuneiform, and first MT (Fig. 8-7). The bony, ligamentous, and muscular arrangement of the medial arch allows a greater amount of motion than the other arches of the foot. Serving as the keystone,

Ray The series of bones formed by the metatarsal and phalanges

Table 8-3 Intrinsic Foot and Toe Muscles

Muscle	Action	Origin	Insertion	Innervation	Root
Abductor Digiti Minimi	Flexion of the 5th MTP joint Abduction of the 5th MTP joint	Lateral portion of the calcaneal tuberosity Proximal lateral portion of the calcaneus	Lateral portion of the 5th proximal phalanx	Lateral plantar	S1, S2
Abductor Hallucis	Abduction of the 1st MTP joint Assists in flexion of the 1st MTP joint Assists in forefoot adduction	Medial calcaneal tubercsity Flexor retinaculum Plantar aponeurosis	Plantar surface of the medial base of the 1st toe's proximal phalanx	Medial plantar	L4, L5, S1
Adductor Hallucis	Adduction of the 1st MTP joint Assists in flexion of the 1st MTP joint	Oblique head • Bases of 2nd through 4th MTs • Tendon sheath of peroneus longus Transverse head • Plantar surface of 3rd, 4th, and 5th MT heads	Lateral surface of the base of the 1st toe's proximal phalanx	Lateral plantar	S1, S2
Flexor Digiti Minimi Brevis	Flexion of the 5th MTP joint	Plantar surface of the cuboid Base of the 5th MT	Plantar aspect of the base of the 5th proximal phalanx	Lateral plantar	S1, S2
Flexor Digitorum Brevis	Flexion of the 2nd through 5th PIP joints Assists in flexion of the 2nd through 5th MTP joints	Medial calcaneal tuberosity Plantar fascia	Via four tendons, each having two slips, into the medial and lateral sides of the proximal 2nd through 5th phalanges	Medial plantar	L4, L5, S1
Flexor Hallucis Brevis	Flexion of 1st MTP joint	Medial side of the cuboid's plantar surface Slip from the tibialis posterior tendon	Via two tendons into the medial and lateral sides of the proximal phalanx of the 1st toe	Medial plantar	L4, L5, S1
Interossei, Dorsal	Abduction of the 3rd and 4th digits Assists in flexion of the MTP joints Assists in extension of the 3rd, 4th, and 5th IP joints	Via two heads to the contiguous sides of the MTs	Bases of proximal phalanges and associated dorsal extensor mechanism of medial 2nd toe and the lateral 2nd, 3rd, and 4th toes	Lateral plantar	S1, S2
Interossei, Plantar	Adduction of the 3rd, 4th, and 5th digits Assists in MTP joint flexion Assists in extension of the 3rd, 4th, and 5th IP joints	Base and medial aspect of the 3rd, 4th, and 5th MTs	Medial portion of the bases of the 3rd, 4th, and 5th proximal phalanges	Lateral plantar	S1, S2
Lumbricals	Flexion of the 2nd through 5th MTP joints Assists in extension of the 2nd through 5th IP joints	Tendons of flexor digitorum longus	Posterior surfaces of the 2nd through 5th toes via the flexor digitorum longus tendons	1st: Medial plantar 2nd to 5th lateral plantar	1st: L4, L5, S1 2nd to 5th: S1, S2
Quadratus Plantae	Modifies the flexor digitorum longus' angle of pull Assists in flexion of the 2nd through 5th MTP joints	Medial head Medial calcaneus Lateral head Lateral calcaneus	Dorsal and plantar surfaces of the flexor digitorum longus	Lateral plantar	S1, S2

Flexor Digitorum Longus	Flexion of 2nd through 5th PIP and DIP joints Flexion of 2nd through 5th MTP joints Assists in ankle plantarflexion Assists in foot supination	Posterior medial portion of the distal two-thirds of the tibia From fascia arising from the tibialis posterior	Plantar base of distal phalanges of the 2nd through 5th toes	Tibial	L5, S1
Flexor Hallucis Longus	Flexion of 1st IP joint Assists in flexion of 1st MTP joint Assists in foot supination Assists in ankle plantarflexion	Posterior distal two-thirds of the fibula Associated interosseous membrane and muscle fascia	Plantar surface of the proximal phalanx of the 1st toe	Tibial	L4, L5, S1
Gastrocnemius	Ankle plantarflexion Assists in knee flexion	Medial head • Posterior surface of the medial femoral condyle • Adjacent portion of the femur and knee capsule Lateral head • Posterior surface of the lateral femoral condyle • Adjacent portion of the femur and knee capsule	To the calcaneus via the Achilles tendon	Tibial	S1, S2
Peroneus Brevis	Pronation of foot Assists in ankle plantarflexion	Distal two-thirds of the lateral fibula	Styloid process at the base of the 5th MT	Superficial peroneal	L4, L5, S1
Peroneus Longus	Pronation of foot Assists in ankle plantarflexion	Lateral tibial condyle Fibular head Upper two-thirds of the lateral fibula	Lateral aspect of the base of the 1st MT Lateral and dorsal aspect of the 1st cuneiform	Superficial peroneal	L4, L5, S1
Plantaris	Ankle plantarflexion Assists in knee flexion	Distal portion of the supracondylar line of the lateral femoral condyle Adjacent portion of the femoral popliteal surface Oblique popliteal ligament	To the calcaneus via the Achilles tendon	Tibial	L4, L5, S1
Soleus	Ankle plantarflexion	Posterior fibular head Upper one-third of the fibula's posterior surface Soleal line located on the posterior tibial shaft Middle one-third of the medial tibial border	To the calcaneus via the Achilles tendon	Tibial	S1, S2
Tibialis Posterior	Supination of the foot Assists in ankle plantarflexion	Length of the interosseous membrane Posterior, lateral tibia Upper two-thirds of the medial fibula	Navicular tuberosity Via fibrous slips to the sustentaculum tali; cuneiforms; cuboid; and bases of the 2nd, 3rd, and 4th MTs	Tibial	L4, S1

DIP = distal interphalangeal; IP = interphalangeal; MT = metatarsal; MTP = metatarsophalangeal; PIP = proximal interphalangeal

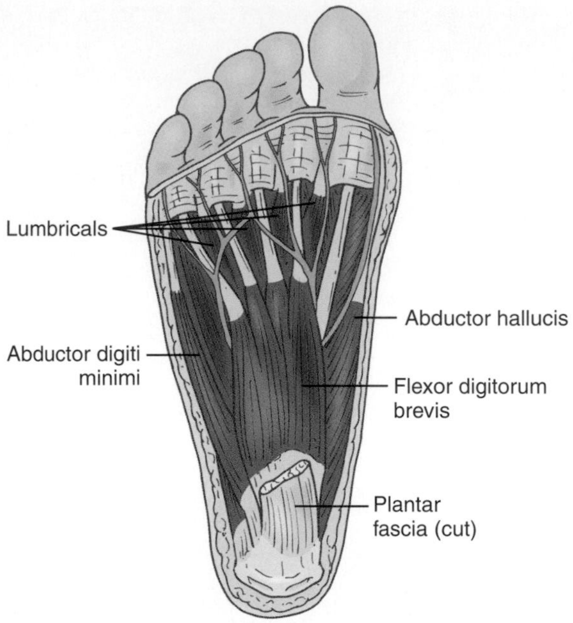

FIGURE 8-6 ■ The superficial layer of the foot's intrinsic muscles is formed by the abductor digiti minimi, the abductor hallucis, and the flexor digitorum brevis muscles. The lumbrical muscles are a component of the middle muscle layer.

the navicular is the stabilizing element between the proximal and distal sides of the arch. Because the navicular plays an important role in supporting the medial longitudinal arch, dysfunction of this bone or the structures that support or attach to it leads to dysfunction of the entire arch.

Ligamentous support of the medial arch is obtained from the plantar calcaneonavicular (spring) ligament, the long and short plantar ligaments, the deltoid ligament, and the plantar fascia. A **slip** from the spring ligament to the ankle's deltoid ligament also assists in supporting the navicular. A second slip supports the talus.

Primary support of the medial longitudinal arch is obtained from the three slips of the plantar fascia.[8] The central slip, originating off the medial calcaneal tubercle and inserting into the distal plantar aspects of each of the five digits, is the longest and thickest (Fig. 8-8). As the central slip progresses down the length of the foot, it gives rise to medial and lateral slips. The function of the plantar fascia is complemented by most of the foot's intrinsic muscles and ligaments.

The plantar fascia supports the medial and lateral longitudinal arches similar to the way a bow string functions to give the bow a curve. By longitudinally supporting the calcaneus to the MT heads, the plantar fascia bows the foot's long arches. Because of the fascia's attachment on the phalanges, extending the toes draws the calcaneus toward the MT heads. As a result, the arches become further accentuated because of the **windlass effect** (Fig. 8-9).

During static weight bearing, muscles provide little support to the medial arch. However, during walking, a **force couple** is formed between the tibialis anterior and the tibialis posterior, drawing the arch proximally and superiorly to supinate the foot. Dysfunction of this force couple can place additional stress on the foot's bony and soft tissue structures, possibly leading to lower leg pathologies such as medial tibial stress syndrome or tibialis posterior tendinopathy.

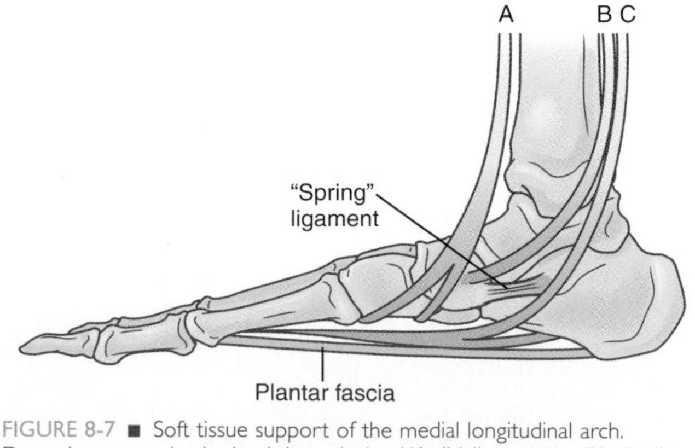

FIGURE 8-7 ■ Soft tissue support of the medial longitudinal arch. Dynamic support is obtained through the (A) tibialis anterior, (B) tibialis posterior, and (C) flexor hallucis longus muscles. The calcaneonavicular (spring) ligament is assisted by the plantar fascia and intrinsic foot muscle in bowing the arch.

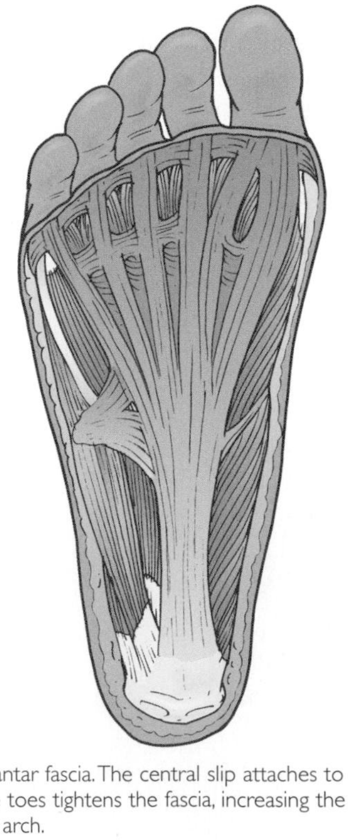

FIGURE 8-8 ■ Plantar fascia. The central slip attaches to each of the five toes. Extending the toes tightens the fascia, increasing the curvature of the medial longitudinal arch.

Slip A distinct band of tissue arising from the main portion of a structure

Table 8-4 Posterior Leg Muscles Acting on the Ankle, Foot, and Toes

Muscle	Action	Origin	Insertion	Innervation	Root
Flexor digitorum longus	Flexion of 2nd through 5th PIP and DIP joints Flexion of 2nd through 5th MTP joints Assists in ankle plantarflexion Assists in foot supination	Posterior medial portion of the distal two-thirds of the tibia From fascia arising from the tibialis posterior	Plantar base of distal phalanges of the 2nd through 5th toes	Tibial	L5, S1
Flexor hallucis longus	Flexion of 1st IP joint Assists in flexion of 1st MTP joint Assists in foot supination Assists in ankle plantarflexion	Posterior distal two-thirds of the fibula Associated interosseous membrane and muscle fascia	Plantar surface of the proximal phalanx of the 1st toe	Tibial	L4, L5, S1
Gastrocnemius	Ankle plantarflexion Assists in knee flexion	Medial head • Posterior surface of the medial femoral condyle • Adjacent portion of the femur and knee capsule Lateral head • Posterior surface of the lateral femoral condyle • Adjacent portion of the femur and knee capsule	To the calcaneus via the Achilles tendon	Tibial	S1, S2
Peroneus brevis	Pronation of foot Assists in ankle plantarflexion	• Distal two-thirds of the lateral fibula	Styloid process at the base of the 5th MT	Superficial peroneal	L4, L5, S1
Peroneus longus	Pronation of foot Assists in ankle plantarflexion	Lateral tibial condyle Fibular head Upper two-thirds of the lateral fibula	Lateral aspect of the base of the 1st MT Lateral and dorsal aspect of the 1st cuneiform	Superficial peroneal	L4, L5, S1
Plantaris	Ankle plantarflexion Assists in knee flexion	Distal portion of the supracondylar line of the lateral femoral condyle Adjacent portion of the femoral popliteal surface Oblique popliteal ligament	To the calcaneus via the Achilles tendon	Tibial	L4, L5, S1
Soleus	Ankle plantarflexion	Posterior fibular head Upper one-third of the fibula's posterior surface Soleal line located on the posterior tibial shaft Middle one-third of the medial tibial border	To the calcaneus via the Achilles tendon	Tibial	S1, S2
Tibialis posterior	Supination of the foot Assists in ankle plantarflexion	Length of the interosseous membrane Posterior, lateral tibia Upper two-thirds of the medial fibula	Navicular tuberosity Via fibrous slips to the sustentaculum tali; cuneiforms; cuboid; and bases of the 2nd, 3rd, and 4th MTs	Tibial	L4, S1

DIP = distal interphalangeal; IP = interphalangeal; MT = metatarsal; MTP = metatarsophalangeal; PIP = proximal interphalangeal

Table 8-5 Anterior Leg Muscles Acting on the Ankle, Foot, and Toes

Muscle	Action	Origin	Insertion	Innervation	Root
Extensor Digitorum Brevis	Extension of the 1st through 4th MTP joints Assists in extension of the 2nd, 3rd, and 4th PIP and DIP joints	Distal portion of the superior and lateral portion of the calcaneus Lateral talocalcaneal ligament Lateral portion of the inferior extensor retinaculum	To the dorsal surface of the base of the 1st phalanx (termed the *extensor hallucis brevis*) Proximal phalanges of the 2nd, 3rd, and 4th toes and to the distal phalanges via an attachment to the extensor digitorum longus tendon	Deep peroneal	L5, S1
Extensor Digitorum Longus	Extension of the 2nd through 5th MTP joints Assists in extending 2nd through 5th PIP and DIP joints Assists in foot pronation Assists in ankle dorsiflexion	Lateral tibial condyle Proximal three-fourths of anterior fibula Proximal portion of the interosseous membrane	Via four tendons to the distal phalanges of the 2nd through 5th toes	Deep peroneal	L4, L5, S1
Extensor Hallucis Longus	Extension of the 1st MTP joint Extension of the 1st IP joint Assists in ankle dorsiflexion	Middle two-thirds of the anterior surface of the fibula Adjacent portion of the interosseous membrane	Base of the distal phalanx of the 1st toe	Deep peroneal	L4, L5, S1
Peroneus Tertius	Pronation of the foot Dorsiflexion of the ankle	Distal one-third of the anterior surface of the fibula Adjacent portion of the interosseous membrane	Dorsal surface of the base of the 5th MT	Deep peroneal	L4, L5, S1
Tibialis Anterior	Dorsiflexion of the ankle Supination of the foot	Lateral tibial condyle Upper one-half of the tibia's lateral surface Adjacent portion of the interosseous membrane	Medial and plantar surface of the 1st cuneiform Medial and plantar surfaces of the 1st MT	Deep peroneal	L4, L5, S1

DIP = distal interphalangeal; IP = interphalangeal; MT = metatarsal; MTP = metatarsophalangeal; PIP = proximal interphalangeal

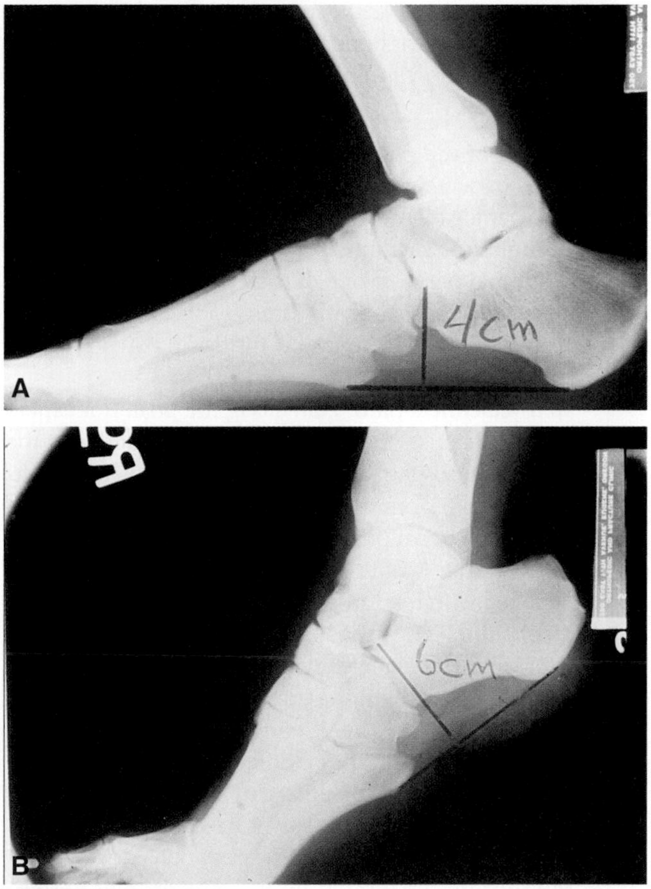

FIGURE 8-9 ■ Windlass effect of the plantar fascia on the medial longitudinal arch of the right foot. (A) The height of the medial arch when the foot is fully weight bearing. (B) Extending the toes causes the plantar fascia to tighten, resulting in an increase in the height of the arch.

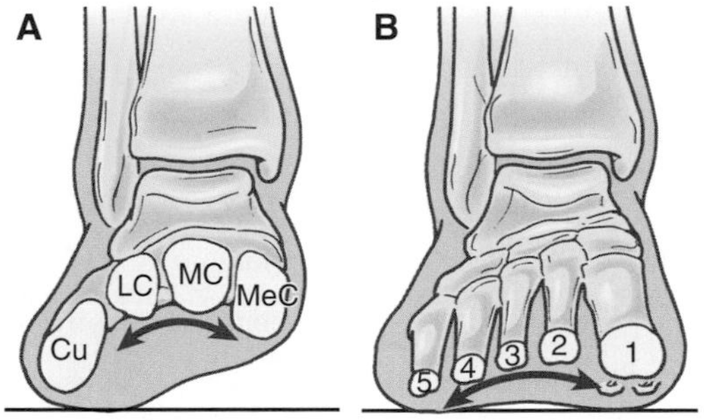

FIGURE 8-10 ■ Transverse metatarsal arch. (A) At the midtarsal joints. (B) At the distal metatarsals. CU = cuboid, LC = lateral cuneiform, MC = middle cuneiform, MeC = medial cuneiform.

Lateral Longitudinal Arch

Lower and more rigid than the medial longitudinal arch, the lateral arch, a continuation of the medial longitudinal arch, is composed of the calcaneus, the cuboid, and the fifth MT. The arch itself is rarely the site of injury.

Transverse Metatarsal Arch

The transverse MT arch is formed by the lengths of the MTs and tarsals and is shaped by the concave features along the inferior surface of the MTs. The arch originates at the MT heads and remains present until the point where it fades on the calcaneus (Fig. 8-10). The first and fifth MT heads are the primary weight-bearing structures of the transverse arch. The second MT forms the apex of the arch.

Architecturally, the transverse MT arch is supported through a buttress formed by the medial and lateral longitudinal arches, with dynamic support provided by the peroneus longus muscle as it runs from lateral to medial along the plantar surface of the foot.[9] Normally, the transverse MT arch is only slightly visible during non–weight bearing, being obscured by the fat pad covering the plantar aspect of the MT heads.

The presence of a functional transverse metatarsal arch as a uniquely identified structure of the foot is controversial. The tripod theory (weight distributed between the first MT head, fifth MT head, and the calcaneus) has been questioned as a result of ultrasonic analysis and studies of the forces on the plantar surface of the foot when weight bearing.[10]

Neurological Anatomy

The sensory and motor nerve supply to the foot is a continuation of the compartmental innervation of the leg described in Chapter 9. The lateral foot is supplied by the **sural nerve**, the dorsal surface of the foot by branches of the **deep and superficial peroneal nerve**, the medial aspect by the **saphenous nerve**, the plantar surface by the **lateral and medial plantar nerves**, and the posterior aspect by the calcaneal branches of the sural nerve and the **tibial nerve**. The tibial nerve branches into the medial and lateral plantar branches. Each of these peripheral nerves represents more than one nerve root; therefore, neurological sensory testing must be specific to both nerve root dermatomes and peripheral nerve dermatomes.

Vascular Anatomy

The foot's dorsal structures receive their blood supply from the **dorsalis pedis artery**, a continuation of the anterior tibial artery. After crossing the anterior talocrural joint line, a branch off the dorsalis pedis artery forms the **lateral tarsal artery**. Other branches off the dorsalis pedis artery form the **arcuate artery**, which supplies the lateral four rays and the **first dorsal metatarsal artery**, supplying the first ray (Fig. 8-11).

The blood supply to the plantar structures is received from the **posterior tibial artery** that gives rise to several branches. The **medial tibial artery** branches from the posterior tibial artery to supply the medial structures and first ray. The posterior tibial artery terminates in a collateral loop formed with the **deep plantar artery**, the **plantar arch**.

Venous drainage occurs via a dorsal and plantar network that exits the foot via the medial marginal vein that drains into the great saphenous vein and the lateral marginal vein, which drains into the small saphenous vein.

Clinical Examination of the Foot and Toes

An examination of the foot will also include the ankle and may include the entire lower extremity and lumbar region. Having the patient dressed in shorts during the examination expedites the evaluation of these structures.

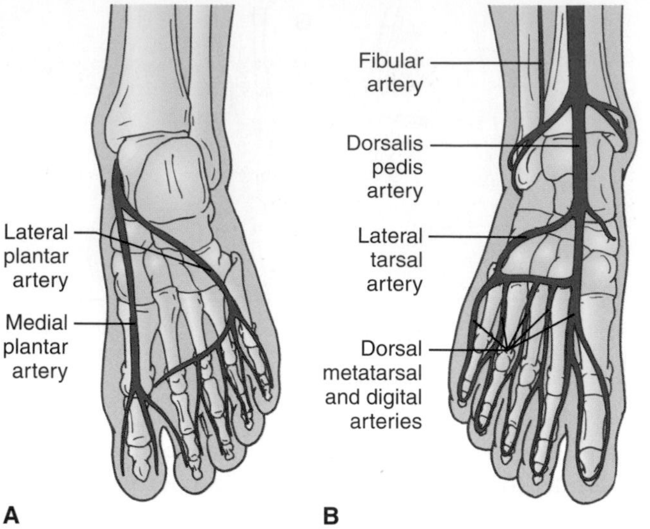

FIGURE 8-11 ■ Foot vasculature: (A) plantar view and (B) dorsal view.

History

A detailed and accurate history of recent and prior incidence of foot pain is required for an accurate evaluation of this body area. An acute onset of symptoms should lead the examiner to suspect bony or soft tissue trauma. Insidious pain may arise from soft tissue degeneration, inflammation of ligamentous or muscular structures, or a stress fracture.

Past Medical History

Many factors contribute to the development and resolution of foot pain. During the exam, consider these potential causative factors:

- **Seronegative spondyloarthropathies:** Conditions such as rheumatoid arthritis, reactive arthritis, psoriatic arthritis, or inflammatory bowel disease can produce swelling in the foot and ankle. Rheumatoid arthritis can lead to osteophytic growth.[11]
- **Gout:** Associated with elevated levels of uric acid, gout attacks tend to localize in the extremities, particularly the great toe. Symptoms include a rapid onset of redness, swelling, and exquisite pain. Risk factors for gout include obesity, weight gain, alcohol intake, and impaired renal function. Attacks may be precipitated by dehydration. Gout affects males nine times more often than females.[12]
- **Diabetes: Peripheral neuropathy** and/or **peripheral arterial disease** affect approximately 27% of people with diabetes who are older than 40.[13] Decreased sensory function can cause the patient to underrecognize the magnitude of the condition. Vascular dysfunction can inhibit the healing process. People with diabetes should be educated regarding the need to frequently inspect their feet for tissue breakdown and infections.
- **Chronic heel pain:** Heel pain with no discernible origin could be indicative of **Ewing's sarcoma** or other metastatic tumors.[11]
- **Open wounds:** Has the patient suffered any recent cuts, punctures, or open sores (including soft corns) of the foot, possibly indicating infection?

History of the Present Condition

- **Location of the pain:** Pain in the foot may arise from trauma or occur secondary to compensation for abnormal lower leg biomechanics. Pain may be referred from the lumbar or sacral nerve roots, the sciatic nerve, or the femoral nerve or one of their branches (Table 8-6). Other neurological symptoms such as numbness, burning, or tingling may be the result of peripheral nerve entrapment.[11]
  - **Retrocalcaneal pain:** Pain along the posterior aspect of the calcaneus may result from inflammation of the subtendinous bursa, degeneration of the Achilles tendon, or os trigonum pathology (see Chapter 9). Subtendinous bursa pain tends to be isolated to the area between the Achilles and the calcaneus; the pain associated with tendon pathology is more diffuse.
  - **Heel pain:** Pain in the heel may be the result of **plantar fasciitis** or a **heel spur**, especially if the pain is located on the medial plantar aspect. Different from plantar fasciitis, heel pad syndrome results in bruise-like pain in the middle of the plantar surface of the heel that worsens with weight bearing and walking on firm surfaces.[11] In the absence of a mechanism of injury to this area, consider pain referred from the lumbar nerve roots or their peripheral nerves.
  - **Medial arch pain:** The medial arch can be the site of pain for tarsal tunnel syndrome (TTS), a midfoot sprain, plantar fasciitis, navicular stress fracture, or tibialis posterior tendinopathy. Compression of the posterior tibial nerve, TTS, radiates a sharp, burning pain and paresthesia to the medial and/or lateral arch.
  - **Metatarsal pain:** Pain specifically isolated to a MT that worsens over time can indicate a stress fracture. This pain should be differentiated from pain arising from between the MTs, possibly the result of impingement of the intermetatarsal nerves. The pain caused by both conditions carries the common trait of worsening with activity. Pain of unknown origin arising from the MTs is termed metatarsalgia.
  - **Great toe pain:** Pain and dysfunction in the great toe can be disabling, causing the patient to walk on the lateral foot to avoid pushing off on the great toe. Pathology within the MTP joint, such as hallux rigidus or hallux valgus, is characterized by diffuse pain throughout the joint during extension and flexion. Pain localized to the plantar surface of the joint may be caused by a sesamoid fracture or inflammation of

---

Ewing's sarcoma A cancerous tumor that forms in the shaft of long bones or, less frequently, in soft tissue; it is most prevalent in children and teenagers

Examination Map

HISTORY

Past Medical History

History of Present Condition

FUNCTIONAL ASSESSMENT

Gait analysis
Tasks that increase symptoms

INSPECTION

General Inspection of the Foot

General foot type classifications
Feiss line

Inspection of the Toes

Toe postures
Posture of the first ray

Inspection of the Medial Structures

Medial longitudinal arch

Inspection of the Lateral Structures

Fifth MT

Inspection of the Dorsal Structures

Long toe tendons

Inspection of the Plantar Surface

Plantar fascia
Medial calcaneal tubercle
Callus/blister formation

Inspection of the Posterior Structures

Achilles tendon
Calcaneus
Retrocalcaneal exostosis

Inspection of Foot and Calcaneal Alignment

Assessment of STJN
Common foot postures assessed in STJN
Position of first tarsometatarsal joint

PALPATION

Palpation of the Medial Structures

First MTP joint
First MT
First cuneiform
Navicular
Talar head
Sustentaculum tali
Calcaneonavicular ligament
Medial talar tubercle
Calcaneus
Tibialis posterior
Flexor hallucis longus
Flexor digitorum longus
Posterior tibial pulse

Palpation of the Lateral Structures

Fifth MTP joint
Fifth MT
Styloid process
Cuboid
Lateral calcaneal border
Peroneal tubercle
Peroneal tendons

Palpation of the Dorsal Structures

Rays
Cuneiforms
Navicular
Dome of the talus
Sinus tarsi
Extensor digitorum brevis
Inferior extensor retinaculum
Tibialis anterior
Extensor hallucis longus
Extensor digitorum longus
Dorsalis pedis pulse

Palpation of the Plantar Structures

Medial calcaneal tubercle
Plantar fascia
Intermetatarsal neuromas
Lateral four MT heads
Sesamoids

JOINT AND MUSCLE FUNCTION ASSESSMENT

Goniometry

Rearfoot inversion and eversion
First MTP abduction
MTP flexion and extension

Active Range of Motion

Toe flexion
Toe extension

Manual Muscle Tests

Toe flexion
Toe extension

Passive Range of Motion

Toe flexion
Toe extension
Mobility of first ray

JOINT STABILITY TESTS

Stress Testing

MTP and IP joints

- Valgus and varus stress testing of the MTP and IP joints

Joint Play Assessment

Intermetatarsal joints
Tarsometatarsal joints
Midtarsal joints

NEUROLOGICAL EXAMINATION

L4–S2 Nerve Roots

Tarsal Tunnel Syndrome

Interdigital Neuroma

VASCULAR EXAMINATION

Dorsalis Pedis Pulse

Posterior Tibial Pulse

Capillary Refill

REGION-SPECIFIC PATHOLOGIES AND SELECTIVE TISSUE TESTS

Foot Type

Navicular drop test

Pes Cavus

Plantar Fasciitis

Test for supple pes planus

Plantar Fascia Rupture

Heel Spur

Tarsal Coalition

Tarsal Tunnel Syndrome

Dorsiflexion–eversion test

Metatarsal Fractures

Acute fractures
Stress fractures

Lisfranc Injury

Phalangeal Fractures

Intermetatarsal Neuroma

Mulder sign

Hallux Rigidus

Hallux Valgus

First MTP Joint Sprains

Sesamoiditis

Table 8-6 Differential Diagnosis Based on the Location of Pain

	Location of Pain					
	Proximal (Calcaneus)	Distal (Toes)	Plantar	Dorsal	Medial	Lateral
Soft Tissue Pathology	Calcaneal bursitis	Corns	Callus	MTP sprain	Spring ligament sprain	Peroneal tendinopathy*
	Retrocalcaneal bursitis	IP sprain	Fat pad syndrome	Forefoot sprain	Plantar fasciitis	
	Achilles tendinopathy*	MTP sprain	Plantar fasciitis		Plantar fascia rupture or sprain	
		Ingrown toenail	Plantar fascia rupture		Posterior tibial nerve entrapment (tarsal tunnel syndrome)	
			Plantar warts		Tibialis posterior tendinopathy*	
			Intermetatarsal neuroma		1st MTP sprain	
			Tarsal tunnel syndrome			
Bony Pathology	Calcaneal fracture	Phalanx fracture	Sesamoiditis	MT stress fracture	Navicular stress fracture	Cuboid fracture
	Calcaneal spur	Arthritis	Sesamoid fracture	Lisfranc fracture-dislocation	Bunion	Fifth MT fracture (especially at the base)
	Calcaneal cyst		Heel spur	Talus fracture	Hallux rigidus	Bunionette
				Tarsal coalition	Hallux valgus	

IP = interphalangeal; MT = metatarsal; MTP = metatarsophalangeal

*Discussed in Chapter 9.

the sesamoids (sesamoiditis). The first MTP joint is often the first part of the body to demonstrate the signs and symptoms of gout, characterized by swelling, redness, and severe pain. Dorsal pain can originate from an ingrown toenail.

- **Lateral arch pain:** Acutely, pain may be isolated to the lateral arch after fractures of the fifth MT or cuboid. Pain arising from peroneal tendon pathology may radiate into the lateral foot (see Chapter 9). Lateral pain may be the result of neuropathy or entrapment of the S1 nerve root and its branches (e.g., deep peroneal).

■ **Onset and mechanism of injury:** The duration of the symptoms and the presence of pain that worsens or diminishes with specific activities provide insight about the nature of the injury and the tissues involved.

- **Acute onset:** The acute onset of foot symptoms can occur from a rotational force as the foot lands on an uneven surface. These irregular positions place an increased force across the bones and ligamentous structures as they are stressed beyond their end ROM. A direct blow to the phalanges or MTs may result in their fracture. Ligaments can be avulsed from their attachment site if the joint is forced beyond its normal ROM. Although rare, avulsion of muscle attachments may result from forceful contractions as the patient attempts to control motion during activity.
- **Insidious onset**
  - **Playing surface:** In athletic activities, changing from a playing surface of one density to a surface with a different density may precipitate injury. For example, a change from running on an indoor rubberized track to running outdoors on pavement alters the ground reaction forces and stabilizing requirements so that different forces are distributed through the foot, ankle, and lower leg. Moving to a harder surface places an increased load on these structures. Moving to a softer or rubberized surface increases eccentric demand of the muscles because of the surface's rebounding effect.
  - **Distance and duration:** Altering the components of the training regimen may increase or otherwise change the forces placed on the body and hinder the foot's ability to accommodate, resulting in overuse injuries. Ask the patient if he or she has significantly increased the distance, duration, or intensity of training. With increased stresses, the muscles providing dynamic support to the foot become fatigued, resulting in altered biomechanics.
  - **Shoes:** Training shoes that no longer provide adequate support may produce injury-causing forces at the foot. Changing either competitive or casual footwear (such as high heels) may alter the biomechanics of the lower extremity and redistribute forces in the foot. Ask the patient if he or she has been wearing shoes that are showing signs of wear-and-tear or if the patient has changed to a shoe with different stabilization (e.g., minimalist shoe). Determine if the patient has a new pair of shoes for competition or daily wear. Question the patient regarding the use of orthotics, the reason for their use, the activities during which they are worn, and the last time they were changed.

*** Practical Evidence**

Wearing high-heeled shoes significantly redistributes the weight-bearing forces on the foot and alters muscular activity up the kinetic chain. The gastrocnemius, especially the lateral portion, fatigues, shifting the center of pressure laterally on the foot.[14] Plantar-flexion strength and ROM is reduced, increasing hip flexor muscle activity and increasing forces on the MTP joints and forefoot.[15]

Functional Assessment

The assessment of patients' function involves observing both their typical daily movement patterns and any functional tasks that cause or worsen the primary symptoms. The goal of this portion of the examination is to identify abnormal movement patterns and their potential impairments to direct the physical examination.

For patients with foot pain, the functional assessment usually begins by watching them approach. Note whether the patient had help entering the facility, is using crutches or a cane, or has any obvious gait dysfunction. Subtle gait deviations, described in Chapter 7, may also be problematic. Observe for prolonged pronation as evidenced by a navicular that is still plantarflexing when the heel rises.[16] Walking on the heel to avoid push-off may indicate a metatarsal or phalanx fracture, plantar fasciitis, or great toe pathology. Walking on the lateral foot may indicate pathology to the medial foot structures, and walking only on the toes may reflect pathology in the calcaneal or ankle region.[17] Any observed functional limitations serve as the basis for further examination to identify the underlying impairments.

Inspection

During the history-taking process, note any bilateral gross or subtle deformity, swelling, or redness in the foot, toes, and ankle (Fig. 8-12).

Inspect the patient's feet while non–weight bearing, weight bearing, and during gait. Note changes (see Chapter 7). When non–weight bearing, the foot normally assumes its natural alignment. When weight bearing, the foot reveals the way it compensates for structural abnormalities of the foot, the lower extremity, and the body as a whole. Also inspect the patient's daily casual and participation footwear for irregular wear patterns and for the appropriateness relative to the activity.

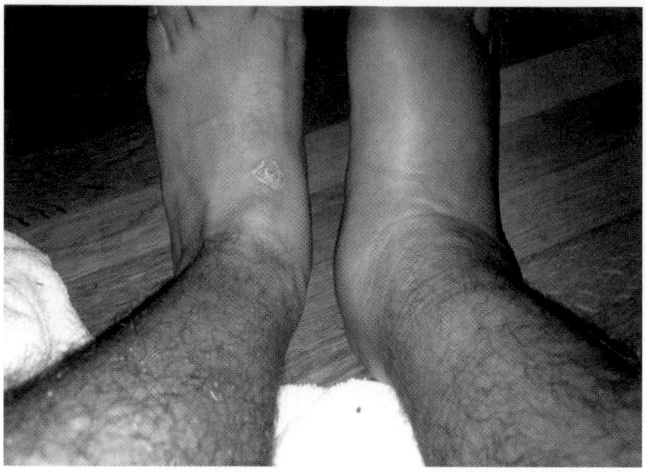

FIGURE 8-12 ■ Swelling of the foot. Without first gathering a history of the injury, it cannot be determined whether this swelling is caused by trauma to the foot or ankle or from a lower leg or knee injury. If the leg is kept in a gravity-dependent position, edema will migrate distally.

General Inspection of the Foot

- **Foot type:** Foot structure is classified as **cavus**, **planus**, or **neutral** through observing the weight-bearing foot from the anterior and posterior views (Inspection Findings 8-1).

A cavus foot is characterized by a high medial longitudinal arch, an adducted forefoot, and an inverted rearfoot. A planus foot has a low and bulging medial longitudinal arch, an abducted forefoot, and an everted rearfoot. Planus foot structure is further classified as either supple or rigid. A rigid planus foot maintains its weight-bearing shape when non–weight bearing. The medial longitudinal arch of a supple planus foot becomes more prominent when non–weight bearing or during a heel raise (see Plantar Fasciitis, p. 215). A normal foot is neither cavus nor planus.

Although a useful classification strategy, this system must be considered relative to the resulting kinematics and pathology. Deviation of a foot from normal represents either a structural foot abnormality or the foot's adaptation to a structural deficit in the leg, pelvis, or spine. Abnormal foot posture may also be the result of neurological or disease states.

*** Practical Evidence**

The shape of the plantar surface of the foot during weight bearing is frequently used to determine the foot type to make subsequent footwear recommendations. This type of visual assessment results in misclassification up to 35% of the time, with accuracy decreasing in those with a higher body mass index (BMI).

- **Feiss line:** This technique provides a gross assessment of the foot type. A line is drawn from the apex of the medial malleolus to the plantar aspect of the base of the first MT, and the position of the navicular tuberosity is marked. If the tuberosity is above the line, a cavus foot is suggested. A planus foot is present if the tuberosity is inferior to the line, and, if the line intersects with the tuberosity, a normal foot alignment is determined. The Feiss line is assessed with the foot weight bearing and non–weight bearing.
- **The Longitudinal Arch Angle:** This technique uses landmarks similar to the Feiss line but provides more quantifiable results (Selective Tissue Test 8-1).
- **Calluses and blisters:** Inspect the foot and toes for blisters and calluses, possibly indicating improperly fitting shoes, poor biomechanics, or underlying bony- or soft tissue dysfunction. Blisters may be the result of dermatologic conditions such as **tinea pedis** or indicate areas of increased friction or irritation from the foot rubbing against the shoe. Calluses develop as the result of long-term pressures. The presence of callus under the MT heads may indicate a biomechanical abnormality. Those under the calcaneus are usually the result of an atypical gait pattern.[18]
- **Skin conditions:** Skin conditions can provide evidence of the nature of pain or alteration in gait. Some open skin lesions are contagious and require the use of Standard Precautions.
  - **Tinea pedis: "Athlete's foot"** is a common dermatophyte infection of the toes, primarily affecting athletes, men, and boys (Fig. 8-13). Proper bathing, regularly changing socks, and keeping the area dry help prevent the buildup of fungi.[19] Treatment includes topical antifungal agents such as terbinafine and clotrimazole. When multiple sites of outbreak occur, systemic oral medication may be prescribed.[19]
  - **Corns:** Also referred to as a clavus, a corn is a thickening of the **stratum corneum** and tends to occur in non–weight-bearing areas. Corns may be sensitive to the touch. Corns should be differentiated from calluses in that a callus does not have a central core.
    - **Hard corns** (heloma dura), located in areas that receive excessive pressure, appear as hard, granular nodules on the skin with a hard central core and a defined margin. Hard corns tend to form on the toes and PIP joints.
    - **Soft corns** (heloma molle) form between the toes, most frequently the web space between the fourth and fifth toes.[20] Dampness in the web space moistens the corn, thus keeping it soft and giving it a **macerated** appearance. The moisture together with the dark, warm environment predispose the lesion to infection and **ulceration**.
  - **Plantar warts:** Plantar warts (verruca plantaris), a common dermatologic condition affecting the foot's plantar aspect, have a different appearance than

Tinea pedis A fungal infection of the foot and toes

Stratum corneum The outermost horny layer of the epidermis

Macerated Soft and soaked with fluid

Ulceration An open sore or lesion of the skin or mucous membrane that is accompanied by inflamed and necrotic tissue

Inspection Findings 8-1
General Foot Type Classifications (Weight Bearing)

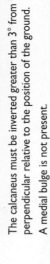

	Pes Planus	Neutral	Pes Cavus
	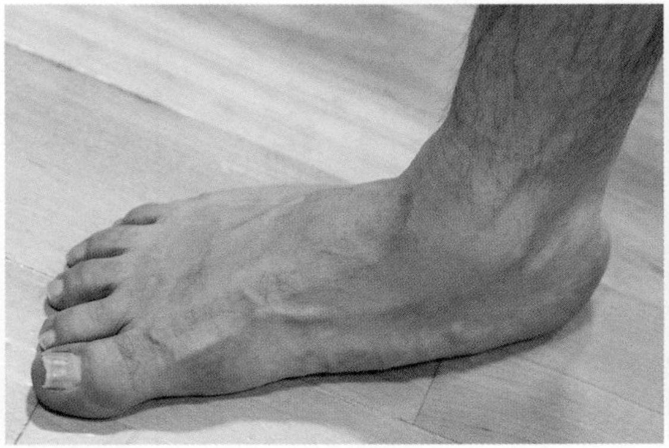	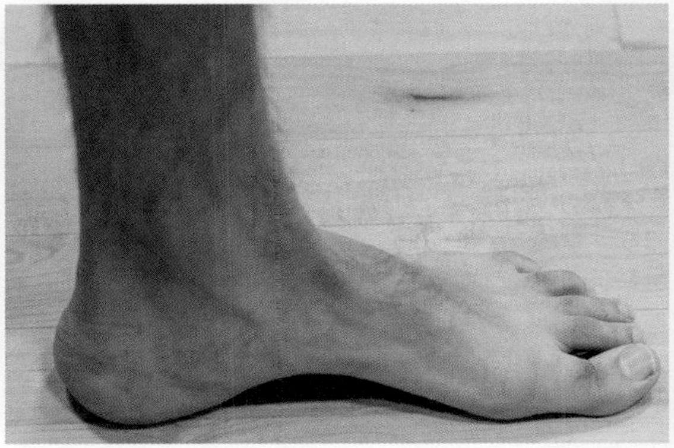	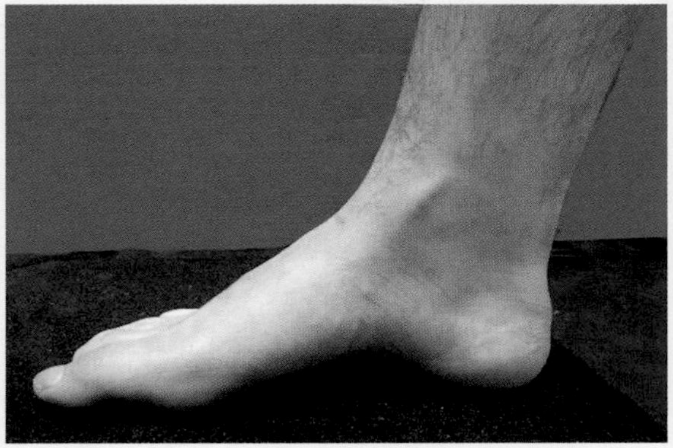
Description	Medial bulge; abducted forefoot, everted calcaneus A medial bulge must be present at the talonavicular joint, indicating excessive talar adduction. The medial arch must be low. This is determined by the Feiss line, formed by connecting the points formed by the head of the 1st MT, the navicular tubercle, and the medial malleolus.	The calcaneus is slightly everted. A medial bulge is not present. Feiss line indicates that the most prominent aspect of the navicular is in line with the apex of the medial malleolus and the plantar surface of the 1st MTP joint.	The calcaneus must be inverted greater than 3° from perpendicular relative to the position of the ground. A medial bulge is not present. The Feiss line indicates that the most prominent aspect of the navicular is above the line.

MT = metatarsal; MTP = metatarsophalangeal

Selective Tissue Test 8-1
Longitudinal Arch Angle

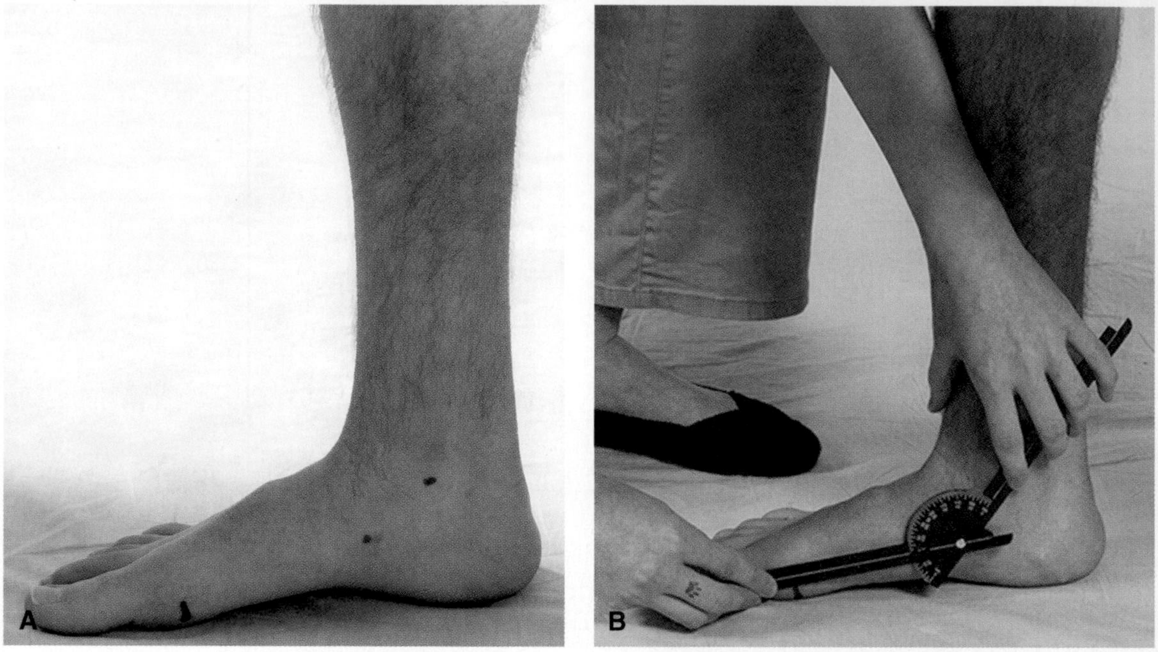

Patient Position
Seated with the foot in STJN

Position of Examiner
Positioned at the patient's feet

Evaluative Procedure
(A) Identify and mark the head of the 1st MT, the navicular tuberosity, and the apex of the medial malleolus.
(B) Measure the angle created by these lines with a goniometer.
Repeat the measurement with the patient standing with weight evenly distributed.
Calculate the difference between the first and second measurements to assess ROM.

Positive Test
Foot posture is based on the resulting angle:[21]

Static position	Range of motion
Severely low arch: <120°	>19° = very flexible
Low arch: 121°–130°	19° to 13° = flexible
Normal: 131°–152°	13° to −1° = normal
High arch: 153°–162°	−1° to −7° = rigid
Severely high arch: >162°	<−7° = very rigid

Evidence

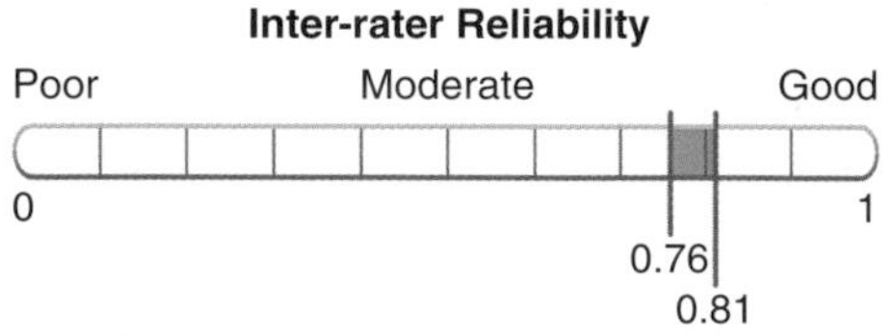

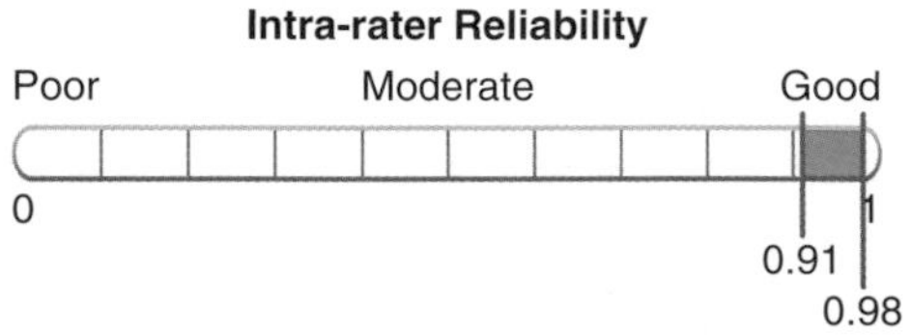

MT = metatarsal; ROM = range of motion; STJN = subtalar joint neutral

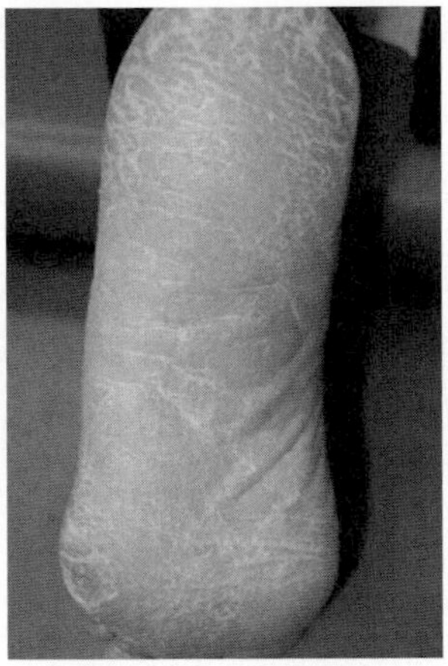

FIGURE 8-13 ■ "Moccasin" type of tinea pedis. Dryness, scaling, and erythema of the plantar and/or lateral foot. *(From Barankin B and Freiman A. Derm Notes: Clinical Dermatology Pocket Guide. Philadelphia, FA Davis, 2006.)*

common warts (verruca vulgaris) (Fig. 8-14). Weight bearing and the thick callus cause plantar warts to appear to grow inward, creating a dark core within a depression on the bottom of the foot. The central **petechiae** mask the normal **whorls** and skin markings, thus differentiating them from callus. Caused by exposure to the human papilloma virus, usually found in a moist environment (e.g., public showers), plantar warts are often localized to areas of excessive weight-bearing stresses. However, they may develop anywhere on the plantar aspect of the foot.

Plantar warts are more focal than an ordinary callus, are point tender, and can cause pain during weight-bearing activities and disrupt gait. The patient often complains of the sensation of "stepping on a pebble." Warts may spontaneously appear and disappear, so initial care is generally watchful. Persistent warts can be successfully treated using over-the-counter wart medication containing salicylic acid but need up to 12 weeks of consistent treatment. Physicians or podiatrists may use liquid nitrogen to freeze the wart, a treatment option that requires fewer treatments. Unrelenting warts may be removed by a physician or podiatrist using laser, injection of medication, or electrocautery.[22]

Inspection of the Toes

- **General toe alignment:** The common toe malalignments are presented in Inspection Findings 8-2.
- **Morton's alignment:** This condition, also referred to as **Morton's toe**, results in a greater amount of force transmitted along the second ray during push-off. A callus may be present under the second MT head. Morton's toe has been associated with increased callus formation, pain, stress fracture, and hallux rigidus.[23,24] Hypertrophy of the second MT was once believed to be a consequence of Morton's toe, but this relationship has not been substantiated.[25]

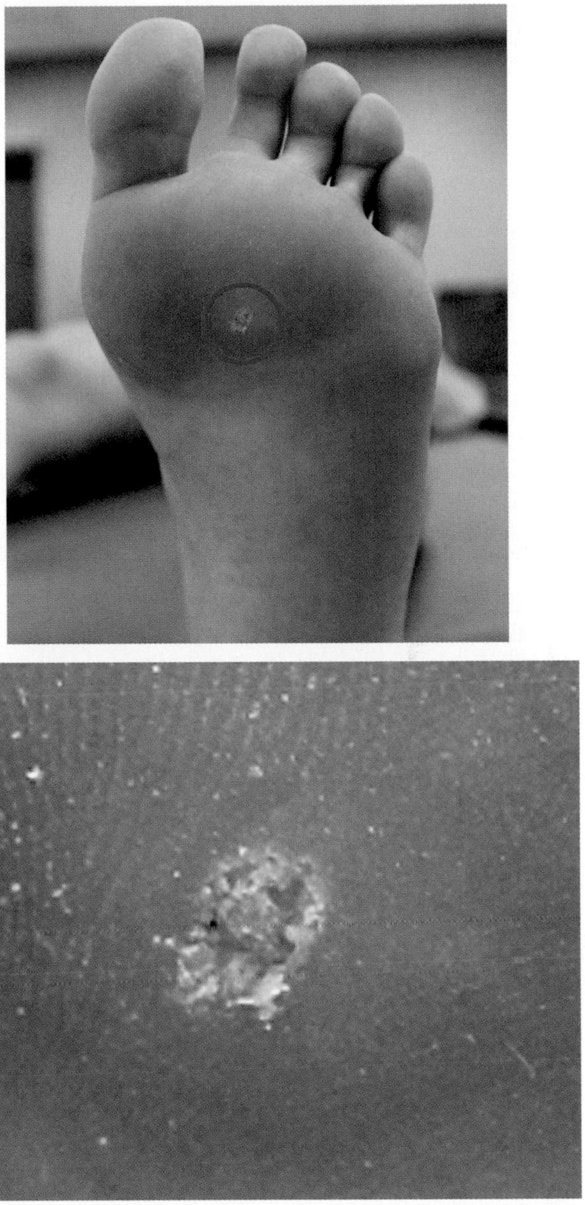

FIGURE 8-14 ■ Plantar warts. This condition results in point tenderness and masks the normal skin markings, thus distinguishing it from callus.

- **Claw toes:** Claw toes are commonly associated with pes cavus. A callus may be found over the dorsal portion of the PIP joint and on the plantar surface of the MTP joint and, in some cases, on the tips of the toes.
- **Hammer toes:** Hammer toes may develop as either the long toe extensors or long toe flexors substitute for weakness of the primary dorsiflexors or plantarflexors. They often occur after injury, such as a rupture of the plantar fascia, or with neuromuscular disease states. A

Petechiae Small, purplish, hemorrhagic spots on the skin

Whorls Swirl markings in the skin; fingerprints are images formed by the whorls on the fingertips

Inspection Findings 8-2
Pathological Toe Postures

	Claw Toe	Hammer Toe
Observation	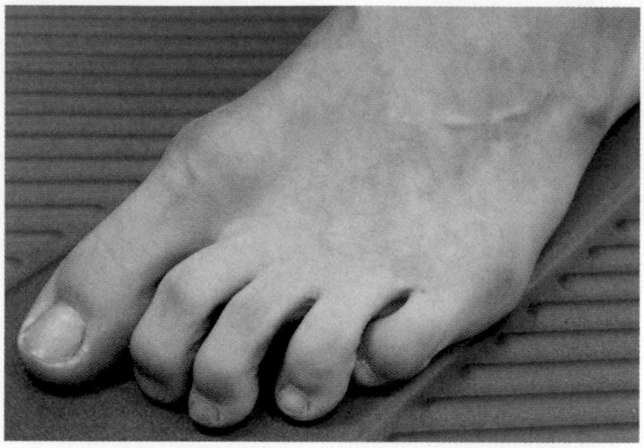	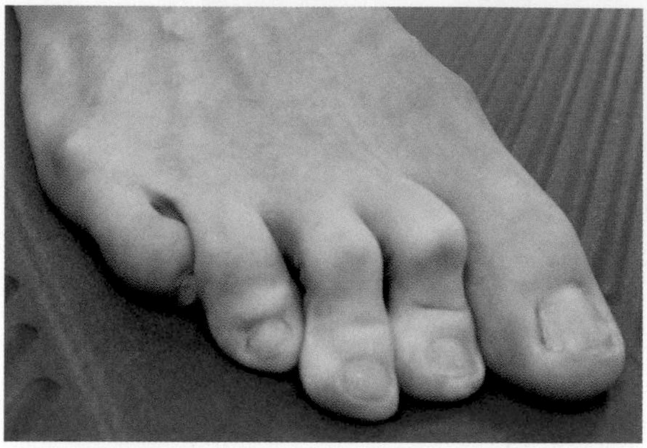
Illustration	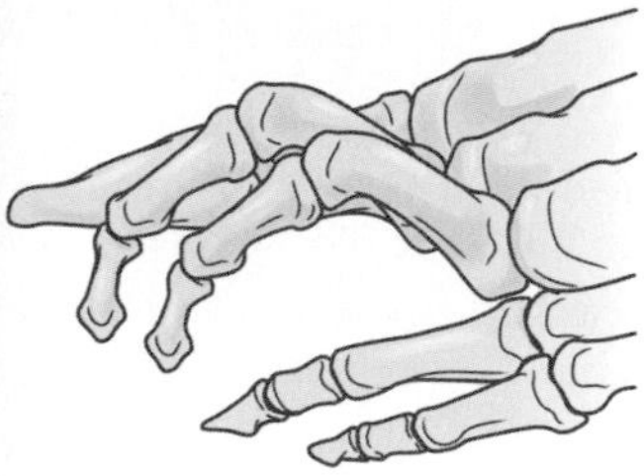	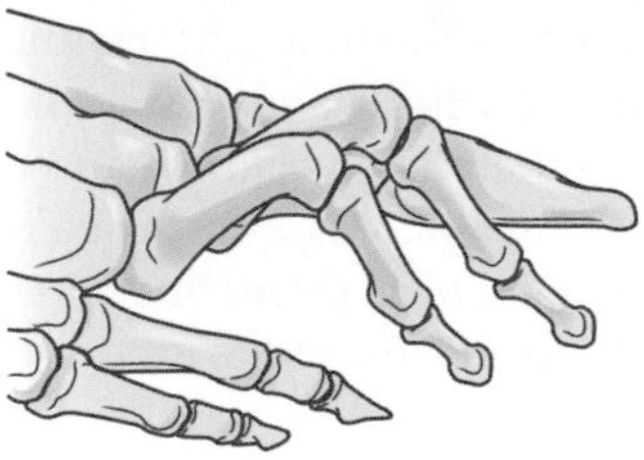
Deviation	Progressive contracture of the interosseous and/or lumbrical muscles	Contractures of the associated toe extensors and flexors; inability of the interosseous muscles to hold the proximal phalanx in the neutral position
Description	Hyperextension of the MTP joint and flexion of the PIP and DIP joints. Claw toes affect the lateral four toes.	Hyperextension of the MTP and DIP joints and flexion of the PIP joints of the lateral four toes

DIP = distal interphalangeal; PIP = proximal interphalangeal; MT = metatarsal; MTP = metatarsophalangeal

callus may be located on the dorsal surface of the PIP joint, resulting from friction against the shoe. In most cases, this deformity affects only one ray and may be caused by improperly fitting shoes (especially during the growth years), hereditary factors, elongation of the plantar fascia, or hallux valgus.[26]

- **Hallux valgus:** Hallux valgus is characterized by an abducted first ray at the MTP joint and is associated with a pes planus foot type.[27] Pain and dysfunction may also result from a bunion over the first MTP joint that forms secondary to the valgus deformity or secondary to the dislocation of the first MTP joint's sesamoid bones. The subsequent toe deformity can cause footwear to fit improperly and alter biomechanics (see Hallux Valgus, p. 230).[28]
  - **Bunion:** Formed by the development and subsequent inflammation of a bursa, bunions are characterized by inflammation on the medial aspect of the first MTP joint. Causes of bunions include hallux valgus and poorly fitting shoes. A smaller bunionette, or tailor's

Morton's Toe	Hallux Valgus
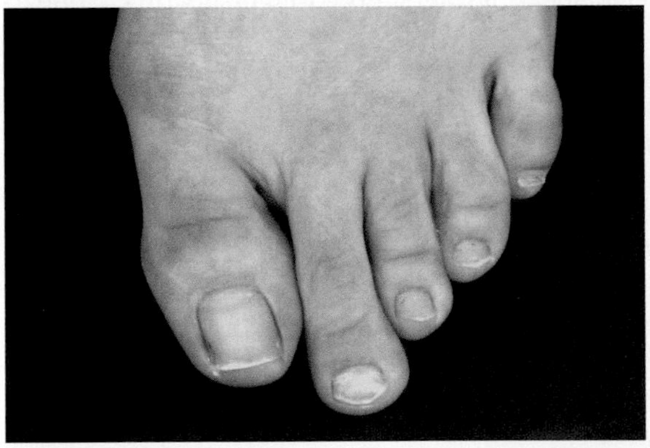	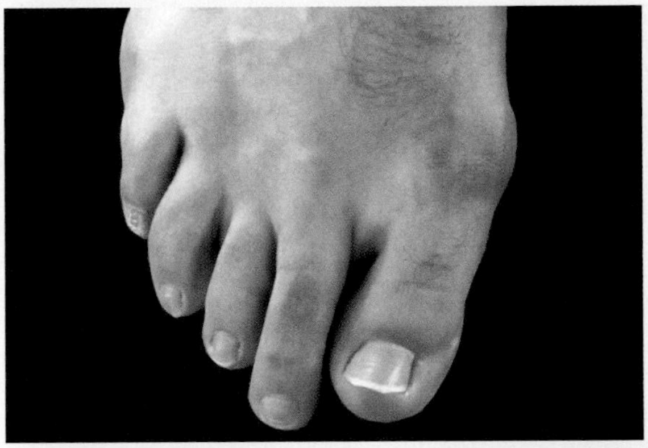
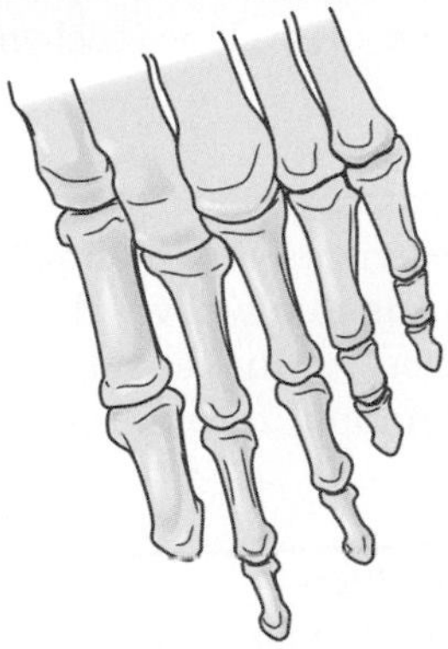	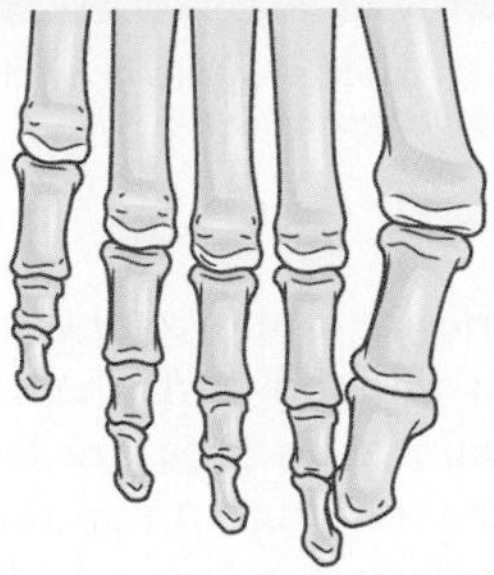
Although it appears that the 2nd toe is longer than the 1st, Morton's toe is formed by the 1st MT being shorter than the 2nd.	Over time, there is a gradual subluxation of the 1st MTP joint. A bunion will develop on the medial border of the 1st MTP joint. Lateral displacement of the great toe may interfere with the function of the 2nd toe.[28]
The posture of the foot is normal, but the 2nd toe extends beyond the great toe.	The 1st MTP joint exceeds an angle of 20° in the frontal plane. The 1st and 2nd toes may overlap.

bunion, may form on the lateral aspect of the fifth MTP joint.

- **Ingrown toenail (onychocryptosis):** Most often involving the great toe, the medial and/or lateral aspect of the nail grows into the bed (Fig. 8-15). The areas of ingrowth cause disruption and subsequent infection of the skin surrounding and beneath the nailbed, causing it to appear red and swollen, warranting physician referral.
- **Onychomycosis:** Fungal infections of the toenail cause the nail to appear yellow and brittle. Although often the result of aging, factors such as poor hygiene, poor blood circulation, and tinea pedis (athlete's foot) may predispose an outbreak. Onychomycosis is often successfully treated using a topical antifungal agent.[29]
- **Subungual hematoma:** Localized trauma to the toe can result in the formation of a hematoma beneath

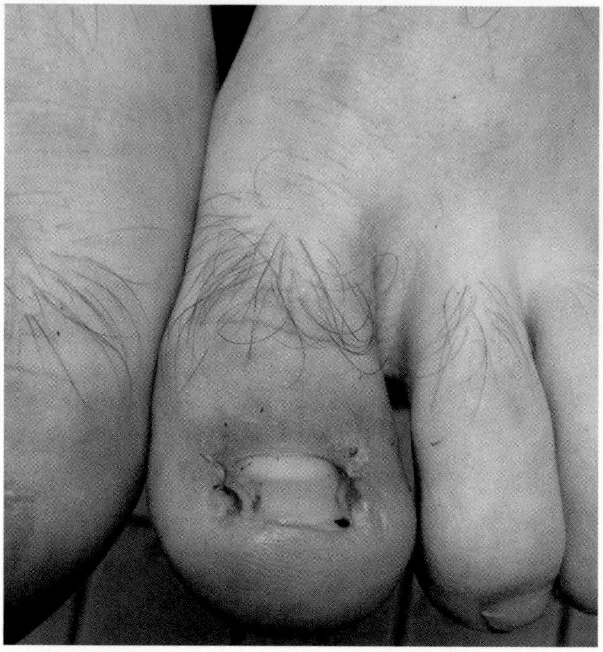

FIGURE 8-15 ■ Ingrown toenail. This painful condition results from abnormal growth patterns of the nail, causing it to imbed within the skin.

the nail (Fig. 8-16). Commonly found in the great toe, the resulting collection of blood turns the nail a dark purple and causes pain from pressure being placed on the involved nerve endings. A subungual hematoma may form secondary to a fracture of the distal phalanx and may be caused by a falling object or other compressive forces. If the lumina is no longer visible, the nail will eventually fall off.

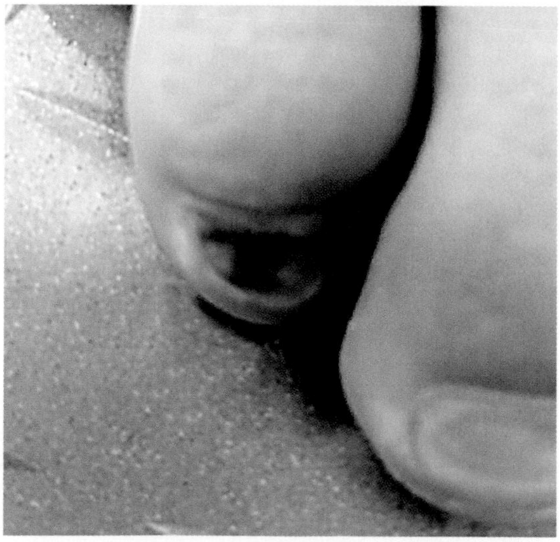

FIGURE 8-16 ■ Trauma to the toe can result in bleeding under the nail, a subungual hematoma. Draining the blood from beneath the nail often provides substantial pain relief.

Inspection of the Medial Structures

- **Medial longitudinal arch:** Spanning from the calcaneus to the first MTP joint, the medial longitudinal arch is more prominent when the foot is non–weight bearing. The relationship between weight-bearing and non–weight-bearing appearance gives a subjective measure of the amount of the foot's flexibility. In the non–weight-bearing position, observe if the arch assumes a planus or cavus posture. A detailed evaluation of the arch is presented in the Region-Specific Pathologies section of this chapter.

Inspection of the Lateral Structures

- **Fifth metatarsal:** Normally, the foot's lateral border is relatively straight, especially along the shaft of the fifth MT. A deviation of the bone's contour is indicative of a fracture.
- **Lateral ankle:** Observe the structures of the lateral ankle, primarily the distal fibula, lateral malleolus, and joint line, for the presence of swelling, ecchymosis, and/or gross deformity.

Inspection of the Dorsal Structures

The tendons of the long toe extensors and the small mass of the extensor digitorum brevis thinly cover the dorsal surface of the foot laterally. Observe the dorsal aspect of the foot for swelling, discoloration, or abnormal bony alignment.

Inspection of the Plantar Surface

When inspecting the length of the plantar surface of the foot, pay particular attention to the condition of the skin and the presence of callus formation or blisters, as previously noted. Mild swelling may be present at the medial calcaneal tubercle in the presence of plantar fasciitis or at the head of the first metatarsal if the sesamoids are pathologically involved. Observe for callus formation. Calluses under the head of the second MT are typical in the presence of a rearfoot varus due to instability at push-off. A "pinch" callus at the medial great toe is associated with a forefoot varus.[30]

Inspection of the Posterior Structures

- **Achilles tendon:** With the patient weight bearing, observe the relationship of the Achilles tendon to the tibia. Normally these two structures are aligned. Bowing of the tendon may be an indication of pes planus (Fig. 8-17). Achilles tendon pathology is discussed in Chapter 9.
- **Calcaneus:** Retrocalcaneal exostosis (also referred to as Haglund deformity or "pump bumps") can be associated with rearfoot varus, retrocalcaneal bursitis, and/or Achilles tendinopathy (Fig. 8-18).[31]

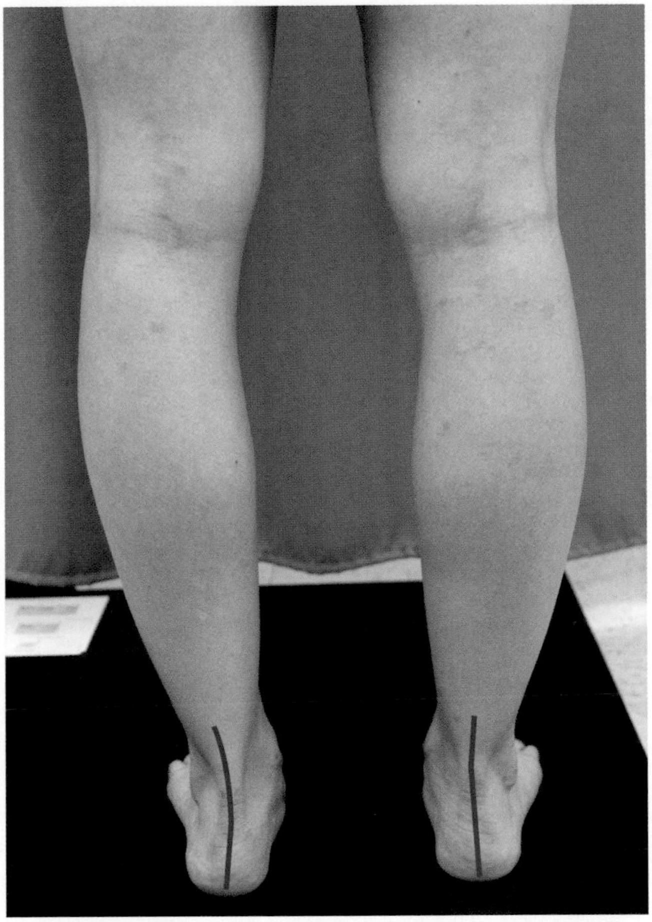

FIGURE 8-17 ■ Achilles tendon alignment in an individual with pes planus. Note the valgus alignment of the calcaneus as noted by the inward bowing of the Achilles tendon.

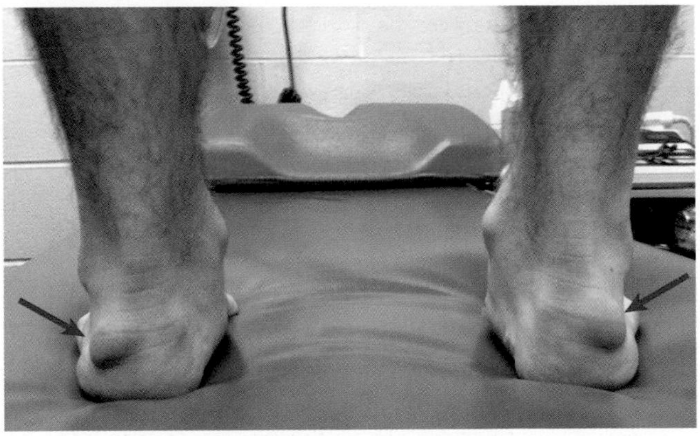

FIGURE 8-18 ■ Retrocalcaneal exostosis, "pump bumps."

Inspection of Foot and Calcaneal Alignment

The controversial concept of a neutral foot position—in which the subtalar joint is neither pronated nor supinated—provides a method to examine the static foot. Establishing a **subtalar joint neutral** (STJN) position allows the observation of frontal plane deviations in the rearfoot and forefoot (Selective Tissue Test 8-2). These deviations alter the gait cycle and place abnormal stress on the foot and proximally along the extremity and into the spine.

Although widely used, the validity of assessing foot alignment has been questioned because it accounts for only frontal plane movement of the more complex subtalar joint, and the interrater reliability is consistently low, making the usefulness of the quantitative results questionable.[32-34] Calcaneal position in STJN is more reliably measured in weight bearing than in non–weight bearing, but it may improve with extensive training.[33,35]

Compare the alignment of the foot when it is weight bearing to when it is non–weight bearing to determine functional adaptations or compensation. Perform the non–weight-bearing assessment with the patient prone and the subtalar joint in neutral to provide a standardized position from which the relative alignment of the rearfoot and forefoot can be observed. Each can be classified as varus, valgus, or neutral (Inspection Findings 8-3).

With the subtalar joint still in the neutral position, assess the tarsometatarsal joint and the first MT for position and mobility (Selective Tissue Test 8-3). A first ray that is plantarflexed at the tarsometatarsal joint results in the first ray being located inferior to the remaining four rays. Plantar-flexed first rays are associated with a cavus foot or can be acquired in the presence of genu varum and may be confused with forefoot valgus. Pes planus is often marked by hypermobility of the first ray at the tarsometatarsal articulation; pes cavus may result in a rigid ray.

- Following assessment of foot position in STJN, observe for compensations with the patient in relaxed stance. For example, an individual with a rearfoot varus assessed in STJN may compensate into a valgus calcaneal position in weight bearing as the medial calcaneal tubercle makes contact with the ground. Use the findings from this static assessment in concert with the findings from the gait assessment.

Selective Tissue Test 8-2
Assessment of Subtalar Joint Neutral

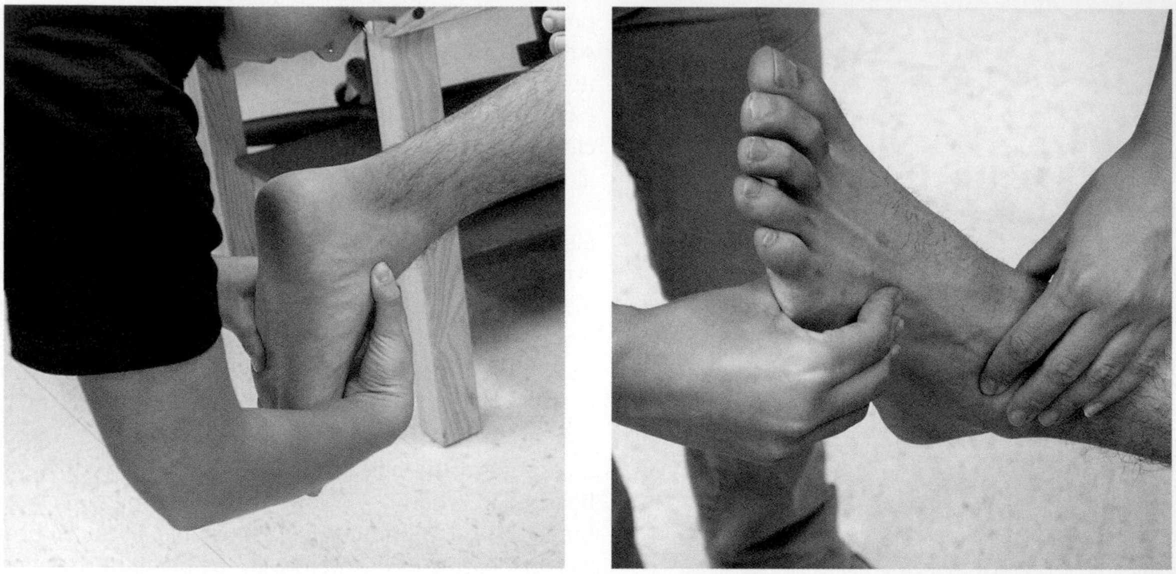

Patient Position

Prone with foot off the end of the table

The nontest leg is positioned with the hip flexed, abducted, and externally rotated and the knee flexed (figure 4 position).

Position of Examiner

At the patient's feet

The thumb and index finger are at the anterior talocrural joint, palpating the medial and lateral aspects of the talar head.

The thumb and index finger of the distal hand grasp the heads of the 4th and 5th MTs, gently applying a dorsiflexion pressure until soft tissue resistance is noted.[36]

Evaluative Procedure

The examiner passively supinates and pronates the foot using the distal hand while palpating the talar position with the proximal hand.

Neutral position is found when the talus is symmetrically aligned between the proximal thumb and forefinger. From this position, the postures of the forefoot and rearfoot are noted (see Inspection Findings 8-3).

A goniometric measurement provides an objective assessment of calcaneal position with the STJ in neutral:

- Align the fulcrum over the proximal calcaneus.
- Position the proximal stationary arm bisecting the lower leg.
- Position the distal movement arm bisecting the calcaneus.

Modification

STJN can be assessed with the patient standing or sitting and the examiner kneeling in front of the patient. The assessment can also be performed with the patient in the supine position.

Comments

Findings from a static foot posture assessment must be interpreted in conjunction with functional assessment.

Evidence

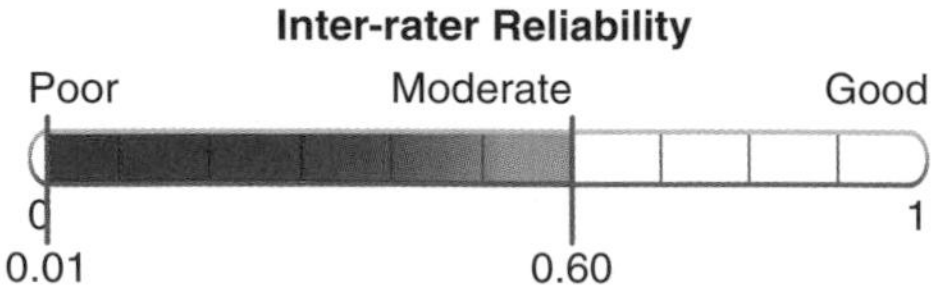

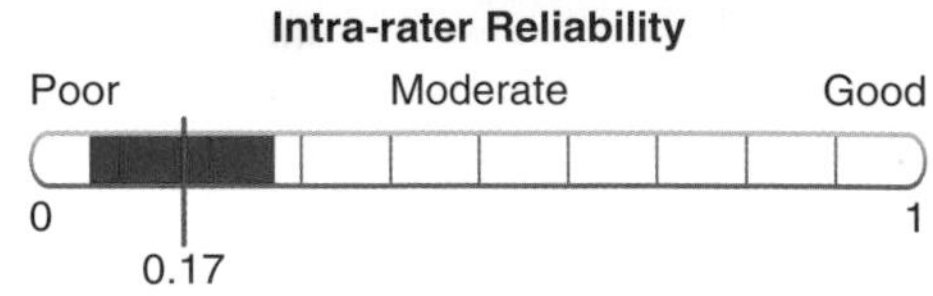

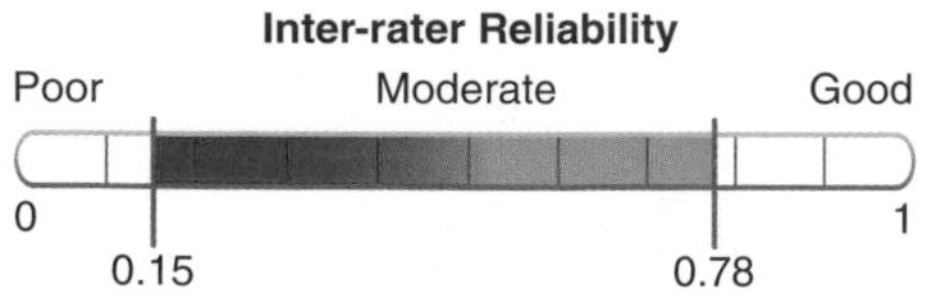

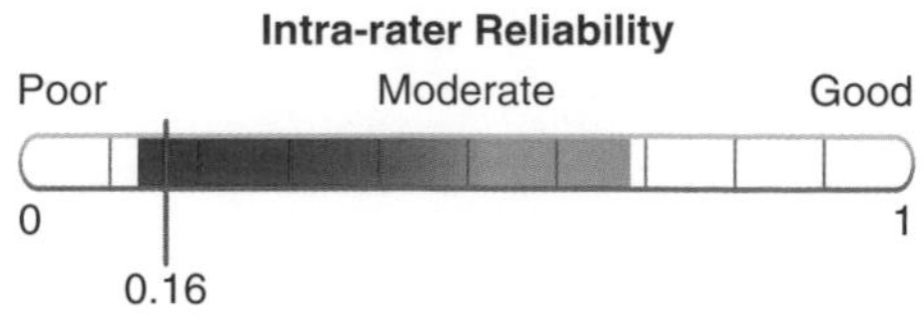

MT = metatarsal; STJ = subtalar joint; STJN = subtalar joint neutral

Inspection Findings 8-3
Common Foot Postures Assessed in Non–Weight-Bearing Subtalar Joint Neutral

	Forefoot Varus	Forefoot Valgus	Rearfoot Varus	Rearfoot Valgus
Illustration	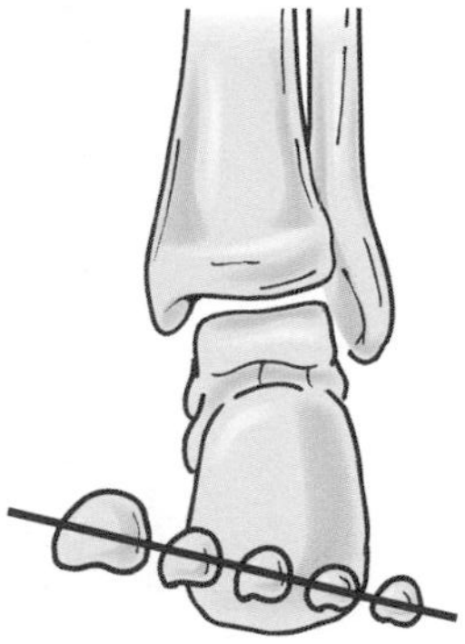	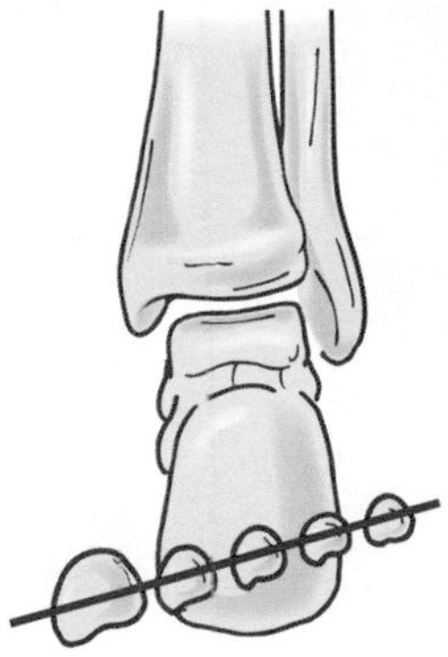	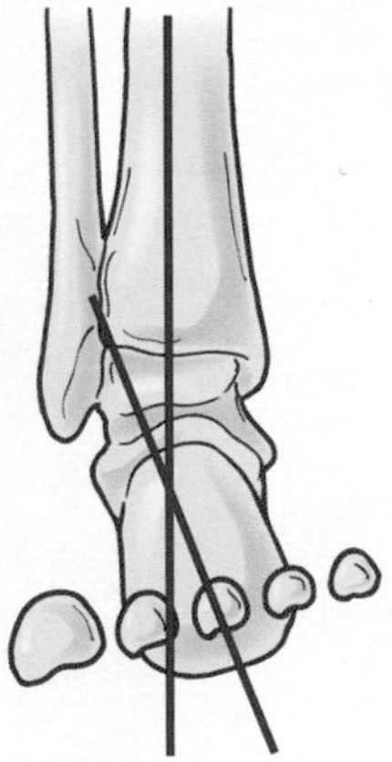	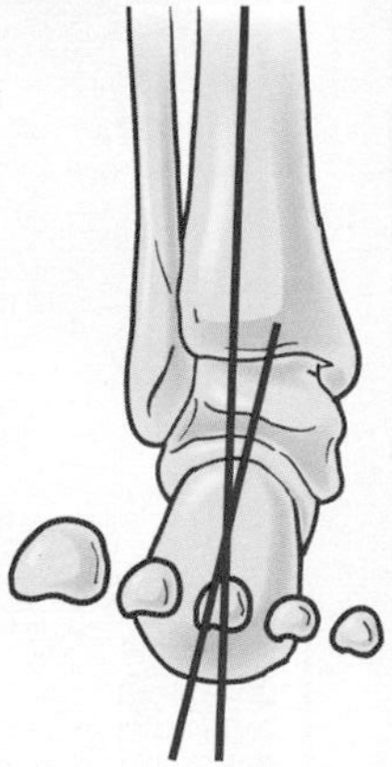
Posture Calcaneus is vertical or slightly (<3°) inverted (varus) relative to the long axis of the bisected lower leg. MT heads are perpendicular to calcaneus.	MT heads are inverted relative to the rearfoot. Varus of 1°–8° is considered normal.[35]	MT heads are everted relative to the rearfoot. A plantar-flexed first ray will also give the appearance of a forefoot valgus.	Calcaneus is inverted relative to the long axis of the bisected lower leg and may be related to a varus alignment of the tibia or a calcaneus that does not completely derotate during development.	Calcaneus is everted relative to the long axis of the tibia and can be associated with a valgus tibial alignment. Rearfoot valgus is rarely observed.
Compensation	During static weight bearing, the forefoot compensates by abducting and everting, resulting in a more planus foot. During gait, pronation is excessive and prolonged, as the 1st MT has farther to travel before contacting the ground.	During static weight bearing, the midfoot supinates as the 1st MT contacts the ground. During gait, the 1st MT strikes the ground prematurely, resulting in early supination, reducing the shock-absorbing capacity of the limb.	With sufficient subtalar joint mobility, the rearfoot will rapidly and excessively pronate during the early stages of gait.	The rearfoot becomes hypermobile, resulting in increased pronation.

Evidence

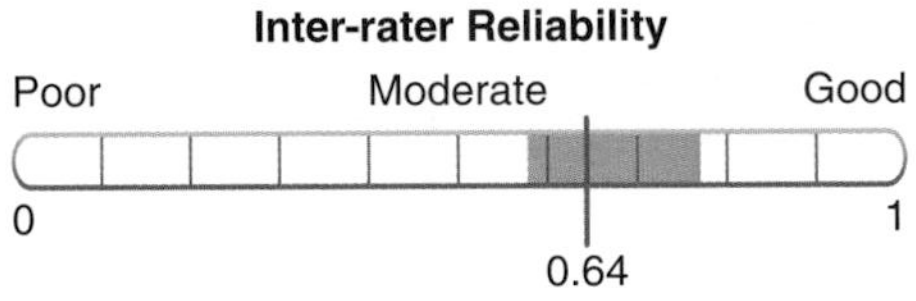

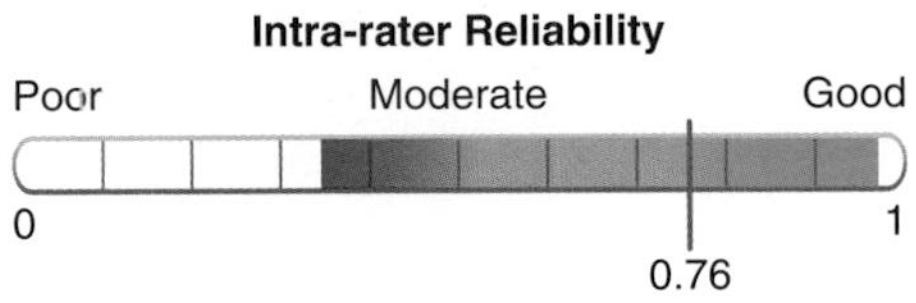

MT = metatarsal

Selective Tissue Test 8-3
Position and Mobility of First Tarsometatarsal Joint

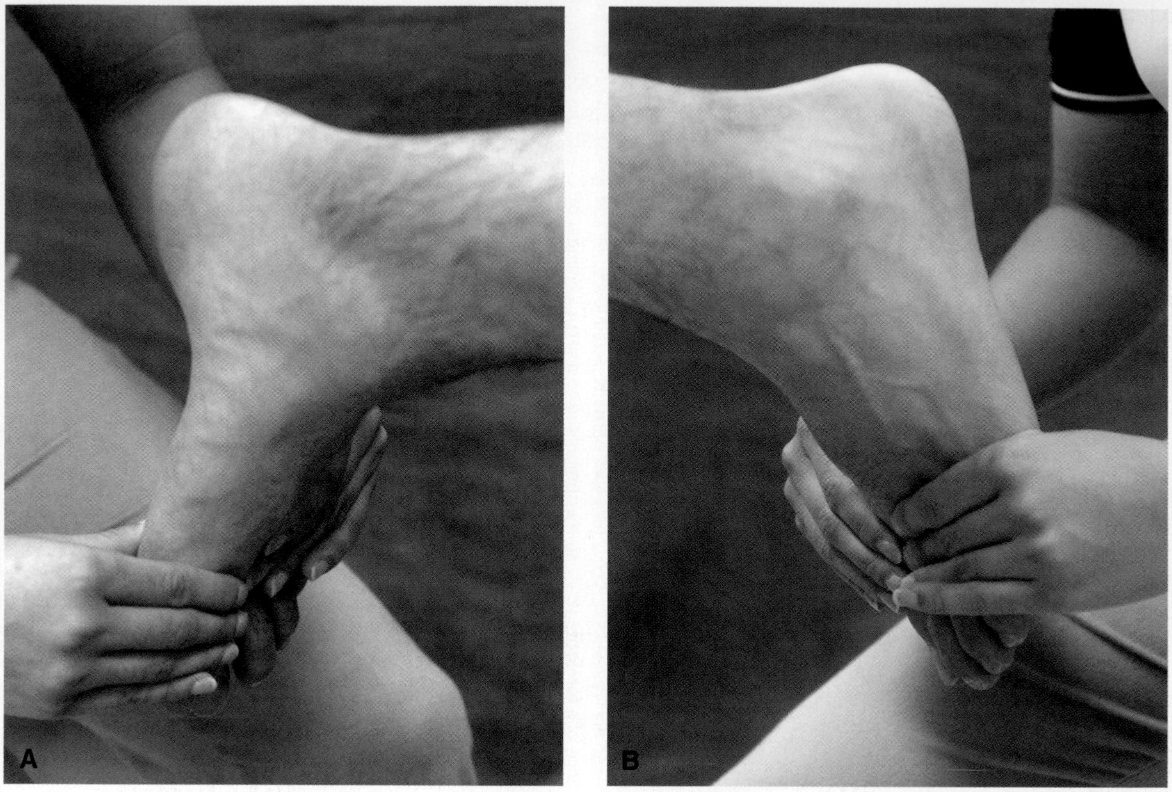

The static position and mobility of the 1st MT can influence foot mechanics and should be assessed from a non–weight-bearing position with the subtalar and talocrural joints in neutral. (A) Medial view (B) Lateral view.

Patient Position	Prone with foot off the end of the table with subtalar and talocrural joints in neutral (see Selective Tissue Test 8-2) The nontest leg is positioned with the hip flexed, abducted, and externally rotated and the knee flexed (figure 4 position).
Position of Examiner	Using a lumbrical grip on the lateral four MT heads while grasping the first MT head allows examination of the MT position.
Evaluative Procedure	Note the resting position of the first MT. Plantarflex and dorsiflex the first ray, noting the amount of mobility in each direction.
Positive Test	A rigid or stiff plantarflexed first ray cannot be brought into a neutral alignment, while a supple plantar-flexed first ray has sufficient mobility to realign. The head of a plantar-flexed first ray is inferior compared with the lateral four MT heads.
Implications	A rigid plantarflexed first ray creates early supination, resulting in less shock absorption during gait. Stress fractures or sesamoid pathology may result. A hypermobile first ray may contribute to general MT pain (metatarsalgia) and hallux valgus deformity.[7]
Modification	Use of a ruler for a quantitative assessment is associated with poor interrater reliability (ICC = 0.05; SEM = 1.2 mm).[37]
Comments	A forefoot valgus alignment is easily confused with a plantar-flexed first ray.
Evidence	Assessment of first-ray mobility has poor interrater reliability [k = 0.16]. The low relationship between results of the manual technique and a more reliable mechanical device indicates that the technique's validity is also suspect.[38] Mechanical measurement of dorsal first-ray mobility has poor reliability. (ICC = 0.05).[37]

MT = metatarsal

PALPATION

To make palpation easier, position the patient so the foot and ankle extend off the end of the table. Palpate structures proximal to the foot as warranted.

Palpation of the Medial Structures

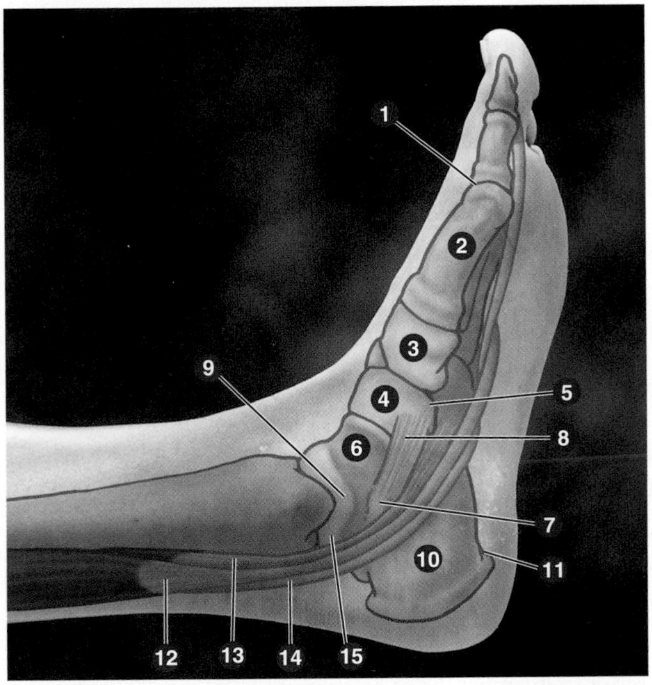

1 First MTP joint: Begin palpating the medial foot by locating the articulation between the proximal phalanx of the first toe and the first MT. Palpate the area for tenderness or increased skin temperature that may indicate acute injury to the ligamentous structures, chronic inflammatory conditions of the tendons or articular structures, or disease states such as **gout**. In the presence of hallux valgus or hallux rigidus, thickening of the synovial capsule, sesamoid pain (see Palpation of the Plantar Structures, p. 200), callus, crepitus, and, possibly, a bunion may be noted. These symptoms may also involve the second toe.[28]

2 First metatarsal: From the first MTP joint, palpate the length of the first MT, noting crepitus, bony deformity, or pain elicited along the shaft. Because the dorsal and medial surfaces and part of the plantar surface of this bone are easily palpated, gross fractures can be identified with relative ease.

3 First cuneiform: Identify the base of the first MT as it articulates with the first cuneiform by the attachment of the tibialis anterior muscle. To make this bone more palpable, ask the patient to actively plantarflex the ankle. The motion causes the base of the first MT to be depressed on the cuneiform, making this junction more palpable.

4–5 Navicular and (5) navicular tuberosity: Palpate proximally from the first cuneiform to locate its articulation with the medial border of the **navicular**. The navicular serves as the keystone of the medial longitudinal arch. As such, any dysfunction of this bone results in dysfunction of the arch as a whole. The **navicular tuberosity:** Move posteriorly from the articulation to find the prominent medial navicular tuberosity. The tuberosity may detach from the bone as the result of trauma or a congenital malformation, forming an **accessory navicular**.

6 Talar head: Palpate the talar head, immediately proximal and superior to the navicular. This structure is more easily located by pronating and supinating the midfoot. When the midfoot is pronated, the talar head is more prominent medially.

7 Sustentaculum tali: Palpate the sustentaculum tali, a protrusion off the calcaneus, inferior to the medial malleolus. Serving as an attachment site for the calcaneonavicular ligament and providing inferior support to the talus, the sustentaculum tali is not always easily identifiable.

8 Calcaneonavicular ligament: Palpate the plantar calcaneonavicular ligament from its origin on the sustentaculum tali to its insertion on the navicular. This ligament, with its very limited extensibility, is the base of the joint capsule of the calcaneotalonavicular joint. In cases of pes planus or midfoot sprains, this ligament may become very tender to the touch or feel thickened.

9 Medial talar tubercle: Palpate proximally and superiorly from the calcaneonavicular ligament to locate the small projection off the proximal-medial border of the talus, immediately adjacent to the anterior margin of the medial malleolus. The medial talar tubercle serves as a site of attachment for a segment of the deltoid ligament.

10–11 Calcaneus and (11) medial calcaneal tubercle: From the medial talar tubercle, palpate inferiorly to locate the posterior flare of the **calcaneus**; continue to palpate to the site of the plantar fascia attachment, the **medial calcaneal tubercle**.

Medial Tendons (12–14):

12 Flexor hallucis longus: The bulk of this muscle, hidden beneath the gastrocnemius and soleus muscles, is not palpable until its tendon begins its path posterior to, and around, the medial malleolus. It is difficult to distinguish this tendon from the other structures in the area. As the tendon begins its course along the plantar aspect of the foot, it again is no longer palpable until it inserts on the distal phalanx of the great toe. Resisting flexion of the great toe makes this tendon more prominent as it passes across the plantar aspect of the first MTP joint and courses to its attachment site.

13 Tibialis posterior: Palpate the tibialis posterior from its insertion on the medial aspect of the navicular. The tendon will become more prominent if the patient actively supinates the foot.

14 Flexor digitorum longus: Similar to the flexor hallucis longus, the mass of the flexor digitorum longus is not identifiable as it lies beneath the bulk of the gastrocnemius and soleus muscles. Its tendon is palpable, although not uniquely identifiable, as it passes posterior to, and around, the medial malleolus. As it passes along the plantar aspect of the foot, the tendon is no longer palpable until it inserts on the plantar aspect of the second through fifth toes.

15 Posterior tibial pulse: Locate the pulse associated with the posterior tibial artery just behind the medial malleolus.

Palpation of the Lateral Structures

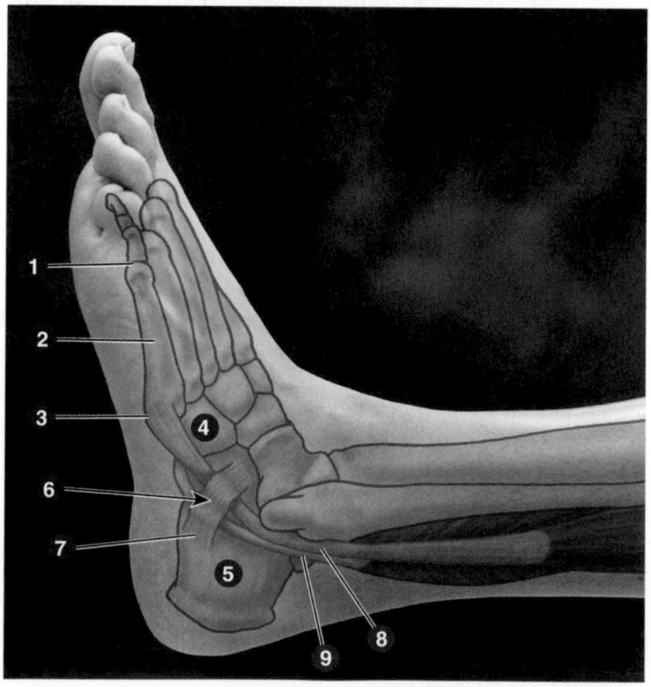

1 Fifth MTP joint: Locate the articulation between the fifth toe and fifth MT. Palpate the joint for tenderness arising from ligament or articular damage.

2 Fifth metatarsal: From the fifth MTP joint, palpate the length of the fifth MT, noting pain or discontinuity in the bone's shaft. This structure, especially at its proximal end, is a frequent site of acute fractures and stress fractures.

3 Styloid process: The base of the fifth MT is marked by a laterally projecting styloid process (tuberosity), the site where the peroneus brevis tendon attaches. Covered by a bursa, this structure is commonly avulsed as the peroneus brevis tendon is pulled from its attachment.

4 Cuboid: Locate the cuboid by palpating immediately proximal to the styloid process. The groove through which the peroneus longus begins to pass on the plantar aspect of the foot is located on the cuboid just proximal to the styloid of the fifth metatarsal.

5 Lateral calcaneal border: From the cuboid, continue to palpate towards the rearfoot. The junction between the cuboid and the calcaneus is often indistinct.

6–7 Peroneal tubercle and (7) interior peroneal retinaculum: The **peroneal tubercle** is the most prominent bony landmark on the lateral calcaneus, located inferior and anterior to the most distal portion of the lateral malleolus and beneath the **inferior peroneal retinaculum.** The peroneal tubercle marks the point where the peroneus longus and brevis tendons diverge after passing posterior and inferior to the lateral malleolus.

8–9 Peroneal tendons: Locate the bony lateral portion of the distal one-third of the fibula. The tendons of the **(8) peroneus brevis** and **(9) longus** are palpated as a single structure as they course posterior to the distal third of the fibula and pass on the inferior aspect of the lateral malleolus. The tendons' paths split at the peroneal tubercle, with the brevis superiorly and the longus inferiorly. From this point, the peroneus brevis tendon can be palpated to its insertion on the styloid process of the fifth MT. The peroneus longus tendon can be palpated to the point where it passes through the peroneal groove between the fifth MT's styloid process and the anterior margin of the cuboid. Here it disappears on the plantar aspect of the foot. The peroneus longus' insertion can be palpated on the medial and inferior surface of the first cuneiform and proximal portion of the first MT. Injury to these structures may result in pain at the base of the fifth MT and cuboid.

Palpation of the Dorsal Structures

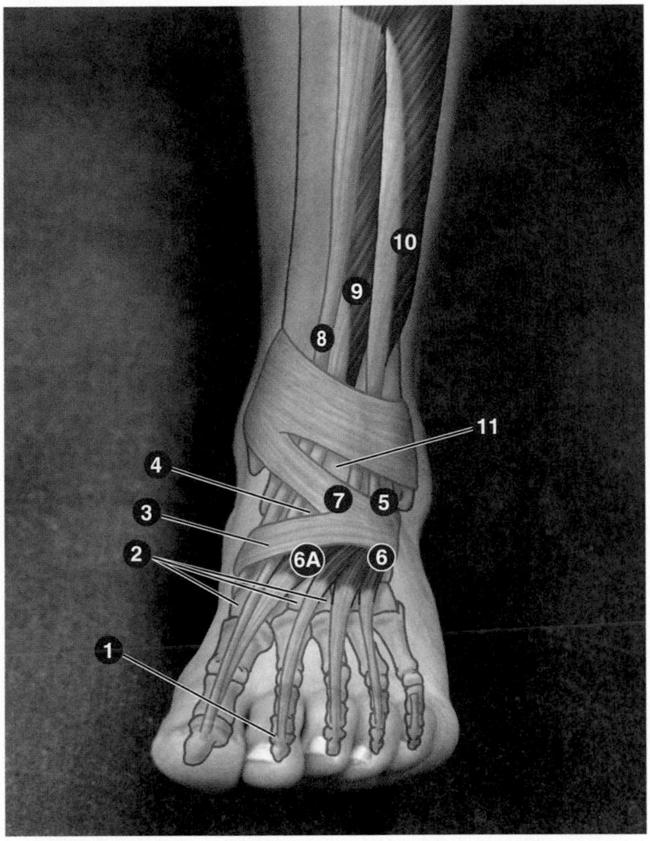

1 Rays: Starting with the distal phalanx, palpate the toes and the length of their associated MTs, noting any deformity, crepitus, or pain elicited during the process.

2 Cuneiforms: Although the cuneiforms are indistinguishable from each other to the touch, their locations can be approximated relative to the first three MTs. In general, the three cuneiforms each articulate with the first three MTs. The individual cuneiforms can be identified by palpating the length of the medial three MTs to their bases (see Fig. 8-3).

3 Navicular: Palpate posteriorly from the cuneiforms to locate the navicular and its prominent medial tuberosity.

4 Dome of the talus: Palpate posteriorly and somewhat laterally from the navicular to find the dome of the talus. This structure is more easily located if the foot and ankle are placed in supination and plantarflexion, allowing the dome's lateral border to become palpable from under the ankle mortise.

5 Sinus tarsi: Locate the sinus tarsi anterior to the lateral malleolus. Normally, this landmark appears as a depression just anterior to the lateral malleolus, marking the site of the extensor digitorum brevis muscle. With chronic conditions such as arthritis or after acute trauma, including ankle sprains, tarsal fractures, or dislocations, the sinus may become obscured by swelling (see Fig. 9.16).

6 Extensor digitorum brevis: Palpate the origin and proximal muscle belly of the extensor digitorum brevis in the sinus tarsi while the patient is actively extending the toes. The tendinous slips to each of the toes become indistinguishable as they pass under the long toe extensor tendons. The most medial portion of the extensor digitorum brevis muscle and its tendon attaching on the first toe are often referred to as a separate muscle, the **(6A) extensor hallucis brevis.**

7 Inferior extensor retinaculum: Palpate the inferior extensor retinaculum along its entire length as it traverses the entire upper portion of the foot. As the tendons of tibialis anterior, extensor hallucis longus, and extensor digitorum longus pass over the talus and tarsals, their proximity to the bones during dorsiflexion is maintained by the retinaculum.

8 Tibialis anterior: Ask the patient to supinate the subtalar joint and dorsiflex the ankle to make the tibialis anterior tendon more palpable at the point where it inserts on the first cuneiform. As the tendon crosses the talocrural joint, it is easily palpable but quickly loses its identity as it flares into its musculotendinous junction.

9 Extensor hallucis longus: Locate the extensor hallucis longus tendon by palpating laterally from the tibialis anterior tendon. With the great toe actively extended, palpate the tendon's length from the tibialis anterior to its flare into the distal phalanx. Continue to palpate the length of the EHL to its origin on the middle half of the anterior fibula and adjacent interosseous membrane.

10 Extensor digitorum longus: Palpate lateral to the extensor hallucis longus for the tendon of the extensor digitorum longus. Although the central portion of the tendon is difficult to palpate, palpate its individual slips to the lateral four toes, prominent on the dorsal aspect of the foot when the patient extends the toes.

11 Dorsalis pedis pulse: Locate the dorsalis pedis artery lying between the tendons of extensor hallucis longus and extensor digitorum longus. With the ankle in the neutral position, palpate the dorsalis pedis pulse and compare it with the opposite extremity. A unilateral absence or decreased pulse may indicate a proximal vascular obstruction such as anterior compartment syndrome (see Chapter 9).

Palpation of the Plantar Structures

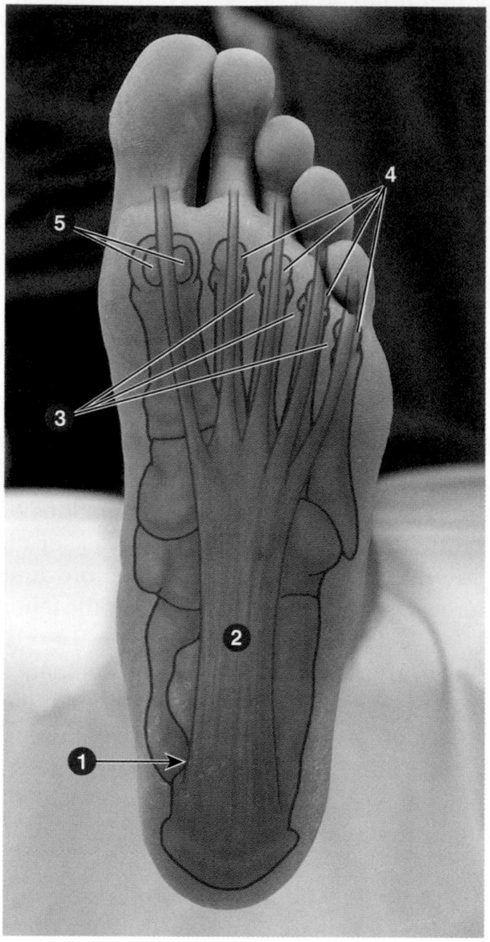

The plantar surfaces of the calcaneus and the MT heads are padded by fatty deposits and overlying thick skin, making it difficult to identify specific bony structures and muscles. The examiner must rely on approximations and functional tests in identifying and determining the source of pain.

1 Medial calcaneal tubercle: Locate the medial calcaneal tubercle by identifying the point where the heel pad begins to thin and merge into the medial longitudinal arch. From this point, move to the medial ridge and apply pressure upward and toward the calcaneus. The medial calcaneal tubercle can also be located by dorsiflexing the ankle and extending the toes to make the plantar fascia more prominent. Then trace the fascia back to its origin on the medial calcaneal tubercle. The anterior ridge of the medial calcaneal tubercle is the attachment site of the plantar fascia and the flexor digitorum brevis muscle. The medial border of this structure is the origin of the abductor hallucis. Pain elicited during palpation of this area may indicate a plantar fasciitis, heel spur, or fat pad pathology.

2 Plantar fascia: Palpate the plantar fascia from its origin on the calcaneus through its length and breadth to its attachment on each of the MT heads, noting any painful areas within this structure. An increase in tissue density along the length of the fascia may be noted.

3 Intermetatarsal neuroma: Apply gentle pressure to the area between the MTs. Nerves located in this area can become compressed and painful.

4 Lateral four metatarsal heads: Beginning with the first MTP joint, palpate each of the MT heads, noting for the presence and integrity of the transverse arch. The pads under the first and fifth MT heads should be the thickest because they are the primary weight-bearing areas of the forefoot.

5 Sesamoid bones of the great toe: Palpate along the plantar surface of the first MT to reach the first MTP joint. At this point, two small sesamoid bones can be felt in the flexor hallucis brevis tendon. Inflammatory conditions of these bones, **sesamoiditis**, or fractures elicit pain to the touch or while weight bearing, especially during the toe-off phase of gait, when pressure is applied to the ball of the foot and the MTP joint is extended. The onset of sesamoiditis has been linked to rigidity of the first ray (often associated with a cavus foot structure).

Joint and Muscle Function Assessment

The relatively limited amount of motion available to the small IP joints makes it difficult to measure their ROM in a clinically meaningful way. This section describes ROM assessment for the MTP and subtalar joints only. The results should be compared bilaterally and considered in light of the functional examination to determine pathology at these joints or their possible contribution to pathologies further up the kinematic chain.

The frontal plane measurement of calcaneal inversion and eversion is frequently used to approximate the amount of pronation and supination, even though it captures only a single plane of these complex motions. The reliability of this measurement is generally poor, improving somewhat when performed in weight bearing.[39] Goniometric measurement of rearfoot inversion and eversion is presented in Goniometry 8-1. Flexion/extension and abduction of the great toe are presented in Goniometry 8-2 and 8-3. Assessment of talocrural plantarflexion and dorsiflexion is described in Chapter 9.

Goniometry 8-1
Rearfoot Inversion and Eversion

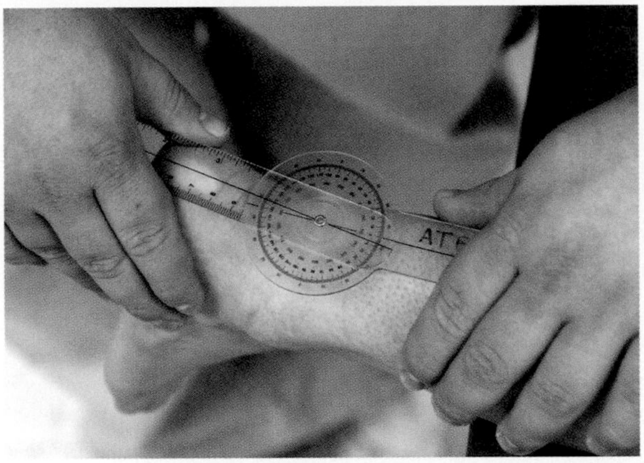

Inversion to eversion (30°–0°–5°)

Patient Position	Prone with ankle in neutral and STJ in neutral
Goniometer Alignment	
Fulcrum	Center the axis over the Achilles tendon with the axis bisecting the malleoli.
Proximal Arm	Center the stationary arm over the midline of the lower leg.
Distal Arm	Center the movement arm over the midline of the calcaneus.
Evidence	

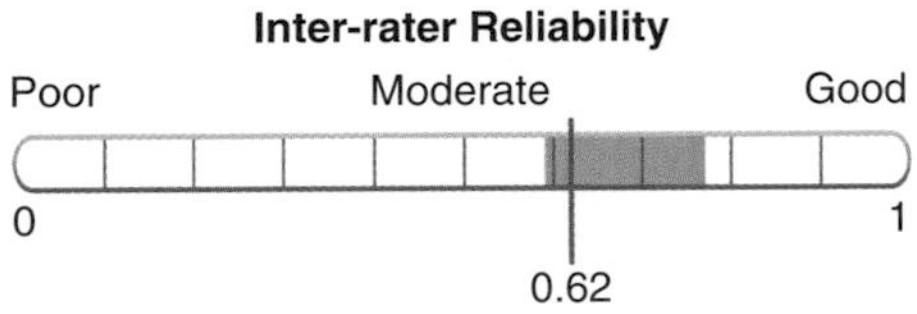

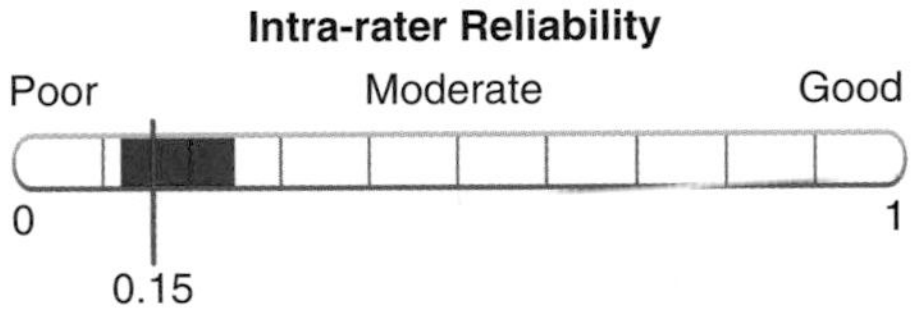

STJ = subtalar joint

Active Range of Motion

The greatest ROM occurs at the first MTP joint, allowing 75 to 85 degrees of extension and 35 to 45 degrees of flexion. To prevent compensatory motion of excessive pronation, the first MTP joint must permit at least 60 to 65 degrees of extension. The ROM available to the MTP joints decreases at each subsequent lateral joint. Active motion at the fifth MTP joint is negligible. Few people have volitional control of the abductor hallucis, making visible active great toe abduction minimal. In the presence of a valgus deformity of the great toe, the muscle is less able to abduct the great toe. It is not clear if this is a cause or a result of the deformity.

Manual Muscle Tests

Strength testing of the great toe musculature is conducted separately from that of the muscles of the lateral four toes (Manual Muscle Tests 8-1 and 8-2). When manual muscle testing, the strength of the long toe flexors and extensors (flexor hallucis longus, flexor digitorum longus, extensor hallucis longus, and extensor digitorum longus) should be assessed repetitively to determine the impact of fatigue on the onset of symptoms and/or weakness. Manual muscle testing for the primary movers of the ankle is discussed in Chapter 9.

Passive Range of Motion

An assessment of passive ROM (PROM) for each MTP joint can identify tendinous or capsular restrictions to movement (Table 8-7). The position of the talocrural joint affects the amount of motion and the firmness of the MTP joint's end-feel because the position of the ankle influences the length of the tendons of the long toe extensors and flexors.

Goniometry 8-2
First Metatarsophalangeal Alignment

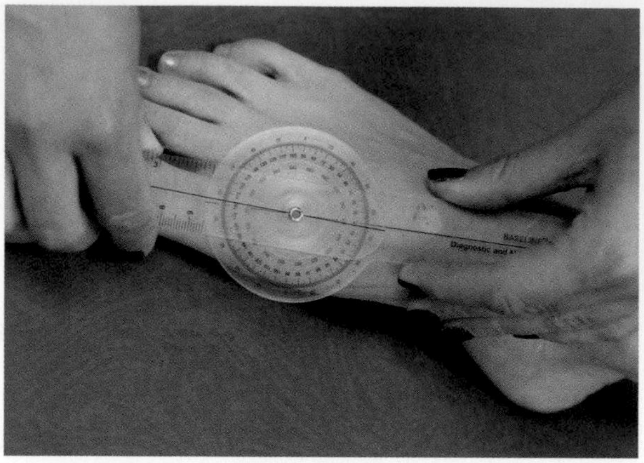

Normal Alignment

Patient Position	Supine or sitting with the STJ and ankle in neutral

Goniometer Alignment

Fulcrum	Place the axis of the goniometer over the dorsal aspect of the MTP joint.
Proximal Arm	Center the stationary arm over the first metatarsal.
Distal Arm	Center the movement arm over the proximal phalanx.
Comments	This measure may be performed with the 1st MTP passively abducted (relative to the 2nd toe).

MTP = metatarsophalangeal; STJ = subtalar joint

In the anatomical position, the talocrural joint is situated at 90 degrees. This is different from the resting position (biomechanical joint neutral). Although the resting position of the talocrural joint differs from person to person, it tends to be 15 to 20 degrees of plantarflexion from the anatomical position and represents the point where the anterior talofibular (ATF) ligament is most taut.

- **Flexion:** Stabilize the forefoot proximal to the MT heads. To prevent contribution from the IP joints, apply pressure on the dorsal portion of the proximal phalanx (Fig. 8-19). The normal end-feel for flexion is firm owing to tension of the dorsal fibers of the joint capsule and the collateral ligaments.
- **Extension:** Maintain stabilization as described for assessment of passive flexion, but apply pressure to the proximal phalanx's plantar aspect (Fig. 8-20). If passive MTP extension is performed with the ankle at 90°, a firm end-feel will develop early, owing to stretching of the long toe flexors. To determine the full joint ROM and capsular end-feel, perform the test with the ankle relaxed. A firm end-feel arises from the capsule's plantar fibers and the short flexor muscles. Limitation in extension of the first MTP can increase the stresses on the medial structures of the foot and lower leg, including the plantar fascia, flexor hallucis longus, and flexor digitorum longus.

Joint Stability Tests

Identifying subtle hyper- and hypomobilities of the individual foot articulations is difficult. This section describes how to isolate stresses to the ligaments stabilizing the toes and the general integrity of the midfoot's soft tissues.

Stress Testing

- **Metatarsophalangeal and interphalangeal joints:** The MTP and IP joints are supported by the medial and lateral collateral ligaments (MCL and LCL). The dorsal and plantar surfaces of these articulations are reinforced by the joint capsule. Passive **overpressure** in

Overpressure A force that attempts to move a joint beyond its normal ROM

Goniometry 8-3
Metatarsophalangeal Flexion and Extension

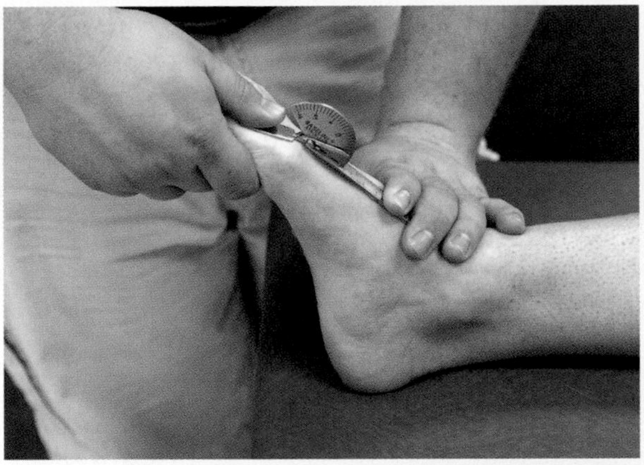

Flexion to extension (30°–0°–70°)

Patient Position	Supine with ankle in neutral
Goniometer Alignment	
Fulcrum	Flexion: Position the axis of the goniometer over the dorsal aspect of the MTP joint being tested. Extension: Place the goniometer on the plantar surface to test MTP extension.
Proximal Arm	Center the stationary arm on the midline of the MT.
Distal Arm	Center the movement arm on the midline of the proximal phalanx.

MT = metatarsal; MTP = metatarsophalangeal

flexion, as described in the Passive Range of Motion section of this chapter, is used to determine the integrity of the dorsal joint capsule; passive overpressure in extension evaluates the integrity of the plantar capsule and plantar plate.

- The application of a valgus force stresses the MCL of the joint. A varus force stresses the LCL (Stress Test 8-1). Compare the results of this examination with those obtained when the test is repeated on the same joint on the opposite extremity.

Joint Play Assessment

- **Intermetatarsal joints:** The deep transverse MT ligaments and the interosseous ligaments secure the MT heads in a relatively stable alignment. Forces causing an abnormal amount of glide between any two MT heads can result in trauma to these ligaments. Likewise, immobilization or degenerative changes can result in hypomobility. Testing intermetatarsal glide, thus duplicating the mechanism of injury, can be used to evaluate the available motion (Joint Play 8-1). Compare the amount of glide bilaterally.
- **Tarsometatarsal joints:** The tarsometatarsal joints are evaluated by assessing the amount of motion during dorsal and plantar glide (Joint Play 8-2). The fourth and fifth MTs have more mobility with the cuboid than the remaining proximal MT-cuneiform articulations.
- **Midtarsal joints:** Evaluate the stability of the midtarsal joints using dorsal and plantar glide of the cuneiforms (Joint Play 8-3).

Neurological Examination

The foot and toes are supplied by the L4 to S2 nerve roots. Neurological dysfunction of the nerve roots or individual nerves can cause radicular symptoms in the foot. When neurological signs or symptoms (e.g., paresthesia, muscle weakness, hyperreflexia , or hyporeflexia) are present, the source of the dysfunction, such as if the lesion involves a spinal nerve root, peripheral nerve, or a branch of the peripheral nerve, must be determined.

To identify nerve root pathology, refer to the Lower Quarter Neurological Screen in Chapter 1 (Neurological

Manual Muscle Test 8-1
Toe Flexion

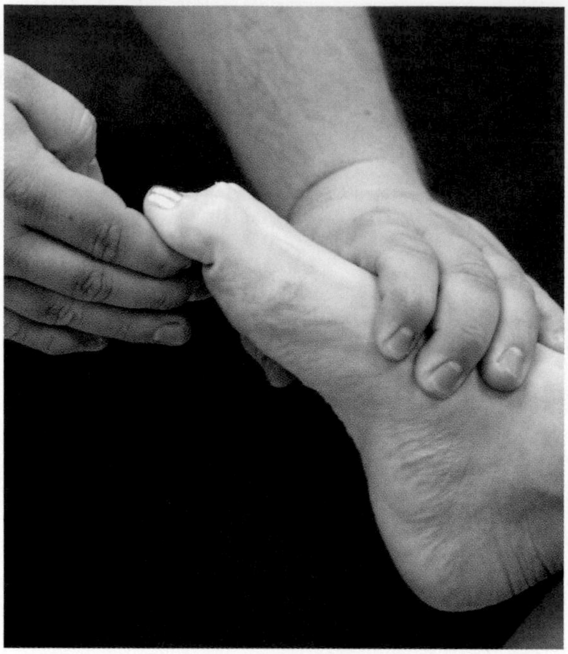

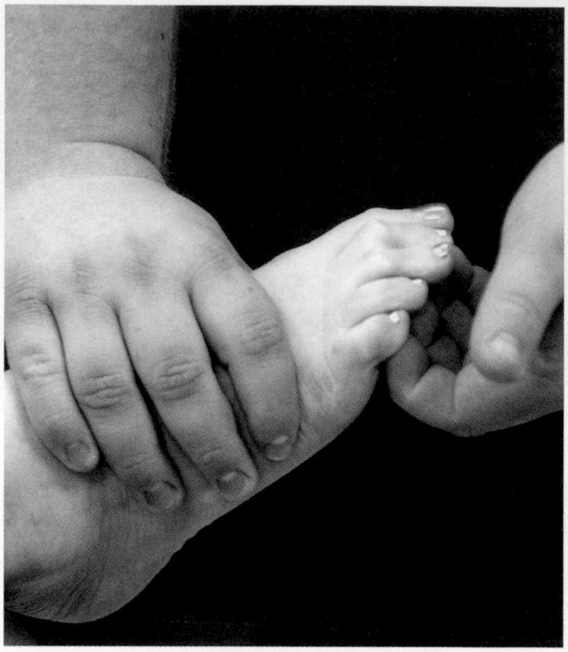

	Great Toe MTP Flexion	Lateral Four Toes Flexion
Patient Position	Long-sitting with the ankle in the neutral position	
Test Position	The toes are in the neutral position.	
Stabilization	Stabilize the forefoot by grasping the MTs proximal to their heads.	
Resistance	Along the entire length of the toe's plantar aspect	On the plantar aspect of the lateral four toes
Primary Movers (Innervation)	Flexor hallucis longus: IP joint (L4, L5, S1) Flexor hallucis brevis: MTP joint (L4, L5, S1)	Flexor digitorum longus: DIP joint (L5, S1) Flexor digitorum brevis: PIP joint (L4, L5, S1) Flexor digiti minimi: MTP joint of the 5th toe (S1, S2)
Secondary Movers (Innervation)		Dorsal interossei: MTP joint flexion (S1, S2) Plantar interossei: MTP joint flexion (S1, S2) Lumbricals: MTP flexion (1st MTP: L4, L5, S1; 2nd to 5th: S1, S2) Talocrural plantarflexion
Substitution		The toe flexors collectively flex the MTP joints.
Comments	IP joint flexion, talocrural plantarflexion	

DIP = distal interphalangeal; IP = interphalangeal; MTP = metatarsophalangeal; PIP = proximal interphalangeal

Manual Muscle Test 8-2
Toe Extension

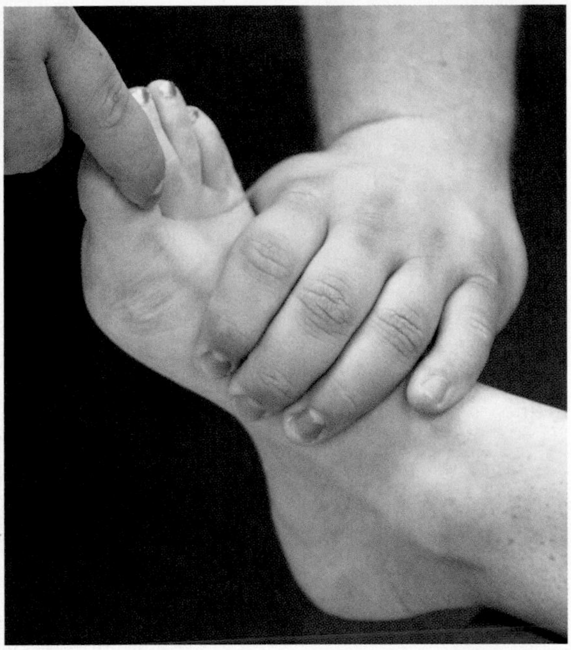

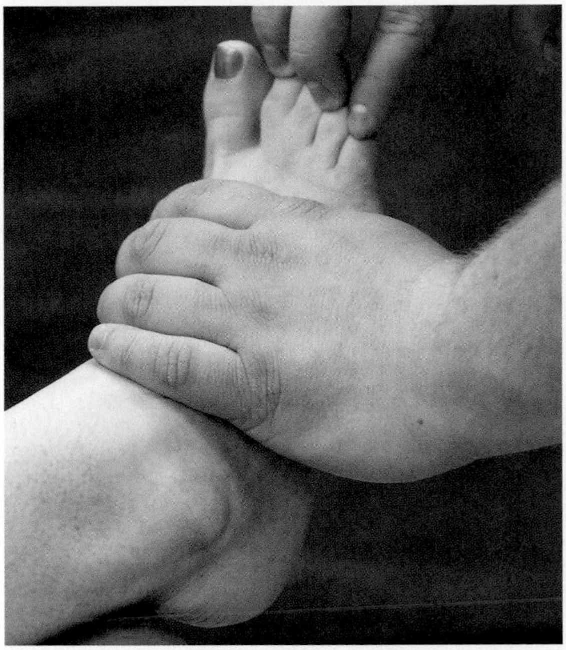

	Great Toe Extension	Toe Extension
Patient Position	Long-sitting with the ankle in the neutral position	
Test Position	The toes are in the neutral position.	
Stabilization	Stabilize the forefoot by grasping the MTs proximal to their heads.	
Resistance	Dorsal aspect of the proximal phalanx of hallux	Dorsal aspect of the proximal phalanges of toes 2–5
Primary Movers (Innervation)	Extensor digitorum longus (L4, L5, S1) Extensor digitorum brevis (L5, S1)	Extensor hallucis longus (L4, L5, S1) Extensor hallucis brevis (L5, S1) Dorsal interossei: IP joint extension (S1, S2) Plantar interossei: IP joint extension (S1, S2) Lumbricals (IP joint extension)
Substitution	Talocrural dorsiflexion	Talocrural dorsiflexion

IP = interphalangeal; MT = metatarsal

Table 8-7 Foot and Toe Capsular Patterns and End-Feels

Capsular Patterns	
Midtarsal joint	Dorsiflexion, plantarflexion, adduction, internal rotation
MTP joint: Great toe	Extension, flexion
MTP joints: 2nd–5th toes	Flexion, extension
End-Feels	
Flexion of the toes	Firm: Tightness of the toe extensors
Extension of the toes	Firm: Tightness of the toe flexors
Abduction of the toes (MTP)	Firm: Soft tissue stretch (intrinsic muscles, capsule, and ligaments)
Adduction of the toes (MTP)	Firm: Soft tissue stretch (intrinsic muscles, capsule, and ligaments)

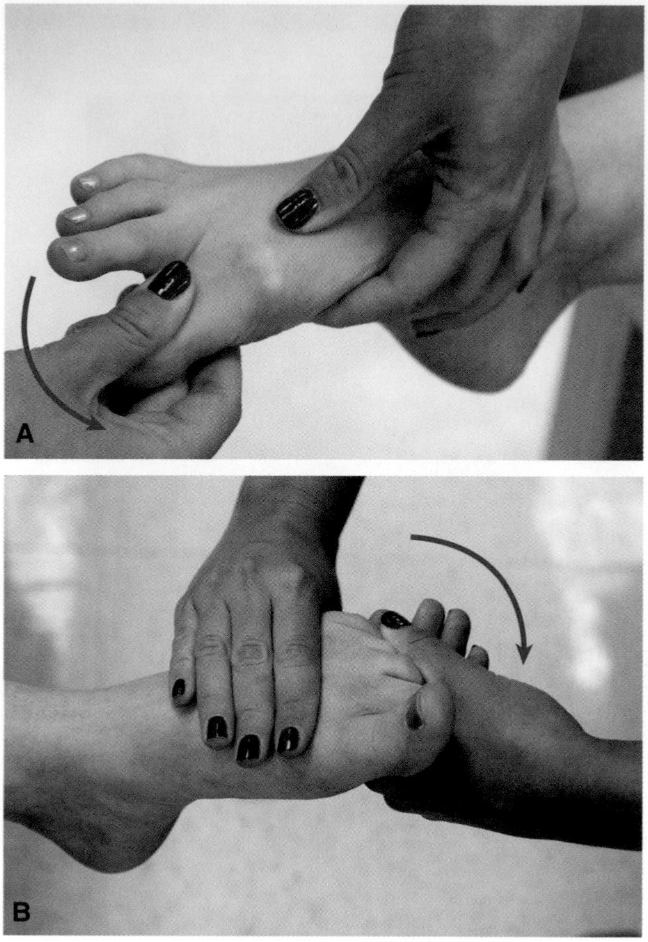

FIGURE 8-19 ■ Passive flexion of the (A) great toe and (B) lateral four toes.

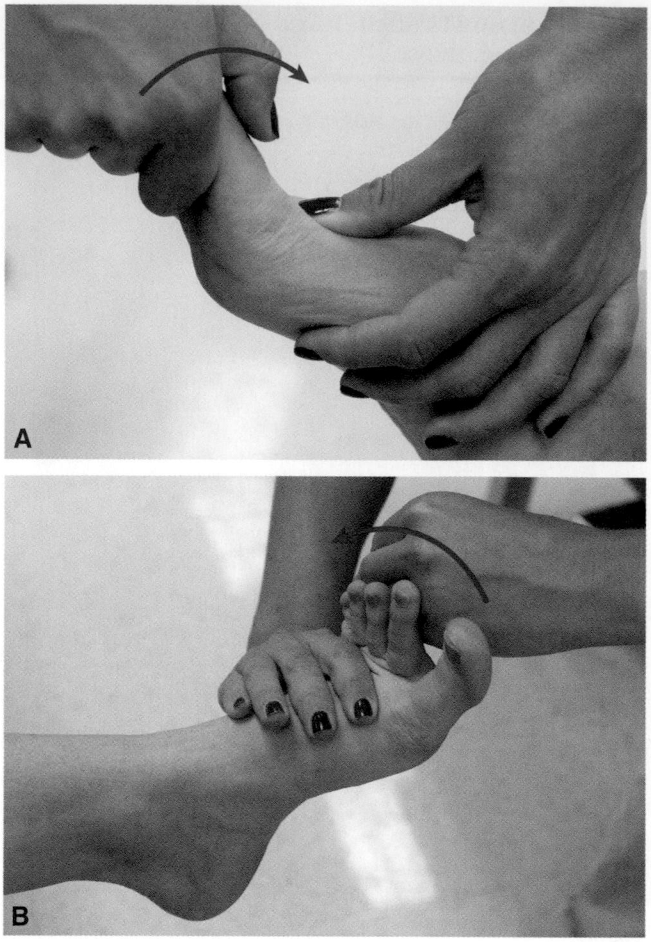

FIGURE 8-20 ■ Passive extension of the (A) great toe and (B) lateral four toes.

Screening Box 1-1). Pathologies that can result in local neurological dysfunction include entrapment of the posterior tibial nerve (TTS) and interdigital neuroma. Peroneal nerve trauma, disk herniations, and anterior compartment syndrome can also provoke symptoms into the foot (Fig. 8-21).

Vascular Examination

The posterior tibial pulse can be palpated just posterior to the medial malleolus. Identifying the pulse is easier when the patient's foot is supinated. Palpate the dorsalis pedis pulse just lateral to the extensor hallucis longus tendon as the artery crosses the talocrural joint line. These pulses, especially the posterior tibial pulse, are frequently undetectable in a young, healthy population. In this case, confirm arterial supply by checking capillary refill in the nailbed or on the skin on the dorsum of the foot. Refer to pages 198, 199, and 269 for more information on palpation of the foot and ankle pulses.

In the absence of trauma, absent or diminished pulses are indicative of peripheral arterial disease. Unexplained edema can be the result of peripheral vascular disease, diabetes, or other disease states.

Region-Specific Pathologies and Selective Tissue Tests

Many of the conditions affecting the normal function of the foot may be traced to improper biomechanics of the foot itself or be the result of compensation by the foot for biomechanical abnormalities elsewhere in the lower extremity.

Influence of Foot Structure on Pathology

Although abnormalities of foot structure may be caused by acute trauma or disease states, they more commonly occur congenitally. Many people function normally with pes planus or pes cavus. Increasing or decreasing the height of the arch alters the biomechanical function of the subtalar and midtarsal joints. These conditions are a concern when they result in pathological biomechanical dysfunction elsewhere in the lower extremity. Possible consequences of pes planus include plantar fasciitis, heel spurs, and patellofemoral pain. Pes cavus can predispose an individual to claw toes, MT stress fractures, or a plantar fascia rupture. Abnormal foot posture also increases the patient's risk of developing overuse injuries,

Stress Test 8-1
Valgus and Varus Stress Testing of the MTP and IP Joints

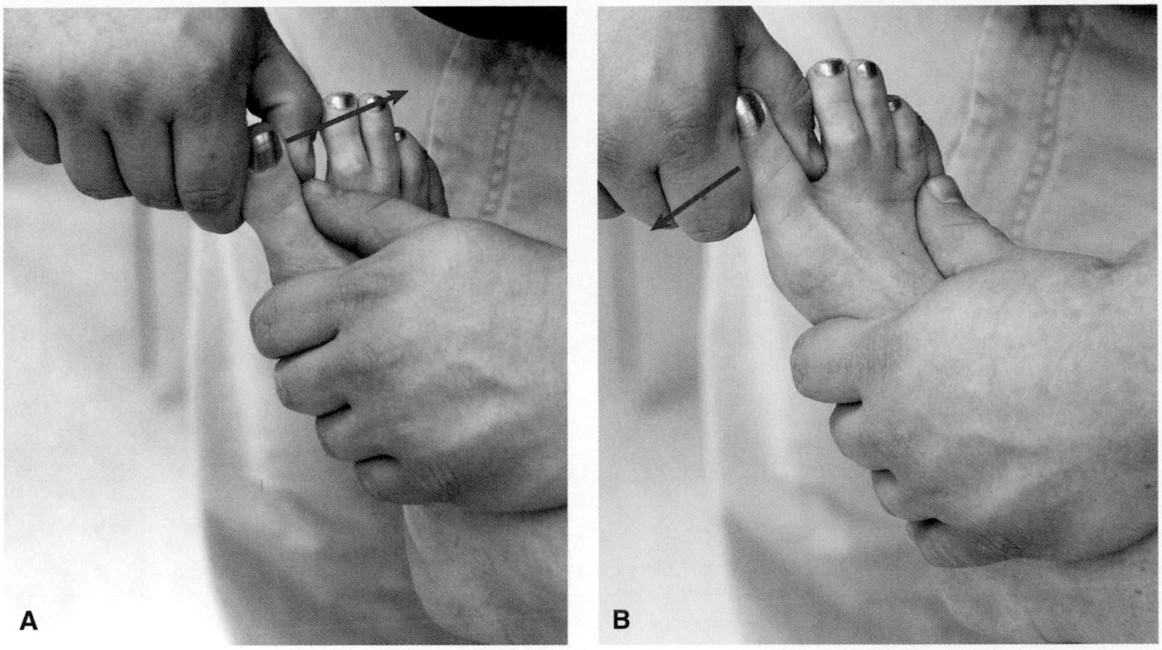

Stress testing of the toe's capsular ligaments: (A) Valgus stress applied to the IP joint; (B) varus stress applied to the MTP joint.

Patient Position	Supine or sitting
Position of Examiner	Standing The proximal bone stabilized close to the joint to be tested Grasp the bone distal to the joint being tested near the middle of its shaft. Care is necessary to isolate the joint being tested while not overlapping the ligament being stressed.
Evaluative Procedure	*Valgus testing (A):* The distal bone is moved laterally, attempting to open up the joint on the medial side. *Varus testing (B):* The distal bone is moved medially, attempting to open up the joint on the lateral side.
Positive Test	Pain or increased laxity or decreased laxity when compared with the same joint on the opposite extremity
Implications	*Valgus test (A):* MCL sprain, avulsion fracture, or adhesions of the involved joint *Varus test (B):* LCL sprain, avulsion fracture, or adhesions of the involved joint
Comments	Increased joint laxity, especially with an empty end-feel, may reflect an associated fracture.
Evidence	Absent or inconclusive in the literature

LCL = lateral collateral ligament; MCL = medial collateral ligament

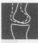

Joint Play 8-1
Intermetatarsal Glide Assessment

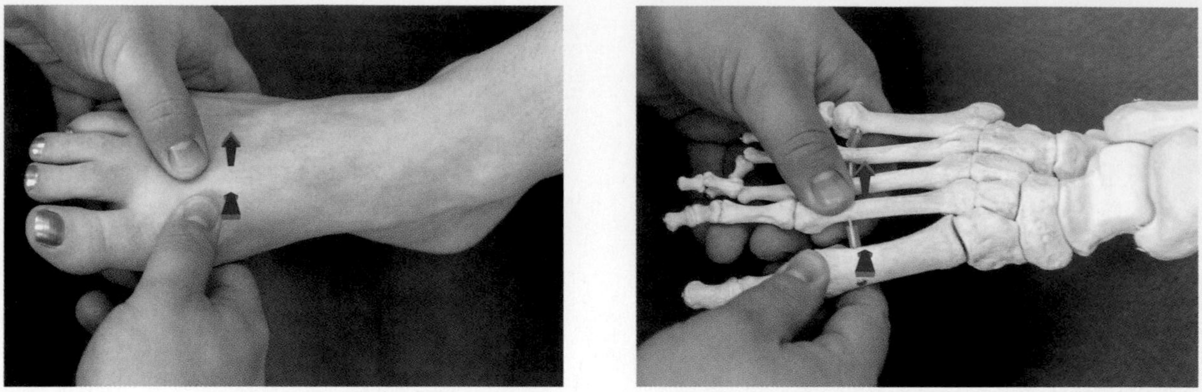

Assessment of the amount of intermetatarsal glide between the 1st and 2nd MT heads. Perform this test for each of the four articulations formed between the five MTs.

Patient Position	Supine or sitting on the table with the knees extended
Position of Examiner	Standing in front of the patient's feet One hand grasping the first MT head; the other grasping the second MT head
Evaluative Procedure	Stabilize one of the MT heads while moving the other in a plantar and dorsal direction. Repeat this procedure by moving to the lateral MT heads until all four intermetatarsal joints have been evaluated.
Positive Test	Pain or increased glide or decreased glide compared with the opposite extremity
Implications	Trauma to the deep transverse MT ligament, interosseous ligament, or both Pain without the presence of laxity may indicate the presence of a neuroma.
Evidence	Absent or inconclusive in the literature

MT = metatarsal

especially when the stress is compounded by a rapid increase in activity.[18]

There are several ways to compute arch height. The most accurate (and most expensive) is a lateral weight-bearing radiograph of the foot from which the (1) height of the medial longitudinal arch, (2) height-to-length ratio, and (3) calcaneal-first MT angle are determined (Fig. 8-22).[40] The height of the arch itself is a less significant finding than the actual change in height that occurs when the foot goes from non–weight bearing to weight bearing as measured by navicular drop (refer to Selective Tissue Test 8-4).

*** Practical Evidence**

Excessive navicular drop is associated with an increased risk for patellofemoral pain. Navicular drop causes increased internal rotation of the tibia on the foot. This rotation creates femoral internal rotation when the knee extends, resulting in lateral pressure in the patellofemoral joint.[41]

Pes Planus

Pes planus is characterized by the lowering of the medial longitudinal arch, giving this condition its colloquial name, "flat feet" (Fig. 8-23). The onset of pes planus can be traced to a congenital origin, biomechanical changes, or acute trauma. Pes planus results in biomechanical changes in all three planes of foot and ankle movement, and those with pes planus are more at risk to develop lower extremity pathology.[45] The lowered arch causes the talus to tilt medially and the navicular to displace inferiorly, making the talus more prominent (talar beaking).

Acute pes planus can occur after trauma to the structures supporting the medial longitudinal ligament, including rupture of the plantar fascia, tears of the plantar ligaments, calcaneonavicular (spring) ligament sprains, or the rupture of the tibialis posterior or tibialis anterior tendon.[43-46] Traumatic, symptomatic pes planus can also be related to a fracture of the navicular tuberosity, including

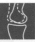

Joint Play 8-2
Tarsometatarsal Joint Play

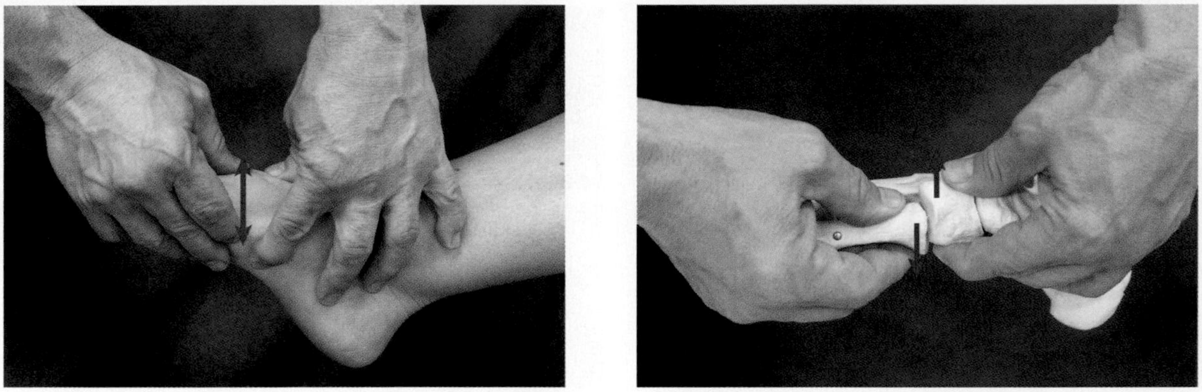

Assessment of the amount of glide between the tarsals and the base of the MTs. Perform this test on each of the five tarsometatarsal joints.

Patient Position	Supine or seated Foot pronated Knee flexed and the heel stabilized by the edge of the table
Position of Examiner	Standing or sitting in front of the patient's foot One hand grasping the proximal tarsal (e.g., cuneiform, cuboid) The opposite hand grasping the MT being glided
Evaluative Procedure	The MT is glided dorsally and plantarly on the tarsal. Repeat for each joint.
Positive Test	Pain associated with movement Increased or decreased glide relative to the opposite foot
Implications	*Increased glide:* Ligamentous laxity *Decreased glide:* Joint adhesions, articular change causing coalition of the joint
Modification	Wedges or balls may be needed to achieve sufficient proximal stabilization.
Evidence	

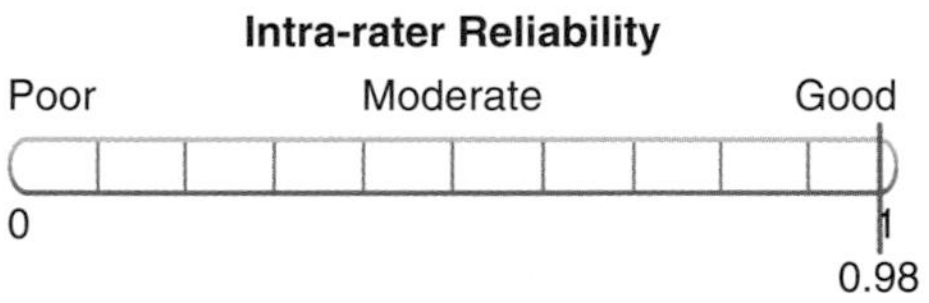

MT = metatarsal

an accessory navicular (Fig. 8-24). The accessory navicular is an abnormal osseous outgrowth on the navicular that, when present, serves as a partial attachment site for the tibialis posterior. Loss of the union between the accessory navicular and the navicular itself results in a decrease in the effectiveness of the tibialis posterior in supporting the medial arch.

*** Practical Evidence**

There are three types of accessory naviculars: a sesamoid bone in the distal tibialis posterior tendon (type I), an accessory center of ossification (type II), and the cornuate navicular, an enlarged navicular tuberosity (type III). When the accessory navicular is symptomatic, the patient will be able to precisely locate the source of pain.[47]

Joint Play 8-3
Midtarsal Joint Play

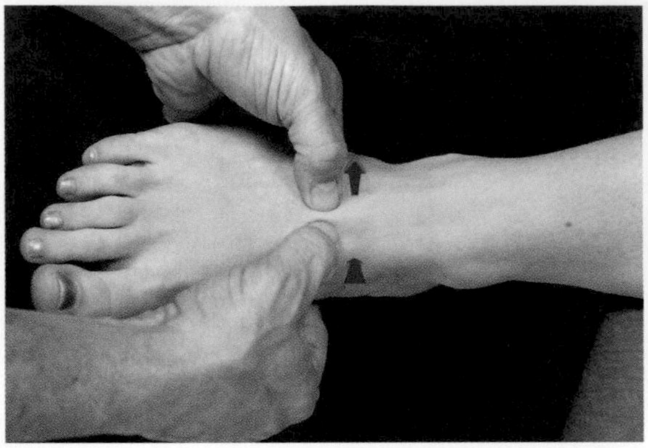

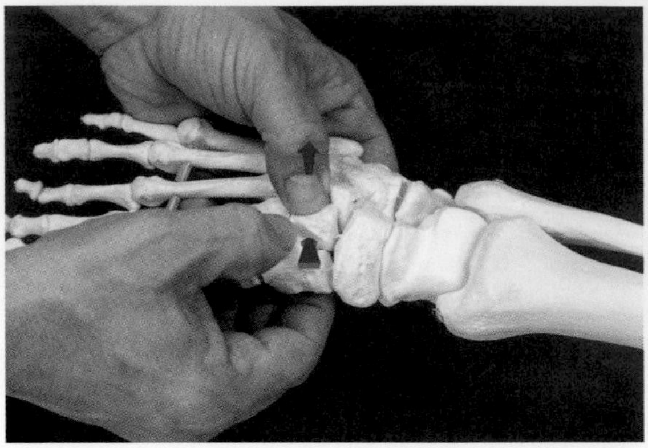

Assessment of the amount of joint glide between the tarsals

Patient Position	Supine or seated Knee flexed and the heel stabilized by the edge of the table
Position of Examiner	Standing or sitting in front of the patient's foot Grasp the plantar and dorsal aspect of one tarsal with the stabilizing hand and grasp the adjacent tarsal in a similar manner with the opposite hand.
Evaluative Procedure	One tarsal is glided dorsally and then plantarly on the stabilized adjacent tarsal. Repeat for each tarsal joint.
Positive Test	Pain associated with movement Increased or decreased glide relative to the opposite foot
Implications	*Increased glide:* Ligamentous laxity *Decreased glide:* Joint adhesions, articular changes causing coalition of the joint
Modification	Wedges or balls may be needed to achieve sufficient proximal stabilization.
Evidence	Absent or inconclusive in the literature

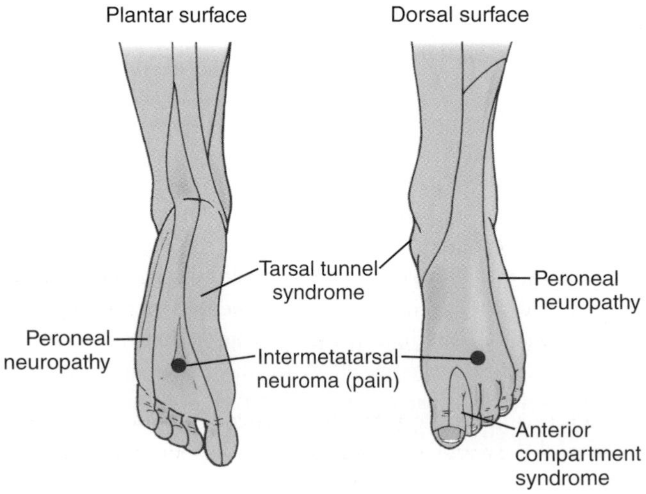

FIGURE 8-21 ■ Peripheral neurological symptoms in the foot.

Mechanical factors leading to pes planus include weakness of the tibialis posterior, the tibialis anterior, and the toe flexors. Stretching or weakness of the supporting ligaments, especially the calcaneonavicular ligament, results from the plantar-medial displacement of the talus, further increasing the amount of weight-bearing pronation. This weakness may be triggered or exacerbated by compensatory postures to structural abnormalities of the spine and lower extremity. Also, compensation may increase over time after injury of the posterior tibialis tendon.

Pes planus is classified as being either rigid (structural) or flexible (supple). Rigid pes planus, sometimes associated with tarsal coalition, is marked by the absence of the medial longitudinal arch when the foot is both weight bearing and non–weight bearing. A rigid pes planus foot has less shock-absorbing capacity. In supple pes planus, the arch appears normal during non–weight

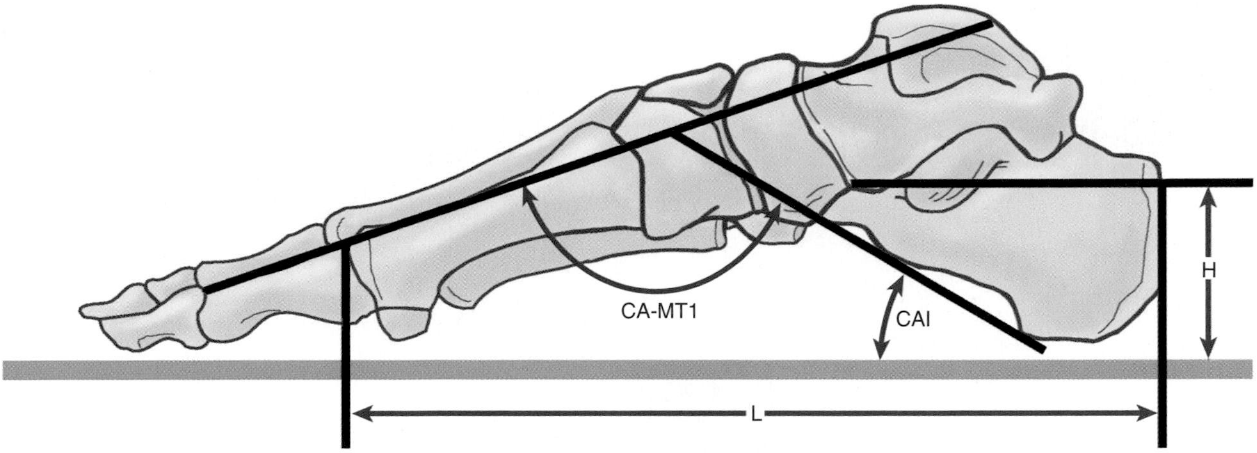

FIGURE 8-22 ■ Calculation of arch height and length taken from a weight-bearing radiograph. H = height; L = length; CA-MT1 = calcaneal 1st metatarsal angle; CAI = calcaneal inclination.

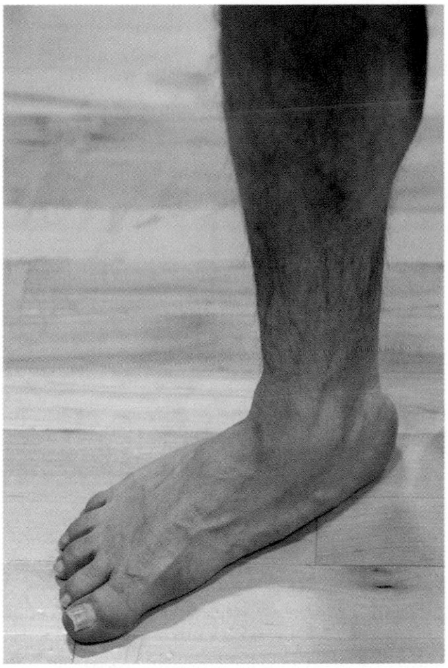

FIGURE 8-23 ■ Pes planus. Note the absence of the medial longitudinal arch.

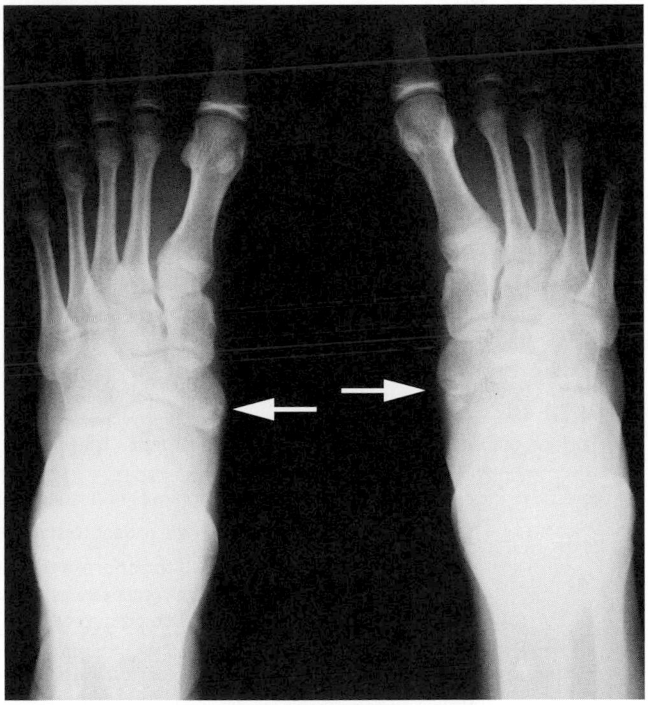

FIGURE 8-24 ■ Accessory navicular. The arrows identify the bony outgrowths associated with an accessory navicular.

bearing but disappears when the foot is weight bearing (Selective Tissue Test 8-4).

Various assessment techniques can be used to determine the position of the navicular and the extent of its displacement when the foot transitions from non–weight-bearing to weight-bearing status. Measurement of the navicular height in a relaxed stance provides a valid estimate of arch height when compared with a radiograph, especially when normalized to the length of the foot.[48] The **Feiss line** provides an estimation of the position of the navicular relative to a line spanning the distance of the plantar aspect of the first MTP joint and the apex of the medial malleolus. A quantitative measure of pronation can be calculated via the **navicular drop test** (Selective Tissue Test 8-5).[50] Navicular drop is the distance between the original height of the navicular (in subtalar joint neutral position) to the final weight-bearing position of the navicular in a relaxed stance.[51]

*** Practical Evidence**

A forefoot varus of greater than 8 degrees is associated with an increased navicular drop, indicating the relationship of forefoot varus to increased pronation.[35]

Selective Tissue Test 8-4

Test for Supple Pes Planus Windlass Test

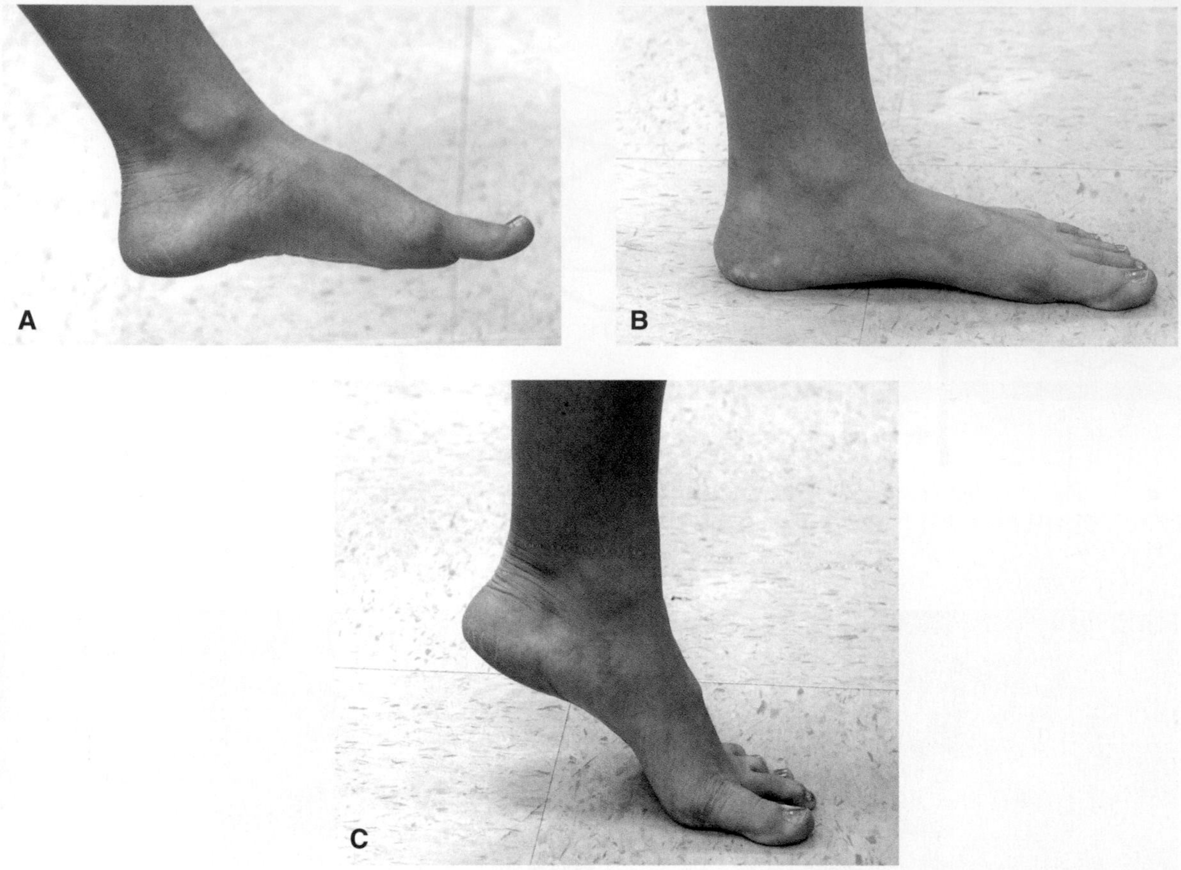

Supple pes planus. (A) The patient displays a normal arch in the non–weight-bearing position. (B) In weight bearing, the arch disappears. (C) When the patient performs a toe raise, the arch returns by means of the windlass effect. In the presence of plantar fasciitis, the windlass test will produce pain. Positive findings are highly related to the presence of plantar fasciitis, but a negative finding is less helpful in ruling out the condition.[49]

Patient Position	Sitting on the edge of the examination table
Position of Examiner	Positioned at the patient's foot
Evaluative Procedure	With the patient in a non–weight-bearing position, the examiner notes the presence of a medial longitudinal arch **(A).** The examiner instructs the patient to stand so that the body weight is evenly distributed **(B).** The patient is then asked to perform a single-leg heel raise on the limb being tested **(C).** In the presence of supple pes planus, note if the arch reappears as the patient performs a toe raise. For the windlass test (used to identify plantar fasciitis), pain may be produced.
Positive Test	The presence of a medial longitudinal arch when non–weight bearing disappears when the patient is weight bearing. The windlass test is positive if pain is reproduced during part C.
Implications	If the medial longitudinal arch disappears when weight bearing, a supple pes planus is present. If no arch is present while in a non–weight-bearing position, a rigid pes planus is present. Windlass test: Pain during the single-leg heel raise
Comments	This test for supple pes planus is meaningful only when the medial longitudinal arch is present with the patient in a non–weight-bearing position.
Evidence	

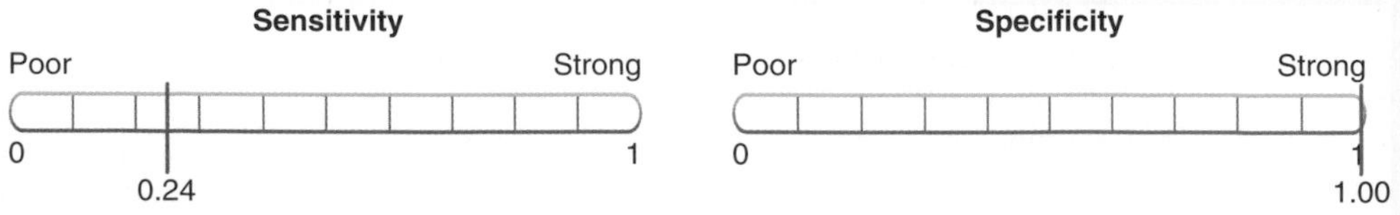

LR−: 0.076

Selective Tissue Test 8-5
Navicular Drop Test

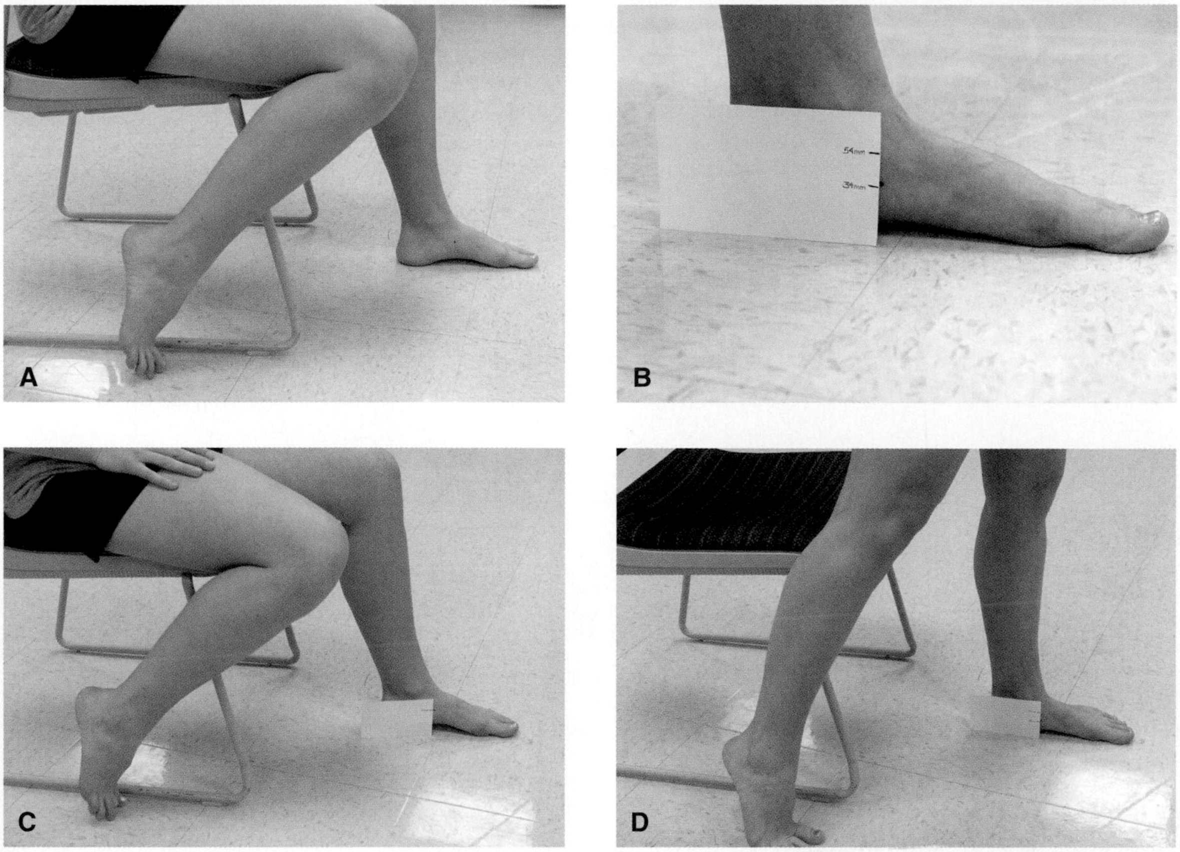

The navicular drop test, considered to be an estimate of the extent of pronation, assesses the change in navicular position between weight-bearing and non–weight-bearing positions. Note that the body weight should be evenly distributed between the two feet (nontest leg above was moved for clarity).

Patient Position	Sitting with both feet on a noncarpeted floor
Position of Examiner	Kneeling in front of the patient
Evaluative Procedure	**(A)** The STJ is placed in the neutral position with the patient's foot flat against the ground, but non–weight bearing. With the patient non–weight bearing, a dot is placed over the navicular tuberosity. **(B)** While the foot is still in contact with the ground, but non–weight bearing, an index card is positioned next to the medial longitudinal arch. A mark is made on the card corresponding to the level of the navicular tuberosity. **(C)** The patient stands with the body weight evenly distributed between the two feet, and the foot is allowed to relax into pronation. Palpate the navicular tuberosity and mark it with a dot. Indicate this level on the index card. **(D)** The relative displacement (drop) of the navicular is determined by measuring the distance between the two marks in millimeters.
Positive Test	Foot flexibility is classified using the relative navicular displacement between the seated and standing positions:[29] >2.3 cm = very flexible 1.8 to 2.3 cm = flexible 0.6 to 1.8 cm = normal 0.0 to 0.6 cm = rigid <0.0 cm = very rigid Limited or excessive pronation

Continued

Selective Tissue Test 8-5
Navicular Drop Test—cont'd

Implications	The relatively static measurement of navicular drop is associated with the amount of pronation during gait.
Comments	A strong relationship exists between excessive forefoot varus (>8°) and an increased navicular drop.[35] The low interrater reliability associated with the navicular drop test is related to the low reliability of assessing subtalar joint neutral. The height of the navicular in weight bearing (the second measurement of the navicular drop test) is highly correlated with radiographic measurements of navicular height in weight bearing.[48]
Evidence	 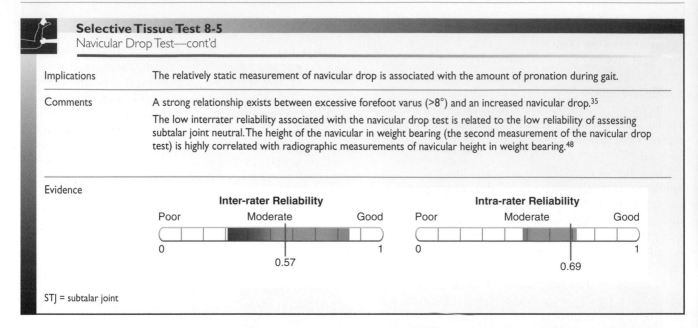

STJ = subtalar joint

Pes planus can lead to MT stress fractures, low back pain, and other musculoskeletal problems in the lower extremity and spine.[52,53] Evidence of a relationship between pes planus (with a related increased navicular drop) and a predisposition to anterior cruciate ligament (ACL) injury is ambiguous, with some research suggesting a connection and other research refuting it.[54]

Pes Planus Intervention Strategies

A pes planus foot type rarely requires surgical correction. Associated pathology frequently responds to proximal muscle strengthening and/or stretching, orthotics, or changes in footwear.

Pes Cavus

Appearing as a high medial longitudinal arch, pes cavus is often a congenital foot deformity. Certain neurological or disease states such as upper motor neuron lesions or **cerebral palsy**: may also result in the acquisition of a cavus foot type.[55] Hypertrophy of the peroneus longus muscle relative to the tibialis anterior has also been associated with cavus deformities.[56] This foot type is associated with a generalized stiffness and impaired ability to absorb ground contact forces. During running, pes cavus results in increased pressure loads on the forefoot and rearfoot.[18] A hypomobile plantarflexed first ray may also contribute to the limited shock absorbing capability of the cavus foot.

A spreading and apparent drop of the forefoot relative to the rearfoot caused by the depression of the MT heads is noted during inspection of the area (Fig. 8-25). The dorsal pads under the calcaneus and the MT heads appear smaller than in a "normal" foot. The lateral four toes may be clawed. Over time, calluses form over the PIP joints.

A cavus foot tends to have decreased ground contact area and be more rigid and have less shock-absorbing characteristics than normal or planus foot types.

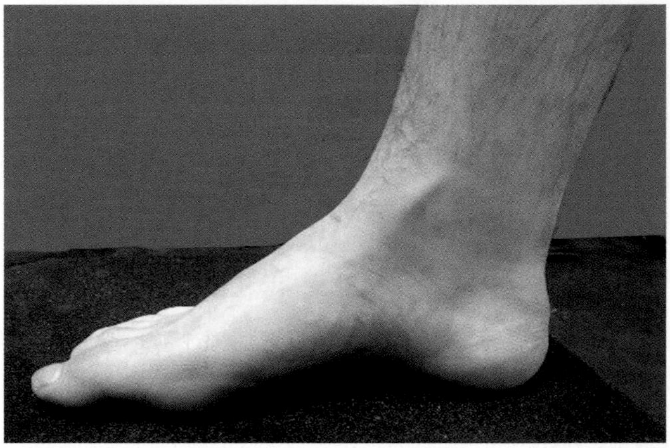

FIGURE 8-25 ■ Pes cavus, abnormally high medial arches.

✱ Practical Evidence

Individuals with cavus feet also tend to experience foot pain more frequently than those with a normal foot type, with the most frequent diagnoses being metatarsalgia and plantar fasciitis.[57] Increased height of the medial longitudinal arch may be a predisposing condition to MT as well as tibial and femoral stress fractures.[50] Pes cavus may also be associated with spinal scoliosis, although the cause-and-effect relationship has not been established.[56]

Pes Cavus Intervention Strategies

In the case of problematic pes cavus, treatment approaches are often symptomatic, and soft orthotics or shoes with soft midsoles may be used to maximize available motion and to dissipate forces. Advanced conditions may be corrected through a plantar fascial release, a surgical technique in which the plantar fascia is sectioned, allowing for increased foot mobility.[58]

Cerebral palsy A birth-related neurological defect that results in motor dysfunction

Plantar Heel Pain

Aggravation of the plantar fascia or the junction between the fascia and the first layer of intrinsic muscles can be traced to a single traumatic episode, repeated stress, biomechanical deficits, the presence of a heel spur, nerve entrapment, or Achilles tendon tightness.[3,59] Most cases of plantar fascia pathology are not inflammatory but rather a degenerative process that is better described as plantar **fasciosis**.[60]

The onset of plantar fasciitis—the most common foot condition—is weakly associated with increasing age.[61] It is also associated with significant changes in activity intensity and duration, prolonged standing, weight gain (in nonathletic populations), or the presence of limited ankle dorsiflexion ROM.[61] Bilateral fasciitis may be caused by nerve, vascular, muscular, or connective tissue disease.[62] Biomechanical dysfunction can also be the result of medial heel pain caused by the entrapment of the medial calcaneal nerve or the lateral plantar nerve, which innervates the abductor digiti minimi muscle.[59]

Plantar fasciitis and heel spurs were once thought to be closely related. It was believed that shortening of the plantar fascia caused an outgrowth (i.e., a heel spur) to appear on the medial calcaneal tubercle, a bony response to prolonged tension. Although heel spurs and plantar fasciitis may occur concurrently, their presence may be coincidental (see the Heel Spurs section of this chapter). Regardless of the relationship between these two conditions, a heel spur has the potential for negatively impacting the foot's biomechanics, leading to plantar fasciitis.

Ongoing stress and subsequent degenerative changes to the plantar fascia lead to a functional shortening of the tissues. Over time, tightness of the triceps surae muscle group occurs, resulting in an everted heel position at heel strike and early heel raise during the latter stages of gait. During push-off, dorsiflexion and supination are restricted, further increasing the tension placed on the plantar fascia. As a result, the triceps surae is less able to produce power.[63]

✱ Practical Evidence

Of the proposed predispositions for plantar fasciitis, limited ankle dorsiflexion and a high BMI in nonathletic populations are the most predictive for the development of this condition.[8]

The clinical diagnosis of plantar fasciitis is based on the patient's history and physical examination findings.[64] Typically, pain is centralized around the plantar fascia's origin on the medial calcaneal tubercle although the fascia may be tender along its entire length. A common symptom of plantar fasciitis is pain when stepping out of bed in the morning or stepping on the foot after a period of non-weight bearing. Initially, the patient's chief complaint is pain in the heel when resting after activity. When assessing function, patients often describe pain with the push-off phase of gait or during a single-leg heel raise task. Dorsiflexion may be painful and decreased with restricted talocrural joint play in the anterior to posterior direction.[64] Pain increases when the ankle is dorsiflexed and the toes are extended.[63] Increased symptoms may also be described when walking barefoot, on the toes, or when climbing stairs.[64] As the condition progresses, the patient experiences pain with the onset of activity, which subsides during activity because of stretching of the tissues and increased blood flow to the area. In the chronic stage, the pain is usually constant (Examination Findings 8-1).

Radiographs are not useful in determining the presence of plantar fasciitis.[61,63] Heel spurs are more common in people with plantar fasciitis, but the presence or absence of heel spurs is not diagnostic.[54,61] Magnetic resonance imaging (MRI) or ultrasonic imaging is more useful in the diagnosis of plantar fasciitis. Each of these methods can identify thickening of the proximal portion of the fascia, localized soft tissue edema, and edema within the calcaneus, in addition to ruling out other conditions such as fibromas.[61]

Chronic plantar fasciitis can lead to tightness of the triceps surae muscle group and vice versa. Tightness of the triceps surae results in premature plantarflexion during the latter stages of gait, increasing and prolonging the tension on the plantar fascia as it attaches at the calcaneal tubercle.[8]

Plantar Fascia Rupture

Forced ankle dorsiflexion and toe extension exerts a tensile force on the plantar fascia.[65] If the force of this stretch is sufficient, the fascia can avulse from its bony attachment on the calcaneus or rupture its central or medial slip.

A low (shallow) calcaneal pitch angle can increase the risk of plantar fascia rupture (see Fig. 8-22)[68,69] and may be associated with a history of plantar fasciitis.[65] The risk of rupture increases further after corticosteroid injections.[26,65,70]

The patient has immediate difficulty bearing weight secondary to pain and may describe a "tearing" sensation on the plantar aspect of the foot.[65] The terminal stance, midstance, and preswing phases of gait are painful. The area around the medial calcaneal tubercle may be swollen and discolored secondary to soft tissue swelling and bleeding. A palpable defect may be noted on the medial calcaneal tubercle.[6] Soon after the rupture, the patient may demonstrate an acute hammer toe deformity on the involved foot (see Examination Findings 8-1).[26]

Heel Spur

A heel spur is a hook-shaped bony outgrowth (exostosis) located on the medial calcaneal tubercle (Fig. 8-26). This condition was once thought to be the result of increased tension from a shortened plantar fascia, leading to exostosis of its attachment on the calcaneus. However, surgical and radiographic investigations have determined that heel spurs are commonly located at the origin of the short toe flexor muscles rather than on the fascia's attachment site.[62]

Fasciosis The noninflammatory degeneration of fascia

Examination Findings 8-1
Plantar Fasciitis

Examination Segment	Clinical Findings
History of Current Condition	*Onset:* Acute or insidious *Pain characteristics:* Pain centralized near the medial calcaneal tubercle that can spread throughout the fascia Pain may be described when weight bearing and is worsened after being in a non–weight-bearing position. Symptoms may increase when barefoot, walking on the toes, or when climbing stairs. Initial steps in the morning or after prolonged sitting may be particularly symptomatic. *Other symptoms:* Complaints of stiffness after periods of non–weight bearing *Mechanism:* **Acute:** Forced dorsiflexion of the ankle combined with toe extension **Insidious:** Increased activity, additional distance when running, changing surface, or using a new or different shoe type or brand *Risk factors:* Pes cavus, pes planus, heel spur, hallux rigidus, forefoot valgus, excessive and prolonged foot pronation, decreased subtalar and/or talocrural joint mobility, triceps surae tightness, leg length discrepancy, weight gain (including pregnancy), middle age
Functional Assessment	Increased symptoms with push-off phase of gait; may present with heel-only (calcaneal) gait; may observe limited or excessive pronation or early heel raise Increased symptoms with single-leg heel raise
Inspection	Postural changes associated with leg length discrepancy, pes planus, or pes cavus may be noted. In some cases, swelling may be noted on the plantar aspect near the calcaneus.
Palpation	Pain is at or near the origin of the plantar fascia that, on occasion, runs the length of the plantar fascia. Tissue thickening may be palpable in chronic cases.
Joint and Muscle Function Assessment	Pain may be experienced during both active and passive ankle dorsiflexion and toe extension because of the stretch placed on the plantar fascia. *AROM:* Decreased ankle dorsiflexion *MMT:* Increased pain with test of flexor digitorum brevis and/or flexor hallucis longus *PROM:* Decreased ankle dorsiflexion with pain at end-range; pain experienced during passive extension of the MTP joints
Joint Stability Tests	*Stress tests:* Not applicable *Joint play:* STJ, talocrural, and/or midtarsal hypomobility (see Chapter 9)
Selective Tissue Tests	Navicular drop; test for supple pes planus
Neurological Screening	Tinel's sign to rule out posterior tibial nerve entrapment (TTS)
Vascular Screening	No remarkable findings
Imaging Techniques	MRI may reveal soft tissue edema and/or heel spur[70] MRI and ultrasonic imaging may be used for early identification of plantar fasciitis by the associated thickening of the proximal structure.[71] Radiographic imaging is used to rule out other conditions. Heel spurs may be noted on 50% of symptomatic patients and 20% of patients without plantar fasciitis.[68,71]
Differential Diagnosis	Heel spur, calcaneal fracture/stress fracture, TTS, fat pad syndrome

AROM = active range of motion; MMT = manual muscle test; MRI = magnetic resonance imaging; PROM = passive range of motion; STJ = subtalar joint; TTS = tarsal tunnel syndrome

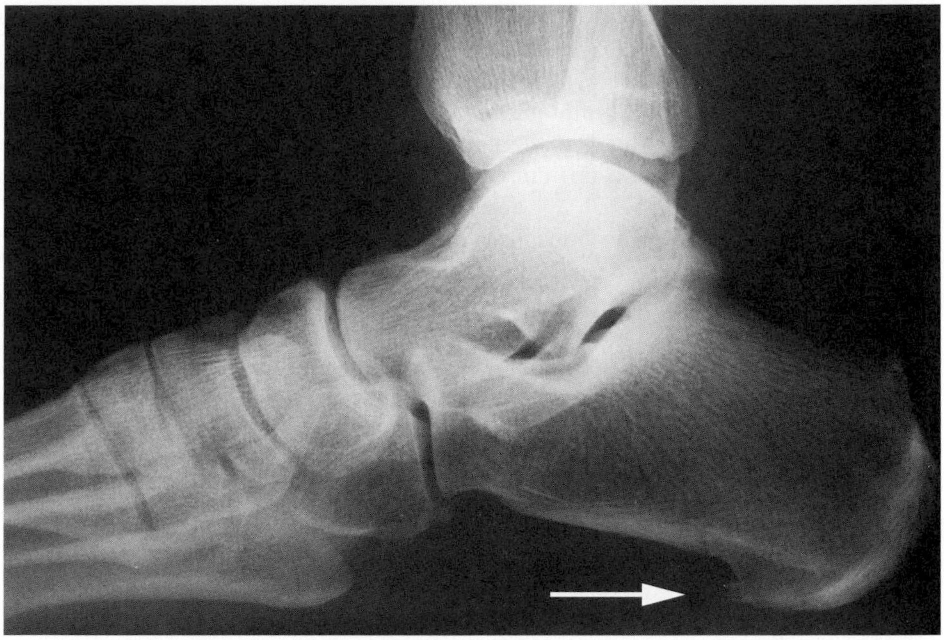

FIGURE 8-26 ■ Radiograph of a heel spur (medial view of the right foot). A form of exostosis, heel spurs are an abnormal bony outgrowth of the calcaneus. Note the hooklike projection arising from the anterior border of the calcaneal tuberosity.

Practical Evidence

Radiographic evidence of heel spurs is noted in around 30% of asymptomatic adults and in 89% of symptomatic cases of plantar fasciitis.[75]

Although plantar fasciitis and a heel spur can occur simultaneously, the cause-and-effect relationship between the two conditions is unclear.[71] Calcaneal pitch angle may be a predictor of heel spurs and plantar fasciitis,[68,69] and, similar to plantar fasciitis, the prevalence of heel spurs increases with age.[72]

The impairments associated with a heel spur are similar to those of plantar fasciitis (refer to Examination Findings 8-1). However, heel spurs tend to have a gradual onset, and the chief complaint is pain during the heel-strike phase of gait. Evaluate the triceps surae muscle group for tightness associated with plantar fasciitis and heel spurs.

Heel Pain Intervention Strategies

Conservative treatment of heel pain is effective in 80% of cases, but those suffering from bilateral inflammation respond less favorably.[20,62,73] There are several management options. A stretching regimen may provide short-term relief. Dorsiflexion splints may be beneficial for those with prolonged symptoms. These devices sustain the ankle in dorsiflexion (such as when sleeping) to passively maintain the length of the triceps surae and the plantar fascia. Taping, orthotics, footwear that addresses the biomechanical needs of the patient's foot, and iontophoresis using dexamethasone or acetic acid may also provide relief.[8]

Manual therapy consisting of soft tissue mobilization of the plantar fascia and flexor hallucis longus combined with restoration of restricted arthrokinematics (e.g., mobilization to increase rearfoot eversion and talocrural dorsiflexion) is more effective than an intervention of pulsed ultrasound, iontophoresis, and stretching.[73] A systematic review comparing the effectiveness of customized foot orthotics and corticosteroid injection in treating plantar heel pain revealed that both might be effective, although evidence is limited. A limiting feature of injections is post-injection pain.[74] Another systematic review of conservative treatments revealed orthotics, stretching, botulinum toxin (BOTOX®) injection, and steroid injections provided consistent reductions in pain and/or improvements in function. Extracorporeal shock therapy results for the management of plantar fascial pain are inconsistent.[75]

With heel spurs, conservative treatments including restoration of dorsiflexion and changes in footwear are the first line of intervention. Surgery may be required for plantar fasciitis or heel spurs that do not respond to conservative treatment. Fascial surgery involves a release where the plantar fascia is sectioned, allowing for increased foot mobility.[58]

Tarsal Coalition

A hereditary condition, tarsal coalition is a bony, fibrous, or cartilaginous union between two or more tarsal bones. Tarsal coalition most often affects the calcaneonavicular, talonavicular, or talocalcaneal joints, with 50% of the cases occurring bilaterally.[20,76,77] The resulting impairments and functional limitations depend on the joints involved. Tarsal coalition clinically resembles rigid pes planus when diagnosed in the adolescent. Joint play assessment reveals restricted subtalar joint motions leading to further stress at the midtarsal area with eventual collapse of the longitudinal arches.

Rigidity of the coalesced bones results in compensatory forces distal and proximal to the subtalar joint. The calcaneus assumes a valgus position relative to the tibia; and the forefoot abducts, the arch flattens, and the navicular overrides the talus to cause **talar beaking** (Fig. 8-27).[76,78] On occasion, spasm and pain in the lower leg result as the peroneals contract, especially the peroneus longus.[76]

Tarsal coalition becomes symptomatic in preteens and teenagers as the bones ossify. The initial finding often follows an inversion ankle sprain, an injury that is predisposed by subtalar joint coalition.[17,76,79] Age appears to be related to the period during which the joints fuse: the talonavicular joint for children aged 3 to 5 years; the calcaneonavicular joint for those aged 8 to 12 years; and the talocalcaneal joint for those aged 12 to 16 years.[76]

Clinically, tarsal coalition is exhibited as a rigid flatfoot with calcaneal valgus and abduction of the forefoot that is unchanged when the patient is in a weight-bearing position (rigid pes planus) (see Selective Tissue Test 8-4).[76] In adults, the foot alignment may appear neutral.[80] Palpation over the involved joint may cause pain.

Tarsal coalition is differentiated from other foot pathologies by the limitations in subtalar motion (see Joint Play 9-1 and 9-2). A definitive diagnosis of tarsal coalition is made via radiographs showing bony fusion, computed tomography (CT), or MRI for cartilaginous or fibrous coalition.[76] Any rigidity in the rearfoot may indicate tarsal coalition, warranting referral to a physician for further evaluation.

Tarsal Coalition Intervention Strategies

If detected in its early stages, tarsal coalition usually responds well to immobilization, the use of orthotics, or both.[76,81] When surgery is performed to release the coalition before any secondary degenerative changes occur, the prognosis is excellent.[82] Fusion is the treatment of choice if degenerative changes are present.

Tarsal Tunnel Syndrome

Tarsal tunnel syndrome (TTS) is caused by the entrapment of the posterior tibial nerve or one of its medial or lateral branches as it passes through the tarsal tunnel. The definition of TTS also includes compressive lesions of the posterior tibial nerve proximal to the retinaculum, under the deep fascia of the leg, and distally under the abductor hallucis muscle.[83]

Anatomically, the tarsal tunnel is bordered anteriorly by the tibia and the talus and laterally by the calcaneus. The flexor retinaculum forms a fibrous roof that is attached to the sheaths of the tibialis posterior, flexor hallucis longus, and flexor digitorum longus tendons (Fig. 8-28). The tunnel itself is compartmentalized by fascial membranes, or septa, which tightly bind the posterior tibial nerve, predisposing it to compressive forces.[83]

Several different factors can cause TTS. Acute TTS may be caused by trauma, including tarsal fracture or dislocation, hyperplantarflexion, or eversion. It can also be the result of overuse injuries. Predisposing conditions include ganglion formation, fibrosis, arthritis, or disease states such as diabetes.[83-86] Anatomic factors that may lead to TTS include nonunion fractures of the sustentaculum tali, tarsal coalition, muscle anomalies, or anterior entrapment of the nerve by the extensor hallucis brevis muscle.[87-90] Biomechanically, rearfoot varus coupled with excessive pronation, increased internal rotation of the tibia, and the resulting hypermobility of the medial longitudinal arch place an increased stress on the posterior tibial nerve, predisposing it to TTS.[5,91]

The primary patient complaints are diffuse pain, burning, paresthesia, or numbness along the plantar and medial aspect of the foot that increases with activity and decreases with rest. Approximately one-third of patients report pain arising from the medial malleolus and radiating into the medial lower leg, midcalf, and, occasionally, the medial heel (Examination Findings 8-2). Cold intolerance and increased pain when wearing low-cut or high-heel shoes may also be described.[68] Muscle function is often normal. A positive **Tinel's sign** may be elicited along the path of the nerve inferior and distal to the medial malleolus (Fig. 8-29). The **dorsiflexion–eversion test** may also reproduce the symptoms of TTS (Selective Tissue Test 8-6).[87]

TTS may be confused with the symptoms produced by plantar fasciitis, but close examination of the symptoms can differentiate between the two.[84] Pain produced by TTS is located along the medial portion of the heel and arch;

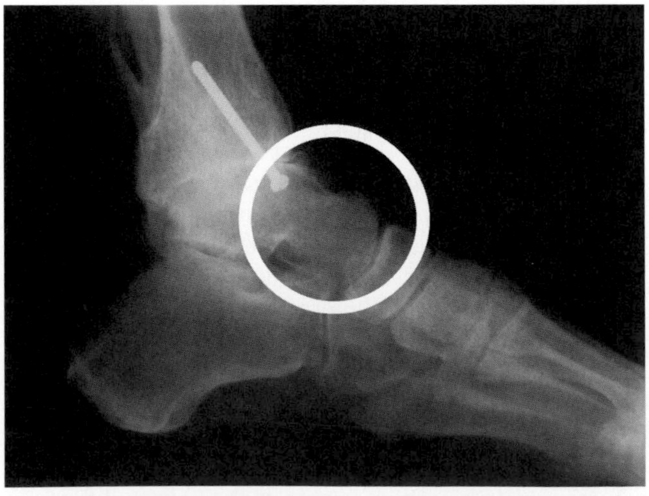

FIGURE 8-27 ■ Talar beaking associated with tarsal coalition (medial view of the left foot). The screw implanted in the tibia is for an unrelated condition.

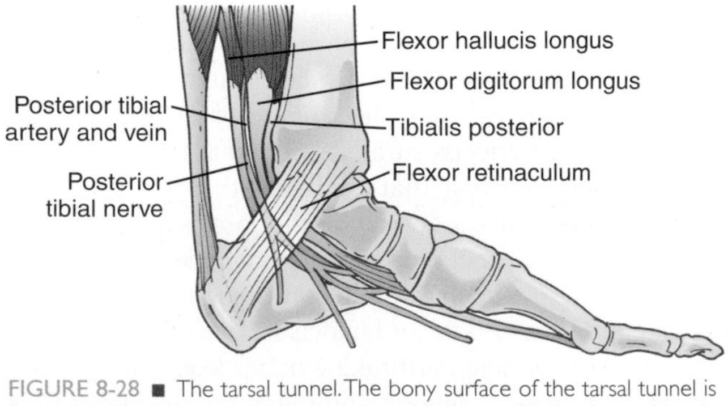

FIGURE 8-28 ■ The tarsal tunnel. The bony surface of the tarsal tunnel is formed by the tibia, talus, and calcaneus, with the roof being formed by the flexor retinaculum.

Examination Findings 8-2
Tarsal Tunnel Syndrome

Examination Segment	Clinical Findings
History of Current Condition	*Onset:* Acute or insidious *Pain characteristics:* Pain, numbness, and paresthesia occur along the plantar or medial aspects of the foot. Symptoms increase with increased activity and may be more troubling at night. *Other symptoms:* The patient may describe cold intolerance of the involved foot. *Mechanism:* Compression of the posterior tibial nerve (or its branches) within the tarsal tunnel. This pressure may also involve the vascular structures within the tunnel. The patient may describe a history of a plantarflexion–eversion mechanism injury to the ankle. TTS is also possibly associated with fracture, dislocation, or inflammation of the tarsals or local ganglion formation. *Risk factors:* Prior tarsal fracture or dislocation; rearfoot varus; history of eversion ankle injury; excessive pronation during gait; arthritis; nonunion fracture of the sustentaculum tali; inflammation of the extensor retinaculum; tarsal coalition; diabetes
Functional Assessment	Increased pain or symptoms during period of maximum pronation such as the midstance phase of gait. Patient may walk on lateral foot to avoid pronation.
Inspection	Rearfoot varus in non–weight-bearing STJN; pes planus; in chronic cases, trophic changes of the foot and nails Inspection of the medial longitudinal arch reveals pes planus, a condition often associated with TTS.
Palpation	Palpation over the tibial nerve and its branches results in reproduction of symptoms, especially in the area of the tarsal tunnel behind the lateral malleolus and beneath the flexor retinaculum.
Joint and Muscle Function Assessment	*AROM:* Motor function of the intrinsic and extrinsic muscles is often normal. *MMT:* Weakness of the toe flexors may be noted in advanced cases. *PROM:* Forced dorsiflexion and eversion may increase symptoms secondary to pressure from the flexor retinaculum and tension on the nerve.
Joint Stability Tests	*Stress tests:* No remarkable findings *Joint play:* Possible medial subtalar hypermobility (see Chapter 9)
Selective Tissue Tests	Dorsiflexion–eversion test for TTS
Neurological Screening	Paresthesia of the posterior tibial nerve distribution Medial plantar nerve: Medial plantar surface Lateral plantar nerve: Lateral plantar surface Medial calcaneal branch (tibial nerve): Medial calcaneus Tinel's sign may be positive inferior and distal to the medial malleolus. Sharp or dull and two-point discrimination may be decreased along the medial and plantar aspects of the foot.
Vascular Screening	No remarkable findings
Imaging Techniques	CT, MRI, and ultrasonic imaging can identify space-occupying lesions within the tarsal tunnel.[91]
Differential Diagnosis	Plantar fasciitis, posterior tibialis tendinopathy, talocalcaneal coalition, calcaneal stress fracture
Comments	Symptoms of TTS closely resemble those of other foot maladies, especially plantar fasciitis. Proximal nerve compression may mimic the signs and symptoms of TTS.

AROM = active range of motion; CT = computed tomography; MMT = manual muscle test; MRI = magnetic resonance imaging; PROM = passive range of motion; STJN = subtalar joint neutral; TTS = tarsal tunnel syndrome

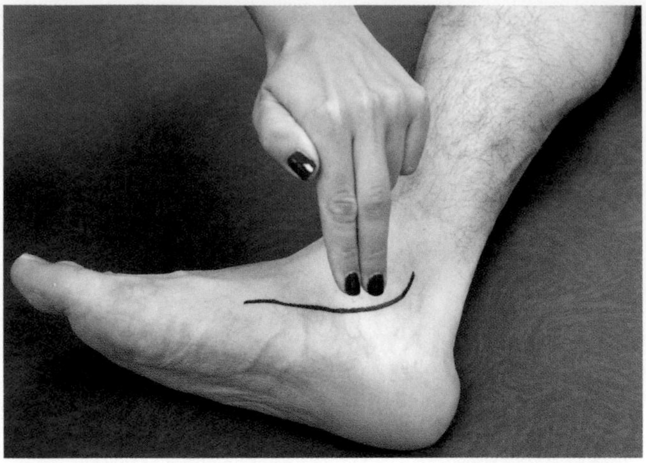

FIGURE 8-29 ■ Location of Tinel's sign for tarsal tunnel syndrome. Tapping over the path of the posterior tibial nerve radiates symptoms into the foot and toes.

with plantar fasciitis, pain is localized near the fascia's insertion on the calcaneus. The straight-leg-raise test can assist in the differential diagnosis between plantar fasciitis and TTS (see Selective Tissue Test 8-6). Stretching and exercise often decrease plantar fasciitis symptoms, but activity increases the pain caused by TTS. A definitive diagnosis of TTS is made via electrodiagnostic studies, MRI, or ultrasonic imaging.[68,83,92]

A complete evaluation of the lower extremity is required to identify the cause of TTS. A common finding is pes planus in which excessive pronation increases the traction stress placed on the nerve.

Tarsal Tunnel Syndrome Intervention Strategies

The use of an orthotic or motion-control shoe to limit the amount and speed of pronation is recommended.[93] Surgical intervention may be needed to release the compressive forces placed on the posterior tibial nerve. Results of this surgery are most successful when the compression occurs within the tarsal tunnel itself.[68]

Metatarsal Fractures

Fracture of the MTs can result from direct trauma or overuse; the location of pain and crepitus are indicative of the type of fracture (Fig. 8-30). Acute fractures occur secondary to compressive, tensile, rotational, or crushing forces. Stress fractures have a more insidious onset. The toe flexors assist the foot in dissipating the forces placed on the MTs. Fatigue or general weakness of the toe flexors increases the amount of strain placed on the MTs, increasing the risk of fracture.[94] People with diabetes are also at an increased risk for an MT fracture.[95]

Acute Fractures

The fifth MT is the most frequently fractured metatarsal, with the proximal segment at the highest risk of acute fracture.[96] The base of the fifth MT is particularly prone to avulsion fractures (Fig. 8-31). Inadvertent inversion of the foot and ankle creates tension on the base of the fifth metatarsal from the lateral cord of the plantar fascia. The body counters against inadvertent inversion of the foot and ankle by contracting the peroneals, everting the foot and bringing it back to its proper orientation. The force of the contraction of the peroneus brevis creates still further tension and displaces the fracture, avulsing from its attachment on the styloid process of the fifth MT.[96] This mechanism, when associated with pain, crepitus, and swelling over the insertion site, strongly suggests a fracture. The location of pain is also indicative of the type of fracture. The signs and symptoms of an avulsion fracture of the fifth MT's styloid process are clinically similar to those of a **Jones fracture**, a transverse fracture of the fifth MT between the metaphysis and diaphysis sections of bone (Examination Findings 8-3).[96]

The signs and symptoms of an acute fracture may include obvious deformity and the presence of a **false joint** over the fracture site. The suspicion of acute fractures may be further substantiated by the long bone compression test (Fig. 8-32). ROM of the joints above and below the fracture site may be limited because of pain. Patients who have pain at the base of the fifth MT combined with an inability to walk four steps both immediately following injury and at the time of examination should be referred for radiographs, in accordance with the Ottawa Ankle Rules (see p. 279).

Metatarsal Fracture Intervention Strategies

Management depends on the type and location of the fracture. Any suspected acute fracture to the MTs requires immediate immobilization and non–weight bearing while the patient is referred to a physician. Avulsion fractures with minimal displacement of the avulsed bone fragment may be managed nonsurgically with compression and partial weight bearing and typically require 3 to 4 weeks for recovery.[96,98,99] Fragment displacement of greater than 2 mm is generally managed with surgical fixation.[96] With the exception of the fifth MT, fractures of the shaft or neck typically require immobilization and weight bearing to tolerance for 4 to 6 weeks.

In an active population, early surgical fixation of Jones fractures has a superior outcome over immobilization alone.[100] Because of their propensity for a nonunion, Jones fractures require surgical fixation with return to competition expected in 8 weeks.[96] Conservative treatment consists of 8 weeks of immobilization followed by weight bearing in a cast as tolerated.[99]

Stress Fractures

Metatarsal, tarsal, and ankle stress fractures are related to biomechanical abnormalities of the foot.[101] Predisposing conditions include dysfunction of the first MTP joint, neuropathy, metabolic disorders (including diabetes and osteoporosis), and rearfoot malalignment.[102] Because of the prevalence of

False joint Abnormal movement along the length of a bone caused by a fracture or incomplete fusion

Selective Tissue Test 8-6

Dorsiflexion–Eversion Test for Tarsal Tunnel Syndrome

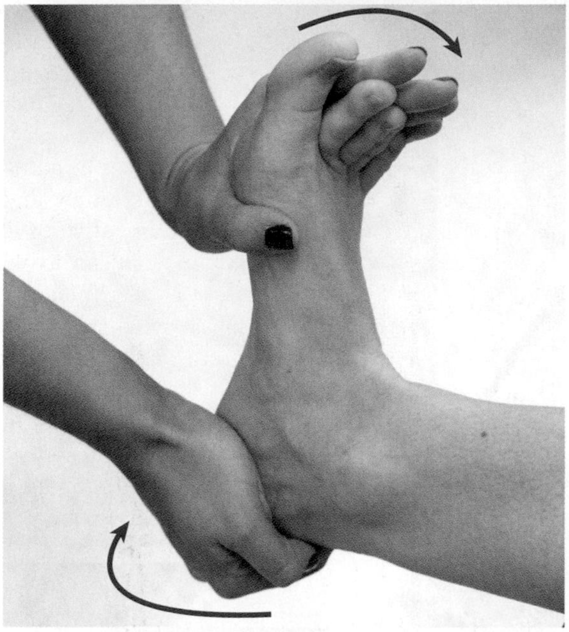

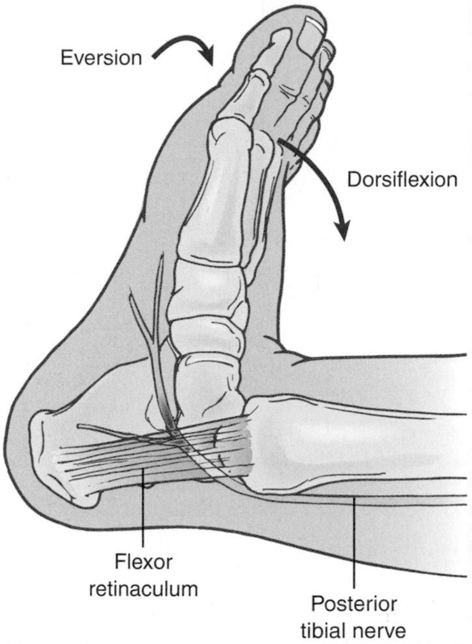

This test places tension on the posterior tibial nerve by replicating the mechanics of excessive and/or prolonged pronation during gait.[91]

Patient Position	Sitting with the legs off the table
Position of Examiner	At the patient's feet
Evaluative Procedure	Passively evert the heel (calcaneus and talus) and dorsiflex the foot and toes. Hold this position for 5 to 10 seconds.
Positive Test	Provocation of pain and/or paresthesia radiating into the foot
Implications	Posterior tibial nerve dysfunction
Modification	The Tinel's sign can be performed over the course of the nerve during this procedure.
Comments	A cadaver study comparing the windlass test with the dorsiflexion–eversion test increased strain on both the tibial nerve and the plantar fascia. Neither test may be helpful in differentiating between the two conditions.[101]

Evidence

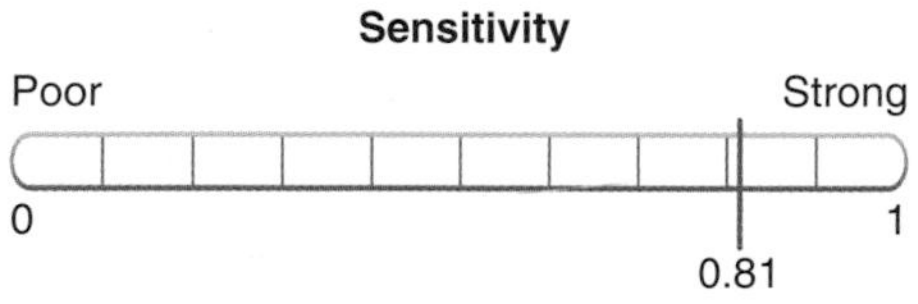

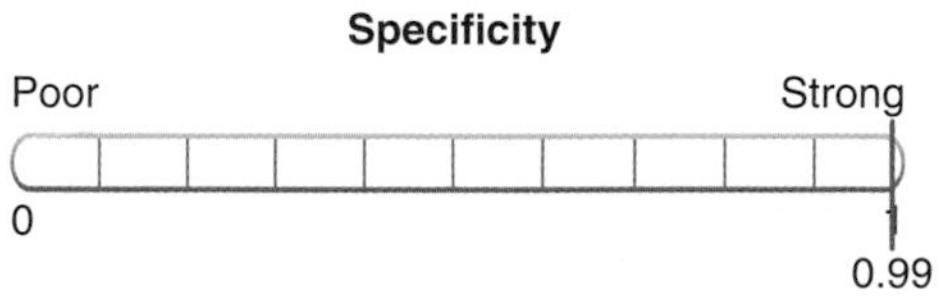

LR+: 81.00

LR−: 0.19

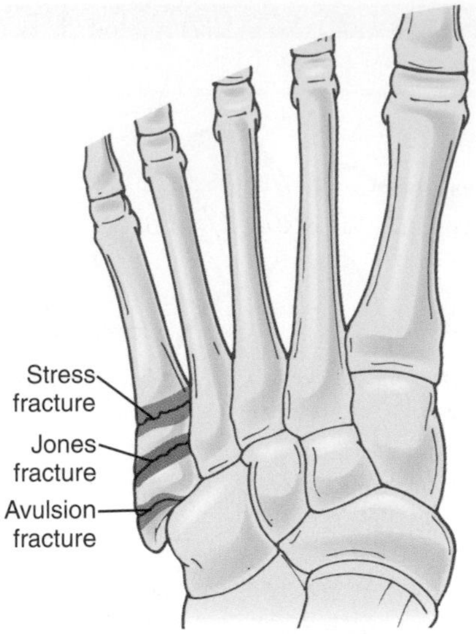

FIGURE 8-30 ■ Fractures of the proximal fifth metatarsal. Avulsion fractures involve the styloid process, "Jones fractures" occur 1 cm distal to the proximal diaphysis, and stress fractures tend to occur distal to that demarcation.

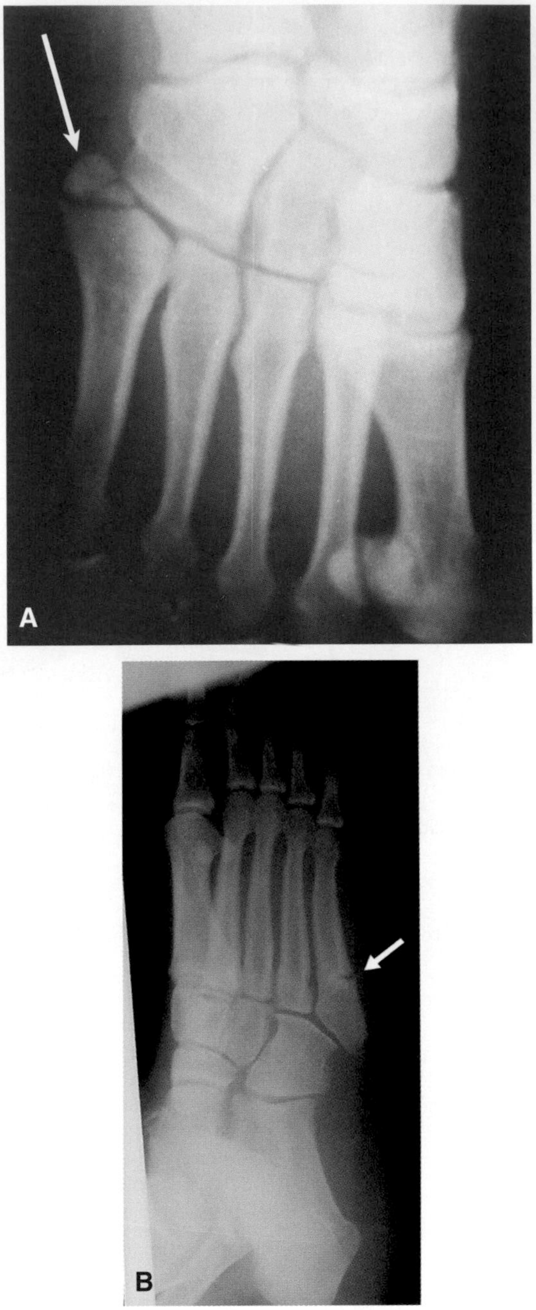

FIGURE 8-31 ■ Metatarsal fractures (A) Fracture of styloid process of the fifth metatarsal (dorsal view of the right foot). (B) Radiograph of a Jones fracture, a transverse fracture of the fifth MT located at the junction between the metaphysis and diaphysis (oblique view of the right foot).

decreased bone density, postmenopausal and amenorrheic women are at increased risk of stress fractures.[107]

During weight bearing, hypomobility of any of the foot articulations increases the stress placed on the midfoot, and hypermobility increases the amount of stress placed on the forefoot. Over time, the individual begins to experience local pain associated with activity. Stress fractures of the MTs have been termed "march fractures" because of their prevalence in new military recruits. If unrecognized and untreated, a stress fracture can progress to a gross fracture.

Stress fractures are characterized by a dull pain over the fracture site that increases with activity and decreases with rest. This condition must be differentiated from other foot conditions. Pain may be referred to the MTs secondary to TTS or an intermetatarsal neuroma. In addition, pain may arise from irritation of the interosseous muscles, be caused by an inflammatory condition such as periostitis, or have a vascular origin. In the case of multiple stress fractures or a stress fracture that fails to heal, the possibility of underlying or contributory pathology such as **osteopenia** must be ruled out.

Metatarsal Stress Fracture Intervention Strategy

Stress fractures are managed symptomatically. The patient is withheld from activities that aggravate the fracture site and either fitted with a walking boot or instructed to wear stiff-soled shoes.

Lisfranc Injuries

Injury to the Lisfranc joint can include sprains, dislocations, fractures, or fracture-dislocations through the tarsometatarsal joints (Fig. 8-33). Lisfranc fractures represent less than 1% of fractures, and up to one-third of these debilitating injuries are not detected upon initial examination.[108] Clinically the signs and symptoms of these conditions may range from subtle to obvious, and frequently the injury is dismissed as a "sprain." Because long-term outcomes are poor, a high index of suspicion is necessary for any acute midfoot injury.[108]

Fracture-dislocations are often the result of a high-energy mechanism; sprains result from lower-energy forces.[107] Lisfranc fracture-dislocations are commonly the result of an axial load being placed on the foot while

Osteopenia Decreased bone density, but less severe than osteoporosis

Examination Findings 8-3
Metatarsal Fractures

Examination Segment	Clinical Findings
History of Current Condition	*Onset:* Acute, or in the case of stress fractures, insidious *Pain characteristics:* Localized pain occurring along the shaft of the MT, radiating into the intermetatarsal space *Other symptoms:* Not applicable *Mechanism:* **Acute:** Direct trauma to the MT (e.g., being stepped on), dynamic overload (e.g., avulsion of the peroneus brevis tendon), or rotational (e.g., inversion of the foot) **Insidious:** Repetitive stresses placed along the shaft of the MT or compression arising from the contiguous MTs (e.g., "march fracture"); symptoms typically increase with activity and decrease with rest; often associated with abrupt increase in activity (e.g., sudden increases in training volume) *Risk factors:* Long-term diabetes, forefoot valgus, rearfoot varus, rearfoot valgus, pes planus, pes cavus, Morton's toe, change in footwear, increased intensity or duration of training, changing running surfaces, and conditions associated with decreased bone density such as menopause or amenorrhea
Functional Assessment	Inability to bear weight or walk Pain during toe-landing or push-off phase of gait
Inspection	In acute injuries, gross deformity and/or swelling may be visible along the shaft of the bone.
Palpation	Stress fractures may reveal no significant signs, but localized swelling and point tenderness around the painful area may be present. A false joint may be present with acutely fractured MTs.
Joint and Muscle Function Assessment	Joint and muscle function assessments are contraindicated if acute fracture is suspected. *AROM:* Movements that compress the bone, mainly dorsiflexion of the ankle or rotation of the foot, typically result in pain. *MMT:* May or may not identify weakness and pain *PROM:* Movements that compress the bone, mainly dorsiflexion of the ankle or rotation of the foot, typically result in pain.
Joint Stability Tests	*Stress tests:* Not applicable *Joint play:* Contraindicated if acute fracture is suspected Hypomobility at an adjacent joint may predispose to stress fracture.
Selective Tissue Tests	Long bone compression test
Neurological Screening	No remarkable findings
Vascular Screening	No remarkable findings
Imaging Techniques	A bone scan or MRI is required to definitively diagnose stress fractures in its early stages. The presence of acute fractures must be confirmed via radiographic examination.
Differential Diagnosis	*Stress fracture:* Interdigital neuromas, TTS *Acute fracture:* Sprain, dislocation

AROM = active range of motion; MMT = manual muscle test; MRI = magnetic resonance images; MT = metatarsal; PROM = passive range of motion; TTS = tarsal tunnel syndrome

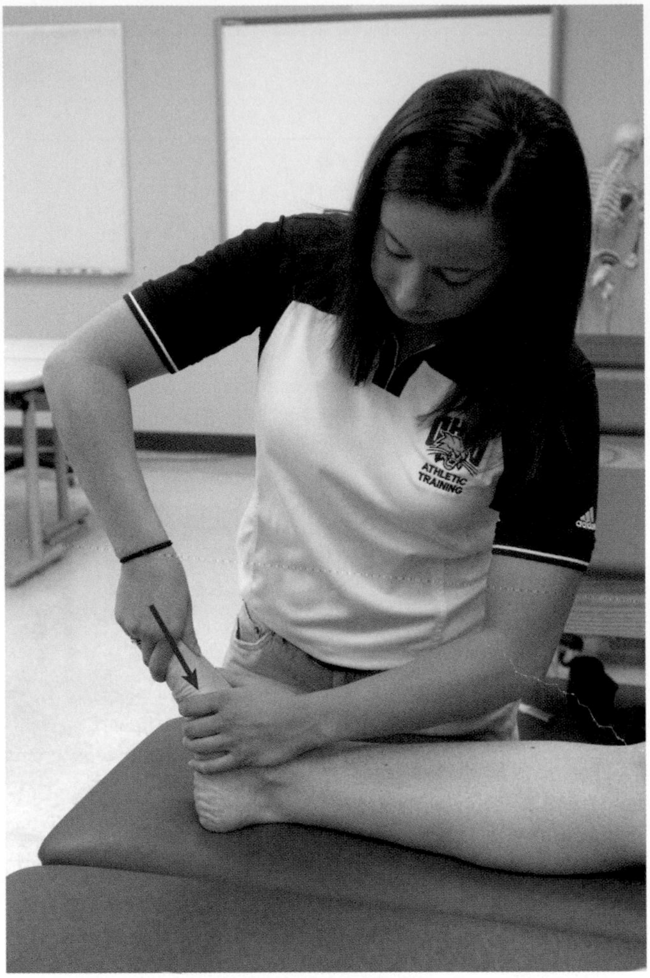

FIGURE 8-32 ■ Long bone compression test for suspected fractures of the metatarsals. A longitudinal force is placed along the shaft of the bone. In the presence of a fracture, compression of the two fragments results in pain and possibly the presence of a "false joint." Do not perform this test if a gross fracture is apparent.

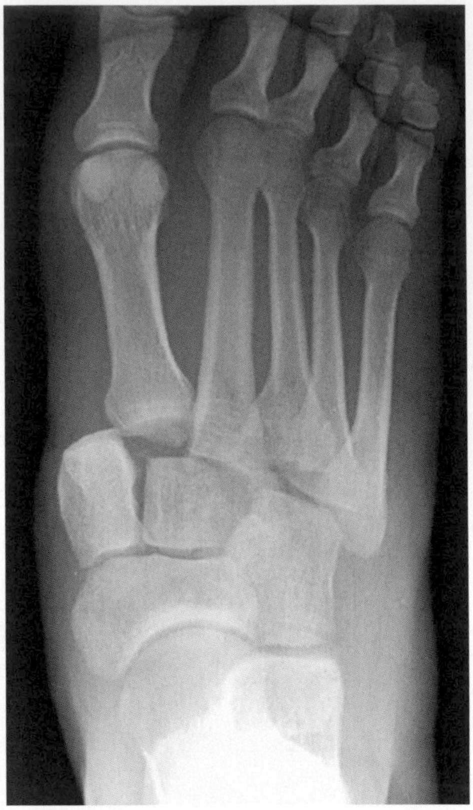

FIGURE 8-33 ■ Lisfranc fracture (dorsal view, right foot). Note the lateral displacement of the metatarsals relative to the tarsals.

the toes are extended (Fig. 8-34). Attempting to rotate (pronate or supinate) the foot while the distal segment is fixed—as in being stepped on—is also a common mechanism. A fracture-dislocation is characterized by severe pain and palpable and potentially visible deformity immediately following the injury. The deformity is quickly obscured by the rapid onset of swelling (Examination Findings 8-4). Radiographs are used to identify the type of fracture and the displacement of the bony surfaces. The injury is classified by the direction and magnitude of displacement of the tarsals using the modified Hardcastle classification system.[104] Unrecognized or untreated Lisfranc joint injury has a high morbidity rate of post-traumatic arthritis and nonunion, malunion, and/or malalignment in bone healing.

* Practical Evidence

Following a loading or crushing mechanism to the foot, plantar ecchymosis is indicative of a possible Lisfranc joint injury.[109]

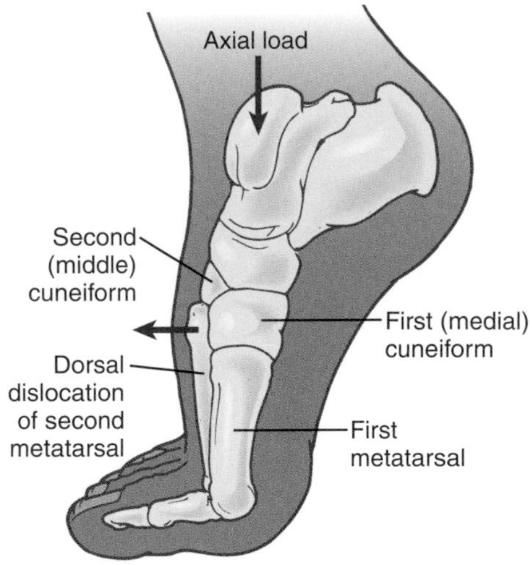

FIGURE 8-34 ■ A mechanism of injury resulting in a Lisfranc fracture-dislocation, an axial load being placed on the rearfoot while weight bearing on extended toes.

Lisfranc Joint Injury Intervention Strategies

Conservative treatment consisting of prolonged non–weight bearing is warranted when weight-bearing radiographs reveal no displacement.[104] Operative reduction and internal fixation is the typical course of treatment for Lisfranc injuries with bony displacement. Postoperative treatment consists of 6 weeks of non–weight bearing in a cast or splint followed by 4 to 6 weeks of progressively increasing weight bearing.[104]

Examination Findings 8-4
Lisfranc Injury

Examination Segment	Clinical Findings
History of Current Condition	*Onset:* Acute *Pain characteristics:* Generally severe pain at the time of injury[108] *Other symptoms:* The patient may report a snapping, popping, or tearing sensation at the time of injury. *Mechanism:* Sudden rotational loading of the TMT joints or axial loading that forces the toes into extension and the foot and ankle into dorsiflexion (e.g., landing from a jump) Rotational loading on a fixed forefoot Crushing force
Functional Assessment	Inability to bear weight or antalgic gait to minimize weight bearing on involved side
Inspection	Swelling over the dorsum of the foot In some instances, displacement of the MTs may be noted. Ecchymosis on the plantar surface of the foot Fracture-dislocations are marked by an apparent shortening and widening of the involved foot.
Palpation	Point tenderness over the TMT joints and fractured MTs
Joint and Muscle Function Assessment	Joint and muscle function assessments are contraindicated in the presence of a suspected fracture. *AROM:* All decreased secondary to pain *MMT:* Decreased strength secondary to pain is found during pronation, supination, dorsiflexion, and plantarflexion. *PROM:* Pain at end-range of all motions
Joint Stability Tests	*Stress tests:* Not applicable *Joint play:* Do not perform if fracture is suspected. Increased glide may represent manual displacement of the fracture line.
Selective Tissue Tests	Not applicable
Neurological Screening	Local branches of peripheral nerve may be damaged secondary to tensile or compression forces.
Vascular Screening	A crushing mechanism of injury may result in vascular compromise including a compartment syndrome.[109]
Imaging Techniques	AP, lateral, and oblique radiographs in standing[108]
Differential Diagnosis	Tarsal fracture, MT fracture
Comments	If a compartment syndrome develops, immediate surgical decompression and repair is needed. Because of the poor long-term outcomes and complications of unrecognized, untreated Lisfranc injuries, any suspected Lisfranc joint involvement should be immediately referred to a physician.[108]

AP = anteroposterior; AROM = active range of motion; MMT = manual muscle test; MT = metatarsal; PROM = passive range of motion; TMT = tarsometatarsal

Phalangeal Fractures

Phalangeal fractures are the result of a longitudinal force applied to the bone, such as kicking an immovable object, or they occur secondary to a crushing force, such as a weight falling on the toes (Fig. 8-35). Impairments associated with a fractured phalanx include deformity, pain, and crepitus. Pain is experienced during toe-off when running or walking.

Phalangeal Fracture Intervention Strategies

Although phalangeal fractures result in pain and an **antalgic gait**, few treatment options exist. After a fracture has been confirmed via radiographic examination, the treatment consists of rest, the use of a hard-soled shoe to prevent extension

Antalgic gait A limp or unnatural walking pattern

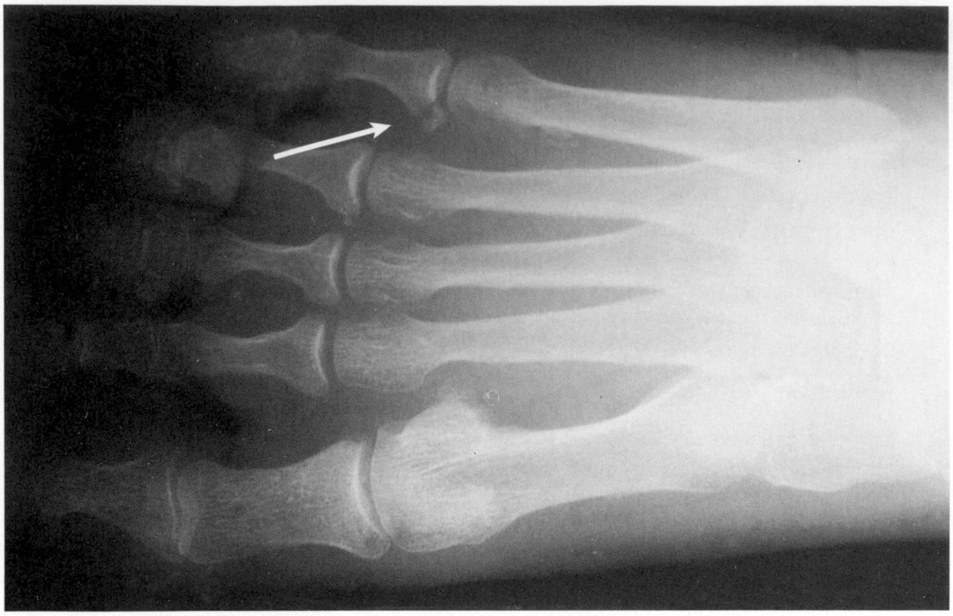

FIGURE 8-35 ■ Fracture of the proximal phalanx of the fifth toe of the right foot.

of the toes, and possibly the use of crutches. Surgical intervention may be required if the fracture disrupts the articular surface.

Intermetatarsal Neuroma

Intermetatarsal neuromas, also referred to as plantar neuromas, interdigital neuromas, or **Morton's** neuromas, are caused by the entrapment of a nerve between two MT heads.[106] The third common digital (plantar) nerve is most commonly affected.[107,108] The communicating branch of the lateral plantar nerve has also been implicated with Morton's neuroma.[107]

Prolonged pressure on the involved nerve results in a degenerative neuropathy and formation of fibrotic nodules and edema around the nerve. The exact relationship of this buildup and the diagnosis of a neuroma is unclear.[106] Over time, **demyelination** of the nerve occurs.[106]

Excessive motion, a thickened and shortened transverse intermetatarsal ligament, and excessive pronation predispose individuals to intermetatarsal neuromas. Activities that increase weight-bearing pressure or compressive pressure in the forefoot, such as wearing pointed-toed and high-heeled shoes, can trigger the signs and symptoms.[106] Middle-aged women are more likely to be affected with this condition. Also, a high likelihood exists for reoccurrence in the same foot.[108,109]

The chief impairments, closely resembling those of a MT stress fracture, include pain in the anterior transverse arch radiating to the toes, the plantar aspect of the foot, and, occasionally, projecting up the ankle and lower leg. Patients may also describe numbness and paresthesia in the digits. An increase in intermetatarsal pressure during weight bearing on the forefoot increases pain.[106,110] The symptoms increase when the patient is wearing shoes, especially if the shoes are tight fitting. Patients report relief of the symptoms when they remove the footwear. A nodule may be palpated between the involved MT heads. Clinical examination is effective in detecting intermetatarsal neuromas. Web space tenderness (Fig. 8-36), a positive foot squeeze test (Mulder sign), a positive plantar percussion test (increased symptoms when extending the digits and tapping over the involved area), and a sensory deficit in the toe are all indicative of an intermetatarsal neuroma (Selective Tissue Test 8-7).[106,110] Tenderness may be increased by extending the digits and dorsiflexing the foot during palpation (Examination Findings 8-5). Squeezing the transverse arch, thus compressing the MT heads, replicates the symptoms.

The definitive diagnosis is based on the clinical symptoms and imaging. Ultrasonography is highly reliable in

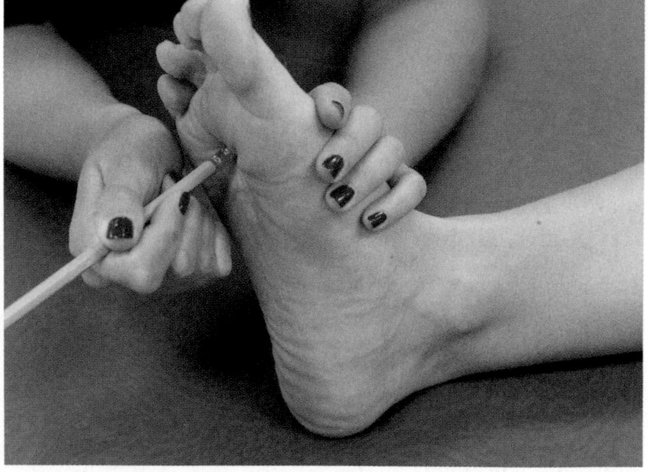

FIGURE 8-36 ■ Determining the presence of an intermetatarsal neuroma via web space tenderness. The intermetatarsal space is palpated with the side of the thumb.

Demyelination Loss of a nerve's fatty lining

Selective Tissue Test 8-7
Mulder Sign for Intermetatarsal Neuroma

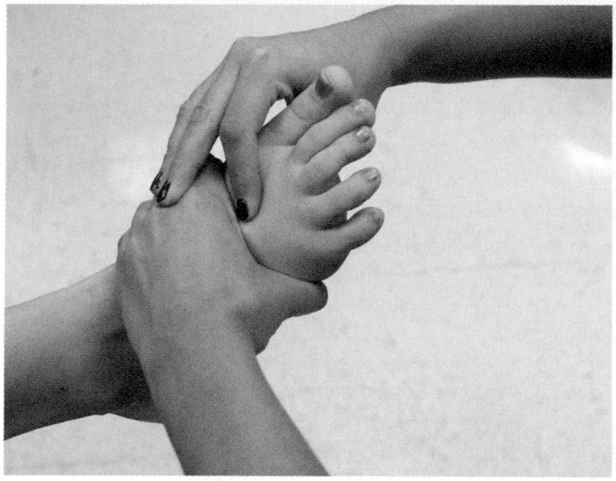

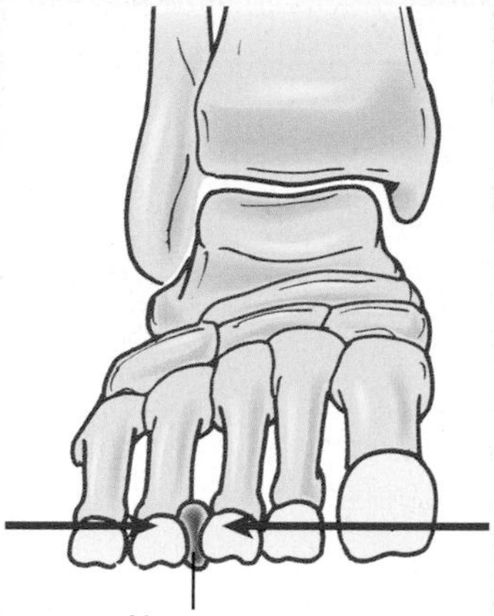

The Mulder sign involves manual compression of the transverse metatarsal arch with pressure applied over the interdigital nerve to reproduce the symptoms associated with an intermetatarsal neuroma.

Patient Position	Long- or short-sitting
Position of Examiner	Standing at the patient's feet
Evaluative Procedure	Position one hand along the distal 5th MT and the opposite hand along the distal 1st MT. Apply pressure to compress the transverse arch. Use the thumb and forefinger to apply pressure over the symptomatic interspace between the metatarsals.
Positive Test	A click, pain, and/or reproduction of symptoms
Implications	Intermetatarsal neuroma
Evidence	

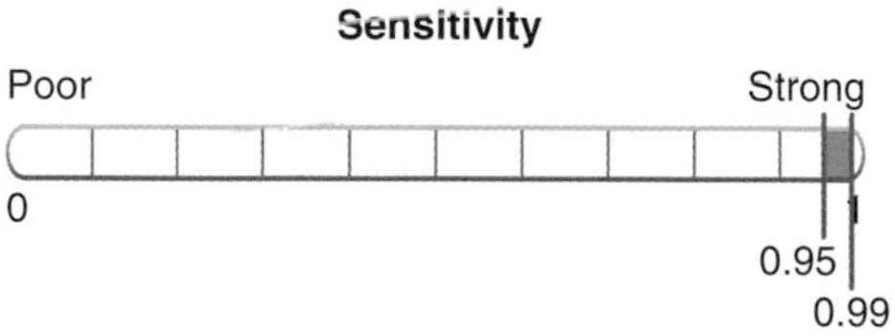

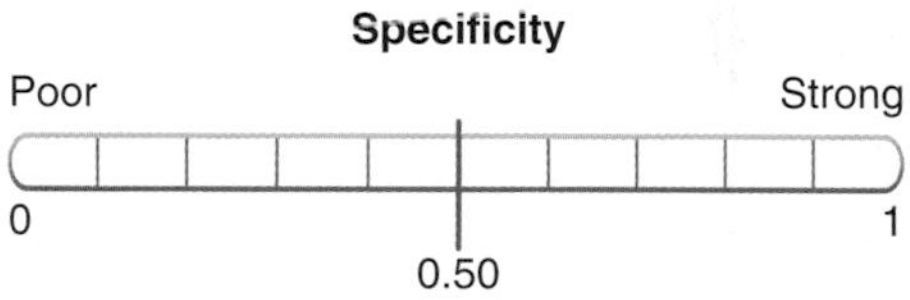

LR+: 0.90 **LR−: 0.05**

MT = metatarsal

identifying the location and size of intermetatarsal neuromas.[110] The temporary alleviation of symptoms following an injection of lidocaine aids in the diagnostic accuracy.

Intermetatarsal Neuroma Intervention Strategies

Initial treatment includes modification of footwear (i.e., the patient should avoid wearing shoes that increase symptoms), the use of orthotics to decrease intermetatarsal pressure, and the use of oral anti-inflammatory medication. Corticosteroid injections may be used for symptomatic relief and are likely more effective if provided early. Surgical excision of the neuroma provides dramatic relief of the symptoms for most patients.[111]

Hallux Rigidus

Literally meaning "stiff great toe," hallux rigidus is the progressive degeneration of the first MTP joint's articular surfaces, with consequences ranging from limited motion (hallux limitus) to complete **ankylosis** (hallux rigidus) that causes the loss of extension at the first MTP joint.[112, 113] The joint degeneration is caused by osteoarthritis; rheumatoid arthritis; gout; and advanced hallux valgus, synovial effusion, or other chondral erosions affecting the articular surfaces.[114-117] The

Ankylosis Immobility of a joint

Examination Findings 8-5
Intermetatarsal Neuroma

Examination Segment	Clinical Findings
History of Current Condition	*Onset:* Pain increases with time. *Pain characteristics:* Pain originating in the forefoot. As symptoms progress, the pain may radiate proximally. *Other symptoms:* The patient may report numbness and paresthesia in the forefoot and toes. *Mechanism:* Inflammation of—or around—a plantar nerve *Risk factors:* Hypermobility, adhesions in the transverse intermetatarsal ligament, pronated foot type
Functional Assessment	Antalgic gait may be noted.
Inspection	Often unremarkable. Swelling may be noted in the forefoot.
Palpation	Point tenderness in the web space between the MT heads Increased pain when squeezing the transverse arch, compressing the MT heads (Mulder sign) A palpable nodule may be noted.
Joint and Muscle Function Assessment	*AROM:* Unremarkable findings *MMT:* Possible increased pain with toe flexion *PROM:* Unremarkable findings
Joint Stability Tests	*Stress tests:* Not applicable *Joint play:* Hypermobility of the intermetatarsal joints
Selective Tissue Tests	Plantar percussion test
Neurological Screening	Lower quarter screen to rule out proximal nerve compression
Vascular Screening	No remarkable findings
Imaging Techniques	MRI using a contrast medium; ultrasonic imaging
Differential Diagnosis	Stress fracture, arthritis, metatarsalgia, proximal nerve compression
Comments	Symptoms increase when the patient is wearing footwear, especially pointed-toed shoes, and decrease when non–weight bearing or walking barefoot.

AROM = active range of motion; MMT = manual muscle test; MRI = magnetic resonance imaging; MT = metatarsal; PROM = passive range of motion

etiology of hallux limitus and rigidus may be related to an irregularly flattened MT head, hypermobility of the first tarsometatarsal joint, or a long first MT leading to degeneration-causing forces on the joint.[113] Hallux rigidus is frequently bilateral and has a strong genetic component.[118] Morton's toe has been associated with hallux rigidus, especially in female dancers.[24]

As the condition progresses, the MT head erodes (chondritis dissecans) or a fracture occurs through the articular surface (osteochondritis dissecans).[118] The axis of joint motion shifts from the center of the MTP to its plantar aspect. If untreated, spastic contractures and fusion of the joint (ankylosis) occur.[117,118] In some cases, the sesamoids located under the first MTP joint may hypertrophy, further decreasing ROM.[115] Irregularity of the joint surfaces results in pain at the first MTP, and vague complaints of lateral foot pain may be present secondary to compensatory forces. The subsequent loss in ROM affects the terminal stance and preswing phases of gait, which is visible during the functional assessment (see Fig. 8-1). With time, atrophy and associated weakness of the triceps surae will develop (Examination Findings 8-6).

A palpable and painful exostosis may develop on the dorsal aspect of the joint. Extension of the first MTP joint is limited by the phalanx striking the exostosis. Similar to what happens with arthritis, the joint is prone to pain and swelling, especially after activity. Radiographs can definitively diagnose this condition (Fig. 8-37).

Hallux Rigidus Intervention Strategies

Conservative treatment includes the use of passive ROM exercises to maintain extension in the joint and the use of orthotics to decrease hyperextension forces on the first

Examination Findings 8-6
Hallux Rigidus

Examination Segment	Clinical Findings
History of Current Condition	*Onset:* Insidious *Pain characteristics:* Pain arising from the first MTP joint *Mechanism:* Degeneration of the articulating surfaces secondary to repetitive stress *Risk factors:* Flattened MT head, long first MT, hypermobility of the first MTP joint, Morton's alignment
Functional Assessment	Restriction of first MTP extension alters terminal stance and the preswing phases of gait.
Inspection	Swelling of the first MTP joint, especially after activity Atrophy of the triceps surae may be noted.
Palpation	Exostosis may be palpable on the dorsal and/or medial aspects of the joint. Hypertrophy of the sesamoids may be noted.
Joint and Muscle Function Assessment	*AROM:* MTP extension is restricted and painful. *MMT:* Extensor hallucis longus: Strength reduced secondary to pain In chronic conditions, weakness of the triceps surae group may be noted (see Chapter 9). *PROM:* MTP extension is restricted and painful.
Joint Stability Tests	*Stress tests:* Hypomobile with valgus and varus stress *Joint play:* MTP hypomobility will be noted.
Selective Tissue Tests	Not applicable
Neurological Screening	No remarkable findings
Vascular Screening	No remarkable findings
Imaging Techniques	Radiographs may reveal osteophytes.
Differential Diagnosis	Arthritis; sesamoiditis; sprain; hallux valgus; gout
Comments	Hallux rigidus often occurs bilaterally.

AROM = active range of motion; MMT = manual muscle test; MT = metatarsal; MTP = metatarsophalangeal; PROM = passive range of motion

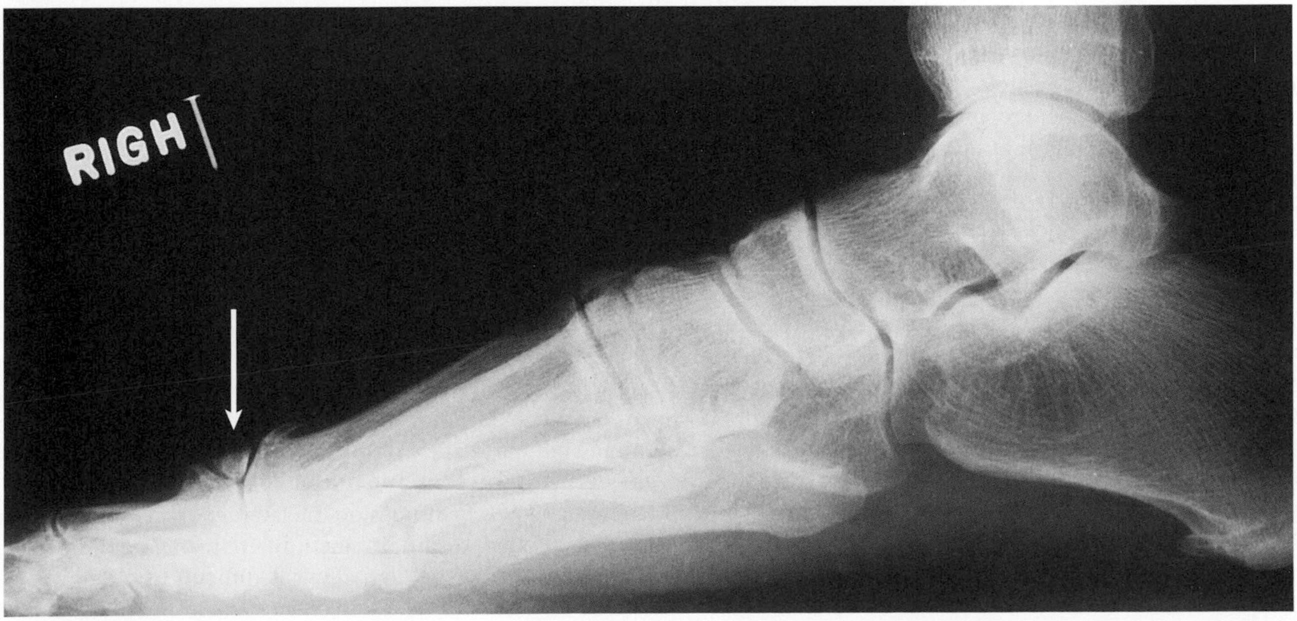

FIGURE 8-37 ■ Radiograph of hallux rigidus (medial view, right foot). The wedge-shaped bony formation over the first metatarsophalangeal joint serves as a mechanical block in limiting extension.

MTP joint. Fit the patient with shoes having adequate depth and width to accommodate the increased bulk of the forefoot. A walking boot may be prescribed to decrease joint motion when the patient is symptomatic.[28]

Corticosteroid injections assist in decreasing inflammation. If the condition progresses to the point where extension is limited and gait is affected, surgical intervention may be required. The most common surgical procedure, a cheilectomy, involves the removal of the distal dorsal aspect of the first MT and the superior half of the joint surface and other areas of exostosis.[119,120] Removal of the bone decreases pain and restores extension to the joint, allowing a more normal gait pattern.

Hallux Valgus

A progressive degeneration and subluxation of the first MTP joint, hallux valgus is characterized by the joint angle being greater than 20 degrees in the frontal plane. As a result, the distal end of the first toe angles laterally, placing a valgus load on the MTP joint (see Inspection Findings 8-2). The valgus deformity may interfere with the function of the second toe. With time, a bunion, the enlargement of the underlying bursa, will develop over the medial aspect of the joint, causing further pain and dysfunction (Examination Findings 8-7).[2]

Along with a genetic predisposition, several biomechanical aberrations may contribute to the development of hallux valgus. A limitation in passive MTP extension, a flexible forefoot valgus, a planterflexed first ray, and an everted calcaneus all place an increased functional load on the first MT.

Hallux Valgus Intervention Strategies

Initial management of hallux valgus involves instructing the patient to wear shoes that can accommodate the deformity without increasing pressure on the medial toe.[122] A felt or foam pad can be inserted between the first and second toe to maintain normal alignment. Anti-inflammatory medications may be helpful in further reducing the symptoms.

In the presence of hallux valgus, the amount of passive first MTP flexion and extension available is indicative of the potential success of surgical repair. Restriction into passive extension while manually maintaining the normal alignment of the great toe suggests that normal ROM could not be restored by surgical realignment.[28]

First Metatarsophalangeal Joint Sprains

Sprains of the first MTP joint usually occur when the foot is planted and the ankle is subsequently dorsiflexed. The friction between the shoe and playing surface, combined with body weight and forward momentum, forces the first MTP joint into hyperextension. Sprains of the plantar MTP joint capsule and/or the subsequent inflammatory response caused by repetitive hyperextension has been termed "turf toe" because of the reportedly high instance of this injury during competition on artificial turf.[123]

Common complaints of patients with first MTP joint sprains are pain in the joint during the push-off phase of gait, active joint motion, or manual resistance, or when attempting quick stops. The joint is painful to the touch, and ROM is limited. A radiograph is needed to rule out fracture to the MT or phalanx.

Athletes, especially those who compete barefooted, are also susceptible to varus and valgus sprains of the MTP joints. A varus force is applied to the joint capsule and collateral ligaments when the toes are bent toward the body's midline. An outward bending results in a valgus force being placed on the capsule. On rare occasions, the MTP joint may dislocate.

First Metatarsophalangeal Joint Sprain Intervention Strategies

Management of sprains of the first MTP involves removing aggravating stresses through the use of crutches, a firm shoe insole, or other immobilization device. The physician may prescribe the use of oral or injectable anti-inflammatory medications.

Sesamoiditis

Two sesamoids lie within the tendon of the flexor hallucis brevis. These bones provide a mechanical advantage to great toe flexion and absorb and redirect weight-bearing forces. Each of the two FHB sesamoids lies in its own groove on the head of the first MT. As great toe extension increases, the sesamoids become less stable in their grooves, subjecting them to greater stresses.

Sesamoiditis, an irritation of the bones and soft tissue in the area, and sesamoid fractures are associated with both cavus and planus foot types. In the cavus foot, the sesamoids are subjected to increased forces from the more acute angle of the MT. In the planus foot, the sesamoids are compressed for prolonged periods while the foot attempts to push off on the relatively unstable surface (Examination Findings 8-8).

Acute fractures occur through direct trauma or forced dorsiflexion of the MTP joint. As a result of multiple ossification centers during development, bipartite sesamoids are present in up to 10% of the population and should not be confused with sesamoid fractures on radiographs.[4] With their ability to detect irregular margins, CT scans may be useful to differentiate between bipartite sesamoids and acute fractures or stress fractures in their early stages.[4]

Sesamoid Fracture

Acute sesamoid fractures are usually the result of eccentric loading during extension and are often accompanied by a popping sensation followed by immediate inability to push off on the involved great toe.[3] Localized swelling is evident on the plantar surface of the first MTP joint. Exquisite point tenderness is present, and the patient's gait is altered to keep the weight-bearing forces on the lateral portion of the foot.

The medial sesamoid fracture may fragment into as many as four parts. Clinically it is difficult to differentiate

Examination Findings 8-7
Hallux Valgus

Examination Segment	Clinical Findings
History of Current Condition	*Onset:* Insidious *Pain characteristics:* Arising from the first MTP joint *Mechanism:* A prolonged valgus stress being placed on the first MTP joint *Risk factors:* Improperly fitting shoes; wearing high heels Pes planus Congenital development Diseases such as cerebral palsy, rheumatoid arthritis, or osteoarthritis[121]
Functional Assessment	Gait, especially toe-off, may be affected.
Inspection	Valgus angulation of the first toe The 1st and 2nd toe may overlap. Bunion formation over the medial border of the first MTP joint
Palpation	The medial joint and sesamoids may be tender to the touch. Thickening of the synovial capsule may be noted.
Joint and Muscle Function Assessment	*AROM:* Pain may be produced during flexion and extension. *PROM:* Pain may be produced during flexion and extension. *MMT:* Extensor hallucis longus is weak secondary to pain.
Joint Stability Tests	*Stress tests:* Valgus and varus stress test *Joint play:* Hypermobility of the first ray
Selective Tissue Tests	Not applicable
Neurological Screening	No remarkable findings
Vascular Screening	No remarkable findings
Imaging Techniques	Weight-bearing radiographs
Differential Diagnosis	Osteoarthritis; septic arthritis;[122] sesamoiditis; sprain; hallux rigidus; gout
Comments	The sesamoid bones on the plantar surface of the MTP joint may also dislocate. The deformity can cause footwear to fit improperly and change biomechanics.[28]

AROM = active range of motion; MMT = manual muscle test; MTP = metatarsophalangeal; PROM = passive range of motion

between a symptomatic bipartite sesamoid and a sesamoid fracture.[124] The definitive diagnosis of a fractured sesamoid is usually determined via CT scans. The shape and magnitude of comminuted fractures can be determined using 3-D CT scans.[3]

Sesamoid Pathology Intervention Strategies

Patients with sesamoid pathology complain of increased symptoms when on their toes, such as during dance or wearing high-heeled shoes, and during the push-off phase of gait. Passive MTP extension is painful at end-range. Walking on the lateral aspect of the foot to avoid push-off is a typical gait strategy used by those with sesamoid pain. Use of orthotics, a metatarsal pad, and appropriate footwear to dissipate forces is the initial intervention for individuals with sesamoid pain. If conservative treatment fails, surgical excision of the sesamoids—sesamoidectomy—is the next intervention and results in good outcomes.[4]

On-Field Examination of Foot Injuries

Although it is possible for an athlete to walk off the playing area with a fracture, especially if it involves the toes, significant trauma to the foot and toes usually results in the athlete's inability to bear weight without pain. The location of the pain and mechanism of injury act as a guide for on-field injury evaluation. Not all of the steps described in this section apply to all injuries.

With any sign or symptom indicating a bony fracture or joint dislocation , splint the foot and ankle, and refer the

Examination Findings 8-8
Sesamoiditis

Examination Segment	Clinical Findings
History of Current Condition	*Onset:* Acute or insidious *Pain characteristics:* Patients may describe pain as local to the sesamoids, or they may report more general complaints of pain arising from the great toe. *Other symptoms:* The patient may report pain or snapping as the hallux extends during gait. The patient may report a sensation of snapping or cracking in the event of a sesamoid fracture. *Mechanism:* Repetitive MTP extension, especially when weight bearing *Risk factors:* Cavus or planus foot type; activities such as dancing or sprinting
Functional Assessment	Alteration of gait to avoid weight bearing on the sesamoids; gait may be modified to avoid extending the great toe during toe-off.
Inspection	Swelling may be noted, especially on the plantar and medial aspects of the joint. A planterflexed first ray
Palpation	Point tenderness over the involved sesamoid(s)
Joint and Muscle Function Assessment	*AROM:* Pain moving into MTP extension *MMT:* The test for flexor hallucis brevis and longus produces pain and weakness secondary to irritation of the sesamoids. *PROM:* Pain moving into MTP extension
Joint Stability Tests	*Stress tests:* Not applicable *Joint play:* Decreased MTP joint glide may be present secondary to joint effusion.
Selective Tissue Tests	Not applicable
Neurological Screening	Tinel's sign along the medial branch of the plantar digital nerve is used to rule out nerve entrapment.
Vascular Screening	No remarkable findings
Imaging Techniques	AP, medial, and medial and lateral oblique radiographs to rule out fracture CT scans can help differentiate between bipartite and fractured sesamoids and also identify post-traumatic degeneration. MRI helps differentiate between a bony stress reaction, fracture, or soft tissue inflammation.[4]
Differential Diagnosis	Sesamoid fracture; hallux valgus; capsular/plantar plate sprain; arthritis; gout; avascular necrosis; chondromalacia[4]
Comments	Edema, inflammation, or displacement of a bipartite sesamoid may place pressure on a digital nerve, producing radicular symptoms.

AP = anteroposterior; AROM = active range of motion; CT = computed tomography; MMT = manual muscle test; PROM = passive range of motion

athlete to a physician. Positive findings consistent with the Modified Ottawa Ankle Rules warrant initial fracture management and referral for imaging. After the athlete is moved to the sideline or the sports medicine facility, the remaining evaluation proceeds, as described earlier in this chapter.

Equipment Considerations

Only the most severe cases, based on the degree of pain, reports of a "crack" or "pop," or obvious trauma such as bleeding through the shoe, warrant removal of the shoe or sock while the patient is on the playing surface. (Chapter 9 provides a description of removing footwear and ankle braces.)

On-Field History

Question athletes about their history relating to the mechanism of injury, the location of the pain, any sounds associated with its onset, and their willingness and ability to bear weight on the injured limb. Pain may also radiate to the foot from the lumbar or sacral plexus or after anterior compartment syndrome or trauma to the peroneal nerve.

On-Field Inspection

Observe the posture of the athlete. Is the individual remaining down on the field or court or is the athlete hopping off or being assisted off the playing surface? The shoe itself will prohibit a direct inspection of the foot. If the footwear is removed while the athlete is still on the field, note the integrity of the joints, any gross deformity of the long bones, or the presence of gross swelling or discoloration.

If a significant injury such as a fracture or dislocation is evident during the initial inspection, perform a secondary survey to rule out the presence of unrecognized trauma. Then immobilize the body part and refer the athlete for medical evaluation.

On-Field Palpation

With the exceptions of the plantar and superior aspects of the calcaneus and the talus, the bones of the foot are relatively subcutaneous, assisting in the identification of crepitus or other deformities through palpation.

- **Bony palpation:** The presence of a fracture or dislocation must be ruled out:
  - Palpate the lengths of the five rays to rule out discontinuity in the bony shafts or joints.
  - Palpate the tarsals, calcaneus, talus, and the medial and lateral malleoli for point tenderness or crepitus that may indicate a gross or avulsion fracture or dislocation.
- **Soft tissue palpation:** The forces placed on the foot can be sufficient to significantly tear or rupture its tendons, fascia, or ligaments.
  - **Plantar fascia:** Palpate the length of the plantar fascia to identify areas of point tenderness. Pain arising from the medial calcaneal tubercle may signify a rupture of the plantar fascia.
  - **Anterior musculature:** Palpate the anterior musculature. Hyperplantarflexion of the ankle or an eccentric contraction of the tibialis anterior can result in a strain, rupture, or avulsion of its tendon, leading to tenderness of these structures. This mechanism may also result in a fracture of an accessory navicular.
  - **Medial musculature:** Palpate the tibialis posterior, flexor hallucis longus, and flexor digitorum longus, which pass posterior to the medial malleolus. These tendons may be impinged by supination of the foot and ankle.
  - **Posterior musculature:** Palpate the posterior musculature. Achilles tendon ruptures are common in activities that require explosive starts or eccentrically load the triceps surae muscles. (Refer to Chapter 9 for more information on this condition.)
  - **Lateral musculature:** Palpate the peroneal tendons as they pass posterior to the lateral malleolus. An inversion and planterflexion mechanism followed by contraction of the peroneals can result in an avulsion of the styloid process of the fifth MT.

On-Field Joint Function Tests

ROM testing during this phase of the evaluation is most likely limited to active flexion and extension of the toes, pronation and supination of the foot, and plantarflexion and dorsiflexion of the ankle. If these can be performed without pain or signs of a fracture or dislocation, the athlete can attempt to bear weight, as described in Chapter 3.

On-Field Management of Foot Injuries

Except in rare circumstances, most foot injuries do not require the athlete to be transported directly from the playing field to the hospital. Acute trauma such as Achilles tendon ruptures, ankle fractures, and ankle dislocations are discussed in Chapter 9.

Plantar Fascia Ruptures

Splint suspected plantar-fascia ruptures with the foot and ankle in a slightly planterflexed position or instruct the athlete not to bear weight. Fit athletes with crutches and refer them to a physician or doctor of podiatric medicine.

Fractures and Dislocations

Remove athletes from the field in a non–weight-bearing manner if a fracture or dislocation is suspected. After further evaluating them on the sideline, immobilize their foot, fit them for crutches, render appropriate immediate treatment, and refer them to a physician.

RFFERENCES

1. Lohman, EB, Sackiriyas, KSB, and Swen, RW: A comparison of the spatiotemporal parameters, kinematics, and biomechanics between shod, unshod, and minimally supported running as compared to walking. *PhysTher Sport*, 12:151, 2011.
2. Wainner, RS, et al: Regional interdependence: a musculoskeletal examination model whose time has come. *J Orthop Sports Phys Ther*, 38:616, 2007.
3. Mouhsin, E, et al: Acute fractures of medial and lateral great toe sesamoids in an athlete. *Knee Surg Sports Traumatol Arthrosc*, 12:463, 2004.
4. Kadakia, AR, and Molloy, A: Current concepts review: traumatic disorders of the first metatarsophalangeal joint and sesamoid completex. *Foot Ankle Int*, 32:834, 2011.
5. Martin, RL: The ankle and foot complex. In Levangie, PK, and Norkin, CC (eds): *Joint Structure and Function: A Comprehensive Analysis*, ed 5. Philadelphia, PA: FA Davis, 2011, p 442.
6. Aldridge, T: Diagnosing heel pain in adults. *Am Fam Physician*, 70:332, 2004.
7. Van Beek, C, and Greisberg, J: Mobility of the first ray: review article. *Foot Ankle Int*, 32:917, 2011.
8. McPoil, TG, et al: Heel pain – plantar fasciitis: clinical practice guidelines linked to the International Classification of Function, Disability, and Health from the orthopaedic section of the American Physical Therapy Association. *J Orthop Sports Phys Ther*, 38:A1, 2008.
9. Thordarson, DB, et al: Dynamic support of the human longitudinal arch: a biomechanical evaluation. *Clin Orthop*, 316:165, 1995.
10. Kanatli, U, Yetkin, H, and Bolukbasi, S: Evaluation of the transverse metatarsal arch of the foot with gait analysis. *Arch Orthop Trauma Surg*, 123:148, 2003.

11. Tu, P, and Bytomski, JR: Diagnosis of heel pain. *Am Fam Physician*, 84:909, 2011.
12. Hamburger, M, et al: 2011 recommendations for the diagnosis and management of gout and hyperuricemia. *Postgrad Med*, 122:157, 2010.
13. Gregg, EW, et al: Prevalence of lower extremity diseases associated with normal glucose levels, impaired fasting glucose, and diabetes among U.S. adults aged 40 or older. *Diabetes Res Clin Pract*, 77:485, 2007.
14. Gefen, A, et al: Analysis of muscular fatigue and foot stability during high-heeled gait. *Gait Posture*, 15:56, 2002.
15. Esenyel, M, et al: Kinetics of high-heeled gait. *J Am Podiatr Med Assoc*, 93:27, 2003.
16. Payne C: Sensitivity and specificity of the functional hallux limitus test to predict foot function. *J Am Podiatr Med Assoc*, 92:269, 2002.
17. Morrison, KE, and Kaminski, TW: Foot characteristics in association with inversion ankle injury. *J Athl Train*, 42:135, 2007.
18. Sneyers, CJL, et al: Influence of malalignment of feet on the plantar pressure patterns in running. *Foot Ankle Int*, 16:624, 1995.
19. Pecci, M, Comeau, D, and Chawla, V: Skin conditions in the athlete. *Am J Sports Med*, 37:406, 2009.
20. Freeman, DB: Corns and calluses resulting from mechanical hyperkeratosis. *Am Fam Physician*, 65:2277, 2002.
21. Nilsson, MK, et al: Classification of the height and flexibility of the medial longitudinal arch of the foot. *J Foot Ankle Res*, 5:3, 2012.
22. Mulhem, E, and Pinelis, S: Treatment of nongenital cutaneous warts. *Am Fam Physician*, 84:288, 2011.
23. Krivickas, LS: Anatomical factors associated with overuse sports injuries. *Sports Med*, 24:132, 1997.
24. Ogilvie-Harris, DJ, Carr, MM, and Fleming, PJ: The foot in ballet dancers: the importance of second toe length. *Foot Ankle Int*, 16:144, 1995.
25. Grebing, BR, and Coughlin, MJ: Evaluation of Morton's theory of second metatarsal hypertrophy. *J Bone Joint Surg*, 86(A): 1375, 2004.
26. Acevedo, JI, and Beskin, JL: Complications of plantar fascia rupture associated with corticosteroid injection. *Foot Ankle Int*, 19:91, 1998.
27. Klaue, K, Hansen, ST, and Masquelet, AC: Clinical, quantitative assessment of first tarsometatarsal mobility in the sagittal plane and its relation to hallux valgus deformity. *Foot Ankle*, 15:9, 1994.
28. Mann, RA: Disorders of the first metatarsophalangeal joint. *J Am Acad Orthop Surg*, 3:34, 1995.
29. Rotta, I, et al: Efficacy and safety of topical antifungals in the treatment of dermatomycosis: a systematic review. *Br J Dermatol*, 166:927, 2012.
30. Tiberio, D: Pathomechanics of structural foot deformities. *Phys Ther*, 68:1840, 1988.
31. Heckman, DS, Gluck, GS, and Parekh, SG: Tendon disorders of the foot and ankle, part 2: Achilles tendon disorders. *Am J Sports Med*, 37:1223, 2009.
32. Razeghi, M, and Batt, ME: Foot type classification: a critical review of current methods. *Gait Posture*, 15:282, 2002.
33. Smith-Oricchio, K, and Harris, BA: Interrater reliability of subtalar neutral, calcaneal inversion and eversion. *J Orthop Sports Phys Ther*, 21:10, 1990.
34. Picciano, AM, Rowlands, MS, and Worrell, T: Reliability of open and closed kinetic chain subtalar joint neutral positions and navicular drop test. *J Orthop Sport Phys Ther*, 18:553, 1993.
35. Buchanan, KR, and Davis, I: The relationship between forefoot, midfoot, and rearfoot static alignment in pain-free individuals. *J Orthop Sports Phys Ther*, 35:559, 2005.
36. Elveru, RA, et al: Methods for taking subtalar joint measurements. *Phys Ther*, 68:678, 1988.
37. Glascoe, WM, et al: Criterion-related validity of a clinical measure of dorsal first ray mobility. *J Orthop Sports Phys Ther*, 35:589, 2005.
38. Glasoe, WM, et al: Comparison of two methods used to assess first-ray mobility. *Foot Ankle Int*, 23:248, 2002.
39. Sell, KE, et al: Two measurement techniques for assessing subtalar joint position: a reliability study. *J Orthop Sports Phys Ther*, 19:162, 1994.
40. Incel, NA, et al: Muscle imbalance in hallux valgus: an electromyographic study. *Am J Phys Med Rehabil*, 82:345, 2003.
41. Boling, MC, et al: A prospective investigation of biomechanical risk factors for patellofemoral pain syndrome: the joint undertaking to monitor and prevent ACL injury (JUMP-ACL) cohort. *Am J Sports Med*, 37:2108, 2009.
42. Levy, JC, et al: Incidence of foot and ankle injuries in West Point cadets with pes planus compared to the general cadet population. *Foot Ankle Int*, 27:1060, 2006.
43. Huang, CK, et al: Biomechanical evaluation of longitudinal arch stability. *Foot Ankle*, 14:353, 1993.
44. Borton, DC, and Saxby, TS: Tear of the plantar calcaneonavicular (spring) ligament causing flatfoot: a case report. *J Bone Joint Surg Br*, 79:641, 1997.
45. Rule, J, Yao, L, and Seeger, LL: Spring ligament of the ankle: normal MR anatomy. *Am J Roentgenol*, 161:1241, 1993.
46. Kitaoka, HB, Luo, Z, and An, K: Three-dimensional analysis of flatfoot deformity: cadaver study. *Foot Ankle Int*, 19:447, 1998.
47. Miller, TT: Painful accessory bones of the foot. *Semin Musculoskel Imaging*. 6:153, 2002.
48. Menz, HB, and Munteanu, SE: Validity of 3 clinical techniques for the measurement of static foot posture in older people. *J Orthop Sport Phys Ther*, 35:279, 2005.
49. De Garceau, D, et al: The association between diagnosis of plantar fasciitis and windlass test. *Foot Ankle Int*, 24:251, 2003.
50. Hewett, TE, Myer GD, and Ford, KV: Anterior cruciate ligament injuries in female athletes. Part 1, mechanisms and risk factors. *Am J Sport Med*, 34:299, 2006.
51. Brody, D: Techniques in the evaluation and treatment of the injured runner. *Orthop Clin North Am*, 13:542, 1982.
52. Saltzman, CL, Nawoczenski, DA, and Talbot, KD: Measurement of the medial longitudinal arch. *Arch Phys Med Rehabil*, 76:45, 1995.
53. Shultz, SJ, et al: Intratester and intertester reliability of clinical measures of lower extremity anatomic characteristics: implications for multicenter studies. *Clin J Sports Med*, 16:155, 2006.
54. Alentorn-Geli, E, et al: Prevention of non-contact anterior cruciate ligament injuries in soccer players. Part 1: Mechanisms of injury and underlying risk factors. *Knee Surg Sports Traumatol Arthrosc*, 17:705, 2009.
55. Ramcharitar, SI, Koslow, P, and Simpson, DM: Lower extremity manifestations of neuromuscular diseases. *Clin Podiatr Med Surg*, 15:705, 1998.
56. Carpintero, P, et al: The relationship between pes cavus and idiopathic scoliosis. *Spine*, 19:1260, 1994.
57. Burns, J, et al: The effect of pes cavus on foot pain and plantar pressure. *Clin Biomech*, 20:877, 2005.
58. Kitaoka, HB, Luo, ZP, and An, K: Effect of plantar fasciotomy on stability of arch of foot. *Clin Orthop*, 344:307, 1997.
59. Sammarco, GJ, and Helfrey, RB: Surgical treatment of recalcitrant plantar fasciitis. *Foot Ankle Int*, 17:520, 1996.
60. Lemont, H, Ammirati, KU, and Usen, N: Plantar fasciitis: a degenerative process (fasciosis) without inflammation. *J Am Podiatr Med Assoc*, 93:234, 2003.
61. McNally, EG, and Shetty, S: Plantar fascia: imaging diagnosis and guided treatment. *Semin Musculoskelet Radiology*, 14:334, 2010.
62. Powell, M, et al: Effective treatment of plantar fasciitis with dorsiflexion night splints: a crossover prospective randomized outcomes study. *Foot Ankle Int*, 19:10, 1998.
63. Kibler, WB, Goldberg, C, and Chandler, TJ: Functional biomechanical deficits in running athletes with plantar fasciitis. *Am J Sports Med*, 19:66, 1991.
64. Cole, C, Seto, C, and Gazewood, J: Plantar fasciitis: evidence-based review of diagnosis and therapy. *Am Fam Physician*, 72:2237, 2005.

65. Saxena, A, and Fullem, B: Plantar fascia rupture in athletes. *Am J Sports Med*, 32:662, 2004.
66. Zhu, F, et al: Chronic plantar fasciitis: acute changes in the heel after extracorporeal high-energy shock wave therapy—observations at MR imaging. *Radiology*, 234:206, 2005.
67. Akfirat, M, Sen, C, and Gunes, T: Ultrasonic appearance of the plantar fasciitis. *J Clin Imaging*, 27:353, 2003.
68. Bailie, DS, and Kelikian, AS: Tarsal tunnel syndrome: diagnosis, surgical technique, and functional outcome. *Foot Ankle Int*, 19:65, 1998.
69. Prichasuk, S, and Subhadrabandhu, T: The relationship of pes planus and calcaneal spur to plantar heel pain. *Clin Orthop*, 306:192, 1994.
70. Kitaoka, HB, Luo, ZP, and An, K: Effect of plantar fasciotomy on stability of arch of foot. *Clin Orthop*, 344:307, 1997.
71. Johal, KS, and Milner, SA: Plantar fasciitis and the calcaneal spur: fact or fiction? *Foot Ankle Surg*, 18:39, 2012.
72. Riepert, T, et al: Estimation of sex on the basis of radiographs of the calcaneus. *Forensic Sci Int*, 77:133, 1996.
73. Cleland, JA, et al: Manual physical therapy and exercise versus electrophysical agents and exercise in the management of plantar heel pain: a multicenter randomized clinical trial. *J Orthop Sports Phys Ther*, 39:573, 2009.
74. Uden, H, Boesch, E, and Kumar, S: Plantar fasciitis – to jab or to support? A systematic review of the current best evidence. *J Multidiscip Healthc*, 4:155, 2011.
75. Tatli, YZ, and Kapasi, S: The real risks of steroid injection for plantar fasciitis, with a review of conservative therapies. *Curr Rev Musculoskelet Med*, 2:3, 2009.
76. Kulik, SA, and Clanton, TO: Tarsal coalition. *Foot Ankle Int*, 18:286, 1996.
77. Stormont, DM, and Peterson, HA: The relative incidence of tarsal coalition. *Clin Orthop*, 181:24, 1983.
78. Clarke, DM: Multiple tarsal coalitions in the same foot. *J Pediatr Orthop*, 17:777, 1997.
79. Kelo, MJ, and Riddle, DL: Examination and management of a patient with tarsal coalition. *Phys Ther*, 78:518, 1998.
80. Varner, KE, and Michelson, JD: Tarsal coalition in adults. *Foot Ankle Int*, 21:669, 2000.
81. Vincent, KA: Tarsal coalition and painful flatfoot. *J Am Acad Orthop Surg*, 6:274, 1998.
82. Bonasia, DE, et al: Arthroscopic resection of talocalcaneal coalitions. *Arthroscopy*. 27:430, 2011.
83. Frey, C: Magnetic resonance imaging and the evaluation of tarsal tunnel syndrome. *Foot Ankle Int*, 14:159, 1993.
84. Jackson, DL, and Haglund, B: Tarsal tunnel syndrome in athletes: case reports and literature review. *Am J Sports Med*, 19:61, 1991.
85. Stefko, RM, Lauerman, WC, and Heckman, JD: Tarsal tunnel syndrome caused by an unrecognized fracture of the posterior process of the talus (Cedell fracture). *J Bone Joint Surg Am*, 76:116, 1994.
86. Sammarco, GJ, Chalk, DE, and Feibel, JH: Tarsal tunnel syndrome and additional nerve lesions in the same limb. *Foot Ankle*, 14:71, 1993.
87. Kinoshita, M, et al: The dorsiflexion-eversion test for diagnosis of tarsal tunnel syndrome. *J Bone Joint Surg*, 83(A):1835, 2001.
88. Myerson, MS, and Berger, BI: Nonunion of a fracture of the sustentaculum tali causing a tarsal tunnel syndrome: a case report. *Foot Ankle Int*, 16:740, 1995.
89. Sammarco, GJ, and Conti, SF: Tarsal tunnel syndrome caused by an anomalous muscle. *J Bone Joint Surg Am*, 76:1308, 1994.
90. Kanbe, K, et al: Entrapment neuropathy of the deep peroneal nerve associated with the extensor hallicus brevis. *J Foot Ankle Surg*, 34:560, 1995.
91. Daniels, TR, Lau, JT, and Hearn, TC: The effects of foot position and load on tibial nerve tension. *Foot Ankle Int*, 19:73, 1998.
92. Masciocchi, C, Catalucci, A, and Barile, A: Ankle impingement syndromes. *Eur J Radiol*, 27(S1):S70, 1998.
93. Mann, RA, and Baxter, DE: Diseases of the nerves. In Mann, RA, and Coughlin, MJ (eds): *Surgery of the Foot and Ankle*, ed 6. St Louis, MO: Mosby, 1992, p 543.
94. Sharkey, NA, et al: Strain and loading of the second metatarsal during heel-lift. *J Bone Joint Surg Am*, 77:1050, 1995.
95. Wolf, SK: Diabetes mellitus and predisposition to athletic pedal fracture. *J Foot Ankle Surg*, 37:16, 1998.
96. Zwitser, EW, and Breederveld, RS: Fractures of the fifth metatarsal; diagnosis and treatment. *Injury*, 41:555, 2010.
97. Alshami, AM, et al: Biomechanical evaluation of two clinical tests for plantar heel pain: the dorsiflexion-eversion test for tarsal tunnel syndrome and the windlass test for plantar fasciitis. *Foot Ankle Int*, 28:499, 2007.
98. Weiner, BD, Linder JF, and Giattini, JF: Treatment of fractures of the fifth metatarsal: a prospective study. *Foot Ankle Int*, 18:267, 1997.
99. Clapper, MF, O'Brien, TJ, and Lyons, PM: Fractures of the fifth metatarsal: analysis of a fracture registry. *Clin Orthop*, 315: 238, 1995.
100. Mologne, TS, et al: Early screw fixation versus casting in the treatment of acute Jones fractures. *Am J Sports Med*, 33:970, 2005.
101. Brukner, P, et al: Stress fractures: a review of 180 cases. *Clin J Sport Med*, 6:85, 1996.
102. Weinfeld, SB, Haddad, SL, and Myerson, MS: Metatarsal stress fractures. *Clin Sports Med*, 16:319, 1997.
103. Kaye, RA: Insufficiency stress fractures of the foot and ankle in postmenopausal women. *Foot Ankle Int*, 19:221, 1998.
104. van Rijn, J, et al: Missing the Lisfranc fracture: a case report and review of the literature. *J Foot Ankle Surg*. 51:270, 2012.
105. Perron, AD, Brady, W, and Keats, TE: Orthopedic pitfalls in the ED: Lisfranc fracture-dislocation. *Am J Emerg Med*, 19:71, 2001.
106. Owens, R, et al: Morton's neuroma: clinical testing and imaging in 76 feet, compared to a control group. *Foot Ankle Surg*, 17:197, 2011.
107. Frank, PW, Bakkum, BW, and Darby, SA: The communicating branch of the lateral plantar nerve: a descriptive anatomic study. *Clin Anat*, 9:237, 1996.
108. Wu, KK: Morton's interdigital neuroma: a clinical review of its etiology, treatment, and results. *J Foot Ankle Surg*, 35:112, 1996.
109. Levine, SE, et al: Ultrasonographic diagnosis of recurrence after excision of an interdigital neuroma. *Foot Ankle Int*, 19:79, 1998.
110. Pastides, P, El-Sallakh, S, and Charalambides, C: Morton's neuroma: a clinical versus radiological diagnosis. *Foot Ankle Surg*, 18:22, 2012.
111. Markovic, M, et al: Effectiveness of ultrasound-guided corticosteroid injection in the treatment of Morton's neuroma. *Foot Ankle Int*, 29:483, 2008.
112. Elveru, RA, et al: Methods for taking subtalar joint measurements. *Phys Ther*, 68:678, 1988.
113. Vanore, JV, and Corey, SV: Hallux limitus, rigidus, and metatarsophalangeal joint arthrosis. In Marchinko, DE (ed): *Comprehensive Textbook of Hallus Abducto Valgus Reconstruction*. Chicago, IL: Mosby, 1993, pp 209-221.
114. Ahn, TK, et al: Kinematics and contact characteristics of the first metatarsophalangeal joint. *Foot Ankle Int*, 18:170, 1997.
115. Camasta, CA: Hallux limitus and hallux rigidus: clinical examination, radiographic findings, and natural history. *Clin Podiatr Med Surg*, 13:432, 1996.
116. Weinfeld, SB, and Schon, LC: Hallux metatarsophalangeal arthritis. *Clin Orthop*, 349:9, 1998.
117. Lichniak, JE: Hallux limitus in the athlete. *Clin Podiatr Med Surg*, 14:407, 1997.

118. Coughlin, M, and Shurnas, P: Cheilectomy vs. fusion for hallux rigidus. Presentation at the Advanced Foot and Ankle Course, San Francisco, May 23-25, 2002.
119. Mackay, DC, Blyth, M, and Rymaszewski, LA: The role of cheilectomy in the treatment of hallux rigidus. *J Foot Ankle Surg*, 36:337, 1997.
120. Iqbal, MJ, and Chana, GS: Arthroscopic cheilectomy for hallux rigidus. *Arthroscopy*, 14:307, 1998.
121. Marchinko, DE: The complex deformity known as hallux abducto valgus. In Marchinko, DE (ed): *Comprehensive Textbook of Hallus Abducto Valgus Reconstruction*. Chicago, IL: Mosby, 1993, pp 1-5.
122. Paige, NM, and Nouvong, A: The top 10 things foot and ankle specialists wish every primary care physician knew. *Mayo Clin Proc*, 81:818, 2006.
123. Tewes, DP, et al: MRI findings of acute turf toe: a case report and review of anatomy. *Clin Orthop Relat Res*, 304:200, 1994.
124. Richardson, EG: Hallucal sesamoid pain: causes and surgical treatment. *J Am Acad Orthop Surg*, 7:270, 1999.

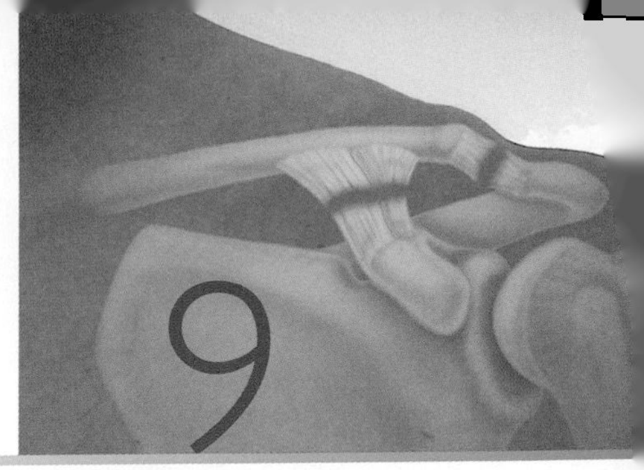

CHAPTER 9

Ankle and Leg Pathologies

The ankle's muscular, capsular, and bony structures must absorb and dissipate normal and abnormal forces. Ankle sprains are frequently cited as the most common sports-related injuries and have a high reinjury rate, secondary to chronic laxity of the ligaments and/or the subsequent loss of the joint's sense of position caused by injury to proprioceptors.[1,2] Seemingly minor injuries, such as contusions, can have severe consequences resulting from compression of the neurovascular structures of the ankle, foot, and toes. Trauma or dysfunction of the ankle and leg muscles can lead to biomechanical changes, causing gait deviations that lead to further injury. Different foot types are associated with gait pattern deviations that may redistribute stresses on bones and demands on the muscles of the lower extremity. Examination of the ankle must also include the trunk and lower extremity to capture potential proximal influences on the ankle and leg.

Clinical Anatomy

The leg is formed by the tibia and fibula (Fig. 9-1). A normal anatomic relationship between the tibia and fibula is required for proper biomechanics of the knee proximally and the ankle and foot distally. These bones function to distribute the weight-bearing forces along the limb, allowing the junction of the distal tibia, fibula, and talus (the **ankle mortise**) to produce the range of motion (ROM) needed for walking and running (Fig. 9-2).

The motions of the subtalar and talocrural joints are described either by their individual single cardinal plane nature (inversion/eversion, dorsiflexion/plantarflexion, or abduction/adduction) or by the composite motions of pronation and supination that occur around an oblique axis. Pronation comprises dorsiflexion, abduction, and eversion, with supination resulting from plantarflexion, adduction, and inversion (see Table 8-1). Closed-chain pronation causes internal tibial rotation, knee flexion, and internal rotation of the hip. Closed-chain supination results in external tibial rotation, knee extension, and external rotation at the hip.

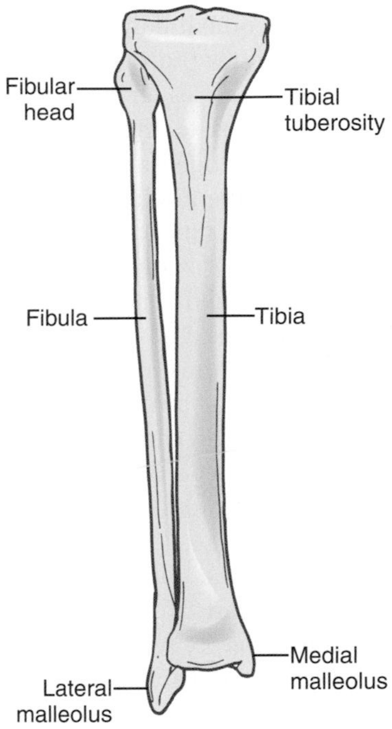

FIGURE 9-1 ■ Long bones of the lower leg and their primary bony landmarks.

The **tibia** is the primary weight-bearing bone of the leg. Its slightly concave distal articular surface forms the roof of the ankle mortise; the medial malleolus forms the shallow medial border of the mortise and provides a broad site for the attachment of the **deltoid ligaments**.

Many of the muscles acting on the ankle, foot, and toes originate off the anterolateral and posterior borders of the tibial shaft. The relatively flat anteromedial portion is covered only by skin, predisposing the richly-innervated periosteum to contusions in this area. The periosteum of

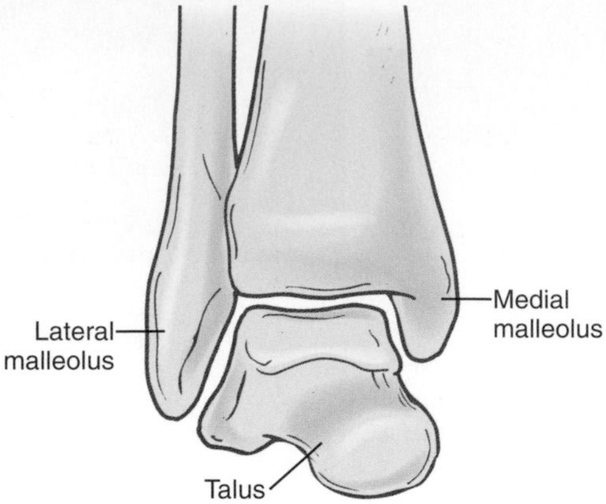

FIGURE 9-2 ■ Ankle mortise—the articulation formed by the distal articular surface of the tibia and its medial malleolus, the fibula's lateral malleolus, and the talus.

the tibial shaft may become inflamed at the sites of muscular attachment secondary to overuse syndromes. The **interosseous membrane** arises off the length of the lateral tibial border and attaches to the length of the medial fibula, binding the bones together.

Lateral to the tibia is the **fibula**. A long, thin bone, the fibula provides lateral stability to the ankle mortise and serves as (1) a site of muscular origin and attachment, (2) a site of ligamentous attachment, and (3) a pulley to increase the efficiency of the muscles that run posteriorly to it.

The amount of force transmitted through the fibula ranges from 0% to 12% of the total body weight.[3] Clinically, the percentage of body weight carried along this bone is inconsequential because the end result is that trauma to the fibula decreases its ability to serve in its previously described roles.

With the exception of the fibular head, the upper two-thirds of the fibular shaft are protected by overlying muscle. The peroneal nerve, which innervates the leg's anterior and lateral compartments, is located close to the fibular head (Fig. 9-3). Protected only by skin, the common peroneal nerve passes posterior to the fibular head, making it vulnerable to injury at this site. The distal one-third of the fibula, a common fracture site, becomes more superficial and begins to thin immediately proximal to the lateral malleolus.

The lateral malleolus provides a site of attachment for the lateral ankle ligaments. The lateral malleolus extends farther distally than the medial malleolus does, forming the lateral wall of the ankle mortise. The lateral malleolus mechanically limits eversion better than the medial malleolus limits inversion due to its greater length and anterior position. The lateral ankle is a common site for sprains, possibly resulting in avulsion of the ligaments from the lateral malleolus, especially when the ankle inverts.

The **talus** is the bony interface between the leg and the foot. The superior articulating portion of the **talus**, the **trochlea**, is quadrilateral in shape and almost entirely covered with articular cartilage. Its anterior surface is broader than its posterior surface (Fig. 9-4). The medial and lateral borders of the talus articulate with the corresponding malleoli. The superior talar surface is concave, creating a snug articulation with the slightly convex shape of the distal tibia.[4] Its inferior surface articulates with the calcaneus, forming the subtalar joint.

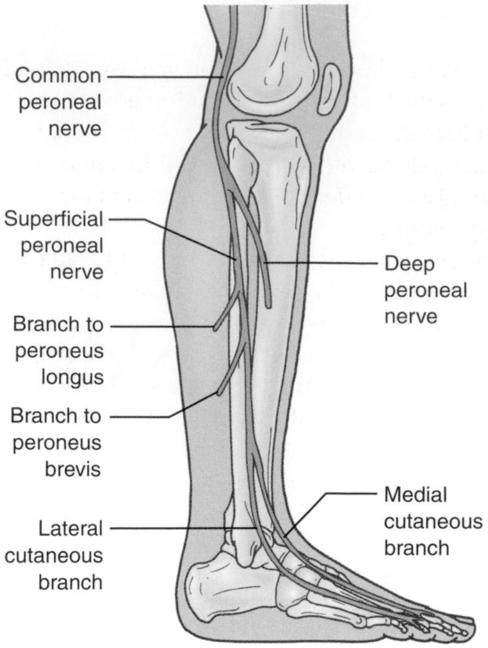

FIGURE 9-3 ■ Path of the peroneal nerve. The common peroneal nerve courses behind the fibular head, exposing it to potential injury. Trauma at this site causes a weakness in eversion and dorsiflexion.

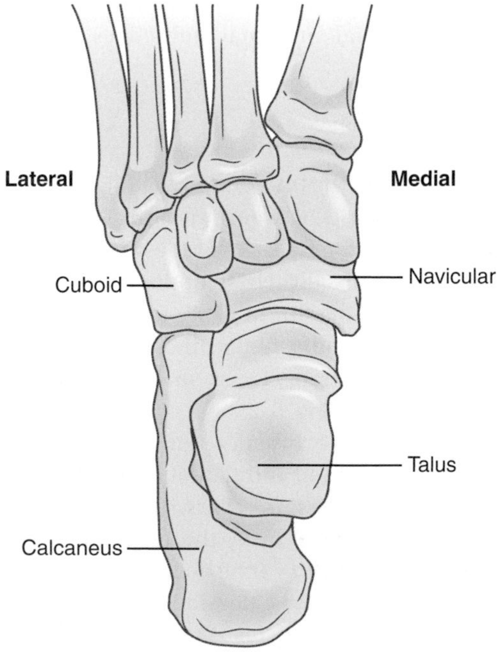

FIGURE 9-4 ■ View of the superior articular surface of the talus (left foot). Its wide anterior edge fits tightly in the mortise when the ankle is dorsiflexed.

Related Bony Structures

The insertion of the Achilles tendon on the **calcaneal tubercle** provides the foot with a mechanical advantage. The calcaneal tuberosity forms a lever arm for the Achilles tendon to increase gait power (see Fig. 8-1). The large body of the calcaneus also provides a site of attachment for some of the ankle's ligaments.

The **navicular** is located anterior to the talus along the foot's medial arch. This bone serves as one of the insertion sites for the tibialis posterior muscle. It also supports the medial longitudinal arch via the plantar calcaneonavicular (spring) ligament. Positioned along the lateral longitudinal arch, the **cuboid** articulates with the anterior calcaneus. The **peroneus longus** (fibularis longus) travels around the cuboid as it passes to the medial aspect of the foot on the plantar surface. The bases of the **fourth** and **fifth metatarsals** articulate with the anterolateral portion of the cuboid. The base of the fifth metatarsal (MT) serves as the site of attachment for the **peroneus brevis** (fibularis brevis).

Articulations and Ligamentous Support

Isolated movements of a single joint in a single plane do not occur during functional movements of the ankle complex. Pure uniplanar injuries are almost nonexistent because of the ankle's intimate anatomic relationship with the structures of the foot. The majority of acute injuries to the ankle involve the lateral structures, resulting from an inversion stress accompanied by plantarflexion of the foot.

Talocrural Joint

Formed by the articulation between the talus, tibia, and fibula, the talocrural joint is a close-fitting articulation, especially as it nears its **closed-packed position** of full dorsiflexion. A modified **synovial hinge joint**, the talocrural articulation has one degree of freedom of movement: dorsiflexion and plantarflexion. The axis of rotation runs obliquely, connecting the points just distal to the inferior tips of the lateral and medial malleoli (Fig. 9-5).

The talocrural joint is surrounded by a joint capsule that is thicker posteriorly than anteriorly. Most of the ligaments described in this section are actually thickened areas in the capsule. Tearing of the ankle ligaments usually results in damage to the joint capsule and irritation of the synovial lining, with the exception of the extracapsular calcaneofibular ligament.

When non–weight bearing, the ankle's ligamentous and tendinous structures are the primary restraints limiting rotation and translation of the talus within the ankle mortise. When weight bearing, the architecture of the joint's articular surfaces limits these motions.[5]

Closed-packed position The point in a joint's range of motion at which its bones are maximally congruent; the most stable position of a joint

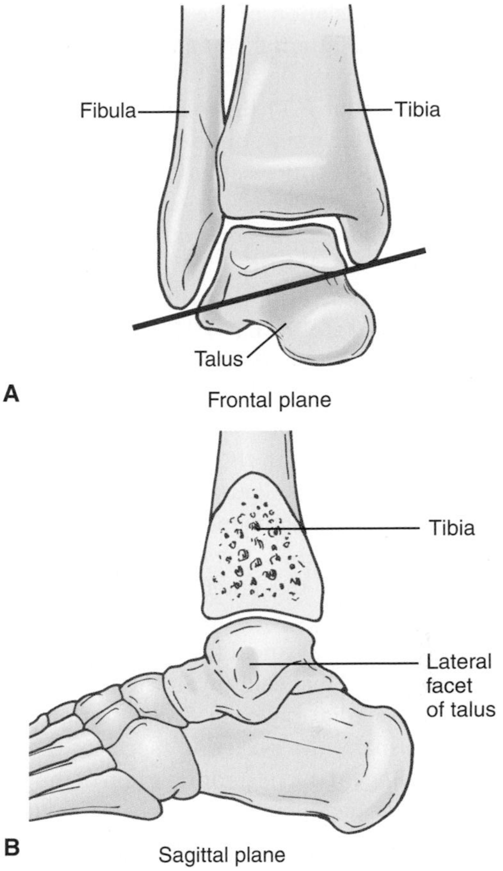

FIGURE 9-5 ■ The right talocrural joint in the (A) frontal and (B) sagittal planes. The axis of motion in the frontal plane is indicated.

Lateral ankle ligaments. Three ligaments provide lateral support to the talocrural joint. At least one is taut regardless of the relative position of the talocalcaneal unit (Fig. 9-6). The **anterior talofibular (ATF) ligament** originates off the anterolateral surface of the lateral malleolus, following a path to the talus near the sinus tarsi. The ATF is oriented parallel to the long axis of the leg when the foot is plantarflexed.[6] This ligament is tight during plantarflexion,

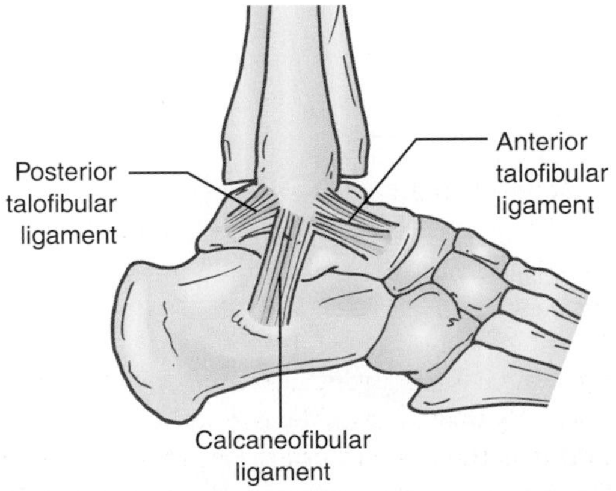

FIGURE 9-6 ■ Lateral ankle ligaments. The calcaneofibular ligament is an extracapsular structure; the anterior and posterior talofibular ligaments are thickenings in the joint capsule.

limiting anterior translation of the talus on the tibia, and resists inversion and internal rotation of the talus within the mortise.

The **calcaneofibular (CF) ligament** is an extracapsular structure with an attachment on the outermost portion of the lateral malleolus. It courses inferiorly and posteriorly to its insertion on the calcaneus.[7] The CF ligament is the primary restraint of talar inversion within the midrange of talocrural motion.

Arising from the posterior portion of the lateral malleolus, the **posterior talofibular (PTF) ligament** takes an inferior and posterior course to attach on the talus and calcaneus. This is the deepest and strongest of the three lateral ligaments and is responsible for limiting posterior displacement of the talus on the tibia.

Medial ankle ligaments. Four individual ligaments collectively form the **deltoid ligament** that supports the medial aspect of the ankle (Fig. 9-7). The **anterior tibiotalar (ATT) ligament** originates off the anteromedial portion of the tibia's malleolus and inserts on the superior portion of the medial talus. The **tibiocalcaneal (TC) ligament** arises from the apex of the medial malleolus to attach on the calcaneus directly below the medial malleolus. The **posterior tibiotalar (PTT) ligament** spans the posterior aspect of the medial malleolus, attaching on the posterior portion of the talus. As a group, these three ligaments prevent eversion of the talus. The **tibionavicular (TN) ligament** runs beneath and slightly posterior to the ATT ligament, inserting on the medial surface of the navicular to limit lateral translation and lateral rotation of the tibia on the foot. The ATT and TN ligaments are taut when the talocrural joint is plantarflexed. The TC and PTT ligaments tighten during dorsiflexion.

SubtalarJoint

The subtalar, or talocalcaneal, joint is a uniaxial, synovial gliding joint that allows 1 degree of freedom of movement around a single oblique axis. The motions of the subtalar joint, the talocrural joint, and the midtarsal joints combine to produce the functional motions of pronation and supination. The incongruent nature of the subtalar joint makes isolated cardinal plane movement impossible, although calcaneal motion is frequently described as either inversion or eversion, the most observable component of pronation and supination. (Chapter 8 provides more information about the subtalar joint.)

Distal Tibiofibular Syndesmosis

The integrity of the ankle mortise relies on the functional relationship between the tibia and fibula. This union is a **syndesmosis joint** in which a convex facet on the fibula is buffered from a concave tibial facet by dense, fatty tissue. The tibia's anterior and posterior bony prominences help maintain the relationship between the tibia and fibula.[8] The syndesmosis is maintained by the inferior **anterior and posterior tibiofibular (tib-fib) ligaments**, the **inferior transverse ligament**, and an extension of the interosseous membrane—the **crural interosseous (CI) ligament** (Fig. 9-8).[4,8,9] The deltoid ligament is the primary stabilizer against talar instability.[9] The syndesmotic ligaments play a secondary role in the stability of the talus by maintaining stability of the mortise.

This structural arrangement allows for rotation and slight spreading of the mortise while still maintaining joint stability and allowing the fibula to glide inferiorly during weight bearing, deepening the ankle mortise and tightening the interosseous membrane.[4] The CI ligament functions as a fulcrum to motion at the lateral malleolus, so a small amount of malleolar movement results in a large amount of movement at the tib-fib joint.[10] During dorsiflexion, the distal fibula moves laterally away from the tibia and glides superiorly, bringing the interosseous membrane and tib-fib ligaments into a more horizontal alignment. When the ankle is plantarflexed, the fibula is pulled inferiorly and medially toward the tibia, and the ligamentous structures take a vertical alignment. [4,11] Forced eversion or dorsiflexion can

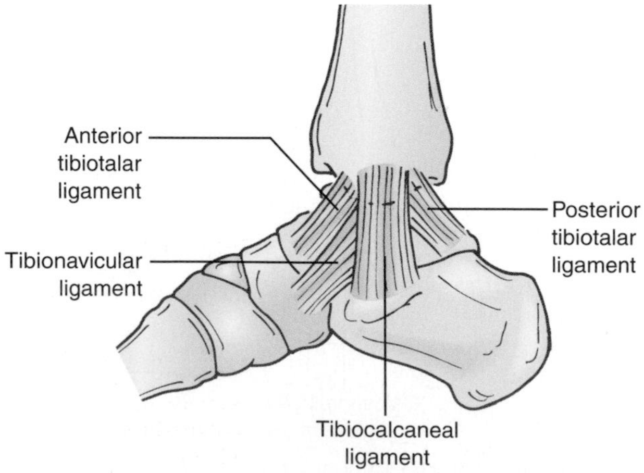

FIGURE 9-7 ■ Medial deltoid ankle ligament group showing the four individual ligaments.

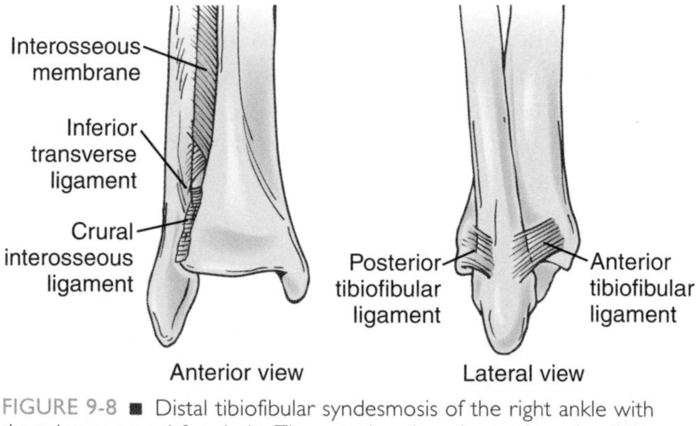

FIGURE 9-8 ■ Distal tibiofibular syndesmosis of the right ankle with the talus removed for clarity. The anterior view shows the role of the interosseous membrane and the crural interosseous ligament in lateral restraint of the fibula. The lateral view shows the role of the tibiofibular ligaments in preventing anterior and posterior displacement of the fibula on the tibia.

Syndesmosis joint A relatively immobile joint in which two bones are bound together by ligaments widen the ankle mortise, with possible injury to the ligaments supporting the syndesmosis.

Interosseous Membrane

The interosseous membrane, a strong fibrous tissue acting to fixate the fibula to the tibia, also serves as part of the origin for many of the muscles acting on the foot and ankle. A small proximal opening allows passage of the deep peroneal nerve and anterior tibial artery. Distally, the membrane blends into the anterior and posterior tib-fib ligaments to support the distal tib-fib syndesmosis joint.

Muscles of the Leg and Ankle

The leg is divided into four compartments: the anterior, lateral, superficial posterior, and deep posterior (Fig. 9-9). Each compartment contains muscles, nerves, and blood vessels that are tightly encased by fascial linings. Because of this fixed volume, intracompartmental injury can result in the accumulation of fluids that increase the pressure within the compartment, obstructing the flow of blood to and from the area and placing pressure on the nerves. The action, origin, insertion, and innervation of each muscle are described in Table 9-1.

Anterior Compartment Structures

The muscles of the anterior compartment—the tibialis anterior, the extensor hallucis longus (EHL), the extensor digitorum longus (EDL), and the peroneus tertius—all act as dorsiflexors at the ankle (Fig. 9-10). The most superficial of these muscles, the **tibialis anterior**, is the prime mover for ankle dorsiflexion and supination, providing approximately 80% of the ankle's dorsiflexion power.[12] In addition to their functions at the toes, the **EHL** assists during supination, and the **EDL** contributes to pronation. The **peroneus tertius** runs parallel with the fifth tendon of the EDL, but its attachment on the dorsal surface of the fifth MT causes this muscle to make a stronger contribution to pronation than dorsiflexion.

Crossing the anterior portion of the ankle mortise is the extensor retinaculum, whose superior and inferior bands give it a Z shape (see Fig. 9-10). The retinaculum secures the distal tendons of the muscles of the anterior compartment as they cross the talocrural joint, preventing a bowstring effect during dorsiflexion or toe extension. The medial portion of the inferior band holds the tibialis anterior and extensor hallucis longus close to the dorsum of the foot. A loop on the lateral border of the retinaculum wraps around the four tendinous slips of the extensor digitorum longus, holding them laterally and against the dorsum of the foot.

Branching off the **common peroneal nerve** near the fibular head and into the anterior compartment, the **deep peroneal nerve** runs from the upper portion of the fibula along the interosseous membrane behind the tibialis anterior. This nerve and its subsequent branches innervate the muscles located within the anterior compartment and most muscles on the dorsum of the foot. Supplying the anterior compartment with blood, the **anterior tibial artery** passes through the superior portion of the interosseous membrane to follow the path taken by the deep peroneal nerve. A branch of the anterior tibial artery, the **dorsalis pedis artery**, supplies blood to the dorsum of the foot.

Lateral Compartment Structures

The peroneus longus and peroneus brevis form the bulk of the lateral compartment. As a group, these muscles are strong evertors of the ankle and contribute to plantarflexion (Fig. 9-11). The **peroneus longus** is the most superficial of these muscles, with its belly covering all but the most inferior portion of the peroneus brevis and its tendon. The **peroneus brevis** lies beneath the peroneus longus as the tendons pass behind the lateral malleolus where they share a common synovial sheath. The peroneal tendons are held in position posterior to the malleolus primarily by the **superior peroneal retinaculum** and, to a lesser extent, the **inferior peroneal retinaculum**.[2] Their paths diverge as they clear the retinaculum and approach the peroneal tubercle. At this point, each tendon has its own synovial sheath.[2] The peroneus brevis tendon courses to the styloid process on the base of the fifth MT, while the peroneus longus tendon runs a more inferior path along the plantar aspect of the

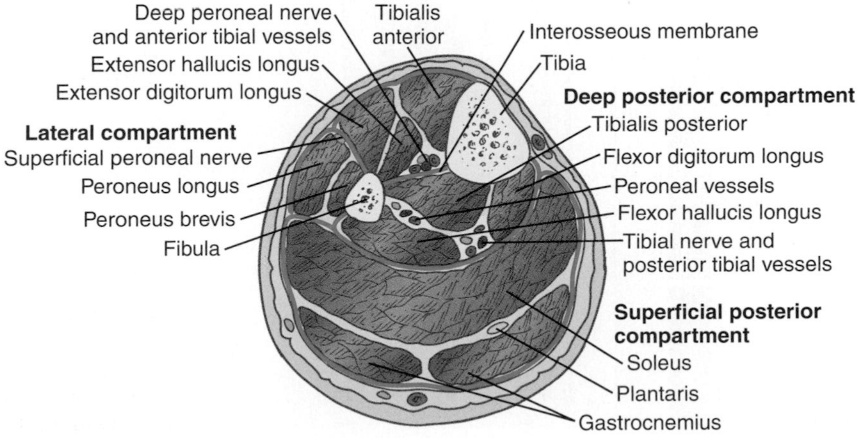

FIGURE 9-9 ■ Cross section of the left leg, indicating the muscles and neurovascular structures located in each of the four compartments. "Vessels" refer to the associated artery, vein, and lymphatic vessel. Note that the peroneus tertius is located below the level of this cross-section.

Table 9-1 Lower Leg Muscles Acting on the Foot and Ankle (Organized by Compartment)

Muscle	Action	Origin	Insertion	Nerve	Root
Anterior Compartment					
Extensor Digitorum Longus	Extension of the 2nd through 5th MTP joints Assists in extending the 2nd through 5th PIP and DIP joints Assists in STJ and midtarsal pronation Assists in ankle dorsiflexion	Lateral tibial condyle Proximal three-fourths of anterior fibula Proximal portion of the interosseous membrane	Via four tendons to the distal phalanges of the 2nd through 5th toes	Deep peroneal	L4, L5, S1
Peroneus Tertius	STJ and midtarsal pronation Assists in ankle dorsiflexion	Distal one-third of the anterior surface of the fibula Adjacent portion of the interosseous membrane	Dorsal surface of the base of the 5th MT	Deep peroneal	L4, L5, S1
Extensor Hallucis Longus	Extension of the 1st MTP joint Extension of the 1st IP joint Assists with dorsiflexion Assists with supination	Middle two-thirds of the anterior surface of the fibula Adjacent portion of the interosseous membrane	Base of the distal phalanx of the 1st toe	Deep peroneal	L4, L5, S1
Tibialis Anterior	Ankle dorsiflexion STJ and midtarsal supination	Lateral tibial condyle Upper one-half of the tibia's lateral surface Adjacent portion of the interosseous membrane	Medial and plantar surfaces of the 1st cuneiform Medial and plantar surfaces of the 1st MT	Deep peroneal	L4, L5, S1
Lateral Compartment					
Peroneus Brevis	STJ and midtarsal pronation Assists in ankle plantarflexion	Distal two-thirds of the lateral fibula	Styloid process at the base of the 5th MT	Superficial peroneal	L4, L5, S1
Peroneus Longus	STJ and midtarsal pronation Assists in ankle plantarflexion	Lateral tibial condyle Fibular head Upper two-thirds of the lateral fibula	Lateral aspect of the proximal 1st MT Lateral and dorsal aspect of the 1st cuneiform	Superficial peroneal	L4, L5, S1
Deep Posterior Compartment					
Flexor Hallucis Longus	Flexion of the 1st IP joint Assists in 1st MTP joint flexion Assists in STJ and midtarsal supination Assists in ankle plantarflexion	Posterior distal two-thirds of the fibula Associated interosseous membrane and muscular fascia	Plantar surface of the proximal phalanx of the 1st toe	Tibial	L4, L5, S1

Flexor Digitorum Longus	Flexion of the 2nd through 5th PIP and DIP joints Flexion of the 2nd through 5th MTP joints Assists in ankle plantarflexion Assists in STJ and midtarsal supination	Posterior medial portion of the distal two-thirds of the tibia From fascia arising from the tibialis posterior	Plantar base of distal phalanges of the 2nd through 5th toes	Tibial	L5, S1
Tibialis Posterior	Assists in ankle plantarflexion STJ and midtarsal supination	Length of the interosseous membrane Posterior, lateral tibia Upper two-thirds of the medial fibula	Navicular tuberosity Via fibrous slips to the sustentaculum tali, cuneiforms, cuboid, and bases of the 2nd, 3rd, and 4th MTs	Tibial	L4, L5, S1
Superficial Posterior Compartment					
Gastrocnemius	Ankle plantarflexion Assists in knee flexion	Medial head • Posterior surface of the medial femoral condyle • Adjacent portion of the femur and knee capsule Lateral head • Posterior surface of the lateral femoral condyle • Adjacent portion of the femur and knee capsule	To the calcaneus via the Achilles tendon	Tibial	S1, S2
Plantaris	Ankle plantarflexion Assists in knee flexion	Distal portion of the supracondylar line of the lateral femoral condyle Adjacent portion of the femoral popliteal surface Oblique popliteal ligament	To the calcaneus via the Achilles tendon	Tibial	L4, L5, S1
Soleus	Ankle plantarflexion	Posterior fibular head Upper one-third of the fibula's posterior surface Soleal line located on the posterior tibial shaft Middle one-third of the medial tibial border	To the calcaneus via the Achilles tendon	Tibial	S1, S2

DIP = distal interphalangeal; IP = interphalangeal; MT = metatarsal; MTP = metatarsophalangeal; PIP = proximal interphalangeal STJ = subtalar joint neutral

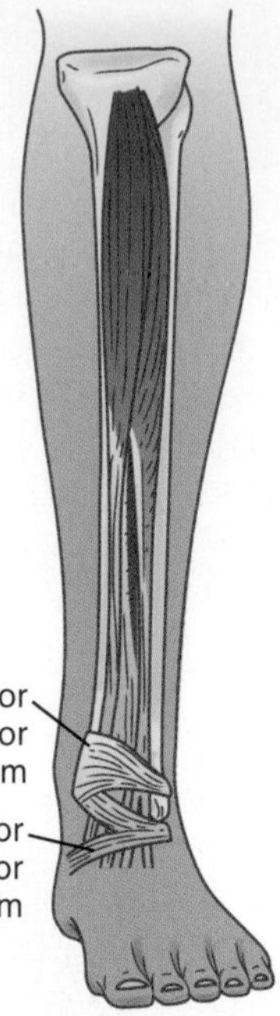

FIGURE 9-10 ■ Muscles of the anterior compartment of the left leg: the tibialis anterior, extensor hallucis longus, and extensor digitorum longus (the peroneus tertius is not shown). These tendons are held in place across the anterior joint line by the extensor retinaculum.

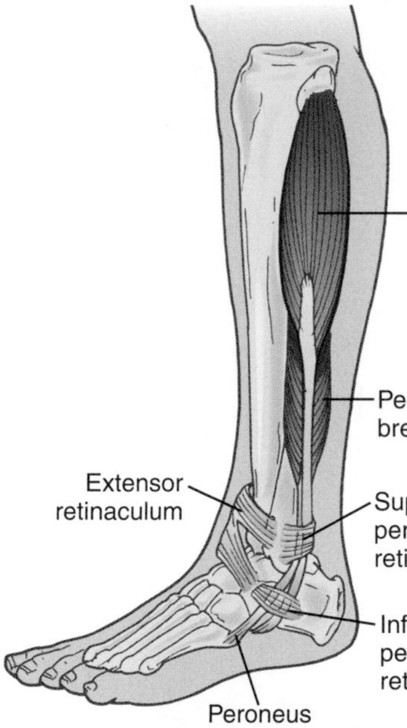

FIGURE 9-11 ■ Muscles of the lateral compartment: the peroneus longus and brevis. The superior and inferior peroneal retinacula maintain the alignment of the peroneal tendons so that their angle of pull plantarflexes and everts the ankle.

foot to attach to the proximal end of the first MT and first cuneiform. A small sesamoid bone, the **os peroneum**, may be located in the peroneus longus tendon just proximal to and at the level of the cuboid.[2] The **peroneus quartus**, a small muscle that arises from the peroneus brevis and inserts on the retrotrochlear eminence on the calcaneus, is present in less than 7% of the population.[13] It adds little to foot and ankle function and is often injured concurrently with other structures.[2,13]

The lateral compartment contains the **superficial peroneal nerve**, which innervates the peroneus longus and brevis. Arising off the **posterior tibial artery**, the peroneal artery runs lateral to the interosseous membrane, supplying blood to the lateral compartment and lateral ankle.

Superficial Posterior Compartment Structures

The **gastrocnemius** and **soleus** form the **triceps surae muscle group**, so called because of the three heads of the two muscles (the gastrocnemius has two heads) (Fig. 9-12). The **gastrocnemius** (arising from the posterior medial and lateral femoral condyles) and **plantaris** (arising from the posterior lateral femoral condyle), the third muscle in the superficial posterior compartment, are two-joint muscles. The **soleus**, arising off the posterior tibia, crosses only one joint. The gastrocnemius, soleus, and plantaris have a common insertion on the calcaneus via the Achilles tendon. The gastrocnemius and soleus are prime movers during plantarflexion. The gastrocnemius is most active in plantarflexing the ankle when the knee is extended.

The longest branch of the sciatic nerve, the tibial nerve runs between the medial and lateral heads of the gastrocnemius to lie deep between the soleus and the tibialis posterior (located in the deep posterior compartment). Supplying the innervation for all of the muscles in the superficial and deep posterior compartments, branches of the tibial nerve continue to the plantar aspect of the foot after coursing around the medial malleolus. The posterior tibial artery, arising

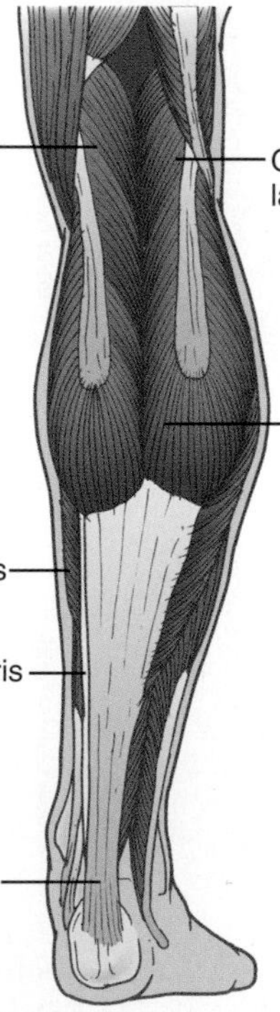

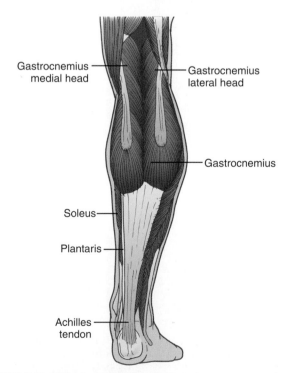

FIGURE 9-12 ■ Muscles of the superficial posterior compartment: the gastrocnemius, soleus, and plantaris. The gastrocnemius and soleus muscles are collectively referred to as the "triceps surae" because of the three heads they form.

from the tibial artery, follows the same course as the tibial nerve.

Deep Posterior Compartment Structures

The **tibialis posterior** is the only muscle of the deep posterior compartment that does not act on the toes (Fig. 9-13). Because of its angle of pull, this muscle is a primary adductor of the forefoot while also assisting in plantarflexion and inversion, and, since it controls pronation, it generates significant tension during running.[12] The remaining two muscles of the deep posterior compartment, the **flexor digitorum longus** and the **flexor hallucis longus**, act primarily to flex the toes and secondarily to plantarflex and invert the ankle. These muscles pass through the tarsal tunnel formed behind the medial malleolus, predisposing them to repetitive mechanical irritation and inflammation (see Tarsal Tunnel Syndrome, p. 218).

Bursae

Two major bursae are associated with the lower leg and ankle. The **subtendinous calcaneal** (retrocalcaneal) **bursa** is found between the Achilles tendon and the calcaneus, decreasing friction between these two structures. Lying between the posterior aspect of the Achilles tendon and the skin is the **subcutaneous calcaneal bursa**, which protects the Achilles tendon from direct trauma and decreases friction from the skin and footwear.

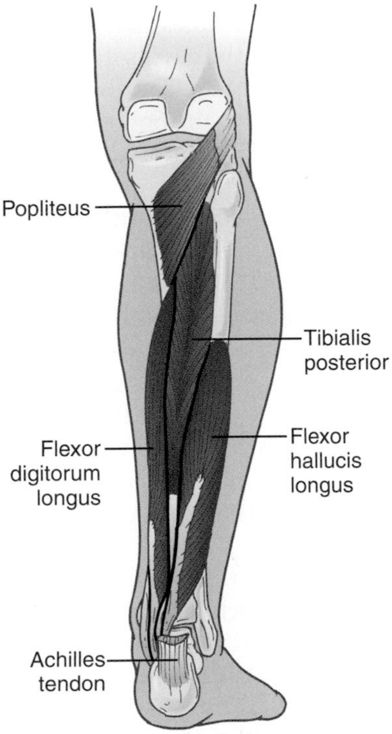

FIGURE 9-13 ■ Muscles of the deep posterior compartment: the tibialis posterior, flexor hallucis longus, and flexor digitorum longus. The muscles of the superficial posterior compartment have been removed to show the deep compartment. A common mnemonic, "Tom, Dick, And Nervous Harry," is used to describe the structures that pass behind the medial malleolus: **t**ibialis posterior, flexor **d**igitorum longus, tibial **a**rtery, tibial **n**erve, and the flexor **h**allucis longus.

Neurological Anatomy

The neurological innervation described for each of the four compartments arises from the lumbar and sacral plexuses (see Chapter 13). The motor nerves supplying the leg muscles are presented in Table 9-1. The common peroneal nerve diverges at the fibular head, with the deep peroneal nerve innervating the muscles of the anterior compartment and the superficial peroneal nerve innervating the muscles of the lateral compartment (see Fig. 9-3). The tibial nerve, deep and well-protected until it becomes superficial at the medial ankle, passes through the deep posterior compartment and divides into the medial and lateral plantar nerves at the flexor retinaculum at the medial ankle. These branches innervate the foot.

The sural nerve, arising from both the common peroneal and tibial nerves, provides sensory input from the posterior and lateral leg and the lateral foot. The saphenous nerve, branching off of the femoral nerve, innervates the skin on the medial ankle and foot. The motor nerves and the sural and saphenous nerves (sensory nerves) contribute to the ankle's proprioception (Fig. 9-14).

Vascular Anatomy

Arterial and venous systems of the leg are described for each of the four compartments. The leg's venous system is divided into superficial and deep components. The deep veins are associated with the major arteries and are

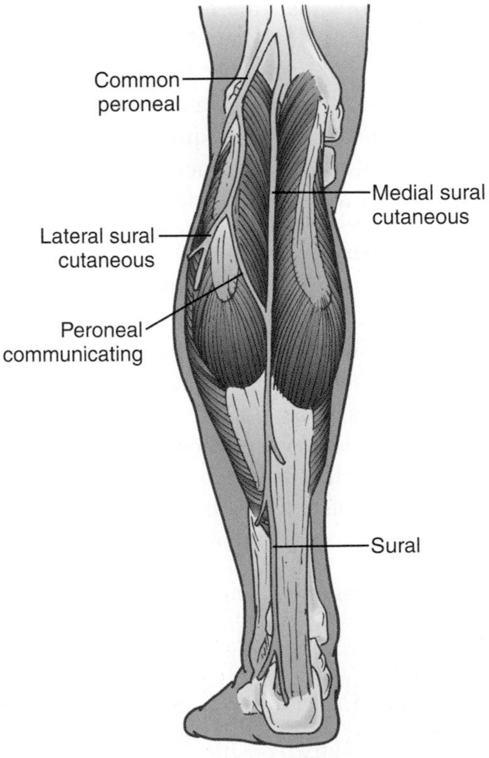

FIGURE 9-14 ■ Motor nerves and the sural and saphenous nerves (sensory nerves) of the foot and ankle.

described in each of the compartmental anatomy portions of this section.

The superficial venous return network is formed by two large veins, the **great** and **small saphenous veins**. Originating in the area of the foot's medial longitudinal arch, the great saphenous vein accepts tributaries that primarily sprout from the foot and posterior leg. Once passing the knee joint and traversing the length of the thigh, the great saphenous vein empties into the femoral vein. Originating near the fifth toe, the small saphenous vein courses up the posterior aspect of the leg and primarily receives blood from the superficial posterior compartment.

Assisted by **perforating veins**, most of the veins in the legs are positioned to allow muscle contractions to squeeze venous blood through a series of one-way valves from the distal extremity toward the heart.

Clinical Examination of the Ankle and Leg

The ankle and leg are influenced by joints distal and proximal, necessitating possible inclusion of the foot, knee, hip, and spine in the examination process. The lower extremities must be exposed to facilitate this examination.

History

When taking a history for a patient with an ankle or leg injury, establish the pain location, the onset and mechanism of injury, the duration of symptoms, and any previous history of injury to the involved or uninvolved limb. For patients reporting a history of chronic ankle instability, the use of a self-reporting instrument such as the **Foot and Ankle Ability Measure (FAAM)** provides a reliable descriptor of how the condition affects daily life and can be used to measure the effectiveness of interventions (see p. 167).[14] The patient's responses to this questioning guide the remainder of the history-taking process and form the framework for the rest of the examination.

Past Medical History

Question the patient and, if available, review the patient's medical file regarding the history of injury to both the involved and uninvolved extremities and the lumbar spine. Patients with a history of previous ankle sprains may demonstrate excess laxity and decreased proprioception. Osteoarthritis may develop secondary to repetitive stresses. **Peripheral vascular disease** can cause swelling in the foot and ankle. Individuals with diabetes may have associated neuropathy and prolonged tissue healing times.

History of the Present Condition

Other injuries to the lower extremities or lumbar spine may present with biomechanical changes in gait, predisposing different tissues to abnormal stresses. For example, patients with lateral ankle sprains often ambulate with a toe-only gait on the involved side to position the talocrural joint in its resting position. This, in turn, causes adaptive shortening of the Achilles tendon, predisposing it to injury when the patient assumes a more normal gait.

- **Location of the pain** (Table 9-2)**:** Ask the patient to specifically identify the location of pain so that the subsequent portions of the evaluation emphasize the suspected structures involved (Fig. 9-15). In the leg, a well-localized, specific pain may be indicative of bone pathology while more diffuse pain points to soft tissue. The leg and ankle may also be areas of radicular symptoms arising from anterior compartment syndrome, tarsal tunnel syndrome (TTS), the peroneal nerve, and root impingement of the sciatic or lumbar nerve.
- **Injury mechanism:** In the case of macrotrauma, determine the mechanism of injury to identify the general area of the structures affected and the type of injury involved (Table 9-3). Disorders of a gradual onset require more in-depth questioning to determine the factors surrounding the cause of pain.
- **Type and severity of pain:** Determine the patient's rating of pain at its extremes using a visual analog or numeric rating scale (see p. 12). Question the patient regarding the type of pain. Burning pain may indicate nerve involvement. Sharp, localized pain may be associated with bone pathology.
- **Pain pattern:** Pose specific questions to determine how certain activities aggravate the symptoms. How are these symptoms affecting athletic participation or normal daily activities? Does the pain pattern change throughout the day? Is the onset of pain associated with fatigue? Leg pain that begins during activity and increases to the point that activity must be discontinued is consistent with exertional compartment syndrome.
- **Changes in activity and conditioning regimen:** Gain an understanding of the patient's recent activity, or changes in activity, to understand better the cause of chronic or insidious conditions. For overuse injuries, establish whether the patient has:
  - Significantly increased the duration, intensity, frequency, or type (i.e., added hills) of exercise. When available, the athlete's training log is useful in determining excessive increases in exercise intensity.
  - Changed shoe brands or styles or is wearing old, worn-out shoes
  - Switched from participating on a surface of one texture and density to one of a different type
  - Recently begun wearing orthotics, changed the type of orthotic worn, or discontinued using orthotics

Functional Assessment

Observe the patient performing the tasks or activities that produce symptoms or recreate typical functional demands to begin to identify the underlying impairments. Gait abnormalities frequently contribute to or result from

Examination Map

HISTORY

Past Medical History
History of the Present Condition
- Location of pain
- Mechanism of injury

FUNCTIONAL ASSESSMENT

Gait

INSPECTIONS

Inspection of the Lateral Structures
- Peroneal muscle group
- Distal one-third of fibula
- Lateral malleolus

Inspection of the Anterior Structures
- Sinus tarsi
- Malleoli
- Talus

Inspection of the Medial Structures
- Medial malleolus
- Medial longitudinal arch

Inspection of the Posterior Structures
- Gastrocnemius and soleus
- Achilles tendon
- Bursae
- Calcaneus

PALPATION

Palpation of the Fibular Structures
- Common peroneal nerve
- Peroneal muscle group
- Fibular shaft
- Anterior tibiofibular ligament
- Posterior tibiofibular ligament
- Interosseous membrane
- Superior peroneal retinaculum

Palpation of the Lateral Ankle
- Lateral malleolus
- Calcaneofibular ligament
- Anterior talofibular ligament
- Posterior talofibular ligament
- Inferior peroneal retinaculum
- Peroneal tubercle
- Cuboid
- Base of 5th MT
- Peroneus tertius

Palpation of the Anterior Structures
- Anterior tibial shaft
- Tibialis anterior
- Extensor hallucis longus
- Extensor digitorum longus
- Dome of the talus
- Extensor retinacula
- Sinus tarsi

Palpation of the Medial Structures
- Medial malleolus
- Deltoid ligament
- Sustentaculum tali
- Spring ligament
- Navicular
- Navicular tuberosity
- Tibialis anterior
- Tibialis posterior
- Flexor hallucis longus
- Flexor digitorum longus

Palpation of the Posterior Structures
- Gastrocnemius and soleus
- Achilles tendon
- Subcutaneous calcaneal bursa
- Calcaneus
- Subtendinous calcaneal bursa

JOINT AND MUSCLE FUNCTION ASSESSMENT

Goniometry
- Plantarflexion/dorsiflexion

Active Range of Motion
- Plantarflexion
- Dorsiflexion
- Inversion
- Eversion

Manual Muscle Tests
- Dorsiflexion and supination
- Eversion and pronation
- Plantarflexion
- Rearfoot inversion

Passive Range of Motion
- Plantarflexion
- Dorsiflexion
- Inversion
- Eversion

JOINT STABILITY TESTS

Stress Testing
- Inversion stress test
- Eversion stress test

Joint Play Assessment
- Medial talar glide
- Lateral talar glide (Cotton test)
- Distal tibiofibular glide

NEUROLOGICAL ASSESSMENT

- Lower Quarter Screen
- Common peroneal nerve
- Tibial nerve

VASCULAR EXAMINATION

- Dorsalis pedis pulse
- Posterior tibial pulse
- Capillary refill

REGION-SPECIFIC PATHOLOGIES AND RELATED SELECTIVE TISSUE TESTS

Ankle Sprains
- Lateral ankle sprain
  - Anterior Drawer test
- Distal tibiofibular syndesmosis
  - Squeeze test
- Medial ankle sprain

Ankle and Leg Fractures

Os trigonum injury

Achilles Tendon Pathology
- Achilles tendon tendinopathy
- Sever's disease
- Achilles tendon rupture
  - Thompson test

Peroneal Tendon Pathology

Medial Tibial Stress Syndrome

Stress Fractures

Compartment Syndromes

Table 9-2 Differential Diagnosis Based on the Location of Pain

	Location of Pain			
	Lateral	**Anterior**	**Medial**	**Posterior**
Soft Tissue	Lateral ankle ligament sprain Syndesmosis sprain Capsular impingement Subluxating peroneal tendons Peroneal muscle tear Peroneal tendinopathy Interosseous membrane trauma Peroneal nerve trauma	Extensor retinaculum sprain Syndesmosis sprain Tibialis anterior or long toe extensor tear Tibialis anterior or long toe extensor tendinopathy Anterior compartment syndrome Interosseous membrane trauma Anterior tib-fib ligament sprain	Deltoid ligament sprain Capsular impingement Tibialis posterior tear or tendinopathy Tibialis posterior tendinopathy Posterior tibial nerve compression (TTS)	Triceps surae tear Achilles tendinopathy Achilles tendon rupture Subtendinous calcaneal bursitis Subcutaneous calcaneal bursitis Deep vein **thrombophlebitis** Posterior tib-fib ligament sprain
Bony	Lateral ligament avulsion from malleolus, talus, and/or calcaneus. Lateral malleolus fracture Fibular stress fracture Frank fibular fracture Fifth MT fracture Peroneal tendon avulsion Osteoarthritis	Tibial stress fracture Frank tibial fracture Talar fracture Talar osteochondritis Osteoarthritis Periostitis	Medial ligament avulsion Medial malleolus avulsion Medial malleolus fracture Arthritis	Calcaneal fracture Arthritis Os trigonum trauma

MT = metatarsal; TTS = tarsal tunnel syndrome

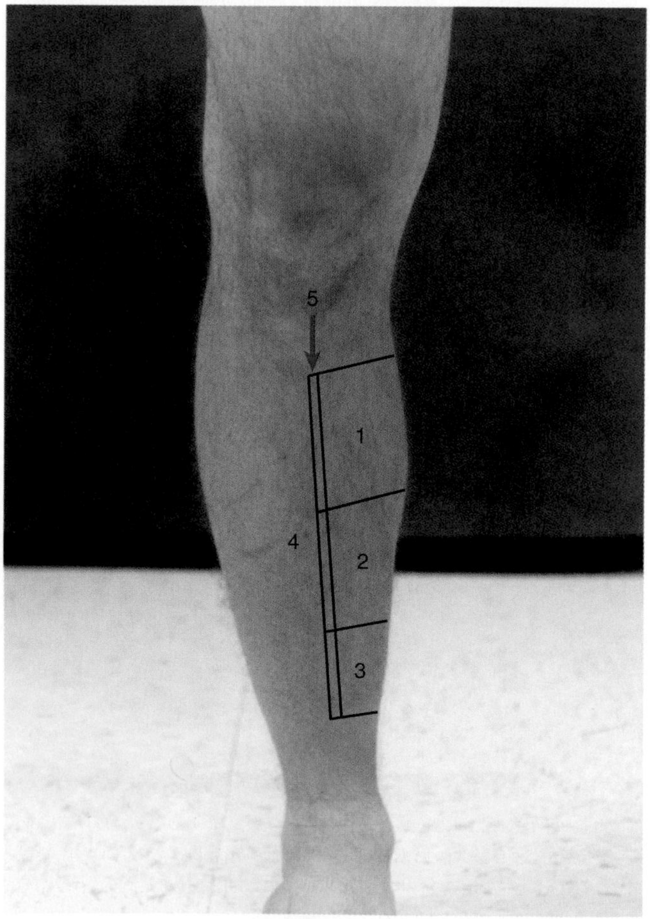

FIGURE 9-15 ■ Pain zones and anatomic correlations. 1 = flexor digitorum longus; 2 = flexor hallucis longus; 3 = tibialis posterior; 4 = tibial crest; 5 = tibial tuberosity.

ankle and leg pathology. The functional assessment that determines willingness to bear weight may begin as the patient enters the facility or walks off the field. Observe for gait deviations such as an antalgic gait or external rotation of the limb on the involved side, suggesting a lack of ankle dorsiflexion caused by pain or restriction. Other functional tasks that may reveal asymmetry or other biomechanical abnormalities contributing to ankle and leg pathology include running and squatting.

Different foot postures also impact gait and the relative demands on the tissues of the leg and foot (see Chapter 8).

Inspection

The observation phase occurs while the patient is both weight bearing and not weight bearing, with a comparison between the two. Begin by observing both lower extremities, noting redness, pallor, tendon discontinuity, or other obvious deformity. If swelling is present, the amount of fluid collection can be quantified using girth or volumetric measurements (see Selective Tissue Test 1-1).[15,16]

Practical Evidence

Both the figure-of-eight and volumetric measurements are reliable methods of determining the amount of ankle swelling. These measurements, however, do not correlate well with the patient's level of function.[17]

Thrombophlebitis Inflammation of a vein and the subsequent formation of blood clots

Table 9-3 Mechanism of Ankle Injury and the Resulting Tissue Damage

Uniplanar Motion	Tensile Forces	Compressive Forces
Inversion	Lateral structures: Anterior talofibular ligament, calcaneofibular ligament, posterior talofibular ligament, lateral capsule, and peroneal tendons; lateral malleolus fracture	Medial structures: Medial malleolus, deltoid ligament, and posterior tibial nerve, tibial artery, tibial vein
Eversion	Medial structures: Deltoid ligament, tibialis posterior, and long toe flexors, posterior tibial nerve, tibial artery	Lateral structures: Lateral malleolus and lateral capsule
Plantarflexion	Anterior structures: Anterior capsule, long toe extensors, tibialis anterior, and extensor retinaculum Lateral structures: Anterior talofibular ligament	Posterior structures: Posterior capsule, subtendinous calcaneal bursa, subcutaneous calcaneal bursa, os trigonum, and talus
Dorsiflexion	Posterior structures: Triceps surae, Achilles tendon, tibialis posterior, flexor hallucis longus, flexor digitorum longus Lateral structures: Posterior talofibular ligament, peroneal tendons	Anterior structures: Anterior capsule, syndesmosis, and extensor retinaculum, anterior talus

Inspection of the Lateral Structures

- **Peroneal muscle group:** Inspect the entire peroneal muscle group. The tendons may be seen as they course posteriorly and inferiorly around the lateral malleolus, being held in position by the superior and inferior peroneal retinacula (see Fig. 9-12). The tendons will become more visible if the patient is able to actively pronate the foot and ankle.
- **Distal one-third of the fibula:** Note the contour and symmetry of the distal one-third of the fibula as it becomes superficial proximal to the lateral malleolus. Any discontinuity in the bone's shaft or the formation of edema over this portion of the shaft may indicate a possible fracture.
- **Lateral malleolus:** The lateral malleolus is covered only by skin, making its shape easily identifiable. Even mild ankle sprains can result in swelling that obscures the malleolus and peroneal tendons (Fig. 9-16). Any formation of ecchymosis around and distal to the lateral malleolus may signify acute trauma such as a sprain or fracture, although it will not occur immediately.

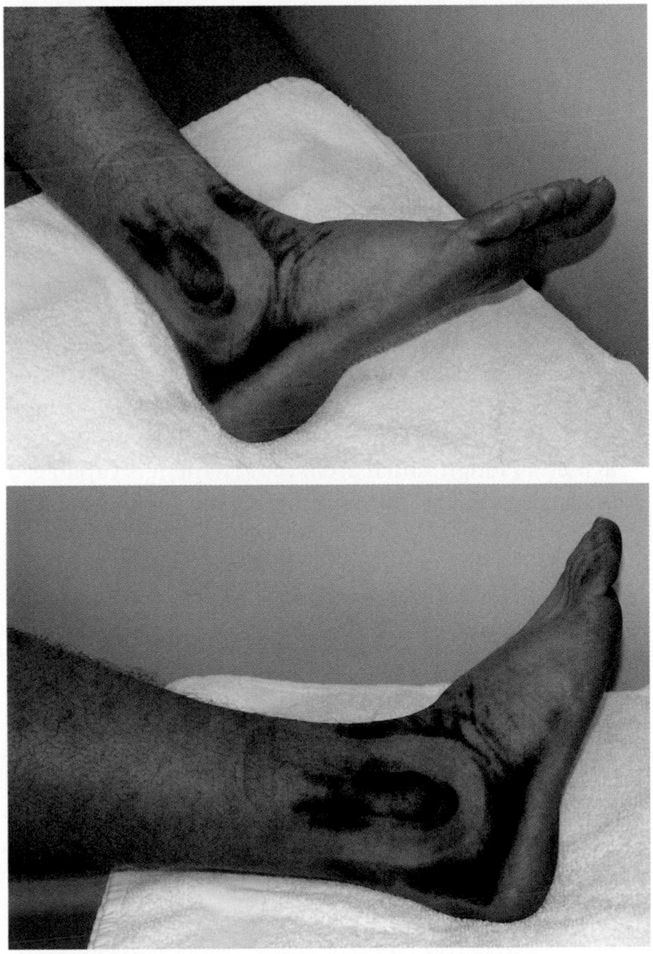

FIGURE 9-16 ■ Damage to the lateral ankle capsule can result in the collection of edema around and distal to the malleolus. Note the distortion of the normal ankle contours and medial formation of ecchymosis.

Inspection of the Anterior Structures

- **Appearance of the anterior leg:** Inspect the anterior leg for skin color and edema. Anterior compartment syndrome may present with reddened or shiny skin or pitting edema. If these signs coincide with paresthesia in the web space between the first and second toes, unremitting pain, decreased dorsiflexion strength, and/or absence of the dorsalis pedis pulse, immediately refer the patient to a physician or emergency room.
- **Sinus tarsi:** Observe the sinus tarsi, an indentation formed over the anterolateral aspect of the talus, looking for its normally concave shape. After injury to the anterior talofibular ligament or fractures about the ankle, the area fills with fluid, resulting in loss of its normal indentation in the proximal foot (Fig. 9-17).[18]
- **Contour of the malleoli:** Observe the malleoli, which should be prominent as they project from the distal tibia and fibula. Swelling can obscure these structures. Edema between the tibia and fibula in the distal one-third of the interosseous membrane may indicate a syndesmotic sprain.
- **Talus:** If possible, observe the bilateral symmetry of the tali while the patient is weight bearing. In the case

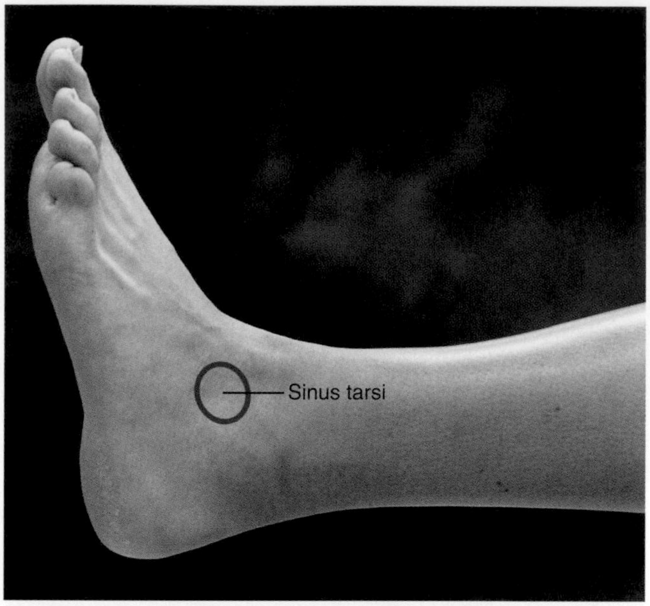

FIGURE 9-17 ■ Location of the left sinus tarsi. This depression may become swollen and painful secondary to trauma to the foot or ankle (see Figure 9-16).

of leg length discrepancies, one foot has a prominent medial talus caused by pronation of the longer leg; the shorter leg maintains a somewhat neutral or supinated position (see Fig. 6-8).

Inspection of the Medial Structures

- **Medial malleolus:** Similar to the lateral malleolus, the medial malleolus is superficial, with little soft tissue covering it. Its appearance should be distinct without obvious deformity or the presence of edema.
- **Medial longitudinal arch:** If the patient is capable of bearing weight, observe the appearance of the medial longitudinal arch, which should be maintained whether the patient is bearing weight or not. If this arch is not adequately supported, the medial aspect of the talus rotates inward, and the navicular drops inferiorly (**pes planus**). Excessive protrusion of the talus can be seen from the anterior and posterior views. Leg pain, such as periostitis or tendinopathy of the tibialis anterior or tibialis posterior muscles, is often associated with this alignment. The supporting muscles may be predisposed to fatigue or pain developing at their tibial origins as they attempt to control excessive medial motion of the talus and the associated increase in amount and/or duration of pronation during gait. On the other hand, **pes cavus**, a high medial arch, results in a supinated foot and a potential predisposition to lateral ankle sprains or stress fractures caused by limited shock-absorbing capacity.

Inspection of the Posterior Structures

- **Gastrocnemius-soleus complex:** Bilateral comparison should indicate calf musculature of approximately equal size, shape, and mass. Atrophy may be present if the leg has been immobilized or the S1 or S2 nerve root or sciatic nerve or tibial nerve portion of the sciatic nerve is impaired. Tearing of the muscle may result in depressions in the skin, especially at the musculotendinous junction with the Achilles tendon. Unexplained redness and swelling of the posterior calf could indicate **deep vein thrombosis** (Box 9-1).
- **Achilles tendon:** The prominent Achilles tendon is visible as it tapers from the musculotendinous junction to its insertion on the calcaneus. Achilles tendon ruptures may present with a visible defect if the tear occurs in its middle or distal portion.
- **Bursae:** Inspect the calcaneal bursae for swelling, redness, or other signs of inflammation or infection.
- **Calcaneus:** The calcaneus is normally very distinct, with little soft tissue covering its medial and lateral borders. The presence of a thickened area at the insertion of the Achilles tendon is sometimes associated with retrocalcaneal pain. This thickening, an exostosis, may be caused by footwear rubbing on this area, possibly associated with subcutaneous calcaneal bursitis (see Chapter 8).

Box 9-1
Deep Vein Thrombosis

Deep vein thrombosis (DVT), a blood clot, is a potentially life-threatening condition because of the associated risk of pulmonary embolism if the clot should dislodge. Clinically, the signs and symptoms of DVT resemble other musculoskeletal conditions such as a triceps surae strain, Achilles tendinopathy, and medial tibial stress syndrome. DVT presents with unexplained warmth, tightness of the calf musculature, and pain during palpation.

Because of the potential for a pulmonary embolism, a high index of suspicion for a DVT is warranted if the patient has any of the risk factors. Strong and moderate risk factors include recent surgery; fracture of the pelvis, femur, or tibia; spinal cord injury; use of oral contraceptives; recent pregnancy; cardiovascular disorders; and periods of prolonged sitting (such as airplane travel).[20]

Given that some signs and symptoms are unreliable in detecting DVT (such as calf tenderness, swelling, and redness), a highly sensitive clinical prediction rule has been developed to help clinicians determine whether or not further testing is necessary.[19] **Homan's sign**, pain in the calf when the foot is passively dorsiflexed, is widely described as an examination technique to detect DVT; however, its low sensitivity and lack of specificity make it an unreliable indicator, and it should not be used in the diagnostic process.[19,20]

The Wells Clinical Prediction Rule is used to determine a score for the patient based on the presence or absence of the following findings:[19]

Box 9-1
Deep Vein Thrombosis—cont'd

Clinical Finding	Score
Active cancer (within 6 months of diagnosis or palliative care)	1
Recent immobilization of lower extremity	1
Recently bedridden >3 days or major surgery within 4 weeks	1
Localized tenderness along distribution of deep venous system	1
Entire lower-extremity swelling	1
Calf swelling >3 cm compared with asymptomatic lower extremity (measured 10 cm below tibial tuberosity)	1
Pitting edema (greater in the symptomatic lower extremity)	1
Collateral superficial veins (nonvaricose)	1
Alternative diagnosis as likely or greater than that of DVT (e.g., cellulitis, calf strain, postoperative swelling)	–2

A score of 1 or 2 is associated with a probability of DVT of 17% while a score of 3 or more increases the probability to 75%. Given the risks of a missed diagnosis, any patient with a score of 1 or more should be referred to a physician for further evaluation. A definitive diagnosis is made via compression ultrasound.[131]

PALPATION

Palpation of the Fibular Structures

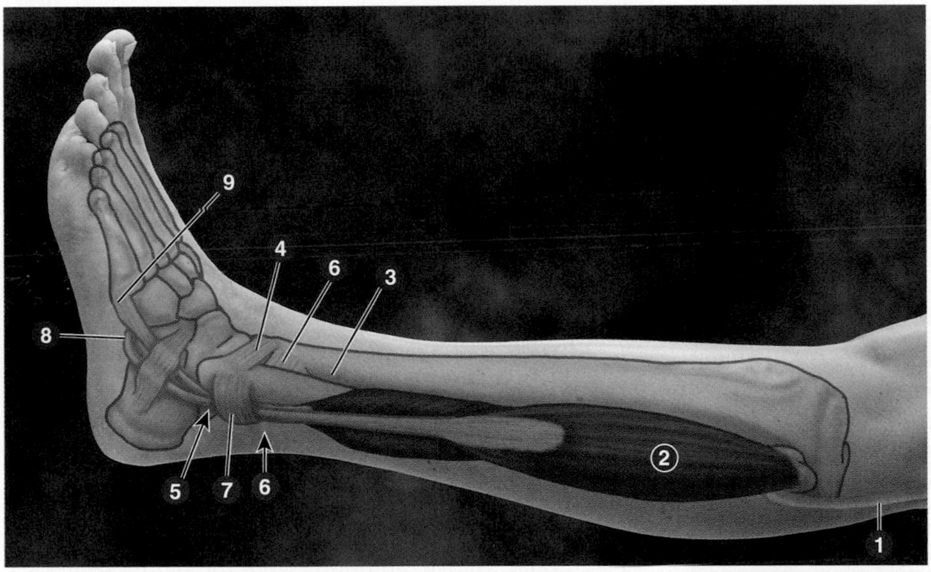

1 Common peroneal nerve: Palpate over the common peroneal nerve as it passes behind the lateral portion of the fibular head and then branches into its deep and superficial branches.

2 Peroneal muscle group: Locate the peroneus longus muscle at its origin on the fibular head and palpate the muscle belly along the upper two-thirds of the lateral fibula. The tendons of both the peroneus longus and brevis are palpable along the distal one-third of the fibula and as they course posterior to the lateral malleolus.

3 Fibular shaft: Begin by locating the fibular head and palpate along the length of the shaft over the bulk of the peroneals until the bone reemerges along its distal third. Apply gentle pressure over the distal one-third of the fibular shaft, noting any pain and discontinuity in the bone, indicative of a fracture.

4 Anterior and 5 posterior tibiofibular ligaments: Locate the attachment of the **anterior** and **posterior tibiofibular ligaments** on the fibula just superior to the lateral malleolus. Palpate anteriorly along the length of the anterior tib-fib ligament to its attachment on the anterolateral portion of the tibia. Direct palpation of the posterior tib-fib ligament is difficult because of the peroneal tendons. Tenderness along these structures or the interosseous membrane may indicate a syndesmotic ankle sprain.

6 Interosseous membrane: A portion of the interosseous membrane may be palpated in the ankle syndesmosis between the distal fibula and tibia. Begin palpating the posterior tibiofibular joint line, just superior to the lateral malleolus and progress superiorly until the fibula becomes covered by the mass of the peroneal muscles.

7 Superior peroneal retinaculum: Palpate the superior peroneal retinaculum as it projects from the superior portion of the lateral malleolus. This structure may be painful after an acute tear or stretching.

8 Peroneus longus tendon and (9) peroneus brevis tendon: As the peroneal tendons approach the peroneal tubercle, they diverge so that the **peroneus longus tendon** passes through the groove in the cuboid and is no longer palpable as it continues to the proximal portion of the first MT and medial cuneiform. The acute angle of the peroneus longus tendon as it changes course at the cuboid is a common site of rupture. The **peroneus brevis tendon** travels a shorter distance to its attachment on the base of the fifth MT.

Palpation of the Lateral Ankle

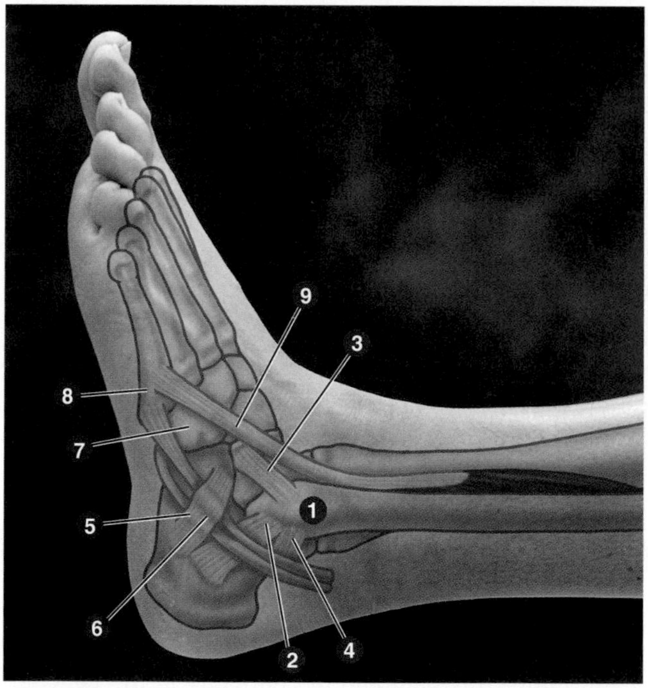

1 Lateral malleolus: The lateral ligamentous structures may be avulsed from their origin on the malleolus or their insertion on the talus or calcaneus through the tensile forces associated with inversion. Avulsion fractures result in point tenderness, swelling, and crepitus. The distal portion of the lateral malleolus may be "knocked off" by the calcaneus or talus during excessive eversion of the calcaneus.

2 Calcaneofibular ligament: Locate the origin of the CF ligament on the distal tip of the malleolus. The ligament becomes palpable as it leaves the malleolus and crosses the joint space, taking an oblique posterior course to the peroneal tubercle. Tenderness of the CF ligament during palpation following ankle injury is highly indicative of a CF sprain.

3 Anterior talofibular ligament: Locate the origin of the CF ligament and move anteriorly on the malleolus to find the origin of the ATF ligament on the inferior portion of the anterolateral malleolus. Running a course somewhat parallel to the foot's plantar surface when it is in neutral position, the ATF ligament attaches on the anterolateral aspect of the talus near the sinus tarsi. The ATF ligament is not normally distinctly palpable. Tenderness tends to be more widespread during the initial examination and becomes more focal to the ATF in the days following an injury.

4 Posterior talofibular ligament: From the origin of the calcaneofibular ligament, move upward and posteriorly around the malleolus to locate the PTF ligament. This ligament is not directly palpable, but pressure should be applied over the point of its insertion on the posterior portion of the talus. Usually, only severe ankle sprains or dislocations result in PTF ligament damage.

5 Inferior peroneal retinaculum: Palpate the space between the posterior portion of the lateral malleolus and the calcaneus for pain elicited over the superior peroneal retinaculum where the peroneal tendons pass beneath it. Follow the length of the tendons to locate the inferior peroneal retinaculum immediately below the lateral malleolus, along the lateral aspect of the calcaneus. Tears in these structures, especially the superior retinaculum, result in dislocating or subluxating peroneal tendons.

6 Peroneal tubercle: Feel for a small nodule located anterior to the attachment of the CF ligament and inferior to the distal tip of the lateral malleolus. The peroneal tubercle marks the point on the calcaneus where the peroneus longus and brevis tendons diverge. In cases of peroneal tendinopathy or rupture of the distal peroneal retinaculum, this area is tender to the touch.

7 Cuboid: Palpate anteriorly from the peroneal tubercle to locate the cuboid as it lies proximal to the base of the fifth MT. The cuboid is rarely injured but may become tender secondary to ligamentous injury such as a cuboid-metatarsal joint sprain or peroneal tendon inflammation.

8 Base of the fifth metatarsal: Palpate anteriorly from the cuboid to find the base of the fifth MT and its laterally projecting flare, the styloid process. This structure may be avulsed from the shaft after the forceful contraction of the peroneus brevis muscle as the muscle attempts to counteract inversion of the ankle.

9 Peroneus tertius: Locate the peroneus tertius where it rises from the distal half of the anterior surface of the fibula. Palpate distally along the length of the muscle belly and tendon to the insertion point on the dorsal aspect of the base of the fifth MT. The tendon is most palpable as it crosses the joint anterior to the lateral malleolus. It is the most lateral of the muscles on the anterior aspect of the lower leg. The peroneus tertius is absent in 5% to 17% of the population, but individuals who are lacking a peroneus tertius are not at an increased risk of experiencing a lateral ankle sprain.[21]

Palpation of the Anterior Structures

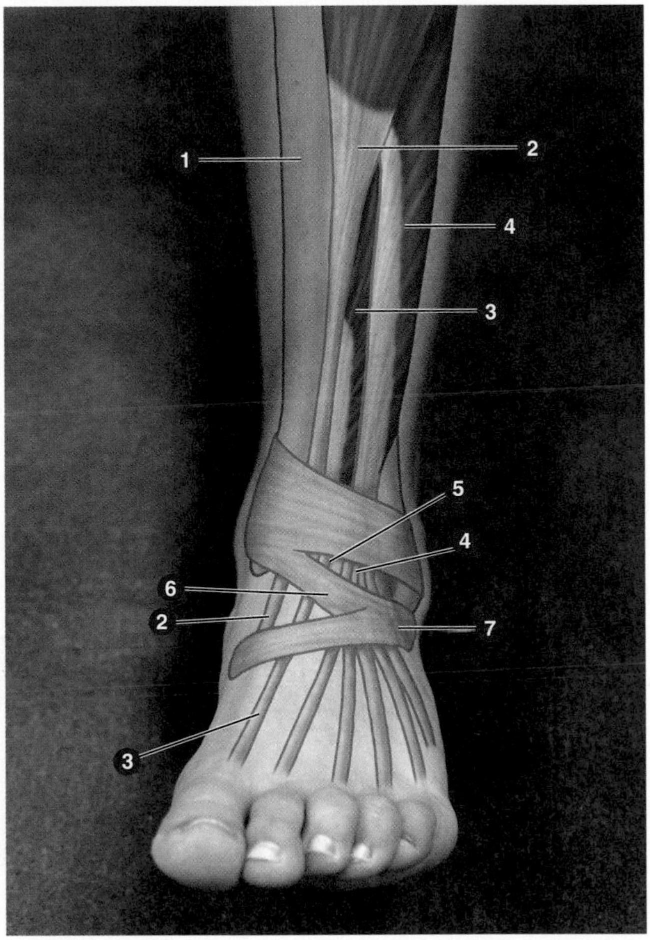

1 Anterior tibial shaft: Locate the patellar tendon's attachment on the tibial tuberosity. The anteromedial portion of the tibia is subcutaneous and therefore palpable along its length to its medial malleolus. Note tenderness arising from the anteromedial ridge of the tibia where the tibialis anterior and long toe extensors originate, as well as to the periosteum and posterior border of the shaft along the origins of the tibialis posterior, flexor hallucis longus (FHL), and flexor digitorum longus (FDL). These areas may become inflamed secondary to overuse and be improperly described as "shin splints" (Box 9-2).

2 Tibialis anterior: Locate the origin of the tibialis anterior on the anterolateral portion of the proximal tibia and palpate distally along the length of the muscle belly. Near the distal one-third of the medial tibia, the belly begins to merge into a thick, round tendon. Palpate the tendon to its insertion on the medial cuneiform and first MT.

Box 9-2
"Shin Splints"

The term "shin splints" has been used to describe nondescript leg pain. Pathologies leading to leg pain include: (1) tibialis anterior and/or long toe extensor tendinopathy, (2) tibialis posterior and/or long toe flexor tendinopathy, (3) periostitis, (4) tibial stress fractures, (5) fibular stress fractures, (6) exertional compartment syndrome, (7) inflammation of the interosseous membrane, (8) popliteal artery entrapment, (9) tear of the tibialis anterior or tibialis posterior, and (10) deep vein thrombosis.

The diagnosis of "shin splints" lacks the accuracy and specificity required to develop a management plan for the patient's condition.[22] Avoid using the term *shin splints*. Rather, identify the underlying pathology that produces the pain and the resulting impairments.

3 Extensor hallucis longus: Have the patient actively extend the great toe to make the EHL tendon palpable at its insertion. Continue to palpate the length of the EHL as it passes lateral to the tibialis anterior to its origin on the middle half of the anterior fibula and adjacent interosseous membrane. The tendon eventually becomes obscured by the tibialis anterior muscle.

4 Extensor digitorum longus: Locate the tendon of the EDL lateral to the extensor hallucis longus. Active extension of the toes causes the EDL tendons to stand out on the dorsal aspect of the toes and foot. Palpate the individual slips on the lateral four toes up through its common tendon.

5 Dome of the talus: Have the patient plantarflex the ankle to allow the anterior dome of the talus to be exposed from under the ankle mortise. Pain along this area is common with ankle synovitis and impact injuries to the ankle joint.

6 Extensor retinacula: Palpate the extensor retinacula for signs of tenderness as the tendons pass under them (see Fig. 9-13). The superior extensor retinaculum is palpated along the anterior aspect of the distal leg, just proximal to the tib-fib joint. The inferior extensor retinaculum is palpated laterally beginning at the area of the inferior peroneal retinaculum and proceeds across the dorsum of the foot to the medial aspect of the midfoot. The retinacula may become traumatically injured during forceful, sudden dorsiflexion, or the tendons passing under it may become inflamed secondary to friction.

7 Sinus tarsi: Locate the sinus tarsi between the lateral malleolus and the neck of the talus. This area may become swollen and painful to the touch following ATF ligament injury, arthritic changes in the ankle, or fracture of the talus (see Fig. 9-17).

Palpation of the Medial Structures

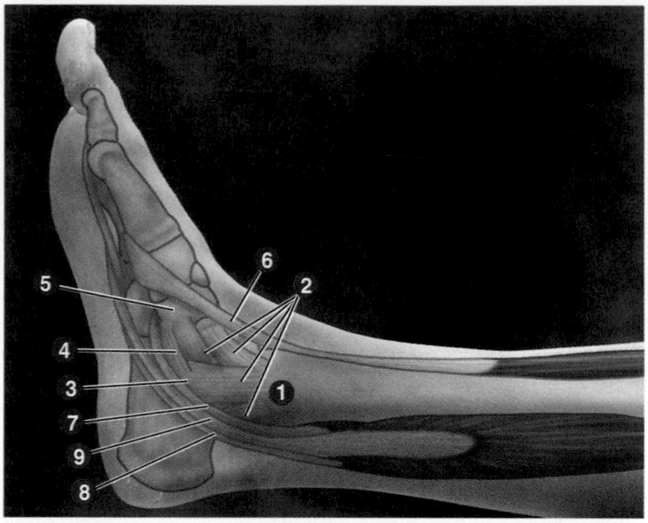

1 Medial malleolus: Palpate the entire border of the medial malleolus, noting any pain that may be elicited at the attachment sites of the medial ligaments or crepitus, possibly indicating a fracture. Continue to palpate up the posteromedial tibial border, noting any pain that arises along the periosteal lining.

2 Deltoid ligament: Palpate the mass of the deltoid ligament as it encircles the distal medial malleolus. Clinically, the individual ligaments forming this complex cannot be distinguished from each other except by their relative location on the joint.

3 Sustentaculum tali: Palpate approximately one finger's width inferior from the medial malleolus to locate the calcaneal sustentaculum tali. This structure supports the talus and is an attachment site for the spring ligament.

4 Spring ligament: Locate the spring ligament's origin on the sustentaculum tali and palpate along its route distally to its insertion on the navicular. The spring ligament becomes stretched in cases of chronic pes planus or torn following acute pronation or rotation of the forefoot.

5 Navicular and navicular tuberosity: Identify the navicular tuberosity (tubercle) by the attachment of the tibialis posterior. Palpate the navicular bone for signs of tenderness that possibly indicate tibialis posterior tendinopathy, a sprain of the spring ligament, or a stress fracture. Pain elicited during palpation of this structure can also indicate an inflamed accessory navicular.

6 Tibialis anterior: From the insertion of the tibialis anterior on the medial and plantar surfaces of the first cuneiform and first metatarsal, identify the tendon and palpate proximally along its length.

7 Tibialis posterior: The belly of the tibialis posterior is not distinctly palpable as it lies under the gastrocnemius and soleus muscles. Its tendon passes behind and around the medial malleolus and becomes most palpable at its insertion on the navicular tuberosity.

8 Flexor hallucis longus: Palpate the FHL tendon as it begins its path behind and around the medial malleolus. Note that it is difficult to distinguish this tendon from the other structures in the area. As the tendon begins its course along the plantar aspect of the foot, it is no longer palpable until it inserts on the distal phalanx of the great toe. The FHL often becomes inflamed in individuals who engage in repetitive push-off activities, such as ballet dancers.[12]

9 Flexor digitorum longus: Similar to the FHL, palpate the FDL tendon, although not uniquely identifiable, as it passes behind and around the medial malleolus. After it passes along the plantar aspect of the foot, the tendon is again palpable as it inserts on the plantar aspect of the second through fifth toes.

Palpation of the Posterior Structures

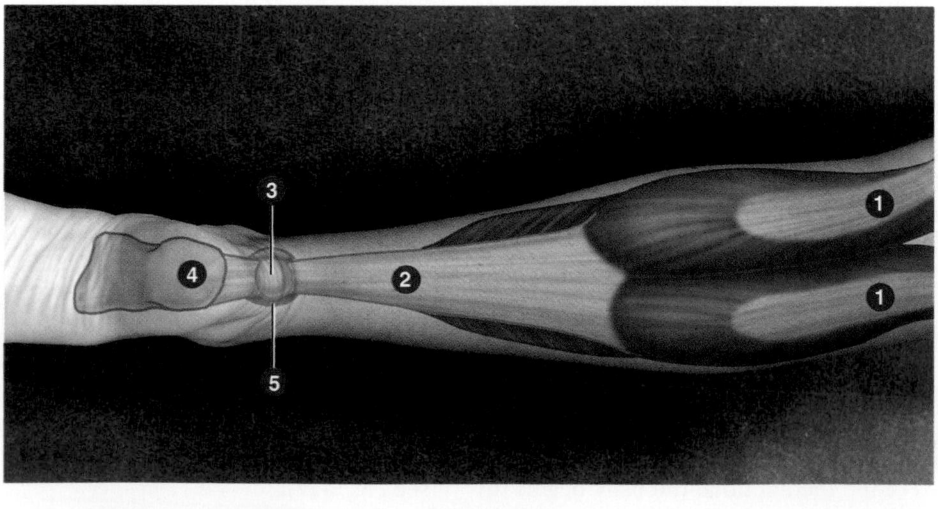

1 Gastrocnemius-soleus complex: Palpate the gastrocnemius from its dual origin on the lateral and medial femoral condyles. Giving rise to a large muscle mass, the belly of the gastrocnemius is palpated in its entirety as it forms the bulk of the posterior calf musculature. The soleus muscle, which is largely covered by the gastrocnemius, is palpable distal to the belly of the gastrocnemius and can be made more prominent by resisting the patient's plantarflexion while the knee is flexed.

2 Achilles tendon: From its attachment on the calcaneus, palpate the length of the Achilles tendon proximally to where it blends with the triceps surae muscle group. This tendon should feel firm and ropelike, with a gradual, symmetrical increase in its width as palpation progresses proximally. Palpate the Achilles tendon and its musculotendinous junction for signs of tendinopathy or an Achilles tendon rupture, in which a gap in the tendon may be felt.

3 Subcutaneous calcaneal bursa: Isolate the subcutaneous calcaneal bursa, located between the posterior aspect of the Achilles tendon and the skin, by pinching the skin that overlies the tendon. In chronic inflammatory conditions, this bursa may be enlarged and thickened, forming "pump bumps" (see Fig. 8-18).

4 Calcaneus: Locate the posterior flare of the calcaneus and continue to palpate to the site of the Achilles tendon attachment. The calcaneal dome is located just anterior to the subtendinous calcaneal bursa. Pain elicited from adolescent patients during palpation of this area may indicate calcaneal apophysitis near the Achilles tendon's insertion on the calcaneus.

5 Subtendinous calcaneal bursa: Isolate this structure between the posterior aspect of the calcaneus and the anterior portion of the Achilles tendon by squeezing the soft tissue on either side of the Achilles tendon. Pain elicited during palpation of the bursa (the two-finger squeeze test) is highly suggestive of retrocalcaneal/subtendinous bursitis.[23]

Joint and Muscle Function Assessment

The ROM available to the talocrural joint can be affected by muscular tightness, bony abnormalities, or soft tissue constraints. To allow for proper gait, the talocrural joint must allow 10° of dorsiflexion during walking and 15° during running as the opposite limb goes from the stance to the swing phase. Limited dorsiflexion can result in increased pronation, increased knee flexion, and resulting internal rotation and adduction of the hip, predisposing the individual to overuse injuries.

For the purposes here, plantarflexion and dorsiflexion are defined as the movement taking place at the talocrural joint, and inversion and eversion describe the single frontal plane calcaneal motion occurring at the subtalar joint (Table 9-4). The shape of the subtalar joint precludes true single cardinal plane motion. Pronation and supination better describe the collective movements of the subtalar and midtarsal articulations. However, the most apparent components of supination and pronation are, respectively, calcaneal inversion and eversion. These terms and measurements are often used to quantify the amount of supination and pronation. Goniometric measurements for plantarflexion and dorsiflexion are described in Goniometry 9-1. Rearfoot inversion and eversion are presented in Goniometry 8-1 (p. 201).

Active Range of Motion

- **Plantarflexion and dorsiflexion:** Spanning a range of 70°, normal active ROM allows 20° of dorsiflexion and 50° of plantarflexion from the neutral position (see Goniometry 9-1).
- **Inversion and eversion:** A component of pronation and supination, rearfoot inversion and eversion accounts for a total of 25°, with the predominant movement being 20° of inversion from the neutral position and 5° of eversion from neutral (see Goniometry 8-1).

Manual Muscle Tests

When the patient's complaint has a gradual onset of symptoms, performing repetitive tests or examining the patient postexercise when the muscles are fatigued may provide more applicable results. Because the ankle plantarflexor group is so powerful, it is often necessary to test these muscles using a unilateral heel raise. The patient is asked to perform a set of 10 toe raises holding onto a sturdy object for balance (Fig. 9-18). Evidence of a weakness in the plantarflexor group is the inability to complete the test, leaning forward, or bending the knee when the gastrocnemius is being isolated.

Table 9-4 Muscles Contributing to Uniplanar Foot and Ankle Movements

Dorsiflexion	Inversion
Extensor digitorum longus	Extensor hallucis longus
Extensor hallucis longus	Flexor digitorum longus
Peroneus tertius	Flexor hallucis longus
Tibialis anterior	Tibialis anterior
	Tibialis posterior
Plantarflexion	**Eversion**
Flexor digitorum longus	Extensor digitorum longus
Flexor hallucis longus	Peroneus brevis
Gastrocnemius	Peroneus longus
Peroneus brevis	Peroneus tertius
Peroneus longus	
Plantaris	
Soleus	
Tibialis posterior	

Goniometry 9-1
Ankle Plantarflexion/Dorsiflexion

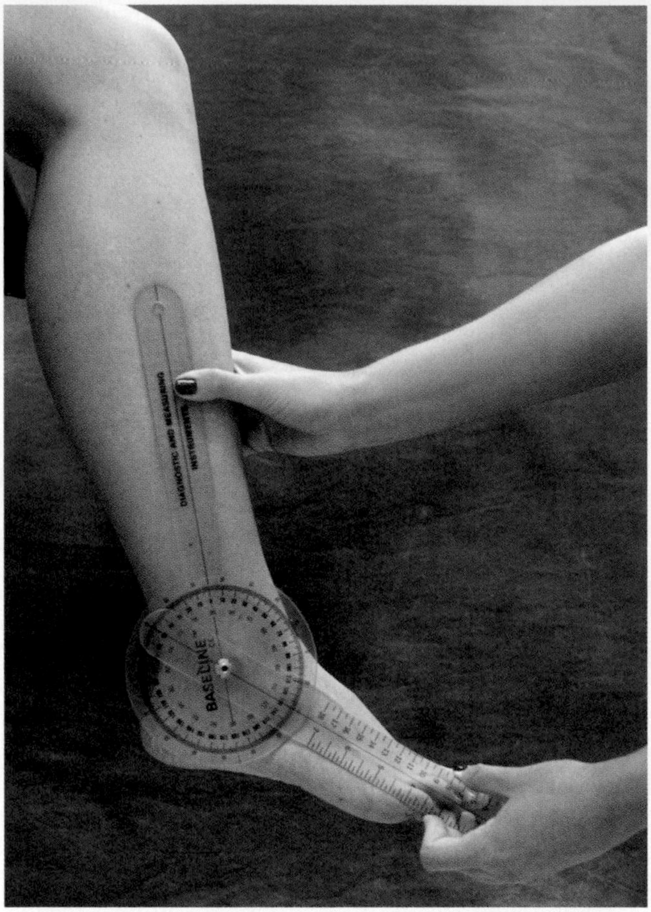

Dorsiflexion to Plantarflexion (20°–0°–50°)

Patient Position	Sitting with the knee flexed to 90° and the ankle in anatomical position

Goniometer Alignment

Fulcrum	Center the axis at the lateral malleolus.
Proximal Arm	Align the stationary arm with the long axis of the fibula.
Distal Arm	Align the movement arm parallel with the bottom of the foot.
Modification	Dorsiflexion may be measured with the patient prone and the knee flexed to 90°.
Comments	Avoid extending the toes or twisting the foot. Measuring dorsiflexion with the knee extended assesses for limitation in dorsiflexion secondary to gastrocnemius tightness, which may be clinically useful. Measurements are relative to the ankle at 90° (anatomical position) on the goniometer, which represents the 0 position.

Evidence

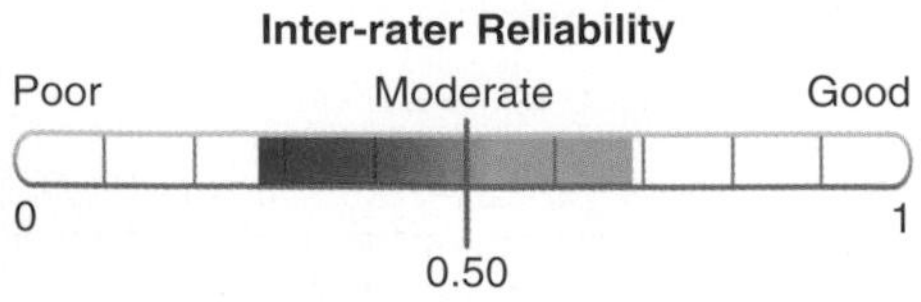

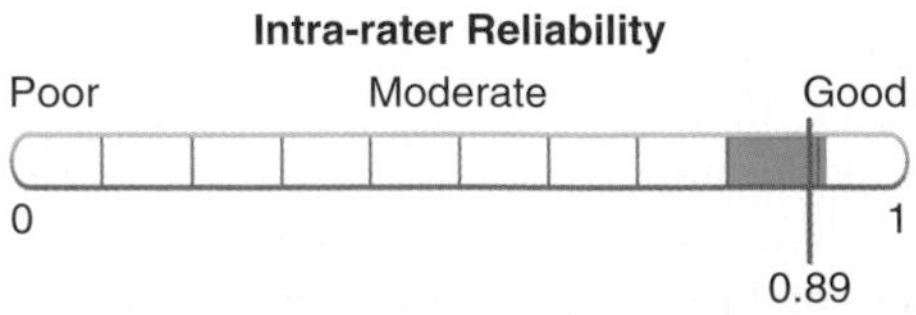

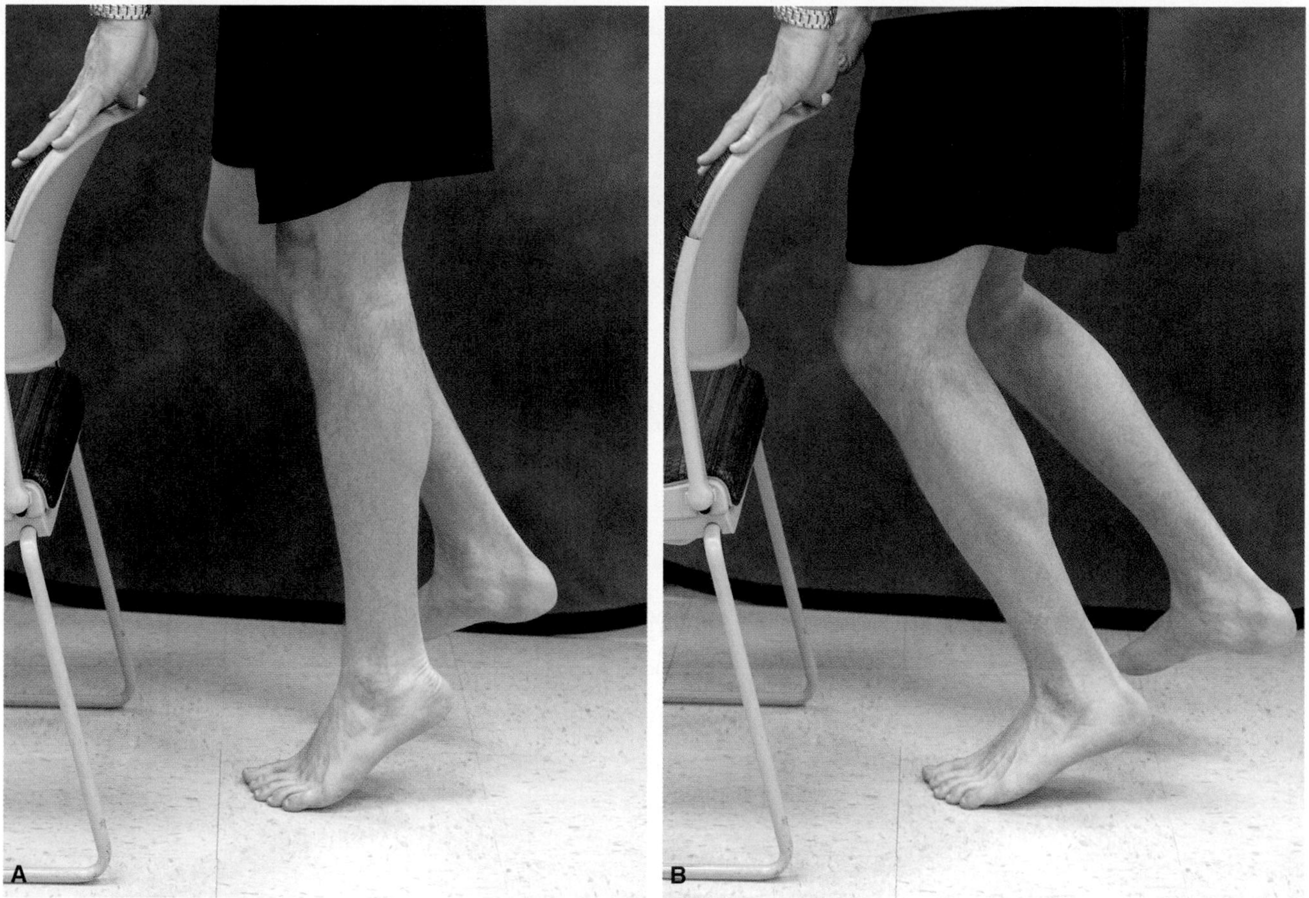

FIGURE 9-18 ■ Heel-raise test for plantarflexion. (A) With the knee extended to include the gastrocnemius. (B) With the knee flexed to isolate the soleus muscle.

Manual Muscle Tests (MMTs) 9-1, 9-2, 9-3, and 9-4 include testing of the muscles originating in the anterior, posterior, and deep posterior compartments. Manual muscle tests of the long toe flexors and extensors are presented in Manual Muscle Tests 8-1 and 8-2 (pp. 204 and 205).

Passive Range of Motion

The extensive soft tissue arrangement of the talocrural and subtalar joint results in a firm end-feel owing to tissue stretch (Table 9-5). Damage to the ligamentous or capsular structures may result in a hard end-feel as bone contacts bone.

- **Plantarflexion and dorsiflexion:** Dorsiflexion is assessed once with the knee extended to determine the overall influence of the triceps surae group and then again with the knee flexed to determine the influence of the soleus. The normal end-feel for both plantarflexion and dorsiflexion is firm, owing to soft tissue stretch of the anterior joint capsule, deltoid ligament, and ATF ligament during plantarflexion and of the Achilles tendon during dorsiflexion. After injury, the amount of ROM lost is greater during plantarflexion than in dorsiflexion. However, loss of dorsiflexion is more debilitating in the long term because of the resultant changes in gait mechanics.
- **Inversion and eversion:** Assess and measure the calcaneal inversion and eversion components of subtalar pronation and supination with the patient prone. Stabilize the tibia and fibula to prevent hip or leg rotation. The normal end-feel during neutral inversion is firm secondary to soft-tissue stretch from the lateral ankle ligaments (especially the CF ligament) and the peroneus longus and brevis muscles. A hard end-feel may be present during eversion if the calcaneus contacts the fibula. The end-feel may be firm because of stretching of the medial joint capsule and musculature. After injury, the capsular pattern loss of motion is greater for inversion than for eversion.

Table 9-5	Talocrural Joint Capsular Patterns and End-Feels
Capsular Pattern Talocrural Joint: Plantarflexion, Dorsiflexion	
Plantarflexion of the talocrural joint	Firm – soft tissue stretch
Dorsiflexion of the talocrural joint	Firm – soft tissue stretch
Capsular Pattern Subtalar Joint: Supination, Pronation	
Inversion of the subtalar joint	Firm – soft tissue stretch
Eversion of the subtalar joint	Firm – soft tissue stretch

Manual Muscle Test 9-1
Dorsiflexion and Supination

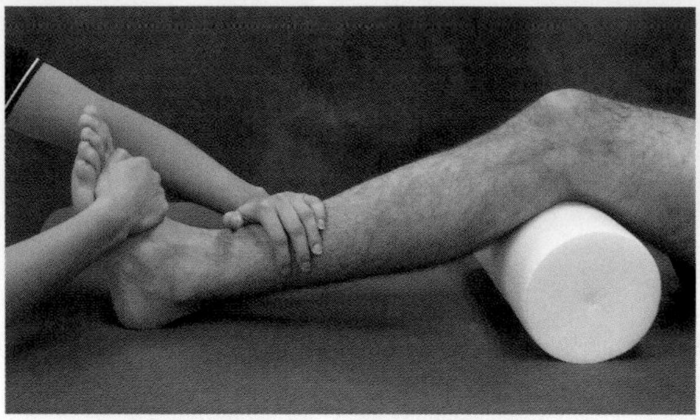

Patient Position	Seated
Test Position	Knee flexed Foot positioned in mid-position of dorsiflexion and supination
Stabilization	Distal tibia, preventing knee extension and femoral external rotation
Resistance	Medial aspect of the dorsum of the foot
Primary Movers (Innervation)	Tibialis anterior (L4, L5, S1)
Secondary Movers (Innervation)	Extensor hallucis longus (L4, L5, S1) Extensor digitorum longus (L4, L5, S1) Peroneus tertius (negligible contribution) (L4, L5, S1)
Substitution	Knee extension Great toe extension
Comments	Ensure that the toes are relaxed to reduce the contribution of the long toe extensors.

Manual Muscle Test 9-2
Eversion and Pronation

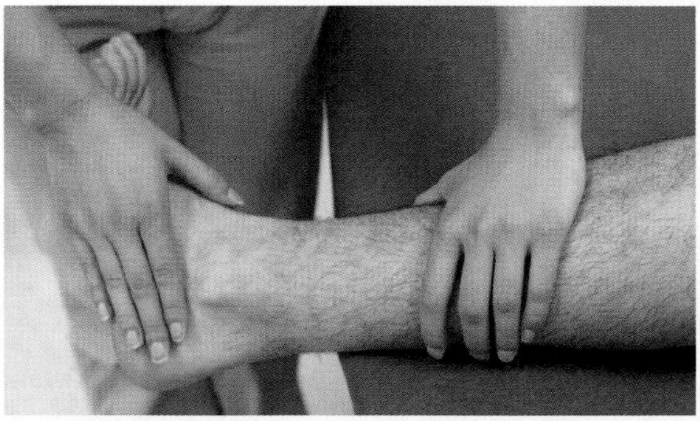

Patient Position	Side-lying on the side opposite the limb being tested Opposite hip flexed
Test Position	Test foot off the end of the table in the mid-position of eversion and pronation
Stabilization	Lower leg
Resistance	Lateral border of the foot
Primary Movers (Innervation)	Peroneus longus (L4, L5, S1) Peroneus brevis (L4, L5, S1)

Manual Muscle Test 9-2
Eversion and Pronation—cont'd

Secondary Movers (Innervation)	Extensor digitorum longus (L4, L5, S1)
Substitution	Plantarflexion Toe extension
Comments	Avoid toe extension to decrease the contribution of the extensor digitorum longus.

Manual Muscle Test 9-3
Plantarflexors

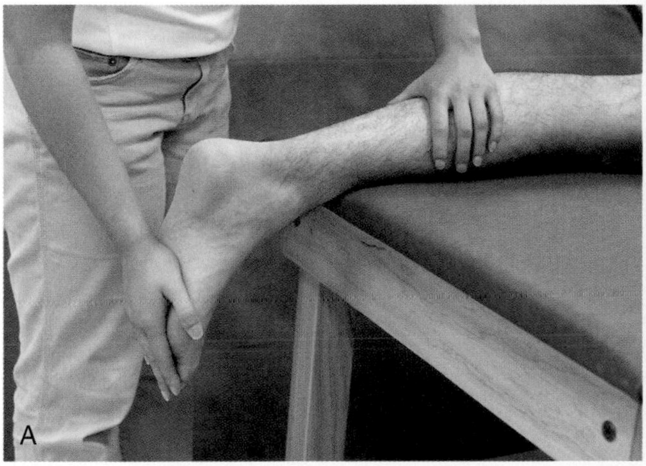

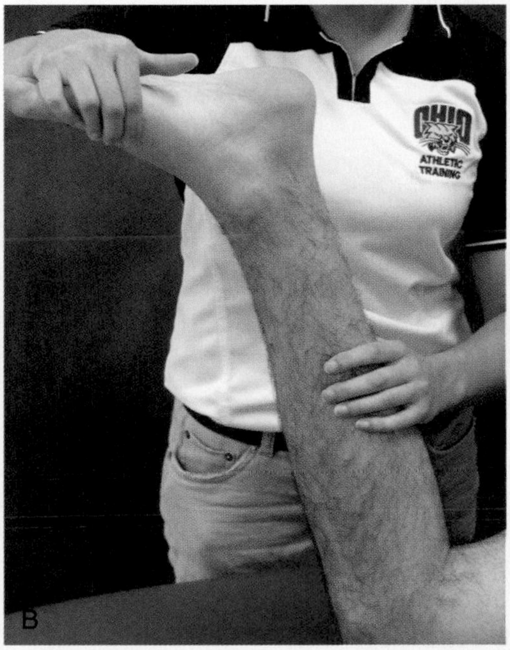

Patient Position	Prone
Test Position	*Gastrocnemius:* **(A)** Knee extended with the foot off the table; ankle in neutral position *Soleus:* **(B)** Knee flexed past 30°
Stabilization	Proximal to the ankle
Resistance	Plantar surface of the foot
Primary Movers (Innervation)	Gastrocnemius (S1, S2) Soleus (S1, S2) Plantaris (S1, S2)
Secondary Movers (Innervation)	Flexor digitorum longus (L5, S1) Flexor hallucis longus (L4, L5, S1) Tibialis posterior (L4, L5, S1)
Substitution	Knee flexion
Comments	Avoid toe flexion to reduce the contribution of the flexor hallucis longus and flexor digitorum longus muscles. Avoid inversion to reduce the contribution of the tibialis posterior muscle. Because the plantarflexors are a strong muscle group, single-leg heel raises may provide a better indicator of strength.

Manual Muscle Test 9-4
Rearfoot Inversion

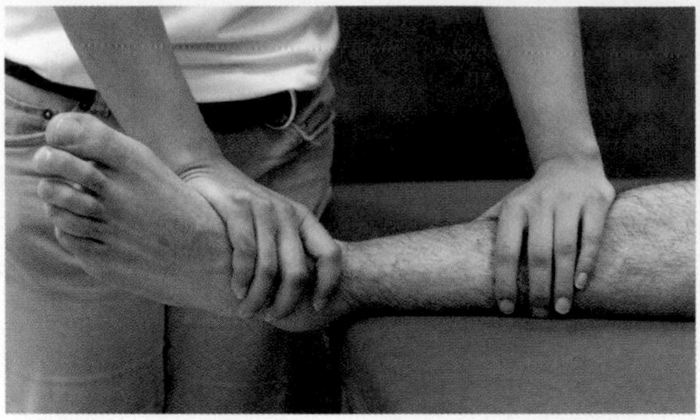

Patient Position	Side-lying on the side opposite being tested Opposite hip flexed
Test Position	Test foot off the end of the table with the ankle in the resting position
Stabilization	Medial aspect of the distal leg
Resistance	Medial border of the foot (navicular, medial cuneiform)
Primary Movers (Innervation)	Tibialis posterior (L4, L5, S1)
Secondary Movers (Innervation)	Flexor digitorum longus (L5, S1) Flexor hallucis longus (L4, L5, S1)
Substitution	Plantarflexion Toe flexion
Comments	Avoid toe flexion to reduce the contribution of the flexor hallucis longus and flexor digitorum longus muscles.

Joint Stability Tests

ROM tests place stress on the ligaments of the ankle complex, especially during passive ROM testing (see Table 9-3). Although several manual stress tests may identify ankle joint laxity, they may lack the specificity to identify which ligaments are involved, owing to individual tissue properties and variations in torque applied during the testing procedure.[24] Ankle arthrometers, instruments designed to quantify the amount of laxity, provide moderate-to-good intrarater reliability, but their validity remains unclear.[24]

Stress Testing

Test for anterior talofibular ligament instability. The combined motions of ankle plantarflexion and subtalar supination strain the ATF ligament as it prevents anterior translation of the talus relative to the ankle mortise. The **anterior drawer test** is used to determine the integrity of the ATF (Stress Test 9-1).[25,26]

Test for calcaneofibular ligament instability. The **inversion stress test** (talar tilt test) is used to determine if the calcaneofibular ligament has been injured (Stress Test 9-2). This test also stresses the anterior and posterior talofibular ligaments and may reveal instability in the subtalar joint.[30]

Tests for deltoid ligament instability. The distal projection of the lateral malleolus limits the amount of ankle eversion, but rotation of the talocrural and/or subtalar joint may injure the deltoid ligament.[31] The **eversion stress test** (Stress Test 9-3) is used to evaluate injury to the deltoid ligament group. The **external rotation test** (Kleiger test) is used to determine injury to the deltoid ligament caused by a rotational stress or injury to the syndesmosis, with the results differentiated by the location of pain (Selective Tissue Test 9-1).

Joint Play Assessment

Joint play assessment is indicated at the proximal (see Chapter 8) and distal tib-fib joints, the talocrural joint, or the subtalar joint. Hypermobility at any of these joints confirms the presence of a sprain. Hypomobility at one articulation may create additional stresses at another.

Talocrural Joint Play

The talocrural joint may become restricted following a period of immobilization (Joint Play 9-1). A restriction in posterior talar glide, common following a period of immobilization, is functionally demonstrated by a limitation in dorsiflexion. A restricted anterior talar glide results in a limitation in plantarflexion.

Stress Test 9-1
Anterior Drawer Test

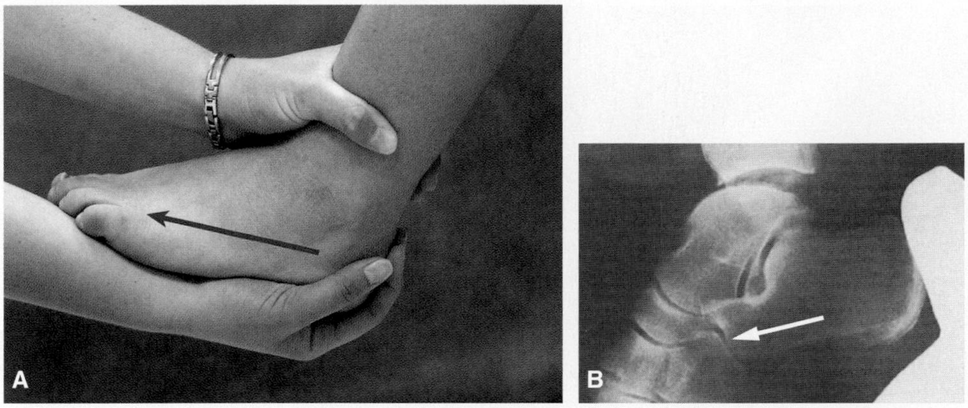

(A) Anterior drawer test to check the integrity of the anterior talofibular ligament. (B) Radiographic view of a positive anterior drawer test. Note the anterior displacement of the talus relative to the tibia. (B Courtesy of Donatelli, RA. *Biomechanics of the Foot and Ankle*. Philadelphia, PA: F.A. Davis Company; 1990.)

Patient Position	Sitting over the edge of the table with the knee flexed to prevent gastrocnemius tightness from influencing the outcome of the test
Position of Examiner	Sitting in front of the patient One hand stabilizes the leg, taking care not to occlude the mortise. The other hand cups the calcaneus, while the forearm supports the foot in a position of slight plantarflexion (10°–20° from the anatomical position).[6,27]
Evaluative Procedure	The calcaneus and talus are drawn forward while providing a stabilizing force to the tibia.
Positive Test	The talus slides anteriorly from under the ankle mortise compared with the opposite side (assuming it is stable). There may be an appreciable "clunk" as the talus subluxates and relocates, and/or the patient may describe pain.
Implications	Sprain of the anterior talofibular ligament and the associated capsule
Modification	The test may be performed with the patient supine, but the knee must be kept in a minimum of 30° flexion to eliminate the influence of the gastrocnemius muscle. The tibia can be pushed posteriorly as the calcaneus is drawn anteriorly.
Comments	Pain or apprehension can result in the patient contracting the triceps surae, thereby producing false-negative results. Do not apply overpressure in an attempt to overcome this response.[28] The anterior drawer test is useful in differentiating an intact ATFL from an isolated ATFL sprain but is less sensitive in differentiating an ATFL sprain from a more diffuse lateral ankle sprain involving the CFL.[29]
Evidence	

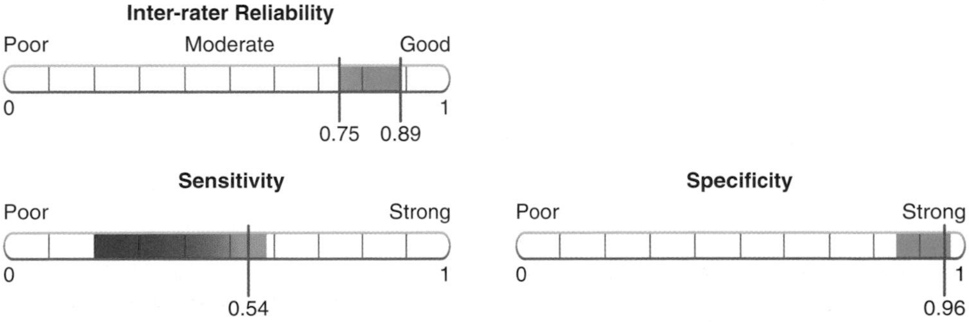

LR+: 1.32–14.50–18.00

LR−: 0.44–0.47–0.94

ATFL = anterior talofibular ligament; CFL = calcaneofibular ligament

Stress Test 9-2
Inversion (Talar Tilt) Stress Test

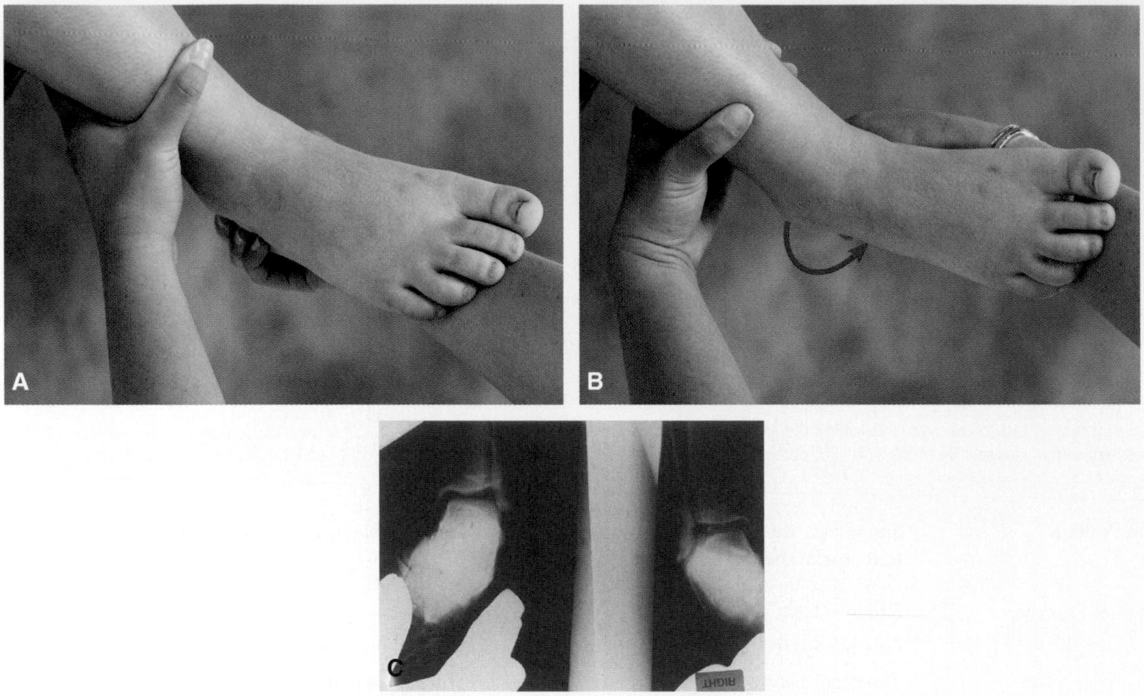

(A and B) Inversion stress test (talar tilt test) to check the integrity of the calcaneofibular ligament. (C) Radiograph of an inversion stress.

Patient Position	Supine or sitting with legs over the edge of a table
Position of Examiner	In front of the patient One hand grasps the calcaneus and talus as a single unit and maintains the foot and ankle in 10° of dorsiflexion to isolate the calcaneofibular ligament.[29] The opposite hand stabilizes the leg; the thumb or forefinger is placed along the calcaneofibular ligament so that any gapping of the talus away from the mortise can be felt.
Evaluative Procedure	The hand holding the calcaneus provides an inversion stress by rolling the calcaneus medially, causing the talus to tilt.
Positive Test	The talus tilts or gaps excessively (i.e., greater than 10°) compared with the uninjured side, and/or pain is produced.
Implications	Involvement of the calcaneofibular ligament, possibly along with the anterior talofibular and posterior talofibular ligaments
Modification	Inversion can be assessed with the ankle in different positions in the ROM to stress different parts of the lateral joint capsule.
Comments	When the severity of injury is being based on the relative laxity, a history of injury and residual laxity to the uninvolved ankle mask the magnitude of the current trauma.[6,29]

Evidence

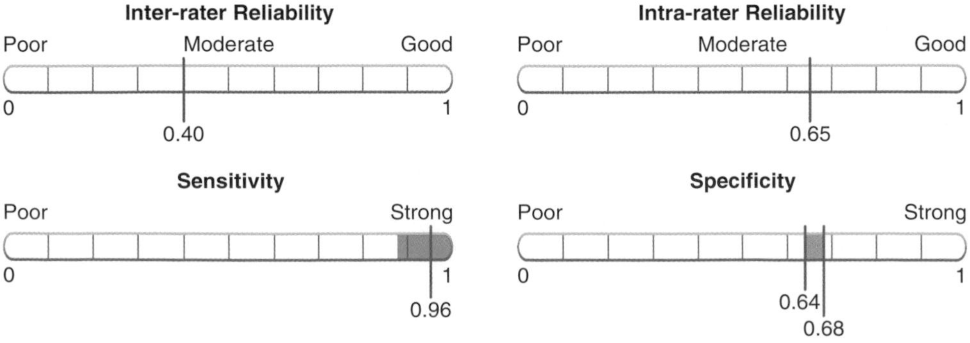

LR+: 2.44–3.00

LR−: 0.06–0.19

ATFL = anterior talofibular ligament; CFL = calcaneofibular ligament

Stress Test 9-3
Eversion (Talar Tilt) Stress Test

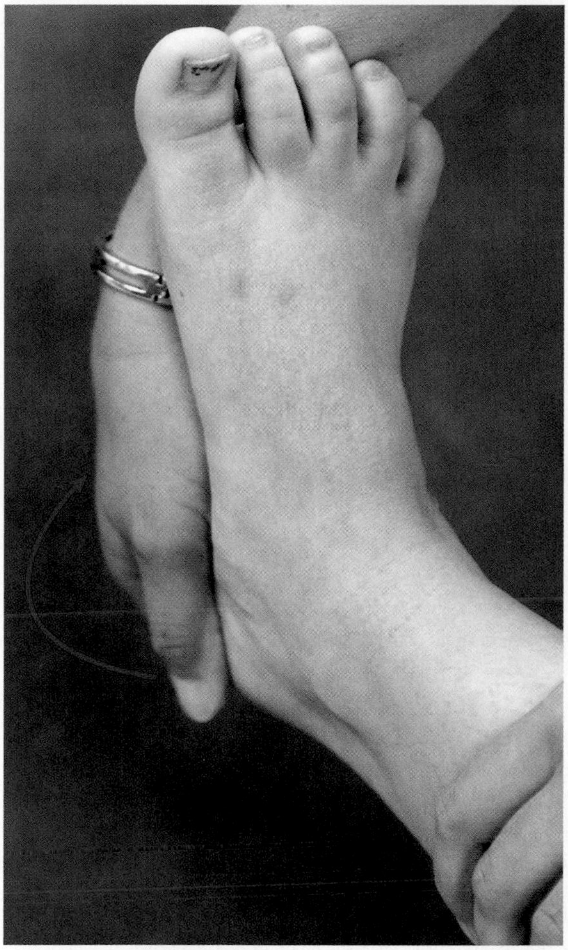

Eversion stress test to determine the integrity of the deltoid ligament, especially the tibiocalcaneal ligament

Patient Position	Supine or sitting with legs over the edge of a table
Position of Examiner	In front of the patient With one hand, grasp the calcaneus and talus as a single unit and maintain the ankle in a neutral position. The thumb or forefinger may be placed along the deltoid ligament so that any gapping of the talus away from the mortise can be felt. The other hand stabilizes the leg.
Evaluative Procedure	The hand holding the calcaneus rolls it laterally, tilting the talus and causing a gap on the medial side of the ankle mortise.
Positive Test	The talus tilts or gaps excessively compared with the uninjured side, and/or the patient describes pain during this motion.
Implications	Deltoid ligament sprain; tib-fib sprain
Comments	The location of the pain determines which structure is injured.
Evidence	Absent or inconclusive in the literature

Selective Tissue Test 9-1
External Rotation Test (Kleiger Test)

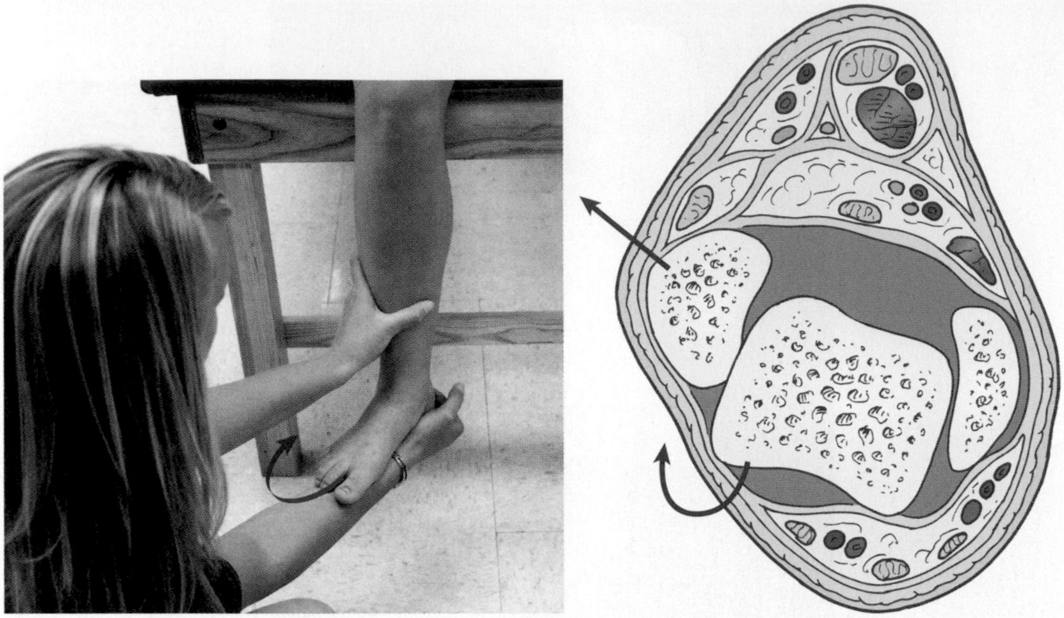

External rotation (Kleiger) test for determination of damage to the deltoid ligament or the distal tib-fib syndesmosis. The tissue implicated is based on the area of pain that is elicited. Externally rotating the talus places a lateral force on the fibula, which spreads the syndesmosis and stretches the deltoid ligament.

Patient Position	Sitting with legs over the edge of the table
Position of Examiner	In front of the patient One hand stabilizes the leg in a manner that does not compress the distal tib-fib syndesmosis. The other hand grasps the medial aspect of the foot while supporting the ankle in a neutral position.
Evaluative Procedure	The foot and talus are externally rotated, while maintaining a stable leg. To stress the syndesmosis, place the ankle in dorsiflexion. To stress the deltoid ligament, place the ankle in a neutral position or in slight plantarflexion.
Positive Test	*Deltoid ligament involvement:* Medial joint pain. The examiner may feel displacement of the talus away from the medial malleolus. *Syndesmosis involvement:* Pain at the anterolateral ankle at the distal tib-fib syndesmosis
Implications	Medial pain is indicative of trauma to the deltoid ligament. Pain in the area of the anterior or posterior tib-fib ligament should be considered syndesmosis pathology unless determined otherwise (e.g., malleolar fracture). Fracture of the distal fibula
Comments	Pain arising from the distal tib-fib syndesmosis during this test is associated with a prolonged recovery time.[30]
Evidence	

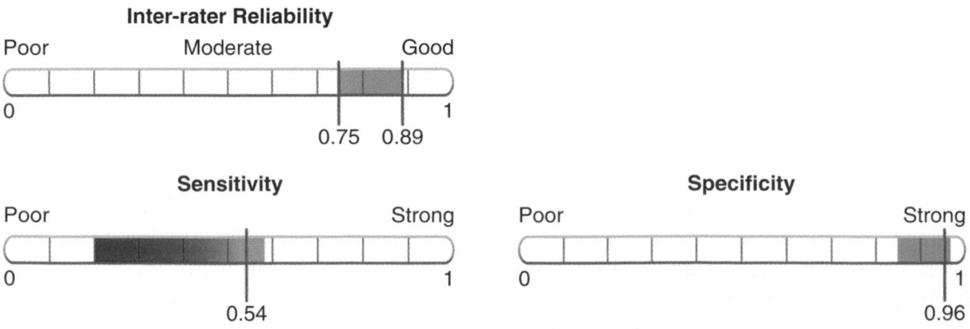

LR+: 1.32–14.50–18.00

LR−: 0.44–0.47–0.94

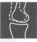

Joint Play 9-1
Talocrural Joint Play

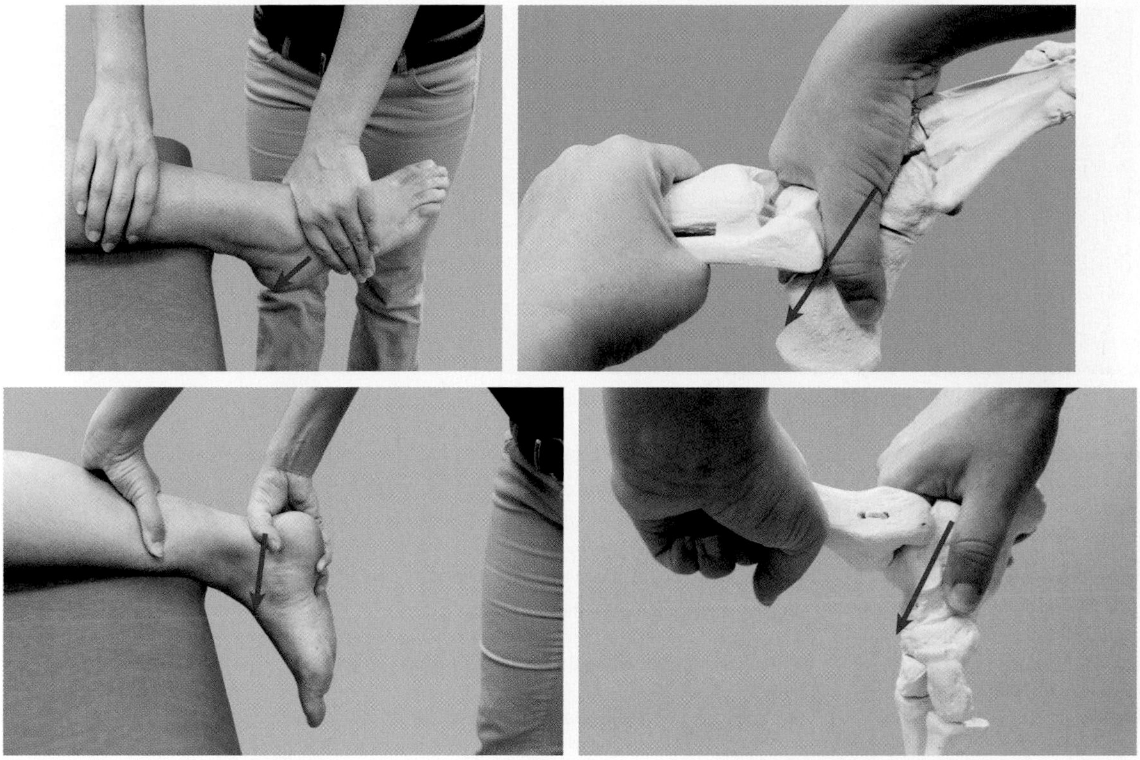

A restriction in posterior talocrural joint play leads to decreased dorsiflexion. A reduction in anterior talocrural joint play restricts plantarflexion.

Patient Position	**Posterior joint play:** Supine; foot over edge of table or elevated with towel; ankle in slight plantarflexion **Anterior joint play:** Prone; foot over edge of table; ankle in slight plantarflexion
Position of Examiner	**Posterior joint play:** At the patient's feet One hand stabilizes the distal leg, cupping the posterior calcaneus. The other hand is positioned over the anterior talus. **Anterior joint play:** At the side of the table The proximal hand stabilizes the distal leg against the table. The distal hand cups the calcaneus.
Evaluative Procedure	**Posterior joint play:** A posteriorly directed force is applied on the talus. **Anterior joint play:** An anteriorly directed force is applied to the talus.
Positive Test	Hypomobility Hypermobility Pain
Implications	Hypomobility: Joint adhesions Hypermobility: Ligamentous and/or capsular laxity
Evidence	Absent or inconclusive in the literature

Subtalar Joint Play
Restricted subtalar medial glide may be a causative factor in limited pronation during ambulation. Subtalar medial glide hypermobility is associated with lateral ankle sprains (Joint Play 9-2).[30] Lateral translation of the talus in the ankle mortise is evaluated using the **Cotton Test** (Joint Play 9-3).

Test for distal tibiofibular syndesmosis instability. Injury to the distal tib-fib syndesmosis, the anterior tib-fib ligament, the interosseous membrane, and the posterior tib-fib ligament may be identified through overpressure at the end of dorsiflexion ROM or by placing an external rotation force on the talus. During forced dorsiflexion,

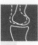

Joint Play 9-2
Medial Subtalar Joint Play

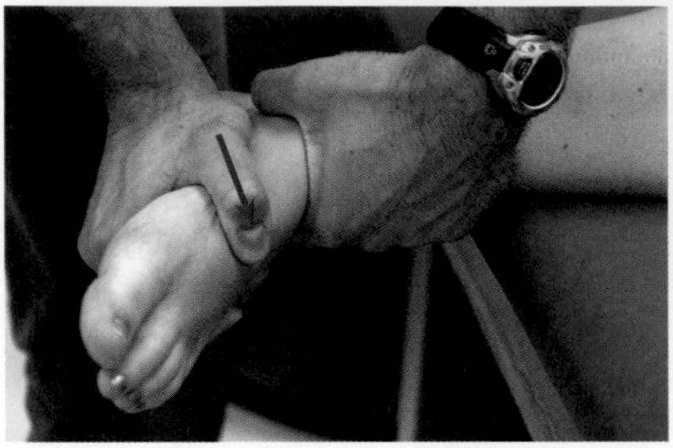
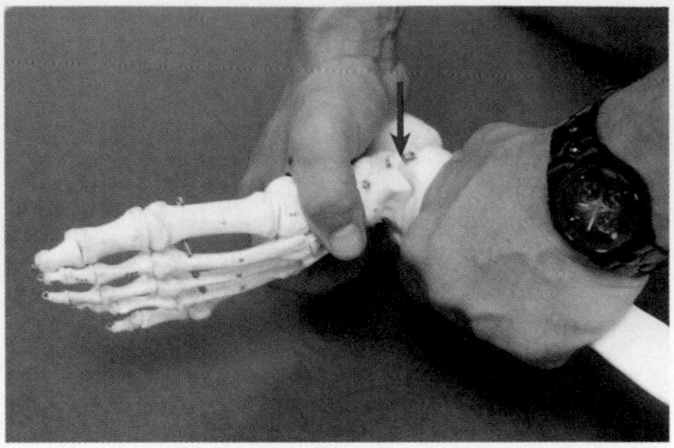

After stabilizing the talus in the mortise, the amount of medial and lateral movement at the STJ is assessed (lateral glide shown).

Patient Position	**Medial glide:** Side-lying on non-test limb; STJ in neutral (see p. 194 for finding STJ neutral position) **Lateral glide:** Side-lying on test limb; STJ in neutral A towel may be placed under the distal tibia.
Position of Examiner	One hand stabilizes the talus in the mortise. The opposite hand cups the calcaneus.
Evaluative Procedure	Force is applied to move the talus medially and laterally.
Positive Test	Increased or decreased medial or lateral translation of the talus relative to the opposite side
Implications	Results are compared relative to the opposite (uninjured) foot: Hypomobile medial glide is associated with decreased pronation/calcaneal eversion. Hypomobile lateral glide is associated with decreased supination/calcaneal inversion.
Comments	Hypermobile medial glide is commonly associated with lateral ankle sprains.[30]
Evidence	Absent or inconclusive in the literature

STJ = subtalar joint

the wider anterior border of the talus is wedged into the talocrural joint, causing the fibula to move slightly away from the tibia. If the syndesmosis has been traumatized, pain will be elicited. **Distal tibiofibular joint play** is used to identify the anterior–posterior stability of the distal syndesmosis (Joint Play 9-4). The external rotation test identifies syndesmosis pathology by forcing the talus and calcaneus against the lateral malleolus, causing it to be displaced laterally and posteriorly, stressing the syndesmosis (see Selective Tissue Test 9-1, p. 264).

Neurological Assessment

Neurological dysfunction can occur secondary to compression proximal to the leg, compartment syndromes, or direct trauma. The common peroneal nerve or its superficial or deep branches is most prone to trauma (Table 9-6). Figure 9-19 presents the distribution of neurological symptoms around the ankle and foot. A lower quarter screen may also be required to rule out neurological symptoms arising from the lumbar or sacral plexus (see Neurological Screening 1-2).

Vascular Assessment

Vascular compromise can result either from an acute or chronic increase in compartmental pressure or from a bony fracture or joint dislocation of a leg structure anywhere proximal to the ankle. Prolonged impaired circulation can result in tissue necrosis.

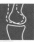

Joint Play 9-3
Cotton Test (Lateral Talar Glide)

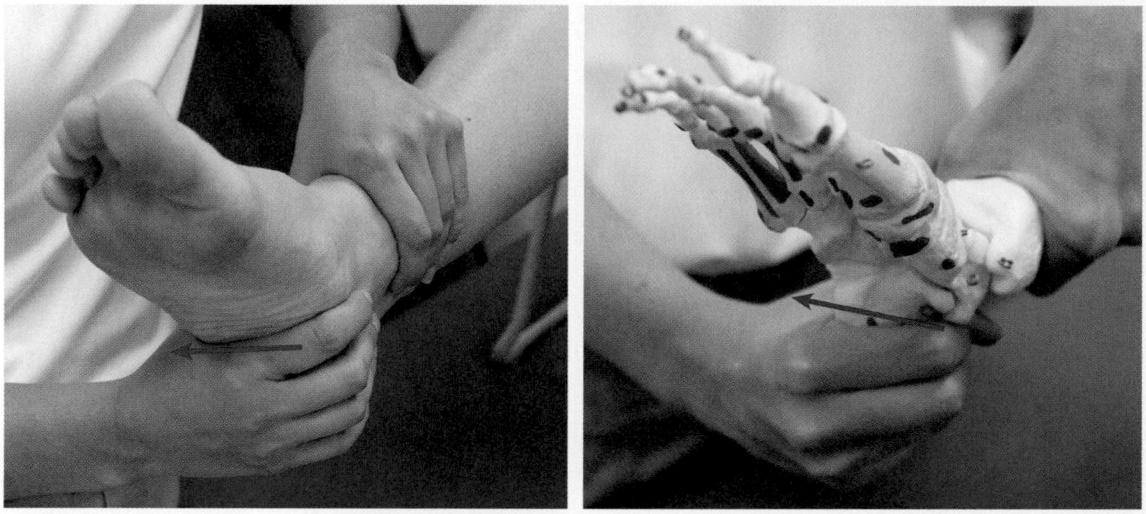

The Cotton test assesses the amount of lateral translation of the talus within the ankle mortise.

Patient Position	Supine or short-sitting with the ankle in the neutral position
Position of Examiner	One hand grasps the ankle mortise just proximal to the tibiotalar joint line, stabilizing the distal leg, but not compressing the distal tib-fib syndesmosis. The opposite hand cups the calcaneus and talus.
Evaluative Procedure	Force is applied to move the talus laterally.
Positive Test	Increased lateral translation of the talus relative to the opposite side Pain[31]
Implications	Distal tib-fib syndesmosis sprain
Comments	There is a relationship between an arthroscopically confirmed diagnosis of tib-fib syndesmosis sprain and a positive Cotton test.[31]
Evidence	Absent or inconclusive in the literature

Table 9-6 Mechanisms of Injury of the Common Peroneal Nerve

Mechanism	Causal Factor
Lesion	Fracture of the fibular head
Concussive	Contusion to the superior lateral portion of the leg
Compression	Knee braces or elastic wraps, especially when combined with cryotherapy
Internal Pressure	Prolonged squatting (e.g., baseball or softball catcher)
Entrapment	Exertional compartment syndromes (branches of the common peroneal nerve)
Traction	Varus stress to the knee, hyperextension of the knee, plantarflexion and inversion of the ankle

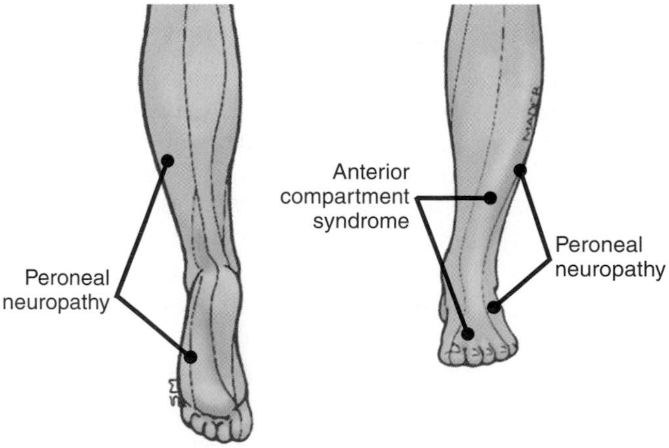

FIGURE 9-19 ■ Local neuropathies of the ankle and leg. These findings should also be matched with those of a lower quarter neurological screen.

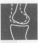

Joint Play 9-4
Distal Tibiofibular Joint Play

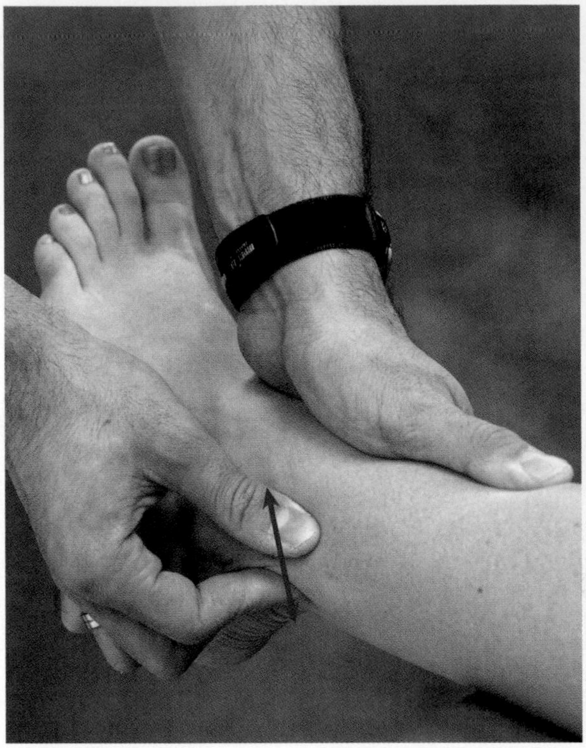

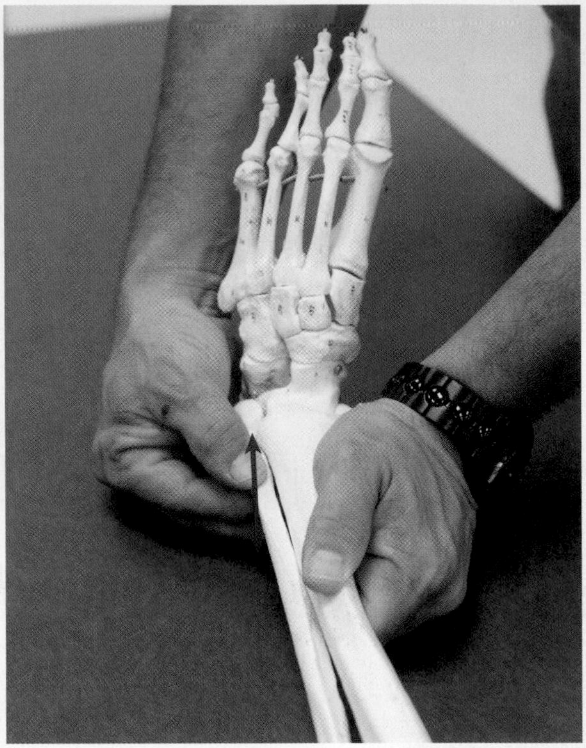

This joint play assessment identifies the amount of anterior–posterior play in the distal tib-fib syndesmosis.

Patient Position	Supine or short-sitting with the ankle relaxed into plantarflexion
Position of Examiner	Grasping the fibula at the lateral malleolus and stabilizing the tibia
Evaluative Procedure	Pressure is applied to obliquely move the fibula anteriorly and then posteriorly relative to the tibia.
Positive Test	Hypomobility Hypermobility Pain
Implications	Sprain of the distal tib-fib syndesmosis
Modification	The distal fibula can be compressed ("squeezed") to identify lateral play based on the amount of movement.
Comments	Pain is a more reliable indicator of syndesmotic trauma than increased motion.[32]
Evidence	Absent or inconclusive in the literature

Palpation of the Pulses

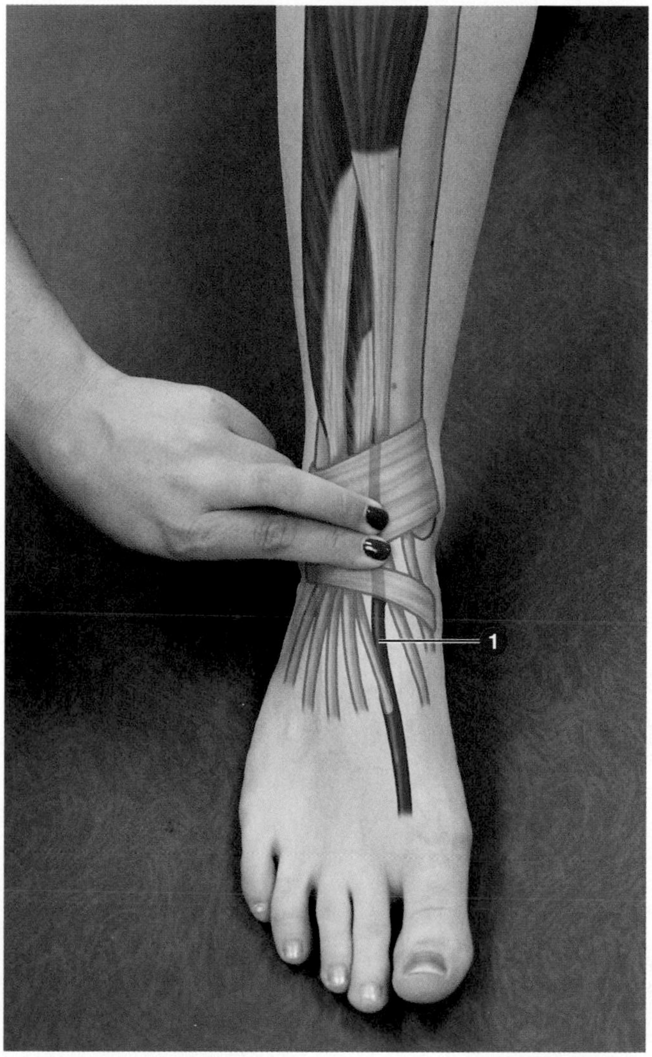

1 Dorsalis pedis artery: A branch of the anterior tibial artery, the dorsalis pedis pulse may be palpated between the extensor digitorum longus and extensor hallucis longus tendons as they pass over the cuneiforms. Establish the presence of this pulse after lower extremity fracture or dislocation and in those individuals suspected of having an anterior compartment syndrome. This pulse is not readily detectable in all people. In the absence of a pulse on the involved side, make sure that the pulse is identifiable on the uninvolved extremity.

- **Posterior tibial artery:** Palpate the posterior tibial artery, located between the flexor digitorum longus and flexor hallucis longus tendons as they pass behind the medial malleolus. As a blood supply to the foot, this pulse must be established after any significant lower extremity bone fracture or joint dislocation. Note that swelling along the medial joint line may mask the presence of this pulse and make its detection difficult.

Region-Specific Pathologies and Selective Tissue Tests

Although sprains are the predominant type of injury suffered by the leg and ankle, the evaluation process must not discount other potential injuries. Other acute injuries to this body area include fractures, dislocations, and tendon ruptures. In addition, many overuse conditions affect the leg. Historically, all emergency room visitations for acute ankle trauma routinely underwent radiographic examination. In many cases, the results were negative for a fracture. The Ottawa Ankle Rules (OAR) were developed to help discriminate among those signs and symptoms that are more highly suggestive of fracture and thus reduce the number of unneeded and costly routine radiographs (see Ankle and Leg Fractures, p. 276).

Ankle Sprains

Most ankle sprains occur secondary to excessive supination, causing trauma to the lateral ligament complex as the calcaneus inverts and the talus abducts in a closed chain. A lesser yet significant percentage of ankle sprains involves the medial ankle ligaments and the distal tib-fib syndesmosis. Because of the close association of many of the ankle ligaments with the joint capsule, ligament injury often results in trauma to the capsule. Ankle sprains are complicated by fractures of the ankle mortise, avulsion of the ligaments from their attachment site, dislocation of the talus, or nerve involvement.[33]

Lateral Ankle Sprains

The ankle complex is least stable when it is in the **open-packed position** (loose-packed position) of plantarflexion and inversion (supination), leaving the lateral ankle ligaments vulnerable in this position. The inversion component of supination is most commonly used to describe mechanism of injury to the lateral ankle ligament complex. Many athletic skills require extreme amounts of supination, thereby predisposing the ankle to injury.

A sudden, forceful supination of the foot and ankle can tear the lateral ligaments. The specific structures injured depend on the position of the talocrural joint and the amount of force applied to the structures. Because it becomes taut when the foot and ankle are supinated, the anterior talofibular ligament is the most commonly sprained ankle ligament. If the amount of supination is sufficient or if the ankle is near its neutral position, the calcaneofibular ligament also may be traumatized. Significantly more force is required to invert the ankle in its dorsiflexed, closed-packed position, primarily stressing the lateral malleolus and posterior talofibular ligament (Examination Findings 9-1).

Examination Findings 9-1
Lateral Ankle Sprains

Examination Segment	Clinical Findings
History of Current Condition	*Onset:* Acute *Pain characteristics:* Lateral aspect of the ankle around the area of the malleolus and sinus tarsi *Other symptoms:* The patient may report an associated "pop." *Mechanism:* Supination (calcaneal inversion), plantarflexion, or talar rotation in any combination *Risk factors:* A history of ankle sprain leading to decreased proprioceptive ability, decreased strength, and/or a lack of muscular coordination[34-36] Achilles tendon and/or triceps surae tightness; tarsal coalition Pes cavus/supinated foot type Overweight as indicated by high body mass index (BMI)[36,37]
Functional Assessment	Gait observation reveals antalgic gait with shortened stance phase on involved side; ankle maintained in resting position of slight plantarflexion The patient's ability to balance on a single leg may be diminished.[1]
Inspection	Findings include swelling around the lateral joint capsule, which may spread to the dorsum of the foot and into the sinus tarsi. Ecchymosis may be present around the lateral malleolus.
Palpation	Pain is elicited along the involved ligaments but may be diffuse during the initial examination.[29] The sinus tarsi may be sensitive. Crepitus at the site of ligamentous origin or insertion may indicate an avulsion fracture.
Joint and Muscle Function Assessment	*AROM:* Pain on the lateral side of the ankle during plantarflexion and inversion indicates stretching of the lateral ligaments. Pain medially indicates a pinching of the medial structures. *MMT:* Peroneals are weak and painful. Extensor digitorum longus is weak and painful. *PROM:* Pain at end range along the ligaments, primarily: –**Inversion and plantarflexion:** Anterior talofibular ligament, calcaneofibular ligament –**Inversion, neutral position:** Calcaneofibular ligament –**Inversion and dorsiflexion:** Posterior talofibular ligament
Joint Stability Tests	*Stress tests:* A positive inversion stress test and/or anterior drawer test results in laxity and/or pain. *Joint play:* Increased medial glide at the subtalar joint; increased talocrural dorsal glide
Selective Tissue Tests	Squeeze test to rule out a fracture of the distal fibula
Neurological Screening	Repeated lateral ankle sprains may result in neuropathy of the peroneal and/or sural nerves.[1] Sensory testing of the peroneal nerve distribution is needed if neurological symptoms are present.
Vascular Screening	Within normal limits
Imaging Techniques	MR images may detect an osteochondral lesion on the superomedial talus or the inferior tibial articulating surface.[38] Ultrasonic imagining is helpful in ruling out a rupture of the lateral ligaments; all imaging techniques offer minimal value in ruling in a rupture: Patients with negative radiographs who still experience pain after 2–4 weeks of conservative rehabilitation should be referred for bone scan, MR, or CT imaging.[38] Ultrasonic images have a LR+ of 2.55 and a LR– of 0.13 in determining lateral ligament ruptures.[26] Stress radiographs have a LR+ of 2.34 and LR–1 of 0.45 in determining lateral ligament ruptures.[26]
Differential Diagnosis	Syndesmotic ankle sprain; subluxating peroneal tendon; tear of the peroneus brevis tendon or muscle; subtalar joint sprain; lateral malleolus fracture; medial malleolus fracture; osteochondral fracture of the talus; Jones fracture
Comments	An avulsion fracture of the lateral ligaments from the malleolus, impingement of the medial joint capsule, impingement of the structures beneath the medial malleolus, and possible fracture of the medial malleolus or base of the 5th MT can occur concurrently with a lateral ankle sprain. A chondral defect may be present in the articulating surfaces of the superior portion of the anteromedial talus and/or the inferior portion of the anteromedial tibia. Adolescents displaying ankle instability should be referred for radiographic examination to rule out the possibility of an epiphyseal injury. Persistent anterolateral ankle pain following lateral ankle sprains may indicate abnormal synovial thickening.[39]

AROM = active range of motion; CT = computed tomography; LR+ = positive likelihood ratio; LR- = negative likelihood ratio; MMT = manual muscle test; MR = magnetic resonance; MT = metatarsal; PROM = passive range of motion

✱ Practical Evidence

Subtalar joint hypermobility is associated with talocrural instability in approximately 66% of cases, although it is unclear if this is causative or a result of pathology.[30]

Anatomic and physiologic factors predisposing individuals to lateral ankle sprains include decreased proprioceptive ability, decreased muscular strength, and a lack of muscular coordination, all factors associated with a history of multiple ankle sprains.[35,40] Tightness of the Achilles tendon or the triceps surae muscle group creates an increased risk of sprains to the lateral ligament complex by placing the ankle complex in a plantarflexed position.

The primary clinical finding of a lateral ankle sprain is a history of inversion, plantarflexion, and/or rotation (see Table 9-3). Patients may also describe a sensation of tearing or "popping." Pain is localized along the lateral ligament complex and sinus tarsi. Because the anterior talofibular and posterior talofibular ligaments are capsular structures, tears of these ligaments can produce rapid, diffuse swelling. Being extracapsular, the calcaneofibular ligament produces relatively little edema when it is damaged. Sprains of the posterior talofibular ligamer rarely occur and are usually associated with an ankle dislocation.[6]

Palpation elicits tenderness along the involved ligament. The associated joint capsule and the sinus tarsi may become tender.[18] Pay special attention to pain and crepitus elicited over the origin and insertion of the ligament, indicating a possible avulsion fracture. Pain is demonstrated during the movements of inversion or plantarflexion, as described in the Joint and Muscle Function Assessment and the Joint Stability Testing sections of this chapter.

✱ Practical Evidence

The accuracy and usefulness of the clinical findings for a lateral ankle sprain improve with time.[29] Five days following the injury, pain elicited during palpation of the ATF ligament, lateral ecchymosis, and a positive anterior drawer is 96% specific in detecting ligament ruptures.[34]

The severity and relative damage associated with moderate ankle sprains is often underestimated, and other trauma caused by the injury mechanism may be overlooked.[41] Excessive inversion can place compressive forces on the medial structures; exert a tensile force on the peroneal tendons and peroneal nerve; and involve the Achilles tendon, tibialis posterior, extensor digitorum brevis, and calcaneocuboid ligament.[33] The subtalar joint is often sprained at the same time as the lateral ankle ligaments.[29]

Inverting the talus can impinge the medial ligaments, medial joint capsule, and the structures passing beneath the medial malleolus, especially the tibialis posterior tendon. Excessive inversion of the talus and calcaneus can result in the fracture of the distal medial malleolus, base, or styloid process of the fifth MT; or avulse the lateral ligaments from their site of origin or insertion (Fig. 9-20).

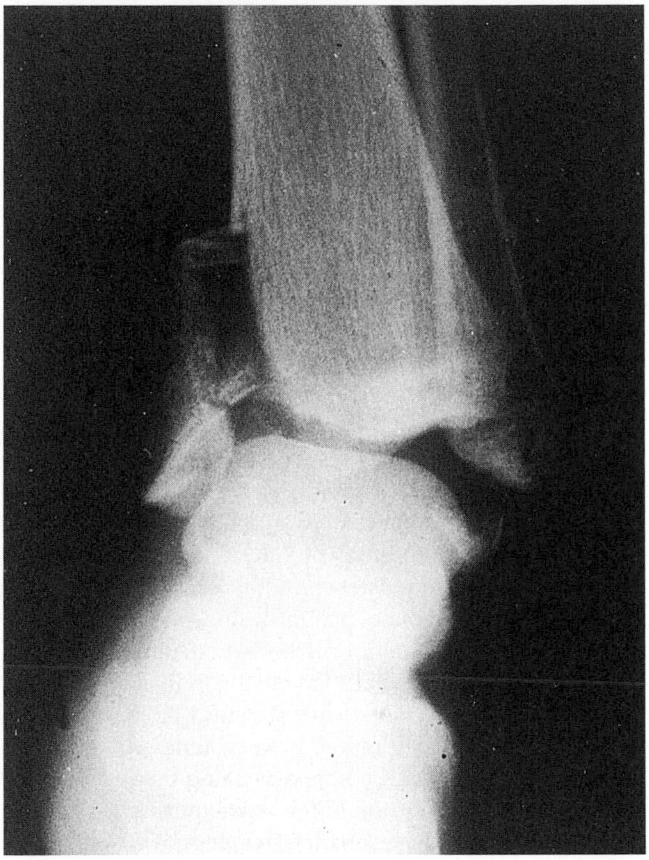

FIGURE 9-20 ■ Posterior view of a fracture of the right medial malleolus caused by excessive inversion of the ankle.

A complete examination of a lateral ankle sprain should also include an examination of the foot.[42] Mobility of the subtalar joint, midtarsal joints, and first ray should be the focus of this segment of the examination.

The risk of recurrent lateral ankle sprains increases when the ankle is both mechanically and functionally unstable.[43] Chronic lateral ankle instability is classified as either mechanical, functional, or both.[1,5] Mechanical instability is characterized by gross laxity to one or more of the ankle's joints or insufficiency of the supporting structures. Functional instability is a self-reported finding that involves repeated ankle sprains in individuals who have normal findings during ligamentous stress tests and is associated with proprioceptive and neuromuscular deficits, decreased strength, and/or postural control.[5]

Moderate to severe ankle sprains result in recurrence rates greater than 70%, with approximately 60% of those affected experiencing residual deficits on athletic performance.[44] Pain and instability are often reported 1 year following the initial injury.[45] Basketball players with a history of ankle sprains are five times more likely to suffer an ankle sprain than players who have no history of sprain.[35] There are two possible explanations for this:[46] (1) the loss of the ligament's ability to passively support and protect the joint in conjunction with a reflex arc that is too slow to evoke a contraction in the peroneal muscles, limiting the force and speed of inversion;[47] and (2) decreased proprioceptive ability of the capsule, ligaments, and peroneal muscles.[48,49]

Chronic or severe lateral ankle sprains often result in a number of secondary conditions. After a sprain of the anterior talofibular and calcaneofibular ligaments, the anterolateral capsule may develop a dense area of thickened connective tissue that becomes impinged between the lateral malleolus and calcaneus when the foot and ankle are dorsiflexed and everted.[50] Bone bruises; accumulations of blood within the talus, navicular, and calcaneus;[51] and longitudinal tears of the peroneus brevis tendon[52] are also associated with lateral ankle sprains. Recurrent pain behind the lateral malleolus following a significant lateral ankle sprain or in the presence of chronic lateral ankle instability is highly suggestive of a peroneal tendon lesion and/or subluxation.

Lateral ankle sprains may produce an associated talar or tibial **chondral lesion** (osteochondral defect) caused by the combination of inversion, plantarflexion, and talar rotation that compress the superior medial articulating cartilage of the talus against the tibia.[38] Patients with these small fractures, not easily identified with standard radiographic examination, commonly report pain of unidentified origin "deep in the ankle" and tenderness along the superior anteromedial (tibial) portion of the ankle mortise (Fig. 9-21). The use of magnetic resonance imaging (MRI) and computed tomography (CT) scans has improved the accuracy in diagnosing chondral lesions.[53,54] If this condition goes unrecognized, osteochondritis dissecans of the talocrural joint is likely to develop.[55,56]

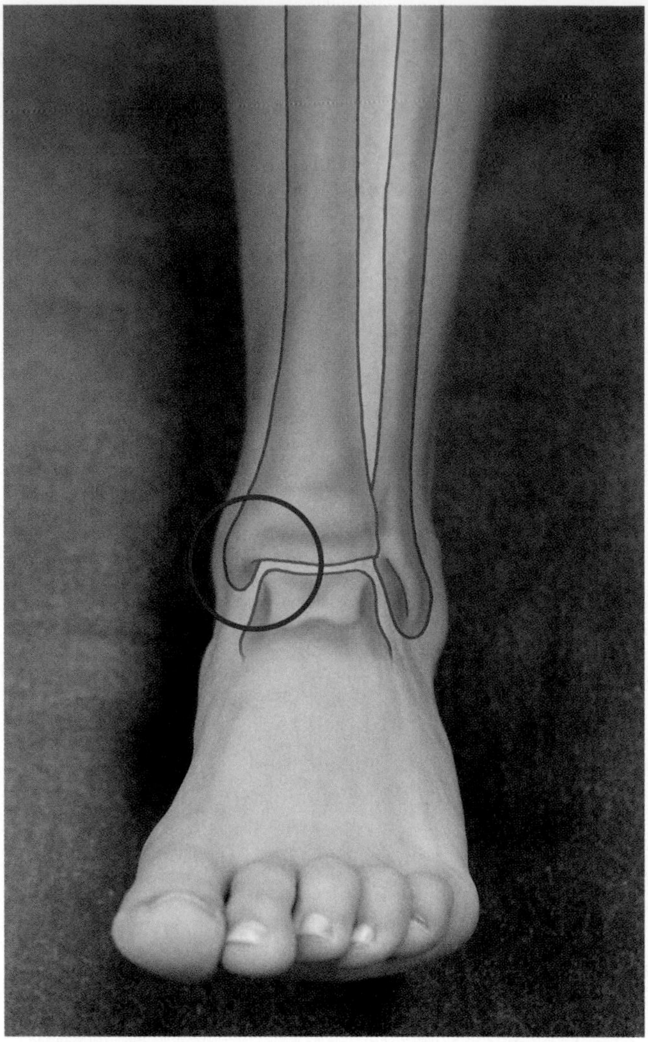

FIGURE 9-21 ■ Location of a tibial osteochondral lesion following an lateral ankle sprain. As the talus inverts, its superomedial border may contact the tibia with sufficient force to cause a bony defect in either the tibia or talus.

Traction injuries to the peroneal nerve can affect the sensory and motor function of the leg and ankle. Decreased sensory function may be present in the involved ankle immediately after forceful plantarflexion and inversion. After a severe sprain, inhibition of sensory and motor function can extend as far as the hip.[57]

Take extra care when evaluating apparent ankle sprains in adolescents. Patients displaying excessive laxity require referral to a physician to rule out epiphyseal fractures.

Syndesmosis Sprains

Injury to the tib-fib syndesmosis accounts for less than 10% of all ankle sprains, but the rate is almost double that in professional football players.[58] Although representing only a small percentage of all ankle sprains, syndesmotic ankle sprains are associated with significantly longer time lost from activity compared with other types of ankle sprains.

During excessive external rotation of the talus or forced dorsiflexion, the talus places pressure on the fibula, causing the distal syndesmosis to spread.[59] The lateral displacement of the distal fibula can result in a sprain of the anterior and posterior tib-fib ligaments, the interosseous membrane, and the crural interosseous ligament (Fig. 9-22).

Syndesmosis sprains, also referred to as "high" ankle sprains, are attributed to playing on artificial surfaces, but research does not substantiate this claim.[11] Other factors contributing to the occurrence of syndesmotic ankle sprains include **collision sports** where the mechanism of injury involves planting the foot and "cutting" so that the talus is externally rotated and the foot is dorsiflexed.[59] Another common mechanism is being fallen on while lying on the ground, causing forced dorsiflexion and external rotation of the foot. Syndesmotic and deltoid ligament sprains often occur concurrently, so deltoid ligament trauma must be ruled out when examining syndesmosis injuries.[11,8] When both the syndesmosis and deltoid ligament are disrupted, the talus becomes inherently unstable within the mortise.[59]

Pain is located primarily on the anterior aspect of the ankle and proximally along the interosseous membrane

Collision sports Individual or team sports relying on the physical dominance of one athlete over another. By their nature, these sports involve violent physical contact.

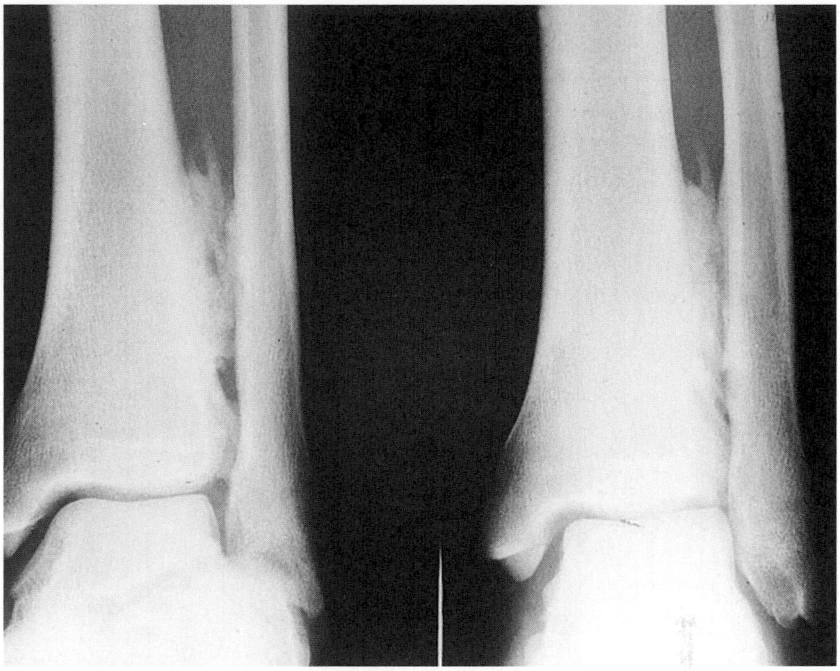

FIGURE 9-22 ■ Radiograph of a syndesmosis sprain. Note the wide gap between the tibia and fibula on the left image versus the image on the right. This injury results from the wide anterior border of the talus being forced into the mortise during hyperdorsiflexion, from external rotation of the foot, or both.

and is intensified during forced dorsiflexion, the **external rotation test** (Selective Tissue Test 9-1), or the **squeeze test** (Selective Tissue Test 9-2).[31,60] Pain is often reported during palpation of the anterior and posterior tib-fib ligaments (Examination Findings 9-2). The widening of the ankle mortise results in instability of the ankle as the talus is allowed a greater amount of glide within the joint. Other clinical findings include provocation of symptoms when the patient is weight bearing and moving the ankle into dorsiflexion and relieved when a compressive force is applied during the same movement (the **dorsiflexion-compression test**). When a syndesmotic sprain is suspected, palpate the entire length of the fibula for pain and crepitus. Forced dorsiflexion and external rotation can result in a Maisonneuve fracture, a spiral fracture of the proximal one-third of the fibula with concurrent disruption of the distal tib-fib syndesmosis (Fig. 9-23).

Medial Ankle Sprains

The strength of the deltoid ligament and the mechanical advantage of the longer lateral malleolus limit eversion. Because of the small amount of eversion (i.e., 5°) normally associated with the subtalar joint, the primary mechanism for damage to this ligament group is external rotation of the talus in the ankle mortise. These anatomic and biomechanical properties result in a low rate of deltoid ligament sprains, with reports from 3% to 15% of all ankle sprains. Deltoid sprains are frequently associated with other ankle pathology including syndesmotic sprains and malleolar fractures.[8,9,62] Because of its close association with the spring ligament, the stability of the medial longitudinal arch requires evaluation when a sprain of the deltoid ligament is suspected.

Physical examination findings can identify trauma to the medial ligaments. Pain is present along the medial joint line, especially the anterior portion, and swelling tends to be more localized than that associated with lateral ankle sprains (Examination Findings 9-3). If an eversion mechanism is described, the lateral malleolus should be carefully evaluated for the presence of a "knock-off" fracture (Fig. 9-24). Stress radiographs are indicated if the anteroposterior radiographs are negative for mortise disruption (less than 4 mm distance between medial malleolus and talus).[63]

Eversion may also cause an avulsion of the medial malleolus. A similar mechanism may cause bimalleolar fracture (**Pott's fracture**) and carries with it the increased potential complication of a nonunion of the medial malleolus unless surgery is performed. Intra-articular trauma to the talus and tibia may also be present.

Ankle Sprain Intervention Strategies

On-field care for individuals with ankle sprains is described later in this chapter. Current management of ankle sprains involves early mobilization in a pain-free range. Research suggests that early ROM exercises and other forms of mobilization decrease pain and swelling while increasing overall ROM.[64,65] Using braces that allow for early exercise may increase the number of adverse effects.[66] While early mobilization results in more residual subjective complaints, it has little long-term detrimental effect on athletic performance.[67] Weight bearing may be limited based on the structures involved or the patient's ability to ambulate normally. A complete rehabilitation program is required for all ankle sprains.

Surgical reconstruction for chronic ankle instability has varying amounts of success and is reserved for those cases where conservative treatment fails.[45,68] For complete ruptures of the lateral ligaments, operative treatment yields improved results relative to conservative treatments.[69]

Selective Tissue Test 9-2
Squeeze Test

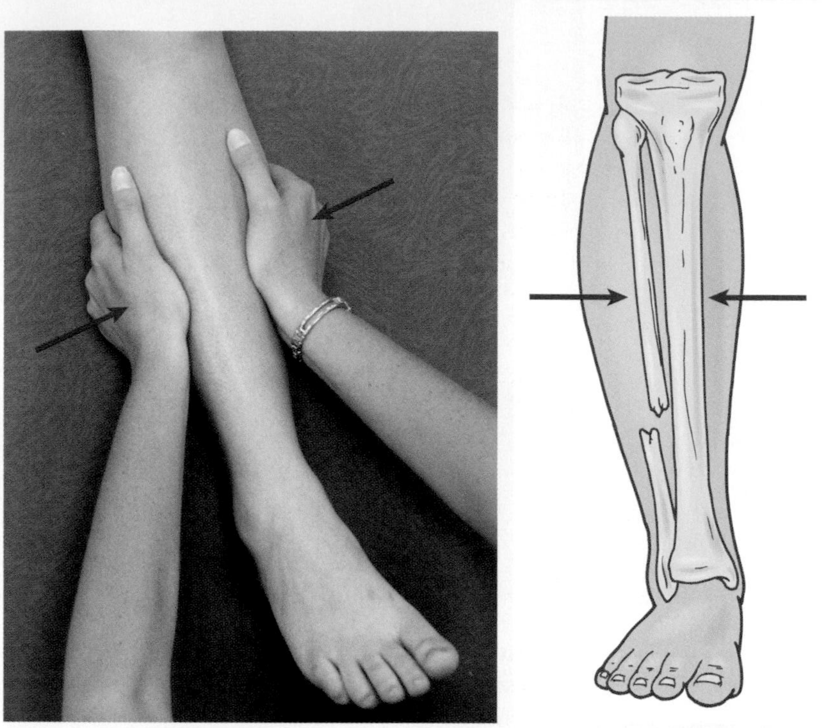

Squeeze test to identify fibular fractures or syndesmosis sprains. Pressure is applied transversely through the leg away from the site of pain. This test is unnecessary if clear fracture findings are present.

Patient Position	Lying with the knee extended
Position of Examiner	Standing next to, or in front of, the injured leg, with the examiner's hands cupped behind the tibia and fibula away from the site of pain
Evaluative Procedure	Gently squeeze (compress) the fibula and tibia, gradually adding more pressure if no pain or other symptoms are elicited. Progress toward the injured site until pain is elicited.
Positive Test	Pain is elicited, especially when it is away from the compressed area.
Implications	(A) Gross fracture or stress fracture of the fibula when pain is described along the fibular shaft (B) Syndesmosis sprain when pain is described at the distal tib-fib joint
Comments	Avoid applying too much pressure too soon into the test. Pressure should be applied gradually and progressively. The test is infrequently positive for syndesmosis sprains, even in the presence for syndesmosis sprains of other clinical findings indicative of a syndesmosis sprains. Its usefulness is limited.[31]
Evidence	

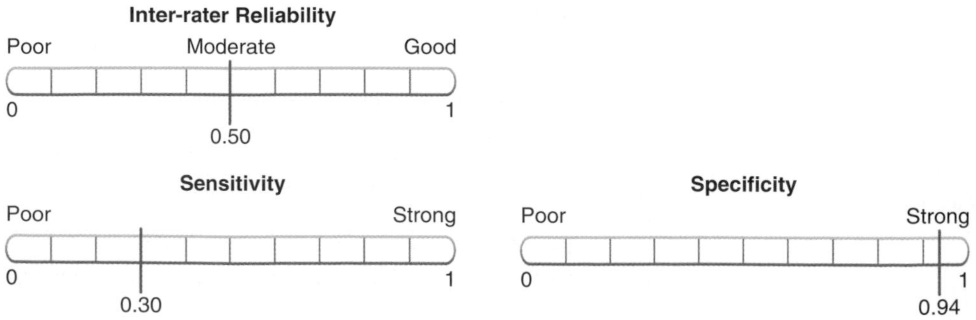

LR+: 4.62

LR−: 0.75

Examination Findings 9-2
Syndesmotic ("High") Ankle Sprains

Examination Segment	Clinical Findings
History of Current Condition	*Onset:* Acute *Pain characteristics:* Anterior portion of the distal tib-fib syndesmosis Pain may also be described on the posteromedial aspect of the ankle at the level of the talus.[8] *Mechanism:* External rotation of the talus within the ankle mortise and/or dorsiflexion Forced hyperdorsiflexion or hyperplantarflexion Internal rotation of the talus *Risk factors:* Activities on surfaces that have a high coefficient of friction between the shoe and playing surface (e.g., artificial turf), especially when sharp cutting or pivoting is required A planus foot type may increase the risk of syndesmosis sprains.[8]
Functional Assessment	Gait assessment may reveal shortened swing on the contralateral side to avoid full dorsiflexion. The patient describes decreased strength or pain when pushing off from the ground.[8] Toe gait may be noted on the involved side.
Inspection	Swelling present over the distal tib-fib syndesmosis, which is less prominent and widespread compared with lateral ankle sprains
Palpation	Pain over the distal tib-fib syndesmosis, especially on the anterior aspect Pain possibly elicited over the anterior and posterior tib-fib ligaments; unremarkable palpation of the ATF and CF ligaments[9] Palpate the deltoid ligament to rule in or rule out possible concurrent trauma.[59] Palpate the length of the fibula to rule out the presence of fibular fracture.[59]
Joint and Muscle Function Assessment	*AROM:* Motion is restricted, and pain is elicited, especially with dorsiflexion and eversion; but pain is also present at the end ranges of plantarflexion and inversion. Rotating the foot increases the pain anteriorly. *MMT:* The tibialis anterior and tibialis posterior may be weak and painful. Resisted testing in all directions can be inhibited by pain in more severe syndesmotic sprains. *PROM:* All motions are limited by pain, with the greatest decreases noted in dorsiflexion and eversion.
Joint Stability Tests	*Stress tests:* No significant findings *Joint play:* Anterior/posterior tib-fib joint play; distal fibular translation test[32] The amount of instability is increased when there is concurrent injury to the deltoid ligament.[8,9]
Selective Tissue Tests	External rotation test Dorsiflexion-compression test Squeeze test Cotton test
Neurological Screening	Within normal limits
Vascular Screening	Within normal limits
Imaging Techniques	Injury to the distal tib-fib syndesmosis may not be apparent in standard radiographs.[9] Standard mortise view to evaluate the talocrural angle and amount of talar tilt Stress test with external rotation of the ankle is better than standard mortise view to detect separation of tib-fib syndesmosis.[61] MRI demonstrates high sensitivity and specificity for the presence of a syndosmotic disruption.[62]
Differential Diagnosis	Lateral ankle sprain; fibular fracture; deltoid ligament sprain
Comments	Heterotopic ossification or synostosis of the interosseous membrane may develop over time. Syndesmosis sprains often occur concurrently with deltoid ligament sprains and/or fractures of the medial malleolus.[9] The presence of a Maisonneuve fracture should be ruled out. Syndesmotic sprains have an increased recovery time relative to other types of ankle sprains.

CF = calcaneofibular; AROM = active range of motion; ATF = anterior talofibular; MMT = manual muscle test; MRI = magnetic resonance imaging; PROM = passive range of motion

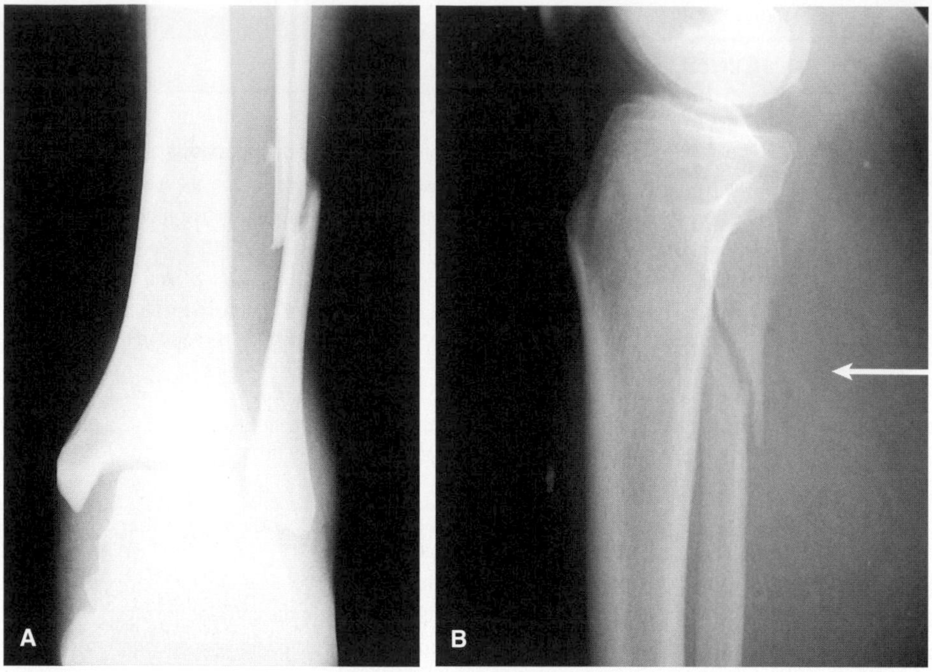

FIGURE 9-23 ■ (A) Fracture of the fibula concurrent with a sprain of the distal tibiofibular syndesmosis. When this fracture occurs proximally on the fibula, it is termed a Maisonneuve fracture (B).

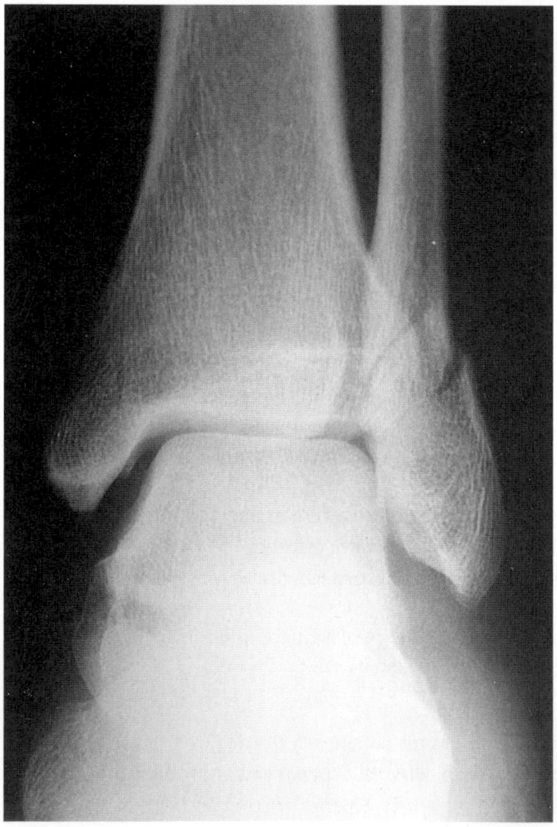

FIGURE 9-24 ■ Fracture of the lateral malleolus caused by excessive eversion of the ankle (anterior view of the left ankle). This type of fracture to the lateral malleolus is more common as it extends farther inferiorly than does the medial malleolus.

Syndesmotic sprains require a longer recovery period than lateral ankle sprains do. The amount of talar instability and pain are increased when the deltoid ligament is also damaged.[8,9] Patients also may benefit from a period of non–weight-bearing activity or immobilization.[11,58] Over time, **heterotopic ossification** or **synostosis** of the interosseous membrane may develop, prolonging pain during the push-off phase of gait.[11] If heterotopic ossification develops, surgery may be required.[70]

Ankle and Leg Fractures

Acute fractures and dislocations of the leg, especially those involving the tibial shaft, often exhibit obvious gross deformity (Fig. 9-25). Significant force is required to fracture the tibial shaft, but inversion, eversion, or rotational forces can fracture the fibula and/or malleoli. Fractures involving the talus and calcaneus will produce more subtle findings and may mimic those of a sprain. Trauma involving the fibula may also disrupt the interosseous membrane, causing a Maisonneuve fracture (see Fig. 9-23B).[71] When only the shaft of the fibula is fractured, it is referred to as a Hugier or high Dupuytren fracture. Fractures of the ankle mortise such as a **trimalleolar fracture**, the concurrent fracture of the medial malleolus, lateral malleolus, and the posterior distal tibia (the

Synostosis The union of two bones through the formation of connective tissue

Examination Findings 9-3
Medial Ankle Sprains

Examination Segment	Clinical Findings
History of Current Condition	*Onset:* Acute *Pain characteristics:* Medial border of the ankle and foot, radiating from the medial malleolus *Mechanism:* Eversion and/or rotation *Risk factors:* Activities such as soccer that load the medial aspect of the foot
Functional Assessment	Decreased strength or medial pain during most motions secondary to stretching of the medial ligaments Gait evaluation reveals shortened midstance phase and/or supinated gait as the patient avoids pronation. Increased pain during midstance phase of gait
Inspection	Swelling around the medial joint capsule
Palpation	Pain around the deltoid ligaments Crepitus at the site of ligamentous origin or insertion may indicate an avulsion fracture.
Joint and Muscle Function Assessment	*AROM:* Pain on the medial side of the ankle during plantarflexion indicates stretching of the anterior tibiotalar and/or or the tibionavicular ligaments. Pain during dorsiflexion indicates trauma to the posterior tibiotalar ligament. Lateral pain may indicate a pinching of the lateral ligaments and/or trauma to the lateral malleolus. *MMT:* Posterior tibialis pain and weakness *PROM:* Motion produces pain along the ligaments (also see Table 9-2).
Joint Stability Tests	*Stress tests:* Eversion stress test *Joint play:* Cotton test Talonavicular joint play (See Joint Play 8.2)
Selective Tissue Tests	External rotation test
Neurological Screening	Posterior tibial nerve
Vascular Screening	Within normal limits
Imaging Techniques	Radiographs are used to rule out bony trauma and evaluate the width of the ankle mortise; stress images may be obtained. MRI may be ordered to ascertain soft tissue trauma.
Differential Diagnosis	Posterior tibialis tear; fibular fracture; distal syndesmosis sprain; medial malleolus fracture; posterior tibial neuropathy
Comments	The anterior fibers of the deltoid ligament tend to be most frequently involved in medial ankle sprains.[6] Excessive calcaneal eversion can result in a fracture of the lateral malleolus or talar dome or a disruption of the syndesmosis. An external rotation mechanism warrants a careful evaluation of the syndesmosis. The possibility of a fracture must be ruled out.

AROM = active range of motion; MMT = manual muscle test; MRI = magnetic resonance imaging; PROM = passive range of motion

posterior malleolus), can result in the rupture of the associated ligaments and talar dislocation.

The patient (or others near where the injury occurred) report an audible snap or crack at the time of injury. The patient reports pain at the fracture site, possibly radiating up the leg and extremity. Palpation, which should not be performed over obvious fractures, may reveal crepitus or discontinuity along the bone shaft (Examination Findings 9-4).

Although long bone fractures normally result in immediate dysfunction and an inability to bear weight, those suffering from fibular fractures may be capable of walking. In cases in which deformity or other signs of a gross

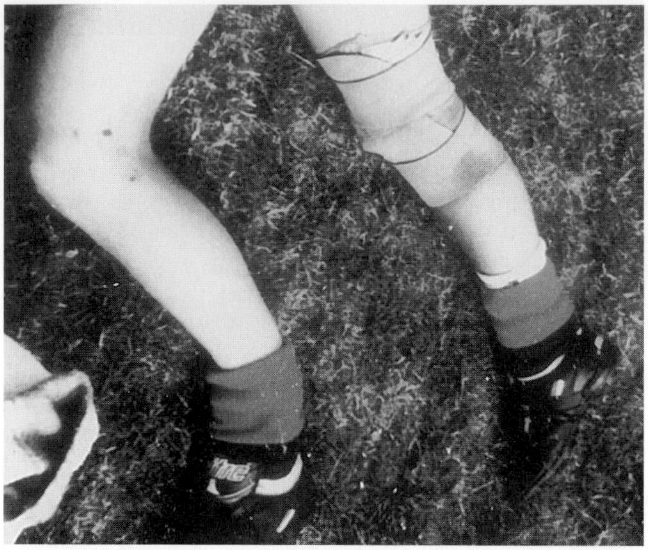

FIGURE 9-25 ■ Obvious deformity caused by a leg fracture and possible ankle dislocation.

fracture are absent, the squeeze test may confirm a fibular fracture.

Historically, emergency room personnel routinely obtain radiographs for all patients with foot and ankle trauma to rule out the presence of a fracture, thereby increasing the costs of the visit. The modified OAR use palpation findings and the patient's ability to bear weight to determine the need for radiographs (Box 9-3).[29,72,73] When the OAR protocol is followed, it is unlikely that a fracture will be missed, especially in children.[74-77]

Anteroposterior and lateral radiographs are used to rule out or more precisely identify fractures involving the tibia and/or fibula. Fractures involving the articular surface, especially the talus, which is difficult to clinically diagnose, are more readily identified using CT or MR imaging.[79] The presence of radiographic stress findings (external rotation force) is not well correlated with physical examination findings such as point tenderness, ecchymosis, and swelling.[63] See Management of Leg Fractures and Ankle Dislocations, p. 296.

Examination Findings 9-4
Ankle and Leg Fractures

Examination Segment	Clinical Findings
History of Current Condition	*Onset:* Acute *Pain characteristics:* Sharp and localized *Mechanism:* A direct blow; inversion or eversion stress
Functional Assessment	None indicated
Inspection	May or may not present with visible deformity Swelling and ecchymosis may be present.
Palpation	Point tender, possible crepitus, possible palpable deformity
Joint and Muscle Function Assessment	*AROM:* Do not perform if a fracture is suspected. *MMT:* Do not perform if a fracture is suspected. *PROM:* Do not perform if a fracture is suspected.
Joint Stability Tests	*Stress tests:* Do not perform if a fracture is suspected. *Joint play:* Do not perform if a fracture is suspected.
Selective Tissue Tests	Squeeze test (do not perform in the presence of an obvious fracture)
Neurological Screening	Within normal limits
Vascular Screening	Within normal limits
Imaging Techniques	Radiograph CT or MRI to detect talar fractures
Differential Diagnosis	Lateral ankle sprain, talocrural joint dislocation, subtalar dislocation, deltoid ligament sprain, compartment syndrome
Comments	Management depends on the involved bone and the extent of deformity. Leg and ankle fractures may be emergent. Management for shock may be required. See "On-Field Examination" for footwear removal instructions.

AROM = active range of motion; CT = computed tomography; MMT = manual muscle test; MRI = magnetic resonance imaging; PROM = passive range of motion

Box 9-3
Ottawa Ankle Rules

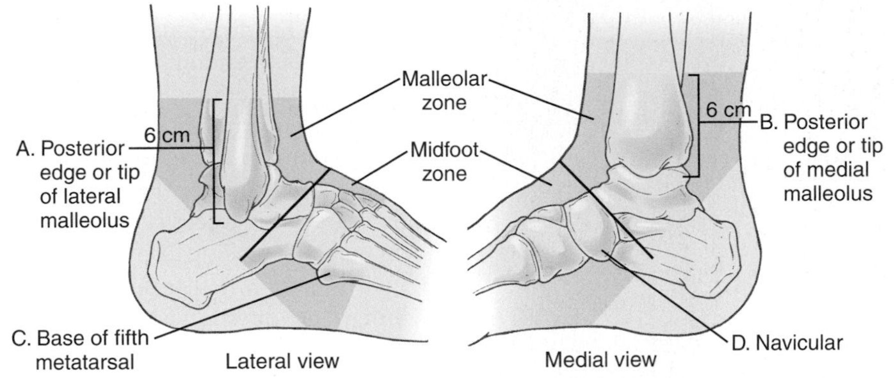

Description

The modified Ottawa Ankle Rules provide evaluative criteria to identify when to refer the patient for radiographs.

Criteria for Radiographic Referral

The patient is unable to walk four steps both immediately following the injury and at the time of examination.

Ankle radiographs should be ordered if pain is elicited during palpation of Zone A or B.

Foot radiographs should be ordered if pain is elicited during palpation of Zone C or D.

Modification

Zones A and B are changed to include pain over the midline of the medial and lateral malleoli.[29,78]

Evidence

Designed to have a high sensitivity so that fractures are not missed, the Ottawa Ankle Rules have a high negative predictive value when applied to a skeletally mature population. The rules have also been validated in children.[76] If the rules are followed, it is highly likely that a fracture will not be missed.[74,75] The conservative nature of the rules results in a relatively low specificity (0.26–0.48), indicating that many patients are still referred for radiographs who do not have a fracture. With the modification relating to the location of the malleolar pain, the specificity is improved to 0.42–0.59.[29,78]

Os Trigonum Injury

An os trigonum is formed when **Stieda's process** separates from the talus (Fig. 9-26).[80,81] Stieda's process first appears between the ages of 8 and 13, normally fusing within 1 year after its appearance.[82,83] Developmentally, an os trigonum occurs in approximately 7% of the population when the secondary center of ossification fails to fuse the process to the talus (Fig. 9-27). A traumatic os trigonum is formed by a nonunion fracture or stress fracture of Stieda's process.[82,83] Athletes, particularly those whose activity requires sustained plantarflexion, such as dancers, are at an increased risk of sustaining an injury to this structure.[84,85]

Symptoms arise when an os trigonum impinges on surrounding tissues. Os trigonum syndrome (also referred to as **talar compression syndrome**) may involve (1) an inflammation of the posterior joint, (2) inflammation of the ligaments surrounding the os trigonum, (3) a fracture of the os trigonum, or (4) pathology involving the Stieda's process.[81] Subtalar and midtarsal joint pronation causes

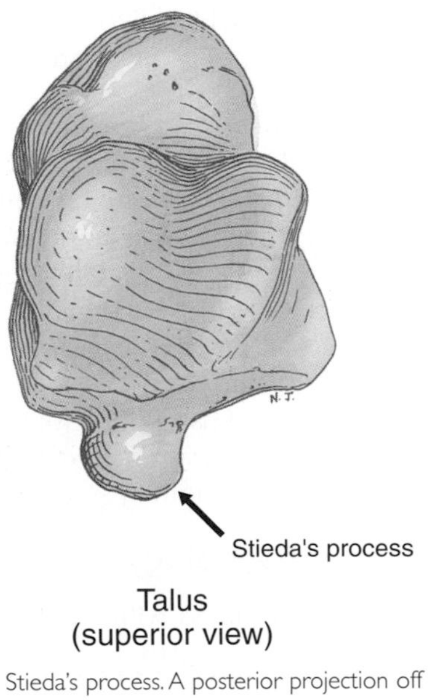

FIGURE 9-26 ■ Stieda's process. A posterior projection off the talus.

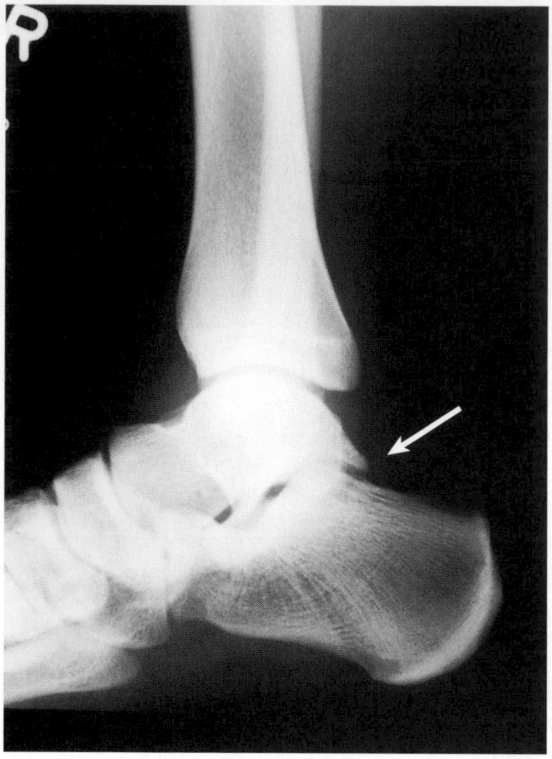

FIGURE 9-27 ■ Radiograph of an os trigonum (medial view of the right ankle). The arrow indicates the location of the os trigonum, a fracture of Stieda's process. A fracture line can be seen at the midpoint on the process.

the os trigonum or Stieda's process to become compressed between the tibia and calcaneus.[81]

Inflammatory conditions of the os trigonum become symptomatic after activity or with repetitive microtrauma.[86] Os trigonum fractures are characterized by the sudden onset of pain after forced plantarflexion or dorsiflexion. Swelling lateral or medial to the Achilles tendon may be noted. During palpation, patients report tenderness anterior to the Achilles tendon and posterior to the talus. Ankle plantarflexion may produce pain during ROM testing (Examination Findings 9-5). Plain film radiographs are used to identify the presence of an os trigonum.[87]

Ankle and Leg Fracture Intervention Strategies

The treatment protocol is based on the patient's symptoms. Patients use a walker boot or cast with no weight bearing or partial weight bearing until they can ambulate without pain and a normal gait pattern. Patients can return to their activities after restoring full pain-free ROM and strength to the leg. The use of a viscoelastic heel insert may be helpful to absorb ground reaction forces. If the condition becomes chronic, the evaluation and use of a permanent orthotic to control foot motion may be warranted or surgical removal of the os trigonum may be required.

Achilles Tendon Pathology

Because of its dual association with the two prime plantarflexors, the gastrocnemius and the soleus, any injury to the Achilles tendon results in decreased plantarflexion strength. This decrease may cause significant changes in gait, impairing the patient's ability to walk, run, and jump normally.

Achilles Tendinopathy

The Achilles tendon receives only a limited blood supply from the posterior tibial artery. The distal avascular zone, 2 to 6 cm proximal to its insertion on the calcaneus, is the most common site of tendon pathology, including inflammation and rupture (Fig. 9-28).[88,89] The tendon's response to aggravating forces is impeded by the poor blood supply in the area, causing delayed healing.

The poor vascular supply of the Achilles tendon itself brings into question whether inflammation is even possible within the tendon's substance, as the available blood supply may not be sufficient to provide a widespread inflammatory response. The tendon is, however, surrounded by a highly vascular structure, the **paratenon**.[23] Inflammation of the paratenon, **peritendinitis**, produces pain and forms adhesions with the underlying tendon.[89,90] In chronic cases, peritendinitis can cause the paratenon to become fibrotic and **stenosed**.[12] **Tendinosis** is the degeneration of the tendon's substance, starting with microscopic tears and necrotic areas within the tendon as the result of decreased blood flow through the paratenon.[12] Although this breakdown is not always a precursor to a tendon rupture, tendinosis represents a progressive degeneration of the tendon:[89]

Peritendinitis → Tendinosis → Tendon rupture

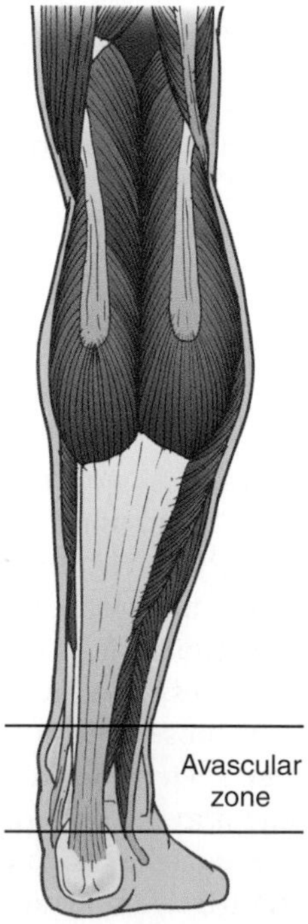

FIGURE 9-28 ■ Achilles tendon avascular zone. The distal 6 cm of the tendon, devoid of a significant blood supply, is a common site of tendinosis.

Stenosed Narrowing of a structure; stenosis

Examination Findings 9-5
Medial Ankle Sprains

Examination Segment	Clinical Findings
History of Current Condition	*Onset:* Acute or insidious: increased pain with activity Sudden onset of pain may suggest a fracture. *Pain characteristics:* Posterior aspect of the talus, anterior to the Achilles tendon *Mechanism:* Acute: forced hyperplantarflexion Chronic or insidious: repetitive activity usually involving plantarflexion *Risk factors:* The presence of an nonunited lateral tubercle on the posterior aspect of the talus (os trigonum)
Functional Assessment	Decreased push-off during ambulation; may demonstrate limited capacity to plantarflex for those activities that require it (e.g., ballet, gymnastics)
Inspection	Swelling possibly observed anteromedial and anterolateral to the Achilles tendon
Palpation	Pain elicited when palpating the posterior talus, anterior to the Achilles tendon
Joint and Muscle Function Assessment	*AROM:* Pain with plantarflexion *MMT:* Gastrocnemius and soleus testing may reproduce symptoms. Pain when performing a heel raise *PROM:* Pain with forced plantarflexion, compressing the structures Pain with forced dorsiflexion, stretching the structures
Joint Stability Tests	*Stress tests:* No significant findings *Joint play:* No significant findings
Selective Tissue Tests	Not applicable
Neurological Screening	Within normal limits
Vascular Screening	Within normal limits
Imaging Techniques	A definitive diagnosis is made with correlation of findings with the presence of an os trigonum on radiographs or MRI.
Differential Diagnosis	Achilles tendinopathy; tibialis posterior tendinopathy; flexor hallucis longus tendinopathy; peroneal tendon subluxation; lateral ankle instability; arthritis, TTS; tarsal coalition; talus fracture; subtendinous bursitis

AROM = active range of motion; MMT = manual muscle test; MRI = magnetic resonance imaging; PROM = passive range of motion; TTS = tarsal tunnel syndrome

Tendon ruptures are not always complete. Approximately 20% of peritendinitis cases are associated with a partial rupture of the Achilles tendon, especially along the tendon's lateral border.[12,89] Unlike frank ruptures, partial ruptures can occur in otherwise young, well-conditioned individuals (see Achilles Tendon Rupture).[89]

Anatomic factors that lead to the onset of Achilles tendon pathology include tibial varum, calcaneovalgus, hyperpronation, and tightness of the triceps surae and the hamstring muscle groups.[89] Running mechanics, an increase in the duration and intensity of running, the type of shoe, running surface, weak plantarflexion strength, and increased dorsiflexion (greater than 9°) can result in Achilles peritendinitis.[91] Achilles tendinopathy may also have an acute onset as the result of a direct blow to the tendon. Certain antibiotic medications such as fluoroquinolones (e.g., ciprofloxacin) have been associated with Achilles tendon pathology, including tendon ruptures.[92] Age and gender are the strongest predictors of Achilles tendon injury. As age increases, so does the risk of Achilles tendon pathology, especially in males, who have three times the risk of developing symptoms than females do.[93,94]

Individuals suffering from Achilles tendinopathy describe pain or "burning" radiating along the length of the tendon, although it is common for the patient to be relatively asymptomatic with the exception of a palpable nodule within the distal tendon. The area may be tender to the touch and crepitus may be elicited, particularly with active ROM. This condition may be the result of or may result in tightness of the triceps surae muscle group (Examination Findings 9-6). MRI is useful in definitively diagnosing the pathology leading to Achilles tendon pain and identifying the predisposition to ruptures.[92]

Inflammation of the Achilles tendon insertion on the calcaneus is categorized as tendinitis (**insertional tendinitis**).[23] The patient complains of posterior heel pain, increased pain during activities such as hill running and interval programs, and awaking with a "stiff" ankle. Physical examination yields tenderness on the tendon's calcaneal insertion and decreased dorsiflexion.

Examination Findings 9-6
Achilles Tendinopathy

Examination Segment	Clinical Findings
History of Current Condition	*Onset:* Insidious or the result of trauma to the Achilles tendon *Pain characteristics:* Along the length of the Achilles tendon *Other symptoms:* The patient may describe a "squeaking" sensation. *Mechanism:* Tendinitis is typically an acute onset relating to a sudden, large increase in load or a blow to the Achilles tendon. Tendinosis results from repetitive stressors and subsequent local tissue degeneration. An improperly fitting shoe rubbing against the tendon may also activate the inflammatory response. *Risk factors:* Tibial varum; calcaneal valgum; hypo- or hypermobile foot type; tightness of the triceps surae muscle group; risk increasing with age, especially in the male population Decreased strength of the plantarflexors and increased dorsiflexion ROM[91] Sudden change in the duration and/or intensity of training Ankle sprains or other foot/ankle pathology resulting in toe-only gait and subsequent shortening of the Achilles tendon
Functional Assessment	Decreased push-off during gait; shortened stride length on contralateral side
Inspection	Possible visible edema along the length of the tendon; tendon on involved leg may appear thicker than on opposite leg A discrete nodule may be seen and felt along the distal tendon.[12]
Palpation	Haglund deformity may be noted (see Fig. 8-18, p 197). Pain elicited during palpation of the tendon, especially 2–6 cm proximal to the tendon's insertion on the calcaneus[12]
Joint and Muscle Function Assessment	*AROM:* Function Assessment Pain and crepitus during plantarflexion and dorsiflexion Dorsiflexion ROM possibly diminished secondary to Achilles tendon tightness *MMT:* Plantarflexion (gastrocnemius and soleus) is painful and/or weak. *PROM:* Pain at end range of dorsiflexion, resulting from stretching the tendon; dorsiflexion may be decreased
Joint Stability Tests	*Stress tests:* Not applicable *Joint play:* Hypomobile lateral glide of the talus
Selective Tissue Tests	None
Neurological Screening	Within normal limits
Vascular Screening	Within normal limits
Imaging Techniques	MR images can identify partial tears or thickening of the tendon.
Differential Diagnosis	Subcutaneous calcaneal bursitis; subtendinous calcaneal bursitis; insertional Achilles tendinitis; Sever's disease
Comments	Achilles tendinopathy may also involve a partial tear of the tendon.

AROM = active range of motion; MR = magnetic resonance; MMT = manual muscle test; PROM = passive range of motion

Most cases of Achilles tendinopathy are traced to overuse syndromes and repeated eccentric loading of the tendon. Individuals with foot rigidity are predisposed to this condition because gait must be modified to compensate for a valgus or varus rearfoot. Improperly fitting footwear may cause friction between the heel counter and the tendon, and shoes with a rigid sole may not permit adequate ROM in the midfoot and forefoot, altering the biomechanics of the foot, ankle, and leg.

Sever's Disease

Calcaneal apophysitis, Sever's disease, involves the inflammation of an unfused **apophysis** in children and is the most common source of heel pain in athletes aged 5 to 11.[95] Foot postures other than normal[96] (e.g., forefoot varus, see Inspection Findings 8-3) and tightness of the triceps surae[97] that affect lower extremity biomechanics appear to be the primary predisposition to this condition. Repetitive tensile forces on the Achilles tendon insertion on the calcaneus cause inflammation.

Patients afflicted with calcaneal apophysitis complain of activity-related pain in the posterior heel that decreases (or resolves) with rest. The patient may assume a touch-toe gait to reduce pressure on the insertion of the Achilles tendon. Palpation and bilateral compression of the calcaneus (squeezing the calcaneus) worsens pain. This condition occurs bilaterally in up to 60% of the population.[96] Although radiographs are often obtained, the diagnosis of calcaneal apophysitis is primarily a clinical determination.[98,99] Those cases that are apparent on radiographs require a more aggressive course of care.[100]

Achilles Tendinopathy Intervention Strategies

Physicians often prescribe anti-inflammatory medications for those with acute or moderate inflammatory conditions, and they may add heel lifts to reduce the stresses placed on the Achilles tendon. In advanced cases, immobilization may be required, but the strength of the triceps surae muscle group is slow to return after this technique.[101] Corticosteroid injections are seldom considered to control chronic or severe inflammation because there is an increased risk of suffering an Achilles tendon rupture for 1 week after the injection.[93,102]

Stretching of the Achilles tendon and triceps surae and hamstrings has long been considered an important component of the therapeutic exercise program. The triceps surae can be strengthened, focusing on eccentric demands, as pain diminishes. A progressive return to activity includes instruction in the proper method of warming up, continued flexibility exercises, monitoring of footwear and activity surfaces, and applying ice after exercise.

Achilles Tendon Rupture

Forceful, sudden contractions, such as when a defensive back or basketball player changes direction or when a gymnast dismounts from an apparatus, results in a large amount of tension developing within the Achilles tendon. If this tension becomes too great, the tendon fails, resulting in an Achilles tendon rupture (Examination Findings 9-7).

Two theories attempt to account for the onset of Achilles tendon ruptures: (1) chronic degeneration of the tendon and (2) failure of the inhibitory mechanism of the musculotendinous unit.[104] As described in the Achilles Tendinopathy section, the Achilles tendon is poorly vascularized, and the body is unable to keep pace with the tendon's breakdown (tendinosis). As a result, the tendon weakens. In the final stages of the degenerative process, a rupture occurs.[89, 104] When the triceps surae's inhibitory mechanism fails, an excessive force (e.g., stepping in a hole) or a forceful muscle contraction (e.g., an explosive push-off) results in the rupture of the tendon. In both types of mechanisms, the rupture tends to occur in the tendon's avascular zone (the distal 2 to 6 cm).[104]

Though this injury can occur in either sex or in any age group, Achilles tendon ruptures tend to be most prominent in men over age 30.[94] Within groups having similar characteristics (e.g., age, sex, body mass), a reported family history of Achilles tendon rupture increases the risk of rupture by a factor of five.[103]

A complete rupture typically occurs in more sedentary individuals who perform episodic strenuous activity. Previous or current tendinosis, age-related changes in the tendon, and **deconditioning** may play roles in the onset of tendon ruptures.[12,105] Healthy and unhealthy tendons can be ruptured through direct trauma or by forceful concentric muscle contraction or eccentric loading of the tendon.[105]

Although there are case reports of Achilles tendon rupture after corticosteroid injections in humans, there are no rigorous long-term studies evaluating the risk of rupture with or without steroid injections.[106] Injections in the paratenon have been demonstrated to be effective without increasing the long-term rate of tendon rupture.[105,106]

Achilles tendon ruptures are characterized by the inability to push off with the injured leg during ambulation or to perform a heel raise. The patient reports the sensation of being "kicked," followed by severe pain, and usually has a stiff-legged gain characterized by external rotation of the extremity.[104] If the lesion occurs in the tendon's midsubstance, the defect may be observable or palpable, although palpation is not a reliable indicator of a tendon defect.[107] As swelling develops, the defect will become difficult to see or palpate (Fig. 9-29). Although the tendon may be completely ruptured, the patient is still able to actively plantarflex the ankle through contraction of the peroneals, long toe flexors, and tibialis posterior muscles, but the strength of the contraction is markedly diminished. Clinically, the presence of a complete Achilles tendon rupture is confirmed through the **Thompson test** (Selective Tissue Test 9-3).[104,108] MRI can be used to identify partial tendon tears.[92]

Apophysis A bony protuberance

Deconditioning The loss of once-existing cardiovascular or muscular endurance and strength

Examination Findings 9-7
Achilles Tendon Rupture

Examination Segment	Clinical Findings
History of Current Condition	*Onset:* Acute *Pain characteristics:* Achilles tendon and/or lower portion of the gastrocnemius *Other symptoms:* The patient often reports the sensation of being kicked. Patient may describe an audible "pop." *Mechanism:* Forceful dorsiflexion or plantarflexion, usually the result of eccentric loading or plyometric contraction of the calf musculature *Risk factors:* A family history of Achilles tendon rupture[103] A possible relationship between a history of Achilles tendinopathy and a rupture of the tendon History of corticosteroid injections to the tendon Advancing age Male
Functional Assessment	Unable to perform a heel raise or push-off during gait
Inspection	A defect may be visible in the Achilles tendon or at the musculotendinous junction, but rapid swelling may obscure this; discoloration may be present around the tendon. The patient is unable to bear weight on the involved extremity because of pain.
Palpation	A palpable defect in the Achilles tendon, although it may quickly become obscured by swelling Pain elicited along the tendon and lower gastrocnemius-soleus muscle group
Joint and Muscle Function Assessment	*AROM:* Plantarflexion may possibly still be present owing to the tibialis posterior, plantaris, peroneals, and long toe flexors, although the patient may complain of pain during this motion and during dorsiflexion (secondary to stretching the Achilles tendon). *MMT:* Weak or absent plantarflexion (gastrocnemius and/or soleus) *PROM:* Pain during dorsiflexion An empty end-feel may be obtained secondary to patient apprehension.
Joint Stability Tests	*Stress tests:* Not applicable *Joint play:* Not applicable
Selective Tissue Tests	Thompson test
Neurological Screening	Within normal limits
Vascular Screening	Within normal limits
Imaging Techniques	MRI Ultrasonic imaging
Differential Diagnosis	Posterior tibial tendon rupture; plantaris tendon rupture; triceps surae tear; Achilles tendinopathy; deep vein thrombosis
Comments	This injury tends to occur more frequently in males older than age 30, but any age group is susceptible. The status of the dorsalis pedis pulse should be monitored.

AROM = active range of motion; MMT = manual muscle test; MRI = magnetic resonance imaging; PROM = passive range of motion

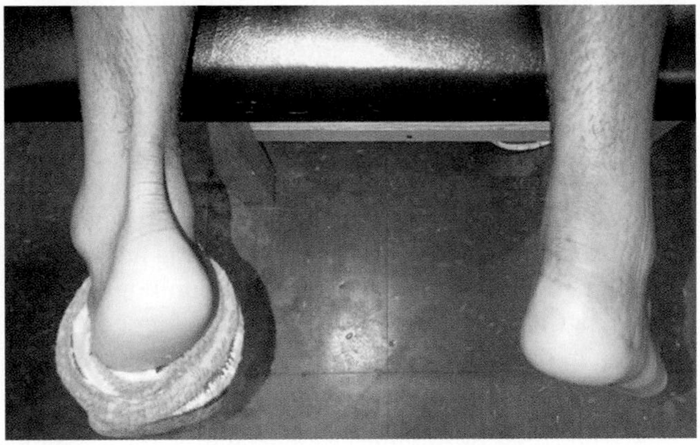

FIGURE 9-29 ■ Ruptured Achilles tendon. The patient's right (far) Achilles tendon has been ruptured. Note the depression proximal to the calcaneus and the involved swelling.

Achilles Tendon Rupture Intervention Strategies

Complete Achilles tendon ruptures can be successfully managed conservatively with casting or dorsiflexion night splints for a minimum of 8 weeks[109] or through open or minimally invasive surgery.[110] The primary advantages of conservative care are decreased wound problems and decreased medical costs. Disadvantages include an increased rate of rerupture, decreased muscle function, and patient dissatisfaction compared with surgical repair.[110,111]

The advantages of surgical repair include a reported rerupture rate of less than 5%; a speedier return to preinjury activity; and a good return of plantarflexion strength, power, and endurance.[110,111] Most disadvantages are caused by surgical complications associated with wound healing. The skin around the Achilles tendon is very thin, with little

Selective Tissue Test 9-3
Thompson Test for Achilles Tendon Rupture

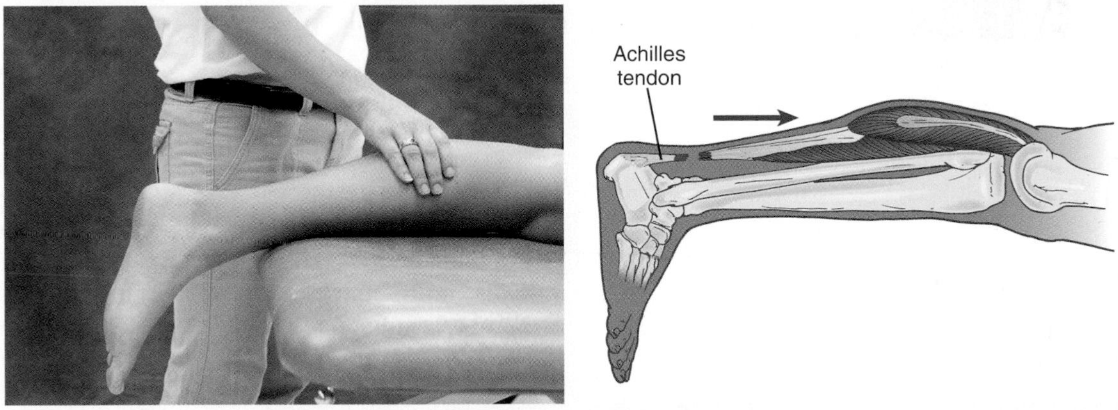

Thompson test for an Achilles tendon rupture. When the Achilles tendon is intact, squeezing the calf muscle results in slight plantarflexion. A positive Thompson test occurs when the calf is squeezed but no motion is produced in the foot, indicating a tear of the Achilles tendon.

Patient Position	Prone, with the foot off the edge of the table
Position of Examiner	At the side of the patient with one hand over the muscle belly of the calf musculature
Evaluative Procedure	The examiner squeezes the calf musculature while observing for plantarflexion of the foot.
Positive Test	When the calf is squeezed, the foot does not plantarflex.
Implications	The Achilles tendon has been ruptured.
Evidence	

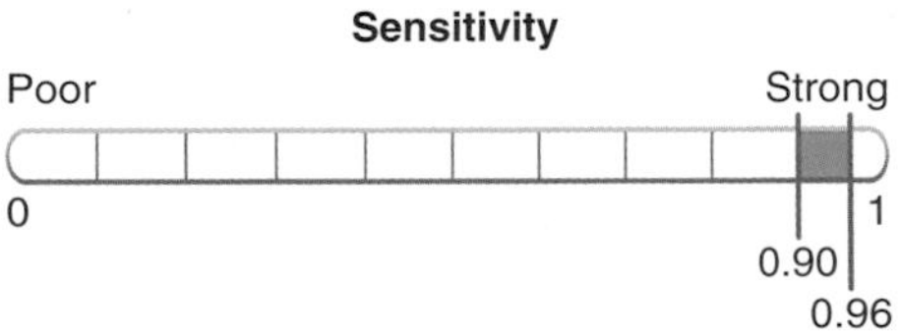

LR+: 48.00–90.00

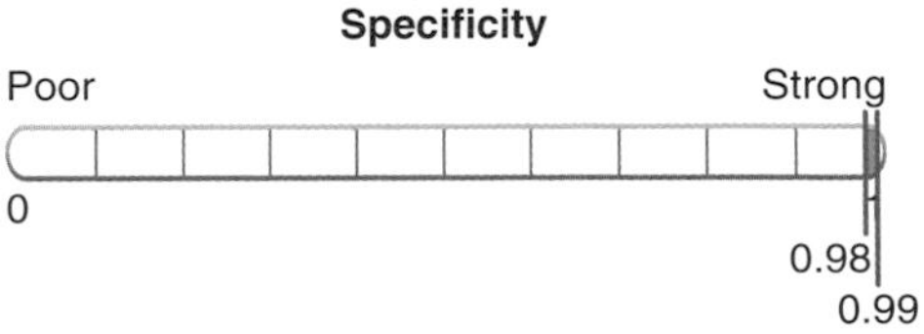

LR−: 0.04–0.10

subcutaneous tissue. Its limited blood supply makes the incision site prone to wound complications.

Peroneal Tendon Pathology

Forceful, sudden dorsiflexion and eversion or plantarflexion and inversion may stretch or rupture the superior peroneal retinaculum, which restrains the peroneal tendons behind the lateral malleolus. All cases of peroneal tendon dislocation are associated with a torn or stretched superior peroneal retinaculum.[2,52] Rare cases also involve the inferior peroneal retinaculum (see Fig. 9-12). When these tendons lose their alignment from behind the lateral malleolus and slip anteriorly, the peroneals, which are normally plantarflexors, become dorsiflexors (Fig. 9-30). The dislocation process starts proximally and, with time, progresses distally.[112]

Anatomically, a flattened or convex fibular groove predisposes peroneal subluxations by decreasing the depth of the bony channel through which the tendons pass.[112,113] Pes planus, rearfoot valgus, recurrent ankle sprains, a shallow fibular peroneal groove, and laxity of the peroneal retinaculum all contribute to the onset of subluxating peroneal tendons (Examination Findings 9-8).[114]

The peroneal tendons may be observed or palpated as they dislocate from the groove behind the lateral malleolus as they snap into and out of position during active plantarflexion and dorsiflexion or active eversion (Fig. 9-31).[114] This change alters the biomechanics of the foot and ankle, resulting in pain and dysfunction. There are four peroneal dislocation classifications:[2]

I. The superior peroneal retinaculum is torn from its fibular insertion.
II. The superior retinaculum and fibrocartilaginous ridge are avulsed from the lateral fibula.
III. The superior retinaculum is torn from the lateral fibula, the fibrocartilaginous ridge is avulsed, and flake fractures occur on the lateral malleolus.
IV. The superior retinaculum is torn from its calcaneal insertion.

Full or partial-thickness longitudinal tears may appear in the tendons.[113,116,117] Longitudinal tears of the peroneus brevis tendon are frequently associated with chronic lateral ankle instability.[52,118] During an inversion mechanism of an ankle sprain, the peroneus longus tendon pulls the anterior portion of the peroneus brevis tendon over the sharp posterior fibular ridge as it snaps out of the groove.[12,52] These ruptures contribute to future subluxations, dislocations, and peroneal tendinopathy.[113,116,117,119] Ultrasonic images can be used to detect chronic subluxation, and kinematic MRIs can be used to identify positional subluxations.[115,120,121] Clinically, peroneus brevis tears and subluxations are differentiated from chronic lateral ankle instability based on the description and location of the symptoms.[52] In the presence of peroneus brevis tendon disorders, the patient will describe lateral instability with associated pain on the posterior portion of the malleolus. Patients with chronic ankle instability will complain of the ankle "giving way" and pain in the anterior aspect of the ankle. Peroneus longus tears tend to afflict older individuals and also result in pain through the foot and lateral ankle.[2]

The peroneus longus' sesamoid, the **os peroneum**, can be the cause of several painful conditions about the foot and ankle. Generally termed as "painful os peroneum syndrome" (POPS), pain and dysfunction can be associated with an acute or chronic fracture, a multipartite os peroneum (the os peroneum being in two or more pieces), or a tear or rupture of the peroneus longus tendon. In rare instances, POPS can be caused by the os peroneum contacting a large peroneal tubercle.[21,22] Clinically, POPS is characterized by increased lateral pain during a single stance heel rise, inversion stress test, and resisted plantarflexion of the first ray.[122]

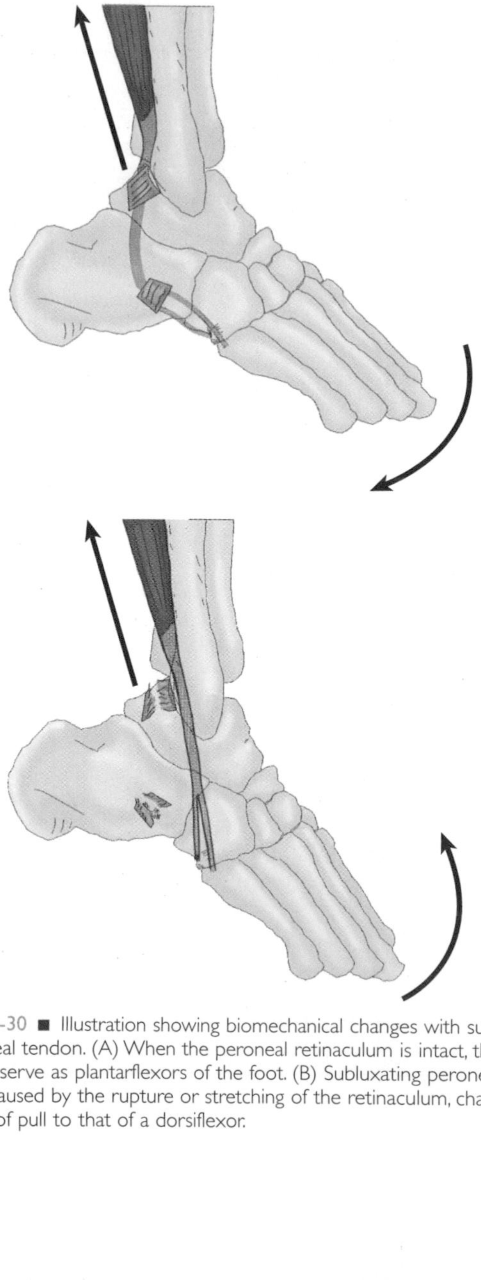

A

B

FIGURE 9-30 ■ Illustration showing biomechanical changes with subluxating peroneal tendon. (A) When the peroneal retinaculum is intact, the peroneals serve as plantarflexors of the foot. (B) Subluxating peroneal tendons, caused by the rupture or stretching of the retinaculum, change the angle of pull to that of a dorsiflexor.

Examination Findings 9-8
Subluxating Peroneal Tendons

Examination Segment	Clinical Findings
History of Current Condition	*Onset:* Acute or insidious In the case of tendon tears, several months may elapse between the initial injury and the report of symptoms.[2] *Pain characteristics:* Behind the lateral malleolus in the area of the superior peroneal retinaculum, across the lateral malleolus, length of the peroneal tendons, and, in rare cases, at the site of the inferior peroneal retinaculum *Other symptoms:* Patients often report ankle instability accompanied by snapping of the tendon.[2,52] *Mechanism:* Forceful dorsiflexion and eversion or plantarflexion and inversion *Risk factors:* A flattened or convex fibular groove, pes planus, rearfoot valgus Recurrent lateral ankle sprain Laxity of the peroneal retinaculum
Functional Assessment	Reproduction of symptoms with movements involving rapid change of direction
Inspection	Swelling and ecchymosis may be isolated behind the lateral malleolus (see functional tests). After 24 hours postdislocation, the swelling becomes diffuse.[2]
Palpation	Tenderness behind the lateral malleolus, over the peroneal tendons, and perhaps over the site of the inferior peroneal retinaculum Involvement of the peroneus longus may result in pain following the tendon's course along the foot. Palpate the area behind the lateral malleolus during peroneal MMT to identify abnormal movement of the peroneal tendons.
Joint and Muscle Function Assessment	*AROM:* The peroneal tendon may be seen, felt, or heard as it dislocates and reduces while the foot and ankle move from plantarflexion and inversion to dorsiflexion and eversion and back. *MMT:* Peroneals: Symptoms may be reproduced. *PROM:* No significant clinical findings
Joint Stability Tests	*Stress tests:* No significant findings *Joint play:* No significant findings
Selective Tissue Tests	None
Neurological Screening	Within normal limits
Vascular Screening	Within normal limits
Imaging Techniques	An avulsion fracture of the lateral ridge of the distal fibula confirms the diagnosis of a peroneal tendon subluxation or dislocation.[12] MRI is used to identify tendon lesions. Tears may be identified by a "boomerang" appearance.[2] Ultrasonic imaging is highly accurate in identifying peroneal tendon lesions.[115]
Differential Diagnosis	Longitudinal tear of the tendon, os peroneum syndrome, lateral ankle sprain, fibular fracture, calcaneal process fracture, talar fracture, osteochondritis dissecans
Comments	Longitudinal tears of the tendon tend to occur concurrently with the onset of dislocation/subluxation.

AROM = active range of motion; MMT = manual muscle test; MRI = magnetic resonance imaging; PROM = passive range of motion

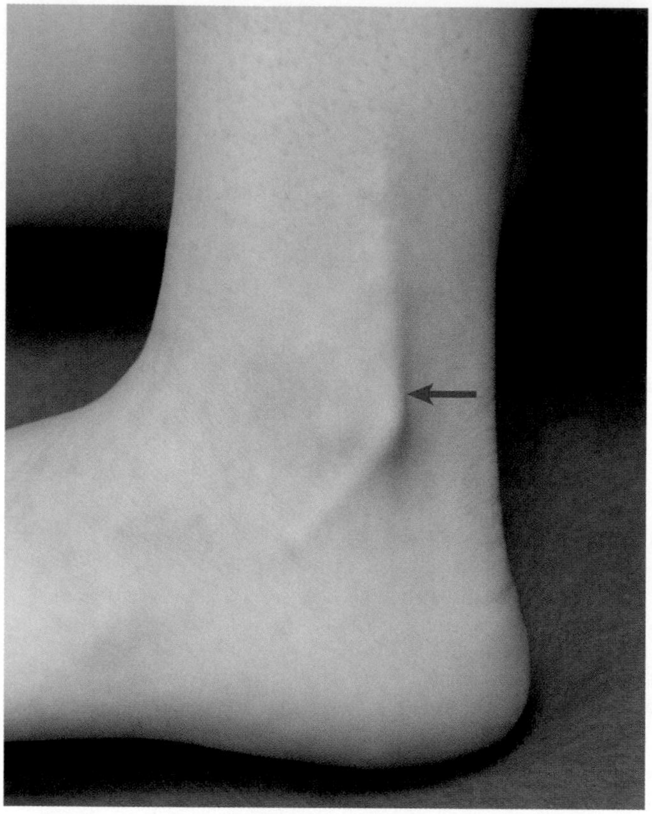

FIGURE 9-31 ■ Observable peroneal dislocation. In some instances the peroneal tendon can be observed as it subluxates from the fibular groove.

Peroneal Tendon Subluxation Intervention Strategies

In cases in which the retinaculum is stretched, the degree of subluxation may be controlled by rehabilitation exercises, taping, and using a felt pad over the peroneal groove to help hold the tendons in place. However, after the retinaculum stretches, it does not return to its original length. When the retinacula have been completely disrupted or pain and dysfunction become great, surgery is required to deepen the fibular groove,[123] repair the involved retinaculum,[114] or both.[112] Surgery to repair the soft tissue structures is usually necessary for patients with recurrent peroneal tendon dislocations.[114,124] If the subluxation is not reduced, chronic ankle instability, pain, and decreased strength impair ankle function.

Medial Tibial Stress Syndrome

Medial tibial stress syndrome (MTSS), a periostitis at the posterior medial border of the tibia, results from repetitive overuse, such as running. Estimated to account for around 15% of all running injuries,[125] the onset of MTSS is attributed to training errors (training on a hard surface, increasing load too quickly), incorrect footwear, muscle fatigue, or biomechanical abnormalities. Women are more susceptible than men.[107,125] Prolonged pronation, indirectly measured via static observation, an excessive navicular drop (see p. 213), or directly using more sophisticated gait measures, is a key feature associated with the development of this condition.[107,125-129] A bone stress reaction, MTSS may be a precursor to stress fractures, and bone scans in individuals with MTSS reveal uptake of the radionucleotide in the involved region (see Chapter 5).[128]

Patients with MTSS describe a gradual onset of symptoms, consistent with many overuse injuries (Table 9-7). Early in the progression, patients describe pain at the beginning of an exercise session that subsides as activity continues but returns when the activity is over. As the condition progresses, pain occurs throughout exercise and leads to a decrease in activity level. The diffuse pain at the posteromedial tibial border covers a broad span (greater than 5 cm), not the localized tenderness associated with stress fractures. Palpation at the medial and distal posteromedial border is painful. Repetitive muscle testing of the long toe flexors, posterior tibialis, or soleus may replicate symptoms that emerge with fatigue of these muscles (Examination Findings 9-9).

Medial Tibial Stress Syndrome Intervention Strategies

Conservative treatment consisting of rest from the offending activities is typically effective. Controlling excessive pronation through adequate footwear or orthotics also provides relief. An examination of lower extremity biomechanics and posture accompanied by appropriate strengthening and ROM exercises may be necessary.

Stress Fractures

Leg stress fractures involve the tibia, fibula, and talus and represent the accumulation of microtraumatic forces. Having symptoms of gradual onset, common complaints include isolated pain along the shaft of the bone. In the case of fibular stress fractures, pain occurs proximal to the lateral malleolus, increases with activity, and subsides with rest. During activity, patients may report decreased muscular strength and cramping. Palpation may reveal crepitus in well-developed stress fractures and point tenderness isolated to a single spot along the shaft of the bone. In many cases, the painful area is visually unremarkable (Examination Findings 9-10). A narrow tibial shaft, high degree of hip external rotation, osteopenia, osteoporosis, and pes cavus are common predisposing factors for stress fractures.[130-133] Immature stress fractures are not visible on standard radiographs until bony callus formation begins, typically around 3 weeks after the onset of symptoms. An early suspicion of a stress fracture requires the use of diagnostic techniques such as bone scans to detect increased bone metabolic activity for definitive diagnosis. In advanced (mature) stress fractures, symptoms may be elicited through the squeeze test although this test has limited value. The signs and symptoms of stress fractures may mimic those of medial tibial stress syndromes and compartment syndromes.

Table 9-7 Differential Findings of Stress Fractures, Medial Tibial Stress Syndrome, Acute Compartment Syndrome, and Chronic Exertional Compartment Syndrome

Finding	Stress Fracture	Medial Tibial Stress Syndrome	Acute Compartment Syndrome	Chronic Exertional Compartment Syndrome
Symptom Characteristics	Localized over the involved area of the bone	More diffuse along the posteromedial border of the middle or distal one-third of the tibia	Severe pain in the involved compartment of the leg Numbness on the dorsum of the foot, especially the web space between the 1st and 2nd toes (anterior) Dorsalis pedis pulse may be diminished (anterior)	Pain in the involved compartment of the leg Numbness on the dorsum of the foot, especially the web space between the 1st and 2nd toes Dorsalis pedis pulse diminished
Onset	Following changes in footwear or playing surfaces or increases in intensity, duration, or frequency of activity	Following changes in footwear or playing surfaces or increases in intensity, duration, or frequency of activity	Acute following trauma to the anterior leg Acute during exercise but symptoms not decreasing with rest	Symptoms increasing in proportion to exercise, resulting in inability to continue Pain possibly limiting activity after symptoms begin
Pain Patterns	Increased with activity and decreased with rest Possibly progressing to constant pain	Initially, pain at the start of activity, possibly diminishing with continued participation; pain possibly increasing again at the end of activity Pain decreasing with rest	Unremitting pain most likely prohibiting activity	Pain increasing with activity Pain decreasing with rest
Positive Findings	Localized pain with palpation	Pain with palpation over the posteromedial tibia Pain during toe raises Pain during resisted plantarflexion, inversion, dorsiflexion, or toe flexion.	Pain with active or resisted motion of the compartment's muscles Pain with passive stretching of the compartment's muscles	Pain after or during exercise
Negative Test Results	AROM MMT PROM	AROM PROM		Most test results negative if the individual has not been exercising recently
Definitive Diagnosis	Bone scan Radiograph MRI	Bone scan may show periosteal irritation	Intracompartmental pressure minus diastolic BP ≥30 mm Hg Pain that does not subside with rest	Increased intracompartmental pressure after activity Pain that subsides with rest

AROM = active range of motion; MRI = magnetic resonance imaging; PROM = passive range of motion; MMT = manual muscle test

Examination Findings 9-9
Medial Tibial Stress Syndrome

Examination Segment	Clinical Findings
History of Current Condition	*Onset:* Insidious *Pain characteristics:* Diffuse posteromedial tibial pain that increases as activity prolongs; may describe pain at rest *Mechanism:* Overuse/repetitive stress *Risk factors:* Increased pronation[126,127]
Functional Assessment	Gait observation reveals excessive pronation.
Inspection	Pes planus Rearfoot and/or forefoot varus when assessed in subtalar joint neutral
Palpation	Diffuse tenderness along posteromedial border of tibia; may have diffuse swelling
Joint and Muscle Function Assessment	*AROM:* Unremarkable *MMT:* Symptoms reproduced with multiple repetitions of testing involved muscle(s): posterior tibialis, soleus, flexor digitorum longus, flexor hallucis longus *PROM:* Increased pain with ankle dorsiflexion, pronation, or toe extension
Joint Stability Tests	*Stress tests:* Not applicable *Joint play:* Not applicable
Selective Tissue Tests	Navicular drop test
Neurological Screening	Within normal limits. Complaints of paresthesia warrant consideration of another diagnosis.
Vascular Screening	Within normal limits
Imaging Techniques	Radiographs and bone scans to differentiate from stress fractures
Differential Diagnosis	Tibial stress fracture, deep posterior exertional compartment syndrome, deep vein thrombosis, popliteal artery entrapment syndrome[128]

*** Practical Evidence**

Medial tibial stress syndrome, the low end of the bone stress–failure continuum, is marked by periostitis or symptomatic periosteal remodeling of the middle and distal third of the medial tibia.[22] The site of early MTSS is often correlated with the long-term development of stress fractures and may be more prevalent in individuals who demonstrate a pronatory foot type.

Dancers and athletes who jump, such as basketball players, are disposed to developing stress fractures in the anterior cortex of the tibia, an area prone to nonunion fractures. The fracture area is visible on radiographs but is "cold" or negative on bone scans, producing "the dreaded black line."[22]

Tuning forks have been advocated as an inexpensive alternative to identifying the presence of stress fractures. A vibrating tuning fork is placed on the shaft of the suspected bone. In the presence of a stress fracture, the vibration would cause pain. This test's low positive likelihood ratio and high negative likelihood ratio mean that its findings add little to the diagnostic decision making.[133]

Stress Fracture Intervention Strategies

Pain guides the management of patients with stress fractures. Many individuals respond to rest and anti-inflammatory medication. Advanced cases may require limited weight bearing, casting or a walker boot (Fig. 9-32).

Compartment Syndromes

Resulting from increased pressure within the compartment, compartment syndromes threaten the integrity of the leg, foot, and toes by obstructing the neurovascular network contained within the involved compartment. The combination of bony borders and dense fibrous fascial lining of the compartments results in poor elastic properties to accommodate for expansion of the intracompartmental tissues. When the compartment pressure exceeds **capillary perfusion pressure**, the local tissues do

Capillary perfusion pressure Pressure within the capillaries that forces blood out into the surrounding tissues

Examination Findings 9-10
Leg and Ankle Stress Fractures

Examination Segment	Clinical Findings
History of Current Condition	*Onset:* Insidious or chronic, secondary to repetitive running and/or jumping *Pain characteristics:* Along the shaft of the tibia or fibula; localized during or after exercise; may be described as a localized "ache" while at rest *Mechanism:* No definitive origin of pain. The history possibly indicates a sudden increase in the duration, frequency, or intensity of exercise or a change in playing surface or footwear. *Risk factors:* Individuals having a narrow tibial shaft, an externally rotated hip, and/or pes cavus/supinated foot type, osteopenia, osteoporosis, and menstrual irregularity.[126]
Functional Assessment	Shortened stance phase on the involved side Restricted or excessive/prolonged pronation may be noted.
Inspection	Normally unremarkable; localized swelling possible in advanced stages Inspect the foot for postural deviations.
Palpation	Pain along the fracture site
Joint and Muscle Function Assessment	*AROM:* All results may be normal in the acute stages of stress fractures. *MMT:* In maturing stress fractures or immediately after exercise, decreased strength may be evident secondary to inflammation of the muscles near the site of the stress fracture. *PROM:* Unremarkable findings
Joint Stability Tests	*Stress tests:* Not applicable *Joint play:* Not applicable
Selective Tissue Tests	The squeeze test is performed for advanced fibular stress fractures. Navicular drop test (see p. 214)
Neurological Screening	Within normal limits
Vascular Screening	Not normally indicated
Imaging Techniques	Radiographic evaluation is typically normal in immature stress fractures. A "V"-shaped defect, the "dreaded black line" visible on tibial radiographs, often determines the need for surgical correction.[114]
Differential Diagnosis	Medial tibial stress syndrome, exertional compartment syndrome Early stages of stress fractures may clinically resemble those of periostitis.
Comments	Early signs of stress fractures appear on bone scans. Stress fractures do not appear on standard radiographic examination for 4–6 weeks after the onset of symptoms. The patient may have a history of disordered eating and/or malnutrition.

AROM = active range of motion; MMT = manual muscle test; PROM = passive range of motion

not receive an adequate supply of oxygen. This lack of oxygen leads to ischemia of the tissues and, if not treated, cell death.[134]

Compartment syndromes are classified as traumatic, acute exertional, or chronic exertional. Traumatic anterior compartment syndrome occurs from intracompartmental hemorrhage caused by a blow to the anterolateral or lateral portion of the leg (Examination Findings 9-11). The subsequent bleeding and edema cause an increased pressure within the compartment, which compresses the deep peroneal nerve, capillaries, and anterior tibial artery and results in ischemic destruction of the involved tissues.

Exertional compartment syndromes can have an acute or chronic onset, with symptoms occurring during or immediately following exercise (Examination Findings 9-12). **Chronic exertional compartment syndrome** (CCS), also referred to as **recurrent compartment syndrome** or

Claudication Pain caused by inadequate venous drainage or poor arterial innervation

Examination Findings 9-11
Traumatic Compartment Syndrome

Examination Segment	Clinical Findings
History of Current Condition	*Onset:* Traumatic *Pain characteristics:* Severe pain Anterolateral portion of the leg, which is described as "achy," "sharp," or "dull" Other complaints such as muscle tightness, cramping, swelling, weakness, or unremitting pain *Other symptoms:* Numbness may develop in the dorsum of the foot, especially in the web space between the 1st and 2nd toes (anterior). *Mechanism:* Direct trauma to the anterolateral or lateral leg Inversion mechanism that avulses peroneals *Risk factors:* Anatomic factors that inhibit the expansion of the involved compartment, tibial fracture, anticoagulant therapy, calcaneal fractures
Functional Assessment	Extreme pain with ambulation; drop-foot gait sometimes observed (anterior)
Inspection	The anterior compartment may appear shiny and swollen. In advanced cases, possible discoloration of the dorsum of the foot may be present.
Palpation	The involved compartment is painful, hard, and edematous to the touch.
Joint and Muscle Function Assessment	*AROM:* Decreased (or absent) ability to dorsiflex the ankle or extend the toes (anterior) Diminished or painful eversion (lateral) *MMT:* Not indicated *PROM:* Pain during passive motion secondary to stretching of the muscles in the involved compartment, creating pressure within
Joint Stability Tests	*Stress tests:* Not applicable *Joint play:* Not applicable
Selective Tissue Tests	There are no clinical tests for these conditions. Compartment syndromes are confirmed by measuring the intracompartmental pressure.
Neurological Screening	Anterior compartment: Paresthesia may be present in the web space between the 1st and 2nd toes and possibly on the dorsum of the foot. Lateral compartment: Paresthesia may be present along the lateral distal leg and dorsum of the foot.
Vascular Screening	The presence of a normal dorsalis pedis pulse should be determined, although pulses are often present throughout the course of this condition.
Imaging Techniques	Radiographic images may be taken to determine the presence of a bony fracture causing the increased compartmental pressure.
Differential Diagnosis	Tibial fracture, fibular fracture
Comments	Do not apply a compression wrap during the treatment of anterior compartment syndrome because the wrap will increase the intracompartmental pressure and exacerbate the condition. Elevation above the heart is also contraindicated as it decreases vascular pressure. Suspicion of acute compartment syndrome warrants immediate referral to a physician or emergency department.

AROM = active range of motion; MMT = manual muscle test; PROM = passive range of motion

Examination Findings 9-12
Chronic Exertional Compartment Syndrome

Examination Segment	Clinical Findings
History of Current Condition	*Onset:* Acute or chronic; gradual presentation of symptoms *Pain characteristics:* Pain in the involved compartment, described as "achy," "sharp," or "dull," that resolves shortly after activity ceases *Other symptoms:* Reports of muscle tightness, cramping, swelling, and weakness The patient may describe transient paresthesia in the dorsum of the foot, especially in the web space between the 1st and 2nd toes (anterior compartment), which resolves when activity stops. *Mechanism:* The patient reports symptoms during or after running or other prolonged activity. *Risk factors:* Anabolic steroid and creatine use (which increase muscle volume); abnormal biomechanics including excessive pronation; eccentric exercise involving leg muscles; abnormal arteriole homeostasis; overtraining
Functional Assessment	The patient reports the inability to continue exercise following the onset of symptoms. Contributing biomechanical abnormalities (e.g., prolonged pronation) may be observed during gait.
Inspection	The anterior compartment may appear swollen with a dull sheen when symptomatic. Deep posterior compartment involvement will have no visible findings.
Palpation	Generally unremarkable if unsymptomatic at time of exam
Joint and Muscle Function Assessment	*AROM:* Decreased function in muscles of the involved compartment Anterior: Inability to dorsiflex the ankle or extend the toes *MMT:* Weakness noted during testing muscles in the involved compartment Anterior: Dorsiflexion, supination/inversion Deep posterior: Plantarflexion, toe flexion, supination/inversion Lateral: Pronation/eversion *PROM:* Increased pain with stretch of muscles in the involved compartment
Joint Stability Tests	*Stress tests:* Not applicable *Joint play:* Not applicable
Selective Tissue Tests	There are no clinical tests for these conditions. Exertional anterior compartment syndrome is confirmed by measuring the intracompartmental pressure before, during, and after activity.
Neurological Screening	Anterior compartment: Numbness may be present in the web space between the 1st and 2nd toes and possibly on the dorsum of the foot. Lateral compartment: Paresthesia may be present along the lateral distal leg and dorsum of the foot. Deep posterior compartment: Paresthesia may be present at the medial calcaneus.
Vascular Screening	Within normal limits if patient is not symptomatic Abnormal pulses are rare with this condition, even when symptomatic.[135]
Imaging Techniques	Angiography may be used to determine the vascular integrity of the extremity.
Differential Diagnosis	Tibial or fibular stress fracture, medial tibial stress syndrome
Comments	Bilateral involvement in exertional compartment syndromes is common. Findings may be unremarkable if the patient is asymptomatic at the time of the examination. Clinical findings are more apparent if the patient exercises until symptoms appear and then the physical examination is conducted.

AROM = active range of motion; MMT = manual muscle test; PROM = passive range of motion

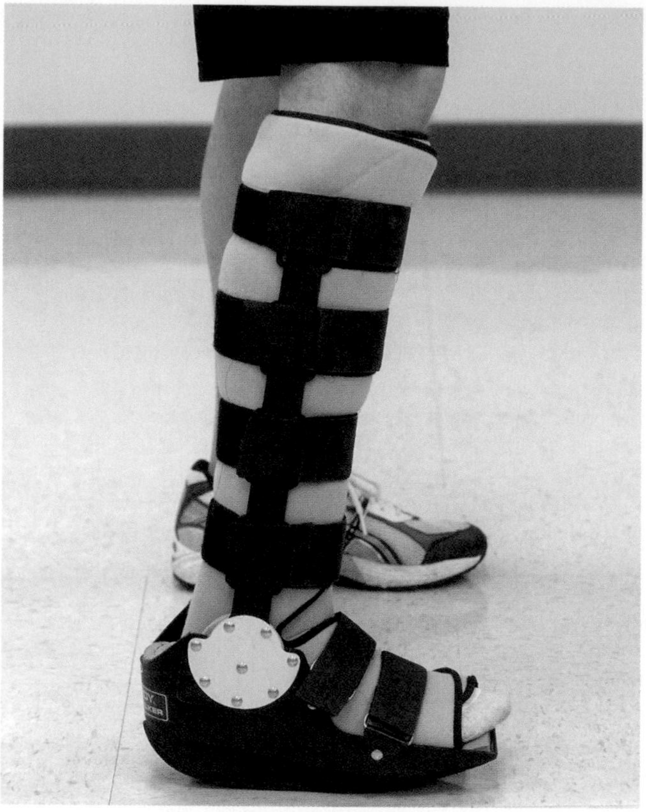

FIGURE 9-32 ■ A walker boot. Walker boots allow for controlled range of motion, earlier stable weight bearing, and the ease of removal for rehabilitation.

intermittent **claudication**, occurs secondary to anatomic abnormalities obstructing blood flow in exercising muscles. Many exertional compartment syndromes are related to an increased thickness of the fascia; exercise exacerbates the condition because muscle volume can increase up to 20% during activity.[135,136] Other risk factors that predispose an individual to CCS include:[135,136]

- Herniation of muscle, occluding the neurovascular network as it transverses the interosseous membrane
- Anabolic steroid or creatine use (which increase muscle volume)
- Abnormal biomechanics including excessive pronation
- Eccentric exercise involving leg muscles
- Abnormal arteriole homeostasis
- Overtraining

Acute compartment syndromes occur most often in young people, possibly because of tighter, stronger fascia and a predisposition to high-energy activities.[137] Other risk factors for acute compartment syndromes include tibial fractures, casts or other braces or wound dressings, diabetes, anticoagulation medication, intense exercise, venomous bites, and direct soft tissue injury.[134,137]

The signs, symptoms, and pathology of acute and chronic exertional syndromes are similar. However, acute exertional compartment syndromes have a distinct onset associated with activity and clearing symptoms shortly after activity stops.[135,136]

The "five P's" may be used to describe the signs and symptoms of compartment syndromes:

- Pain
- Pallor (redness)
- Pulselessness
- Paresthesia
- Paralysis

The identification and management of a compartment syndrome should not be delayed because all of the five P's are not present.[134] Pain is localized within the affected compartment and is often disproportionate with the other findings of the examination. Paresthesia may occur as a result of proximal nerve injury or muscle guarding and is not a reliable indicator. The most germane clinical indications of acute compartment syndrome are pain that increases with motion and increased tissue density to palpation.[134,137]

The presence of the dorsalis pedis pulse must be established in the involved limb (see Vascular Assessment, p. 266); however, pulses often remain intact throughout the progression of the condition. Although the blood pressure within the tibial artery may be sufficient to produce a palpable dorsalis pedis pulse, the pressure increase may be great enough to inhibit flow within the smaller vessels and capillaries.[134] Because this pulse is not detectable in all individuals, both limbs must be examined. If the pulse is present in the uninvolved extremity but not in the involved extremity, it can be deduced that blood flow to the foot has been compromised.

Acute compartment syndromes are emergent conditions requiring immediate referral for medical treatment. Muscle is relatively resilient to ischemic conditions for up to 4 hours; after 8 hours of ischemia, irreversible muscle damage occurs.[138] Exertional compartment syndromes usually present symptoms during exercise that subsequently subside with rest.

The diagnosis of acute compartment syndromes is based on the intracompartmental pressure. An absolute intracompartmental pressure of 30 to 45 mm Hg is an indication for fasciotomy, as is an intracompartmental pressure within 30 mm Hg of the patient's diastolic blood pressure.[137]

To diagnose exertional compartment syndromes, compartmental pressures can also be monitored during exercise, an invasive technique performed in a medical facility. Increases of more than 15 mm Hg when resting, 30 mm Hg 1 minute after exercise, or 20 mm Hg 5 minutes postexercise are diagnostic signs of an exertional compartment syndrome.[135] MRIs may also be used to detect exertional compartment syndromes; however, sequences must be obtained before and after activity, making this a costly enterprise.[135]

Compartment Syndrome Intervention Strategies

For acute compartment syndromes, surgical fasciotomy remains the standard treatment. After surgery, the initial treatment and rehabilitation must allow for adequate healing of the incision site, and complete skin closure may be delayed until after swelling has started to resolve.[137]

After the wound heals, therapeutic exercise to restore ROM and strength to the lower extremity is begun. The patient is progressed through functional activities to return to full activity.

For individuals with exertional compartment syndromes who want to maintain their activity level, conservative treatment using activity modification and correction of biomechanical abnormalities rarely results in complete resolution of symptoms. Operative treatment, especially for the anterior and lateral compartments, is associated with successful outcomes and a return to activity in 6 to 8 weeks. Deep posterior fasciotomies are associated with a higher rate of complications and a less favorable outcome.[135,136]

On-Field Examination of Leg and Ankle Injuries

The goals of the on-field evaluation of patients with these injuries include ruling out fractures and dislocations, determining the athlete's weight-bearing status, and identifying the best method for removing the athlete from the field.

Equipment Considerations

The nature of competitive athletics brings with it ever-more-specialized footwear, braces, and types of tape. Although designed to protect athletes from injury while also improving performance, these devices may hinder the evaluation and management of acute injuries.

Footwear Removal

After a gross fracture or dislocation has been ruled out, the athlete's shoe must be removed so a thorough examination of the injury can be conducted after the athlete has reached the sideline. Most shoes may be easily removed by completely unlacing them, spreading the sides, and pulling the tongue down to the toes (Fig. 9-33). The athlete is asked to plantarflex the foot, if possible. The shoe is removed by sliding the heel counter away from the foot and then lifting the shoe up and off the foot. Apprehensive athletes may be allowed to remove the shoe themselves. If a fracture or dislocation is suspected, the examiner should loosen the shoe enough to allow for palpation of the dorsalis pedis and posterior tibial pulses and transport the athlete with the shoe in place and the leg splinted. Metal cleats or spikes may need to be removed prior to immobilization or transportation.

Tape and Brace Removal

Prophylactic devices such as tape or ankle braces must be removed to allow for the complete examination of the foot and ankle. Braces tightened by laces or Velcro® straps may be removed in a manner similar to shoe removal. Ankle tape can be removed by cutting along a line parallel to the posterior portion of the malleolus on the side of the leg opposite the site of pain. The cut is then continued along the plantar aspect of the foot.

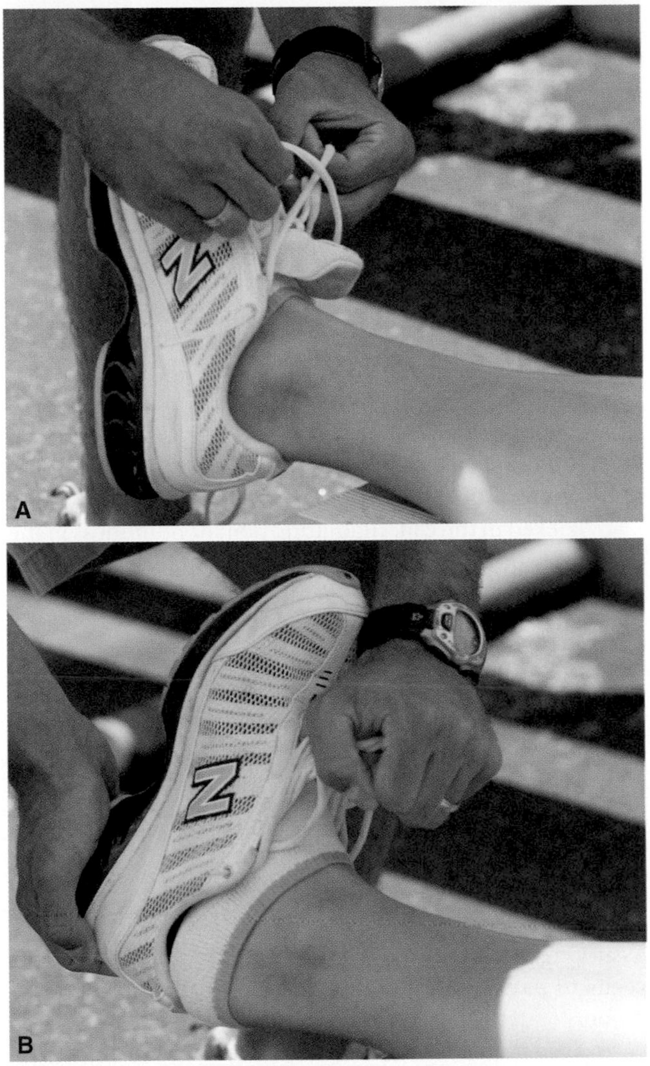

FIGURE 9-33 ■ Removing the shoe following a foot or ankle injury. (A) After completely removing the laces, withdraw the tongue and (B) slide the shoe from the foot.

On-Field History

In the absence of gross deformity, the mechanism of injury and the associated sounds and sensations can help to identify either the underlying pathology or a direct blow to the leg.

- **Mechanism of injury:** Identify the injurious forces placed on the ankle, keeping in mind that the injury may involve multiple forces (e.g., inversion and plantarflexion) or a direct blow to the leg.
  - **Inversion:** Rolling the talus and calcaneus inward exerts tensile forces on the lateral aspect of the ankle and compressive forces on the medial aspect. Lateral ankle sprains, lateral ligament avulsions, and medial malleolar fractures are associated with this mechanism.
  - **Eversion:** Excessive eversion of the talus and calcaneus places tensile forces on the medial aspect of the ankle and compression on the lateral aspect. Syndesmotic ankle sprains and fractures of the

lateral malleolus and fibula are also associated with this mechanism.
- **Rotation:** Rotational forces can lead to syndesmotic sprains or fracture of the tibia, fibula, or both.
- **Dorsiflexion:** Forced dorsiflexion can strain or rupture the Achilles tendon or cause the distal tib-fib syndesmosis to separate.
- **Plantarflexion:** Although this mechanism is rare, forced plantarflexion can traumatize the extensor retinaculum and anterior joint capsule and its associated ligaments.

- **Associated sounds and sensations:** Ascertain for any sounds or sensations. A "snap" or "pop" may be associated with a ligament rupture or bony fracture. An audible snap or pop is also associated with an Achilles tendon rupture and may be described as being "kicked in the calf." Radiating pain or numbness in the anterior ankle and leg can indicate anterior compartment syndrome or trauma to the peroneal nerve.

On-Field Inspection

During on-field inspection of ankle and leg injuries, any gross bony or joint injury must be ruled out before progressing to the other elements of the evaluation. Examine the contour and alignment of the leg, foot, and ankle, noting any discontinuity or malalignment of the structures that may indicate a fracture or dislocation.

On-Field Palpation

Assuming normal alignment of the leg, the evaluation proceeds to palpation of the bony structures and related soft tissue.

- **Bony palpation:** Begin by palpating the length of the tibia and fibula and continuing on to the talus, the remaining tarsals, and the MTs. Note any deformities, crepitus, or areas of point tenderness, especially in areas where pain is described. If a disruption of a long bone or joint is felt, splint the joint and transport the athlete to a hospital.
- **Soft tissue palpation:** Perform a quick yet thorough evaluation of the major soft tissues, emphasizing the ligamentous structures for point tenderness and the tendons for signs of rupture.

On-Field Range of Motion Tests

After the possibility of a gross fracture or dislocation has been ruled out, the athlete's ability to move the limb and subsequently bear weight must be established:

- **Willingness to move the involved limb:** If the athlete displays normal alignment of the limb, observe his or her willingness to move the injured body part through the full ROM. This task should be performed with a minimal amount of discomfort. If the athlete has no ability or is unwilling to move the involved limb, use assistance to remove the athlete from the field.
- **Willingness to bear weight:** If the athlete describes no pain and there are no signs of restriction in the ROM, assist the athlete to the standing position, bearing weight on the uninvolved leg. Assistance is provided by assuming position under the athlete's arm on the involved side, giving some support. The athlete should walk off the field, attempting to place as little weight as possible on the involved limb.

Initial Management of On-Field Injuries

This section describes the emergency management procedures for major trauma occurring to the ankle and lower extremity. Most ankle injuries (e.g., sprains, Achilles tendon ruptures) are managed on the sidelines or in athletic training rooms. On-field care involves ruling out the presence of a fracture or neurovascular deficit, keeping the injured body part from bearing weight, and removing the athlete from the playing field.

Ankle Dislocations

Resulting from excessive rotation combined with inversion or eversion, dislocations of the talocrural joint result in major disruptions of the joint capsule and associated ligaments. Associated fractures of the malleoli, long bones, or talus often occur. Such injuries result in immediate pain in the ankle and leg and loss of function, and the patient may also report an audible snap or crack. The foot and ankle may be grossly malaligned. If the defect is not visible, the superior portion of the talus may be palpated as it protrudes anteriorly and medially from the ankle mortise (Fig. 9-34). The evaluation also must confirm the presence of the distal pulses and include a secondary survey of the ankle mortise and long bones for possible fracture (Fig. 9-35).

Management of Leg Fractures and Ankle Dislocations

Any obvious fracture or joint dislocation should immediately be immobilized using a moldable or vacuum splint (see Box 2-1). In most cases, it is recommended that the shoe be left in place while the athlete is being transported to the hospital. It may be more safely removed in the emergency room after further diagnostic tests, such as radiographic examination, to determine the full extent of the injury (Fig. 9-36). The laces and tongue of the shoe are loosened, and the sock is cut to permit palpation of the dorsalis pedis and the posterior tibial pulses, which are then compared bilaterally and continually monitored.

Management of an open fracture involves controlling bleeding and immobilizing the fracture. The area around the open fracture should be packed with sterile bandages without causing any further disruption at the fracture site. After bleeding is controlled, the extremity can be immobilized in the position in which it is found, the pulses continually monitored, and the athlete transported to a medical facility.

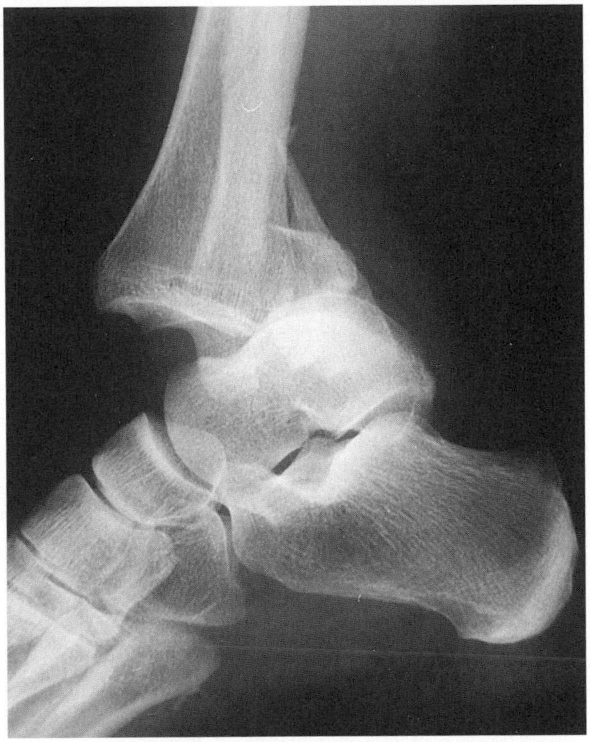

FIGURE 9-34 ■ Posterior ankle dislocation (medial view of the right ankle). Often the talus displaces anteriorly relative to the tibia. This radiograph shows the talus being displaced posteriorly relative to the tibia. Note the fracture of the malleolus caused by the wide anterior talar border's being forced into the mortise.

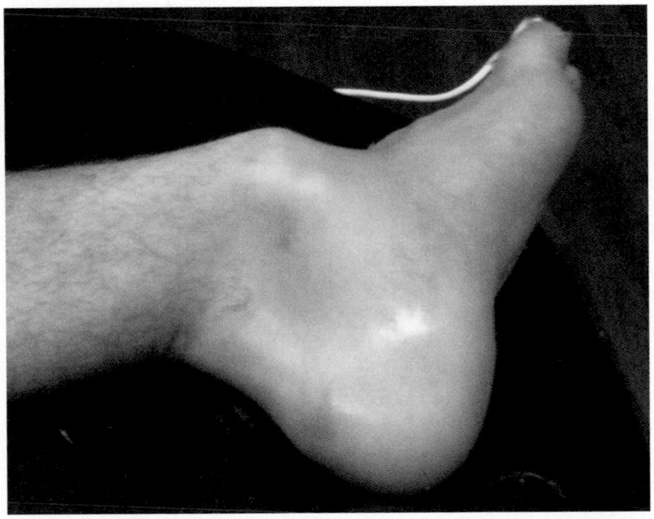

FIGURE 9-35 ■ Ankle fracture–dislocation. Note the irregular contour beneath the lateral malleolus.

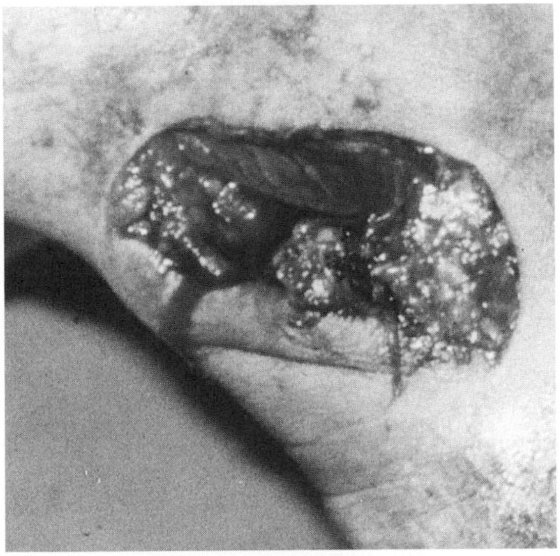

FIGURE 9-36 ■ This apparent laceration is actually an open dislocation of the talus.

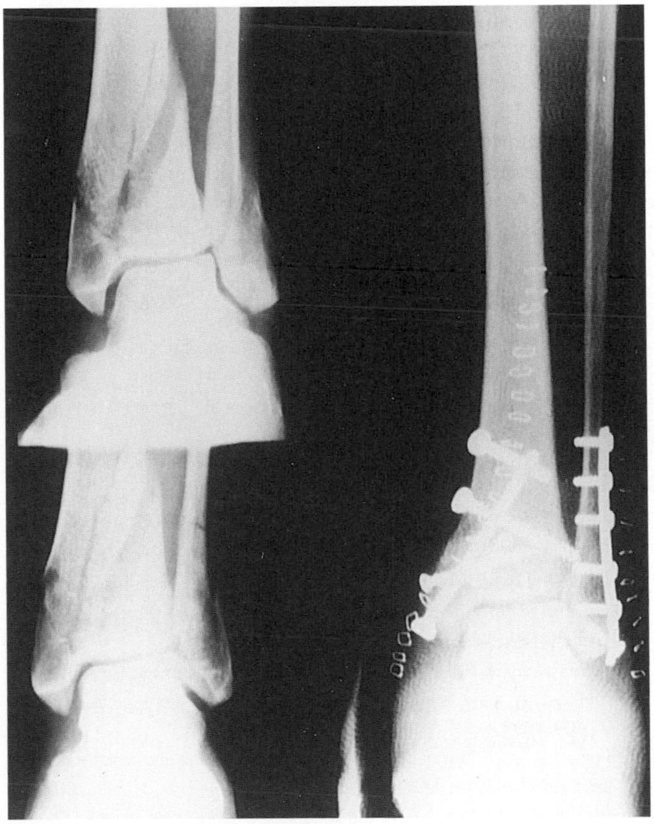

FIGURE 9-37 ■ Radiograph showing screws and plates used to set a fracture of the ankle joint.

Nondisplaced fibular or tibial fractures may be treated by simple casting. Comminuted or displaced fractures often require the use of internal or external fixation devices to realign and stabilize the fracture sites. A fracture of the distal fibula involving the syndesmosis may require an internal fixation device or a screw to maintain the alignment of the fibula with the tibia during the healing process and to prevent subsequent rotational instabilities of the talus (Fig. 9-37).[139]

Compartment Syndrome

Unlike other acute soft tissue injuries, suspected compartment syndromes are not treated with compression. The use of external compression devices, such as wraps or compression boots, increase the pressure within the compartment, exacerbating the condition. If the mechanism of injury combined with symptoms such as unremitting pain, absent distal pulses, or increased tissue density create a suspicion of a compartment syndrome, the athlete must be immediately referred for medical intervention. If, at the time of the injury, the athlete does not display signs of intracompartmental hemorrhage but there is reason to suspect such a response, provide the athlete with a list of the danger signs and symptoms (see Table 9-7) and instruct the athlete about contacting a physician if the symptoms worsen.

REFERENCES

1. Hertel, J: Functional instability following lateral ankle sprain. *Sports Med*, 29:361, 2000.
2. Sammarco, GJ, and Mangone, PG: Diagnosis and treatment of peroneal tendon injuries. *Foot Ankle Surg*, 6:197, 2000.
3. Takebe, K, et al: Role of the fibula in weight-bearing. *Clin Orthop*, 184:2899, 1984.
4. Norkus, SA, and Floyd, RT: The anatomy and mechanisms of syndesmotic ankle sprains. *J Athl Train*, 36:68, 2001.
5. Hertel, J: Functional anatomy, pathomechanics, and pathophysiology of lateral ankle instability. *J Athl Train*, 37:364, 2002.
6. Lynch, SA: Assessment of the injured ankle in the athlete. *J Athl Train*, 37:406, 2002.
7. Burks, RT, and Morgan, J: Anatomy of the lateral ankle ligaments. *Am J Sports Med*, 22:72, 1994.
8. Williams, GN, Jones, MH, and Amendola, A: Syndesmotic ankle sprains in athletes. *Am J Sports Med*, 35:1197, 2007.
9. Zalavras, C, and Thordason, D: Ankle syndesmotic injury. *J Am Acad Orthop Surg*, 15:330, 2007.
10. Mueller, MJ: The ankle-foot complex. In Levangie, PK, and Norkin, CC (eds): *Joint Structure and Function: A Comprehensive Analysis*, ed 4. Philadelphia, PA: FA Davis, 2005, p 437.
11. Doughtie, M: Syndesmotic ankle sprains in football: a survey of National Football League athletic trainers. *J Athl Train*, 34:15, 1999.
12. Jones, DC: Tendon disorders of the foot and ankle. *J Am Acad Orthop Surg*, 1:87, 1993.
13. Zammit, J, and Singh, D: The peroneus quartus muscle: anatomy and clinical relevance. *J Bone Joint Surg*, 85:1134, 2003.
14. Hale, SA, and Hertel, J: Reliability and sensitivity of the Foot and Ankle Disability Index in subjects with chronic instability. *J Athl Trng*, 40:35, 2005.
15. Mawdsley, RH, Hoy, DK, and Erwin, PM: Criterion-related validity of the figure-of-eight method of measuring ankle edema. *J Orthop Sports Phys Ther*, 30:149, 2000.
16. Peterson, EJ, et al: Reliability of water volumetry and the figure of eight method on subjects with ankle joint swelling. *J Orthop Sports Phys Ther*, 29:609, 1999.
17. Pugia, ML, et al: Comparison of acute ankle swelling and function in subjects with lateral ankle injury. *J Orthop Sports Phys Ther*, 31:348, 2001.
18. Breitenseher, MJ, et al: MRI of the sinus tarsi in acute ankle injuries. *J Comput Assist Tomogr*, 21:274, 1997.
19. Riddle, DL, and Wells, PS: Diagnosis of lower-extremity deep vein thrombosis in outpatients. *Phys Ther*, 84:729, 2004.
20. Urbano, FL: Homans' sign in the diagnosis of deep vein thrombosis. *Hosp Physician*, March:22, 2001.
21. Witvrouw, WE, et al: The significance of peroneus tertius muscle in ankle injuries: a prospective study. *Am J Sports Med*, 34:1159, 2006.
22. Reshef, N, and Guelich, DR: Medial tibial stress syndrome. *Clin Sports Med*. 31:273, 2012.
23. Heckman, DS, Gluck, GS, and Parekh, SG: Tendon disorders of the foot and ankle, part 2: Achilles tendon disorders. *Am J Sports Med*. 37:1223, 2009.
24. Fujii, T, et al: The manual stress test may not be sufficient to differentiate ankle ligament injuries. *Clin Biomech*. 15:619, 2000.
25. van Dijk, CN, et al: Physical examination is sufficient for the diagnosis of sprained ankles. *J Bone Joint Surg Br*. 78:958, 1996.
26. van Dijk, CN, et al: Diagnosis of ligament rupture of the ankle joint: physical examination, arthrography, stress radiography and sonography compared in 160 patients after inversion trauma. *Acta Orthop Scand*, 67:566, 1996.
27. Corazza, F, et al: Mechanics of the anterior drawer test at the ankle: the effects of ligament viscoelasticity. *J Biomech*, 38:2118, 2005.
28. Tohyama, H, et al: Anterior drawer test for acute anterior talofibular ligament injuries of the ankle: how much load should be applied during the test? *Am J Sports Med*, 31:226, 2003.
29. Vela, L, Tourville, TW, and Hertel, J: Physical examination of acutely injured ankles: an evidence-based approach. *AthlTher Today*, 8:13, 2003.
30. Hertel J, et al: Talocrural and subtalar instability after lateral ankle sprain. *Med Sci Sports Exer*, 31:1501, 1999.
31. Alonso, A, Khoury, L, and Adams, R: Clinical tests for ankle syndesmosis injury: reliability and prediction of return to function. *J Orthop Sports Phys Ther*, 27:276, 1998.
32. Beumer, A, Swierstra, BA, and Mulder, PG: Clinical diagnosis of syndesmotic ankle instability: evaluation of stress tests behind the curtains. *Acta Orthop Scand*, 73:667, 2002.
33. Fallat, L, Grimm, DL, and Saracco, JA: Sprained ankle syndrome: prevalence and analysis of 639 acute injuries. *J Foot Ankle Surg*, 37:280, 1998.
34. Olmsted-Kramer, LC, Hertel, J: Preventing recurrent lateral ankle sprains: an evidence-based approach. *Athl Ther Today*, 9:19, 2004.
35. McKay, GD, et al: Ankle injuries in basketball: injury rate and risk factors. *Br J Sports Med*, 35:103, 2001.
36. Tyler, TF, et al: Risk factors for noncontact ankle sprains in high school football players: the role of previous ankle sprains and body mass index. *Am J Sports Med*, 34:471, 2006.
37. McHugh MP, et al: Risk factors for noncontact ankle sprains in high school athletes: the role of hip strength and balance ability. *Am J Sports Med*. 34:464, 2007.
38. Stone, JW: Osteochondral lesions of the talar dome. *J Am Acad Orthop Surg*, 4:63, 1996.
39. Molloy, S, Solan, MC, and Bendall, SP: Synovial impingement in the ankle: a new physical sign. *J Bone Joint Surg*, 85:330, 2003.
40. Hertel, J, and Kaminski, T: Second international ankle symposium summary statement. *J Orthop Sports Phys Ther*, 35:A-2, 2005.
41. Frey, C, et al: A comparison of MRI and clinical examination of acute lateral ankle sprains. *Foot Ankle Int*, 17:533, 1996.
42. Morrison, KE, and Kaminski, TW: Foot characteristics in association with inversion ankle injury. *J Athl Train*, 42:135, 2007.
43. Rodriguez-Merchan, EC: Chronic ankle instability: diagnosis and treatment. *Arch Orthop Trauma Surg*, 132:211, 2012.
44. Yeung, MS, et al: An epidemiological survey on ankle sprains. *Br J Sports Med*, 28:112, 1994.
45. van Rijn, RM, et al: What is the clinical course of acute ankle sprains? A systematic literature review. *Am J Med*, 121:324, 2008.
46. Johnson, MB, and Johnson, CL: Electromyographic response of peroneal muscles in surgical and nonsurgical injured ankles during sudden inversion. *J Orthop Sports Phys Ther*, 18:497, 1993.
47. Isalov, E: Response of peroneal muscles to sudden inversion of the ankle during standing. *Int J Sport Biomech*, 2:100, 1986.
48. Hiller, CE, et al: Characteristics of people with recurrent ankle sprains: a systematic review with meta-analysis. *Br J Sports Med*, 45:660, 2011.
49. Hubbard, TJ, and Hertel, J: Mechanical contributions to chronic lateral ankle instability. *Sports Med*, 36:263, 2006.
50. Meislin, RJ, et al: Arthroscopic treatment of synovial impingement of the ankle. *Am J Sports Med*, 21:186, 1993.

51. Pinar, H, et al: Bone bruises detected by magnetic resonance imaging following lateral ankle sprains. *Knee Surg Sports Traumatol Arthrosc*, 5:113, 1997.
52. Karlsson, J, and Wiger, P: Longitudinal split of the peroneus brevis tendon and lateral ankle instability: treatment of concomitant lesions. *J Athl Train*, 37:463, 2002.
53. Taga, I: Articular cartilage lesions in ankles with lateral ligament injury: an arthroscopic study. *Am J Sports Med*, 21:120, 1993.
54. Loomer, R, et al: Osteochondral lesions of the talus. *Am J Sports Med*, 21:13, 1993.
55. Bassett, FH: A simple surgical approach to the posteromedial ankle. *Am J Sports Med*, 21:144, 1993.
56. Verhagen, RAW, et al: Prospective study on diagnostic strategies in osteochondral lesions of the talus. *J Bone Joint Surg*, 87-B:41, 2005.
57. Bullock-Saxton, JE: Local sensations and altered hip muscle function following severe ankle sprain. *Phys Ther*, 74:17, 1994.
58. Yammine, K, and Fathi, Y: Ankle "sprains" during sport activities with normal radiographs: incidence of associated bone and tendon injuries on MR findings and its clinical impact. *Foot*, 21:176, 2011.
59. Kellett, JJ: The clinical features of ankle syndesmosis injuries: a general review. *Clin J Sport Med*, 21:524, 2011.
60. Teitz, CC, and Harrington, RM: A biomechanical analysis of the squeeze test for sprains of the syndesmotic ligaments of the ankle. *Foot Ankle Int*, 19:489, 1998.
61. Candal-Couto, JJ, et al: Instability of the tibio-fibular syndesmosis: have we been pulling in the wrong direction? *Injury*, 35:814, 2004.
62. Oae, Km, et al: Injury of the tibiofibular syndesmosis: value of MR imaging for diagnosis. *Radiology*, 227:155, 2003.
63. McConnell, T, Creevy, W, and Tornetta, P: Stress examination of supination external rotation-type fibular fractures. *J Bone Joint Surg*, 86A:2171, 2004.
64. Dettori, JR, et al: Early ankle mobilization, part I: the immediate effect on acute, lateral ankle sprains (a randomized clinical trial). *Mil Med*, 159:15, 1994.
65. Eiff, MP, Smith, AT, and Smith, GE: Early mobilization versus immobilization in the treatment of lateral ankle sprains. *Am J Sports Med*, 22:83, 1994.
66. Lin, CC, Hiller, CE, and de Bie, RA: Evidence-based treatment for ankle injuries: a clinical perspective. *J Man Manip Ther*, 18:22, 2010.
67. Dettori, JR, and Basmania, CJ: Early ankle mobilization, part II: a one-year follow up of acute, lateral ankle sprains (a randomized clinical trial). *Mil Med*, 159:20, 1994.
68. Schmidt, R, et al: Anatomical repair of lateral ligaments in patients with chronic ankle instability. *Knee Surg Sports Traumatol Arthrosc*, 13:231, 2005.
69. Punenburg, ACM, et al: Treatment of ruptures of the lateral ankle ligaments: a meta-analysis. *J Bone Joint Surg*, 82:761, 2000.
70. Veltri, DM, et al: Symptomatic ossification of the tibiofibular syndesmosis in professional football players: a sequela of the syndesmotic ankle sprain. *Foot Ankle Int*, 16:285, 1995.
71. Nielson, JH: Correlation of interosseous membrane tears to the level of the fibular fracture. *J Orthop Trauma*, 18:68, 2004.
72. Stiell, IG, et al: The "real" Ottawa Ankle Rules. *Ann Emerg Med*, 27:103, 1996.
73. Stiel, I, et al: Multicentre trial to introduce the Ottawa ankle rules for use of radiography in acute ankle injuries. *BMJ*, 311:594, 1995.
74. Bachmann, LM, et al: Accuracy of Ottawa ankle rules to exclude fractures of the ankle and mid-foot: systematic review. *Br J Med*, 326:417, 2003.
75. Nugent, PJ: Ottawa ankle rules accurately assess injuries and reduce reliance on radiographs. *J Fam Pract*, 53:785, 2004.
76. Gravel, J, et al: Prospective validation and head-to-head comparison of 3 ankle rules in a pediatric population. *Ann Emerg Med*, 54:534, 2009.
77. Bachmann, LM, et al: Accuracy of Ottawa ankle rules to exclude fractures of the ankle and mid-foot: systematic review. *BJM*, 326: 417, 2003.
78. Leddy, JJ, et al: Prospective evaluation of the Ottawa ankle rules in a university sports medicine center. With a modification to increase specificity for identifying malleolar fractures. *Am J Sports Med*, 26:158, 1998.
79. Bhanot, A, et al: Fracture of the posterior process of talus. *Injury*, 35:1341, 2004.
80. Abramowitz, Y, et al: Outcome of resection of a symptomatic os trigonum. *J Bone Joint Surg*, 85A:1052, 2003.
81. Mouhsine, E, et al: Post-traumatic overload or acute syndrome of the os trigonum: a possible cause of posterior ankle impingement. *Knee Surg Sports Traumatol Arthrosc*, 12:250, 2004.
82. Yilmaz, C, and Eskandari, MM: Arthroscopic excision of the talar Stieda's process. *Arthroscopy*, 22:225, 2009.
83. Brodsky, AE, and Khalil, M: Talar compression syndrome. *Am J Sports Med*, 14:472, 1986.
84. Paulos, LE, et al: Posterior compartment fracture of the ankles: a commonly missed athletic injury. *Am J Sports Med*, 11:439, 1983.
85. McDougall, A: The os trigonum. *J Bone Joint Surg Br*, 37:257, 1955.
86. Karasick, D, and Schweitzer, ME: The os trigonum syndrome: imaging features. *Am J Roentgenol*, 166:125, 1996.
87. Masciocchi, C, Catalucci, A, and Barile, A: Ankle impingement syndromes. *Eur J Radiol*, 27(S1):S70, 1998.
88. Ahmed, IM, et al: Blood supply of the Achilles tendon. *J Orthop Res*, 16:591, 1998.
89. Scioli, MW: Achilles tendinitis. *Orthop Clin North Am*, 25:177, 1994.
90. Puddu, G, et al: A classification of Achilles tendon disease. *Am J Sports Med*, 4:145, 1976.
91. Mahieu, NN, et al: Intrinsic risk factors for the development of Achilles tendon overuse injury: a prospective study. *Am J Sports Med*, 34:1, 2006.
92. Gillet, P, et al: Magnetic resonance imaging may be an asset to diagnose and classify fluorouinolone-associated Achilles tendinitis. *Fundam Clin Pharmacol*, 9:52, 1995.
93. Astrom, M, and Rausing, A: Chronic Achilles tendinopathy: a survey of surgical and histopathic findings. *Clin Orthop*, Jul:151, 1995.
94. Astrom, M: Partial rupture in chronic Achilles tendinopathy: a retrospective analysis of 342 cases. *Acta Orthop Scand*, 69:404, 1998.
95. Cassas, KJ, and Cassettari-Wayhs, A: Childhood and adolescent sports-related overuse injuries. *Am Fam Physician*, 73:1014, 2006.
96. Scharfbillig, RW, Jones, S, and Scutter, S: Sever's disease: a prospective study of risk factors. *J Am Podiatr Med Assoc*, 101:133, 2011.
97. Becerro de Bengoa Vallejo, R, et al: Plantar pressures in children with and without sever's disease. *J Am Podiatr Med Assoc*, 101:17, 2011.
98. Kose, O, et al: Can we make a diagnosis with radiographic examination alone in calcaneal apophysitis (Sever's disease)? *J Ped Orthop B*, 19:396, 2010.
99. Kose, O: Do we really need radiographic assessment for the diagnosis of non-specific heel pain (calcaneal apophysitis) in children? *Skeletal Radiol*, 39:359, 2010.
100. Rachel, JN, et al: Is radiographic evaluation necessary in children with a clinical diagnosis of calcaneal apophysitis (Sever's disease)? *J Pediatr Orthop*, 31:548, 2011.
101. Alfredson, H: Achilles tendinosis and calf muscle strength: the effect of short-term immobilization after surgical treatment. *Am J Sports Med*, 26:166, 1998.
102. Shrier, I, Matheson, GO, and Kohl, HW 3rd: Achilles tendonitis: are corticosteroid injections useful or harmful? *Clin J Sport Med*, 6:245, 1996.
103. Kraemer, R, et al: Analysis of hereditary and medical risk factors in Achilles tendinopathy and Achilles tendon ruptures: a matched pair analysis. *Arch Orthop Trauma Surg*, 132:847, 2012.
104. Leppilahti, J, and Orava, S: Total achilles tendon rupture: a review. *Sports Med*, 25:79, 1998.

105. Saltzman, C, and Bonar, S: Tendon problems of the foot and ankle. In Lutter, LD, Mizel, MS, and Pfeffer, GB (eds): *Orthopaedic Knowledge Update: Foot and Ankle*. Rosemont, IL: American Academy of Orthopaedic Surgeons, 1994, p 271.
106. Shrier, I, Matheson, GO, and Kohl, HW: Achilles tendonitis: are corticosteroid injections useful or harmful? *Clin J Sports Med*, 6:245, 1996.
107. Bennet, JE, et al: Factors contributing to the development of medial tibial stress syndrome in high school runners. *J Orthop Sports Phys Ther*, 31:504, 2001.
108. Maffulli, N: The clinical diagnosis of subcutaneous tear of the Achilles tendon: a prospective study in 174 patients. *Am J Sports Med*, 26:266, 1998.
109. Kearney, RS, et al: A systematic review of early rehabilitation methods following a partial rupture of the Achilles tendon. *Physiother*, 98:24, 2012.
110. Fierro, NL, and Sallis, RE: Achilles tendon rupture: is casting enough? *Postgrad Med*, 98:145, 1995.
111. Troop, RL, et al: Early motion after repair of Achilles tendon ruptures. *Foot Ankle Int*, 16:705, 1995.
112. Kumai, T, and Benjamin, M: The histological structure of the malleolar groove of the fibula in man: its direct bearing on the displacement of peroneal tendons and their surgical repair. *J Anat*, 203:257, 2003.
113. Schweitzer, ME, et al: Using MR imaging to differentiate peroneal splits from other peroneal disorders. *Am J Roentgenol*, 168:129, 1997.
114. Ferran, NA, Oliva, F, and Maffulli,N: Recurrent subluxation of the peroneal tendons. *Sports Med*, 36:839, 2006.
115. Grant, TH, et al: Ultrasound diagnosis of peroneal tendon tears: a surgical correlation. *J Bone Joint Surg*, 87:1788, 2005.
116. Yao, L: MR Findings in peroneal tendonopathy. *J Comput Assist Tomogr*, 19:460, 1995.
117. Krause, JO, and Brodsky, JW: Peroneus brevis tendon tears: pathophysiology, surgical reconstruction, and clinical results. *Foot Ankle Int*, 19:271, 1998.
118. Steensma, MR, Anderson, JG, and Bohay, DR: Update on diseases and treatment of the peroneal tendon, including peroneal tendon tear, subluxating peroneal tendon, and tendinosis. *Curr Opin Orthop*, 16:60, 2005.
119. Boles, MA, et al: Enlarged peroneal process with peroneus longus tendon entrapment. *Skeletal Radiol*, 26:313, 1997.
120. Magnano, GM, et al: High-resolution US of non-traumatic recurrent dislocation of the peroneal tendons: a case report. *Pediatr Radiol*, 28:476, 1998.
121. Shellock, FG, et al: Peroneal tendons: use of kinematic MR imaging of the ankle to determine subluxation. *J Magn Reson Imaging*, 7:451, 1997.
122. Sobel, M, et al: Painful os peroneum syndrome: a spectrum of conditions responsible for plantar lateral foot pain. *Foot Ankle Int*, 15:112, 1994.
123. Kollias, SL, and Ferkel, RD: Fibular grooving for recurrent peroneal tendon subluxation. *Am J Sports Med*, 25:329, 1997.
124. Karlsson, J, Eriksson, BI, and Sward, L: Recurrent dislocation of the peroneal tendons. *Scand J Med Sci Sports*, 6:242, 1996.
125. Yates, B, and White, S: The incidence and risk factors in the development of medial tibial stress syndrome among naval recruits. *Amer J Sports Med*, 32:772, 2004.
126. Rauh, M, et al: Epidemiology of stress fracture and lower-extremity overuse injury in female recruits. *Med Sci Sports Exer*, 38:1571, 2006.
127. Willems, TM, et al: A prospective study of gait related risk factors for exercise-related lower leg pain. *Gait Posture*, 23:91, 2006.
128. Edwards, PH, Wright, ML, and Hartman, JF: A practical approach for the differential diagnosis of chronic leg pain in the athlete. *Am J Sports Med*, 33:1241, 2005.
129. Willems, TM, et al: Gait-related risk factors for exercise-related lower-leg pain during shod running. *Med Sci Sports Exer*, 39:330, 2007.
130. Giladi, M, et al: Stress fractures: identifiable risk factors. *Am J Sports Med*, 19:647, 1991.
131. Saltzman, CL, Nawoczenski, DA, and Talbot, KD: Measurement of the medial longitudinal arch. *Arch Phys Med Rehabil*, 76:45, 1995.
132. Varner, KE, et al: Chronic anterior midtibial stress fractures with athletes treated with reamed intramedullary nailing. *Am J Sport Med*, 35:1071, 2005.
133. Lesho, EP: Can tuning forks replace bone scans for identification of tibial stress fractures? *Mil Med*, 162:802, 1997.
134. Konstantakos, EK, et al. Diagnosis and management of extremity compartment syndromes: an orthopaedic perspective. *Am Surg*, 73:1199, 2007.
135. Gill, CS, Halstead, ME, and Matava, MJ. Chronic exertional compartment syndrome of the leg in athletes: evaluation and management. *Phys Sportsmed*, 38:126, 2010.
136. Tucker, AK. Chronic exertional compartment syndrome of the leg. *Curr Rev Musculoskelet Med*, 3:32, 2010.
137. Shadgan, B, et al: Current thinking about acute compartment syndrome of the lower extremity. *Can J Surg*, 532:329, 2010.
138. Whitesides, TE, and Heckman, MM: Acute compartment syndrome: update on diagnosis and treatment. *J Am Acad Orthop Surg*, 4:209, 1996.
139. Michelson, J: Controversies in ankle fractures. *Foot Ankle*, 14:170, 1993.

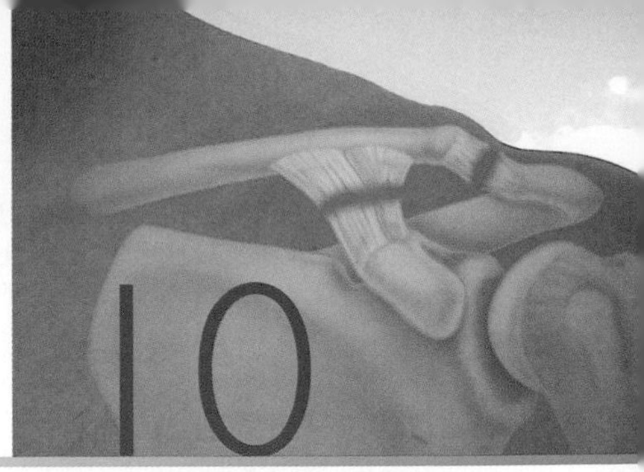

CHAPTER 10

Knee Pathologies

The knee complex, formed by the tibiofemoral, tibiofibular, and patellofemoral joints, has little bony support and must rely on soft tissue structures to control the forces transmitted through the joints. The tibiofemoral joint is located between the body's two longest lever arms, the femur and tibia; these long lever arms exert extreme forces on ligaments and tendons. The knee relies on static stabilizers (ligaments) more so than dynamic support (muscles) and is more stable when the extremity is weight bearing than when it is not.

This chapter discusses injury to the knee and related muscles. The patella as it relates to the function of the tibiofemoral joint is described in this chapter. Conditions that are exclusive to the patellofemoral articulation are described in Chapter 11, and injury to the quadriceps and hamstring muscle groups is addressed in Chapter 12. The knee is functionally interdependent with the foot, ankle, hip, and trunk. Pathomechanics at these joints alter the biomechanical function of the knee. In the case of chronic knee injuries, these areas should also be examined.

Clinical Anatomy

The term "tibiofemoral joint" seems to imply that the knee involves only the articulation between the tibia and femur. In fact, the femur, menisci, and tibia all must function together. The patellofemoral mechanism (**extensor mechanism**) must also function properly to ensure adequate tibiofemoral mechanics. The proximal tibiofibular joint is functionally more influenced by the ankle joint.[1]

The **femur**, the longest and strongest bone in the body, is approximately one quarter of the body's total height.[2] The femur's posterior aspect is demarcated by the **linea aspera**, a bony ridge spanning the length of the shaft (Fig. 10-1). As the femur reaches its distal end, the shaft broadens to form the medial and lateral condyles.

The **medial and lateral condyles** are covered with articular hyaline cartilage and articulate with the tibia via the menisci. These structures have a discrete anteroposterior curvature that is convex in the frontal plane. The articular surface of the medial condyle is longer than that of the lateral condyle and flares outward posteriorly. The condyles share a common anterior surface, then diverge posteriorly, becoming separated by the deep **intercondylar notch**. The

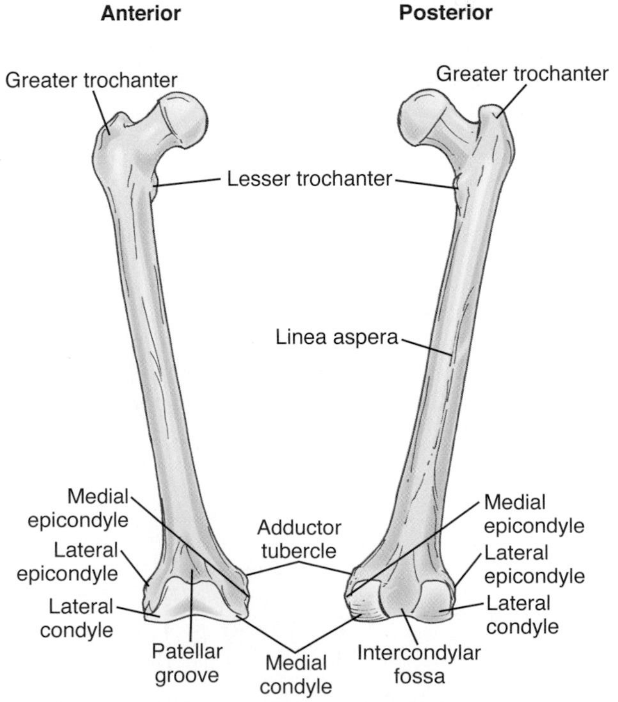

FIGURE 10-1 ■ Anterior and posterior view of the femur. Note that the single anterior articular surface on the condyles of the femur diverges posteriorly to form a lateral and medial compartment of the knee joint.

Extensor mechanism The mechanism formed by the quadriceps and patellofemoral joint responsible for causing extension of the lower leg at the knee joint

femoral trochlea is an anterior depression through which the patella glides as the knee flexes and extends. The lateral and medial epicondyles arise off the condyles. The **lateral epicondyle** is wider and emanates from the femoral shaft at a lesser angle than the **medial epicondyle**. The **adductor tubercle** arises off the superior crest of the medial epicondyle. These prominences serve as attachment sites for tendons to improve the mechanical advantage of the muscle.

The **medial and lateral tibial plateaus** correspond to the femoral condyles. The medial tibial plateau is concave in both the frontal and sagittal planes. The lateral articular plateau is concave in the frontal plane and convex in the sagittal plane. To accommodate for the flare of the femur's medial condyle, the medial tibial plateau is 50% larger than the lateral plateau. Intercondylar eminences, raised areas between the tibial plateaus that match the femur's intercondylar notch, separate the two condyles (Fig. 10-2). The **tibial tuberosity**, the site of the patellar tendon's distal attachment, is located on the proximal portion of the anterior tibia.

Two bones outside the tibiofemoral articulation directly affect the knee's function and stability. The **patella**, a sesamoid bone located in the patellar tendon, improves the mechanical function of the quadriceps during knee extension, dissipates the forces received from the extensor mechanism, and protects the anterior portion of the knee. Several of the soft tissues on the lateral aspect of the knee attach to the fibular head. Fracture of the proximal fibula or injury to the proximal **tibiofibular syndesmosis** can affect the stability of the knee.

Articulations and Ligamentous Support

The presence of the medial and lateral articular condyles classifies the tibiofemoral joint as a double condyloid articulation, capable of 3 degrees of freedom: (1) flexion and extension, (2) internal and external rotation, and (3) abduction and adduction.[1] Anterior and posterior translation also occur between the tibia and the femur. The joint may be hypermobile after a sprain or hypomobile secondary to the formation of scar tissue (arthrofibrosis). Hypomobility may occur if a ligament-replacement graft is placed too tightly or as the result of scar tissue formation. Adhesion or tearing of one or more ligaments significantly affects the function of the remaining ligaments.[3]

Joint Capsule

A fibrous joint capsule surrounds the knee joint. Along the medial, anterior, and lateral aspects of the joint, the capsule arises superior to the femoral condyles and attaches distal to the tibial plateau. Posteriorly, the capsule inserts on the margins of the femoral condyles above the joint line and, inferiorly, to the posterior tibial condyle. Medially, the stability of the joint is reinforced by the medial collateral ligament, medial patellofemoral ligaments, and medial patellar retinaculum; laterally, the joint is augmented by the extra-articular lateral collateral ligament, lateral patellar retinaculum, lateral patellofemoral ligament, and iliotibial band; posteriorly by the posterolateral corner (oblique popliteal ligament and arcuate ligaments); and anteriorly by the patellar tendon. Further support is gained from other tendons that cross the knee joint.

A **synovial capsule** lines the articular portions of the fibrous joint capsule. The synovium surrounds the articular condyles of the femur and tibia medially, anteriorly, and laterally. On the posterior portion of the articulation, the synovial capsule invaginates anteriorly along the femur's intercondylar notch and the tibia's intercondylar eminences, excluding the cruciate ligaments from the synovial membrane (Fig. 10-3). When the anterior cruciate ligament (ACL) is torn, its fibers are exposed to the synovial fluid. The circulating **plasmin** is believed to break down the fibrin clot on the ACL and inhibit fibroblastic activity, both inhibiting healing.[4]

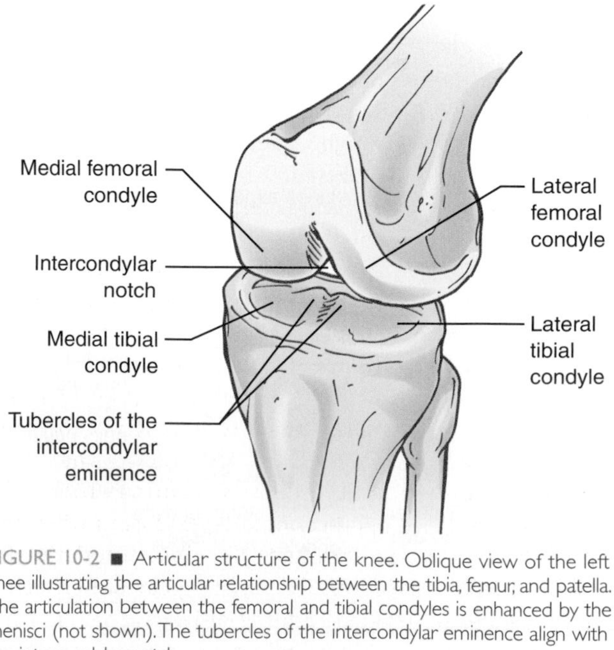

FIGURE 10-2 ■ Articular structure of the knee. Oblique view of the left knee illustrating the articular relationship between the tibia, femur, and patella. The articulation between the femoral and tibial condyles is enhanced by the menisci (not shown). The tubercles of the intercondylar eminence align with the intercondylar notch

Plasmin A blood enzyme that dissolves the fibrin in blood clots

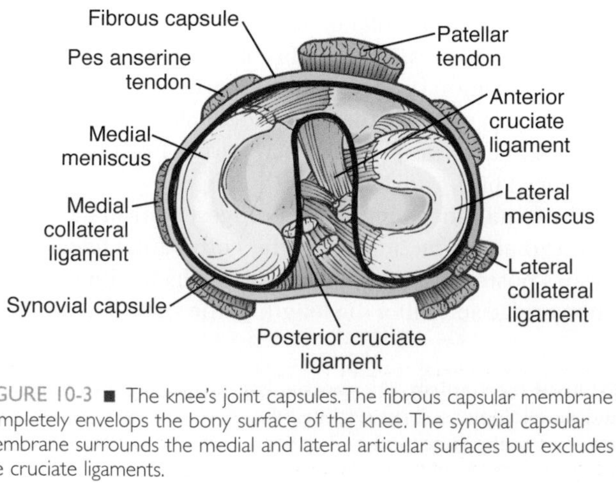

FIGURE 10-3 ■ The knee's joint capsules. The fibrous capsular membrane completely envelops the bony surface of the knee. The synovial capsular membrane surrounds the medial and lateral articular surfaces but excludes the cruciate ligaments.

Collateral Ligaments

The **medial collateral ligament** (MCL) is the primary medial stabilizer of the knee and consists of a deep layer and a superficial layer. The **deep layer** is a thickening of the joint capsule and is attached to the medial meniscus. Separated from the deep layer by a bursa, the **superficial layer**, approximately 1.5 cm wide, arises from a broad band just below the adductor tubercle and follows a superoposterior to inferoanterior path across the joint line deep to the pes anserine tendons (Fig. 10-4).[5] As a unit, the two layers of the MCL are tight in complete extension. As the knee is flexed to the midrange, the anterior fibers of both layers are taut; in complete extension, the posterior fibers are tight. The MCL primarily acts to protect the knee against valgus forces and also provides a secondary restraint against external rotation of the tibia and anterior translation of the tibia on the femur when the ACL is torn.

Unlike the MCL, the **lateral collateral ligament** (LCL) does not attach to the joint capsule or meniscus.[6] This cordlike structure arises from the lateral femoral epicondyle, sharing a common site of origin with the lateral joint capsule, and inserts on the proximal aspect of the fibular head (Fig. 10-5). Considered part of the posterolateral corner, the LCL is the primary restraint against varus forces when the knee is in the range between full extension and 30 degrees of flexion. This structure also provides a primary restraint against external tibial rotation and a secondary restraint against internal rotation of the tibia on the femur.[7] The lateral knee system is stronger than the medial structures because it is subjected to increased stress during the initial contact phase of gait when the knee is extended and weight bearing, placing varus forces on the joint.[7]

Cruciate Ligaments

The cruciate ligaments, although intra-articular, are located outside of the synovial capsule (see Fig. 10-3). Jointly, the cruciates also help to stabilize the knee against valgus and varus forces.

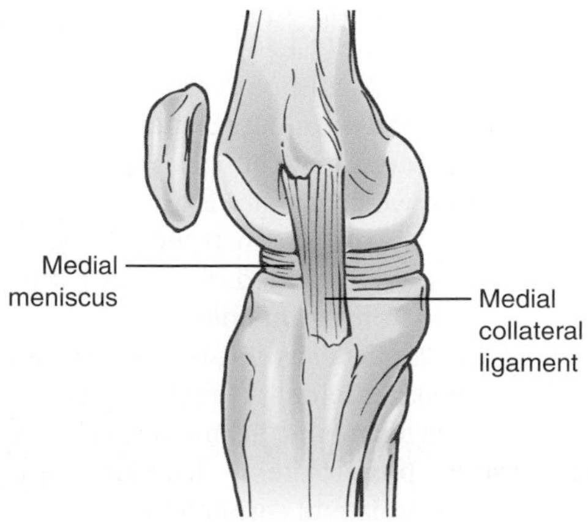

FIGURE 10-4 ■ Medial collateral ligament. Arising from a broad band on the medial femoral epicondyle just below the adductor tubercle, it tapers inward to attach on the medial tibial plateau. Consisting of two layers separated by a bursa, the deep layer is continuous with the medial joint capsule and has an attachment on the medial meniscus

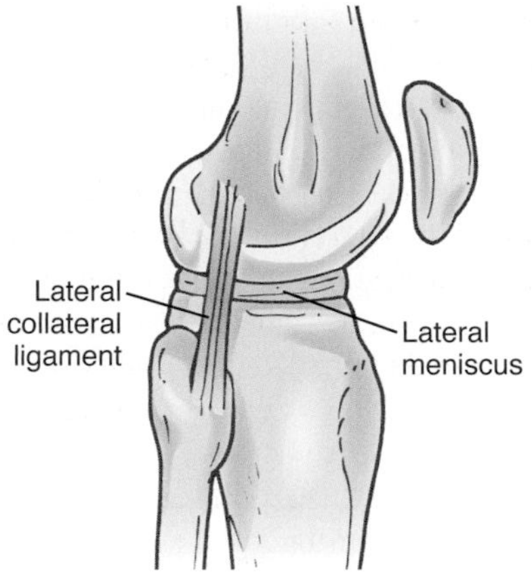

FIGURE 10-5 ■ Lateral collateral ligament. This ropelike structure originates from the lateral femoral epicondyle and attaches to the apex of the fibular head. The lateral collateral ligament is an extracapsular structure.

Anterior cruciate ligament. The ACL arises from the anteromedial intercondylar eminence of the tibia, travels posteriorly, and passes lateral to the posterior cruciate ligament (PCL) to insert on the medial wall of the lateral femoral condyle (Fig. 10-6). The ACL serves as a static stabilizer against:

1. Anterior translation of the tibia on the femur
2. Internal rotation of the tibia on the femur
3. External rotation of the tibia on the femur
4. Hyperextension of the tibiofemoral joint

The ACL has two discrete segments, an **anteromedial bundle** and a **posterolateral bundle**, which are named for their attachment site on the tibia.[8] As the knee moves from extension into flexion, a reversal of the ACL's attachment sites occurs. When the knee is fully extended, the femoral attachment of the anteromedial bundle is anterior to the attachment of the posterolateral bundle. When the knee is flexed, the relative positions switch, causing the ACL to wind upon itself (Fig. 10-7). This leads to varying portions of the ACL being taut as the knee moves through its range of motion (ROM). When the knee is fully extended, the posterolateral bundle is tight; when the knee is fully flexed, the anteromedial bundle is taut.[8]

The amount of strain placed on the ACL is influenced by the type of movement and the subsequent translation of the tibia. During passive ROM (PROM), the amount of strain placed on the ACL is minimized when the tibia remains in the neutral position. In the final 15 degrees of extension, internally rotating the tibia greatly increases the strain placed on the ACL; externally rotating the tibia decreases the strain relative to internal rotation, but it is still greater than the strain with the tibia in neutral. Both valgus and varus stresses increase the strain on the ACL during PROM (Fig. 10-8).[9] During active open-chain knee extension when the pull of the quadriceps translates the tibia anteriorly, the amount of strain placed on the ACL is greatest between 0 and 30 degrees of flexion.[10] Adding resistance through the arc of knee extension significantly increases the amount of

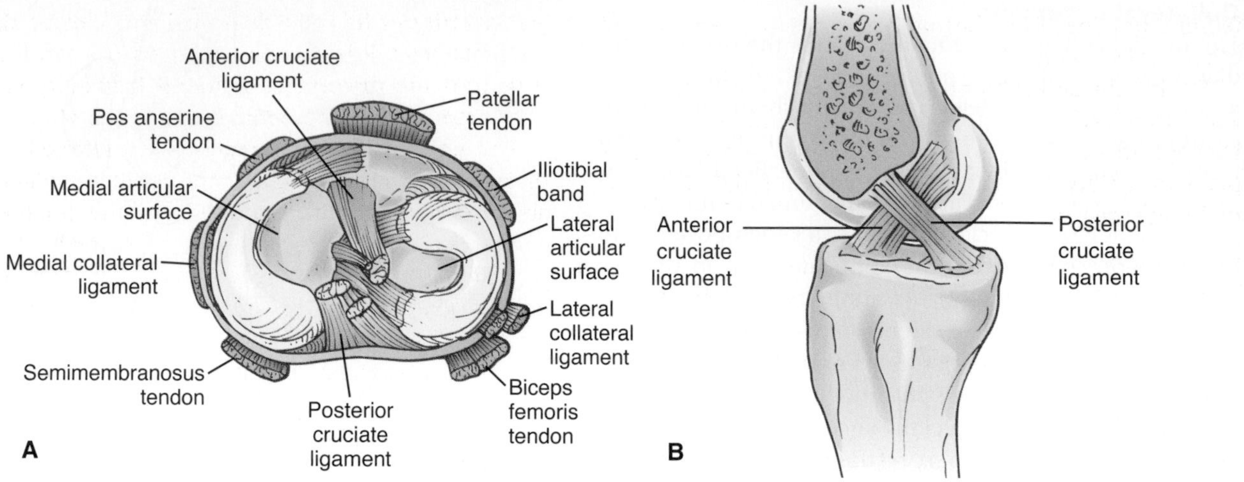

FIGURE 10-6 ■ Cruciate ligaments. The ligaments are named according to their relative attachment on the tibia. (A) Superior view referencing the cruciate ligaments to each other and to other supportive structures about the knee. (B) Lateral view of the cruciate ligaments.

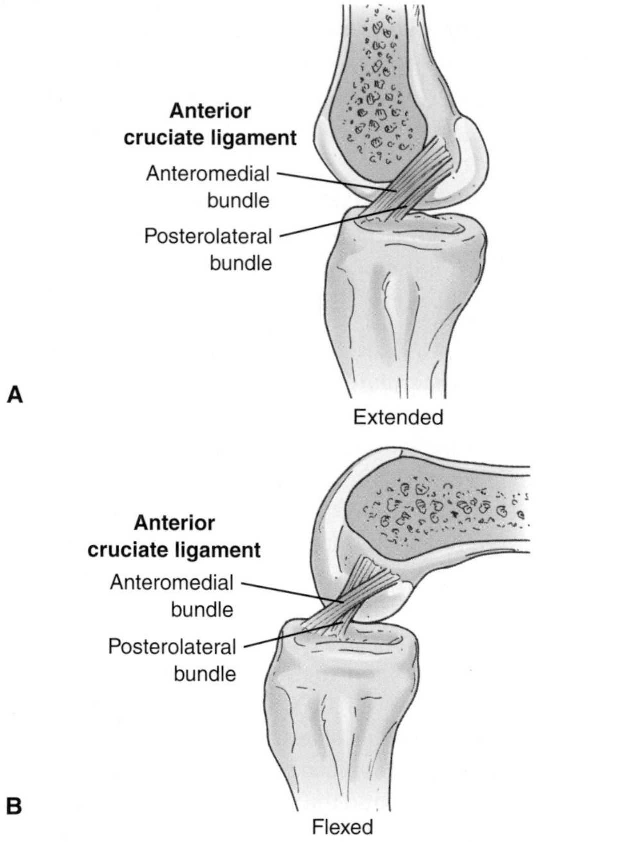

FIGURE 10-7 ■ Biomechanics of the anterior cruciate ligament. (A) When the knee is fully extended, the femoral attachment site of the anteromedial bundle is proximal to the attachment site of the posterolateral bundle. (B) When the knee is flexed, these attachment sites juxtapose their positions, causing the anterior cruciate to wind upon itself.

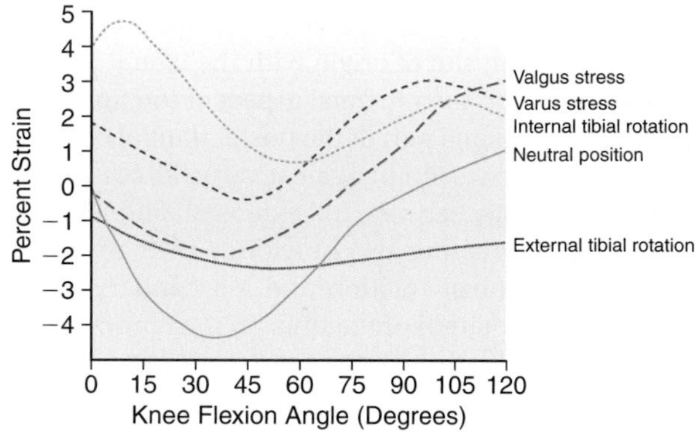

FIGURE 10-8 ■ Strain placed on the anterior cruciate ligament through passive range of motion. Altering the relative alignment of the tibia to the femur increases the strain on the ligament throughout the range of motion.

strain as the knee extends from 45 to 0 degrees of flexion.[10] During closed kinetic chain exercises, the strain on the ACL does not significantly change throughout the ROM.[11]

Posterior cruciate ligament. The PCL arises from the posterior aspect of the tibia and takes a superior and anterior course, passing medially to the ACL, to attach on the lateral portion of the femur's medial condyle. The PCL, stronger and 120% to 150% wider than the ACL, is a primary stabilizer of the knee.[12-15] The PCL has two distinct components: the **anterolateral** and **posteromedial** bundles, bands named relative to their tibial insertions, although three and four bundles have been described in the PCL.[15,16] As an entire unit, the PCL is the primary restraint against posterior displacement of the tibia on the femur and a secondary restraint against external tibial rotation. The anterolateral bundle is taut when the knee is flexed and loosens when the knee is extended; the posteromedial bundle is relatively lax when the knee is flexed and tightens when the knee is extended.[14,15,17] The PCL receives its limited blood supply from the middle geniculate artery.[14]

Although the PCL offers significant support against posterior forces on the knee joint, its function is augmented by the meniscofemoral ligaments (ligaments of Humphrey and Wrisberg) and the posterolateral structures of the knee, specifically the posterolateral corner.[1,18] A combined injury to the PCL and posterolateral structures results in greater posterior laxity than when either structure is affected alone.[19,20] When the knee is near extension, the primary restraint against posterior displacement of the tibia on the femur is obtained from the popliteus, posterior capsule, and other joint structures.[17]

During the **screw home mechanism**, the PCL and ACL wind upon each other in flexion and unwind in extension. Damage to the PCL can result in frontal and transverse plane instability because the stable axis for tibial rotation is no longer present.

Posterolateral Corner

The posterolateral corner (PLC), also known as the lateral complex and posterolateral complex, has been referred to as "the dark side of the knee" for its varied and relatively poorly understood anatomy (Fig. 10-9).[6,21] Consisting of both dynamic and static stabilizers, the PLC is integral in providing stability against varus stress, external tibial rotation, and anterior and posterior forces about the knee. The combined contributions of the anatomical elements of this structure are greater than the sum of the combined parts; the integrity of its individual elements can be disrupted with relatively little joint instability. However, if multiple structures are disrupted, profound instability can result (see Posterolateral Rotational Instability, p. 346).[5]

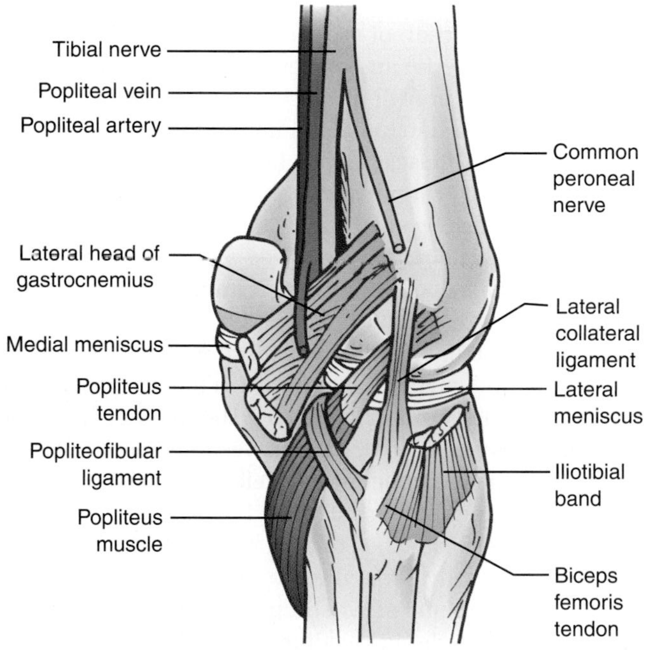

FIGURE 10-9 ■ The posterolateral corner of the knee.

Layer	Structures
I (Superficial)	Lateral fascia
	Iliotibial band
	Biceps femoris tendon
II (Middle)	Patellar retinaculum
	Patellofemoral ligament
III (Deep)	Joint capsule
	Lateral collateral ligament*
	Arcuate ligament
	Popliteofibular ligament
	Fabellofibular ligament
	Popliteus tendon

*Sometimes grouped into the middle layer.

The **popliteofibular ligament** (also referred to as the short external lateral ligament, the popliteofibular fascicles, fibular origin of the popliteus, and the popliteofibular fibers), is a Y-shaped structure with origins from the tibia and fibula. Inserting on the femur, the popliteofibular ligament is a key stabilizer against posterior translation, varus forces, and external rotation.[5,7,21-23]

The **popliteus complex** is formed by the popliteus muscle and its tendon, the popliteofibular ligament, popliteotibial fascicle, and the popliteomeniscal fascicles. The popliteus muscle has attachments to the posterior horn and middle posterior portions of the lateral meniscus and helps resist external tibial rotation between 20 and 130 degrees of knee flexion.[21] The **arcuate ligament** provides further support to the posterolateral joint capsule.[5] Arising from the fibular head, the arcuate ligament passes over the popliteus muscle, where it diverges into the intercondylar area of the tibia and the posterior aspect of the femur's lateral epicondyle. The arcuate ligament assists the cruciate ligaments in controlling posterolateral rotational instability. Injury to this area results in increased external rotation of the tibia on the femur.

The **fabella**, when present, lies within the lateral head of the gastrocnemius muscle. Although its actual significance to the structure and function of the knee is unclear, when the fabella is present, a fabellofibular ligament attaches from the fabella to the fibular head, increasing the thickness of the tissues in the posterolateral corner of the knee.[5,21]

Proximal Tibiofibular Syndesmosis

The proximal tibiofibular syndesmosis is a relatively immobile joint where the proximal tibia and fibula are bound together by ligaments. The proximal syndesmosis is more stable than the distal tibiofibular syndesmosis because of the alignment between the fibular head and the indentation on the proximal tibia. The superior tibiofibular joint is stabilized by the superior anterior and posterior tibiofibular ligaments and, to a lesser degree, by the interosseous membrane. Anterior displacement of the fibula is partially blocked by a bony outcrop from the tibia. Therefore, most fibular instabilities tend to occur posteriorly, possibly affecting the common peroneal nerve because of its proximity to the articulation (Fig. 10-10).

The Menisci

The anatomic incongruities between the articular surfaces of the tibia and femur are partially resolved by the presence of the fibrocartilaginous medial and lateral menisci. The menisci serve to:

1. Deepen the articulation and fill the gaps that normally occur during the knee's articulation, increasing load transmission over a greater percentage of the joint surfaces

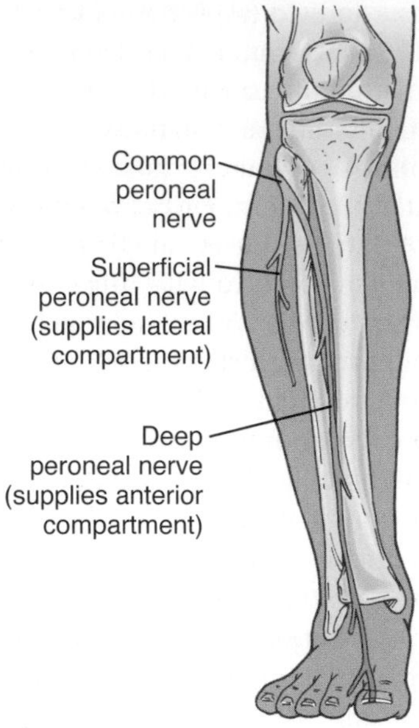

FIGURE 10-10 ■ The common peroneal nerve and its branches.

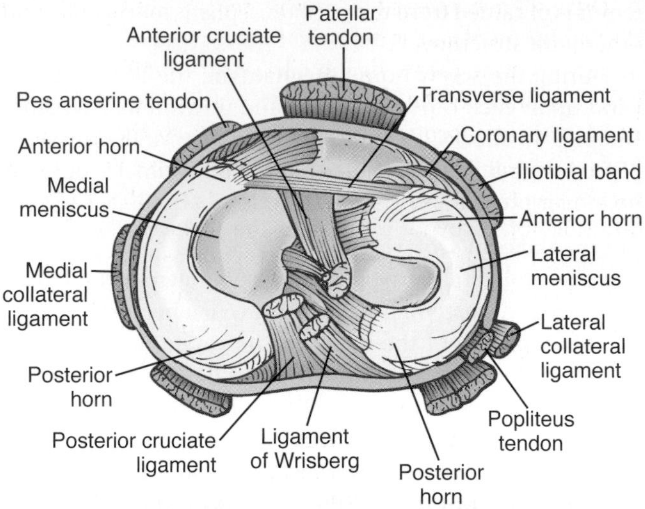

FIGURE 10-11 ■ Superior view of the medial and lateral menisci and their associated ligamentous structures (right knee shown). The peripheral border of the menisci is fixated to the tibia by the coronary ligament.

2. Improve lubrication for the articulating surfaces
3. Provide shock absorption
4. Increase passive joint stability
5. Limit the extremes of flexion and extension
6. Serve as proprioceptive organs

When viewed in cross section, the menisci are wedge shaped, with their outer borders thicker than their inner rims. When viewed from above, this wedge creates a concave area on the tibia to accept the femur's articulating surfaces. Because of this geometry, the knee is more stable when it is bearing weight than when it is not.

At birth, the entire meniscus is vascularized, but by the age of 9 months the inner third becomes avascular. At 10 years of age, the menisci reach the vascular profile seen in adulthood.[24] The menisci also become less resistant to stress with aging due to degeneration and dehydration.

Each meniscus is divided into an anterior, middle, and posterior third (Fig. 10-11). The anterior and posterior portions of the menisci are marked by the horns, the areas of the menisci most frequently torn. Approximately 10% to 25% of the outer portion of the lateral meniscus and 10% to 30% of the medial meniscus is vascularized.[24] The menisci have a narrow **vascular (red) zone** along their outer rim and the anterior and posterior horns and an **avascular (white) zone** formed by the inner portion of the meniscus. There is a thin, lightly vascular **pink zone** between the red and white zones (Fig. 10-12). Because of the presence of an active blood supply via the medial, middle, and lateral geniculate arteries, meniscal tears occurring within the vascular zone have an improved chance of healing compared with tears in the avascular zone, which rely on nutrients being delivered through the synovial fluid. These zones cannot be differentiated via standard or contrast imaging techniques and must be visually identified during surgery.[25]

The central portion of the meniscus is relatively denervated, but the anterior and posterior horns do contain sensory nerves that provide proprioceptive feedback during the extremes of flexion (posterior horns) and extension (anterior horns).[24] Meniscal lesions become painful when the adjacent and richly innervated joint capsule becomes irritated or distended by edema.

The **medial meniscus** resembles a half crescent, or C shape, that is wider posteriorly than it is anteriorly. The **lateral meniscus** is more circular in shape, but the size, thickness, shape, and mobility are different from those of the medial meniscus.[26] Both menisci are attached at their peripheries to the tibia via the **coronary ligament**. The **anterior horns** of each meniscus are joined by the **transverse ligament** and connected to the patellar tendon via **patellomeniscal ligaments**.

The lateral meniscus, smaller and more mobile than the medial meniscus, attaches to the lateral aspect of the medial femoral condyle via the two **meniscofemoral ligaments** (the **ligaments of Wrisberg** and **Humphrey**) and to the popliteus muscle via the joint capsule and coronary ligament. Attaching the **posterior horn** of the lateral meniscus to the femur, the meniscofemoral ligaments are oriented in a way that mimics the PCL.[1]

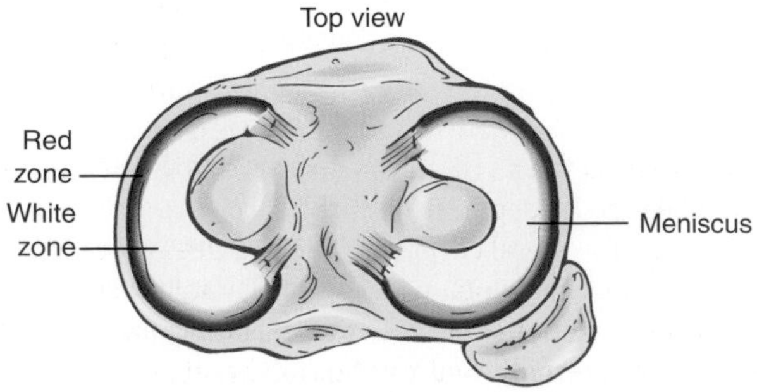

FIGURE 10-12 ■ Vascularity of the menisci.

During knee extension, patellomeniscal ligaments pull the lateral meniscus anteriorly, distorting its shape in the anteroposterior plane. In the early degrees of flexion, the popliteus pulls the lateral meniscus posteriorly; in the later ROM, the meniscofemoral ligament pulls the posterior horn medially and anteriorly.[27] During passive flexion, the menisci are displaced posteriorly and laterally, with the anterior horn moving more than the posterior horn, with maximum displacement occurring at 90 degrees of flexion.[28] Because of its relative lack of mobility and its attachment to the MCL, the medial meniscus tends to be injured from acute trauma, while the lateral meniscus tends to suffer degenerative tears.

Muscles Acting on the Knee

The muscles acting on the knee primarily serve to flex or extend it. The flexor musculature has the secondary responsibility of rotating the tibia. The flexors attaching on the tibia's medial side internally rotate it, and those attaching on the lateral side externally rotate it. The muscles acting on the knee, their origins, insertions, and innervation are presented in Table 10-1.

Anterior Muscles

The **quadriceps femoris** muscle group consists of four muscles: the **vastus lateralis**, **vastus intermedius**, **vastus medialis**, and **rectus femoris**. Each of the quadriceps femoris muscles has a common insertion on the tibial tuberosity via the patellar tendon (Fig. 10-13). The vastus medialis has two discrete groups of fibers arising from the medial femoral condyle and the fascia of the adductor magnus. Separated by a fascial plane, the muscle is divided into the vastus medialis longus and the vastus medialis oblique (VMO). As a group, the quadriceps femoris extends the knee. The rectus femoris, a two-joint muscle, also serves as a hip flexor, especially when the knee is flexed. During knee extension, the VMO guides the patella medially.

Posterior Muscles

The **semitendinosus**, **semimembranosus**, and **biceps femoris** are collectively known as the **hamstrings**. They act as a unit to flex the knee and extend the hip (Fig. 10-14). With attachments to the iliotibial band, Gerdy's tubercle, the LCL, and posterolateral capsule, the biceps femoris serves to rotate the tibia externally and help protect the knee against varus stresses.[7] The semimembranosus and semitendinosus internally rotate the tibia. Because its function is redundant with the semimembranosus, the semitendinosus is a good candidate as a graft source for ACL reconstruction. The hamstring muscles also decrease the anterior shear forces that stress the ACL when the knee is flexed beyond 20 degrees.[29,30]

The posterolateral corner of the knee is reinforced by the **popliteus** muscle, which provides both dynamic and static stabilization to the knee, resisting posterior tibial translation, static external tibial rotation, dynamic internal tibial rotation, and buffers against varus forces (see Fig. 10-6).[7] In an open kinetic chain, the popliteus causes internal rotation of the tibia on the femur; in a closed kinetic chain, the popliteus externally rotates the femur on the tibia. Responsible for unscrewing the knee from its locked position in extension, its remaining influence on knee flexion is slight. However, when the patient is bearing weight with the knee partially flexed, the popliteus assists the PCL in preventing posterior displacement of the tibia on the femur. Because of the close association between the popliteus muscle and the other structures in the posterolateral corner of the knee, injury to this muscle will weaken the entire complex.[7]

A diamond-shaped **popliteal fossa** is formed by the knee's posterior musculature (Fig. 10-15). Although its inner boundaries are largely devoid of muscles (with the exception of the popliteus), the popliteal fossa contains the popliteal artery and vein; the tibial, common peroneal, and posterior femoral cutaneous nerves; and the small saphenous vein.

Pes Anserine Muscle Group

The **gracilis**, **sartorius**, and **semitendinosus** muscles form the pes anserine muscle group. In addition to flexing the knee, the pes anserine group internally rotates the tibia when the foot is not planted on the ground. When the foot is planted, the pes anserine externally rotates the femur on a fixed tibia.

The gracilis and semitendinosus muscles are relatively straightforward in their anatomic orientation. However, the sartorius muscle is unusual. Although its belly is located on the anterior aspect of the femur, it is a flexor of the knee joint because the sartorius muscle crosses the knee posterior to its axis (see Fig. 10-13). With an origin proximal and anterior to the hip joint, the sartorius muscle also assists in flexion, external rotation, and abduction of the hip.

Iliotibial Band

The **iliotibial (IT) band** is an extension of the **tensor fasciae latae** (a small muscle originating from the **anterior superior iliac** crest) and gluteus maximus muscular fascia. The IT band travels down the lateral aspect of the femur to insert on **Gerdy's tubercle** on the anterolateral tibia and attaches to the lateral patellar retinaculum and the biceps femoris tendon through divergent slips.[31] Although the tensor fasciae latae and IT band make a relatively insignificant contribution to knee motion, the deep fibers of the IT band attach to the lateral joint capsule and function as an anterolateral knee ligament, playing a significant role in knee stability and patellofemoral pathology.[7,32]

The angle between the IT band and tibia varies according to the knee flexion angle, which, in turn, alters the knee's biomechanics. When the knee is fully extended, the IT band is anterior to, or located over, the lateral femoral epicondyle. When the knee is flexed past 30 degrees, the IT band shifts behind the lateral femoral epicondyle, giving it an angle of pull as if it were a knee flexor, exerting an external rotation and posterior force on the tibia (Fig. 10-16). This posterior shift is greatly influenced by the biceps femoris, which has a fibrous expanse attaching to the IT band. During contraction of the biceps femoris, the IT band is drawn posteriorly.

Table 10-1 Muscles Acting on the Knee

Muscle	Action	Origin	Insertion	Innervation	Root
Primary Action: Knee Extension					
Biceps Femoris	Knee flexion External tibial rotation Long head • Hip extension • Hip external rotation	Long head • Ischial tuberosity • Sacrotuberous ligament Short head • Lateral lip of the linea aspera • Upper two-thirds of the supracondylar line	Lateral fibular head Lateral tibial condyle	Long head • Tibial Short head • Common peroneal	Long head S1, S2, S3 Short head L5, S1, S2
Gastrocnemius	Assists knee flexion Ankle plantarflexion	Medial head • Posterior surface of the medial femoral condyle • Adjacent portion of the femur and knee capsule Lateral head • Posterior surface of the lateral femoral condyle • Adjacent portion of the femur and knee capsule	To the calcaneus via the Achilles tendon	Tibial	S1, S2
Gracilis	Knee flexion Internal tibial rotation Hip adduction	Symphysis pubis Inferior ramus of the pubic bone	Proximal portion of the anteromedial tibial flare	Obturator (posterior)	L3, L4
Popliteus	Open chain • Internal tibial rotation • Knee flexion Closed chain External femoral rotation	Lateral femoral condyle Oblique popliteal ligament	Posterior tibia superior to the soleal line Fascia covering the soleus	Tibial	L4, L5, S1
Sartorius	Knee flexion Knee flexion Internal tibial rotation Hip flexion Hip abduction Hip external rotation	Anterior superior iliac spine	Proximal portion of the anteromedial tibial flare	Femoral	L2, L3

Semimembranosus	Knee flexion Internal tibial rotation Hip extension Hip internal rotation	Ischial tuberosity	Posteromedial portion of the tibia's medial condyle	Tibial	L5, S1
Semitendinosus	Knee flexion Internal tibial rotation Hip extension Hip internal rotation	Ischial tuberosity	Medial portion of the tibial flare	Tibial	L5, S1, S2
Primary Action: Knee Extension					
Rectus Femoris	Knee extension Hip flexion	Anterior inferior iliac spine Groove located superior to the acetabulum	To the tibial tubercle via the patella and patellar ligament	Femoral	L2, L3, L4
Vastus Intermedius	Knee extension	Anterolateral portion of the upper two-thirds of the femur Lower one-half of the linea aspera	To the tibial tubercle via the patella and patellar ligament	Femoral	L2, L3, L4
Vastus Lateralis	Knee extension	Proximal intertrochanteric line Greater trochanter Gluteal tuberosity Upper one-half of the linea aspera	To the tibial tubercle via the patella and patellar ligament	Femoral	L2, L3, L4
Vastus Medialis	Knee extension Oblique portion • Patellar stabilization	Longus portion • Distal one-half of the intertrochanteric line • Medial portion of the linea aspera Oblique portion • Tendons from adductor longus and adductor magnus	To the tibial tubercle via the patella and patellar ligament	Femoral	L2, L3, L4

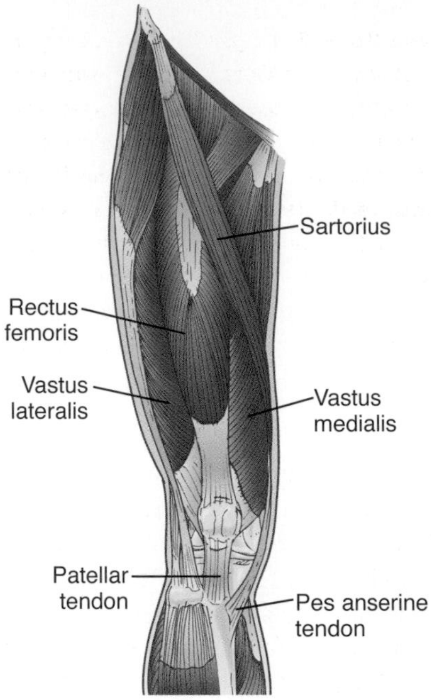

FIGURE 10-13 ■ Anterior muscles acting on the knee. The vastus lateralis, rectus femoris, vastus intermedius (hidden beneath the rectus femoris), and vastus medialis share a common insertion via the patellar tendon.

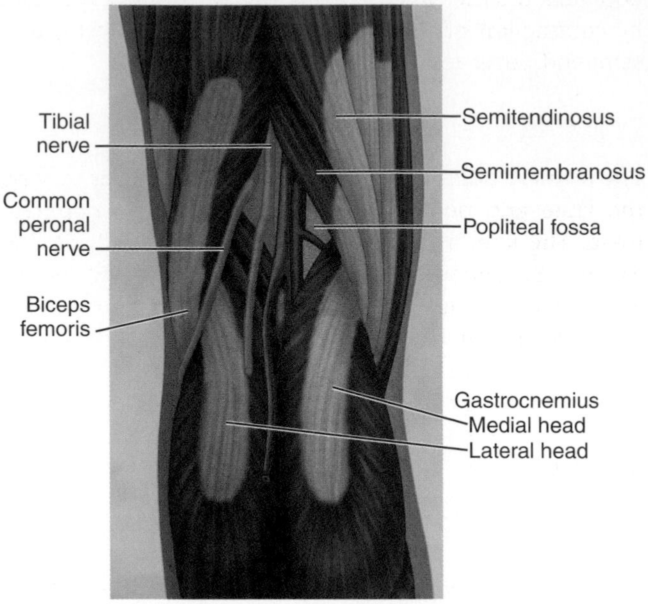

FIGURE 10-15 ■ Popliteal fossa of the right knee.

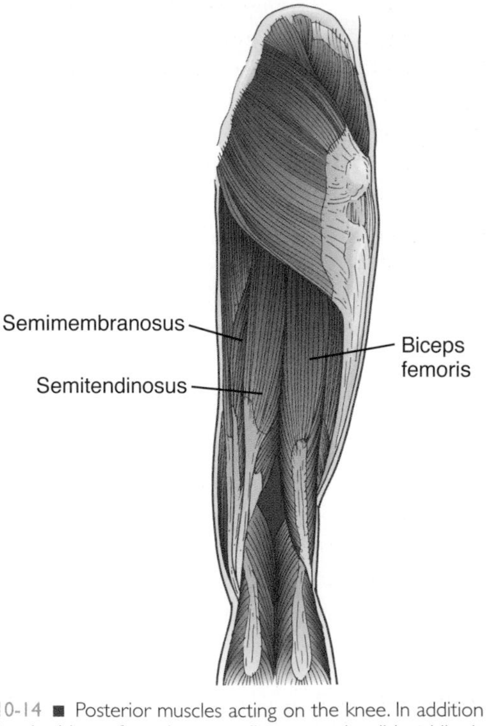

FIGURE 10-14 ■ Posterior muscles acting on the knee. In addition to flexing the joint, the biceps femoris externally rotates the tibia, while the semimembranosus and semitendinosus internally rotate it.

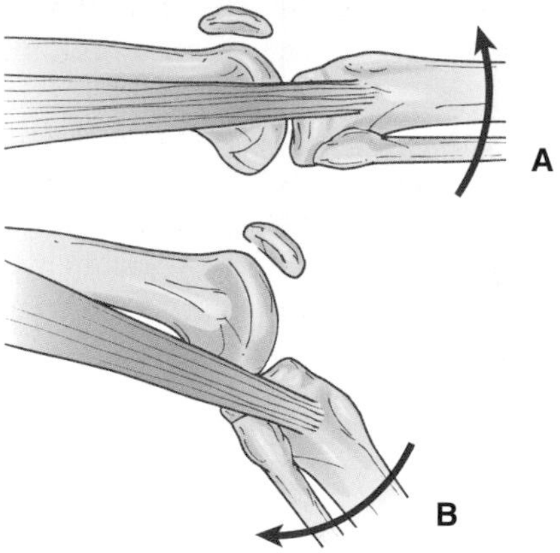

FIGURE 10-16 ■ The iliotibial band's dynamic line of pull in flexion and extension. (A) When the knee is fully extended, the iliotibial band's angle of pull is that of a knee extensor. (B) When it is flexed past 30°, it assumes an angle of flexor.

The Screw Home Mechanism

The unequal sizes of the femoral condyles and the tightening of the cruciate ligaments as they wind upon themselves during flexion necessitates a locking mechanism as the knee nears its final degrees of extension.[33] The medial femoral condyle has a larger surface area than the lateral condyle. As the knee straightens, the articular distance on the lateral femoral condyle is extended, and the medial articulation continues to glide, resulting in external rotation of the tibia with the lateral meniscus serving as the pivot point.

During extension of a non–weight-bearing knee, complete motion is achieved by the tibia externally rotating 5 to 7 degrees on the femur. However, when bearing weight, the tibia is relatively fixed, so the terminal ROM is accomplished by a combination of tibial external rotation and femoral internal rotation. For flexion to occur, the tibia must internally rotate relative to the femur. When not bearing weight, this internal rotation is accomplished by the popliteus muscle; when bearing weight, unlocking occurs by contraction of the popliteus, semimembranosus, and semitendinosus muscles.

Neurological Anatomy

The primary neurological and vascular structures serving the knee and points distal pass through the popliteal fossa. The knee is supplied primarily by the L3, L4, L5, S1, and S2 nerve roots. The knee is innervated by the anterior cutaneous branches of the femoral nerve and the infrapatellar branch of the saphenous nerve anteriorly, the saphenous nerve medially, the posterior cutaneous branches of the cluneal nerve posteriorly, and the sural cutaneous nerve (via the common peroneal nerve) laterally.

Vascular Anatomy

The popliteal artery and vein are separated from the posterior capsule by a layer of adipose tissue. Within the popliteal fossa, the popliteal artery sprouts five geniculate arteries (two superior, two inferior, and one middle) that provide collateral circulation to the knee.[34] The anterior tibial artery and lateral femoral circumflex artery provide further blood supply to the anterior and lateral portions of the knee.

Because of the intimacy of the neurovascular structures to the knee joint proper, damage to these structures must be ruled out in the presence of a tibiofemoral dislocation. The popliteal artery is attached to the adductor hiatus proximal to the knee and to the soleus muscle distal to the knee, making it particularly prone to trauma.[34]

Clinical Examination of Knee Injuries

The patient is evaluated while wearing shorts to permit inspection and palpation of the muscles originating off the femur and pelvis. The patella is described in this section only as it relates to tibiofemoral function. The examination of patients with patellofemoral conditions is presented in Chapter 11.

History

Blows to the knee place compressive forces on the joint structures at the point of the blow, tensile forces on the side opposite the blow, and shear forces across the joint. Rotational forces about the knee, such as those experienced when an athlete cuts to change direction, place tensile forces about the joint capsule and cruciate ligaments. The menisci may also be torn by this mechanism secondary to impingement and shearing between the articular condyles. The need for radiographs of the knee to rule out fracture can be determined using the **Ottawa Knee Rules** (OKR).[35-37]

> ✻ Practical Evidence
>
> The **Ottawa Knee Rules** are used to identify individuals who should be referred for radiographic examination of the knee. Following acute knee trauma, a patient who meets any of the following five criteria should be referred for radiographs: (1) age 55 or older; (2) demonstrates tenderness of the fibular head; (3) has palpable, isolated tenderness of the patella; (4) is unable to flex the knee to 90°; or (5) is unable to bear weight for four steps immediately after the trauma and/or during clinical examination. Designed to be highly sensitive, the use of these rules could reduce the need for plain knee radiographs by approximately 25%.[35-37]

Past Medical History

- **Past history of injury:** A past history of injury for both the involved and uninvolved knee must be established. Previous injury can result in chronic inflammation secondary to internal derangement or biomechanical dysfunction. Nonsurgical ligament and capsule sprains may have healed with a great deal of scar tissue, restricting the ROM, or with excess laxity, both of which predispose the knee to reinjury. Surgical conditions involving grafts or **primary repairs** are also subject to reinjury.
- **Injury to related body areas:** Previous injury to the low back, lower leg, foot, and/or ankle may alter mechanics at the knee, inviting pathological changes. Consider the gait adapted by the individual with a sprained ankle. This type of sustained ankle plantarflexion during ambulation places the knee in a prolonged flexed position, altering compressive forces. In children, hip pathology such as slipped capital femoral epiphysis may refer pain to the knee.
- **General medical conditions:** For conditions of chronic or insidious onset, determine if the patient has a history of systemic or local inflammatory diseases such as osteoarthritis (OA), rheumatoid arthritis, or gout.[38] Knee OA is a common source of knee pain in post-college aged individuals (see Chapter 4).

> ✻ Practical Evidence
>
> Aging itself puts certain knee tissues at risk. Articular cartilage reaches its maximum tensile strength between the ages of 20 and 30, and its strength dramatically declines with increasing age, making it more susceptible to shearing injury with rotational forces.[39]

History of the Present Condition

- **Location of pain:** Tears of the collateral ligaments or the anteromedial or anterolateral capsule normally result in pain directly corresponding to the area of trauma. Pain arising from the ACL may be described as being "beneath the kneecap" or "inside the knee," and pain from the PCL may mimic that caused by a tear of the medial or lateral origin of the gastrocnemius. Tears

---

Primary repair The process of surgically repairing a soft tissue injury, usually by suturing the ends together

Examination Map

HISTORY

Past Medical History
History of the Present Condition
Mechanism of Injury

FUNCTIONAL ASSESSMENT

Gait Assessment

INSPECTION

Girth Measurements

Inspection of the Anterior Structures

Patella
Patellar tendon
Quadriceps muscle group
Tibiofemoral alignment
Tibial tuberosity

Inspection of the Medial Structures

General medial aspect
Vastus medialis

Inspection of the Lateral Structures

General lateral structure
Fibular head
Posterior sag of tibia
Hyperextension

Inspection of the Posterior Structures

Hamstring muscle group
Popliteal fossa
- Baker's cyst

PALPATION

Palpation of the Anterior Structures

Patella
Patellar tendon
Tibial tuberosity
Quadriceps tendon
Quadriceps muscle group
- Vastus medialis
- Rectus femoris
- Vastus lateralis

Sartorius

Palpation of the Medial Structures

Medial meniscus and joint line
Medial collateral ligament
Medial femoral condyle and epicondyle
Medial tibial plateau
Pes anserine tendon and bursa
Semitendinosus
Gracilis

Palpation of the Lateral Structures

Joint line
Fibular head
Lateral collateral ligament
Popliteus
Biceps femoris
Iliotibial band

Palpation of the Posterior Structures

Popliteal fossa
Hamstring muscle group
- Biceps femoris
- Semimembranosus
- Semitendinosus

Determination of Intracapsular versus Extracapsular Swelling

JOINT AND MUSCLE FUNCTION ASSESSMENT

Goniometry

Flexion
Extension

Active Range of Motion

Flexion
Extension

Manual Muscle Tests

Knee extension
Knee flexion
Isolating the sartorius

Passive Range of Motion

Flexion
Extension

JOINT STABILITY TESTS

Stress Testing

Anterior instability
- Anterior drawer test
- Lachman test
- Prone Lachman test

Posterior instability
- Posterior drawer test
- Godfrey's test

Medial instability
- Valgus stress test: 0° flexion
- Valgus stress test: 25° flexion

Lateral instability
- Valgus stress test: 0° flexion
- Valgus stress test: 25° flexion

Joint Play Assessment

Proximal tibiofibular syndesmosis

NEUROLOGICAL ASSESSMENT

Lower Quarter Screen

Common Peroneal Nerve

VASCULAR ASSESSMENT

Distal Capillary Refill

Distal Pulse

Posterior tibial artery
Dorsal pedal artery

REGION-SPECIFIC PATHOLOGIES

Uniplanar Knee Sprains

Medial collateral ligament
- Valgus stress test

Lateral collateral ligament
- Varus stress test

Anterior cruciate ligament
- Anterior drawer test
- Lachman test
- Prone Lachman test
- Quadriceps active test

Rotational Knee Instabilities

Anterolateral rotational instability
- Pivot shift test
- Jerk test
- Slocum drawer test
- Crossover test
- Slocum ALRI test
- Flexion-rotation drawer test

Anteromedial rotational instability
- Slocum drawer test
- Crossover test
- Lachman test
- Valgus stress test

Posterolateral rotational instability
- External rotation (dial) test
- External rotation recurvatum test
- Posterolateral drawer test
- Reverse-pivot shift test
- Dynamic posterior shift test

Meniscal Tears

McMurray test
Apley compression/distraction test
Thessaly test

Osteochondral Lesions

Wilson's test

Iliotibial Band Friction Syndrome

Noble compression test
Ober test

Popliteus Tendinopathy

Tibiofemoral Joint Dislocations

to the vascular zone of the menisci can present with joint line pain. Tears in the avascular zone may be described as pain or, more commonly, as popping, clicking, or locking within the knee. Posterior knee pain can represent a PCL tear or popliteal (Baker's) cyst (Table 10-2).[38] Individuals with knee OA commonly report medial and lateral joint line pain.[40]

- **Mechanism of injury:** Forces delivered to the knee in the frontal or sagittal plane when the knee is extended have less of a rotational component than blows received at an angle or when the knee is flexed. Forces delivered in a straight planar motion usually result in more isolated ligamentous injuries. Rotational stresses may more commonly injure multiple ligamentous and meniscal tissues. A description of an acute, non–contact-related onset most likely reflects a rotational stress that was placed on the knee, as occurs when a person changes directions while running or pivoting (Table 10-3).
- **Weight-bearing status at the time of injury:** Rotational injuries may further be identified by establishing the weight-bearing status of the involved limb. A foot that was planted at the time of injury fixates the tibia, allowing the femur to rotate on it. This effect is magnified by an increased shoe-surface friction.
- **Associated sounds or sensations:** Determine the sensations and any associated sounds (e.g., "pop" or "snap") experienced at the time of the injury. After ruling out a patellar dislocation, subluxation, or fracture, these sounds may indicate a tear of one of the cruciate ligaments.[41,42] Patients often report the knee "giving way." With true giving way, the knee buckles during weight bearing, likely indicating ligamentous instability. The buckling as the result of pain is often related to meniscal injury or patellofemoral joint disease.

True locking, the inability to passively fully extend the knee, indicates an unstable meniscal tear or subluxation of the posterior horn of the meniscus[43] or a loose body such as an osteochondral fragment within the joint that wedges between the femur and tibia. Patients may report catching or crepitation as locking. These symptoms often more accurately indicate patellofemoral joint disease.

- **Onset of injury:** Ligamentous injuries most often present with an acute onset related to a specific episode. Injuries having an insidious onset are most likely to involve inflammation of the muscles and tendons acting on the knee, may be the result of patellar maltracking, or may represent degenerative changes within the knee. As with chronic foot and ankle injuries, chronic knee pain

Table 10-2 Differential Diagnosis Based on the Location of Pain

Location of Pain	Lateral	Anterior	Medial	Posterior
Soft Tissue	LCL sprain Lateral joint capsule sprain Proximal tibiofibular syndesmosis sprain Lateral patellar retinaculum irritation* Biceps femoris tear Biceps femoris tendinopathy Popliteal tendinopathy IT band friction syndrome Lateral meniscus tear	ACL sprain (emanating from "inside" the knee) Patellar tendinopathy* Patellar tendon rupture (partial or complete)* Patellar bursitis* Patellofemoral joint dysfunction* Quadriceps contusion Fat pad irritation* Quadriceps tendon rupture*	MCL sprain Medial joint capsule sprain Medial patellar retinaculum irritation* Pes anserine bursitis or tendinopathy Semitendinosus tear Semitendinosus tendinopathy Semimembranosus tear Semimembranosus tendinopathy Medial meniscus tear	PCL sprain Posterior capsule sprain Gastrocnemius tear Hamstring tear Popliteus tendinopathy Popliteal cyst Medial/lateral meniscal tear (posterior horn)
Bony	Fibular head fracture Osteochondral fracture Osteochondritis dissecans Lateral femoral condyle contusion Lateral tibial plateau contusion Epiphyseal fracture Osteoarthritis	Patellar fracture Tibial plateau fracture Sinding-Larsen-Johansson disease* Osgood-Schlatter disease Patellar dislocation or subluxation* Chondromalacia	Osteochondral fracture Osteochondritis dissecans Medial femoral condyle contusion Medial tibial plateau contusion Epiphyseal fracture Osteoarthritis	

*Discussed in Chapter 11.

ACL = anterior cruciate ligament; IT = iliotibial; LCL = lateral collateral ligament; MCL = medial collateral ligament; PCL = posterior cruciate ligament

Table 10-3 Mechanism of Knee Injuries and the Resultant Soft Tissue Damage

Force Placed on the Knee	Tensile Forces	Compressive Forces
Valgus	Medial structures: MCL, medial joint capsule, pes anserine muscle group, medial meniscus	Lateral meniscus
Varus	Lateral structures: LCL, lateral joint capsule, IT band, biceps femoris	Medial meniscus
Anterior Tibial Displacement	ACL, IT band, LCL, MCL medial and lateral joint capsules	Posterior portion of the medial and lateral meniscus
Posterior Tibial Displacement	PCL, meniscofemoral ligament(s), popliteus, medial and lateral joint capsules	Anterior portion of the medial and lateral meniscus
Internal Tibial Rotation	ACL, anterolateral joint capsule, posteromedial joint capsule, posterolateral joint capsule, LCL	Anterior horn of the medial meniscus Posterior horn of the lateral meniscus
External Tibial Rotation	Posterolateral joint capsule, anteromedial joint capsule, MCL, PCL, LCL, ACL	Anterior horn of the lateral meniscus Posterior horn of the lateral meniscus
Hyperextension	ACL, posterior joint capsule, PCL	Anterior portion of the medial and lateral meniscus
Hyperflexion	ACL, PCL	Posterior portion of the medial and lateral meniscus

ACL = anterior cruciate ligament; IT = iliotibial; LCL = lateral collateral ligament; MCL = medial collateral ligament; PCL = posterior cruciate ligament

may arise secondary to training errors, foot type, shoe type, postural deviations, hip pathology, and foot biomechanics. Meniscal injuries may be acute or occur gradually in association with degenerative changes, as is often the case with the lateral meniscus.

Functional Assessment

The patient is observed while performing those tasks that are problematic or part of the daily routine. Gait observation is a standard component of the functional assessment. Following a capsular or ligamentous knee injury, there is a natural inclination to shorten the stance phase of gait and maintain the knee in the resting position of 30 degrees of flexion. Shortening of the stride length may also indicate functional shortening of the hamstrings. With knee sprains and resulting joint instability, the patient may display and describe apprehension and/or decreased speed with tasks requiring abrupt change of direction. OA symptoms may be associated with any weight-bearing activity or after periods of prolonged sitting. Limitations in knee motion may manifest themselves with abnormal movement patterns in tasks such as going upstairs. The results of this task analysis are then used during the remainder of the examination process to identify the underlying impairments.

Inspection

As much of the inspection process as possible is performed while the patient is weight bearing to detect postural abnormalities and resulting compensations. Acute injuries with an associated **hemarthrosis** will result in visible swelling of the knee.

Hemarthrosis Blood within a joint cavity

Girth Measurements

Ongoing reexamination of existing conditions must include a determination of the amount of fluid in and around the knee joint and atrophy of the quadriceps muscle groups. To be objective, these measurements must be made in a consistent and reproducible manner (Selective Tissue Test 10-1). Following disuse secondary to trauma, including surgery, the volume of the quadriceps muscles significantly decreases relative to the uninvolved limb, but this reduction is not typically seen in the hamstring or adductor muscles. Within the quadriceps group, all muscles tend to atrophy at the same rate, but the vastus medialis and rectus femoris lose slightly more volume.[44] Note that the muscles of the dominant thigh may naturally be hypertrophied relative to the nondominant thigh, and measurements are more accurate in lean individuals, especially when performed by the same examiner.[45,46]

Inspection of the Anterior Structures

- **Patella:** Observe the patella, normally found resting above the femoral trochlea, evenly aligned with the medial and lateral aspects of the knee. Shifting of the patella away from its central position on the trochlea may indicate **patellar malalignment or dislocation**. Patellar dislocations normally occur laterally. A unilaterally high-riding patella, when accompanied by spasm of the quadriceps muscle group, indicates a **ruptured patellar tendon** (see Chapter 11). The actual tendon defect may be obliterated by swelling.
- Normally there are concave depressions on both sides of the patella when the patient is supine with the knee extended. A loss of these depressions is indicative of intra-articular effusion.[38]
- **Patellar tendon:** Note any swelling over or directly around the patellar tendon, possibly indicating tendinopathy or bursitis. Swelling on both sides that

Selective Tissue Test 10-1
Girth Measurements

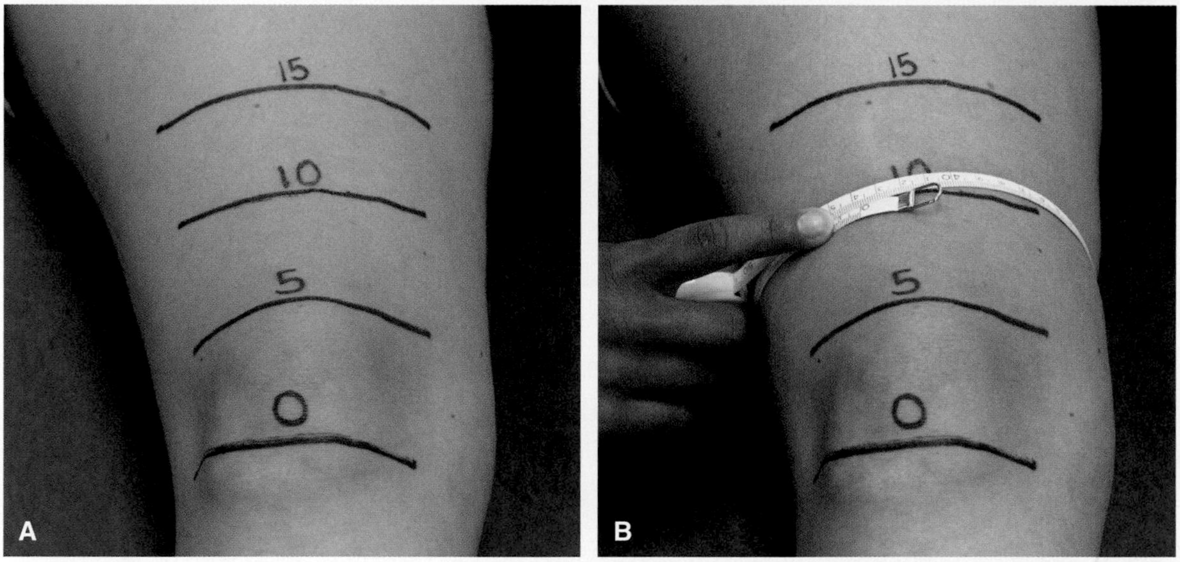

Knee girth is determined by (A) identifying the joint line (0 mark) and (B) measuring above and below the joint line. Measurements are made around the joint line and then at consistent intervals up the quadriceps group.

Patient Position	Supine or standing (The patient should be in the same position each time a measurement is taken.)
Position of Examiner	Standing next to the patient
Evaluative Procedure	The joint line is identified and measured at the 0-inch mark. Measurements are taken at 5-, 10-, and 15-cm intervals above the joint line. Measurements are taken at 15 cm below the joint line.
Positive Test	A difference of ±1 cm compared bilaterally
Implications	Increased girth on the injured side across the joint line: Edema Decreased muscular girth on the injured side: Atrophy
Modification	The measurement increments can be increased for taller individuals and decreased for shorter people.
Comments	Standardization of the measurements is required for accurate results (e.g., the patient in the same position, same landmarks). The muscular girth of the dominant leg may be naturally hypertrophied relative to the nondominant leg. In the case of migrating edema, ankle and calf girth measurements should also be taken. There is only a slight to moderate relationship between strength and girth in the overall population.
Evidence	

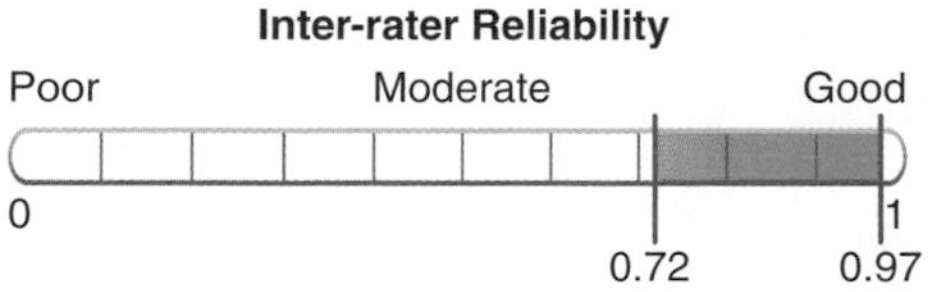

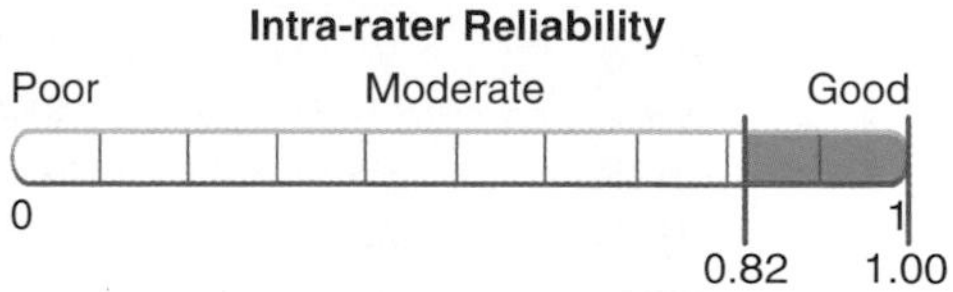

masks the definition of the tendon may indicate inflammation of the underlying fat pad.

- **Quadriceps muscle group:** Compare the mass and tone of the quadriceps muscle groups bilaterally and confirm any apparent deficits through girth measurements. Note any discoloration, swelling, or loss of continuity within the quadriceps group.
- **Alignment of the femur on the tibia:** Observe the angle at which the medial tibia and femur articulate (do not confuse this with the Q-angle) (Inspection Findings 10-1). In older individuals, varus deformity may be associated with osteoarthritis of the medial articulating surfaces, and a valgus alignment can suggest osteoarthritis of the lateral articulating surfaces (see p. 366).[47]

Inspection Findings 10-1
Tibiofemoral Alignment

	Normal	Genu Valgum	Genu Varum	Genu Recurvatum
	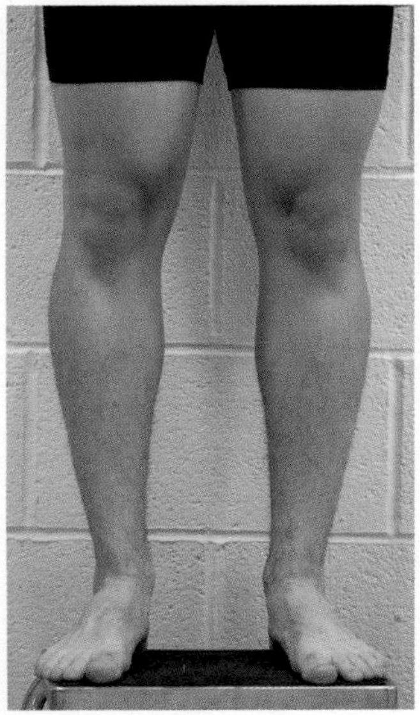	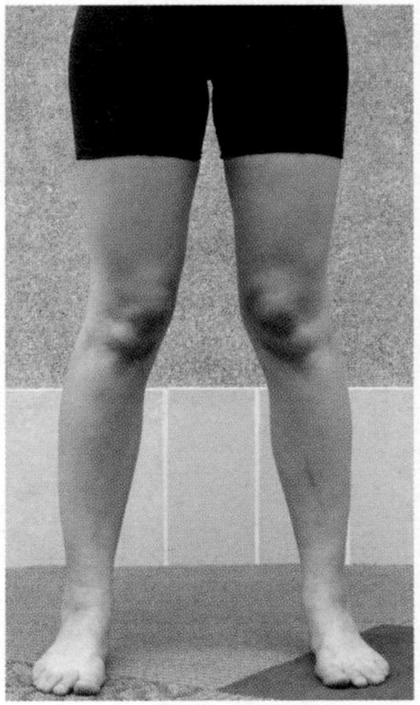	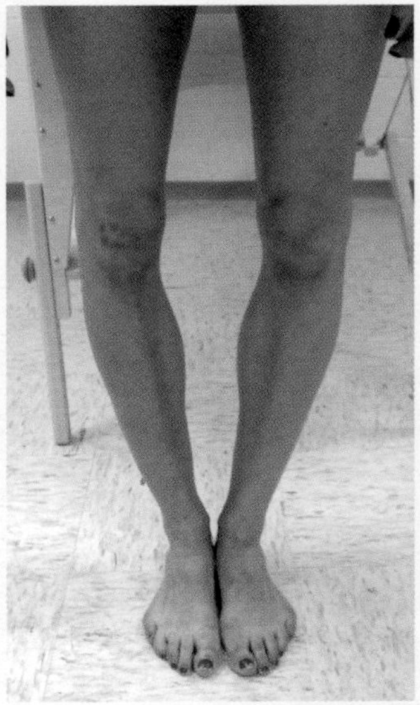	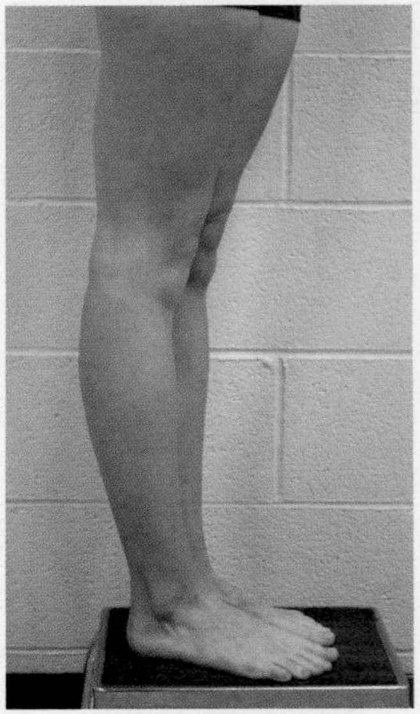
Description		The proximal tibia is angled toward the midline more than 5° relative to the femur	The proximal tibia is angled away from the midline more than 5° relative to the femur	Tibiofemoral extension greater than 0°
Potential Causes		Structural or acquired hip abnormalities	Structural or acquired hip abnormalities	Rupture of the ACL or PCL
Consequences		Increased compressive forces on the lateral joint structures Degeneration of the lateral meniscus Increased tensile forces on the medial joint structures Increased/prolonged pronation Internal tibial rotation Lateral patellar position Internal femoral rotation	Increased tensile forces on the lateral joint structures Increased compressive forces on the medial joint structures Degeneration of the medial meniscus Increased foot supination External tibial rotation Medial patellar position External femoral rotation	Increased strain on the ACL and/or PCL Increased contact pressure between the patella and femur

ACL = anterior cruciate ligament; PCL = posterior cruciate ligament

- **Tibial tuberosity:** Look for enlargement of the tibial tuberosity. In adolescent patients, enlargement could indicate Osgood-Schlatter disease (see Chapter 11). A history of this condition may result in residual enlargement of the tibial tuberosity into adulthood, but it is not typically implicated in future pathology (Fig. 10-17).

Inspection of the Medial Structures

- **Medial aspect:** Inspect the medial aspect of the knee joint, noting any swelling or discoloration along the tibia, knee joint line, femur, or pes anserine tendon.
- **Vastus medialis:** Observe the vastus medialis with particular attention to the oblique fibers. The VMO should display normal muscle tone and girth compared with that of the opposite limb. This muscle group is the first to atrophy after a knee injury, possibly as the result of disuse or increasing intracapsular fluid that inhibits its normal function.[48]

Inspection of the Lateral Structures

- **Lateral aspect:** Inspect the lateral aspect of the tibia, joint line, and femur for swelling or discoloration.
- **Fibular head:** Note the head of the fibula, normally aligned at an equal height compared with the opposite side. With the knee flexed, the biceps femoris tendon and LCL may be visible. Swelling around the fibular head may encroach on the common peroneal nerve.
- **Posterior sag of the tibia:** With the patient lying supine and the knees flexed to 90 degrees, observe the relative positions of the tibia. In PCL-deficient knees, the tibia on the involved side drops or "sags" posteriorly (Fig. 10-18). The influence of gravity is increased by flexing the patient's hips to 90 degrees (**Godfrey's test**). A straightedge placed along the patella and the anterior aspect of the tibia helps to bilaterally compare the amount of sagging. If the involved tibial tuberosity sits in a more lateral position than on the uninvolved side, damage to the posterolateral corner may be present.

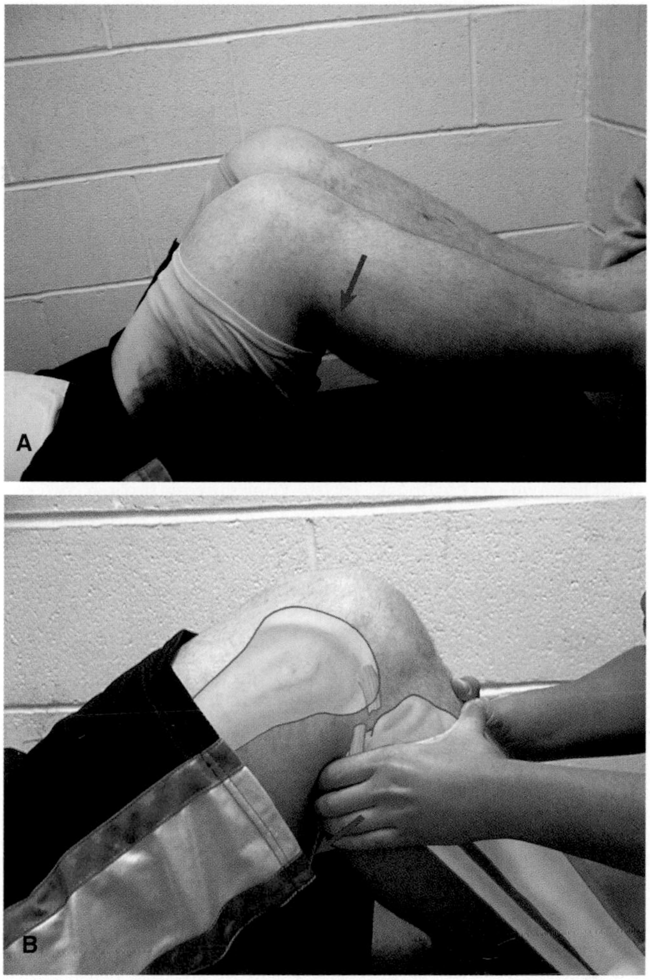

FIGURE 10-18 ■ Posterior cruciate ligament sprain of the right (facing) knee. (A) Posterior tibial sag indicating posterior cruciate ligament deficiency. Note the posterior (downward) displacement of the tibia. (B) Illustration showing the posterior displacement of the tibia demonstrated during the posterior drawer test (see Stress Test 10.4).

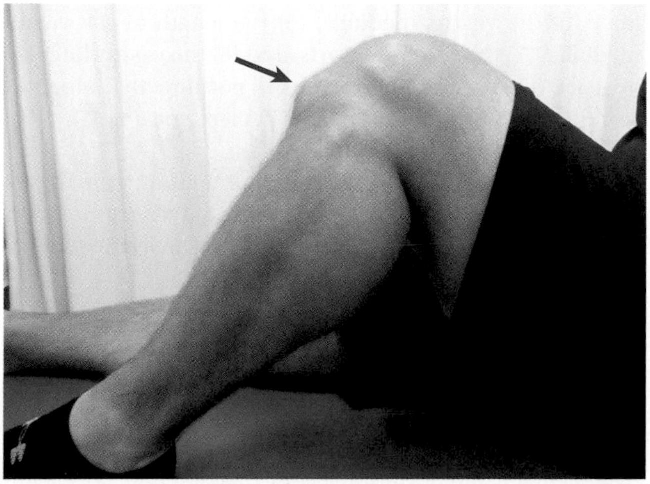

FIGURE 10-17 ■ Residual enlargement of the tibial tuberosity caused by Osgood-Schlatter disease as a child.

- **Hyperextension:** View the standing patient from the side. Hyperextension, or **genu recurvatum**, is indicated by the posterior bowing of the knee (see Inspection Findings 10-1). Acquired genu recurvatum, especially when occurring unilaterally, can indicate an ACL sprain or PCL sprain.

Inspection of the Posterior Structures

- **Hamstring muscle group:** Observe the hamstring group for signs of a contusion, such as ecchymosis and edema. These signs may also be associated with strains, which are described in Chapter 8.
- **Popliteal fossa:** Inspect the popliteal fossa for signs of swelling or discoloration that can indicate capsular trauma, tears of the distal hamstring tendon or the heads of the gastrocnemius muscle, or a cyst.

Medially the bursae associated with the semimembranosus tendon and the medial head of the gastrocnemius may be interconnected to the synovial lining of the knee. The structure of this junction allows fluids to flow from the joint capsule into the bursa, but not in the reverse direction, forming a **Baker's cyst.**[49] By definition, Baker's cysts involve only the bursa of the semimembranosus and medial head of the gastrocnemius. Other cysts may form in the popliteal fossa, often involving the popliteus muscle. Popliteal cysts may not be grossly visible and could require magnetic resonance imaging (MRI) for positive identification.

The cyst itself is often not the cause of a patient's problem but is more indicative of pathology within the knee itself. Popliteal cysts tend to develop in the presence of OA, meniscal tears (in particular, the posterior horn of the medial meniscus), ligament sprains, or other conditions that produce synovitis in the joint capsule.[49,50] Patients may describe these cysts as "coming and going," a cycle explained by the relative amount of knee effusion, resulting in aching in the fossa, and they may report "fullness" in the knee during flexion and extension. When the cyst extends into the triceps surae muscles (the gastrocnemius and soleus), the signs and symptoms may mimic those of phlebitis (pseudothrombophlebitis).[49,51]

PALPATION

Palpation is performed to confirm the findings of the inspection portion of the evaluation process and further identify traumatized tissues, although many of the most-often-injured tissues cannot be palpated.

Palpation of the Anterior Structures

1 Patella: Begin palpating the patella at its superior patellar pole where the quadriceps muscle group inserts, noting for areas of point tenderness. Progress centrally down the patella to reach the inferior pole and the origin of the patellar tendon. Return to the starting point on the superior pole by palpating up the medial and lateral patellar borders. In the adolescent, pain at the inferior border may be associated with **Sinding-Larsen-Johansson disease** (see Chapter 11).

With the knee extended and the quadriceps relaxed, palpate the patella to ensure its proper alignment in the femoral trochlea and its freedom of movement. A dislocated patella can occur with or without a rupture of the patellar tendon. A rigid, displaced patella accompanied by the inability or unwillingness to extend the knee indicates a patellar dislocation.

2 Patellar tendon: Palpate the length of the patellar tendon from its insertion at the tibial tuberosity to the inferior aspect of the patella. The patellar tendon normally feels broad and ropelike. A chronic tendinopathy often results in palpable nodules within the mass of the tendon. The tendon can also be palpated while the patient performs active ROM of the knee, noting any crepitus indicating patellar tendinopathy.

3 Tibial tuberosity: Palpate the patellar tendon's attachment site on the tibia. The tibial tuberosity is normally a smooth, rounded protrusion. With adolescent patients, sensitivity and roughness of the tuberosity indicate an inflammation of the tibial tuberosity's growth center: **Osgood–Schlatter disease**. Pain in mature patients may be caused by a contusion or inflammation.

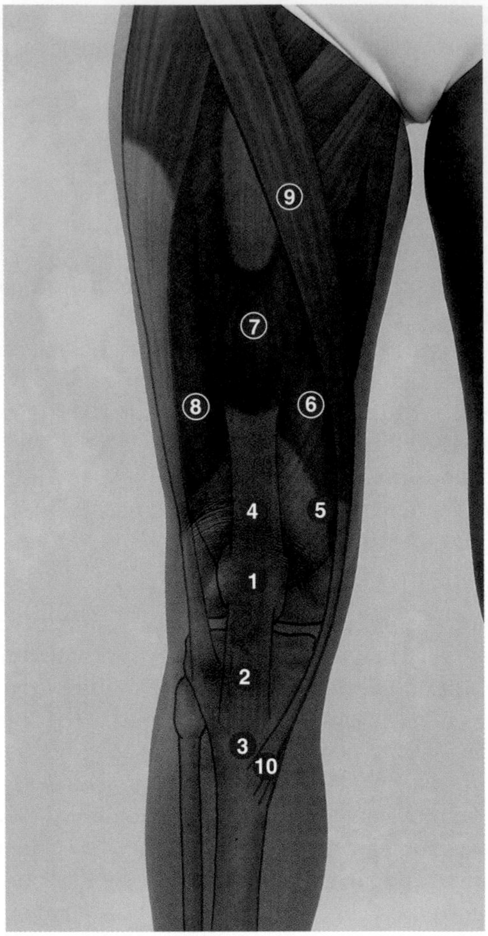

Palpation of the Anterior Structures

4 Quadriceps tendon: From the superior aspect of the patella, palpate the quadriceps tendon as it attaches across the width of the patella's superior pole. Note that the suprapatellar pouch of the joint capsule and the suprapatellar fat pad lie deep to the quadriceps tendon. Fluid tends to accumulate here because of the large capsular redundancy.

5-8 Quadriceps muscle group: Palpate (5) the oblique fibers of the **vastus medialis,** (6) the length of the **vastus medialis,** (7) the **rectus femoris,** and (8) the **vastus lateralis** muscles (the vastus intermedius is not directly palpable), searching for point tenderness, defect, or spasm.

9 Sartorius and (10) pes anserine tendon: Palpate the **sartorius** muscle from its origin on the anterior superior iliac spine (ASIS) to its insertion via the **pes anserine tendon**.

Palpation of the Medial Structures

1 Medial meniscus and joint line: Place the knee in at least 45 degrees of flexion to locate the joint lines. Palpate on either side of the proximal aspect of the patellar tendon until the indentation formed by the femur and tibia is located. Palpate medially and posteriorly along the joint line, noting any crepitus or pain that may indicate possible meniscal, ligamentous, or capsular trauma. Externally rotating the tibia makes the border of the medial meniscus more palpable.

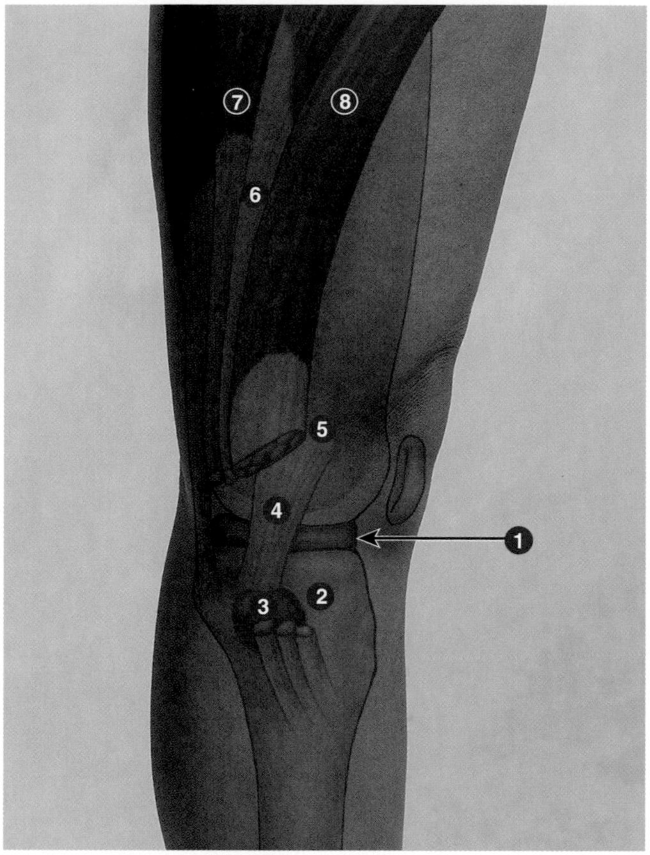

Palpation of the Medial Structures

2 Medial tibial plateau: Locate the medial tibial plateau inferior to the joint line. After palpating along its length, proceed inferiorly to locate the medial tibial flare, a structural necessity to disperse compressive forces at the articulation.

3 Pes anserine tendon and bursa: Locate the medial tibial flare, the site of attachment for the gracilis, sartorius, and semitendinosus muscles. Palpate the common insertion of these tendons located just medial to the tibial tuberosity. The **pes anserine bursa** may be more easily identified midway between the tibial tuberosity and the anterior aspect of the medial joint line if the tibia is slightly internally rotated.[38] Direct blows or overuse may cause these structures and the overlying pes anserine bursa to be inflamed.

4 Medial collateral ligament: Many sprains of the MCL occur at the origin or insertion of the ligament. Palpate the length of the MCL from its origin on the medial femoral condyle, just below the adductor tubercle, progressing inferiorly to its insertion on the medial tibial flare that can be located up to 7 cm distal to the joint line. The medial portion of the joint line is covered by the MCL. Note the close relationship between the tendons of the pes anserine group and the MCL.

5 Medial femoral condyle and epicondyle: Flex the knee beyond 90 degrees to better expose the articulating surface of the condyle immediately above the anteromedial joint line. The adductor tubercle, the attachment site for the adductor longus, projects off the medial femoral condyle. Injuries with rotational or loading mechanisms may cause bone bruising or osteochondral fracture, leading to pain in the condyles.

6 Gracilis: Palpate the thin, ropelike gracilis, located immediately anterior to the semitendinosus tendon, from its insertion to the point that it is lost in the mass of the adductor group.

7 Semitendinosus tendon: From the pes anserine attachment, palpate the semitendinosus tendon, the most medial tendon of the hamstring group, to its muscular belly.

8 Sartorius: Palpate the length of the sartorius across the anterior portion of the quadriceps group to the point where it passes over the medial joint line and attaches to the anteromedial tibia as a part of the pes anserine tendon.

Palpation of the Lateral Structures

1 Joint line: Position the knee in at least 45 degrees of flexion to locate the anterolateral joint line. Begin palpating the joint line lateral to the patellar tendon and progress posteriorly. Pain along the joint line may indicate meniscal pathology. Internally rotating the tibia makes the periphery of the lateral meniscus more palpable.

2 Fibular head: Locate the fibular head below and slightly posterior to the lateral joint line. Two ropelike structures may be felt arising from the fibular head. The LCL projects off its superior portion; slightly posterior to this structure is the insertion of the biceps femoris tendon.

3 Lateral collateral ligament: Place the knee in 90 degrees of flexion and externally rotate and abduct the hip (i.e., cross the ankle of the involved leg over the opposite leg) to make the LCL more identifiable. Because it is a separate structure from the joint capsule, the LCL is easily identified as it arises from the fibular head and courses to the lateral femoral condyle.

4 Popliteus: Palpate a small portion of the anterior popliteus tendon, posterior to the LCL just above the joint line. Provide slight resistance to knee flexion to make the tendon more prominent.

5 Biceps femoris: Flex the knee to 25 degrees and ask the patient to externally rotate the lower leg to make the biceps tendon easily palpable (note that as the tendon crosses the joint line, it may become confused with the IT band). The biceps femoris tendon inserts on the fibular head, posterior to the insertion of the LCL. Continue palpating the biceps femoris tendon to its muscular belly.

6 Iliotibial band, (7) Gerdy's tubercle, and (8) lateral femoral condyle: Palpate the **IT band** located anterior to the biceps femoris tendon at its insertion on **Gerdy's tubercle** just lateral to the tibial tuberosity. The IT band becomes more identifiable during resisted flexion past 30 degrees. Palpate the IT band upward to the tensor fasciae latae, noting any increased

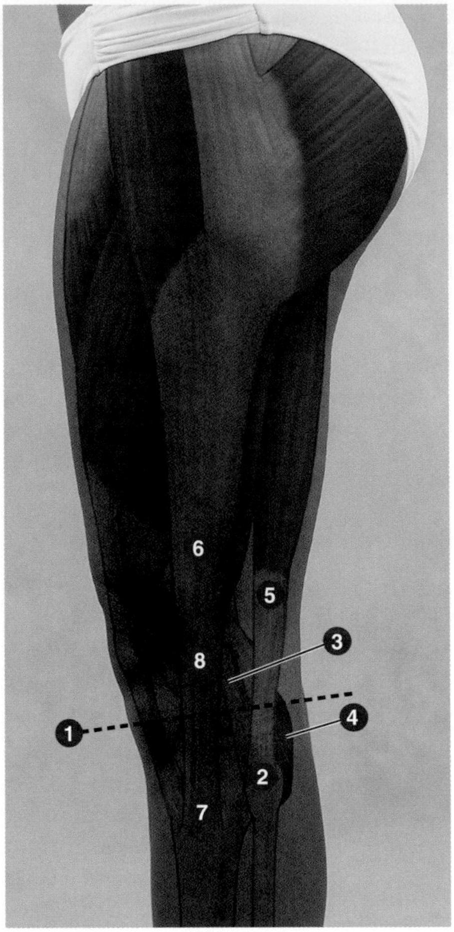

Palpation of the Lateral Structures

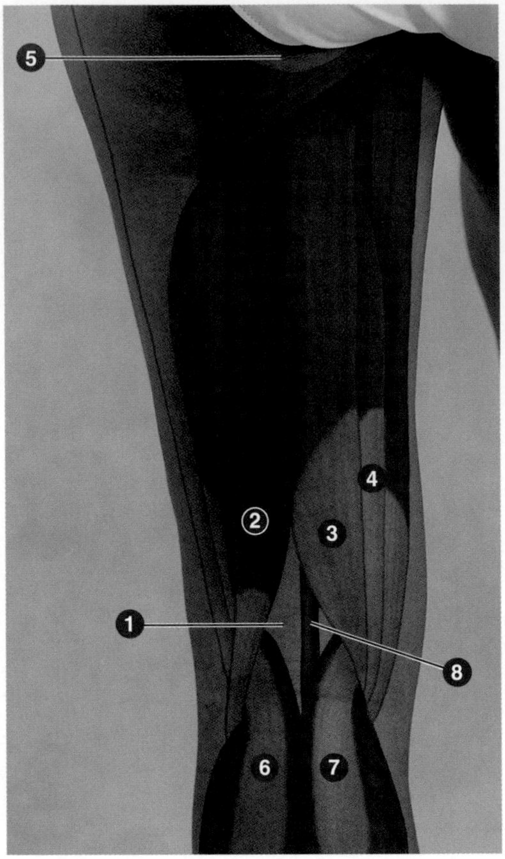

Palpation of the Posterior Structures

sensitivity, especially as it passes over the **lateral femoral condyle**, possibly indicating IT band friction syndrome.

Palpation of the Posterior Structures

1 Popliteal fossa: Trauma to this area or edema within this space can occlude neurovascular structures, resulting in radicular pain, inhibition of nerve transmission, or disruption of blood flow to or from the lower leg, possibly mimicking the signs and symptoms of thrombophlebitis.[49,50]

With the patient prone, palpate the popliteal fossa for the presence of a cyst, most commonly found on the medial aspect of the fossa under the medial head of the gastrocnemius and semimembranosus tendon (Baker's cyst). The cyst is usually more prominent during palpation with the knee extended. The cyst may feel firm with the knee extended and soft when the knee is flexed, **Foucher's sign.**[49] Cysts may also be found laterally and are associated with the popliteus tendon (see Inspection of the Posterior Structures, p. 317).

2-5 Hamstring muscle group: Palpate the length of the (2) **biceps femoris** on the lateral aspect of the knee and the (3) **semitendinosus** and (4) **semimembranosus** muscles on the medial side of the knee to their common origin on the (5) **ischial tuberosity**, noting any point tenderness, spasm, or defect.

6-7 Heads of the gastrocnemius: Palpate the (6) **lateral** and (7) **medial heads** of the gastrocnemius muscle.

8 Popliteal artery: Palpate the pulse associated with this artery. This pulse is most notable in the inferior portion of the popliteal fossa with the knee flexed.

Determination of Intracapsular versus Extracapsular Swelling

Pathology to the knee can result in a collection of fluid within the joint capsule (effusion) or outside of the capsule (extracapsular swelling/edema). The onset of effusion, generally associated with internal derangement, provides important insight to the nature of the underlying condition. The rapid onset of effusion suggests a tear of one of the knee's major ligaments or a fracture of the knee's articular surface. More slowly forming edema is indicative of a meniscal tear, inflammatory conditions, or a less significant ligamentous sprain.[38]

Joint effusion is definitively identified by MRI. Effusion may also be identified by patient self-report; by the ability to manually move ("milk") the fluid from one side of the knee to the other via the **Sweep test** (also known as the peripatellar fluctuation test) (Selective Tissue Test 10-2); or by the **ballottable patella test** (Selective Tissue Test 10-3), which assesses the extent to which the patella is "floating"

Selective Tissue Test 10-2

Sweep Test (or Peripatellar Fluctuation Test) for Intracapsular Swelling/Effusion

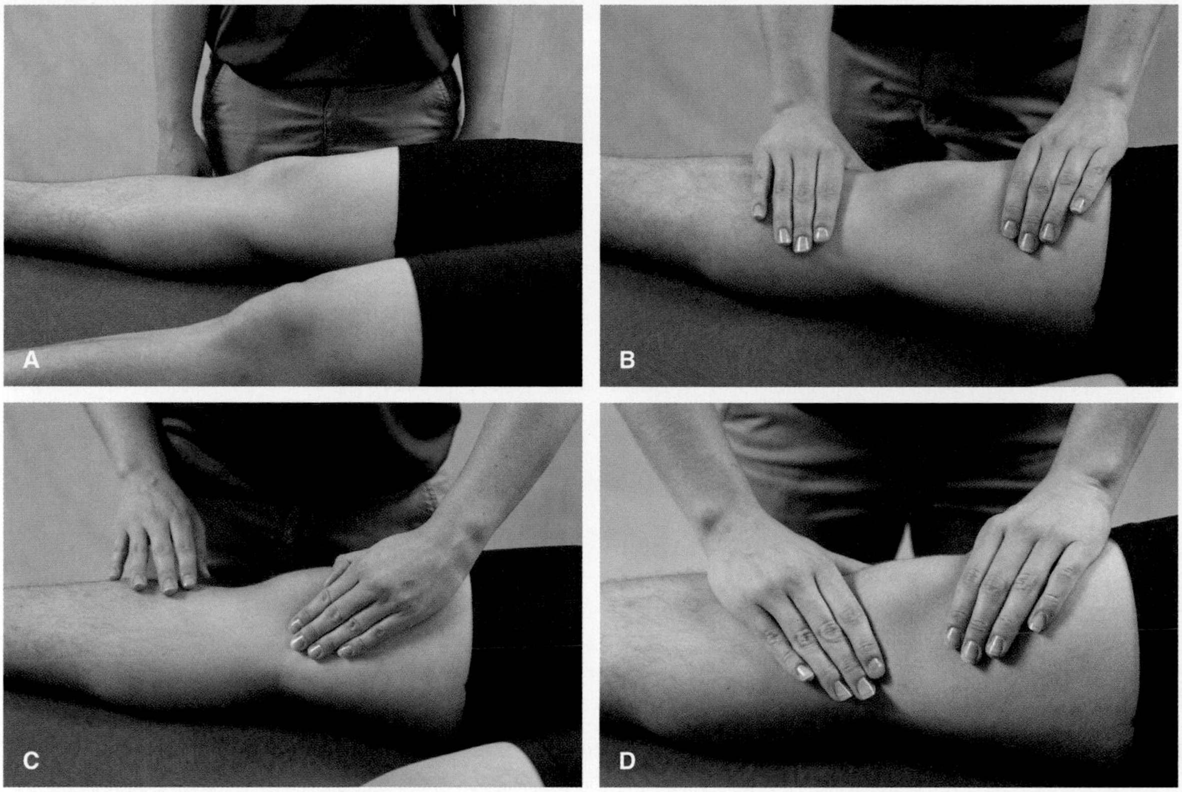

Sweep test to determine the presence of intracapsular swelling

Patient Position	Lying supine with the knee extended
Position of Examiner	Standing lateral to the patient
Evaluative Procedure	Assuming that the fluid is on the medial side of the knee **(A):** **(B)** The edema is stroked ("milked") proximally and laterally towards the middle. **(C)** The normal contour of the knee is restored. **(D)** When pressure is applied on the lateral aspect of the knee, a fluid bulge immediately appears on the medial aspect.
Positive Test	Reformation of edema on the medial side of the knee when pressure is applied to the lateral aspect
Implications	Swelling within the joint capsule, indicating possible ACL trauma, osteochondral fracture, synovitis, meniscal lesion, or patellar dislocation
Modification	If swelling is more prevalent on the lateral aspect of the knee, the steps are performed on the lateral side of the knee joint.
Comments	When compared with ballottment and patient report of swelling, this assessment is not helpful in determining the presence or absence of effusion as diagnosed by MRI.[52]
Evidence	

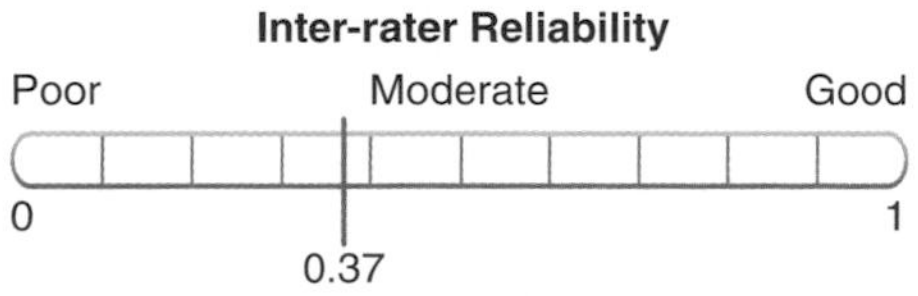

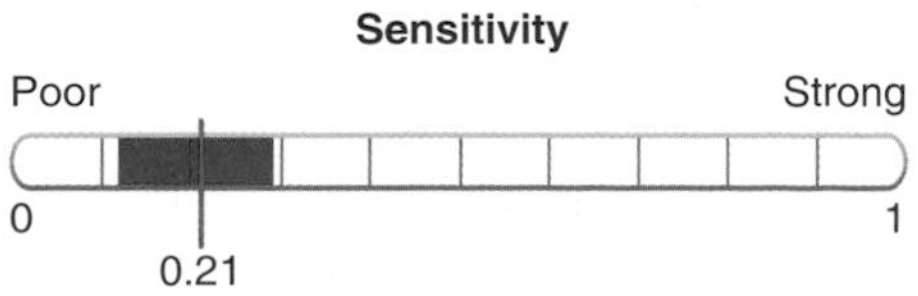

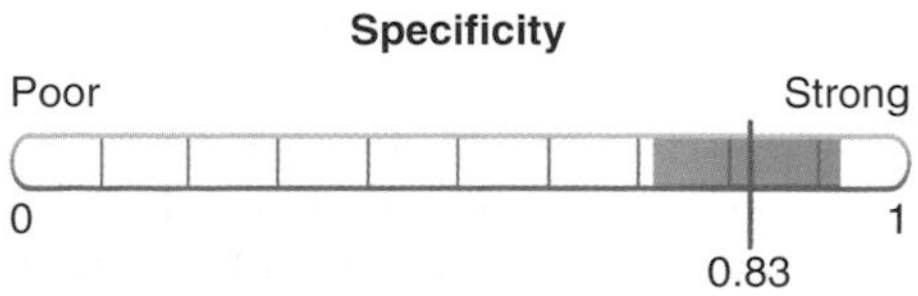

LR+: 0.61–1.53–2.44

LR−: 0.80–0.97–1.10

ACL = anterior cruciate ligament

Selective Tissue Tests 10-3
Ballotable Patella

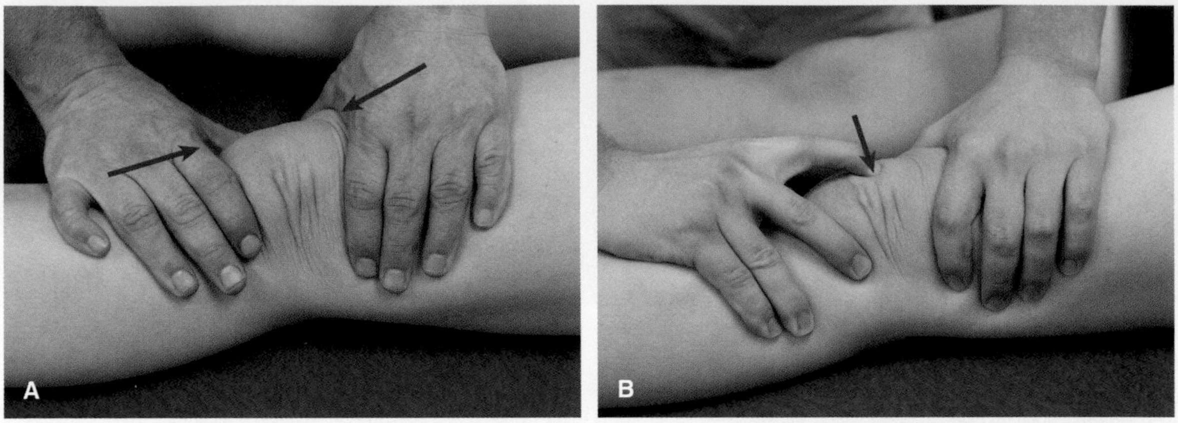

(A) Excess fluid is manually moved superiorly and inferiorly towards the middle of the knee. (B) In the presence of knee effusion, the patella will "float" over the femoral trochlea when the knee is extended.

Patient Position	Supine The knee is extended, and the quadriceps are relaxed.
Position of Examiner	Standing to the side being tested
Evaluative Procedure	**(A)** The superior hand pushes any fluid in the superior portion of the knee inferiorly toward the patella. The opposite hand pushes any fluid in the inferior portion of the knee superiorly toward the patella. **(B)** A finger is used to press the patella down towards the patellar groove.
Positive Test	The patella depresses and strikes the patellar groove (femoral trochlea) and returns back to its former position.[52]
Implications	Effusion within the joint capsule
Comments	Knee effusions, especially those of rapid onset, are associated with fractures, patellar dislocations, or cruciate ligament sprains.
Evidence	

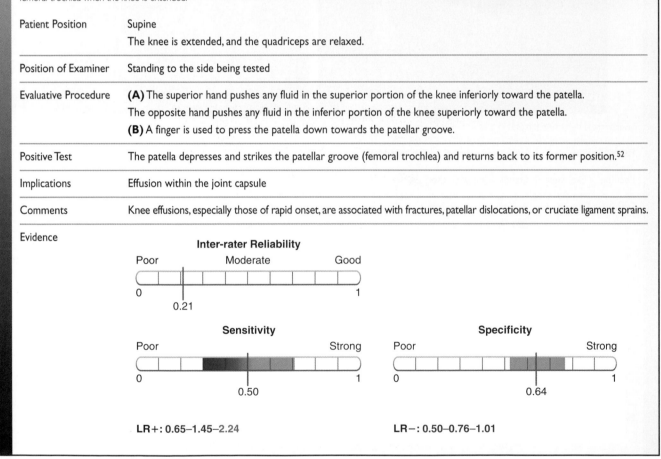

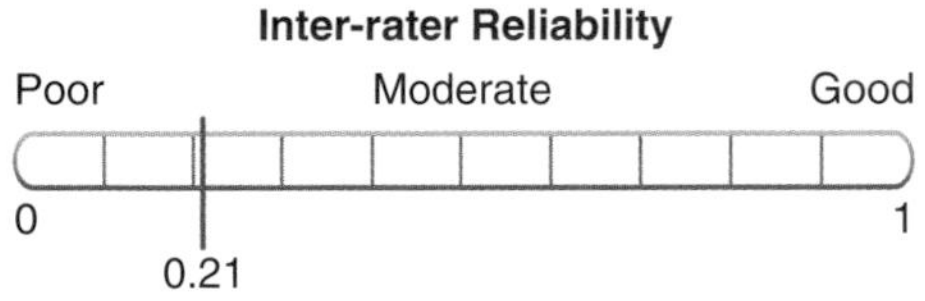

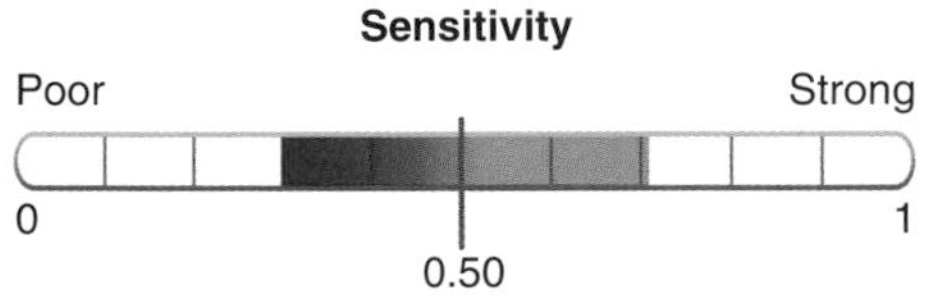

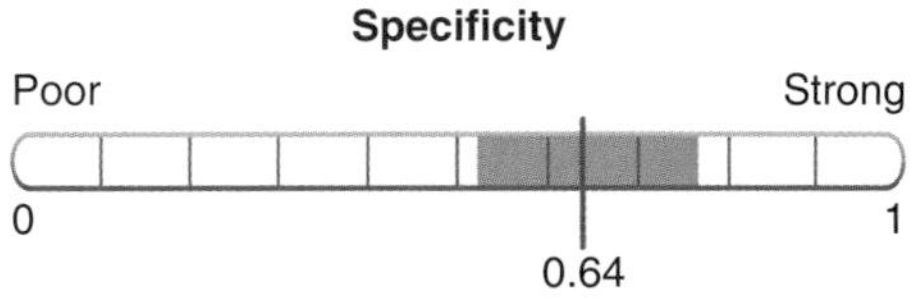

LR+: 0.65–1.45–2.24

LR−: 0.50–0.76–1.01

over the femoral trochlea.[52] Localized edema tends to represent extra-articular swelling.[38]

Acute injuries leading to rapid-onset effusion usually indicate a sprained ACL or capsule possibly resulting from the dislocation of the patella, a fractured tibial plateau, or an osteochondral fracture. If aspirated, the fluid would most likely be dark red because of bleeding from these structures (**hemarthrosis**). Knee joint effusion of more gradual onset is also caused by the inflammatory response producing excess synovial fluid such as in arthritic knees, a mensical tear in the avascular zone, or with chondromalacia patella. Aspiration yields a clear and straw-colored fluid. If the joint were infected, the fluid would be cloudy.

*** Practical Evidence**

The rapid onset of effusion, indicating a hemarthrosis, is strongly associated with an ACL sprain, a patellar dislocation, or an osteochondral fracture.[53]

Extracapsular edema is often caused by inflammation of the soft tissues surrounding the joint, possibly indicating inflamed bursae or a contusion. Venous insufficiencies may affect the knee in addition to the entire lower extremity, causing the buildup of edema.

Joint and Muscle Function Assessment

The only voluntary movements available at the knee joint are flexion and extension and tibial internal and external rotation. The motions of flexion and extension are easily measured and quantified, but tibial rotation is less accurately measured. The use of a goniometer to measure knee flexion and extension is described in Goniometry 10-1. Loss of knee extension can occur following ACL surgery, and flexion may be lost following PCL reconstruction.[54] Extension loss may be the result of scar tissue formation in the anterior intercondylar notch ("cyclops lesion"), fibrous nodules creating a mechanical block, or capsulitis (Fig. 10-19). Focal

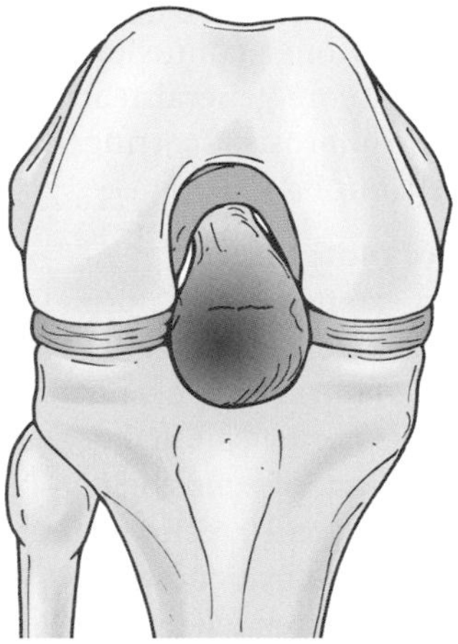

FIGURE 10-19 ■ Cyclops lesion. This is a form of arthrofibrosis where a fibrous nodule forms in the tibial tunnel following an ACL lesion. The nodule impinges on the intracondylar notch, limiting extension.

Goniometry 10-1
Knee Flexion/Extension

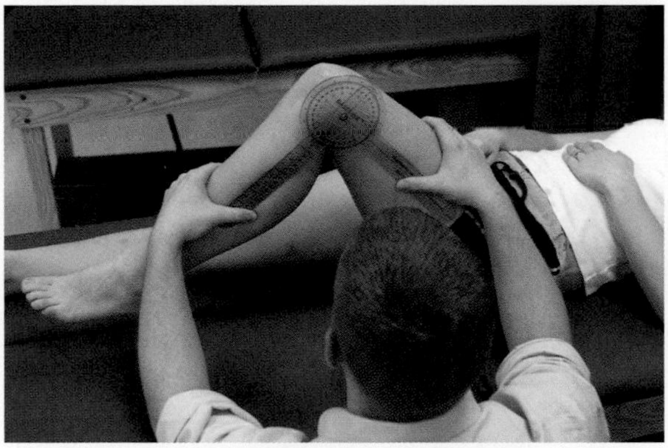

Extension to Flexion (10°– 0°– 135° to 145°)

Patient Position	Lying supine. Place a bolster under the distal tibia for the extension measurement.

Goniometer Alignment

Fulcrum	Centered over the lateral femoral epicondyle
Proximal Arm	The stationary arm is centered over the midline of the femur, aligned with the greater trochanter.
Distal Arm	The movement arm is centered over the midline of the fibula, aligned with the lateral malleolus.
Comments	Knee flexion can be assessed with the patient prone and using the same landmarks to assess the influence of the two-joint rectus femoris length on knee flexion.

Evidence

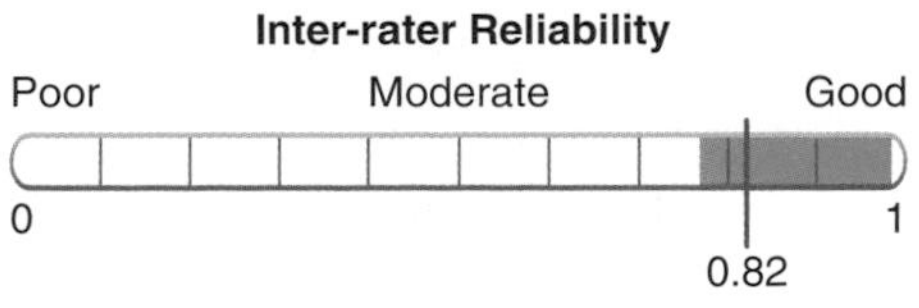

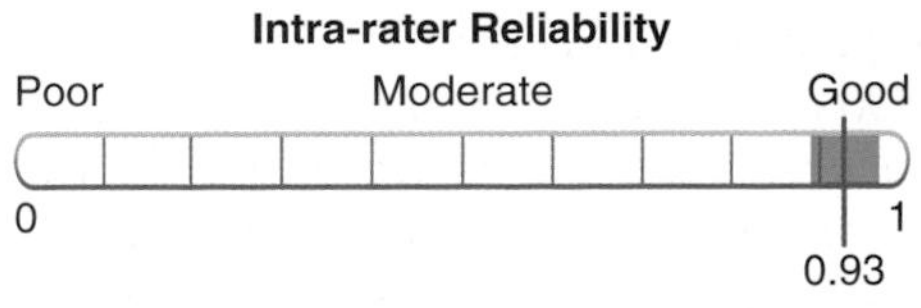

capsulitis may take the form of a synovial plica (see Chapter 7) or result from a contusion or MCL sprain. Diffuse capsulitis is a more general reaction to trauma and may lead to arthrofibrosis, scarring that restricts both flexion and extension.[56]

Active Range of Motion

- **Flexion and extension:** The normal arc of motion for knee flexion and extension is 135 to 145 degrees, with the majority of the motion occurring as flexion. A fully extended knee normally is at 0 degrees, but in certain cases the end range of extension may be as great as 10 or more degrees beyond 0 (genu recurvatum). Knee flexion may be limited by tightness of the rectus femoris, in which case an extended hip can limit the amount of flexion available at the knee.
- **Internal and external rotation:** To allow for full ROM during knee flexion and extension, the tibia must internally and externally rotate on the femur. Observe and bilaterally compare the rotation of the tibial tuberosity to estimate the amount of internal and external rotation that occurs during active knee flexion and extension.

Manual Muscle Testing

The leg muscles must be relaxed when manual muscle testing the hamstring group to minimize contributions from the gastrocnemius as a knee flexor. Performing the same test with the tibia internally and externally rotated magnifies contributions from the semimembranosus/semitendinosus and biceps femoris, respectively. The quadriceps (Manual Muscle Test 10-1) and hamstrings (Manual Muscle Test 10-2)

Manual Muscle Test 10-1
Knee Extension

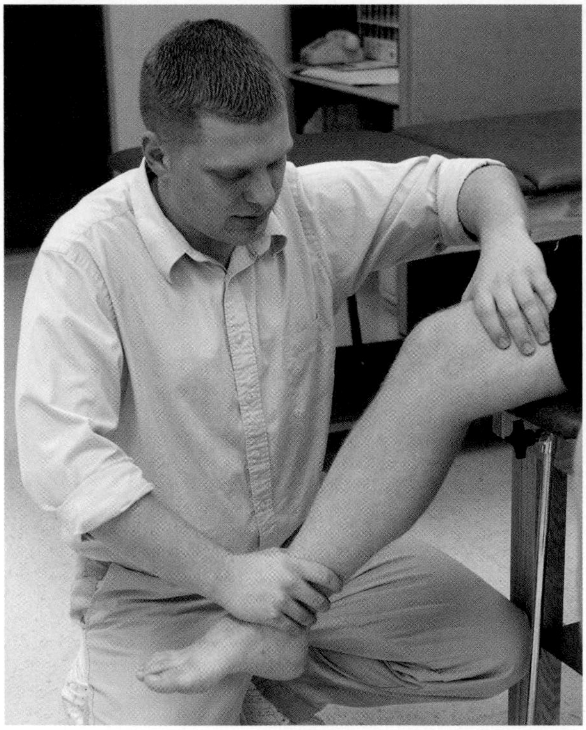

Patient Position	Seated
Test Position	Midway between flexion and extension
Stabilization	Distal femur
Resistance	Distal tibia, proximal to the ankle
Primary Movers (Innervation)	Vastus lateralis (L2, L3, L4) Vastus medialis (L2, L3, L4) Vastus intermedius (L2, L3, L4) Rectus femoris (L2, L3, L4)
Secondary Mover (Innervation)	Not applicable
Substitution	Ankle dorsiflexion Hip extension

Manual Muscle Test 10-2
Knee Flexion

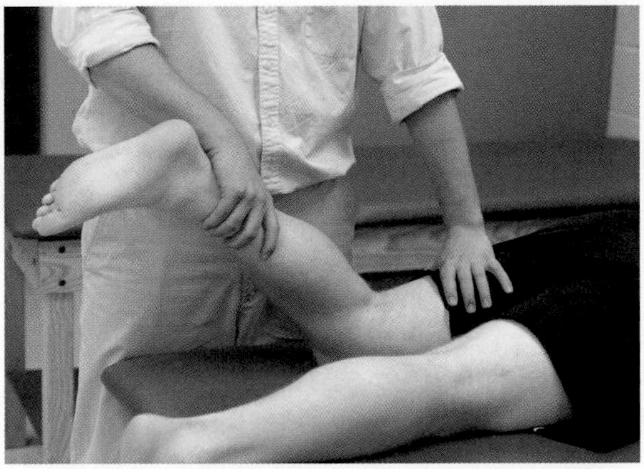

Patient Position	Prone
Test Position	Midway between flexion and extension
Stabilization	Femur
Resistance	Distal tibia
Primary Movers (Innervation)	***Biceps femoris:*** Long head—tibial (S1, S2, S3); Short head—common peroneal (L5, S1, S2) ***Semimembranosus:*** Tibial (L5, S1) ***Semitendinosus:*** Tibial (L5, S1, S2)
Secondary Mover (Innervation)	Gastrocnemius
Substitution	Hip flexion Ankle plantarflexion
Comments	Internally rotating the leg will emphasize contributions from the semimembranosus and semitendinosus muscles. Externally rotating the leg will emphasize contribution from the biceps femoris.

are tested as a group. The function of the sartorius can be relatively isolated (Manual Muscle Test 10-3).

Passive Range of Motion

An equal amount of flexion and extension is lost with capsular involvement (Table 10-4).

- **Extension:** Extension is measured with the tibia slightly elevated by placing a **bolster** under the distal tibia with the patient in the supine position. Extension produces a firm end-feel because the posterior capsule and the cruciate ligaments are taut. Tightness of the hamstring group may limit extension, especially in cases in which the knee has been flexed for extended periods because of stiffness, swelling, or immobilization. A flexion contracture may also limit extension as evidenced by an early firm end-feel.
- **Flexion:** Flexion is assessed with the patient supine and the hip flexed to remove the influence of rectus femoris tightness. Restrictions in flexion ROM in the supine position suggest joint capsule adhesions or effusion or may be a normal postoperative finding. Flexion measured in the prone position with the rectus femoris stretched over the hip and knee joints more closely reflects the effect of muscular tightness on the joint. The normal end-feel for flexion is soft because of the approximation of the gastrocnemius group with the hamstrings or the heel striking the buttock.

Joint Stability Tests

Ligamentous stability of the knee may occur in one plane, either as anteroposterior instability in the frontal plane or as valgus-varus instability in the sagittal plane. It may also occur as a multidirectional rotational instability. This section presents tests for uniplanar instabilities. Tests for rotational

Bolster A support used to maintain the position of a body part

Manual Muscle Test 10-3
Isolating the Sartorius

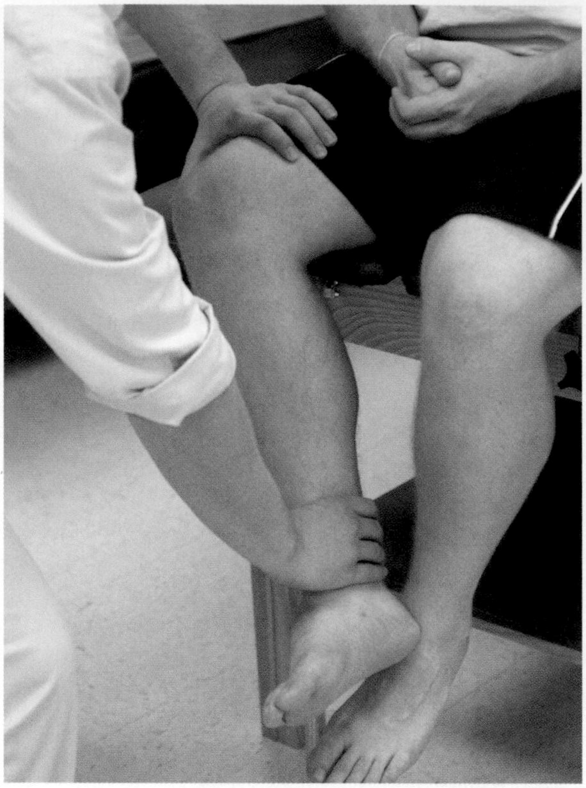

Patient Position	Seated
Test Position	The hip is slightly flexed and externally rotated. The foot of the limb being tested is on the medial tibia of the opposite leg.
Stabilization	See "Resistance" below
Resistance	Medial aspect of the distal tibia and medial ankle and distal femur to prevent hip flexion, hip abduction, hip external rotation, and knee flexion
Primary Mover (Innervation)	Sartorius (L2, L3)
Secondary Movers (Innervation)	Secondary movers include the hamstring muscle group, hip external rotators, gracilis, and hip flexors.
Substitution	Hip flexion without external rotation or abduction indicates substitution by the rectus femoris and/or iliopsoas.[55]

instabilities are discussed in the Region-Specific Pathologies section of this chapter.

Stress Testing

Tests for anterior instability: Two basic tests attempt to displace the tibia anteriorly on the femur, thus assessing the relative stability of the ACL. The ACL provides 86% of the restraint against anterior translation.[8,56] In the case of a complete ACL disruption, further displacement is limited by the posterior capsule, the deep layer of the MCL, and the posterolateral complex.

The anterior drawer test involves placing the knee in 90 degrees of flexion and attempting to translate the tibia anteriorly (Stress Test 10-1). The line of pull from the hamstrings complements the function of the ACL, possibly masking an otherwise-positive test result (Fig. 10-20). The hamstrings, however, do not replicate the function of the ACL as the knee nears extension.[30]

Factors limiting the anterior drawer test include:

1. The need to overcome the effects of gravity while moving the tibia anteriorly

Table 10-4 Knee Capsular Pattern and End-Feels

Capsular Pattern: Flexion, Extension	
End-Feel	
Extension	Firm: Stretch of the posterior capsule; ACL; PCL
Flexion	Soft: Soft tissue approximation between the triceps surae and the hamstrings Firm: Stretch of the rectus femoris
Internal tibial rotation	Firm: Capsular stretch; LCL; IT band
External tibial rotation	Firm: Capsular stretch; MCL; LCL; pes anserine

ACL = anterior cruciate ligament; IT = iliotibial; LCL = lateral collateral ligament; MCL = medial collateral ligament; PCL = posterior cruciate ligament

2. Guarding by the hamstring group, masking anterior displacement of the tibia on the femur
3. Effusion within the capsule, providing resistance to movement or the inability to flex the knee to 90 degrees
4. The geometry of the articular condyles, causing the triangular shape of the menisci to form a block against anterior movement of the tibia, similar to a doorstop's wedging against the bottom of a door
5. Flexing the knee to 90 degrees, causing anterior displacement of the tibia, masking the amount of further displacement during the drawer test[8,57]
6. Reduced sensitivity to lesions located in the posterolateral bundle[8,58]

A modification of the anterior drawer test, the **Lachman test** assesses the ACL when both the anteromedial and posterolateral portions of the ligament are taut (Stress Test 10-2) (see Fig. 10-8). Several modifications of the Lachman test have been proposed to help accommodate for differences in size, strength, and stature between the clinician and patient (Fig. 10-21). When compared with the gold standard of viewing the ACL through an arthroscope, the Lachman test's combined sensitivity and specificity makes it the best examination technique for detecting whether or not an ACL sprain is present.[59]

*** Practical Evidence**

A positive anterior drawer test with a history of effusion, "popping sensation" at the time of injury, and giving way significantly increases the probability of an ACL sprain.[60]

Performing the Lachman test requires a firm grasp to manipulate the tibia and femur. In many cases, athletes or other large patients have heavy, muscular legs, making it difficult to perform this test. In these cases, the femur may be rested on a tightly rolled towel to maintain the knee in flexion. Another method is to abduct the patient's leg off the side of the table and flex the knee to 25 degrees.

In each of these modifications, the tibia is drawn forward in a way similar to the drawer test procedure. Manual ACL and PCL testing can be quantified by instrumented **arthrometers** (Fig. 10-22). Arthrometers measure the amount of tibial translation in a more accurate, quantitative, reproducible manner and are less prone to the physical limitation faced by the clinician when performing the anterior drawer or Lachman test.[61-65] However, as with other clinical testing procedures, the reliability of instrumented arthrometers is correlated with the skill and experience of the individual performing the test.[65-67]

When examination findings include an apparently positive Lachman test or anterior drawer test, the knee must also be screened for PCL insufficiency. If the PCL is deficient, tests for ACL insufficiency may appear positive, since the tibia is relocated anteriorly from its posteriorly subluxed position on the femur.[68]

The **prone Lachman test** (also called reverse Lachman or alternate Lachman) can be used to differentiate abnormal tibiofemoral glide caused by tears of the ACL from that caused by PCL deficiencies.[69] This test places the patient in the prone, rather than the supine, position, preventing the posterior tibial sag resulting from the supine position (Stress Test 10-3).

Tests for posterior instability: Tests for damage of the PCL attempt to determine the amount of posterior displacement of the tibia on the femur relative to the uninvolved side. This motion places stress primarily on the PCL, followed by the arcuate ligament complex and the anterior joint capsule.

A posterior sag of the tibia may be evidenced when the flexed knee is viewed from the lateral side (see Fig. 10-18). Using the same positioning as the anterior drawer test, the **posterior drawer test** attempts to displace the tibia posteriorly (Stress Test 10-4). **Godfrey's test** uses gravity to increase the posterior sag as noted during the inspection process (Selective Tissue Test 10-4). The following grading system is used for PCL sprains[70,71]

Grade	Clinical Signs	Posterior Displacement
I	Palpable but diminished step-off between tibia and femur	0 mm–5 mm
II	Step-off is lost; the tibia cannot be pushed beyond the medial femoral condyle.	5 mm–10 mm
III	Step-off is lost; the tibia can be pushed beyond the medial femoral condyle.	>10 mm

Tests for medial instability: When the knee is fully extended, the MCL is assisted in limiting valgus stress by the posterior oblique ligament, posteromedial capsule, cruciate

Stress Test 10-1
Anterior Drawer Test for Anterior Cruciate Ligament Laxity

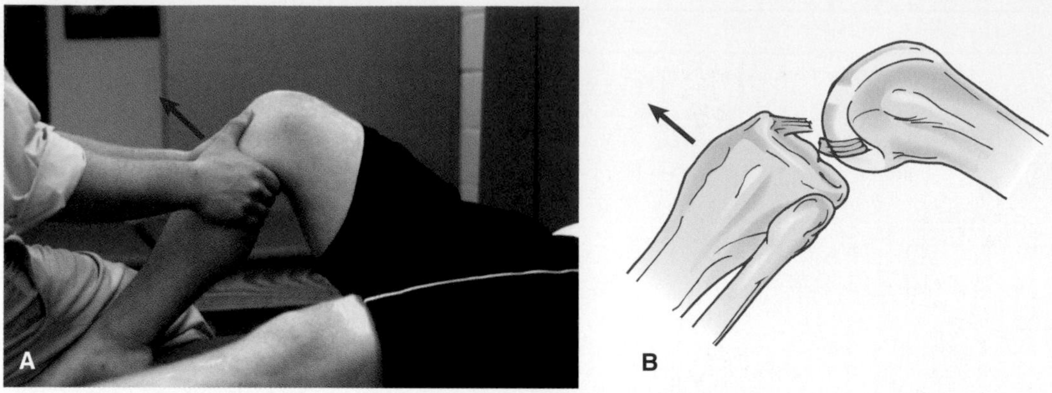

The anterior drawer test for anterior cruciate laxity (A). Schematic representation of tibial displacement in a positive test (B).

Patient Position	Lying supine Hip flexed to 45° and the knee to 90°
Position of Examiner	Sitting on the examination table in front of the involved knee, the examiner grasps the tibia just below the joint line of the knee with the thumbs placed along the joint line on either side of the patellar tendon. The index fingers are used to palpate the hamstring tendons to ensure that they are relaxed.
Evaluative Procedure	The tibia is drawn anteriorly.
Positive Test	An increased amount of anterior tibial translation compared with the opposite (uninvolved) limb or the lack of a firm endpoint
Implications	A sprain of the ACL
Modification	The patient is seated to remove the posterior sag of the tibia that would be caused by PCL injury. The examiner is kneeling with the patient's lower leg stabilized between the examiner's knees. The tibia is translated anteriorly.
Comments	The anterior drawer test is better at detecting anterior laxity in patients with older ACL sprains than in those who are acutely injured.[6] The hamstring muscle group must be relaxed to ensure proper test results. Too much flexion can result in a false-negative result due to tibial plateau and the posterior horns of the menisci contacting the femoral condyle.
Evidence	

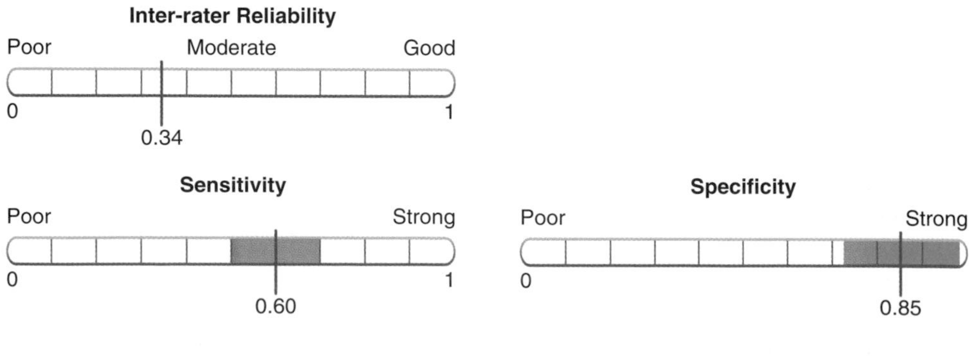

LR+: 2.86–9.50–16.14

LR−: 0.22–0.52–0.83

ACL = anterior cruciate ligament; PCL = posterior cruciate ligament

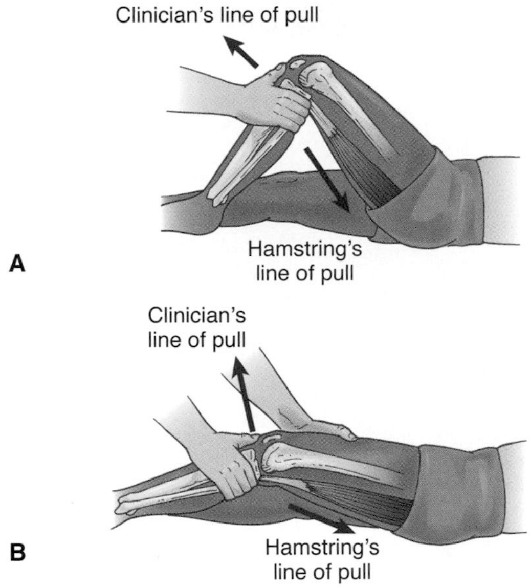

FIGURE 10-20 ■ Biomechanics of the (A) anterior drawer test and (B) Lachman test for anterior cruciate laxity. (A) During the drawer test, contraction of the hamstring group pulls the tibia posteriorly, the direction opposite the line of pull, potentially masking a positive result. (B) The joint position used during the Lachman test (20° of flexion) alters the hamstring's force vector, thereby reducing the possibility of a false-negative result.

ligaments, and the muscles crossing the medial joint line. The **valgus stress test** is performed once with the knee fully extended and again with the knee flexed to 25 degrees (Stress Test 10-5). Valgus laxity demonstrated on a fully extended knee indicates a major disruption of the medial supportive structures, and the presence of an empty end-feel indicates a possible rupture of the cruciate ligaments or fracture of the distal femoral epiphysis in younger patients.[72] Placing the knee in approximately 25 degrees of flexion isolates the stress to the MCL.[1]

Tests for lateral instability: The **varus stress test** is used to determine the integrity of the LCL, lateral joint capsule, IT band, posterior lateral complex, cruciate ligaments, and lateral musculature when it is performed in complete extension (Stress Test 10-6). When the knee is flexed to 25 degrees and the varus stress reapplied, the LCL is better isolated. A positive varus stress test result when the knee is fully extended may also indicate a distal femoral epiphysis fracture in a younger patient.

Joint Play Assessment

The anterior and posterior drawer tests also are used to identify the amount of anteroposterior glide between the tibia and femur (see Stress Tests 10-1 and 10-4).

Assessment of proximal tibiofibular syndesmosis stability: The proximal tibiofibular syndesmosis is of concern because of the attachment of the LCL and biceps femoris to the fibular head. Instability of the syndesmosis most commonly caused by a glancing blow to the superior fibula results in altered biomechanics and decreased lateral stability secondary to abnormal movement between the fibula and tibia (Joint Play 10-1).

Neurological Assessment

A neurological examination is required when referred pain to the knee is suspected, the proximal tibiofibular joint displays laxity, the patient demonstrates posterolateral instability, or after a dislocation of the tibiofemoral joint. In addition, knee pain can be radicular in nature, arising from proximal nerves such as the sciatic nerve or obturator nerve that refers to the medial knee. Neurological involvement may also be associated with swelling within the popliteal fossa or lateral joint line. In addition, local or distal neurological involvement may occur after surgery (Fig. 10-23). (Refer to Box 1-1 for a lower quarter screen.)

Tibiofibular trauma can also damage the common peroneal nerve, which is superficial at the fibular head. Distal symptoms include paresthesia along the dorsum of the foot and the lateral leg and foot and an inability or weakness in active dorsiflexion and eversion.

Vascular Testing

An examination of distal pulses (posterior tibial artery, dorsal pedal artery) is indicated if a dislocation of the tibiofemoral joint is suspected.

Region-Specific Pathologies and Selective Tissue Tests

Trauma to the knee may result from a contact-related mechanism, through rotational forces placed on the knee while bearing weight, or secondary to overuse. Knee injuries suffered by school-aged athletes (including college students) are most likely to be the result of a single traumatic episode. A small portion of this population and a larger percentage of older athletes are likely to suffer from degenerative changes within the knee.

Uniplanar Knee Sprains

Uniplanar knee sprains present with instability in only one of the body's cardinal planes. Damage to the MCL or LCL leads to valgus or varus instability in the frontal plane. Trauma to the ACL or PCL results in instability in the sagittal plane where the tibia shifts anteriorly or posteriorly relative to the femur. This type of injury involves damage that is isolated to a single structure. When multiple structures are involved (e.g., the ACL and lateral joint capsule), a multiplanar or rotational instability results.

Medial Collateral Ligament Sprains

The MCL is damaged as the result of tensile forces, most commonly a valgus stress caused by a blow to the lateral aspect of the knee. Noncontact valgus loading or a rotational force being placed on the knee can also injure the MCL (Examination Findings 10-1). The valgus stress test (see Stress Test 10-5) performed in complete extension and 25 degrees of flexion is used to manually determine the integrity of the MCL. When the knee is fully extended, the valgus force is

Stress Test 10-2
Lachman Test for Anterior Cruciate Ligament Laxity

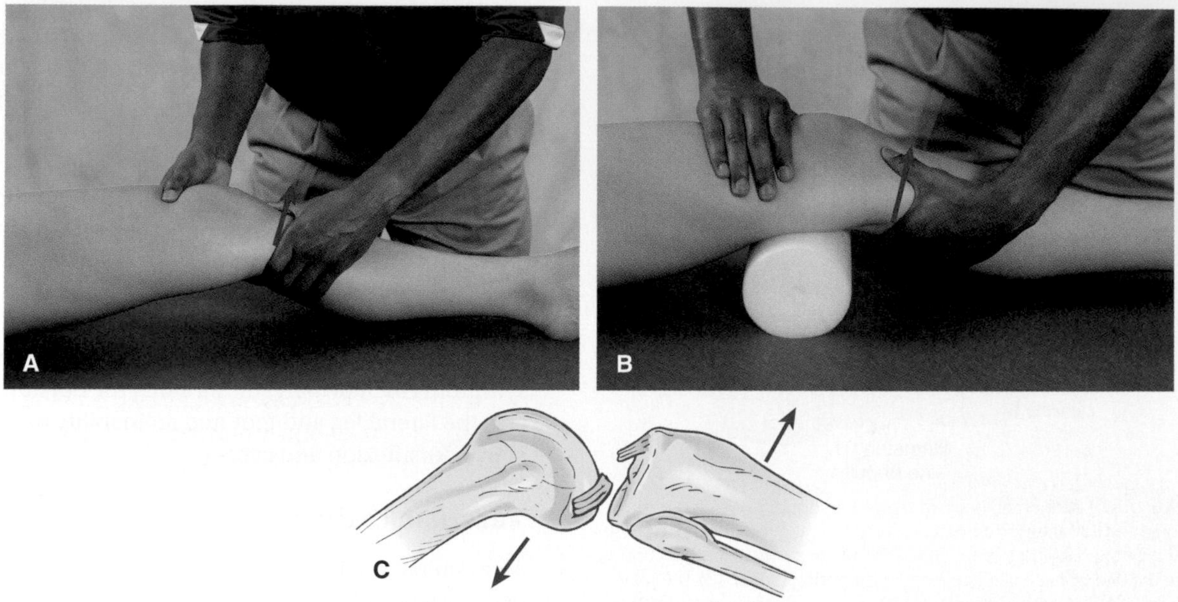

The Lachman test (A) and modification of the Lachman test (B). Schematic representation of tibiofemoral translation in the presence of ACL deficiency (C).

Patient Position	Lying supine The knee passively flexed 20°–25°
Position of Examiner	One hand grasps the tibia around the level of the tibial tuberosity, and the other hand grasps the femur just above the level of the condyles.
Evaluative Procedure	With the patient's leg relaxed, the examiner's distal hand draws the tibia anteriorly while the proximal hand stabilizes the femur.
Positive Test	An increased amount of anterior tibial translation compared with the opposite (uninvolved) limb or the lack of a firm endpoint
Implications	Sprain of the ACL
Modification	As shown in **B** above, placing a bolster under the knee may assist in stabilizing the femur.
Comments	See Stress Test 10-3, Prone Lachman Test.
Evidence	

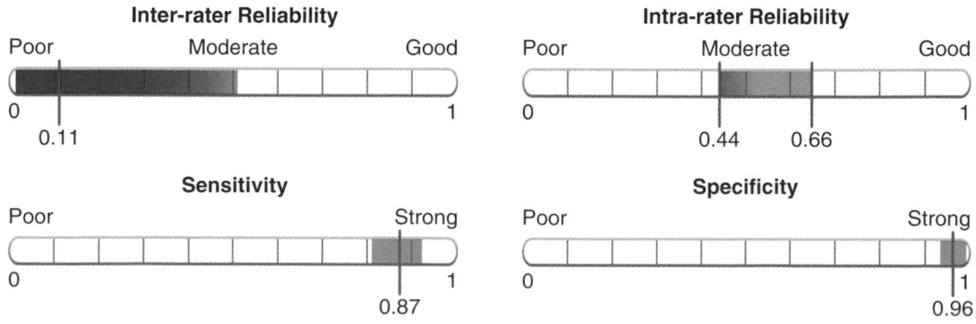

LR+: 4.16–28.00–51.86

LR−: 0.07–0.15–0.23

ACL = anterior cruciate ligament

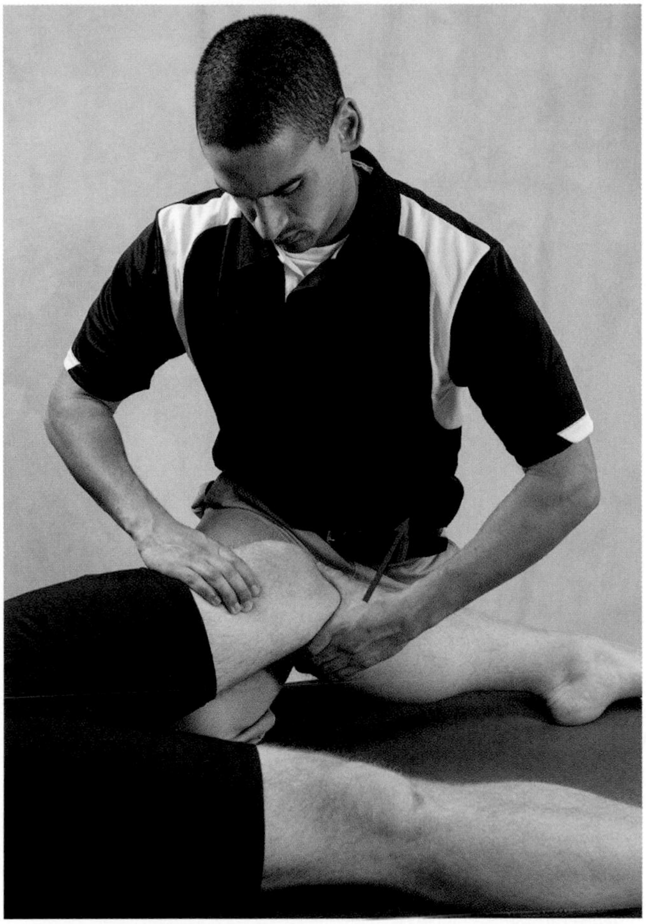

FIGURE 10-21 ■ Modification of the Lachman test.

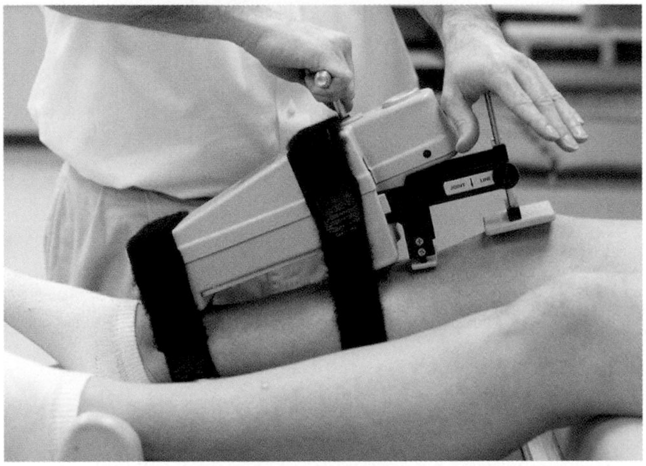

FIGURE 10-22 ■ Instrumented testing of the anterior cruciate ligament using the KT-2000™ arthrometer.

dissipated by the superficial and deep layers of the MCL, the anteromedial and posteromedial joint capsule, and the tendons of the pes anserine group. When the knee is flexed beyond 20 degrees, the superficial layer of the MCL becomes more responsible for resisting valgus forces. Ruptures of the deep layer of the MCL are almost always associated with a rupture of the superficial layer.[74]

Medial collateral ligament sprains may occur in isolation, but, because of the deep layer's communication with the medial joint capsule and medial meniscus, concurrent injury to these structures must always be suspected. Fluid escaping from the knee joint to the area around the MCL is an indirect sign of a complete rupture of the deep layer of the MCL.[5]

✱ Practical Evidence

A complete tear of the MCL, marked by the medial joint line opening 8 mm to 15 mm and marked by an empty end-feel strongly suggests that the ACL and/or PCL have also been ruptured.[72] Complete ruptures of the MCL are associated with ACL sprains in about 80% of cases.[74]

Extreme valgus forces or rotational forces placed on the knee at the time of injury may also lead to the involvement of the ACL or the posteromedial corner.[75] Fractures of the distal femoral physis can mimic a third-degree MCL sprain in growing patients.[76] As described in Chapter 11, patellar dislocations can occur secondary to a valgus force placed on the knee. Therefore, all MCL sprains must include an evaluation of the patella for lateral instability before stress testing.

Medial Collateral Ligament Sprain Intervention Strategies

Most MCL injuries are managed nonoperatively, even when surgical repair of other structures, including the ACL, is warranted.[74,77] The ligament lies within the soft tissue matrix of the medial aspect of the knee and enjoys an adequate blood supply for healing. An aggressive functional rehabilitation program provides long-term stability against valgus forces.[78] Successful nonoperative rehabilitation of the MCL includes protecting the joint from valgus stress while healing, providing an optimal healing environment within the MCL through a controlled restoration of ROM, and adequate strengthening and proprioceptive training of the lower extremity. Use of a knee brace with the ability to limit ROM may be indicated in grade II and III injuries to control further injurious stress and provide the restoration of motion without compromising healing within the ligament.[73,79]

If a period of conservative treatment does not restore valgus stability, the physician may opt to reconstruct the MCL with a third-degree sprain when an associated ACL injury is present.[74]

Lateral Collateral Ligament Sprains

Resulting from a blow to the medial knee that places tensile forces on the lateral structures or by internal rotation of the tibia on the femur, LCL sprains result in varus laxity of the knee. The extracapsular nature of the LCL gives it a normally "springy" end-feel. A varus stress test result that feels empty when compared with the contralateral side should be considered a positive result for an LCL sprain (Examination Findings 10-2).

Examination Findings 10-1
Medial Collateral Ligament Sprain

Examination Segment	Clinical Findings
History of Current Condition	*Onset:* Acute *Pain characteristics:* Medial aspect of the knee, on, above, or below the joint line, depending on the location of the damage *Mechanism:* A valgus force to the knee or, less commonly, external rotation of the tibia with the foot planted *Predisposing conditions:* Increased foot fixation on the ground (e.g., cleats)
Functional Assessment	Increased pain during midstance phase of gait secondary to femur internally rotating on tibia, increasing valgus forces Acute: Antalgic gait secondary to pain and instability Chronic instability: Decreased ability to quickly change direction (cut) to the opposite side
Inspection	Immediate inspection of an MCL injury may produce unremarkable findings. Over time, swelling may be present along the medial aspect of the knee.
Palpation	Tenderness along the length of the MCL from its origin below the adductor tubercle to the insertion on the medial tibial flare
Joint and Muscle Function Assessment	*AROM:* Pain with possible loss of motion during the terminal ranges of flexion and extension; greater loss of ROM when the MCL is torn proximal to the joint line because of greater capsular involvement[75] *MMT:* Decreased flexion and extension strength secondary to pain, with flexion being more painful than extension *PROM:* Pain and possible loss of motion at the end ranges of flexion and extension
Joint Stability Tests	*Stress tests:* Valgus laxity in complete extension indicates involvement of the MCL and medial capsular structures. An empty end-feel strongly suggests an associated sprain of the ACL and/or PCL. Valgus laxity and/or pain in 25° of flexion indicates involvement of the MCL. *Joint play:* No remarkable findings
Selective Tissue Tests	Slocum drawer test for laxity of the anteromedial capsule (see p. 349)
Neurological Screening	Common peroneal nerve and its branches (L4/L5)
Vascular Screening	Within normal limits
Imaging Techniques	T1- and T2-weighted MRI[5] Plain film radiographs may be ordered to rule out epiphyseal fractures in children or avulsion fractures in adults.
Differential Diagnosis	ACL, PCL, medial meniscal tear, semimembranosus tear, pes anserine tear, pes anserine bursitis, common peroneal neuropathy, distal femoral epiphyseal fracture
Comments	Adolescent patients displaying the valgus laxity should be referred to a physician to rule out injury to the epiphysis. If a rotational force is suspected, laxity is displayed in complete extension, or the Slocum drawer test result is positive, pathology of the ACL and PCL should be ruled out. The patella should be checked for lateral stability prior to valgus stress testing (see Selective Tissue Test 11-2). An associated bone bruise, OCD, or common peroneal nerve contusion may occur secondary to lateral compressive forces.

ACL = anterior cruciate ligament; AROM = active range of motion; MCL = medial collateral ligament; MMT = manual muscle test; OCD = osteochondral defect; PCL = posterior cruciate ligament; PROM = passive range of motion

Examination Findings 10-2
Lateral Collateral Ligament Sprain

Examination Segment	Clinical Findings
History of Current Condition	*Onset:* Acute *Pain characteristics:* Lateral joint line of the knee, fibular head, or femoral condyle, depending on the location of the sprain *Mechanism:* Varus force placed on the knee or excess internal tibial rotation
Functional Assessment	Antalgic gait secondary to pain
Inspection	Swelling, if present, is likely to be localized, especially when trauma is isolated to the LCL, because it is an extracapsular structure.
Palpation	Palpation eliciting tenderness along the length of the LCL and possibly the lateral joint line
Joint and Muscle Function Assessment	*AROM:* Pain and loss of motion may be experienced during knee flexion and at terminal extension. *MMT:* Pain and weakness when assessing knee flexion and extension *PROM:* Pain and loss of motion may be experienced during the terminal ROMs, although lack of such pain does not conclusively rule out LCL trauma.
Joint Stability Tests	*Stress tests:* Varus laxity in complete extension indicates involvement of the lateral capsular structures and possibly the cruciate ligaments.[21] Varus laxity in 25°-30° of flexion isolates the LCL. *Joint play:* Tibiofibular joint play
Selective Tissue Tests	Slocum drawer test for laxity of the anterolateral capsule (see p. 349)
Neurological Screening	Common peroneal nerve and its branches (L4/L5)
Vascular Screening	Within normal limits
Imaging Techniques	A T2-weighted MRI can demonstrate tearing of the LCL and/or associated meniscal injury.
Differential Diagnosis	Posterolateral corner injury, posterolateral rotational instability, lateral meniscus tear, lateral head of gastrocnemius tear, biceps femoris tear, IT band inflammation, proximal tibiofibular sprain, fibular head fracture, distal femoral epiphysis fracture
Comments	The LCL has a normal "spring" when a varus force is applied, making bilateral comparison essential. Adolescent patients displaying varus laxity require a referral to a physician to rule out possible epiphyseal injury. For patients who have reported a rotational mechanism of injury or who display LCL laxity through either a varus stress or a positive Slocum drawer test result, anterolateral rotational instability must be suspected. LCL injuries are frequently associated with damage to the posterolateral corner.[80]

AROM = active range of motion; LCL = lateral collateral ligament; MRI = magnetic resonance image; PROM = passive range of motion

Stress Test 10-3
Prone Lachman Test

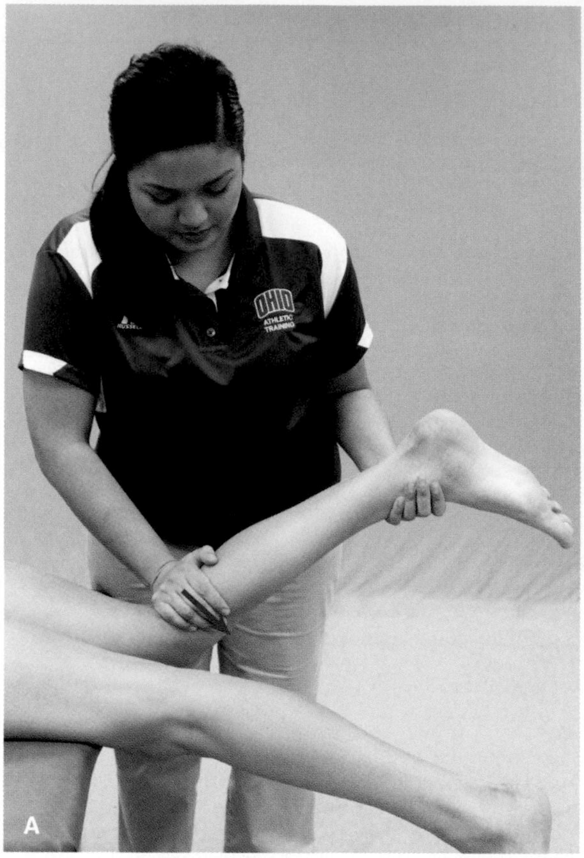

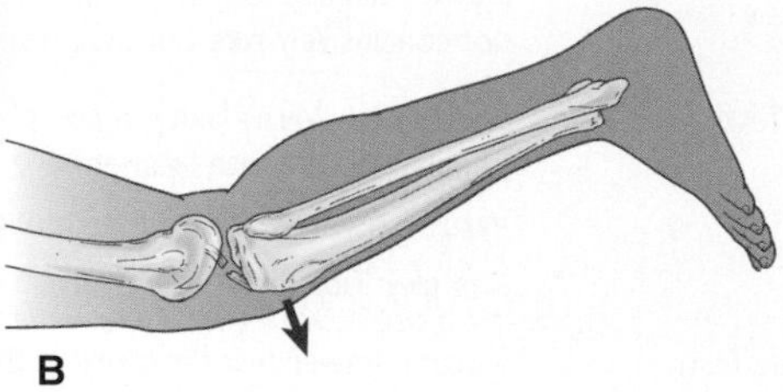

The prone Lachman test is used to differentiate between anterior tibial glide caused by ACL versus PCL laxity and may be easier to perform than the Lachman test for clinicians with small hands or patients with large legs.

Patient Position	Prone, with the leg hanging off the table The knee passively flexed 20°-25°
Position of Examiner	Positioned at the legs of the patient so that the examiner supports the ankle The opposite hand is placed on the posterior aspect of the proximal leg.
Evaluative Procedure	A downward pressure is placed on the proximal portion of the posterior tibia.
Positive Test	Excessive anterior translation relative to the uninvolved knee indicates a sprain of the ACL.
Implications	Positive test results found in the anterior drawer and/or Lachman test and in the alternate Lachman test indicate a sprain of the ACL. A positive anterior drawer test and/or Lachman test result and a negative alternate Lachman test result implicate a sprain in the PCL.

Evidence

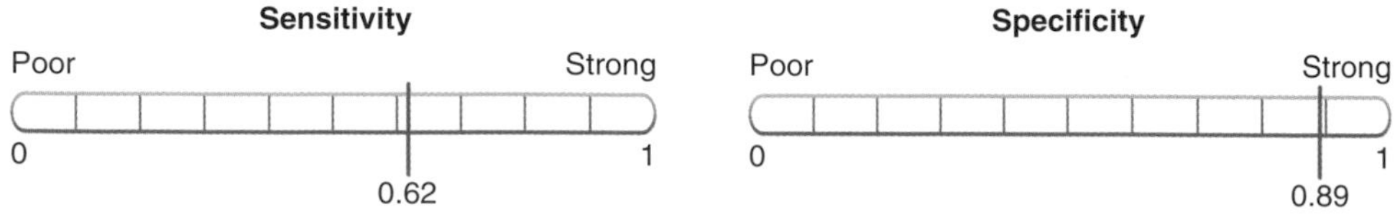

LR+: 5.64

LR−: 0.43

ACL = anterior cruciate ligament; PCL = posterior cruciate ligament

Stress Test 10-4
Posterior Drawer Test for Posterior Cruciate Ligament Laxity

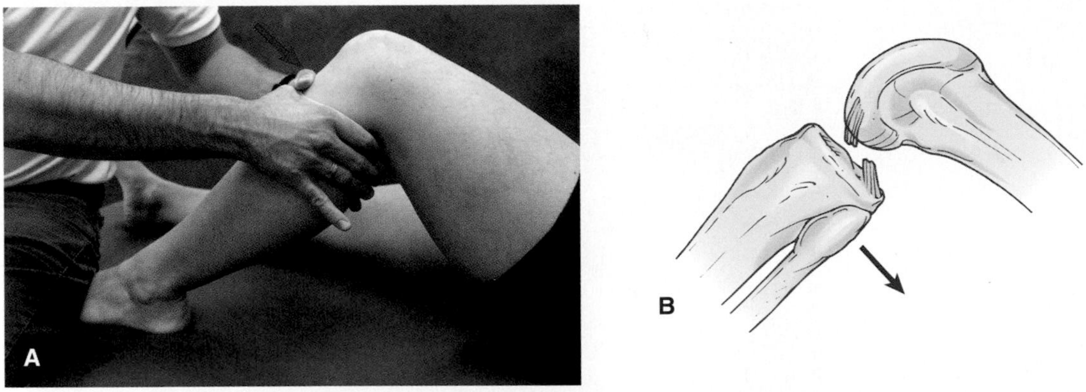

Posterior drawer test for PCL laxity instability. (A) The tibia is moved posteriorly relative to the femur. (B) Translation of the tibia on the femur in the presence of a PCL tear. The posterior drawer test is also used to assess posterior joint play.

Patient Position	Lying supine The hip flexed to 45° and the knee flexed to 90°
Position of Examiner	Sitting on the examination table in front of the involved knee The patient's tibia stabilized in the neutral position
Evaluative Procedure	The examiner grasps the tibia just below the joint line of the knee with the fingers placed along the joint line on either side of the patellar tendon. The proximal tibia is pushed posteriorly.
Positive Test	An increased amount of posterior tibial translation compared with the opposite (uninvolved) limb or the lack of a firm endpoint
Implications	PCL sprain
Modification	To identify injury to the posterolateral corner of the knee, perform the posterior drawer test at 30° of flexion. The drawer test may also be performed with the tibia internally and externally rotated. In isolated PCL tears, there will be decreased tibial translation with the tibia internally rotated.[15]
Comments	Increased posterior translation relative to the uninvolved knee at 30° but not at 90° implicates injury to the posterolateral corner. Increased posterior translation relative to the uninvolved knee at 30° and at 90° indicates injury to the PCL.[6]
Evidence	

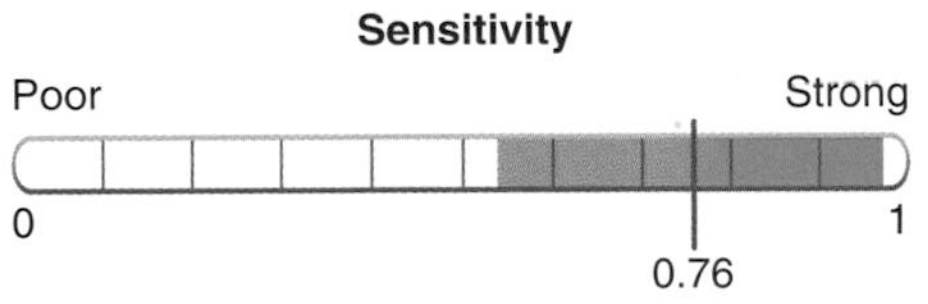

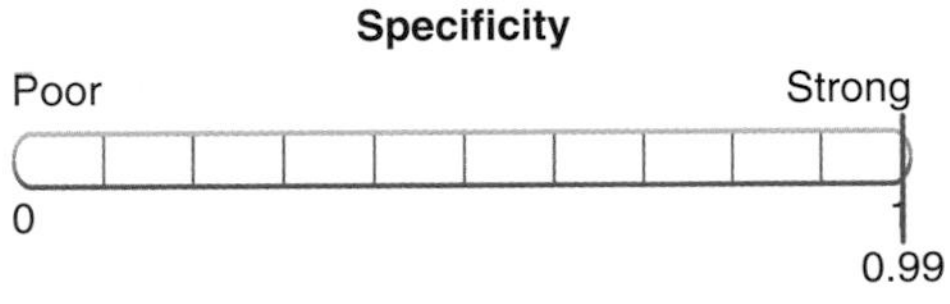

LR+: 90.00

LR−: 0.10

PCL = posterior cruciate ligament

Because a varus force with concurrent tibial rotation can cause damage to other structures, injuries to the posterolateral corner, ACL, and/or PCL as well as posterolateral rotational instability must be suspected in patients suffering from LCL injury. Because of the relative proximity of the peroneal nerve, patients suspected of having suffered an injury to the lateral or posterolateral aspect of the knee require careful evaluation of distal function of the common and superficial peroneal nerve, especially if an associated fracture of the fibular head is suspected.[81]

Selective Tissue Tests 10-4
Godfrey's Test for Posterior Cruciate Ligament Laxity

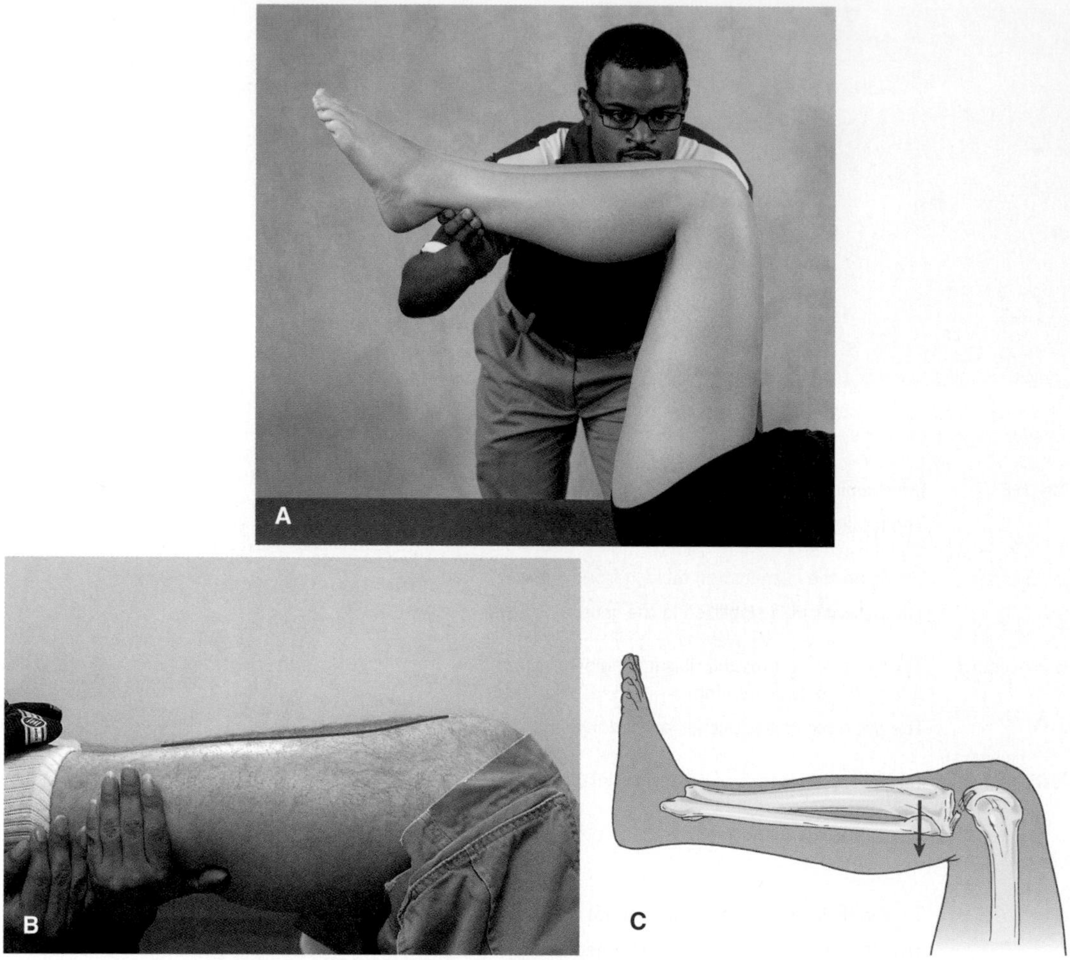

(A) Clinical procedure; (B) Photograph depicting a posterior sag; (C) Illustration showing associated ligamentous damage.

Patient Position	Lying supine with the knees extended and legs together
Position of Examiner	Standing next to the patient
Evaluative Procedure	Lift the patient's lower legs and hold them parallel to the table so that the knees are flexed to 90°. Observe the level of the tibial tuberosities.
Positive Test	A unilateral posterior (downward) displacement of the tibial tuberosity
Implications	PCL sprain
Modification	A straightedge (such as a ruler) can be placed between the patella and tibia to better visualize the posterior sag. Ask the patient to raise the foot against resistance. Anterior translation of the proximal tibia indicates a tear of the PCL.
Comments	The lower leg must be stabilized as distally as possible; supporting the tibia proximally prevents it from sagging posteriorly. An assistant may be used to hold the distal legs.
Evidence	**Sensitivity**: Poor 0 – Strong 1; 0.79 – 1.00 **Specificity**: Poor 0 – Strong 1; 1.00 **LR−:** 0.21

PCL = posterior cruciate ligament

Stress Test 10-5
Valgus Stress Test for Medial Collateral Ligament Laxity

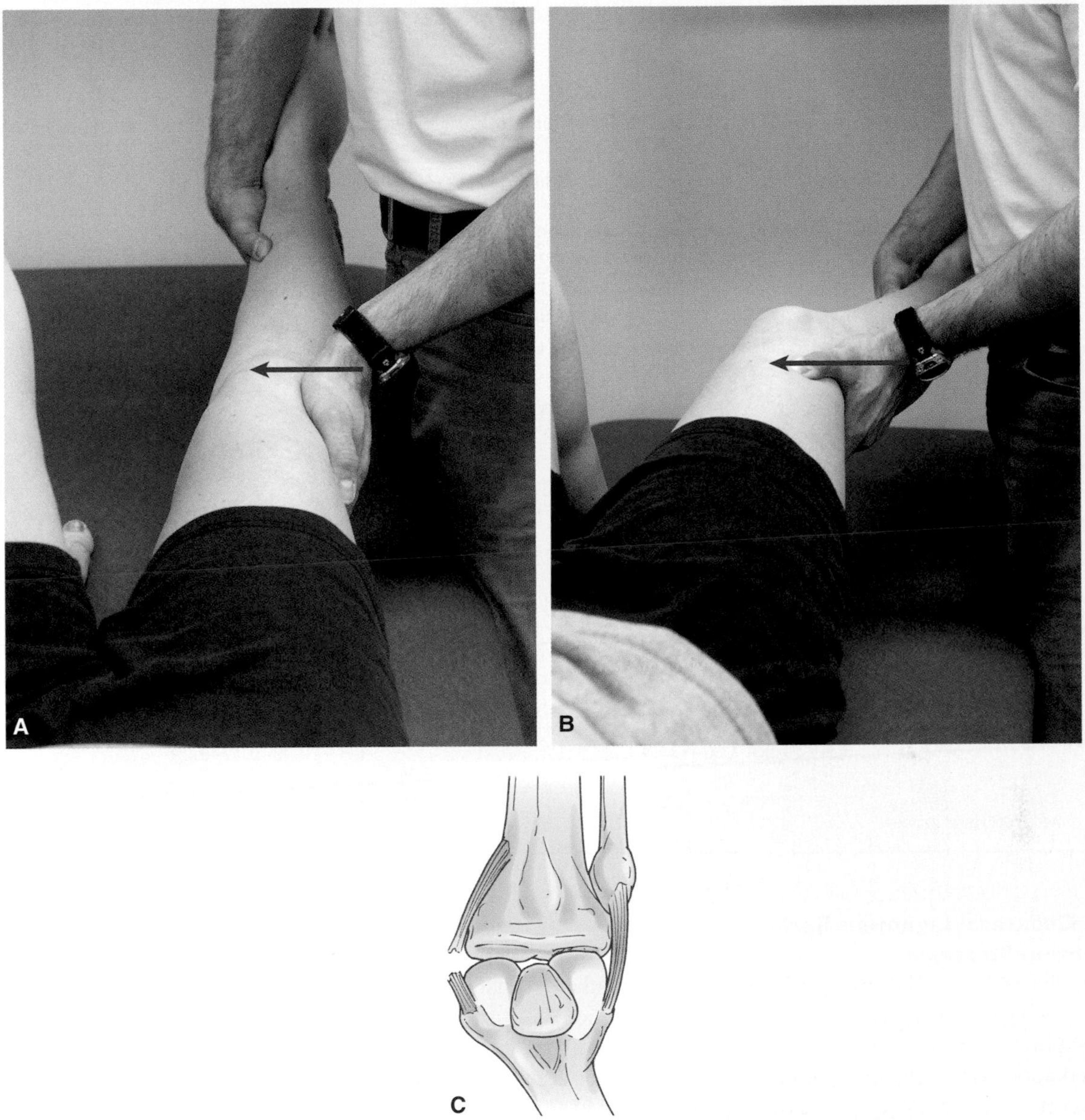

Valgus stress test (A) in full extension to determine the integrity of medial capsular restraints and cruciate ligaments, (B) with the knee flexed to 25° to isolate the medial collateral ligament, and (C) schematic representation of the opening of the medial joint line.

Patient Position	Lying supine with the involved leg close to the edge of the table
Position of Examiner	Standing lateral to the involved limb One hand supports the medial portion of the distal tibia, while the other hand grasps the knee along the lateral joint line. To test the entire medial joint capsule and other restraining structures, the knee is kept in complete extension. To isolate the MCL, the knee is flexed to 25°.
Evaluative Procedure	A medial (valgus) force is applied to the knee while the distal tibia is moved laterally.
Positive Test	Increased laxity, decreased quality of the endpoint, and/or pain compared with the uninvolved limb

Continued

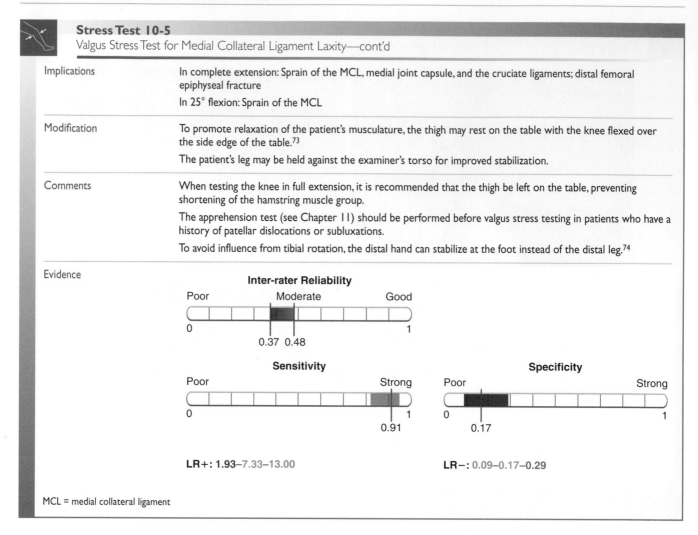

Stress Test 10-5
Valgus Stress Test for Medial Collateral Ligament Laxity—cont'd

Implications	In complete extension: Sprain of the MCL, medial joint capsule, and the cruciate ligaments; distal femoral epiphyseal fracture In 25° flexion: Sprain of the MCL
Modification	To promote relaxation of the patient's musculature, the thigh may rest on the table with the knee flexed over the side edge of the table.[73] The patient's leg may be held against the examiner's torso for improved stabilization.
Comments	When testing the knee in full extension, it is recommended that the thigh be left on the table, preventing shortening of the hamstring muscle group. The apprehension test (see Chapter 11) should be performed before valgus stress testing in patients who have a history of patellar dislocations or subluxations. To avoid influence from tibial rotation, the distal hand can stabilize at the foot instead of the distal leg.[74]
Evidence	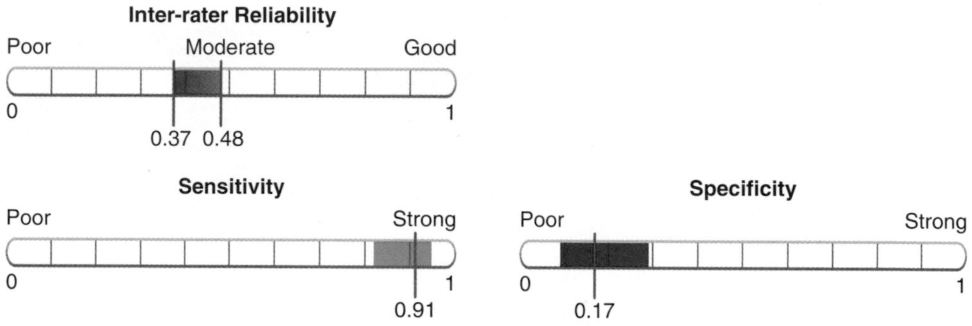 LR+: 1.93–7.33–13.00 LR−: 0.09–0.17–0.29

MCL = medial collateral ligament

Lateral Collateral Ligament Sprain Intervention Strategies

Although the LCL is an extracapsular and extra-articular structure, the ligament still relies on synovial fluid for much of its nutrition.[82] In many cases, even complete LCL ruptures are treated nonoperatively. However, the LCL's relatively poor healing properties and the ligament's importance in providing rotational stability to the knee often necessitate early surgical repair or late reconstruction (also see Posterolateral Corner Injuries).[83]

Anterior Cruciate Ligament Sprains

Injury to the ACL results from a force causing an anterior displacement of the tibia relative to the femur (or the femur being driven posteriorly on the tibia) from rotation or hyperextension of the knee. Unlike injury to other ligaments, the majority of ACL sprains arise from noncontact-related torsional stress, such as what occurs when an athlete cuts or pivots.[84,85]Associated with the injury mechanism, the patient may describe hearing or sensing a "pop" within the knee joint and an immediate loss of knee function (Examination Findings 10-3). Swelling occurs rapidly secondary to trauma of the medial geniculate artery, the ACL's primary blood supply. Normally, this hemarthrosis remains within the fibrous capsule, but trauma to the capsule results in diffuse swelling that may **extravasate** distally over time. Intracapsular swelling combined with the tension placed on the ACL limits the ROM (see Fig. 10-8). Laxity of the ACL may be confirmed through a Lachman test and the anterior drawer test. However, clinical laxity is not a strong predictor of functional ability.[86]

The rotational forces placed on the knee also make structures other than the ACL vulnerable to injury. Instability of the knee is greatly increased when trauma also damages one or more of the other ligaments or the menisci.[53,90] As described in the Rotational Knee Instabilities section of this chapter, the degree of anterior displacement of the tibia increases and an anterior subluxation of the tibial condyles results when the anteromedial or anterolateral joint capsules, pes anserine, biceps femoris, or IT band are also traumatized.

Multiple internal and external risk factors for ACL injury have been suggested (Fig. 10-24).[9,91] Some risk factors can be modified to reduce the risk of injuries, but others are inherent to the person and cannot be modified. The typical mechanism of injury results in tibial rotation and possibly a valgus force on

Extravasate Fluid escaping from vessels into the surrounding tissue

Stress Test 10-6
Varus Stress Test for Lateral Collateral Ligament Laxity

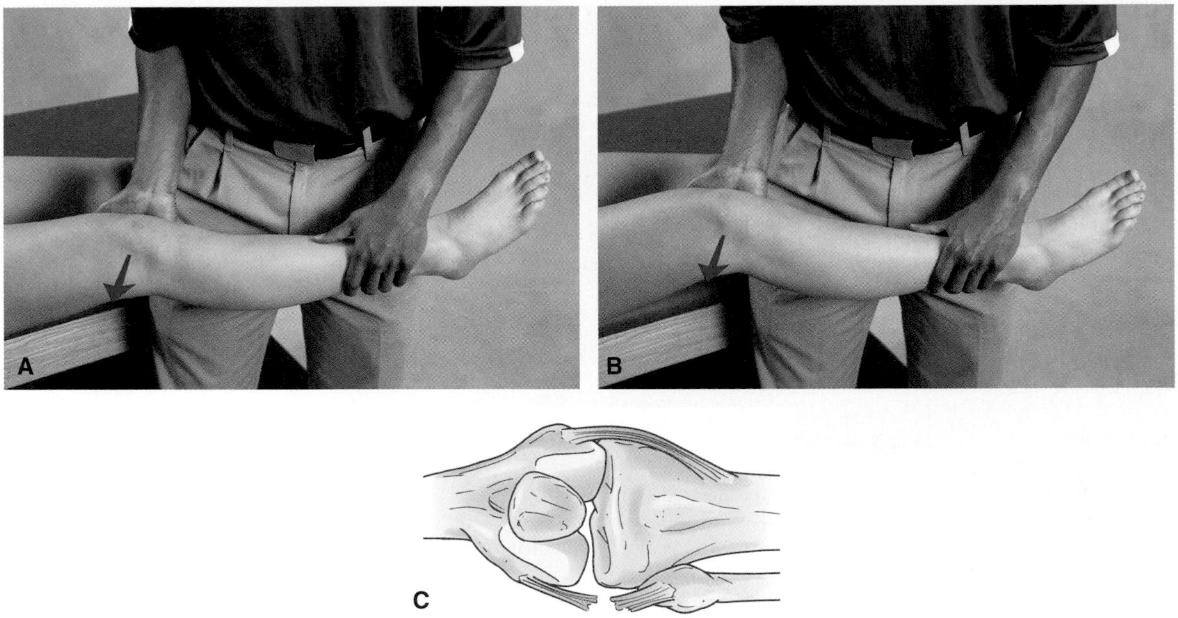

Varus stress test (A) in full extension to determine the integrity of lateral capsular restraints, (B) with the knee flexed to 25°–30° to isolate the lateral collateral ligament, and (C) schematic representation of the opening of the medial joint line.

Patient Position	Lying supine with the involved leg close to the edge of the table
Position of Examiner	Sitting on the table One hand supports the lateral portion of the distal tibia, while the other hand grasps the knee along the medial joint line. To test the entire lateral joint capsule and other restraining structures, the knee is kept in complete extension. To isolate the LCL, flex the knee to 25°.
Evaluative Procedure	A lateral (varus) force is applied to the knee while the distal tibia is moved inward.
Positive Test	Increased laxity, decreased quality of the endpoint, and/or pain compared with the uninvolved limb
Implications	In complete extension: Sprain of the LCL, lateral joint capsule, cruciate ligaments, and related structures, indicating possible rotational instability of the joint, distal femoral epiphyseal fracture In 25° of flexion: Sprain of the LCL
Modification	The patient is supine. The examiner is standing to allow the patient's abducted thigh to rest on the table for improved stabilization and relaxation.
Comments	Avoid hip external rotation during the maneuver. The varus force must be applied perpendicular to the ligament in both testing positions.

Evidence

Sensitivity

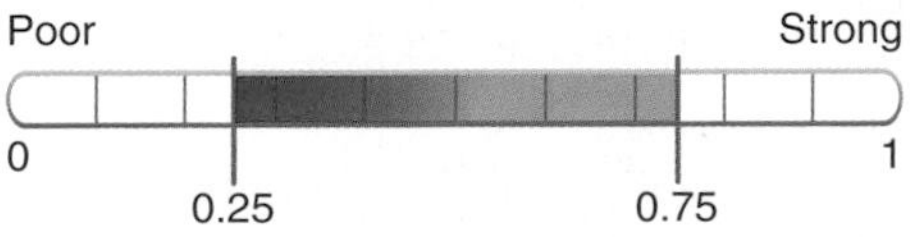

Specificity

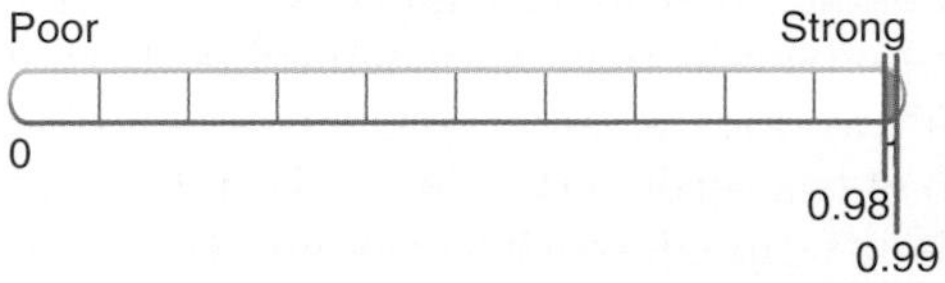

LR+: 25.00–37.50

LR−: 0.26–0.76

LCL = lateral collateral ligament

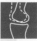

Joint Play 10-1
Proximal Tibiofibular Syndesmosis

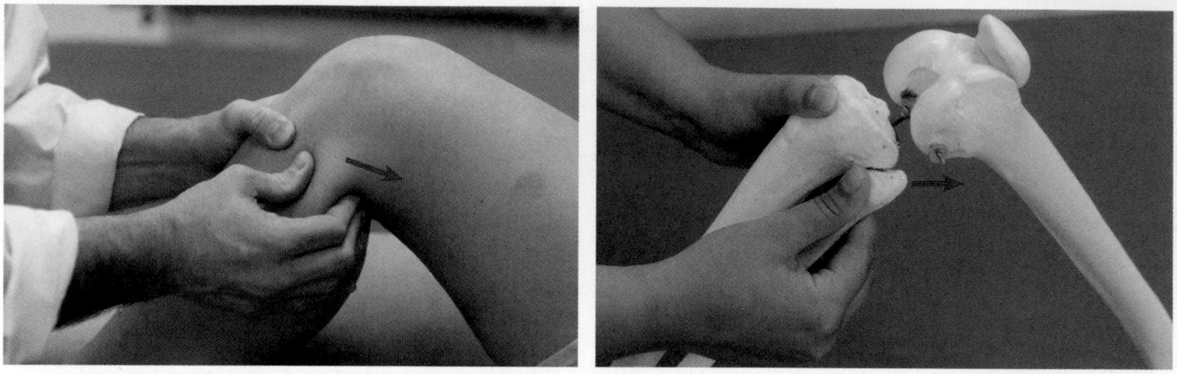

The fibular head is translated to determine its anterior/posterior stability.

Patient Position	Lying supine with the knee passively flexed to approximately 90°
Position of Examiner	Standing lateral to the involved side
Evaluative Procedure	One hand stabilizes the tibia, while the other hand grasps the fibular head. While stabilizing the tibia, the examiner attempts to displace the fibular head perpendicular to the joint surface.
Positive Test	Hyper- or hypomobility of the fibula on the tibia compared with the uninvolved side and/or pain elicited during the test
Implications	An anterior fibular shift indicates damage to the proximal posterior tibiofibular ligament; posterior displacement reflects instability of the anterior tibiofibular ligament of the proximal tibiofibular syndesmosis. Hypomobility may alter proximal and distal joint mechanics.
Comments	Damage to the common peroneal nerve is frequently associated with a proximal tibiofibular syndesmosis sprain.
Evidence	Inconclusive or absent in the literature

the knee, thus placing an additional stress on the ACL. Females are particularly predisposed to ACL injury (Box 10-1).

Because PCL deficiency can replicate positive test results for ACL involvement as the tibia is returned to its normal position, tests for PCL sprains need to be performed to rule out such false-positive results.

The term "partially torn ACL" is a misnomer. Because the bands of the ACL wind upon each other, even partial trauma to an individual band results in biomechanical dysfunction, instability, and increased stress on the remaining fibers, predisposing them to future injury. Knees with incomplete tears of the ACL (typically involving the anteromedial bundle) may initially appear stable during manual stress testing but degrade to demonstrate signs of clinical instability as the remaining ligament fibers adaptively lengthen or tear secondary to increased stress loads.[58]

The long-term consequences of an ACL-deficient knee include instability, meniscal degeneration, chondral surface damage, and OA.[93] Patients who perform physical activities that do not involve cutting or pivoting on a planted foot may not experience pain or dysfunction, although proprioceptive function in a single-limb stance is decreased in the presence of an ACL-deficient knee.[94] Patients who have a history of an ACL tear are seven times more likely to develop moderate to severe clinical OA and have a 105 times greater chance of developing radiographically diagnosed OA than those without a history of an ACL tear.[93]

Anterior Cruciate Ligament Intervention Strategies

The rehabilitation program for a patient with an ACL-deficient knee focuses on restoring ROM, lower extremity strength, and proprioception.[94] The use of a functional knee brace may be helpful, although the efficacy of these devices has not been substantiated.

ACL-deficient patients who perform activities involving cutting and pivoting will most likely benefit from ACL reconstruction. Several donor tissue options are available, including **autografts** and **allografts**. The use of an accelerated rehabilitation program involving early return of

Autograft The tissues used to replace the ligament harvested from the patient's body (e.g., bone-patellar tendon-bone, hamstring tendon)

Allograft The tissues used to replace the ligament obtained from a cadaver

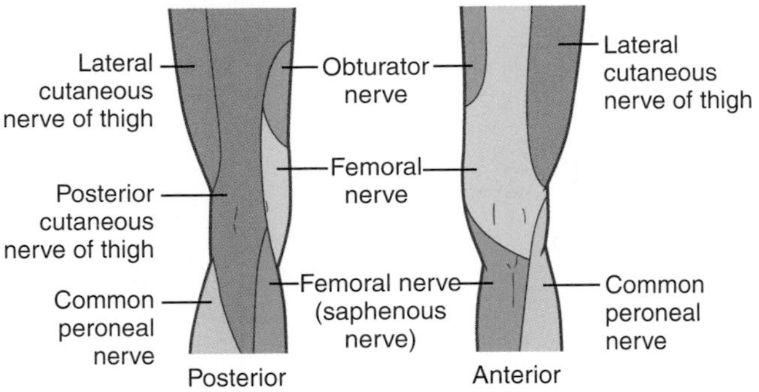

FIGURE 10-23 ■ Local neuropathies of the knee. These findings should also be correlated with a lower quarter neurological screen.

ROM, early weight bearing, and restoration of muscular function decreases the time lost after surgery with no adverse long-term effects.[95] Accelerated programs have also been found to promote early mobility and decrease surgical morbidity including postoperative stiffness and patellofemoral pain.[95] The risk for developing OA remains higher than that in the general population even following reconstruction.[96]

Posterior Cruciate Ligament Sprains

Uniplanar PCL injury results from knee hyperextension or a blow to the anterior tibia as occurs when plantarflexed. If the foot is dorsiflexed when falling on the knee, much of the force is directed toward the patellofemoral joint, thereby sparing the PCL (Examination Findings 10-4). However, if the foot is plantarflexed, the resulting force is delivered to the PCL when the tibial tuberosity makes contact with the ground or another stationary object (Fig. 10-25).[97]

Immediately after the onset of injury, the patient may be relatively asymptomatic or may display the signs and symptoms of a tear of the medial head of the gastrocnemius or a sprain of the posterior capsule.[97] Over time, symptoms such as pain in the posterior knee, weakness of the hamstring and quadriceps muscle groups, and reduced ROM during flexion and extension become evident. Initially, knee ROM may be equal to that of the opposite limb if there is an isolated PCL sprain, but noticeable deficits will be evident if multiple structures are damaged.[98] The posterior drawer and sag tests are highly specific in identifying the presence of chronic PCL sprains.[68] The **quadriceps active test** can identify grade II and III PCL tears (Selective Tissue Test 10-5).[98] Isolated PCL trauma results in greater posterior instability as the knee is flexed from 0 to 90 degrees.[6] The LCL, posterolateral corner, and MCL are secondary restraints to posterior tibial displacement of the tibia on the femur, especially in the presence of a PCL-deficient knee.[98]

PCL tears are often asymptomatic and go unreported and/or undiagnosed. Isolated PCL sprains increase the amount of posterior tibial translation but do not increase the varus rotation or external tibial rotation.[21] Instability is greatest when there is concurrent damage to both the PCL and the knee's posterolateral structures.[6,68] The presence of a partial or complete tear of the PCL can be identified via MRI.[68] PCL sprains must also be evaluated for posterolateral corner deficiencies (see p. 346).

Posterior Cruciate Ligament Sprain Intervention Strategies

Joint loading, joint congruency, and muscular activity can compensate for static PCL deficiency. The strength of the quadriceps muscle group soon returns after a PCL sprain to assist the popliteus in providing muscular compensation against posterior tibial displacement.[18,69,101] Actual posterior laxity does not always result in knee dysfunction.[102] Patients treated nonsurgically can regain full function and independence and may often return to athletic competition unhindered by the ligamentous deficit.[100,102] If the PCL deficiency is not identified or not appropriately treated, changes in the structure and function of the ACL, meniscus, and weight-bearing surfaces will occur over time, potentially leading to chronic joint instability, alteration in the gait pattern, muscle activation patterns, and reduced muscle strength.[100,103,104] The long-term consequence of these conditions is the early onset of OA and increased joint laxity.

Rotational Knee Instabilities

Unlike uniplanar knee instabilities, rotational (multiplanar) instabilities involve abnormal internal or external rotation at the tibiofemoral joint. The four types of instabilities are named based on the relative direction in which the tibia subluxates on the femur and are presented in Box 10-2. When this type of instability occurs, the axis of tibial rotation is shifted in the direction opposite that of the subluxation.

Rotational instabilities result when multiple structures are traumatized, often as the result of rotational forces placed on the knee. The tests for laxity of the individual structures may produce only mildly positive results. However, when the combined laxity of each structure is summed, the degree of instability is marked.

Any injury to the knee's ligaments can cause rotational instability. Therefore, any injury to the cruciate or collateral ligaments, the IT band, the joint capsule, or the biceps femoris must be presumed as potentially resulting in rotational instability.[31] Clinically, patients suffering from rotational instability report the feeling of the knee "giving way," decreased muscle strength, diminished performance, and a lack of confidence in the stability of the joint.

Anterolateral Rotational Instability

The most common rotational instability of the knee, an anterolateral rotary instability (ALRI), results in a greater displacement of the tibia because of trauma to both the ACL and the lateral extra-articular restraints.[105] Disruption of the LCL, IT band, biceps femoris, and lateral meniscus accentuates the amount of anterior tibial displacement and internal tibial rotation. Many selective tissue tests exist for determining the presence of ALRI, each with its own merits and limitations. The large number of tests probably reflects their relatively low reliability.

Examination Findings 10-3
Anterior Cruciate Ligament Sprain

Examination Segment	Clinical Findings
History of Current Condition	*Onset:* Acute *Pain characteristics:* Pain within the knee joint Diffuse pain throughout the joint after injury *Other symptoms:* A "pop" under the kneecap is often described. *Mechanism:* Rotation of the knee while the foot is planted, a blow that drives the tibia anterior relative to the femur or the femur posterior relative to the tibia, or hyperextension *Predisposing conditions:* See Figure 10-24. Footwear and/or playing surfaces that increase foot fixation
Functional Assessment	The extent of disability is influenced by the secondary restraints that are also injured. **Acute:** Antalgic gait (shortened stance time), inability to climb or descend stairs (tending to lead with the uninvolved leg); inability to achieve full extension secondary to quadriceps inhibition resulting from effusion **Chronic:** Complaints of instability with change of direction
Inspection	Rapid effusion, often in the suprapatellar area, that forms within hours after the onset of injury
Palpation	For isolated ACL injuries, pain is not normally reported during palpation (other than that resulting from a contusion caused by the traumatic force). The sweep and ballottable patella test results are positive if an effusion is present.
Joint and Muscle Function Assessment	*AROM:* Pain or intracapsular swelling may prohibit any meaningful ROM tests; pain is expected to be greatest at the extremes of the ROM. *MMT:* Pain and/or weakness during flexion and extension, possibly precluding this portion of the examination's being conducted in the acute stage of injury *PROM:* Pain likely throughout the ROM (especially at the extremes) and possibly intensified when the tibia is internally or externally rotated
Joint Stability Tests	*Stress tests:* Lachman test Anterior drawer test Prone Lachman test *Joint play:* Anterior glide of the tibia on the femur is assessed using the anterior drawer test. Posterior glide of the tibia is assessed using the posterior drawer test.[87]
Selective Tissue Tests	Pivot shift test Flexion-rotation drawer test[88] Slocum drawer test Crossover test Slocum ALRI test

Neurological Screening	Within normal limits
Vascular Screening	Within normal limits
Imaging Techniques	Four-view radiographic series: AP, lateral, skyline, tunnel [89] Coronal and sagittal T1- and T2-weighted MR images
Differential Diagnosis	PCL sprain, meniscus tear, hamstring strain, tear of the proximal gastrocnemius, MCL sprain, osteochondral fracture, patellar dislocation
Comments	The anterior drawer test is more helpful in detecting ACL sprains after the acute injury phase has passed. Trauma to the PCL may produce false-positive results for ACL insufficiency. Chronic instability can lead to meniscal degeneration. Hamstring strains may occur secondary to the sudden eccentric contraction of the muscles in an attempt to restrict anterior translation of the tibia..

ACL = anterior cruciate ligament; AROM = active range of motion; MCL = medial collateral ligament; MMT = manual muscle test; OCD = osteochondral defect; PCL = posterior cruciate ligament; PROM = passive range of motion

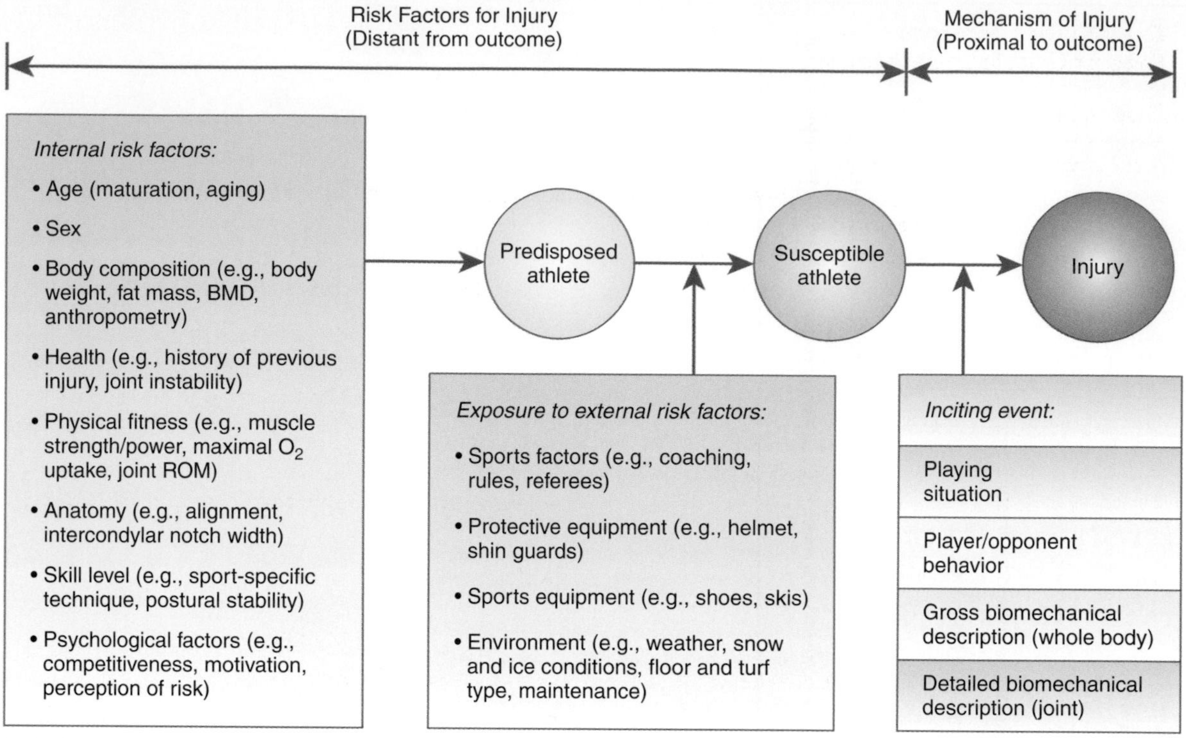

Risk Factors for Injury
(Distant from outcome)
Mechanism of Injury
(Proximal to outcome)
Internal risk factors:
• Age (maturation, aging)
• Sex
• Body composition (e.g., body weight, fat mass, BMD, anthropometry)
• Health (e.g., history of previous injury, joint instability)
• Physical fitness (e.g., muscle strength/power, maximal O2 uptake, joint ROM)
• Anatomy (e.g., alignment, intercondylar notch width)
• Skill level (e.g., sport-specific technique, postural stability)
• Psychological factors (e.g., competitiveness, motivation, perception of risk)
Predisposed athlete
Susceptible athlete
Injury
Exposure to external risk factors:
• Sports factors (e.g., coaching, rules, referees)
• Protective equipment (e.g., helmet, shin guards)
• Sports equipment (e.g., shoes, skis)
• Environment (e.g., weather, snow and ice conditions, floor and turf type, maintenance)
Inciting event:
Playing situation
Player/opponent behavior
Gross biomechanical description (whole body)
Detailed biomechanical description (joint)

FIGURE 10-24 ■ Continuum of risk factors for ACL injury. Internal risk factors are inherent to the individual. External risk factors are imposed on the individual during activity. The inciting event presents the opportunity for the internal and external risk factors to interact, thereby increasing the risk of an ACL tear. *Adapted from: Alentorn-Geli, E, Myer, GD, Silvers, HJ, et al. Prevention of non-contact anterior cruciate ligament injuries in soccer players. Part 1: Mechanisms of injury and underlying risk factors. Knee Surg Sports Traumatol Arthrosc. 17:705, 2009.*

Box 10-1
Anterior Cruciate Ligament Injuries in Females

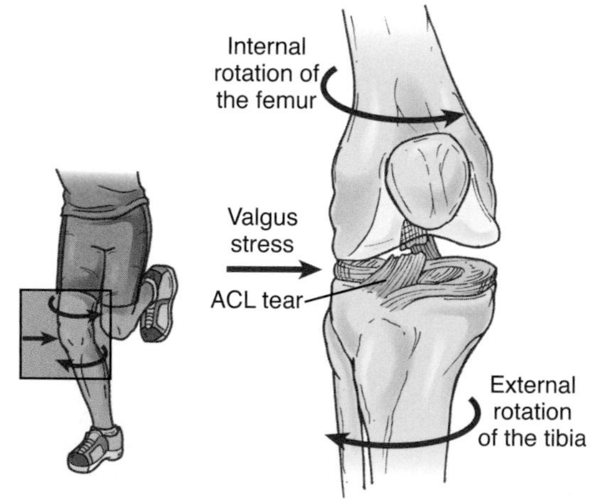

Internal rotation of the femur
Valgus stress
ACL tear
External rotation of the tibia

Women's participation in sports continues to grow. Although the expected increase in participation of female athletes would normally give rise to an increased number of injuries, female athletes have experienced a disproportionately high rate of noncontact ACL injuries relative to their male counterparts.[92]

Although women normally have an increased amount of anterior tibial translation compared with men, this fails to account for the high incidence rate.[29] Changes in muscle activation patterns, increased rates of fatigue, and biomechanical differences in landing from a jump and cutting appear to contribute to the increased rate of ACL injuries in females.[91] Also, females, on average, have narrower intercondylar notch widths, which may partially account for the higher noncontact ACL injury rate in female athletes.[91]

The influence of the menstrual cycle as a predisposition to ACL injury remains under dispute. Hormone-dependent changes occur throughout the menstrual cycle that may alter physical performance, such as decreasing reaction time and viscoelastic tissue properties. The risk of sustaining an ACL injury appears to be increased during the first days of the menstrual period.[91]

Examination Findings 10-4
Posterior Cruciate Ligament Sprain

Examination Segment	Clinical Findings
History of Current Condition	*Onset:* Acute *Pain characteristics:* Within the knee joint radiating posteriorly, although pain may not be immediately experienced Unlike ACL tears, the patient may not report feeling a "pop" at the time of injury.[15] *Mechanism:* Posterior displacement of the tibia on the femur (e.g., falling on the knee with the ankle plantarflexed) Knee hyperflexion Knee hyperextension *Predisposing conditions:* Quadriceps weakness
Functional Assessment	Acute: Antalgic gait secondary to avoidance of full extension Chronic: May avoid full extension during ambulation. With damage to the posterolateral complex, the patient may demonstrate limited push-off on the involved extremity.
Inspection	Effusion may not be present initially but may develop over time. A posterior sag of the tibia may be noted.
Palpation	Tenderness may be elicited in the popliteal fossa if the sprain involves the posterior capsular structures or popliteus muscle; otherwise, no pain or abnormalities are usually noted.
Joint and Muscle Function Assessment	*AROM:* Acutely, normal ROM present; pain and restrictions possible as the knee nears full flexion or extension *MMT:* Quadriceps strength may be diminished in patients with chronic PCL sprains. *PROM:* Pain produced as the knee nears 90° of flexion and with overpressure during flexion, especially in the presence of a partial PCL tear; extension limited over time
Joint Stability Tests	*Stress tests:* Posterior drawer test; Godfrey's sign, external rotation test *Joint play:* Posterior glide of the tibia is assessed using the posterior drawer test. Anterior glide of the tibia on the femur is assessed using the anterior drawer test.
Selective Tissue Tests	Quadriceps active test See also Selective Tissue Tests for posterolateral rotational instability (pp. 357-361)
Neurological Screening	Within normal limits
Vascular Screening	Within normal limits
Imaging Techniques	Anteroposterior, lateral, sunrise, and tunnel views may be ordered. Avulsion fractures may be noted at the PCL tibial insertion.[98] Posterior drawer stress radiograph[99] MR images are accurate in identifying the location of an acute tear and for identifying concomitant trauma about the knee.[98]
Differential Diagnosis	Tear of the medial head of the gastrocnemius, posterior capsule sprain, ACL, posterolateral complex sprain, meniscus tear
Comments	Individuals with moderate PCL sprains as measured by instrumented testing display few functional differences (e.g., during ambulation and landing from a jump) as compared with those with normal knee stability.[100]

AROM = active range of motion; MMT = manual muscle test; MR = magnetic resonance; PCL = posterior cruciate ligament; PROM = passive range of motion

Three tests specific to this pathology are discussed here: the **pivot shift**, the Slocum ALRI test, and the flexion-rotation drawer. In addition, two tests, the Slocum drawer test and the crossover test, may be used to determine the presence of either ALRI or anteromedial rotational instability (AMRI). A positive result for any one of the following techniques is sufficient to warrant further examination by an orthopedic physician.

A derivation of the anterior drawer test, the **Slocum drawer test** attempts to isolate either the anteromedial or the anterolateral joint capsule (Selective Tissue Test 10-6). Internally rotating the tibia checks for the presence of ALRI; externally rotating it checks for AMRI.

The **crossover test** is a semifunctional test used to determine the rotational stability of the knee (Selective Tissue Test 10-7).

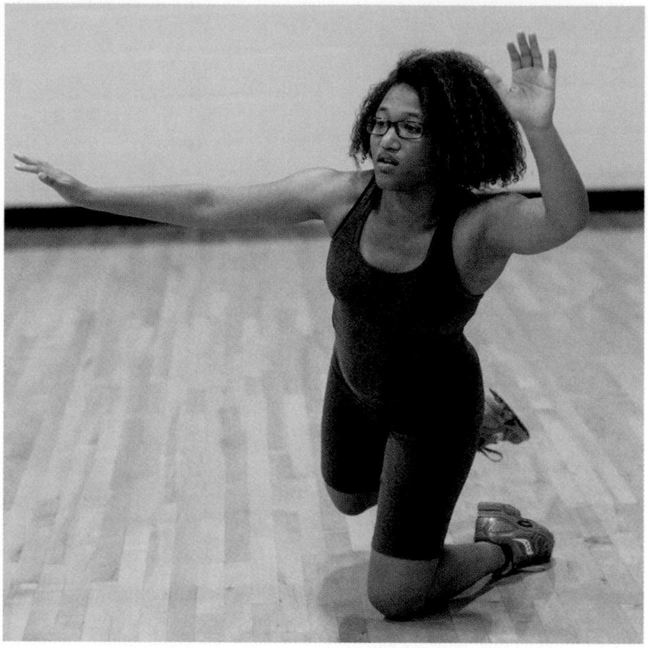

FIGURE 10-25 ■ Mechanism of posterior cruciate ligament sprain. Landing on a bent knee and plantar flexed foot forces the tibia posteriorly relative to the femur.

This test is not as exacting as other tests for ligamentous instability, but it has the advantage of replicating a sport-specific skill, albeit in slow motion. Although primarily used to determine the presence of ALRI, the crossover test may be modified to test for AMRI by stepping behind with the uninvolved leg.

Used to evaluate ALRI, the **pivot shift test** (also known as the lateral pivot shift) duplicates the anterior subluxation and reduction that occurs during functional activities in ACL-deficient knees (Selective Tissue Test 10-8). The tibia is internally rotated, and a valgus force is applied to the joint while the knee is moved from extension into flexion. In the presence of a torn ACL, the tibia is displaced anteriorly when the knee is near full extension. When the knee reaches the range of 30 to 40 degrees of flexion, the IT band changes its line of pull from an extensor to a flexor and causes the tibia to relocate, resulting in an appreciable "clunk." Although positive findings with the pivot shift are associated with an ALRI, the test also has a high positive predictive value for diagnosing an ACL sprain. A positive pivot shift almost always indicates damage to the ACL.[59] The **jerk test** is a variant of the pivot shift test but determines subluxation and reduction as the knee goes from flexion into extension (see Selective Tissue Test 10-8).

✱ Practical Evidence

In consolidating the evidence of examination techniques for the ACL, a positive pivot shift is the most predictive of an ACL tear, and a negative Lachman is most predictive in ruling out a rupture.[59,106]

During the **Slocum ALRI test**, the weight of the patient's limb is used to fixate the femur while the knee is flexed and a simultaneous valgus force is applied (Selective Tissue Test 10-9). As the knee reaches 30 to 50 degrees of flexion, a subluxation of the tibia is reduced. This test is not as sensitive as the lateral pivot shift but is useful when dealing with large or heavy patients.

The **flexion-rotation drawer test** (FRD) involves the stabilization of the tibia, resulting in the relative subluxation of the femur (Selective Tissue Test 10-10). In the presence of ALRI, lifting and supporting the distal lower leg causes the femur to displace posteriorly and rotate externally. The test then identifies the subsequent reduction of the femur relative to the tibia.

Anteromedial Rotational Instability

The O'Donohue triad is an injury involving the ACL, MCL, and medial meniscus, resulting in AMRI. The definition has been changed to include the lateral meniscus rather than the medial meniscus.[107] As described in the ALRI section, the variants of the Slocum drawer test and the crossover test may be used to determine the presence of AMRI. In addition, isolated tests for ACL and MCL insufficiency yield positive test results.

Posterolateral Corner Injuries

While a purely varus force can injure the LCL, a combined mechanism of knee hyperextension and varus stress or hyperextension and external tibial rotation can result in trauma to the structures of the posterolateral corner of the knee (Examination Findings 10-5). The greater the number of structures involved, including the ACL or PCL, the more significant the resulting instability (Table 10-5).

Posterolateral corner injuries are particularly difficult to evaluate in the acute setting and frequently require general anesthesia to produce the most accurate results.[7,108] Because isolated injuries to the posterolateral corner are rare or nonexistent, injury to the ACL and PCL must also be ruled out.

Posterolateral rotational instability involves the anterior displacement of the lateral femoral condyle relative to the tibia (the tibia externally rotating relative to the femur). The amount of external tibial rotation varies greatly from person to person and increases with the amount of knee flexion.[109] This motion is produced when the axis of rotation shifts medially. The patient often reports a history of external tibial rotation or knee hyperextension and describes knee instability. Pain is localized to the posterolateral aspect of the knee, but tension on the medial structures and the change in the rotational axis may produce pain in the medial knee.[110] The patient may describe the sensation of the knee's giving way during activity or static stance. The patient may respond favorably to heel lifts or high-heeled shoes that prevent the knee from fully extending during gait.[7] To prevent subluxation, the tibia may be maintained in a flexed and internally rotated position during gait.

Pain and instability make participation in strenuous activities difficult or impossible. Swelling forms rapidly, and the lack of contained edema strongly suggests a complete posterolateral corner injury.[108]

Selective Tissue Test 10-5
Quadriceps Active Test

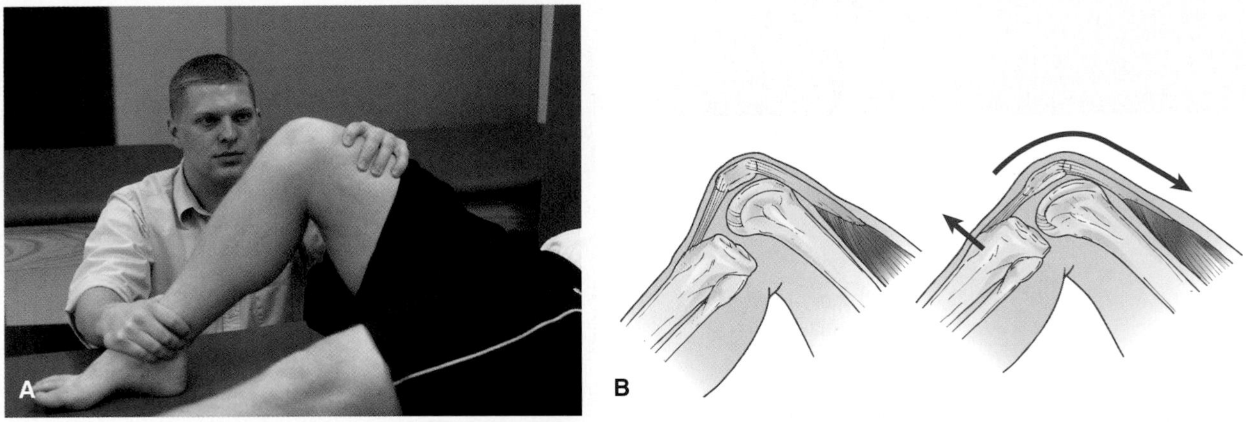

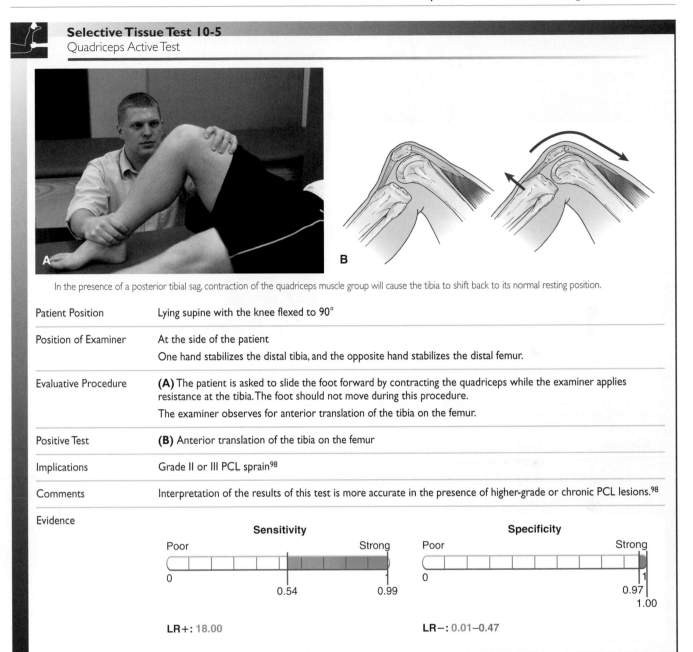

In the presence of a posterior tibial sag, contraction of the quadriceps muscle group will cause the tibia to shift back to its normal resting position.

Patient Position	Lying supine with the knee flexed to 90°
Position of Examiner	At the side of the patient One hand stabilizes the distal tibia, and the opposite hand stabilizes the distal femur.
Evaluative Procedure	**(A)** The patient is asked to slide the foot forward by contracting the quadriceps while the examiner applies resistance at the tibia. The foot should not move during this procedure. The examiner observes for anterior translation of the tibia on the femur.
Positive Test	**(B)** Anterior translation of the tibia on the femur
Implications	Grade II or III PCL sprain[98]
Comments	Interpretation of the results of this test is more accurate in the presence of higher-grade or chronic PCL lesions.[98]
Evidence	

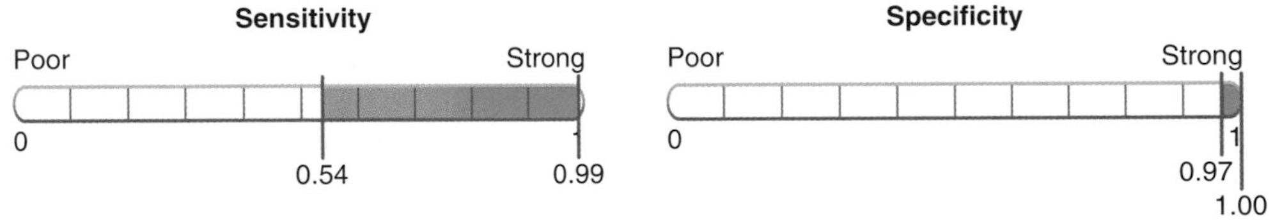

LR+: 18.00

LR−: 0.01–0.47

Non–weight-bearing ROM may be reduced secondary to swelling in the acutely injured knee. With time and as swelling diminishes, the tibia externally rotates on the femur when the knee is extended, resulting in a varus thrust or hyperextended varus thrust of the involved leg during gait.[80]

Several other selective tissue tests have been documented to identify trauma to the posterolateral corner of the knee and/or posterolateral rotary instability (PLRI). These techniques are based on replicating the subluxation and/or reduction of the tibia on the femur. Those tests that reproduce tibial subluxation are the **external rotation (dial) test** (Selective Tissue Test 10-11), the **external rotation recurvatum test** (Selective Tissue Test 10-12), and the **posterolateral drawer test** (Selective Tissue Test 10-13). The **reverse-pivot shift test** (Selective Tissue Test 10-14) and **dynamic posterior shift test** (Selective Tissue Test 10-15) cause reduction of a subluxated tibia.

Rotational Knee Instability Intervention Strategies

Anterolateral and Anteromedial Instability: The decision about conservative versus surgical treatment is based on the structures injured and the resulting impact of the injury on the patient's desired level of activity. Patients who want to participate in activities that require twisting or sudden changes of direction generally opt for surgery followed by rehabilitation to restore the necessary static and dynamic stability. Continued participation on a knee with rotational instability often results in additional meniscal injury. Surgical interventions generally address a reconstruction of the ACL using an allograft or an autograft and repair of other damaged tissues.

Box 10-2
Classification of Rotational Knee Instabilities

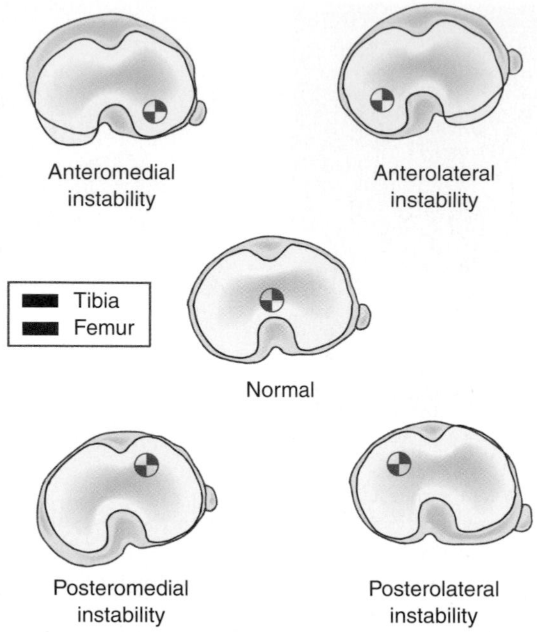

The tibial articulating surface is outlined in black and the femoral articular surfaces are outlined in red. The type of instability is described based on the displacement of the tibia relative to the femur. Note that the axes of rotation are approximated.

Instability	Tibial Displacement	Pathological Axis	Structural Instability
Anteromedial	Medial tibial plateau subluxes anteriorly.	Posterolateral, resulting in abnormal external tibial rotation	ACL, anteromedial capsule, MCL, pes anserine, medial meniscus, posteromedial capsule
Anterolateral	Lateral tibial plateau subluxes anteriorly.	Posteromedial, resulting in abnormal internal tibial rotation	ACL, anterolateral capsule, LCL, IT band, biceps femoris, lateral meniscus, popliteus, posterolateral capsule
Posteromedial	Medial tibial plateau subluxes posteriorly.	Anterolateral, resulting in abnormal internal tibial rotation	Posterior oblique ligament, MCL, semimembranosus, anteromedial capsule
Posterolateral	Lateral tibial plateau subluxes posteriorly.	Anteromedial, resulting in abnormal external tibial rotation	Posterolateral complex, LCL, biceps femoris

ACL = anterior cruciate ligament; IT = iliotibial; LCL = lateral collateral ligament; MCL = medial collateral ligament

Posterolateral Corner: Management of patients with posterolateral corner injuries is directly related to the ensuing activity limitations and participation restrictions. Mild injuries, which are less common, may be managed conservatively with bracing (using OA braces that unload the medial compartment), restoration of normal gait mechanics, and rehabilitation. Most posterolateral corner injuries are managed surgically, with concomitant ACL or PCL reconstruction. The surgical technique used depends on the involved structures, with reconstruction using an allograft technique resulting in improved outcomes over a primary repair.[80]

Meniscal Tears

Acute meniscal tears result from rotation and flexion of the knee, impinging the menisci between the articular condyles of the tibia and femur. Because of its greater mobility, the lateral meniscus may develop tears secondary to repeated stress, presenting with an insidious onset. Historically, the majority of meniscal tears were believed to involve the medial meniscus. However, contemporary research has reversed this thought.[114] Many lateral meniscal tears, often asymptomatic, are associated with ACL sprains. Improved

Selective Tissue Test 10-6

Slocum Drawer Test for Rotational Knee Instability

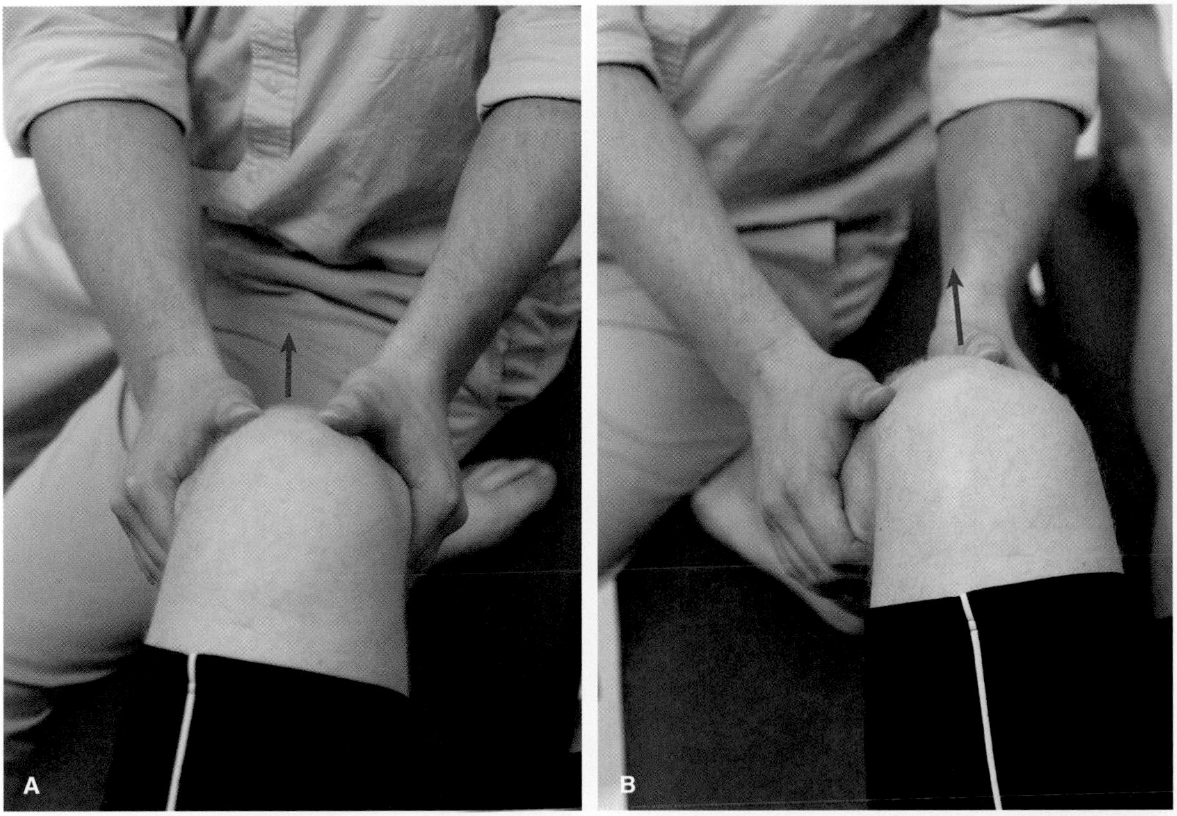

Slocum drawer test (A) with the tibia internally rotated to isolate the lateral capsular structures and (B) with the tibia externally rotated to isolate the medial capsule

Patient Position	Lying supine with the knee flexed to 90°
Position of Examiner	Sitting on the patient's foot: **(A)** The tibia is internally rotated to 25° to test for anterolateral capsular instability. **(B)** The tibia is externally rotated to 15° to test for anteromedial capsular instability.
Evaluative Procedure	The tibia is drawn anteriorly.
Positive Test	An increased amount of anterior tibial translation compared with the opposite (uninvolved) limb or the lack of a firm endpoint
Implications	**(A)** Test for anterolateral instability: Damage to the ACL, anterolateral capsule, LCL, IT band, popliteus tendon, posterolateral complex, lateral meniscus **(B)** Test for anteromedial instability: Damage to the MCL, anteromedial capsule, ACL, posteromedial capsule, pes anserine, medial meniscus
Comments	Excessive tibial rotation can cause a false-negative test due to wedging of the menisci in the joint space.
Evidence	Inconclusive or absent in the literature

ACL = anterior cruciate ligament; IT = iliotibial; LCL = lateral collateral ligament; MCL = medial collateral ligament

Selective Tissue Test 10-7
Crossover Test for Rotational Knee Instability

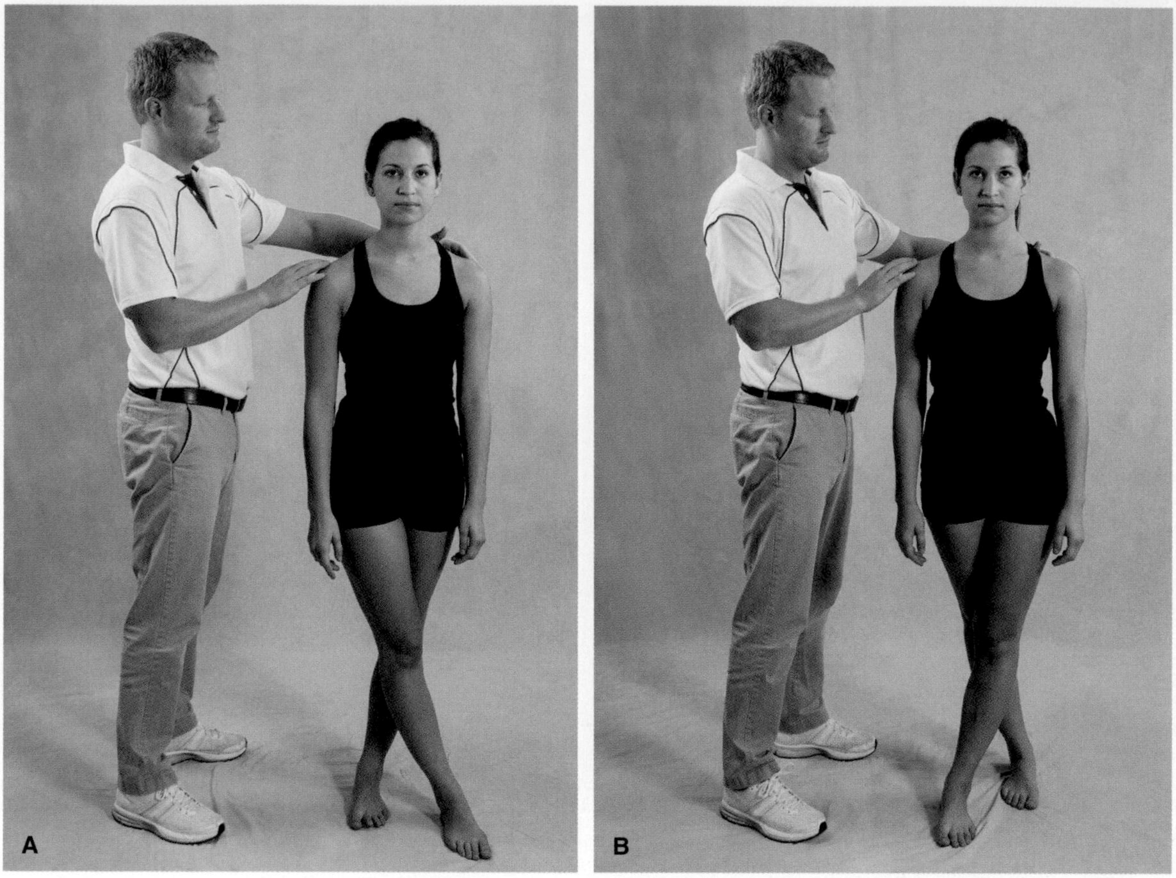

Crossover test: (A) Stepping in front of the injured leg determines the presence of anterolateral rotational instability. (B) Stepping behind the injured leg determines anteromedial rotational instability. Note that patient's left leg is being tested.

Patient Position	Standing with the weight on the involved limb
Position of Examiner	Standing in front of the patient
Evaluative Procedure	**(A) ALRI:** The patient steps across and in front with the uninvolved leg, rotating the torso in the direction of movement. The weight-bearing foot remains fixated. **(B) AMRI:** The patient steps across and behind with the uninvolved leg rotating the torso in the direction of movement. The weight-bearing foot remains fixated.
Positive Test	Patient reports pain, instability, or apprehension.
Implications	**(A) ALRI:** Instability of the lateral capsular restraints **(B) AMRI:** Instability of the medial capsular restraints
Comments	This test can be used as a prelude to assessing the patient's ability to perform a more-functional cutting maneuver.
Evidence	Inconclusive or absent in the literature

ALRI = anterolateral rotational instability; AMRI = anteromedial rotational instability

Selective Tissue Test 10-8
Pivot Shift Test for Anterolateral Knee Instability Jerk Test

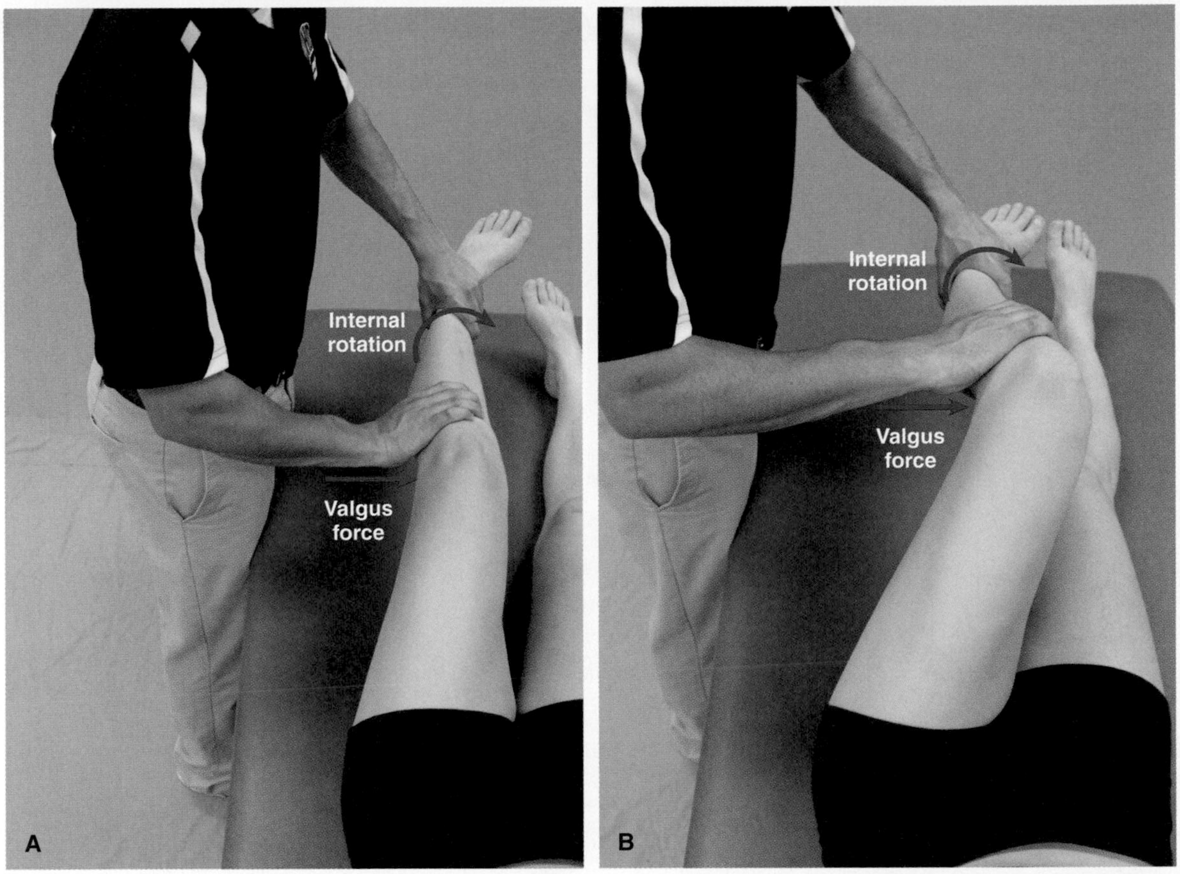

When positive, the pivot shift test (lateral pivot shift) reproduces the subluxation/reduction of the tibia on the femur experienced during functional tasks that involve a change of direction.

Patient Position	Lying supine with the hip passively flexed to 30°
Position of Examiner	Standing lateral to the patient, the examiner grasps the distal lower leg and/or ankle, maintaining 20° of internal tibial rotation. The knee is allowed to sag into complete extension **(A)**. The opposite hand grasps the lateral portion of the leg at the level of the superior tibiofibular joint, increasing the force of internal rotation.
Evaluative Procedure	While maintaining internal rotation, a valgus force is applied to the knee while it is slowly flexed **(B)**. To avoid masking any positive test results, the patient must remain relaxed throughout this test.
Positive Test	The tibia's position on the femur reduces as the leg is flexed in the range of 30°-40°. Jerk test: During extension, the anterior reduction is felt in the same range.
Implications	ACL, anterolateral capsule, LCL, biceps femoris, lateral meniscus, popliteus, posterolateral capsule
Modification	The **jerk test** is a modification of the lateral pivot shift test: The patient's hip is flexed to 45°, and the knee is flexed to 90°. A valgus and internal rotation force is applied as the knee is extended.
Comments	Meniscal involvement may limit ROM to produce a false-negative test result. Muscle guarding can produce a false-negative result. This test is most reliable when performed with the patient under anesthesia.

Evidence

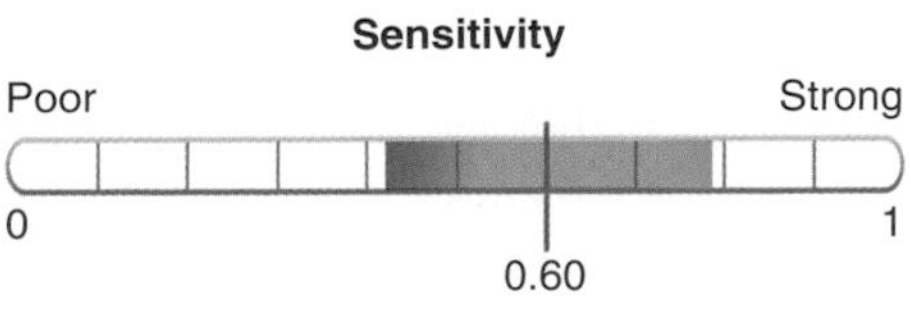

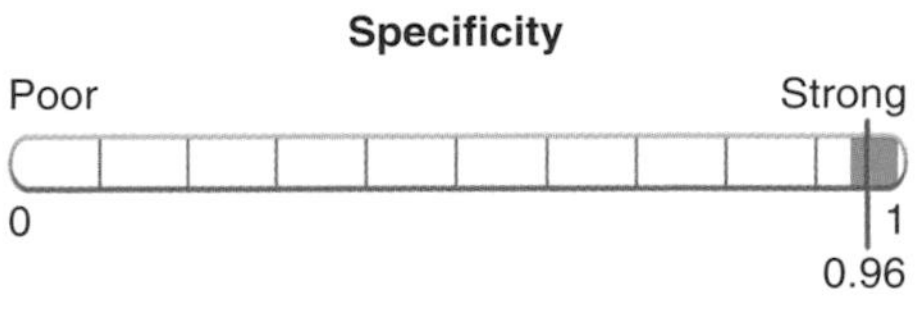

LR+: 7.45–26.29–45.13

LR−: 0.51–0.61–0.71

ACL = anterior cruciate ligament; IT = iliotibial; ROM = range of motion

Selective Tissue Test 10-9

Slocum Anterolateral Rotational Instability (ALRI) Test

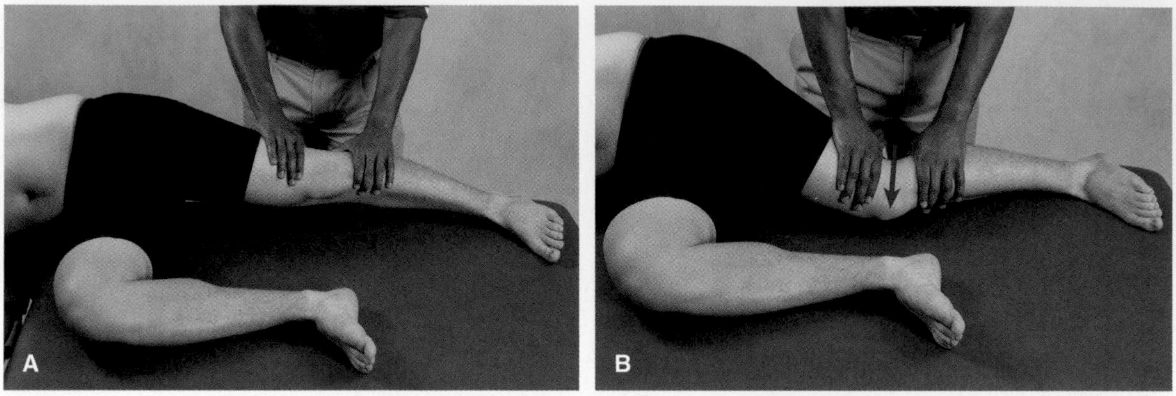

A modification of the valgus stress test, the Slocum ALRI accentuates the amount of internal tibial rotation, causing the tibial plateau to subluxate.

Patient Position	**(A)** Lying on the uninvolved side The uninvolved leg is flexed at the hip and knee, positioning it anterior to the involved extremity. The involved hip is externally rotated. The involved leg is extended with the medial aspect of the foot resting against the table to provide stability.
Position of Examiner	Standing behind the patient, grasping the knee on the distal aspect of the femur and the proximal fibula
Evaluative Procedure	A valgus force is placed on the knee, causing it to move into 30°–50° of flexion **(B)**.
Positive Test	An appreciable "clunk" or instability as the lateral tibial plateau subluxates or pain or instability is reported.
Implications	Tear of the ACL, LCL, anterolateral capsule, arcuate ligament complex, or biceps femoris tendon
Comments	Muscle guarding can produce false-negative results. This test should be performed with caution and, if performed, should be done so only at the end of the examination.
Evidence	Inconclusive or absent in the literature

ACL = anterior cruciate ligament; LCL = lateral cruciate ligament

soft tissue imaging, such as the MRI, is now detecting lateral meniscal tears that once may have gone undetected (Examination Findings 10-6).[62]

Classic symptoms of meniscal tears involve "locking" or "clicking" (or both) in the knee, pain along the joint line, and the knee giving way during activity. Locking can occur secondary to a tear or subluxation (hypermobility) of the posterior horn of the medial or lateral meniscus.[43] Patients may describe a rotational mechanism combined with flexion and a valgus or varus stress. Pain may not be described if the tear occurs in the avascular zone of the meniscus. Meniscal lesions may mimic the symptoms of patellofemoral dysfunction. Chapter 11 discusses the differential diagnosis between these two conditions.

Two evaluative tests, the **McMurray test** (Selective Tissue Test 10-16) and the **Apley compression and distraction test** (Selective Tissue Test 10-17), are frequently used to determine the presence of meniscal tears although their clinical usefulness is debatable because of the degree of inaccuracy when compared with the gold standard of MRI or arthroscopy. The McMurray test was originally intended to identify tears in the posterior horn of the meniscus. Most clinical research has assessed the extent to which the test can identify lesions in any part of the meniscus, possibly explaining its limited clinical value.[116]

The **Thessaly test**, a dynamic weight-bearing procedure, has reported high predictive values for identifying meniscal tears (Selective Tissue Test 10-18).[115] The absence of physical examination findings essentially rules out meniscal pathology, more so for the medial meniscus than for the lateral meniscus.[117]

Joint line pain, and more specifically joint line fullness, is a more accurate predictor of a meniscal tear than either the McMurray test or Apley compression test.[119,120] Because it

Selective Tissue Test 10-10
Flexion-Rotation Drawer Test for Anterolateral Rotational Instability

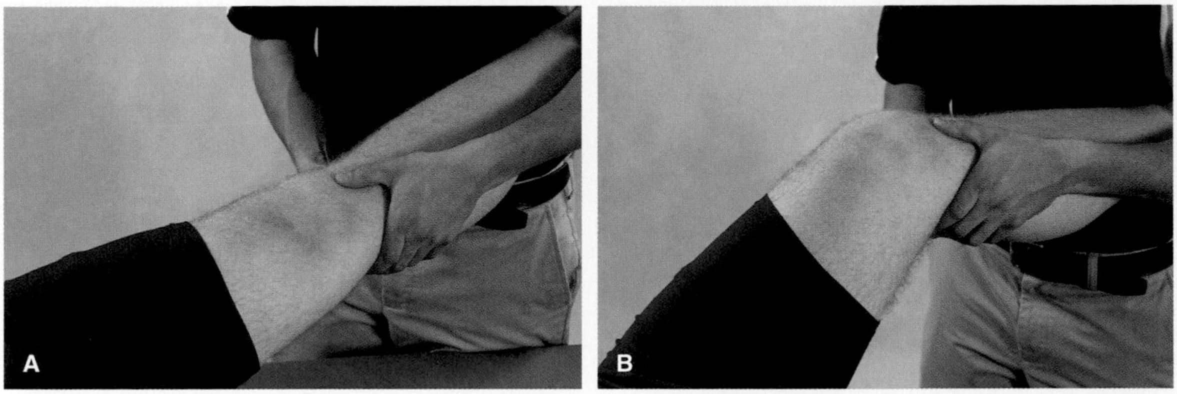

The flexion-rotation drawer test replicates the femur reducing itself on the tibia as seen in a closed kinetic chain. It is also known as the flexion-reduction drawer test.

Patient Position	Lying supine The clinician lifts the calf and ankle so that the knee is flexed to approximately 25°. Heavier patients may require that the tibia be supported between the examiner's arm and torso.
Position of Examiner	Standing lateral and distal to the involved knee
Evaluative Procedure	The tibia is depressed posteriorly to the femur.
Positive Test	The femur is reducing itself on the tibia by moving anteriorly and internally, rotating on the tibia.
Implications	Tears of the ACL, LCL, anterolateral capsule, arcuate ligament complex, biceps femoris tendon
Modification	A valgus stress and axial compression along the tibial shaft can be applied as the knee is slowly flexed.
Evidence	

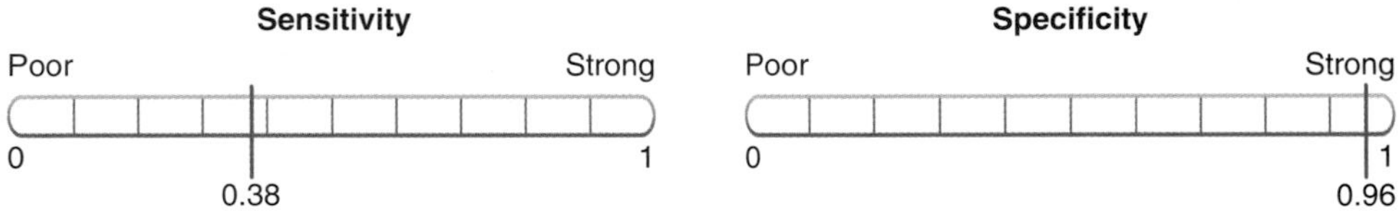

LR+: 3.00

LR−: 0.65

ACL = anterior cruciate ligament; LCL = lateral cruciate ligament

incorporates the weight bearing, the Thessaly may be more valuable in identifying meniscal lesions.

The types of meniscal tears are based on the orientation and etiology of the defect (Fig. 10-26). Tearing can occur as the result of excessive forces being placed on healthy tissues or otherwise normal forces being exerted on a degenerating meniscus. Degenerative tears are most prevalent in the posterior horn. **Meniscal cysts** are frequently associated with longitudinal meniscal tears and become symptomatic because of localized swelling (Fig. 10-27).[24] After a longitudinal tear along the periphery of the meniscus, breaches are formed in the joint capsule that fills with synovial fluid. Meniscal cysts, typically painless and immobile, are often found coincidentally during MRI scanning or arthroscopic examination.[50]

Most commonly involving the lateral meniscus, a **discoid meniscus** has increased thickness and covers a larger area of the tibia.[26] The size, shape, and stability of a discoid meniscus can cause instability leading to catching or locking during movement ("snapping knee syndrome"). A Wrisberg-type discoid meniscus has only the ligament of Wrisberg as a posterior stabilizer, potentially leading to an unstable fixation of the meniscus on the tibia and creating locking or catching of the knee during flexion and extension as the meniscus dislocates.[43]

Meniscal Tear Intervention Strategies

Patients who clinically present with locking or catching of the knee and demonstrate decreased ROM with associated pain and swelling may require surgical to repair or resect

Examination Findings 10-5
Posterolateral Rotational Instability

Examination Segment	Clinical Findings
History of Current Condition	*Onset:* Most have an acute onset, although chronic cases are possible. *Pain characteristics:* Along the posterolateral knee and popliteal area Chronic conditions may produce medial joint line pain. *Other symptoms:* Sensation of the knee "giving way" *Mechanism:* Posterolaterally directed blow to the medial tibia while the knee is in extension, producing hyperextension, tibial external rotation, and varus force Noncontact knee hyperextension and varus force Noncontact knee hyperextension and external tibial rotation *Predisposing conditions:* PCL, LCL sprain Genu varum[15] Tibiofemoral dislocation
Functional Assessment	Possible varus thrust or hyperextension varus thrust during gait[80] Complaints of lateral posterior knee instability Hyperextension results in functional instability when ascending or descending stairs or walking on inclines.[6]
Inspection	Swelling of the posterolateral knee Swelling possibly more diffuse because of tearing in the capsule Possible hyperextension and/or varus alignment of the involved knee when weight bearing The tibia may be held in internal rotation during gait.[7]
Palpation	Tenderness and swelling possible along the posterolateral capsule, lateral knee, and popliteal fossa A palpable defect may be felt in the biceps femoris tendon.[108]
Joint and Muscle Function Assessment	*AROM:* Acutely, normal ROM; pain and restrictions possible as the knee nears full flexion Motions may be inhibited by pain especially as the knee moves back into a flexed position. *MMT:* Knee flexion with the tibia internally rotated, making the popliteus more active, may be painful. Biceps femoris (rule out a secondary tear to the tendon) *PROM:* Pain produced as the knee nears 90° of flexion and with hyperextension
Joint Stability Tests	*Stress tests:* Varus stress test at 0°: PLC, ACL, PCL Varus stress test at 30°: Isolated LCL injury Lachman test Anterior drawer test Alternate Lachman test Posterior drawer test at 30° and 90°

	Joint play: Anterior glide of the tibia on the femur is assessed using the anterior drawer test. Posterior glide of the tibia is assessed using the posterior drawer test.
Selective Tissue Tests	Godfrey's sign Pivot shift test External rotation test (dial test) Posterolateral drawer test External rotation recurvatum test
Neurological Screening	The peroneal nerve may become secondarily involved, resulting in paresthesia along the lateral leg and dorsum of the foot.[80] Manual muscle tests of the tibialis anterior and extensor hallicus longus may be indicated to rule out peroneal nerve trauma.
Vascular Screening	Required after suspected posterolateral dislocation (see p. 375)
Imaging Techniques	T1-weighted coronal oblique MR images can help identify trauma to the posterolateral structures including the fibular head. MRI is also used to rule out bone contusions and trauma to the LCL. Radiographs may be ordered to rule out an avulsion fracture of the capsule from the lateral tibial plateau (Segond fracture), avulsion fracture of the fibular head, or an avulsion fracture of Gerdy's tubercle.[80] Stress radiographs will indicate a widening of the lateral joint line.
Differential Diagnosis	Avulsion fracture of the fibular head; lateral meniscus tear; ACL sprain; LCL sprain; PCL sprain; tibiofemoral dislocation; physeal fracture
Comments	Posterolateral instability is typically found concurrently with a sprain of the ACL or PCL.

ACL = anterior cruciate ligament; AROM = active range of motion; LCL = lateral collateral ligament; MMT = manual muscle test; MR = magnetic resonance; PCL = posterior cruciate ligament; PLC = posterolateral corner; PROM = passive range of motion; ROM = range of motion

Examination Findings 10-6
Meniscal Tears

Examination Segment	Clinical Findings
History of Current Condition	*Onset:* Acute; patients with symptoms involving accumulated microtrauma often still present as having an acute onset. *Pain characteristics:* Along the medial or lateral joint line with possible posterior knee pain *Other symptoms:* The patient may report episodes of the knee "giving out." "Clicking" may be described with chronic meniscal lesions. Snapping or locking may be associated with a discoid meniscus.[26,43] *Mechanism:* Tibial rotation, often in combination with knee flexion and/or a varus or valgus stress Hyperflexion impinges the posterior horns; hyperextension impinges the anterior horns. *Predisposing conditions:* Over time, repetitive motion can degrade the lateral meniscus. ACL injury; PCL injury
Functional Assessment	The patient may complain of clicking or locking during activity in the presence of a chronic tear.
Inspection	Inspection of a patient with an acutely torn meniscus may not present any conclusive initial findings. Over time, or in the case of a peripheral tear of the meniscus, swelling may be seen along the joint or in the popliteal fossa. Joint effusion may develop over 24–48 hours and may recur sporadically with irritation of the meniscus.[115]
Palpation	Possible pain, fullness, and/or crepitus along the joint line A meniscal cyst, highly suggestive of a meniscal tear, may be palpable.[24]
Joint and Muscle Function Assessment	The ROM available may be limited owing to a mechanical block formed by a defect in the meniscus. *AROM:* Possible decrease in ROM A displaced longitudinal ("bucket handle") tear of the meniscus can present a mechanical block to extension.[24] Discoid menisci or other meniscal variants may cause blocks to motion and/or compensatory motion (e.g., increased external rotation) to obtain full extension or flexion.[26] Pain or locking is revealed as the torn portion of the meniscus passes beneath the femur's articular surface. *MMT:* Typically unremarkable *PROM:* Pain is present near the extremes of flexion or extension. Apprehension may be experienced as the knee nears terminal extension if locking is caused by the meniscus' anterior horn.[43]
Joint Stability Tests	*Stress tests:* The integrity of all the knee ligaments must be established. The presence of any ligamentous injury to the knee limits the ability to determine meniscal pathology during the clinical examination. *Joint play:* Unremarkable
Selective Tissue Tests	McMurray test Apley compression/distraction test Thessaly test
Neurological Screening	Within normal limits
Vascular Screening	Within normal limits
Imaging Techniques	MR imaging can be used to identify the presence of a meniscal tear, but its value is debatable, showing approximately equal predictive results as the clinical examination.[24] A widened lateral joint space may be noted on radiographs in the presence of a discoid meniscus.[26]
Differential Diagnosis	Patellofemoral joint dysfunction, synovial plica irritation, osteochondral defect, instability
Comments	All suspected ACL and MCL injuries should be thought to involve a meniscal tear until proven otherwise.

ACL = anterior cruciate ligament; AROM = active range of motion; MMT = manual muscle test; PCL = posterior cruciate ligament; PROM = passive range of motion; ROM = range of motion

Table 10-5	Posterolateral Corner Instabilities Relative to Injured Tissues[6]
Loss of Integrity in These Tissues	**Resulting Instability**
LCL and Posterolateral Complex	Slight increase in posterior tibial translation at all angles of flexion
	Increase in external rotation with posterior force at all angles
	Increased varus displacement at 30° of flexion
PCL, LCL, Posterolateral Complex	Increased posterior translation at all angles of flexion
	Increased varus displacement in response to varus force, especially at 60° of flexion
	Increased external rotation

LCL = lateral collateral ligament; PCL = posterior cruciate ligament

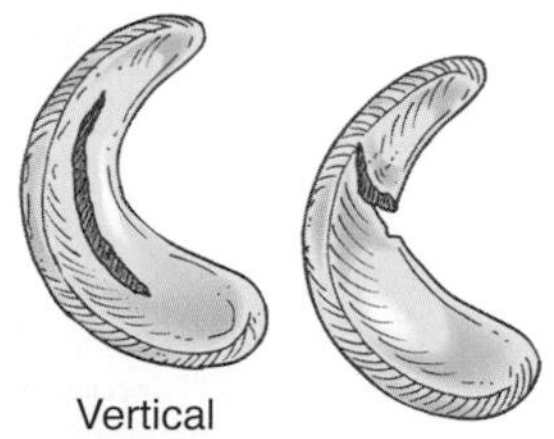

FIGURE 10-26 ■ Classification of meniscal tears.

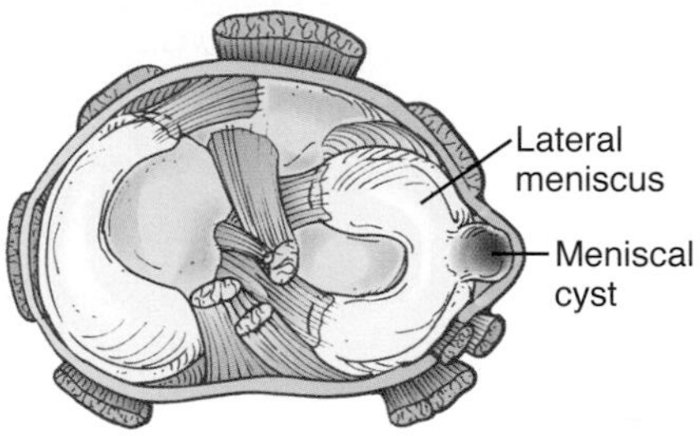

FIGURE 10-27 ■ Types of meniscal cysts.

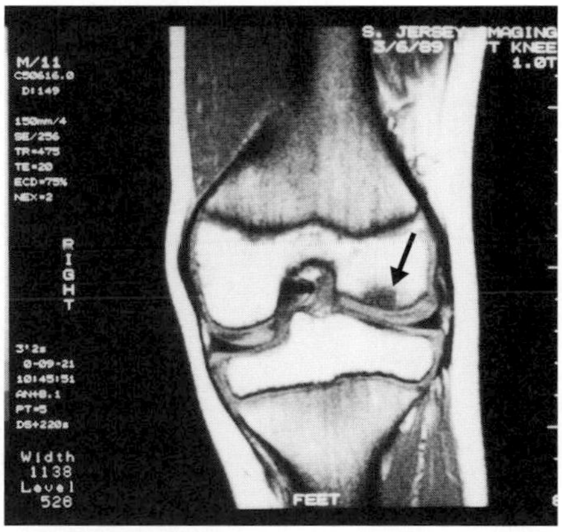

FIGURE 10-28 ■ MRI of an osteochondral defect. The arrow points to an OCD on the lateral femoral condyle.

the torn meniscus.[24] Standard surgical options include a partial meniscectomy, where only the torn fragment is removed, or meniscal repair, where tears in the vascular portion of the meniscus are repaired using sutures, staples, or anchors. Experimental procedures involving grafts, adhesives, and implants are also being performed.[121] Total meniscectomies where the entire meniscus is removed are rarely performed.[122]

Osteochondral Lesions

Osteochondral lesions are used to describe a series of disorders including osteochondral defects (OCDs) and osteochondritis dissecans that involve a joint's articular cartilage and underlying subchondral bone.[123] OCDs are fractures of the articular cartilage and underlying bone that are typically caused by compressive and shear forces (Fig. 10-28). Eighty percent of knee OCDs involve the medial femoral condyle.[124] The lateral femoral condyle, tibial articulating surface, and patella are also susceptible to OCDs.[125] Males are affected more frequently than females.[124,125]

The signs and symptoms of OCDs are often masked by those of a concurrent injury, although the OCD itself is often asymptomatic (Examination Findings 10-7). Symptomatic OCDs are characterized by complaints of diffuse pain within the knee that is worse with weight bearing, a "locking" sensation, and the knee's giving way. A "clunking" sensation may also be described. In addition, an increase in pain and a decrease in strength are noted in closed kinetic chain activities as compared with open-chain motions. **Wilson's test** can be used as a clinical evaluation tool for the presence of OCDs on the knee's articular surface (Selective Tissue Test 10-19). A definitive diagnosis must be made with radiographic examination or MRI.

Osteochondral Defect Intervention Strategies

Osteochondral defects can be managed conservatively, with the outcome largely dependent on the location of the defect with respect to the weight-bearing surface. Activity is modified to reduce painful stresses placed on the knee. When conservative treatment fails, surgical repair of the defect may be required. Surgical intervention can include simple débridement or procedures such as abrasion arthroplasty, subchondral drilling, or microfracture techniques to stimulate fibrocartilage formation in the defect. Other surgical interventions include autogenous chondrocyte transplantation, characterized chondrocyte implantation, or osteoarticular transplantation (OATS procedure).[126] The goals of these techniques are to place newly grown articular cartilage within the defect or to transplant healthy articular cartilage from one area of the knee into the defect.[127] The timing of the procedure relative to the onset is a primary factor in obtaining satisfactory results from these surgical approaches.[126]

After surgery, a 4- to 6-week period of protected weight-bearing activities may be necessary to reduce shearing stresses on the implant. Aquatic therapy can be used in the early active ROM period to provide ROM and strengthening

Selective Tissue Test 10-11

External Rotation Test (Dial Test) for Posterolateral Knee Instability

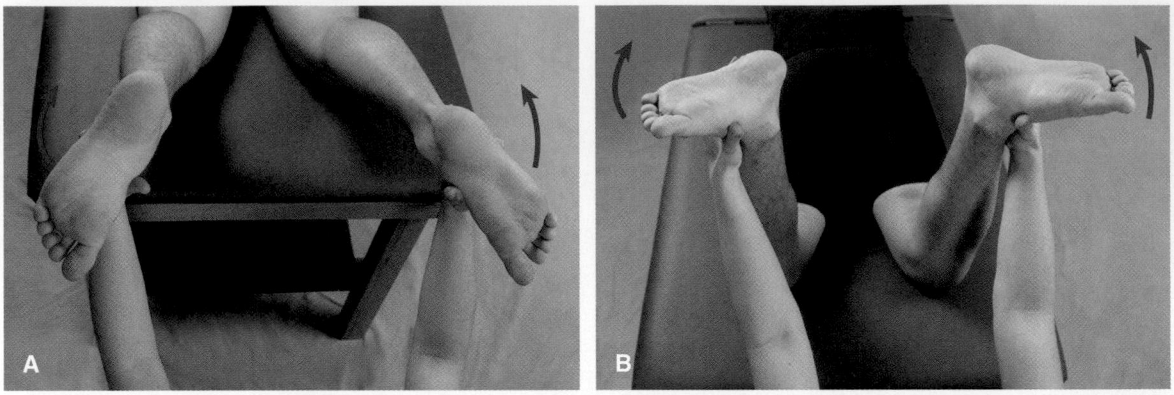

The external rotation test (dial test) for posterolateral knee instability at 30° of knee flexion (A) and at 90° of knee flexion (B).

Patient Position	Prone or supine
Position of Examiner	Standing at the patient's feet
Evaluative Procedure	The knee is flexed to 30°. Using the medial border of the foot as a point of reference, the examiner forcefully externally rotates the patient's lower leg. The position of external rotation of the foot relative to the femur is assessed and compared with the opposite extremity. The knee is then flexed to 90° and the test repeated. Care must be taken to keep the hips from abducting during the examination.[22]
Positive Test	An increase of external rotation greater than 10° compared with the opposite side[21,111]
Implications	Difference at 30° of knee flexion but not at 90°: Injury isolated to the posterolateral corner of the knee Difference at 30° and 90° of knee flexion: Trauma to the PCL, posterolateral knee structures, and the posterolateral corner Difference at 90° of knee flexion but not at 30°: Isolated PCL sprain
Modification	This test can also be performed with the patient in the supine position. A goniometer can be used to quantify the amount of external rotation.[6]
Comments	Normal variations for rotation are expected. The results of one extremity must be compared with those of the opposite leg. If performed with the patient in the supine position, the tibia should be anteriorly translated to its original position by a second examiner.
Evidence	Inconclusive or absent in the literature

PCL = posterior cruciate ligament

while decreasing weight-bearing stresses through the joint. After the early protection phase of rehabilitation, strength, ROM, and proprioceptive exercises are advanced to restore normal function to the knee.

Iliotibial Band Friction Syndrome

Resulting from friction between the IT band and the lateral femoral epicondyle, IT band friction syndrome tends to occur in athletes who are participating in sports that require repeated knee flexion and extension, such as running, rowing, and cycling.[128] A bursa located between the distal IT band and the lateral femoral epicondyle becomes inflamed secondary to overuse. This condition may progress to involve periostitis of the epicondyle (Examination Findings 10-8). The bursa cushioning the IT band from the lateral femoral epicondyle is not a primary bursa, but rather a continuation of the knee joint capsule.[129,130]

Several factors may predispose someone to IT band friction syndrome.[131-134] Genu varum may project the lateral

Selective Tissue Test 10-12

External Rotation Recurvatum Test for Posterolateral Knee Instability

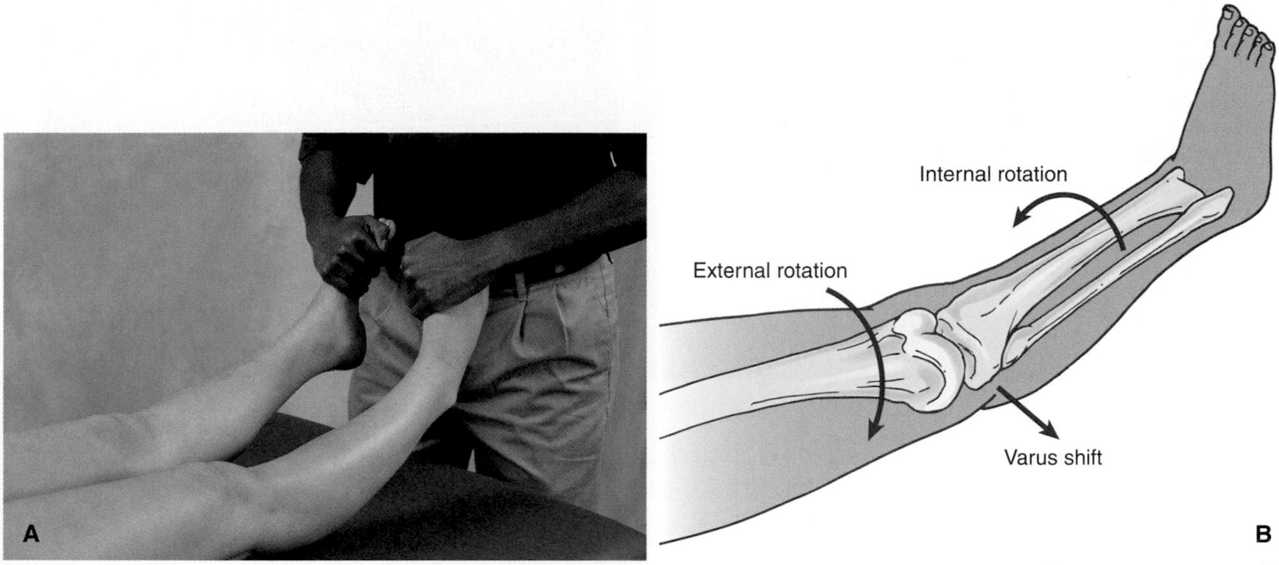

This test is a gross evaluation of the amount of external femoral rotation that occurs when the knee is hyperextended with the femur stabilized.

Patient Position	Lying supine
Position of Examiner	Standing at the side of the patient, with one hand stabilizing the distal femur and the other grasping the great toe/medial foot
Evaluative Procedure	The examiner passively extends the knee while maintaining stabilization of the femur on the table.
Positive Test	A marked difference in hyperextension, external femoral rotation, and varus alignment between the two knees
Implications	Posterolateral corner trauma ACL sprain Posterolateral rotary instability
Modification	While holding the heel, the examiner flexes the knee 40°. The opposite hand grasps the posterolateral aspect of the knee. The examiner passively extends the knee while noting external rotation and hyperextension relative to the opposite extremity.
Evidence	Note that the test is essentially identifying anterior translation of the tibia on the femur. Positive findings are strongly associated with a combined injury to the ACL and the posterolateral corner.[112]

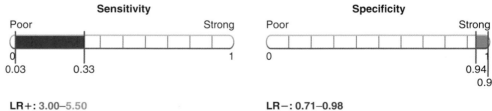

LR+: 3.00–5.50

LR–: 0.71–0.98

ACL = anterior cruciate ligament

Selective Tissue Test 10-13
Posterolateral/Posteromedial Drawer Test for Posterolateral Knee Instability

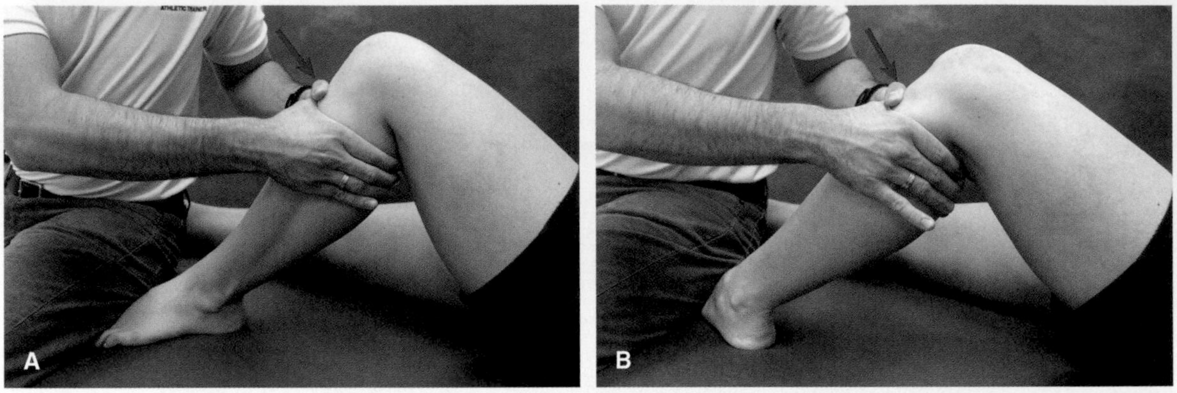

A modification of the posterior drawer test to identify lesions to the posterolateral corner of the knee[113]

Patient Position	Supine with the hip flexed to 45° and the knee flexed to 80° **(A)** The tibia is externally rotated 15° (posterolateral test). **(B)** The tibia is internally rotated 15° (posteromedial test).
Position of Examiner	Sitting on the foot of the limb being tested, the examiner grasps the proximal tibia.
Evaluative Procedure	A posterior force is applied to the proximal tibia.
Positive Test	Increased external rotation of the lateral (posterolateral) or medial (posteromedial) tibial condyle relative to the uninvolved side
Implications	**(A)** Tibia externally rotated 15° (posterolateral test) Trauma to the posterolateral corner and PCL Possible posterolateral rotational instability **(B)** Tibia internally rotated 15° (posteromedial test) PCL tear, oblique ligament, MCL, posteromedial capsule, semimembranosus
Modification	The posterolateral drawer test is sometimes performed with the knee flexed to 90°. This test can be performed with the patient sitting with the knees off the edge of the table.
Comments	Excessive tibial rotation can produce false-negative results, especially in the presence of a meniscal tear.
Evidence	Inconclusive or absent in the literature

MCL = medial collateral ligament; PCL = posterior cruciate ligament

femoral condyle laterally, increasing the friction as the IT band passes over it. Excessive pronation during gait, leg-length differences, a lateral heel strike, and other conditions resulting in internal tibial rotation alter the angle at which the IT band approaches its attachment on Gerdy's tubercle, increasing pressure at the lateral femoral epicondyle. Activities that cause overstriding, such as running downhill, may also increase tension between the distal IT band and the lateral femoral epicondyle. Finally, a large lateral femoral epicondyle may result in increased irritation of the IT band as it passes over the epicondyle.

The patient typically describes a "burning" pain over the lateral femoral condyle that may radiate distally. Point tenderness is displayed at the point where the IT band passes over the epicondyle. Pain may be described during manual muscle testing of the hamstrings or quadriceps with the knee in 30 degrees of flexion. However, no pain may be described during active ROM (AROM) or PROM testing. The presence of IT band friction syndrome may be confirmed through the **Noble compression test** as the IT band passes over the lateral femoral condyle (Selective Tissue Test 10-20). IT band tightness can be identified by the **Ober test** (see Selective Tissue Test 12-5.)

Iliotibial Band Friction Syndrome Intervention Strategies

The initial treatment approach for IT band friction syndrome is to correct any biomechanical faults by modifying

Selective Tissue Test 10-14
Reverse Pivot Shift Test for Posterolateral Knee Instability

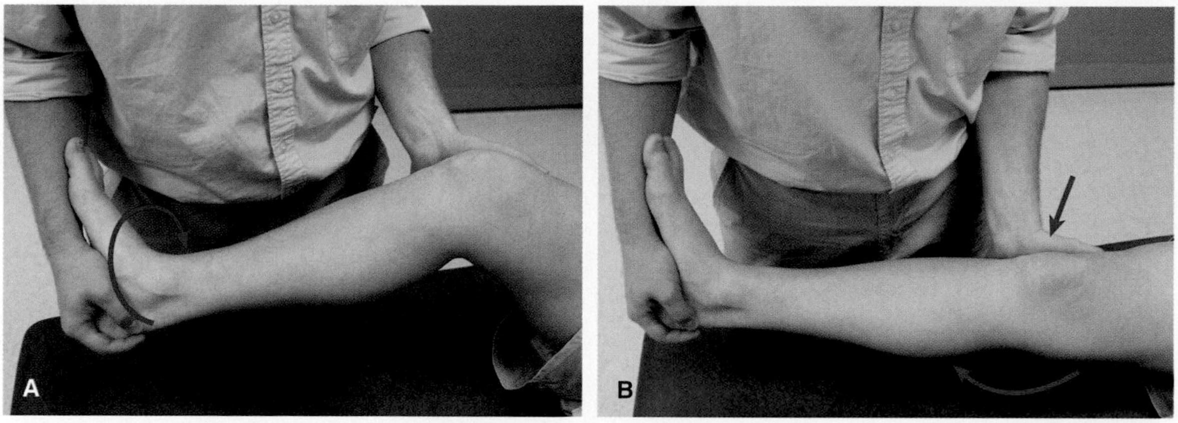

The reverse pivot shift test is used to identify trauma to the PCL or the posterolateral corner of the knee.[21]

Patient Position	Supine
Position of Examiner	Standing to the side of the involved leg
Evaluative Procedure	**(A)** The examiner flexes the knee and externally rotates the tibia of the involved leg. **(B)** The patient's knee is passively extended while a valgus stress is applied to the knee.
Positive Test	Appreciable reduction ("clunk") of the tibia on the femur
Implications	Posterolateral rotational instability and/or trauma to the posterolateral corner
Comments	This test may be positive in 35% of knees examined under anesthesia.[7,21]
Evidence	

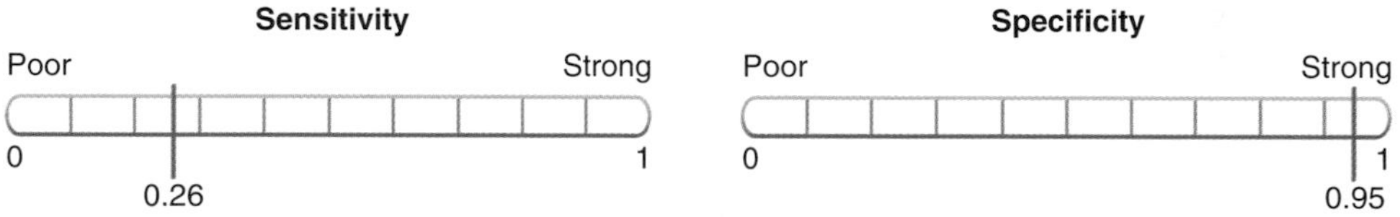

LR+: 5.20 **LR–:** 0.78

footwear, using orthotics to correct hyperpronation, or altering training during athletic activities. The use of nonsteroidal antiinflammatory medication and local modalities to decrease the inflammation at the bursa and IT band as it passes over the lateral epicondyle are usually helpful. Stretching of the tensor fascia latae, the IT band, and any other tight musculature is also warranted. Proprioceptive hip and lower extremity exercises are useful in enhancing the dynamic control of foot pronation.[132,133]

Popliteus Tendinopathy

Popliteus tendinopathy arises secondary to other biomechanical changes in the knee or lower extremity or secondary to repetitive stress. The popliteus muscle is often injured in conjunction with other knee injuries.[135] Popliteus inflammation manifests itself similarly to IT band friction syndrome except that individuals suffering from popliteus tendinopathy describe pain in the proximal portion of the tendon, immediately posterior to the LCL. As with IT band friction syndrome, patients who excessively pronate during gait are predisposed to this condition, which worsens when running downhill (Examination Findings 10-9). The popliteus acts to prevent a posterior shift of the tibia on the femur during midstance; squatting activities and running downhill place increased demand on the tendon.[136] Palpation of the popliteus tendon is easiest when the foot of the involved leg is placed on the uninvolved knee in the figure-4 position, a position that may produce pain in and of itself (Fig. 10-29).

The function of the popliteus muscle changes, albeit slightly, in knees that are ACL deficient[137] and more significantly when the PCL is absent.[18] Because the popliteus helps retract the lateral meniscus during knee flexion, inhibition or dysfunction of this muscle may alter the biomechanics of the lateral meniscus, possibly resulting in an increased load on the cartilage.[27]

Selective Tissue Test 10-15
Dynamic Posterior Shift Test for Posterolateral Knee Instability

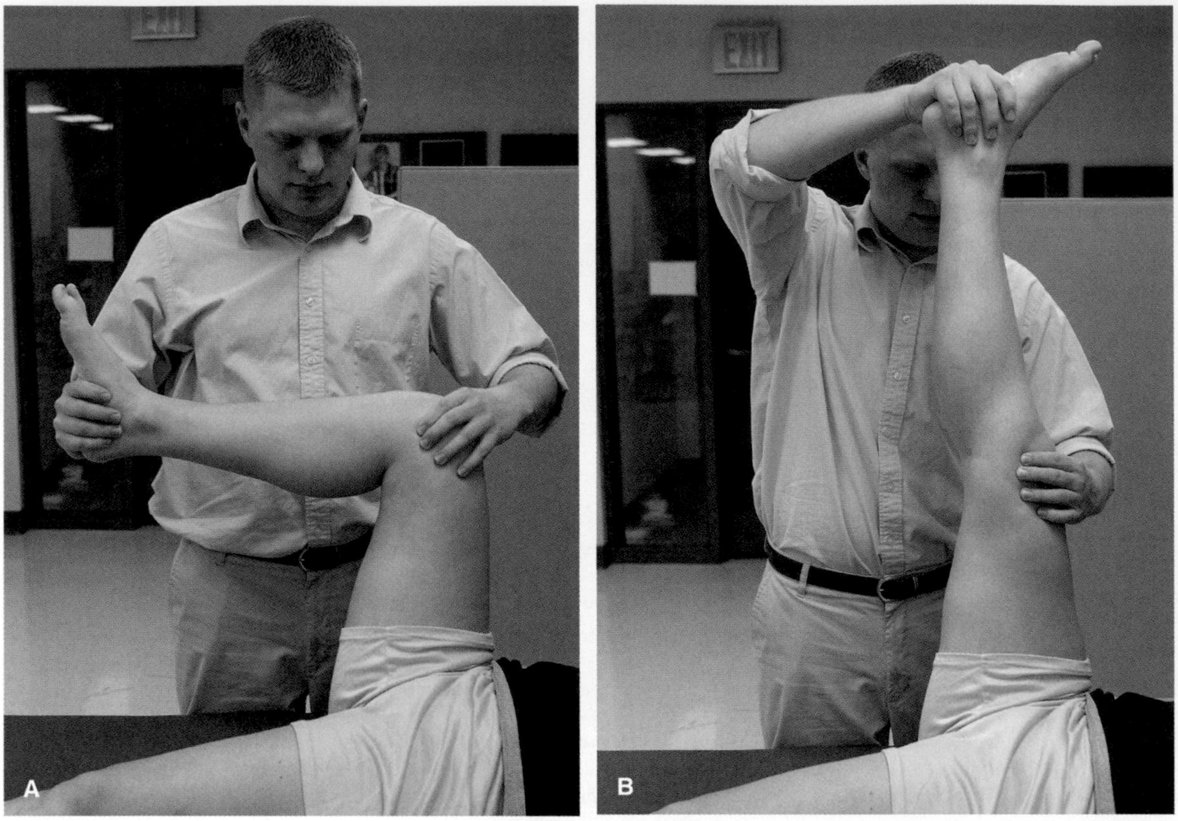

In the presence of posterolateral instability, the lateral tibial plateau is subluxed during knee flexion and reduces during knee extension.[21]

Patient Position	Supine
Position of Examiner	Standing on the side being tested
Evaluative Procedure	**(A)** The examiner passively flexes the patient's hip and knee to 90°. **(B)** The knee is then passively extended.
Positive Test	A "clunk" or "jerk" as the knee nears full extension, representing the subluxated tibia reducing on the femur
Implications	Posterolateral instability
Comments	During knee flexion, the tibia is posteriorly subluxated on the femur. Reduction is noted by an appreciable clunk during extension.[98]
Evidence	**Sensitivity** Poor 0 — Strong 1: 0.58 **Specificity** Poor 0 — Strong 1: 0.94 **LR+:** 9.67 **LR−:** 0.45

Selective Tissue Test 10-16
McMurray Test for Meniscal Lesions

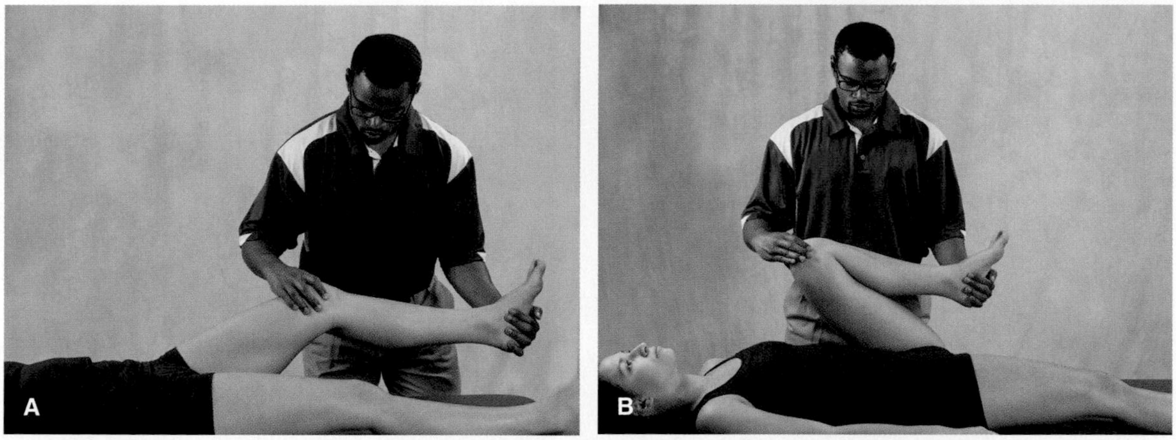

The McMurray test aims to impinge the meniscus, especially the posterior horns, between the tibia and femur.

Patient Position	Lying supine
Position of Examiner	Standing lateral and distal to the involved knee One hand supports the lower leg, while the thumb and index finger of the opposite hand are positioned in the posteromedial and posterolateral joint line **(A)**. The knee is fully flexed and the tibia is rotated.
Evaluative Procedure	**Pass one:** With the tibia maintained in its neutral position, a valgus stress is applied while the knee is flexed through its available ROM. A varus stress is then applied as the knee is returned to full extension. **Pass two:** The examiner internally rotates the tibia and applies a valgus stress while the knee is flexed through its available ROM. A varus stress is then applied as the knee is returned to full extension. **Pass three:** With the tibia externally rotated, the examiner applies a valgus stress while the knee is flexed through its available ROM. A varus stress is then applied as the knee is returned to full extension.
Positive Test	A popping, clicking, or locking of the knee; pain emanating from the menisci; or a sensation similar to that experienced during ambulation
Implications	A meniscal tear on the side of the reported symptoms
Modification	Multiple modifications have been derived from the original test, including variations of additional varus and valgus stress and internally and externally rotating the tibia.
Comments	In acute injuries, the available ROM may not be sufficient to perform this test. Full flexion is required to impinge the posterior horns of the meniscus. Chondromalacia patellae or improper tracking of the patella may produce a click resembling a meniscal tear, leading to false-positive results. Sensitivity is greater for lateral meniscus tears than for tears of the medial meniscus.[115] Different interpretations and methods of performing the test lead to widely varied opinions about the diagnostic usefulness of this test.
Evidence	

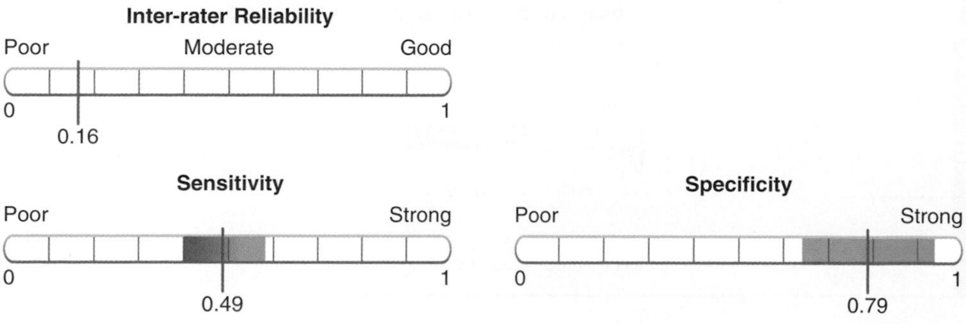

LR+: 2.17–5.20–8.20

LR−: 0.51–0.61–0.71

ROM = range of motion

Selective Tissue Test 10-17
Apley Compression and Distraction Tests for Meniscal Lesions

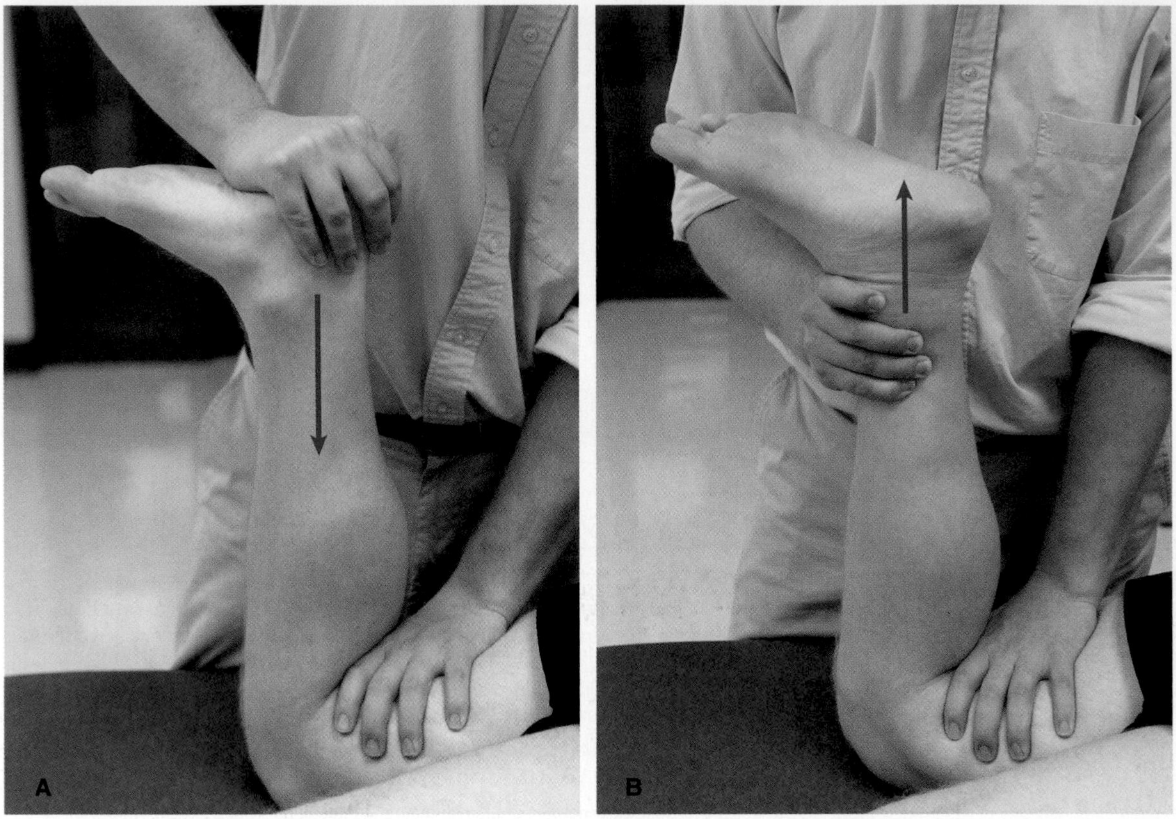

During the compression segment, pain may be caused by the menisci being caught between the tibia and femur (A). During the distraction segment, the joint's ligaments are stressed (B). Also, pain exhibited during compression should be reduced as the tibia is distracted from the femur.

Patient Position	Lying prone with the knee flexed to 90°
Position of Examiner	Standing lateral to the involved side
Evaluative Procedure	**(A)** Compression test: The clinician applies pressure to the plantar aspect of the heel, applying an axial load to the tibia while simultaneously internally and externally rotating the tibia. **(B)** Distraction test: The clinician grasps the lower leg and stabilizes the knee proximal to the femoral condyles. The tibia is distracted away from the femur while internally and externally rotating the tibia.
Positive Test	Pain experienced during compression that is reduced or eliminated during distraction
Implications	Meniscal tear
Comments	To perform this test, 90° of knee flexion is required. Pain that is experienced only during distraction or during both compression and distraction may indicate trauma to the collateral ligaments, joint capsule, or cruciate ligaments.
Evidence	

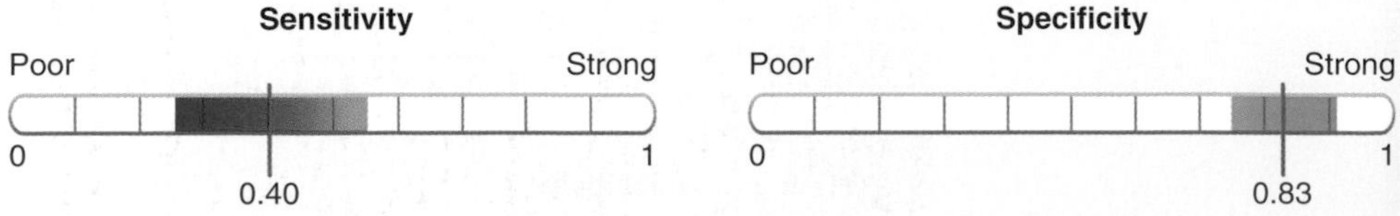

LR+: 0.00–7.69–17.11 **LR−: 0.50–0.76–1.02**

Selective Tissue Test 10-18
Thessaly Test for Meniscal Tears

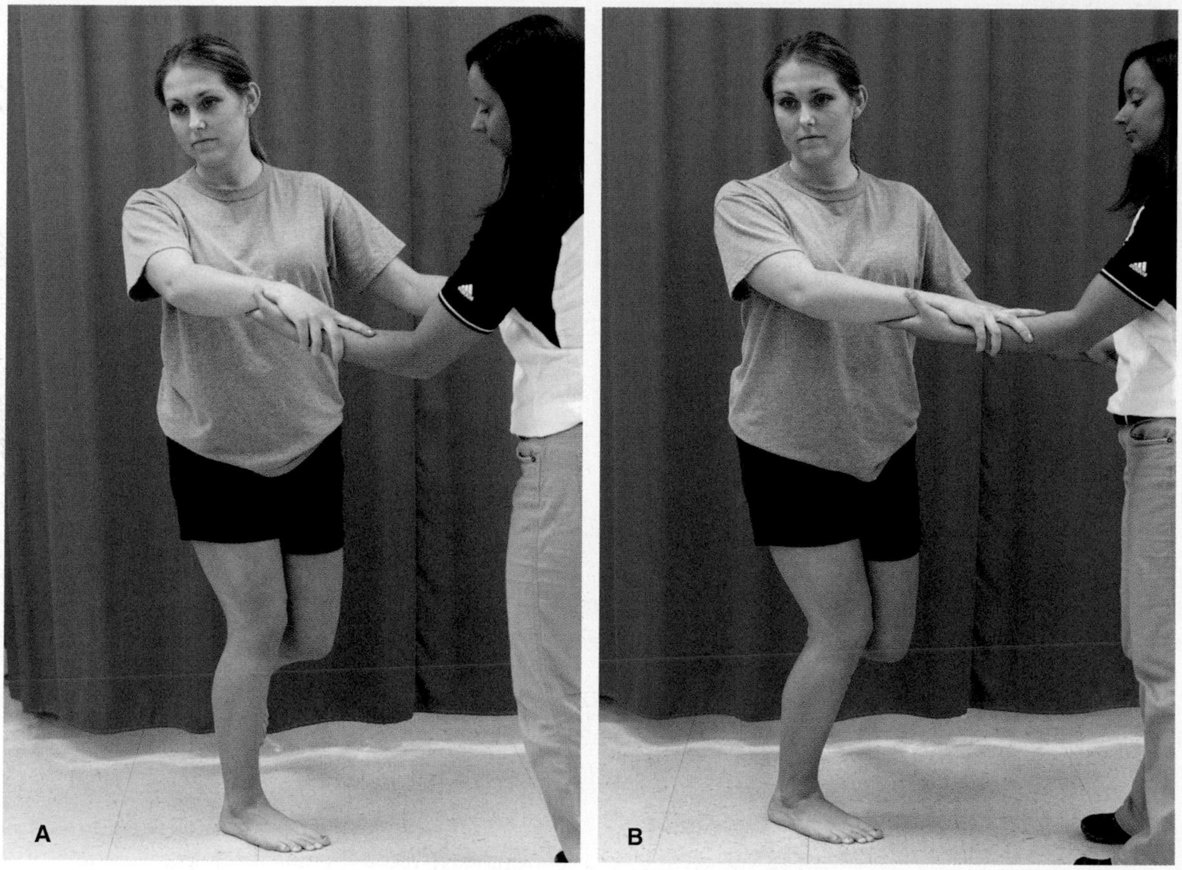

Performed while the patient is weight bearing and with femoral internal and external rotation, the Thessaly test is used to identify meniscal lesions. (A) The patient rotates on a fixed leg with the knee flexed to 5° and again (B) with the knee flexed to 20°.

Patient Position	Standing flatfooted on the involved leg The knee of the opposite leg is flexed to approximately 45°.
Position of Examiner	Standing in front of the patient, supporting the patient's arms
Evaluative Procedure	The uninvolved limb is tested first, allowing the patient to practice the maneuver. *Bout 1* The patient flexes the knee to 5°. The patient rotates the body to internally and externally rotate the femur on the tibia. Repeat three times. *Bout 2* The patient flexes the knee to 20°. The patient rotates the body to internally and externally rotate the femur on the tibia. Repeat three times.
Positive Test	Joint-line discomfort Complaints of "locking" or "catching"
Implications	A lesion of the medial or lateral meniscus, depending on the source of the pain and/or catching sensation
Comments	The diagnostic value of the Thessaly test decreases when the patient has an associated ACL injury.[118]
Evidence	

Sensitivity

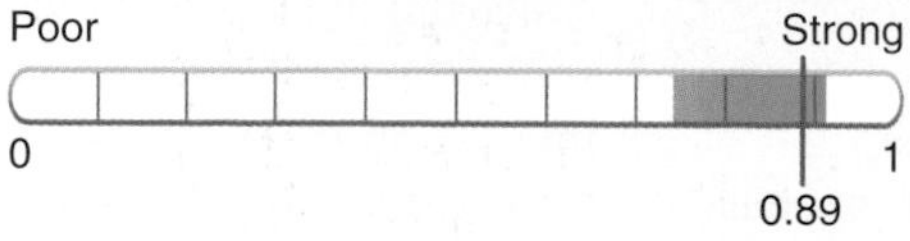

Specificity

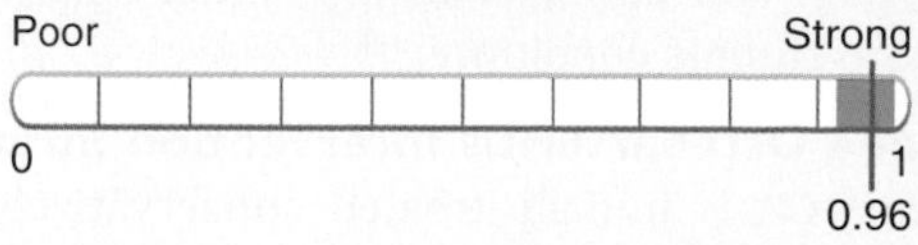

LR+: 9.23–20.25–37.84

LR–: 0.09–0.12–0.29

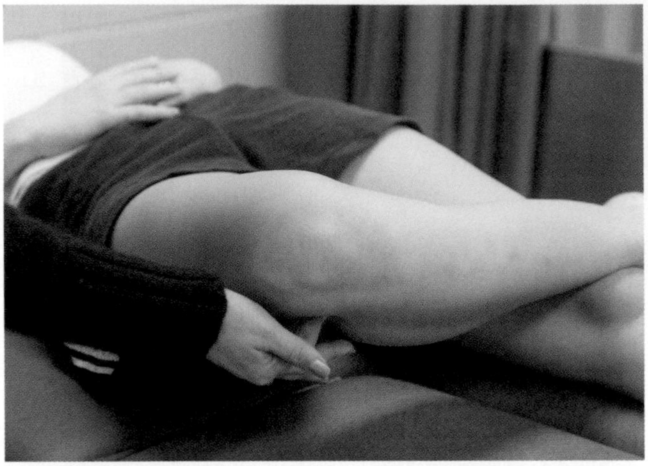

FIGURE 10-29 ■ Figure-4 position for palpating the popliteus tendon, located just posterior to the lateral collateral ligament.

Popliteus Tendinopathy Intervention Strategies

As with other tendinous conditions, correction of abnormal biomechanics, the use of nonsteroidal antiinflammatory agents, and the use of local modalities to decrease inflammation are needed to return the patient to full activity. Improving strength and endurance of the proximal hip musculature is often necessary.

Knee Osteoarthritis

The prevalence of knee OA increases with age. Increasing lifespans have increased the number of individuals affected by this condition. Knee OA involves the degeneration of articular cartilage, subchondral bone, and the synovium (see p. 90). The progressive degeneration of the articular cartilage results in osteophyte formation along the periphery of the joint.[138] The results of these changes are generalized joint stiffness, decreased ROM and strength, and decreased function (Examination Findings 10-10).[138] Women are more susceptible to OA than men. Other risk factors for developing OA include a history of past knee trauma, aging, and obesity.[47] The risk of OA is increased in postsurgical ACL patients when there is an associated chondral or meniscal injury.[139]

✱ Practical Evidence

In patients with knee OA, radiographic evidence of narrowing of the medial or lateral joint space positively correlates with increased patient symptoms.[138]

Pain may be the result of inflammation of the synovial capsule (inflammatory mediated pain) but, more commonly, is triggered by joint loading and joint motions (mechanically mediated pain).[140] The diagnosis of knee OA is made radiographically. Patients often have higher amounts of pain and disability in the earlier stages of OA than in more chronic conditions.[138]

Knee Osteoarthritis Intervention Strategies

Knee OA is initially treated conservatively with exercise and weight loss if necessary. Pharmacologic interventions begin with acetaminophen and, if this is not effective, progress to nonsteroidal antiinflammatory medications (e.g., ibuprofen). The next line of intervention may include steroid injections or supplementation with glucosamine and chondroitin for pain relief. Viscosupplementation using an injection of hyaluronate, essentially attempting to increase joint lubrication, may be effective. For patients whose disability remains following these treatments, arthroplasty is used.[47]

Tibiofemoral Joint Dislocations

Several systems are used to classify and describe the dislocation, including the direction of tibial displacement, complete or partial displacement, open or closed, and whether the trauma was caused by low- or high-velocity forces (athletic-related dislocations are the result of low-velocity forces), although accurate descriptions of the injury include elements from each of these classifications.[34] Tibiofemoral dislocation results in the rupture of at least three of the four primary knee ligaments (ACL, PCL, MCL, LCL).[41] The joint capsule, musculotendinous structures, meniscus, articular surfaces, and neurovascular elements are also disrupted (Examination Findings 10-11). Despite the relative severity of this injury and the magnitude of displacement required to produce widespread tissue damage, many acute tibiofemoral dislocations self-reduce, making a high index of suspicion necessary.[42]

Most tibiofemoral dislocations are the result of uniplanar knee hyperextension, hyperextension combined with tibial rotation, or posterior displacement of the tibia with the knee flexed, but any extreme force applied across the knee joint line can result in dislocation.[141] Most dislocations occur perpendicular to the long axis of the femur, usually with the tibia displacing anterior to the femur, although posterior, medial, lateral, and rotational components or combinations of these directions can result.[42] Anterior or posterior tibial displacement is more likely to produce an open dislocation than other directions.[34,141] Dislocations are also further classified by the direction of the resulting instability.

Dislocations of the tibiofemoral joint present with severe pain, muscle spasm, and obvious deformity of the joint. Unreduced gross dislocations may be marked by obvious deformity and a possible shortening of the involved limb (Fig. 10-30). Posterolateral dislocations can be clinically identified by the presence of a transverse indentation along the medial joint line caused by the capsule being displaced laterally (the dimple sign). The presence of the dimple sign usually indicates that surgical reduction of the dislocation will be required.[34]

Partial dislocations or frank dislocations that have spontaneously reduced may not reveal remarkable findings on initial inspections. A tibiofemoral joint dislocation should be suspected if distal neurovascular symptoms are present and if at least three of the major

Examination Findings 10-7
Osteochondral Lesions

Examination Segment	Clinical Findings
History of Current Condition	*Onset:* Osteochondritis dissecans: Insidious Osteochondral defect: Acute or insidious *Pain characteristics:* Diffuse pain within the knee *Other symptoms:* Locking or catching may be described. Knee instability may be reported. *Mechanism:* Shear or rotational forces across the joint line Compressive force Osteochondritis dissecans may result from repetitive microtrauma. *Predisposing conditions:* Family history, prior injury, and/or repetitive stress may predispose the onset of osteochondritis dissecans.
Functional Assessment	Pain is increased and strength is decreased when the involved extremity is weight bearing. Antalgic gait may be noted. Symptoms decrease with rest.
Inspection	Joint effusion may be noted. Quadriceps atrophy may be noted in chronic cases.
Palpation	Joint effusion
Joint and Muscle Function Assessment	*AROM:* Normal ROM for flexion and extension may be within normal limits when non–weight bearing but decreased when weight bearing. *MMT:* Within normal limits Quadriceps MMT may reveal weakness in chronic cases. *PROM:* Within normal limits
Joint Stability Tests	*Stress tests:* Stress tests may be positive with concurrent injury. *Joint play:* Not applicable
Selective Tissue Tests	Wilson's test
Neurological Screening	Within normal limits
Vascular Screening	Within normal limits
Imaging Techniques	AP and lateral radiographs of the knee and axial views of the patellofemoral joint CT or MRI can visualize the osteochondral defect.
Differential Diagnosis	Osteoarthritis, meniscal tear or cyst, patellofemoral joint dysfunction, tibial or femoral condyle fracture
Comments	Osteochondral defects often occur concurrently with soft tissue trauma, especially ACL sprains.

ACL = anterior cruciate ligament; AP = anteroposterior; AROM = active range of motion; CT = computed tomography; MMT = manual muscle test; MRI = magnetic resonance imaging; PROM = passive range of motion

ligaments (ACL, PCL, MCL, and/or LCL) have been torn.[34,41] Swelling and discoloration may rapidly occur soon after the injury. On palpation, the joint line and surrounding structures are sensitive. Unreduced dislocations will have a palpable deformity across the joint line.

Patients suffering from a tibiofemoral dislocation will be unwilling and unable to move the joint or bear weight on the involved limb. Do not perform ROM and ligamentous, selective tissue tests or functional tests on obvious dislocations.

The popliteal artery's anatomical fixation to the structures proximal and distal to the joint line makes it more predisposed to injury than the tibial artery.[34,141] Vascular injuries occur in 32% to 40% of dislocations, and nerve injuries may occur in as many as 30% of the cases.[34,142]

Selective Tissue Test 10-19

Wilson's Test for Osteochondral Defects of the Knee

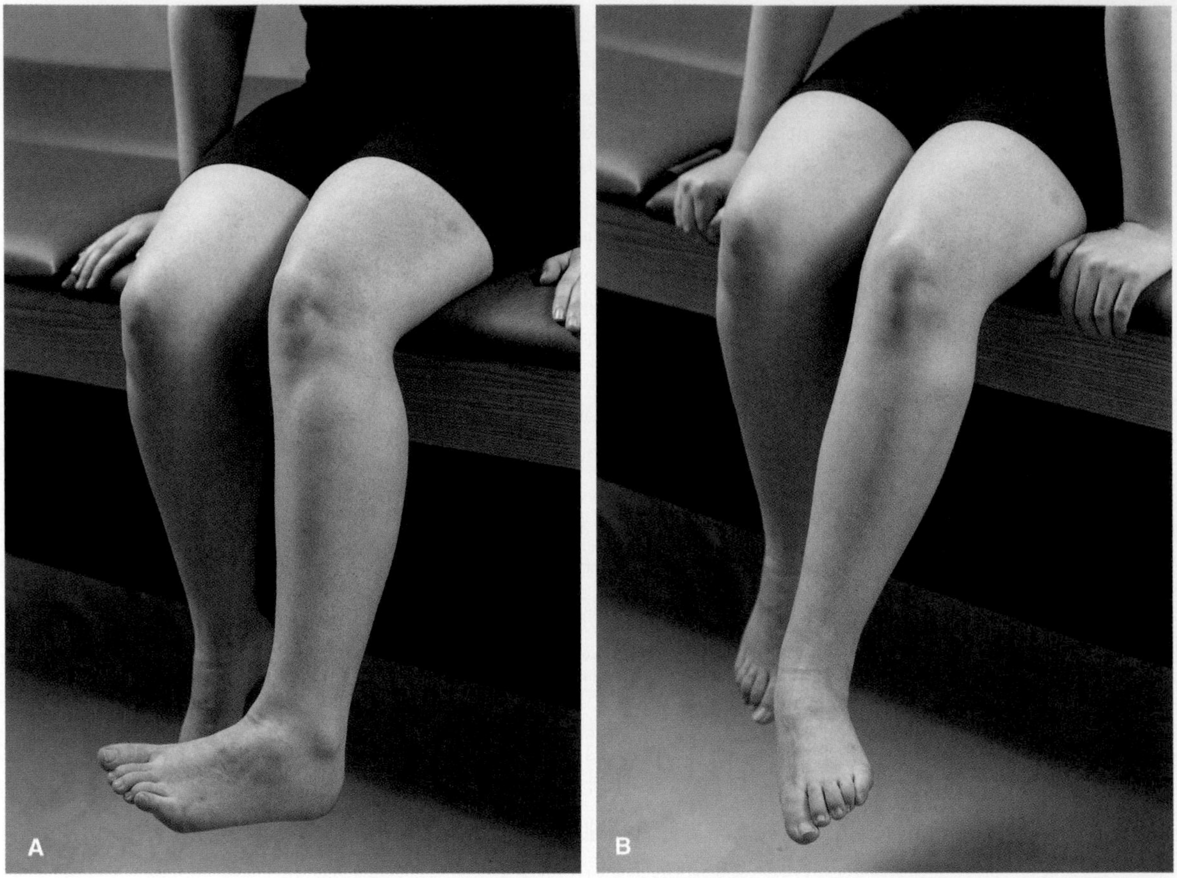

While the tibia is internally rotated, (A) the patient extends the knee. When pain is experienced, the patient externally rotates the tibia (B). In the presence of some OCDs, pain is relieved during the external rotation.

Patient Position	Sitting with the knee flexed to 90°
Position of Examiner	In front of the patient to observe any reactions secondary to pain
Evaluative Procedure	The patient actively extends the knee while maintaining the tibia in internal rotation. The patient is told to stop the motion and hold the knee in the position in which pain is experienced. If pain is experienced, the patient is instructed to externally rotate the tibia while the knee is held at its present point of flexion.
Positive Test	Pain experienced during extension with internal tibial rotation that is relieved by externally rotating the tibia
Implications	OCD or osteochondritis dissecans on the intercondylar area of the medial femoral condyle
Evidence	Inconclusive or absent in the literature

OCD = osteochondral defect

Examination Findings 10-8
Iliotibial Band Friction Syndrome

Examination Segment	Clinical Findings
History of Current Condition	*Onset:* Insidious *Pain characteristics:* Pain over the lateral femoral condyle proximal to the joint line that may radiate distally *Mechanism:* Activities involving repeated knee flexion and extension *Predisposing conditions:* Tightness of the IT band; genu varum, excessive pronation, leg-length discrepancy, excessive lateral heel strike[131]
Functional Assessment	The patient may demonstrate limited ability to control hip motion during a single leg squat. Pain or limitations may be described when decelerating gait, descending stairs, or walking or running down hills. Patient may avoid full knee extension during the push-off phase of gait.
Inspection	Genu varum Excessive pronation during gait; a lateral heel strike may be noted during observation of running and walking gait. Leg-length discrepancy
Palpation	In advanced cases, pain is elicited over the lateral femoral condyle, about 2 cm above the joint line.
Joint and Muscle Function Assessment	*AROM:* Within normal limits Pain may be described as the knee passes 30° during flexion and extension (representing the point where the IT band shifts over the lateral femoral condyle). *MMT:* Tensor fascia latae: May be weak and/or painful (see p. 426) Often associated weakness of hip abductors/external rotators (see p. 426) *PROM:* Within normal limits
Joint Stability Tests	*Stress tests:* None *Joint play:* Tightness of the lateral patellar restraints may be noted during medial patellar glide test (see Joint Play 11.1.
Selective Tissue Tests	Noble compression test Ober test
Neurological Screening	Within normal limits
Vascular Screening	Within normal limits
Imaging Techniques	Anteroposterior and lateral radiographs or CT scans may be ordered to identify enlargement of, or bony outgrowths from, the lateral femoral condyle.
Differential Diagnosis	Lateral meniscus tear; biceps femoris tendinopathy; patellofemoral dysfunction; popliteus tendinopathy
Comments	IT band tightness should be confirmed with an Ober test. IT band tightness may also be noted on the opposite hip.[131]

AROM = active range of motion; IT = iliotibial; MMT = manual muscle test; PROM = passive range of motion; ROM = range of motion

Dislocations caused by low-velocity forces are less likely to result in neurovascular compromise than those caused by high-velocity forces.[34] The posterior tibial and dorsal pedal pulses, distal capillary refill, and skin color and temperature must be carefully assessed bilaterally in any suspected tibiofemoral dislocation.[141] Because the collateral circulation around the knee is not sufficient to maintain the viability of the lower extremity if the popliteal artery is obstructed, the longer the popliteal artery is occluded, the greater the probability of permanent disability or even loss of the leg.[34,143] Circulation must be restored in 6 to 8 hours to minimize the risk of lower leg amputation.[34] Although Doppler blood flow measurements and arteriograms are used to confirm or rule out the presence of vascular trauma, physical examination typically will identify arterial and/or venous occlusion.[41,143]

Tibiofemoral Dislocation Intervention Strategies

The potential for permanent disability or loss of the leg secondary to trauma of the neurovascular structures makes a

Selective Tissue Test 10-20

Noble Compression Test for Iliotibial Band Friction Syndrome Modification: Renne's Test

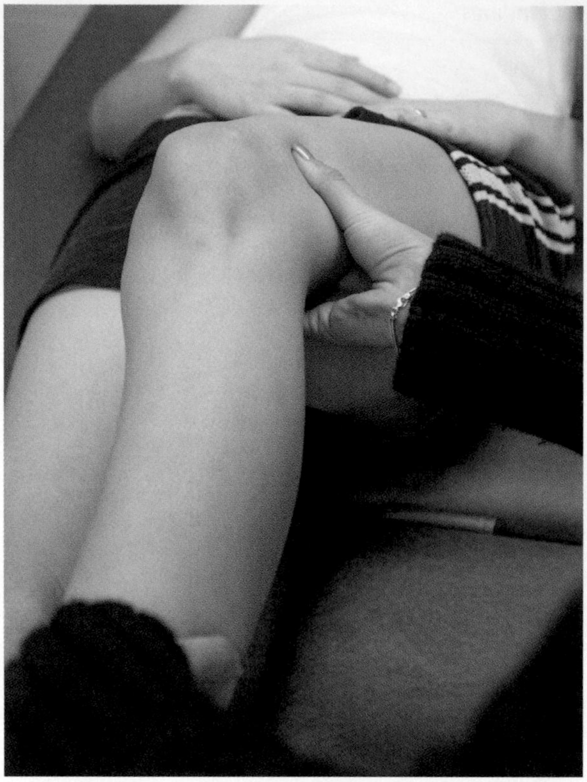

The examiner attempts to compress the distal portion of the IT band against the lateral femoral condyle during passive motion of the knee. In the presence of IT band inflammation, pain will be elicited.

Patient Position	Lying supine with the knee flexed
Position of Examiner	Standing lateral to the side being tested The knee is supported above the joint line with the thumb over or just superior to the lateral femoral condyle. The opposite hand controls the lower leg.
Evaluative Procedure	While applying pressure over the lateral femoral condyle, the knee is passively extended and flexed.
Positive Test	Pain under the thumb, most commonly as the knee approaches 30°
Implications	Inflammation of the IT band or its associated bursa or inflammation of the lateral femoral condyle
Modification	**Renne's test** replicates the mechanics of the Noble compression test but is performed with the patient standing on the involved leg and flexing the knee. No pressure is applied to the lateral femoral epicondyle.
Evidence	Inconclusive or absent in the literature

IT = iliotibial

Examination Findings 10-9
Popliteus Tendinopathy

Examination Segment	Clinical Findings
History of Current Condition	*Onset:* Insidious *Pain characteristics:* Pain in the popliteal fossa radiating along the length of the popliteus tendon posterior to the LCL *Mechanism:* Overuse *Predisposing conditions:* Excessive pronation during gait Posterior knee instability
Functional Assessment	Pain increases when running downhill. Excessive and prolonged pronation during walking and/or running
Inspection	In acute conditions, inspection is unremarkable; in chronic conditions, swelling may be noted along the lateral joint line.
Palpation	Palpation is best performed in the figure-4 position (see Fig. 10-29). Pain and crepitus elicited along the tendon posterior to the LCL
Joint and Muscle Function Assessment	*AROM:* Within normal limits *MMT:* The popliteus cannot be specifically isolated but is active during testing of the hamstrings. Pain is possible during resisted flexion from full extension as the popliteus "unscrews" the tibia. *PROM:* Within normal limits
Joint Stability Tests	*Stress tests:* None *Joint play:* Posterior glide of the tibia is assessed using the posterior drawer test.[87]
Selective Tissue Tests	None
Neurological Screening	Within normal limits
Vascular Screening	Within normal limits
Imaging Techniques	MRI can be used to rule out rupture of the popliteus tendon. Thickening of the tendon may be identified on MR images.
Differential Diagnosis	Biceps femoris tendinopathy, IT band friction syndrome, gastrocnemius tear (lateral head), lateral meniscus tear, LCL sprain, PCL sprain, posterolateral corner instability
Comments	The findings for popliteus tendinopathy are similar to those of IT band friction syndrome, except for the location of the pain.

AROM = active range of motion; LCL = lateral collateral ligament; MMT = manual muscle test; MRI = magnetic resonance imaging; PROM = passive range of motion; ROM = range of motion

tibiofemoral dislocation a medical emergency. Some tibiofemoral dislocations, especially those in the posterolateral direction, require surgical reduction and surgical repair of the damaged ligaments. These repairs may require multiple surgeries.[41] A significant proportion of dislocations are managed nonoperatively and yield outcomes that parallel or exceed those managed with a surgical approach.[41,42]

On-Field Examination of Knee Injuries

The process used during the on-field evaluation of knee injuries is similar to that described for the ankle. The presence of a gross fracture or dislocation of the tibiofemoral joint or the patellofemoral joint (see Chapter 11) must be ruled out before other examination procedures are used. Question the athlete about the mechanism of injury, the fixation of the foot, and any associated sounds and sensations.

Equipment Considerations

Protective devices around the knee include both stabilizing and prophylactic braces, neoprene sleeves, and padding, all of which must be removed before evaluating the knee and patella.

Football Pants

The pants worn for practice and competition in football are tight fitting but, fortunately, are elastic. Expose the knee by reaching under the anterior portion of the pant and locating the kneepad. Hold down the kneepad while the pant leg is pulled up and over the knee or the pad is removed from the pocket. Then remove the pad and flip the pouch up and out of the way (Fig. 10-31). If the pants are extraordinarily tight fitting or inelastic or if a brace is worn beneath the pants, making the preceding procedure difficult, cut the pant leg along one of the seams.

Knee Brace Removal

Both prophylactic and stabilizing knee braces greatly hinder the on-field evaluation of knee injuries. After the pant leg has been pulled over the brace, a prophylactic knee brace can be removed by loosening the lower strap holding it in place or cutting the tape. To remove the upper support, slide a hand under the strap or tape while pulling downward on the brace (see Fig. 10-31).

Because of the complexity of many of the stabilizing knee braces, it is usually easiest to remove or detach all of the tibial straps first and then those on the femur. Detach the femoral ones. If the athlete does not experience pain during knee flexion, slightly flex the knee to allow the lower (tibial) portion of the brace to move away from the leg and then lift the upper portion up and downward, away from the knee.

On-Field History

- **Location of the pain:** Inquire about the location of any pain. Pain localized to the joint line can indicate meniscal tears. Diffuse pain can indicate trauma to the MCL or joint capsule. Pain described as arising from within the knee joint, from "under the kneecap," or in the posterior aspect of the knee is associated with cruciate ligament sprains.
- **Mechanism of injury:** Identify the forces exerted on the knee, keeping in mind that the injury may involve multiple forces (e.g., valgus stress with tibial rotation). To cross-reference the injury mechanism with the possible trauma, refer to Table 10-3.
- **History of injury:** Ascertain if the athlete has suffered any significant prior ligamentous injury that may influence the findings of the current examination.
- **Associated sounds and sensations:** Question the patient about any sounds or sensations. A "snap" or "pop" may be associated with a ligament rupture, most commonly associated with the ACL. True locking of the knee can be associated with an unstable meniscal tear that has lodged between the knee's articular surfaces. A snapping, popping, or giving-way sensation may also be associated with a patellar dislocation or subluxation (discussed in Chapter 11).
- **Associated neurological symptoms:** Inquire about any neurological symptoms. Reports of paresthesia distal to the knee or the inability to dorsiflex the foot indicate trauma to the common peroneal nerve. In the presence of these symptoms, suspect a dislocated tibiofemoral joint until this condition can be ruled out.

On-Field Inspection

- **Patellar position:** Ensure that the patella is properly seated within the femoral trochlea.
- **Alignment of the tibiofemoral joint:** Through concurrent inspection and palpation, identify that the tibia and femur are properly aligned. Note that a normal alignment does not preclude consideration that a tibiofemoral dislocation occurred and subsequently reduced.

On-Field Palpation

- **Extensor mechanism:** Palpate the length of the patellar tendon, patella, quadriceps tendon, and distal quadriceps for incongruity and point tenderness, noting the overall integrity of the extensor mechanism.
- **Medial collateral ligament and medial joint line:** Note any point tenderness along the joint line, indicating meniscal pathology.
- **Lateral collateral ligament and lateral joint line:** Palpate the LCL, an extracapsular structure, for areas of defect or point tenderness. As with the medial meniscus, lateral joint line pain can indicate pathology of the lateral meniscus.
- **Fibular head:** Palpate the fibular head to rule out the presence of a fracture and determine the stability of the proximal tibiofibular syndesmosis.

On-Field Range of Motion Tests

In the absence of gross deformity, suspected fracture, or joint dislocation, have the athlete actively flex and extend the knee throughout the ROM. The inability to perform this motion signifies that the patient should be transported in a non–weight-bearing manner from the field to the sideline for further evaluation. Passive ROM and manual muscle testing may not be indicated during the on-field assessment.

On-Field Ligamentous Tests

If a ligamentous injury is suspected, an apprehension test, valgus stress testing, varus stress testing, Lachman test, and, if possible, a posterior drawer test may be carried out before moving the athlete and the onset of reflexive muscle guarding. If the athlete cannot be properly assessed on the field, transport the individual to the sideline in a non–weight-bearing position. Because of the awkward position that an examiner is placed in when performing on-field ligamentous stress tests, repeat these tests when the athlete has been moved to the sideline.

Examination Findings 10-10
Knee Osteoarthritis

Examination Segment	Clinical Findings
History of Current Condition	*Onset:* Gradual *Pain characteristics:* Diffuse around the knee; may localize to discrete areas within the joint (e.g., medial or lateral joint line) or from beneath the patella Pain and other symptoms may be intermittent based on the level of activity, medicine use, and other factors. *Other symptoms:* Morning pain that resolves in less than 30 minutes; increased pain with activity, especially after a period of rest Stiffness of the knee *Mechanism:* **Acute:** May be the residual secondary to bony or ligamentous injury to the knee or its interdependent areas: the foot, ankle, patellofemoral joint, or hip. Insidious: Repetitive stress, improper biomechanics; These may be related to an acute injury in the patient' past medical history. *Predisposing conditions:* History of ACL tear or other internal knee derangement; conditions that affect the biomechanics of the extremity; family history; female; obesity[47]
Functional Assessment	A compensatory gait that relieves pressure on the knee may be noted.
Inspection	Valgus or varus knee alignment may be noted. Compressive forces are increased on the side to which the malalignment occurs. Generalized swelling; a popliteal or Baker's cyst may develop.
Palpation	The joint may feel warm. The joint line may be tender to the touch. Effusion may be noted.
Joint and Muscle Function Assessment	*AROM:* May be limited by pain *MMT:* The quadriceps group's strength may be limited secondary to pain. *PROM:* Limited relative to ROM
Joint Stability Tests	*Stress tests:* As the condition progresses, varus laxity increases. Underlying instability may be a contributing factor. *Joint play:* Underlying hypermobility may be a contributing factor.
Selective Tissue Tests	As needed to rule in or rule out predisposing factors
Neurological Screening	Within normal limits
Vascular Screening	Within normal limits
Imaging Techniques	Radiographs are obtained with the patient weight bearing and non-weight-bearing. Medial or lateral joint space narrowing is characteristic of OA. Osteophytes may be noted, but their presence does not relate to increased symptoms.
Differential Diagnosis	Rheumatoid arthritis, osteochondral defect, meniscal tear or cyst, patellofemoral joint dysfunction, Lyme disease, gout
Comments	OA may affect multiple joints.

AROM = active range of motion; OA = osteoarthritis; PROM = passive range of motion; ROM = range of motion;

Examination Findings 10-11
Tibiofemoral Joint Dislocations

Examination Segment	Clinical Findings
History of Current Condition	*Onset:* Acute *Pain characteristics:* Severe diffuse pain about the knee The patient will report "popping" and other sensations of tearing at the time of injury. *Mechanism:* Knee hyperextension, rotation, posterior tibial shear force, posterior femoral shear force, valgus stress, varus force, or any combination thereof *Predisposing conditions:* Significant knee instability; Muscular weakness; Morbid obesity
Functional Assessment	The patient will be unwilling and/or unable to bear weight on the involved limb.
Inspection	Frank dislocations will reveal obvious deformity of the joint. Spontaneously reduced or subtly displaced dislocations may not reveal any obvious immediate deformity.[42] Swelling and discoloration may appear soon after the injury. A transverse indentation along the medial joint line ("dimple sign") may indicate an unreduced posterolateral dislocation.
Palpation	Frank and subtle dislocations will have a palpable incongruence of the joint line.
Joint and Muscle Function Assessment	*AROM:* Obvious dislocation: Contraindicated Spontaneously reduced or subtle dislocation: Absent or incomplete; the patient may be unwilling to perform the procedure. *MMT:* Obvious dislocation: Contraindicated Spontaneously reduced or subtle dislocation: Flexion and extension are weak or absent; the patient may be unwilling to perform the procedure. *PROM:* Obvious dislocation: Contraindicated Spontaneously reduced or subtle dislocation: Premature endpoint; the patient may be unwilling to allow the procedure to be performed.
Joint Stability Tests	*Stress tests:* Obvious dislocation: Contraindicated Anterior drawer test Lachman test Posterior drawer test Valgus stress test Varus stress test *Joint play:* Anterior glide of the tibia on the femur is assessed using the anterior drawer test. Posterior glide of the tibia is assessed using the posterior drawer test.[87]
Selective Tissue Tests	Avoided in the presence of an obvious dislocation
Neurological Screening	Peroneal nerve distribution (superficial and deep branches) Tibial nerve distribution

Vascular Screening	Posterior tibial artery Dorsal pedal pulse Distal capillary refill Skin color Skin temperature
Imaging Techniques	Angiograms assist in determining the viability of the popliteal artery.
Differential Diagnosis	Femoral fracture, tibial fracture
Comments	A patient who presents with a mechanism of injury described above has sustained a rupture of at least three of the major ligaments (ACL, PCL, MCL, LCL) and/or who displays distal neurological and/or vascular symptoms should be suspected of a tibiofemoral dislocation. Stress tests and selective tissue tests should not be performed on a knee that is obviously dislocated. Deep vein thrombosis may occur secondary to a tibiofemoral dislocation.[141]

ACL = anterior cruciate ligament; AROM = active range of motion; LCL = lateral collateral ligament; MCL = medial collateral ligament; MMT = manual muscle test; PCL = posterior cruciate ligament; PROM = passive range of motion

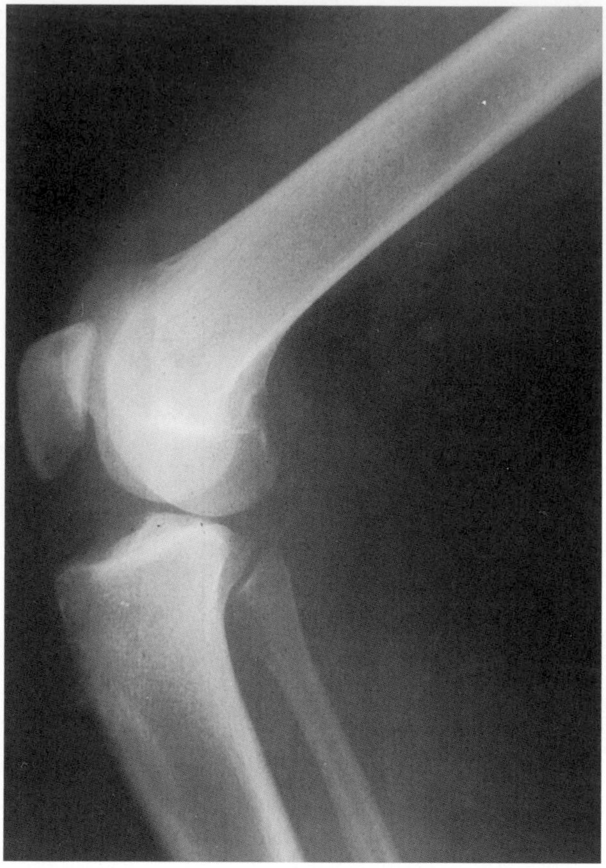

FIGURE 10-30 ■ Radiograph of a tibiofemoral dislocation. Note the anterior displacement of the tibia relative to the femur.

On-Field Management of Knee Injuries

Tibiofemoral Joint Dislocations

Tibiofemoral dislocations must be immediately evaluated by a physician; gross dislocations must be reduced as soon as possible. Prior to transporting the patient, establish the presence of the distal pulses, immobilize the limb in the position it was found, and treat for shock. If an open dislocation has occurred, then the wound must also be managed prior to transportation.

*** Practical Evidence**

The presence of a distal pulse following knee dislocation does not rule out severe arterial damage or blockage. Because of potential catastrophic consequences (amputation), a 79% rate of detecting arterial damage via pulse palpation is not sufficiently sensitive. Angiography is recommended after a dislocation, even with a normal pulse and well-perfused limb. Angiography is not recommended if vascular injury is obvious (diminished pulse; signs of ischemia) because any delay in surgery greatly hurts the outcome.[144]

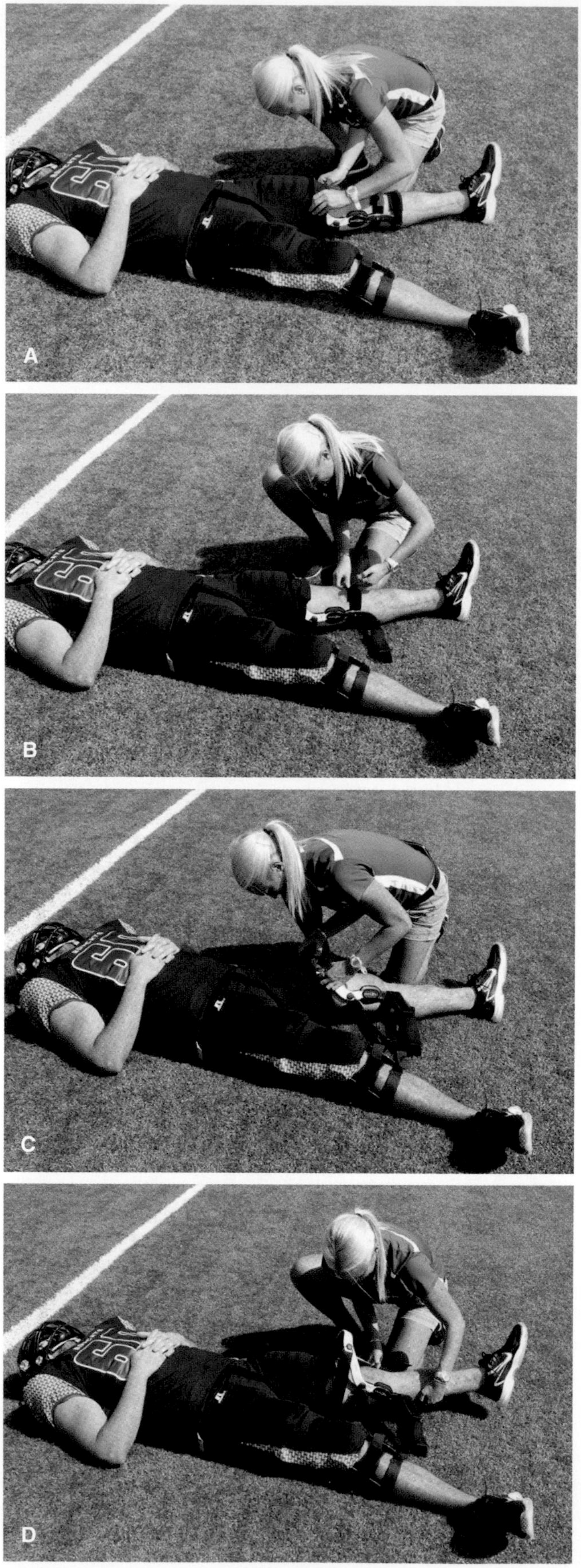

FIGURE 10-31 ■ (A) Remove the knee pad and flip its pouch upward. (B) Remove the Velcro® straps. (C) Displace the distal (tibial) portion of the brace and slide the proximal portion from beneath the pant. (D) Remove any underlying padding.

Collateral and Cruciate Ligament Sprains

While the athlete is still on the playing field or court, only uniplanar ligamentous stress tests for the MCL, ACL, LCL, and PCL are performed. For a basis of comparison and if the situation permits, also evaluate the uninvolved knee at this time. Laxity in the involved knee warrants the athlete's being removed from the field in a non–weight-bearing manner, such as a two-person assist.

After removing the athlete to the sideline and, if significant laxity or pain is demonstrated, treat the knee with ice, compression, and elevation. Place the knee in an immobilizer and refer the athlete to a physician.

Meniscal Tears

The on-field determination of the possibility of a meniscal tear is based on the athlete's description of the injury mechanism. Until otherwise ruled out, suspect a meniscal tear in athletes who describe a "locking" or "giving way" at the time of the injury or who are hesitant to move the knee. Likewise, assume that any rotational mechanism or possible ACL or MCL sprain involves the meniscus.

REFERENCES

1. Martin, RL: The ankle and foot complex. In Levangie, PK, and Norkin, CC: *Joint Structure and Function*, ed 5. Philadelphia, PA: FA Davis, 2011, p 332.
2. Moore, KL, and Dalley, AF: The lower limb. In Moore, KL, and Dalley, AF: *Clinically Oriented Anatomy*, ed 5. Baltimore, MD: Williams & Wilkins, 2006, p 563.
3. Moglo, KE, and Shirazi-Adl, A: On the coupling between anterior and posterior cruciate ligaments, and knee joint response under anterior femoral drawer in flexion: a finite element study. *Clin Biomech (Bristol, Avon)*, 18:751, 2003.
4. Vayken, P, and Murray, MM: The potential for primary repair of the ACL. *Sports Med Arthrosc*, 19:44, 2011.
5. Rasenberg, EIJ, et al: Grading medial collateral ligament injury: comparison of MR imaging and instrumented valgus-varus laxity testing device. A prospective double-blind patient study. *Eur J Radiol*, 21:18, 1995.
6. Davies, H, Unwin, A, and Aichroth, P: The posterolateral corner of the knee: anatomy, biomechanics and management of injuries. *Injury*, 35:68, 2004.
7. Chen, FS, Rokito, AS, and Pitman, MI: Acute and chronic posterolateral rotatory instability of the knee. *J Am Acad Orthop Surg*, 8:97, 2000.
8. Amis, AA: The functions of the fibre bundles of the anterior cruciate ligament in anterior drawer, rotational laxity and the pivot shift. *Knee Surg Sports Traumatol Arthrosc*, 20:613, 2012.
9. Alentorn-Geli, E, et al: Prevention of non-contact anterior cruciate ligament injuries in soccer players, part 1: mechanisms of injury and underlying risk factors. *Knee Surg Sports Traumatol Arthrosc*, 17:705, 2009.
10. Beynnon, BD, et al: Anterior cruciate ligament strain behavior during rehabilitation exercises in vivo. *Am J Sports Med*, 23:24, 1995.
11. Heijne, A, et al: Strain on the anterior cruciate ligament during closed kinetic chain exercises. *Med Sci Sports Exerc*, 36:935, 2004.
12. Van Dommelen, BA, and Fowler, PJ: Anatomy of the posterior cruciate ligament: a review. *Am J Sports Med*, 17:24, 1989.
13. Harner, CD, et al: Comparative study of the size and shape of human anterior and posterior cruciate ligaments. *J Orthop Res*, 13:429, 1995.
14. Hop, J: Anatomy and pathomechanics of the posterior cruciate ligament. *Athl Ther Today*, 6:6, 2001.
15. Wind, WM, Bergfeld, JA, and Parker, RD: Evaluation and treatment of posterior cruciate ligament injuries. *Am J Sports Med*, 32:1765, 2004.
16. Margheritini, F, et al: Posterior cruciate ligament injuries in the athlete: an anatomical, biomechanical and clinical review. *Sports Med*, 32:393, 2002.
17. Race, A, and Amis, AA: Loading of the two bundles of the posterior cruciate ligament: an analysis of bundle function in a-P drawer. *J Biomech*, 29:873, 1996.
18. Harner, CD, et al: The effects of a popliteus muscle load on in situ forces in the posterior cruciate ligament and on knee kinematics: a human cadaveric study. *Am J Sports Med*, 26:669, 1998.
19. Petrigliano, FA, et al. The effect of proximal tibial slope on dynamic stability testing of the posterior cruciate ligament- and posterolateral–corner-deficient knee. *Am J Sports Med*, 40:1322, 2012.
20. Grood, ES, Stowers, SF, and Noyes, FR: Limits of movement in the human knee: effect of sectioning the posterior cruciate ligament and posterolateral structures. *J Bone Joint Surg*, 70A:88, 1988.
21. Covey, DC: Injuries of the posterolateral corner of the knee. *J Bone Joint Surg*, 83(A):106, 2001.
22. Stannard, JP, et al: The posterolateral corner of the knee. Repair versus reconstruction. *Am J Sports Med*, 33:881, 2005.
23. Wadia FD, et al: An anatomic study of the popliteofibular ligament. *Int Orthop*, 27:172, 2003.
24. Greis, PE, et al: Meniscal injury: I. Basic science and evaluation. *J Am Acad Orthop Surg*, 10:168, 2002.
25. Hauger, O, et al: Characterization of the "Red zone" of knee meniscus: MR imaging and histologic correlation. *Radiology*, 217:193, 2000.
26. Makris, EA, Hadidi, P, and Athanasiou, KA: The knee meniscus: structure-function, pathophysiology, current repair techniques, and prospects for regeneration. *Biomaterials*, 32:7411, 2011.
27. Chuncharunee, A, Chanthong, P, and Lucksanasombool, P: The patterns of attachments of the popliteus muscle: form and function. *Med Hypotheses*, 78:221, 2012.
28. Tienen, TG, et al: Displacement of the medial meniscus within the passive motion characteristics of the human knee joint: an RSA study in human cadaver knees. *Knee Surg Sports Traumatol Arthroc*, 13:287, 2005.
29. Rosene, JM, and Fogarty, TD: Anterior tibial translation in collegiate athletes with normal anterior cruciate integrity. *J Athl Train*, 34:93, 1999.
30. Fujiya, H, et al: Effect of muscle loads and torque applied to the tibia on the strain behavior of the anterior cruciate ligament: an in vitro investigation. *Clin Biomech*, 26:1005, 2011.
31. Bryant, AL, et al: Dynamic restraint capacity of the hamstring muscles has important functional implications after anterior cruciate ligament injury and anterior cruciate ligament reconstruction. *Arch Phys Med Rehabil*, 89:2324, 2008.
32. Kennedy, A, et al: Biomechanical evaluation of pediatric anterior cruciate ligament reconstruction techniques. *Am J Sports Med*, 39:964, 2011.
33. Moglo, KE, Shirazi-Adl, A: Cruciate coupling and screw-home mechanism in passive knee joint during extension-flexion. *J Biomech*, 38:1075, 2005.
34. Zhong, H, et al: Role of CT angiography in the diagnosis and treatment of popliteal vascular entrapment syndrome. *AJR Am J Roentgenol*, 197:W1147, 2011.
35. Stiell, IG, et al: Prospective validation of a decision rule for the use of radiography in acute knee injuries. *JAMA*, 275:611, 1996.
36. Emparanza, JI, and Aginaga, JR: Validation of the Ottawa Knee Rules. *Ann Emerg Med*, 38:364, 2001.
37. Bachmann, LM, et al: The accuracy of the Ottawa Knee Rule to rule out knee fractures: a systematic review. *Ann Intern Med*, 140:121, 2004.
38. Smith, CC: Evaluating the painful knee: a hands-on approach to acute ligamentous and mensical injuries. *Adv Stud Med*, 4:362, 2004.
39. Temple, MM, et al: Age- and site-related biomechanical weakening of human articular cartilage of the femoral condyle. *Osteoarthritis Cartilage*, 15:1042, 2007.
40. Thompson, LR, et al: The knee pain map: reliability of a method to identify knee pain location and pattern. *Arthritis Rheum*, 61:726, 2009.

41. Levy, BA, et al: Controversies in the treatment of knee dislocations and multiligament reconstruction. *J Am Acad Orthop Surg*, 17:197, 2009.
42. Rihn, JA, et al: The acutely dislocated knee: evaluation and management. *J Am Acad Orthop Surg*, 12:334, 2004.
43. Garofalo, R, et al: Locking knee caused by subluxation of the posterior horn of the lateral meniscus. *Knee Surg Sports Traumatol Arthroc*, 13:569, 2005.
44. Akima, H, and Furukawa, T: Atrophy of thigh muscles after meniscal lesions and arthroscopic partial meniscectomy. *Knee Surg Sports Traumatol Arthrosoc*, 13:632, 2005.
45. Tothill, P, and Stewart, AD: Estimation of thigh muscle and adipose tissue volume using magnetic resonance imaging and anthropometry. *J Sports Sci*, 20:563, 2002.
46. Soderberg, GL, Ballantyne, BT, and Kestel, LL: Reliability of lower extremity girth measurements after anterior cruciate ligament reconstruction. *Physiother Res Int*, 1:7, 1996.
47. Sinsusas, K: Osteoarthritis: diagnosis and treatment. *Am Fam Physician*, 85:49, 2012.
48. Voight, M, and Weider, D: Comparative reflex response times of vastus medialis oblique and subjects with extensor mechanism dysfunction. *Am J Sports Med*, 19:131, 1991.
49. Neubauer, H, et al: Popliteal cysts in paediatric patients: clinical characteristics and imaging features on ultrasound and MRI. *Arthritis*, 2011:751593, 2011.
50. Yu, WD, and Shapiro, MS: Cysts and other masses about the knee: identifying and treating common and rare lesions. *Phys Sports Med*, 27:59, 1999.
51. Handy, JR: Popliteal cysts in adults: a review. *Semin Arthritis Rheum*, 31:108, 2001.
52. Kastelein, M, et al: Diagnostic value of history taking and physical examination to assess effusion of the knee in traumatic knee patients in general practice. *Arch Phys Med Rehabil*, 90:82, 2009.
53. Frobell, RB, Lohmander, LS, and Roos, HP: Acute rotational trauma to the knee: poor agreement between clinical assessment and magnetic resonance imaging findings. *Scand J Med Sci Sports*, 17:109, 2007.
54. Ahn,JH, et al: Anterior cruciate ligament reconstruction using remnant preservation and a femoral tensioning technique: clinical and magnetic resonance imaging results. *Arthroscopy*, 27:1079, 2011.
55. Hislop, HJ, and Montgomery, J: *Muscle Testing: Techniques of Manual Examination*. Philadelphia, PA: W.B. Saunders, 2002, p 187.
56. Blair, DF, and Willis, RP: Rapid rehabilitation following anterior cruciate ligament reconstruction. *J Athl Train*, 26:32, 1991.
57. More, RC, et al: Hamstrings-an anterior cruciate ligament protagonist. *Am J Sports Med*, 21:231, 1993.
58. Christel, PS, et al: The contribution of each anterior cruciate ligament bundle to the Lachman test: a cadaver investigation. *J Bone Joint Surg*, 94B:68, 2012.
59. Benjaminse, A, Gokeler, A, and van der Schans, CP: Clinical diagnosis of an anterior cruciate ligament rupture: a meta-analysis. *J Orthop Sports Phys Ther*, 36:267, 2006.
60. Brophy, RH, et al: Changes in length of virtual anterior cruciate ligament fibers during stability testing. *Am J Sports Med*, 36:2196, 2008.
61. Harter, RA, et al: A comparison of instrumented and manual Lachman test results in anterior cruciate ligament-reconstructed knees. *J Athl Train*, 25:330, 1990.
62. Kijowski, R, et al: Evaluation of the menisci of the knee joint using three-dimensional isotropic resolution fast spin-echo imaging: diagnostic performance in 250 patients with surgical correlation. *Skeletal Radiol*, 41:169, 2012.
63. Engelen-van Melick, N, et al: Assessment of functional performance after anterior cruciate ligament reconstruction: a systematic review of measurement procedures. *Knee Surg Sports Traumatol Arthrosc*, 21:869, 2013.
64. Webright, WG, Perrin, DH, and Gansneder, BM: Effect of trunk position on anterior tibial displacement measured by the KT-1000 in uninjured subjects. *J Athl Train*, 33:233, 1998.
65. Papandreou, MG, et al: Inter-rater reliability of Rolimeter measurements between anterior cruciate ligament injured and normal contralateral knees. *Knee Surg Sports Traumatol Arthroc*, 13:592, 2005.
66. Berry, J, et al: Error estimates in novice and expert raters for the KT-1000 arthrometer. *J Orthop Sports Phys Ther*, 29:49, 1999.
67. Fleming, BC, et al: Measurement of anterior-posterior knee laxity: a comparison of three techniques. *J Orthop Res*, 20:421, 2002.
68. Rubinstein, RA, et al: The accuracy of the clinical examination in the setting of posterior cruciate ligament injuries. *Am J Sports Med*, 22:550, 1994.
69. Draper, DO, and Schulthies, S: A test for eliminating false positive anterior cruciate ligament injury diagnoses. *J Athl Train*, 28:355, 1993.
70. Lee, BK, and Nam, SW: Rupture of posterior cruciate ligament: diagnosis and treatment. *Knee Surg Relat Res*, 23:135, 2011.
71. Voos, JE, et al: Posterior cruciate ligament: anatomy, biomechanics, and outcomes. *Am J Sports Med*, 40:22, 2012.
72. Sawant, M, Murty, AN, and Ireland, J: Valgus knee injuries: evaluation and documentation using a simple technique of stress radiography. *Knee*, 11:25, 2004.
73. Indelicato, PA: Isolated medial collateral ligament injuries of the knee. *J Am Acad Ortho Surg*, 3:9, 1995.
74. Stannard, JP: Medial and posteromedial instability of the knee: evaluation, treatment, and results. *Sports Med Arthrosc Rev*, 18:1263, 2010.
75. Robbins, AJ, Newman, AP, and Burks, RT: Postoperative return of motion in anterior cruciate ligament and medial collateral ligament injuries: the effects of medial collateral ligament rupture location. *Am J Sports Med*, 21:20, 1993.
76. Veenema, KR: Valgus knee instability in an adolescent: ligament sprain or physeal fracture? *Phys Sportsmed*, 27:62, 1999.
77. Kastelein, M, et al: Assessing medial collateral ligament knee lesions in general practice. *Am J Med*, 121:982, 2008.
78. Laprade, RF, and Wijdicks, CA: The management of injuries to the medial side of the knee. *J Orthop Sports Phys Ther*, 42:221, 2012.
79. Reider, B, et al: Treatment of isolated medial collateral ligament injuries with early functional rehabilitation: a five-year follow-up study. *Am J Sports Med*, 22:470, 1993.
80. Lunden, JB, et al: Current concepts in the recognition and treatment of posterolateral corner injuries to the knee. *J Orthop Sports Phys Ther*, 40:502, 2010.
81. Krivickas, LS, and Wilbourn, AJ: Peripheral nerve injuries in athletes: a case series of over 200 injuries. *Semin Neurol*, 20:225, 2000.
82. Murakami, Y, et al: Quantitative evaluation of nutritional pathways for the posterior cruciate ligament and the lateral collateral ligament in rabbits. *Acta Physiol Scand*, 162:447, 1998.
83. Zorzi, C, et al: Combined PCL and PLC reconstruction in chronic posterolateral instability. *Knee Surg Sports Traumatol Arthrosc*, 21:1036, 2013.
84. Aherns, P, et al: A novel tool for objective assessment of femorotibial rotation: a cadaver study. *Int Orthop*, 35:1611, 2011.
85. Beaulieu, ML, and McLean, SG: Sex-dimorphic landing mechanics and their role within the noncontact ACL injury mechanism: evidence, limitations and directions. *Sports Med Arthrosc Rehabil Ther Technol*, 15:4, 2012.
86. Snyder-Mackler, L, et al: The relationship between passive joint laxity and functional outcome after anterior cruciate ligament surgery. *Am J Sports Med*, 25:191, 1997.
87. Kaltenborn, FM: *Manual Mobilization of the Joints*, Oslo, Norway: Olaf Norlis Bokhandel, 2002, p 286.
88. Anderson, AF, Rennirt, GW, and Standeffer, WC: Clinical analysis of the pivot shift tests: description of the pivot drawer test. *Am J Knee Surg*, 13:19, 2000.
89. Andrish, JT: Anterior cruciate ligament injuries in the skeletally immature patient. *Am J Orthop*, 30:103, 2001.

90. Grant, JA, Tannenbaum, E, and Miller, BS: Treatment of combined tears of the anterior cruciate and medial collateral ligaments. *Arthroscopy*, 28:110, 2012.
91. Alentorn-Geli, E, Myer, GD, Silvers, HJ, et al: Prevention of non-contact anterior cruciate ligament injuries in soccer players, part 1: mechanisms of injury and underlying risk factors. *Knee Surg Sports Traumatol Arthrosc*, 17:705, 2009.
92. Renstrom, P, et al: Non-contact ACL injuries in female athletes: an International Olympic Committee current concepts statement. *Br J Sports Med*, 42:394, 2008.
93. Flynn, RK, et al: The familial predisposition towards the anterior cruciate ligament. *Am J Sports Med*, 33:23, 2005.
94. Ageberg, E, et al: Balance in single-limb stance in patients with anterior cruciate ligament injury: relation to knee laxity, proprioception, muscle strength, and subjective function. *Am J Sports Med*, 33:1527, 2005.
95. Logerstedt, DS, et al: Knee stability and movement coordination impairments: knee ligament sprain. *J Orthop Sports Phys Ther*, 40:A1, 2010.
96. Li, RT, et al: Predictors of radiographic knee osteoarthritis after anterior cruciate ligament reconstruction. *Am J Sports Med*, 39:2595, 2011.
97. Schulz, MS, et al: Epidemiology of posterior cruciate ligament injuries. *Arch Orthop Trauma Surg*, 234:186, 2003.
98. Cosgarea, AJ, and Jay, PR: Posterior cruciate ligament injuries: evaluation and management. *J Am Acad Orthop Surg*, 9:297, 2001.
99. Schulz, MS, et al: Reliability of stress radiography for evaluation of posterior knee laxity. *Am J Sports Med*, 33:502, 2005.
100. Fontboté, CA, et al: Neuromuscular and biomechanical adaptations of patients with isolated deficiency of the posterior cruciate ligament. *Am J Sports Med*, 33:982, 2005.
101. Jonsson, H, and Karrholm, J: Three-dimensional knee kinematics and stability in patients with a posterior cruciate ligament tear. *J Orthop Res*, 17:185, 1999.
102. Shelbourne, KD, Davis, TJ, and Patel, DV: The natural history of acute, isolated, nonoperatively treated posterior cruciate ligament injuries: a prospective study. *Am J Sports Med*, 27:276, 1999.
103. Goyal, K, et al: In vivo analysis of the isolated posterior cruciate ligament-deficient knee during functional activities. *Am J Sports Med*, 40:777, 2012.
104. Ochi, M, et al: Isolated posterior cruciate ligament insufficiency induces morphological changes of anterior cruciate ligament collagen fibrils. *Arthroscopy*, 15:292, 1999.
105. Zantop T, Schumacher, T, and Diermann, N, et al: Anterolateral rotational knee instability: role of posterolateral structures. *Arch Orthop Trauma Surg*, 127:743, 2007.
106. Ostrowski, JA: Accuracy of 3 diagnostic tests for anterior cruciate ligament tears. *J Athl Train*, 41:120, 2006.
107. Shelbourne, KD, and Nitz, PA: The O'Donoghue triad revisited: combined knee injuries involving anterior cruciate and medial collateral ligament tears. *Am J Sports Med*, 19:474, 1991.
108. Ross, G, et al: Evaluation and treatment of acute posterolateral corner/anterior cruciate ligament injuries of the knee. *J Bone Joint Surg*, 86(A):2, 2004.
109. Cooper, DE: Tests for posterolateral instability of the knee in normal subjects: results of examination under anesthesia. *J Bone Joint Surg*, 73(A):30, 1991.
110. Ferrari, DA, Ferrari, JD, and Coumas, J: Posterolateral instability of the knee. *J Bone Joint Surg*, 76-B:187, 1994.
111. Loomer, RL: A test for posterolateral rotatory instability. *Clin Orthop*, 235, 1995.
112. LaPrade, RF, Ly, TV, and Griffith, C: The external rotation recurvatum test revisited: reevaluation of the sagittal plane tibiofemoral relationship. *Am J Sports Med*, 36:709, 2008.
113. Hughston, JC, and Norwood, LA: The posterolateral drawer test and external rotational recurvatum test for posterolateral rotatory instability of the knee. *Clin Orthop*, 147:82, 1980.
114. Yeh, PC, et al: Epidemiology of isolated meniscal injury and its effect on performance in athletes from the National Basketball Association. *Am J Sports Med*, 40:589, 2012.
115. Karachalios, T, et al: Diagnostic accuracy of a new clinical test (the Thessaly test) for early detection of meniscal tears. *J Bone Joint Surg*, 87A:955, 2005.
116. Davis, E: Clinical examination of the knee following trauma: an evidence-based perspective. *Trauma*, 4:135, 2002.
117. Ellis, MR, and Griffin, KW: Clinical inquiry: for knee pain, how predictive is physical examination for meniscal injury? *J Fam Pract*, 53:918, 2004.
118. Mirzatolooei, F, et al: Validation of the Thessaly test for detecting meniscal tears in anterior cruciate deficient knees. *Knee*, 17:221, 2010.
119. Meserve, BB, Cleland, JA, and Boucher, TR: A meta-analysis examining clinical test utilities for assessing meniscal injuries. *Clin Rehabil*, 22:143, 2008.
120. Couture, J, et al: Joint line fullness and meniscal pathology. *Sports Health*, 4:47, 2012.
121. Zaffagnini, S, et al: Prospective long-term outcomes of the medial collage meniscus implant versus partial medial meniscectomy: a minimum 10-year follow-up study. *Am J Sports Med*, 39:977, 2011.
122. Greis, PE, et al: Meniscal injury: II. Management. *J Am Acad Orthop Surg*, 10:177, 2002.
123. Redler, LH, et al: Management of articular cartilage defects of the knee. *Phys Sportsmed*, 40:20, 2012.
124. Cetik, O, Turker, M, and Uslu, M: Bilateral osteochondritis dissecans of lateral femoral condyle. *Knee Surg Sports Traumatol Arthrosc*, 13:468, 2005.
125. Quatman, CE, et al: The clinical utility and diagnostic performance of MRI for identification and classification of knee osteochondritis dissecans. *J Bone Joint Surg Am*, 94(A):1036, 2012.
126. Vanlauwe, J, et al: Five-year outcome of characterized chondrocyte implantation versus microfracture for symptomatic cartilage defects of the knee. *Am J Sports Med*, 39:2566, 2011.
127. Mithoefer, K, et al: Current concepts for rehabilitation and return to sport after knee articular cartilage repair in the athlete. *J Orthop Sports Phys Ther*, 42:254, 2012.
128. Reese, NB, and Bandy, WD: Use of an inclinometer to measure flexibility of the iliotibial band using the Ober test and modified Ober test: differences in the magnitude and reliability of measurements. *J Orthop Sports Phys Ther*, 33:326, 2003.
129. Muhle, C, et al: Iliotibial band friction syndrome: MR imaging findings in 16 patients and MR arthrographic study of six cadaveric knees. *Radiology*, 212:103, 1999.
130. Fairclough, J, et al: Is iliotibial band syndrome really a friction syndrome? *J Sci Med Sport*, 10:74, 2007.
131. Pettitt, R, and Dolski, A: Corrective neuromuscular approach to the treatment of iliotibial band friction syndrome: a case report. *J Athl Train*, 35:96, 2000.
132. Strauss EJ, et al: Iliotibial band syndrome: evaluation and management. *J Am Acad Orthop Surg*, 19:728, 2011.
133. Baker, RL, Souza, RB, and Fredericson, M: Iliotibial band syndrome: soft tissue and biomechanical factors in evaluation and treatment. *PM R*, 3:550, 2011.
134. Ellis, R, Hing, W, and Reid, D: Iliotibial band friction syndrome: a systematic review. *Man Ther*, 12:200, 2007.
135. Quinlan, JF, et al: Isolated popliteus rupture at the musculo-tendinous junction. *J Knee Surg*, 24:137, 2011.

136. Schinhan, M, et al: Electromyographic study of the popliteus muscle in the dynamic stabilization of the posterolateral corner structures of the knee. *Am J Sports Med*, 39:173, 2011.
137. Weresh, MJ, et al: Popliteus function in ACL-deficient patients. *Scand J Med Sci Sports*, 7:14, 1997.
138. Fukui, N, et al: Relationship between radiographic changes and symptoms or physical examination finding in subjects with symptomatic medial knee osteoarthritis: a three-year prospective study. *BMC Musculoskelet Disord*, 11:269, 2010.
139. Murray, JR, et al: Does anterior ligament reconstruction lead to degenerative disease? Thirteen-year results after bone-patellar tendon-bone autograft. *Am J Sports Med*, 40:404, 2012.
140. Chan, KKW, and Chan, LWY: A qualitative study on patients with knee osteoarthritis to evaluate the influence of different pain patterns on patients' quality of life and to find out patients' interpretation and coping strategies for the disease. *RheumatolRep*, 3:9, 2011.
141. Henrichs, A: A review of knee dislocations. *J Athl Train*, 39:365, 2004.
142. Gray, JL, and Cindric, M: Management of arterial and venous injuries in the dislocated knee. *Sports Med Arthrosc*, 19:131, 2011.
143. Chabra, A, et al: Surgical management of knee dislocations. *J Bone Joint Surg*, 87(A) Suppl:1, 2005.
144. Barnes, CJ, Pietrobon, R, and Higgins, LD: Does the pulse examination in patients with traumatic knee dislocation predict a surgical arterial injury? A meta-analysis. *J Trauma*, 53:1109, 2002.

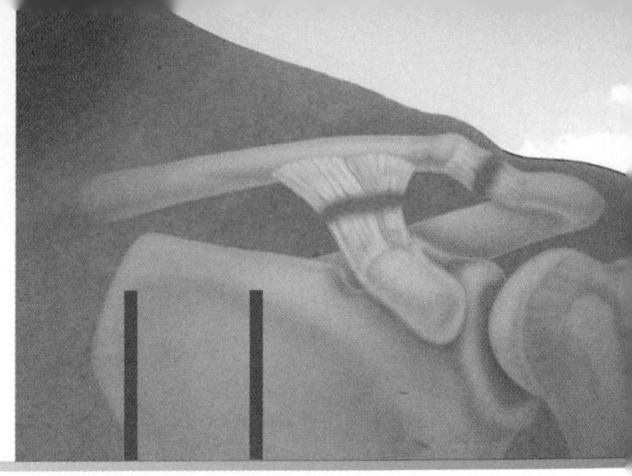

CHAPTER

Patellofemoral Pathologies

Although the patellofemoral (PF) articulation is an integral part of the knee, the two areas are separated in this text because of the differences in the mechanisms and onset of injury. Injury to the patellofemoral articulation is the result of overuse, congenital malalignment, structural insufficiency, impaired motor control, or trauma. The mechanics of the PF joint are interdependent with the foot, ankle, knee, and hip. Examination of individuals with nonacute-onset patellofemoral pathology should include the entire lower extremity, lumbar region, and gait biomechanics.

Clinical Anatomy

Lying within the patellar tendon, the **patella** is the largest sesamoid bone in the body. The patella's anatomical design allows for increased mechanical efficiency of the quadriceps muscle group, protection of the anterior portion of the knee joint, and the absorption and transmission of the **joint reaction forces**. In the frontal and sagittal planes, the patella is triangular. In the frontal plane, the superior portion is wider than its inferior apex; in the sagittal plane, it is marked with an anterior, nonarticulating surface and a narrower posterior articulating surface (Fig. 11-1).

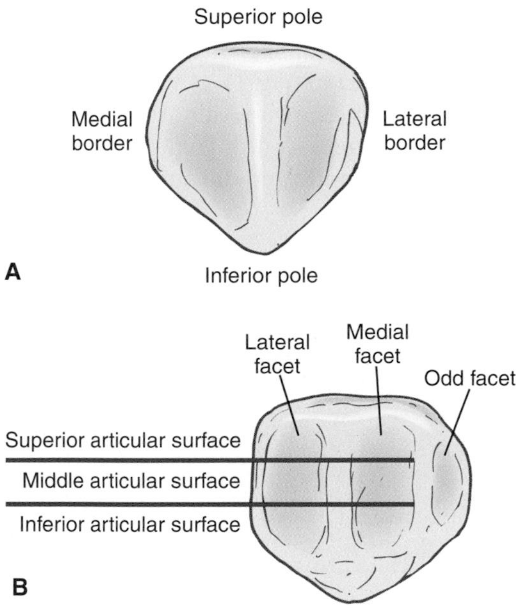

FIGURE 11-1 ■ The left patella. (A) Anterior view identifying the poles; (B) Posterior view identifying the of the articular surfaces and facets. The lateral and medial facets may be conceptualized as having superior, middle, and inferior articular surfaces. The odd facet has no such subdivisions.

Articulations and Ligamentous Support

The patella's articular surface has three distinct facets: the medial, lateral, and odd facets, which create seven unique articular surfaces.[1] Each facet is covered with up to a 5-mm thickness of hyaline cartilage, thicker than the femur's articular cartilage. The medial and lateral facets have superior, middle, and inferior articular surfaces. The odd facet, lying medial to the medial facet, has no articular subdivisions (see Figure 11-1B).

At birth, the patella is cartilaginous, and it ossifies between 3 and 6 years of age. When separate ossification centers fail to join, a **bipartite patella** may result, reducing the efficiency of the extensor mechanism. The superior lateral border is the most common site, with up to 50% of the cases occurring bilaterally.[2,3]

The mechanics of the patellofemoral joint differ when weight bearing and non–weight bearing. When non–weight bearing, the patella moves on the femur. During weight bearing, the femur moves under the patella. This relationship further explains the need to examine the hip (which controls movement of the femur) in individuals with patellofemoral pain.[4]

Joint reaction forces Forces that are transmitted through a joint's articular surfaces

During open-chain knee flexion and extension, the patella tracks within the femoral trochlear groove, the area between the two femoral condyles lined with articular cartilage. As the knee moves from flexion into extension, the patella tracks medially within the range of 45 to 18 degrees. The patella then tracks laterally during the final 18 degrees of extension. During flexion, hamstrings exert a force that causes the patella to increase its angle of lateral tilt and lateral shift, which then decreases during extension.[1,5]

When the knee is fully extended, the patella rests just proximal to the femoral groove, leaving it vulnerable to dislocating forces. When the knee is fully flexed, the odd facet articulates with the medial femoral condyle. When the knee is flexed moving towards extension, the patella initially makes contact with the groove at 10 to 20 degrees of flexion and becomes seated within the groove as the knee approaches 20 to 30 degrees.[6,7] At this point, the lateral border of the femoral trochlea forms a buttress against lateral patellar movement. A shallow trochlear groove is associated with an increased incidence of patellofemoral pain, since it allows increased lateral patellar tilt and displacement as the knee nears full extension (Fig. 11-2).[8]

Joint reaction forces are a result of the amount of contact between the patella and the femur, force vectors between the patellar tendon and the quadriceps, and muscle activity. In general, patellar compressive forces are greater in weight bearing as compared with non–weight bearing, especially as knee flexion increases.[9] These forces range from 0.5 times body weight when walking on a level surface to as much as 7 times body weight when squatting.[10] As the knee moves from extension to flexion, the patella flexes and moves posteriorly, increasing the area in contact with the femur (Fig. 11-3). At the same time, increased compression occurs as a result of the increasing flexion angle, with a resulting overall 4-fold increase in joint reaction force as the knee moves from extension to flexion.[9,10]

The patellar retinaculum and **patellofemoral ligaments** maintain the patella's position through the arc of motion (Fig. 11-4). The **lateral retinaculum** originates as an expansion off the vastus lateralis tendon and the iliotibial (IT) band to insert on the patella's lateral border.[11,12] The thinner **medial retinaculum** originates from the distal portion of the vastus medialis and adductor magnus and inserts on the medial border of the patella. The superior portion of the knee's fibrous capsule thickens and inserts on the patella's superior border, forming the medial and lateral patellofemoral ligaments. With attachments on the medial portion of the upper patella, on the femoral condyle near the adductor tubercle, and on the posteromedial joint capsule, the **medial patellofemoral**

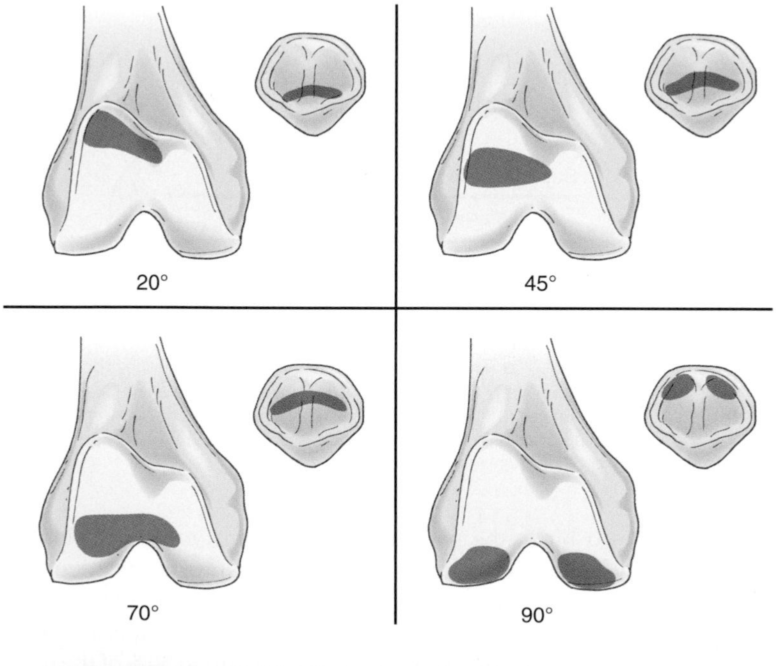

Range of Motion	Patellar Facets in Contact With the Femoral Trochlear Groove
0°	Patella resting on the suprapatellar fat pad on the distal femoral shaft
20°	Inferior portion of facets
45°	Medial and lateral facets
90°	Largest contact area across the medial and lateral facets
135°	Odd facet

FIGURE 11-2 ■ The influence of tibiofemoral joint position and the resulting compressive forces placed on the patella.

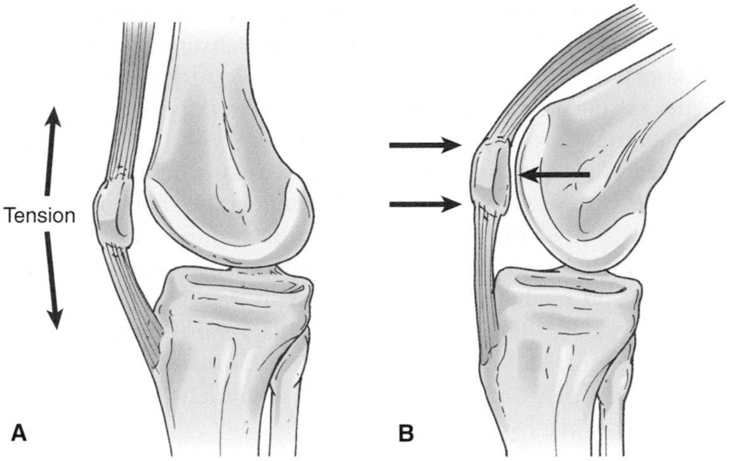

FIGURE 11-3 ■ Loading of the patellofemoral joint during weight bearing. (A) When the knee is extended primarily tensile forces are placed on the patella. (B) As the knee moves into flexion the amount of compression between the patella and femoral trochlea is increased.

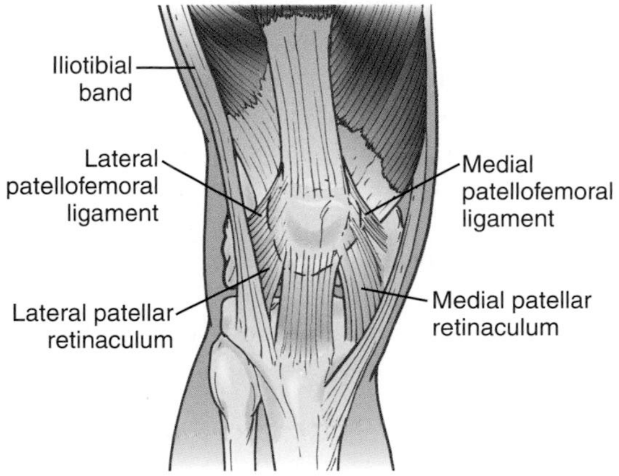

FIGURE 11-4 ■ Patellar retinaculum and the medial and lateral patellofemoral ligaments.

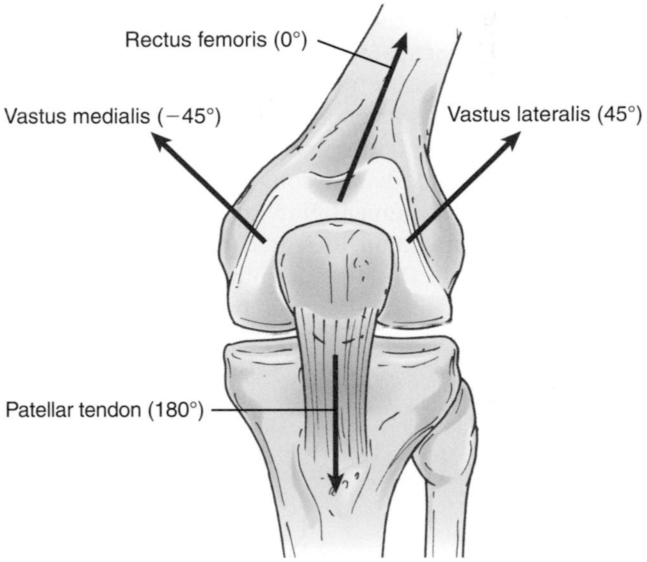

FIGURE 11-5 ■ Line of pull (vectors) placed on the patella during quadriceps contraction.

ligament (MPFL) is a primary restraint against lateral patellar displacement, especially in the lateral inferior direction.[13-15] A band of the MPFL often shares common fibers with the knee's medial collateral ligament.[16]

Muscular Anatomy and Related Soft Tissues

The muscles of the quadriceps femoris merge distally to form the quadriceps tendon and attach on the patella's superior pole. During flexion, the patella is pulled inferiorly by the patellar tendon's attachment to the tibial tuberosity. During extension, the quadriceps femoris and its tendon pull the patella superiorly (Fig. 11-5).

Normally, the length of the patellar tendon is approximately the same as the long axis of the patella (±10%) (Fig. 11-6).[15] Abnormally long or short tendons alter the mechanics, and therefore the strength and associated compressive forces, of the extensor mechanism.

The **vastus lateralis** (VL) is the primary muscle pulling the patella laterally. Further lateral tension is derived from

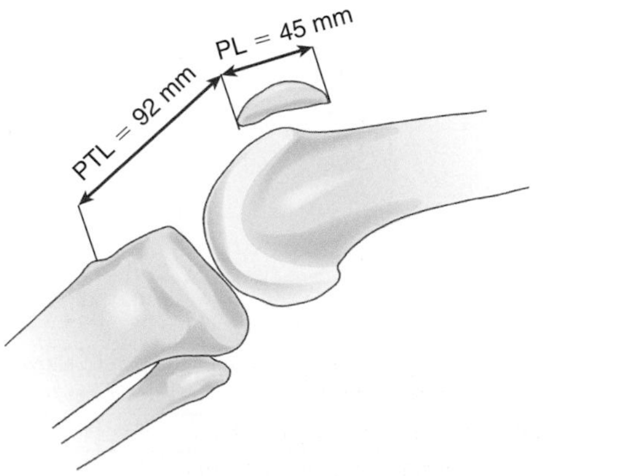

FIGURE 11-6 ■ Calculation of patellar tendon length (drawn from a radiograph) demonstrating a high-riding patella (patella alta). PTL = patellar tendon length; PL = patellar length.

slips arising from the IT band and attaching to the lateral patellar restraints. Tightness of the IT band can accentuate the lateral tracking of the patella because of its attachment to the retinaculum, resulting in subluxations or patellar malalignment.

Medially, the **oblique fibers of the vastus medialis** (VMO) approach the patella at a 55-degree angle, guiding the patella medially and proximally, preventing lateral patellar subluxation. Wide individual differences in the orientation and medial tracking functions of the VMO have been described.[17,18] The adductor magnus, serving as part of the origin of the VMO and medial retinaculum, may have a secondary function in limiting the amount of lateral patellar tracking.[19,20]

Normal flexibility and strength ratios between the quadriceps, triceps surae, and hamstring muscle groups are needed to provide adequate knee ROM and normal patellofemoral mechanics (Box 11-1).[21] Decreased quadriceps length relative to the hamstrings increases the risk factor for developing patellofemoral pain by increasing lateral patellar tilt and causing the patella to track laterally.[5,22] Tightness of the gastrocnemius or soleus muscle may prohibit the 10 degrees of dorsiflexion required while walking and the 15 degrees of dorsiflexion required when running. The most common compensation for a lack of dorsiflexion is excessive foot pronation. Increased foot pronation causes internal rotation of the hip and femur which moves the patella medially. This more medial position of the patella results in an increased dynamic Q-angle and increased lateral force on the patella (refer to Fig. 11-12).[10,23]

Box 11-1
Patellofemoral Mechanics

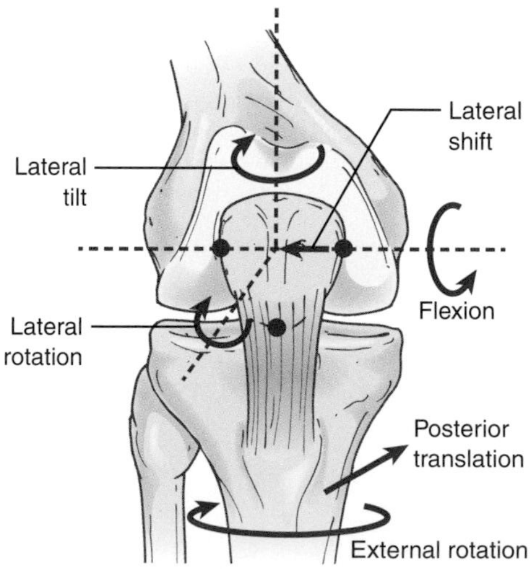

The relatively unconstrained nature of the patella allows it to move in all planes. Patellar glide (or shift) describes medial and lateral movement in the frontal plane. Tilt describes anterior and posterior movement (with the medial side moving posteriorly when the lateral side moves anteriorly and vice versa) around a longitudinal axis. Rotation describes turning around an anterior/posterior axis.

Bursae of the Extensor Mechanism

Anatomic differences and varying biomechanics from individual to individual result in varying numbers of bursae forming within the extensor mechanism. However, four bursae are consistently found throughout the population (Fig. 11-7). Lying deep at the distal end of the quadriceps femoris muscle group and allowing free movement over the distal femur, the **suprapatellar bursa** is an extension of the knee's joint capsule. This bursa is held in place by the articularis genus muscle. The **prepatellar bursa** overlies the anterior portion of the patella and allows the patella to move freely beneath the skin. The distal portion of the patellar tendon and tibial tuberosity receives protection against friction and blows by the **subcutaneous infrapatellar bursa**. The **deep infrapatellar bursa** is located between the tendon and the tibia.

The **infrapatellar fat pad**, one of three fat pads located in the anterior knee compartment, is intracapsular but extrasynovial. Covered by a synovial membrane posteriorly, the infrapatellar fat pad separates the patellar tendon and the deep infrapatellar bursa from the joint capsule of the knee and extends posteriorly to fill the anterior joint line of the tibiofemoral joint.[24] The infrapatellar fat pad can be injured, inflamed, or fibrotic secondary to patellar dislocation, surgery, or synovitis.[24]

Clinical Examination of the Patellofemoral Joint

Patellofemoral joint evaluation often necessitates examination of the back, hip, lower leg, ankle, and foot. Dysfunction of the joints superior or inferior to the knee may result in patellofemoral pain. Pain originating from the lumbar spine can alter posture and gait mechanics, increasing or

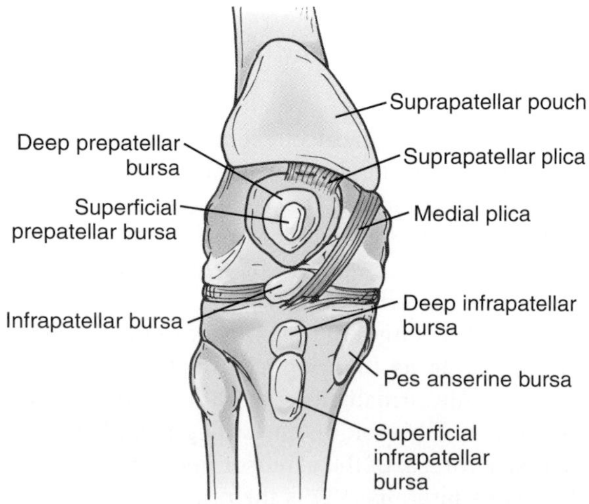

FIGURE 11-7 ■ Bursae and plicae about the knee joint (anterior view, right knee).

Examination Map

HISTORY

Past Medical History

History of the Present Condition

FUNCTIONAL ASSESSMENT

Gait Analysis

INSPECTION

Patella Alignment
- Normal
- Patella alta
- Patella baja
- Squinting
- "Frog eyed"

Patellar Orientation
- Medial/lateral glide
- Spin
- Anterior/posterior tilt
- Medial/lateral tilt

Lower Extremity Posture
- Genu varum
- Genu valgum
- Genu recurvatum

Q-Angle

Patellar Tendon

Tubercle Sulcus Angle

Leg-Length Difference

Foot Posture

PALPATION

Palpation of the Anterior Structures
- Tibial tuberosity
- Patellar tendon
- Patellar bursae
  - Subcutaneous infrapatellar
  - Deep infrapatellar
- Fat pads
- Patellar articulating surface
- Femoral trochlea
- Suprapatellar bursa
- Medial patellofemoral ligament
- Medial patellar retinaculum
- Synovial plica
- Lateral patellar retinaculum
- Pes anserine insertion
- Iliotibial band

JOINT AND MUSCLE FUNCTION ASSESSMENT

Goniometry
- Knee flexion
- Knee extension

Active Range of Motion
- Knee flexion
- Knee extension

Manual Muscle Tests
- Knee extension
- Knee flexion
- Isolating the sartorius

Passive Range of Motion
- Flexion
- Extension

JOINT STABILITY TESTS

Stress Testing

Testing of the major knee ligaments may be indicated.

Joint Play Assessment
- Medial patellar glide
- Lateral patellar glide
- Patellar tilt
- Patellar spin

Selective Tissue Tests
- Ober test
- Navicular drop test

NEUROLOGICAL EXAMINATION

Lower Quarter Screen

Common Peroneal Nerve Assessment

VASCULAR EXAMINATION

Distal Capillary Refill

Distal Pulse
- Posterior tibial artery
- Dorsal pedal artery

REGION-SPECIFIC PATHOLOGIES AND SELECTIVE TISSUE TESTS

Patellofemoral Pain Syndrome

Patellofemoral Instability
- Apprehension test
- Patellar Dislocation

Patellofemoral Tendinopathy
- Apophysitis
- Osgood-Schlatter disease
- Sinding-Larsen-Johansson disease
- Patellofemoral bursitis
- Synovial plica

Traumatic Conditions
- Patellar fracture
- Patellar tendon rupture

altering patellofemoral stresses. To meet this need, have the patient dress in shorts and bring his or her casual and competitive footwear to the examination.

History

Many patellofemoral joint pathologies can be the result of overuse stresses, structural abnormalities, or biomechanical deficiencies of the lower extremity. However, several acute traumatic conditions can affect the patella and the extensor mechanism. The use of region-specific or general outcome measures (see Section Opener, p. 167) help determine the impact of the condition on the patient's life and are critical to establish a baseline and to measure the effectiveness of interventions. For example, patients with patellofemoral pain syndrome (PFPS) who scored worse on the region-specific Kujala Patellofemoral Score were associated with a poorer prognosis regardless of examination findings.[25]

Past Medical History

Question the patient regarding a family history of patellofemoral pain or osteoarthritis (OA). Meniscal tears, anterior cruciate ligament (ACL) tears, posterior cruciate ligament (PCL) tears, and other trauma to the knee may result in tibiofemoral OA, but a history of these conditions may not significantly influence patellofemoral joint degeneration.[26]

- **Relevant past history:** Prior injuries to the lower extremity commonly alter the biomechanics of the extensor mechanism. Question the patient and review the medical file to identify conditions such as foot pathologies, recurrent ankle sprains, Achilles tendon pathology, knee sprains, injury to the hip, OA, or conditions involving the lumbar region. Prior injury to the opposite limb may result in compensatory motion of the currently involved knee.
- **Previous history of patellofemoral conditions:** Question the patient regarding a past history of dislocations, patellofemoral pain, and/or surgery.
- **History of injury to the knee:** Ligamentous and meniscal knee injuries can result in biomechanical changes of the patellofemoral joint. Prior knee surgery can result in inflammation, adhesion, or entrapment of the patella's restraints, resulting in painful movement and reduced ROM.[27] Use of patellar tendon grafts for ACL reconstruction can result in residual changes in patellofemoral joint mechanics.
- **History of hip pathologies:** Pain may also be referred to the knee secondary to **Legg-Calvé-Perthes disease** or a **slipped capital femoral epiphysis** (see Chapter 12).

History of the Present Condition

Identify the duration and intensity of the pain, functional limitations, and resulting disability. Patients describing more subjective symptoms and having more functional limitations are more apt to have an associated cartilage defect.[28]

- **Mechanism and onset of injury:** Determine if the chief complaint is the result of a single traumatic episode or if it stems from a gradual progression of symptoms.
  - **Acute onset:** Contusions and fractures may result from direct blows. A rupture or tearing of the patellar tendon is caused by dynamic overload of the musculotendinous unit. A dislocated patella has an acute onset, but repeated subtle subluxations represent chronic instability.
  - **Chronic or insidious onset:** Low-energy repetitive trauma, such as that associated with walking and running, can magnify the impact of patellofemoral maltracking and also lead to tendinopathy, bursitis, fat pad syndrome (**Hoffa's disease**), or chronic patellar instability (Box 11-2).
- **When pain occurs:** For chronic conditions, questions focus on when the pain occurs throughout the day, which activities cause its onset, and how these symptoms affect the level of activity. Activities such as ascending or descending stairs or open-chain knee extension exercises through the full ROM increase compressive forces of the patella on the knee.[33] Pain occurring after prolonged periods of sitting, the "movie sign" ("theater sign"), may arise from prolonged pressure being placed on one or more articular facets. Descriptions of the knee as "locking" or "giving way" require follow-up for more details to determine the underlying cause. A distinction must be made between true locking of the knee and "clicking" beneath the patella. True locking of the knee is not normally indicative of patellofemoral pathology but, rather, of meniscal tears or an intra-articular loose

Box 11-2
Chondromalacia Patella

Although often referred to and treated as a discernible ailment, chondromalacia patella (CP) is best thought of as a finding related to a more distinct pathology. Chondromalacia patella is the softening and subsequent erosion of the patella's hyaline cartilage. This malady presents itself as grinding beneath the patella and may cause related swelling and pain. It is confirmed only via visual inspection during arthroscopy. CP is nebulous in nature because it is often found incidentally in otherwise normal knees.[6,29] Likewise, many individuals describing these symptoms before surgery have no signs of CP at the time of arthroscopy.[30-32]

CP is most often, if not always, the result of biomechanical changes affecting the lower extremity. As such, chondromalacia may be treated symptomatically, but the key to its remedy is determining and correcting the underlying pathology.

body. Reports of the knee's giving way may be the result of patellar subluxation, inhibition secondary to pain, or internal derangement of the knee.

- **Location of the pain:** Pain radiating medially or laterally from the patella may indicate restricted or excessive glide within the trochlea or an abnormal patellar orientation causing atypical compression of the facets. Insidious patellar pain may also be indicative of knee OA.[34] Posterior knee pain is a common complaint associated with synovitis, but the pain may radiate to any area of the knee.
- **Level of activity:** Any changes in the level of activity, a change in the surface on which the activity occurs, or any other change in physical demand (e.g., as occurs in changing from playing first base to playing catcher or from bicycling to running) must be determined. Each of these may place excessive or unaccustomed forces on the patellofemoral joint.
- **Other biomechanical changes:** Many different factors can influence patellofemoral joint mechanics and resulting compressive forces.
  - Has the patient changed the type of footwear for exercising? For example, switching from a running shoe designed to control pronatory forces to a running shoe with a softer midsole may magnify the impact of excessive pronation.
  - Are the patient's running shoes too old? Excessively worn shoes can lose their orthotic capacity and alter the mechanics of the patellofemoral joint.
  - Has the patient recently gained weight? Weight gain such as seen with obesity or pregnancy is a predisposing factor for secondary arthritis of the knee and increases compressive forces on the patellofemoral articular surfaces during gait.

Functional Assessment

- Ask the patient to replicate those functional tasks that exacerbate the symptoms and observe for compensations, lack of hip control, and strategies to minimize pain.[35] A dynamic valgus force—with its resulting lateral forces on the patellofemoral joint—occurs when the patient cannot control adduction and internal rotation during functional tasks.[10] Patients with patellofemoral pain or patellar tendinopathy pain often complain of pain in the midrange of motion and with eccentric loading, such as when descending stairs, squatting, or landing from a jump.[6,10]
- Patellar motion and function differ between open and closed kinetic chain activities, so the patient may report different complaints when squatting than when kicking a ball. Isokinetic knee testing for patients suffering from acute patellofemoral pain may be contraindicated because of the increased compressive forces placed on the patella at slower speeds.[36]

Inspection

Examine the entire knee complex for signs of gross deformity, including patellar malalignment, dislocation, and the integrity of the patellar tendon. Patellar alignment and orientation should be examined twice, once with the quadriceps relaxed and again with the quadriceps contracted. The patellofemoral joint should also be assessed with the patient weight bearing.

✱ Practical Evidence

Approximately half of the patients describing patellofemoral pain will have normal patellar alignment when the quadriceps are relaxed but will display malalignment when the quadriceps are contracted.[37]

Patellar Position

The extent to which patellar position influences the development of anterior knee pain is debatable, likely to high variability among those with and without pain and the difficulty in obtaining reliable findings.[38-40]

- **Patellar alignment:** With the knee fully extended and the patient weight bearing, observe the patella for alignment, at approximately the center of the femur, with the inferior pole located at the upper margin of the femoral trochlea (Fig. 11-8). Observe for possible malalignment while the lower extremity is weight bearing (Inspection Findings 11-1). Clinically, patella alta—a high-riding patella—may be identified via the camel sign (Fig. 11-9). Atypical alignment or orientation of the patella can increase the rate of erosion of the patellar and/or femoral articulating surfaces.[41]
- **Patellar orientation:** Clinical examination of the resting position of the patella on the femur provides gross evidence of the patella's orientation within the trochlea and on the femur (Inspection Findings 11-2).[38] The clinical examination of static patellar orientation has questionable validity when compared with MRI findings,[42] fair-to-good intrarater reliability, and poor interrater reliability.[37,39] More precise measurements of

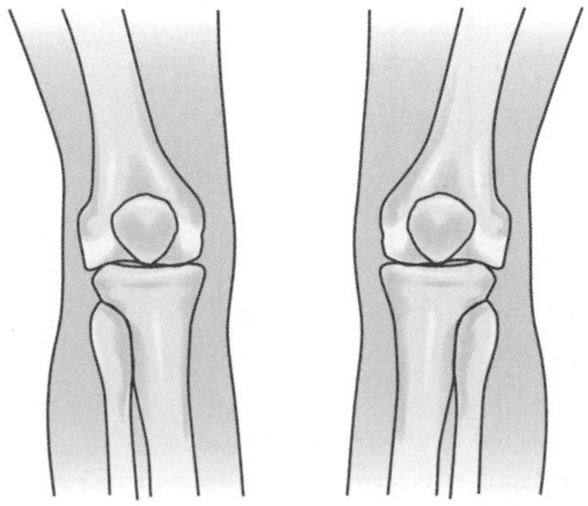

FIGURE 11-8 ■ Normal patellar alignment with the knee extended.

Inspection Findings 11-1
Patellar Alignment

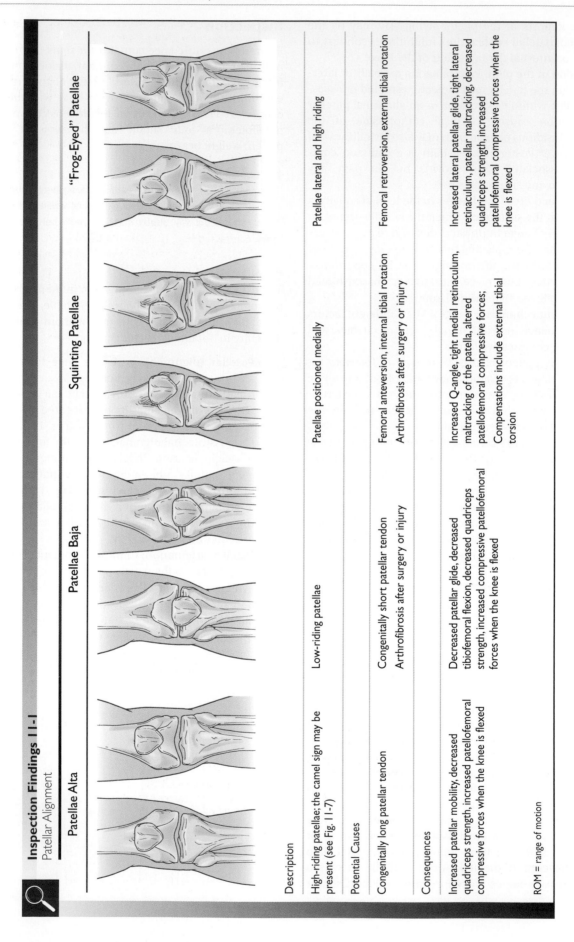

Patellae Alta	Patellae Baja	Squinting Patellae	"Frog-Eyed" Patellae
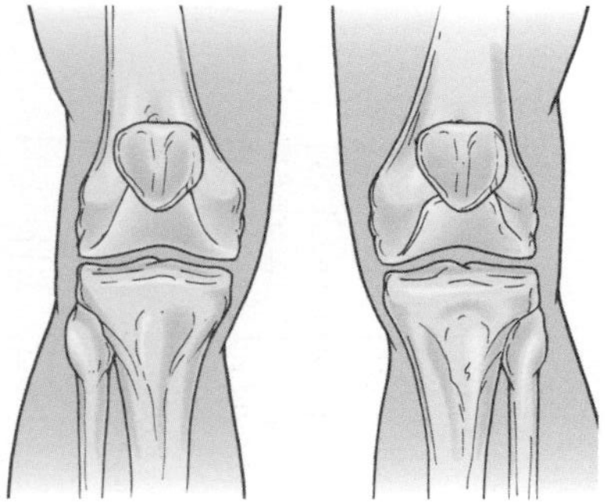	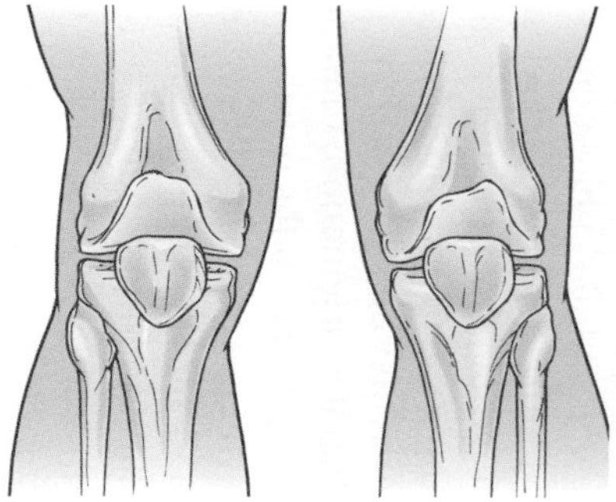	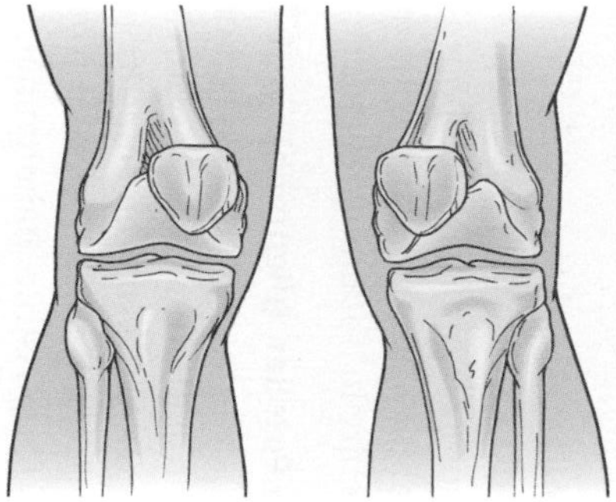	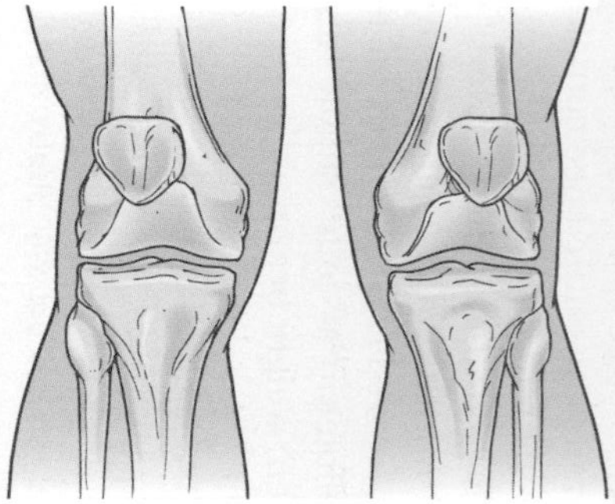
Description			
High-riding patellae; the camel sign may be present (see Fig. 11-7)	Low-riding patellae	Patellae positioned medially	Patellae lateral and high riding
Potential Causes			
Congenitally long patellar tendon	Congenitally short patellar tendon Arthrofibrosis after surgery or injury	Femoral anteversion, internal tibial rotation Arthrofibrosis after surgery or injury	Femoral retroversion, external tibial rotation
Consequences			
Increased patellar mobility, decreased quadriceps strength, increased patellofemoral compressive forces when the knee is flexed	Decreased patellar glide, decreased tibiofemoral flexion, decreased quadriceps strength, increased compressive patellofemoral forces when the knee is flexed	Increased Q-angle, tight medial retinaculum, maltracking of the patella, altered patellofemoral compressive forces; Compensations include external tibial torsion	Increased lateral patellar glide, tight lateral retinaculum, patellar maltracking, decreased quadriceps strength, increased patellofemoral compressive forces when the knee is flexed

ROM = range of motion

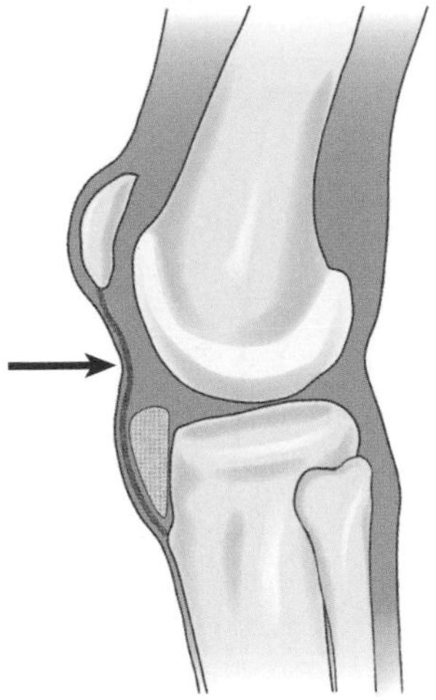

FIGURE 11-9 ■ "Camel sign," a clinical indication of patella alta. The high-riding patella exposes the fat pad, forming a "double hump" when viewed from the lateral side.

patellar orientation can be determined using various radiographic techniques.[42,43]

Inspection of the Lower Extremity

The effects of the surrounding soft tissues on patellar position occur in three dimensions. Changing the tibiofemoral angle causes the patella to rotate about its long axis. A varus alignment causes lateral rotation, increasing pressure between the lateral facet and the lateral femoral trochlea. A valgus alignment causes medial rotation and increased pressure on the odd and medial facets (Table 11-1).

- **Posture of the lower extremity:** Inspect the lower extremities for the presence of the following alignments, which are also described in Chapter 6:
  - **Genu varum** positions the patella more medially.
  - **Genu valgum** causes excessive lateral forces.
  - **Genu recurvatum** places additional pressure on the superior articular surfaces. The articulation may also be hypermobile as the patella distracts from the femur.[44]

Inspection Findings 11-2
Patellar Orientation

Medial/Lateral Patellar Glide	Patellar Rotation (Spin)	Anterior/Posterior Patellar Tilt	Medial/Lateral Patellar Tilt
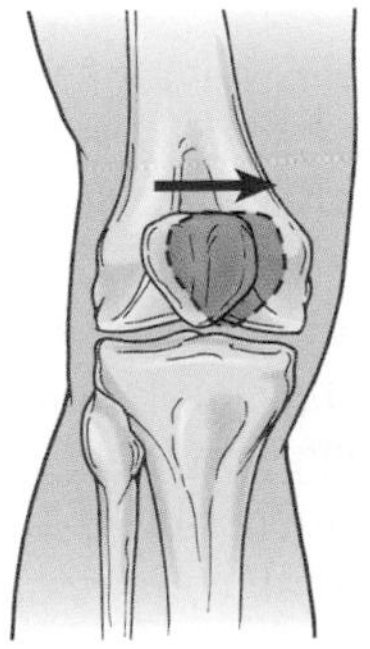	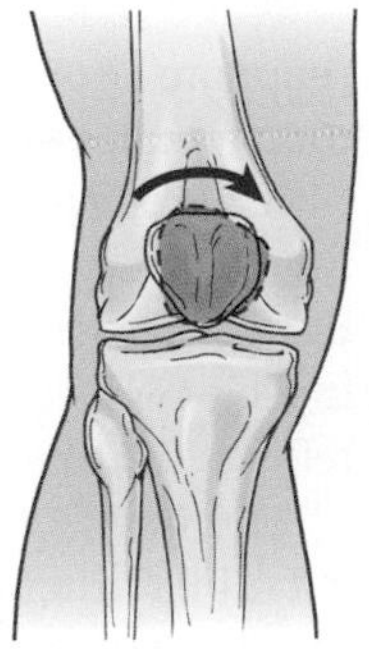	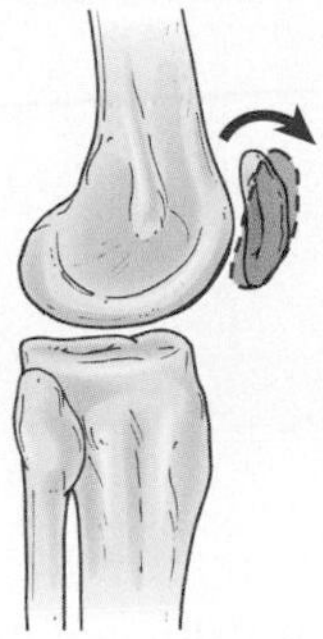	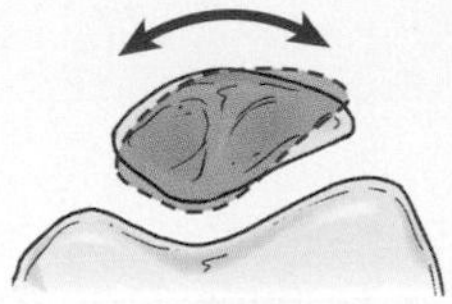
Description			
Position of the patella in the frontal plane	The longitudinal (superior to inferior pole) orientation in the frontal plane	Rotation in the sagittal plane	Rotation in the transverse plane
Evaluation of Alignment			
The patella should be centered between the medial and lateral patellar condyles. Displacement is described in the direction to which the patella is shifted. See Joint Play 11-1.	The long axis of the patella should be directed toward the ASIS. If the long axis is directed lateral to the ASIS, then the patella is laterally rotated and vice versa.	The inferior patellar pole should be palpable when the knee is extended and the quadriceps are relaxed. The patella is anteriorly rotated if the superior pole of the patella must be depressed to make the inferior pole palpable.	See Joint Play 11-2.

ASIS = anterior superior iliac spine

Table 11-1	Structural Alignment and the Resulting Forces and Biomechanical Changes
Alignment	Resulting Forces and Biomechanical Changes
Genu Varum	Increased compressive forces on the medial tibiofemoral articulating surfaces Tensile forces on the lateral tibiofemoral soft tissue structures and LCL Quadriceps exerting medially directed forces on the patella Compressive forces on the lateral facet Stretching of the lateral patellar restraints
Genu Valgum	Increased compressive forces on the lateral tibiofemoral articulating surfaces Tensile forces on the medial tibiofemoral ligaments Quadriceps exerting laterally directed forces on the patella Compressive forces on the odd and medial facets (during knee flexion) Stretching of the medial patellar restraints
Increased Q-Angle or Lax Medial Restraints	Lateral tracking of the patella Compressive forces on the lateral facet Stretching of the medial patellar restraints
Decreased Q-Angle or Lax Lateral Restraints	Medial tracking of the patella Compressive forces on the odd and medial facets Stretching of the lateral patellar restraints
Genu Recurvatum	Decreased compressive forces in terminal knee extension

LCL = lateral collateral ligament

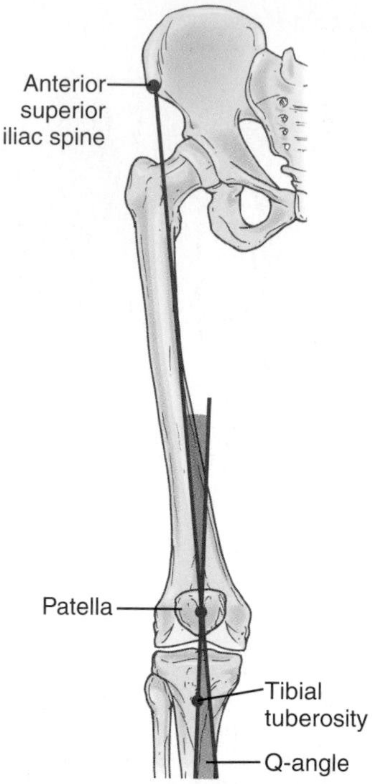

FIGURE 11-10 ■ The Q-angle describes the relationship between the long axis of the femur, measured from the anterior superior iliac spine to the center of the patella, to the long axis of the patella tendon, measured from the midpoint of the patella to the center of the tibial tuberosity.

- **Q-angle:** Determine the approximate tracking of the patella through the measurement of the Q-angle—the relationship between the anterior superior iliac spine, midpoint of the patella, and tibial tuberosity (Fig. 11-10). The Q-angle helps quantify the line of pull of the quadriceps and the patellar tendon and the resultant forces on the patella, but knowing the Q-angle often does little to identify the underlying pathology or influence intervention strategies (Selective Tissue Test 11-1).[45]

The Q-angle typically decreases as the knee is flexed due to the internal tibial rotation that occurs. With the knee extended, the normal Q-angle is approximately 13 degrees for men and 18 degrees for women, although there is variation between studies.[25] The Q-angle appears to be inversely proportional to height. Taller people have lower Q-angles than shorter people. The difference in Q-angle between sexes is therefore probably related to males having longer femurs than females.[49]

A measurement in standing, the functional Q-angle is more representative of the forces that occur in weight bearing.[6] Likewise, isometrically contracting the quadriceps muscle tends to decrease the Q-angle and more accurately reflects the biomechanics of patellar motion.[47]

Multiple factors can cause an increased Q-angle. External tibial rotation increases lateral compression of the patella in the trochlea and causes rotation of the patella in the frontal plane, increasing its susceptibility to subluxation, although evidence suggests that smaller Q-angles may also increase the risk.[50] Internal femoral rotation, resulting from femoral **anteversion**, causes more translational—as opposed to rotational forces—on the patella. Lateral compression of the patellofemoral joint is increased, but the patella is pushed medially.[7] Increased Q-angles increase the forces placed on the lateral patellar facet, medial patellar retinaculum, and lateral border of the femoral trochlea secondary to an increased lateral glide of the patella. The amount of torque produced by the quadriceps muscle group decreases as the Q-angle increases.[51]

A Q-angle that is within normal limits does not necessarily mean that normal forces are present at the patellofemoral

Anteversion A forward bending or angulation of a bone or organ

Selective Tissue Test 11-1
Q-Angle Measurement

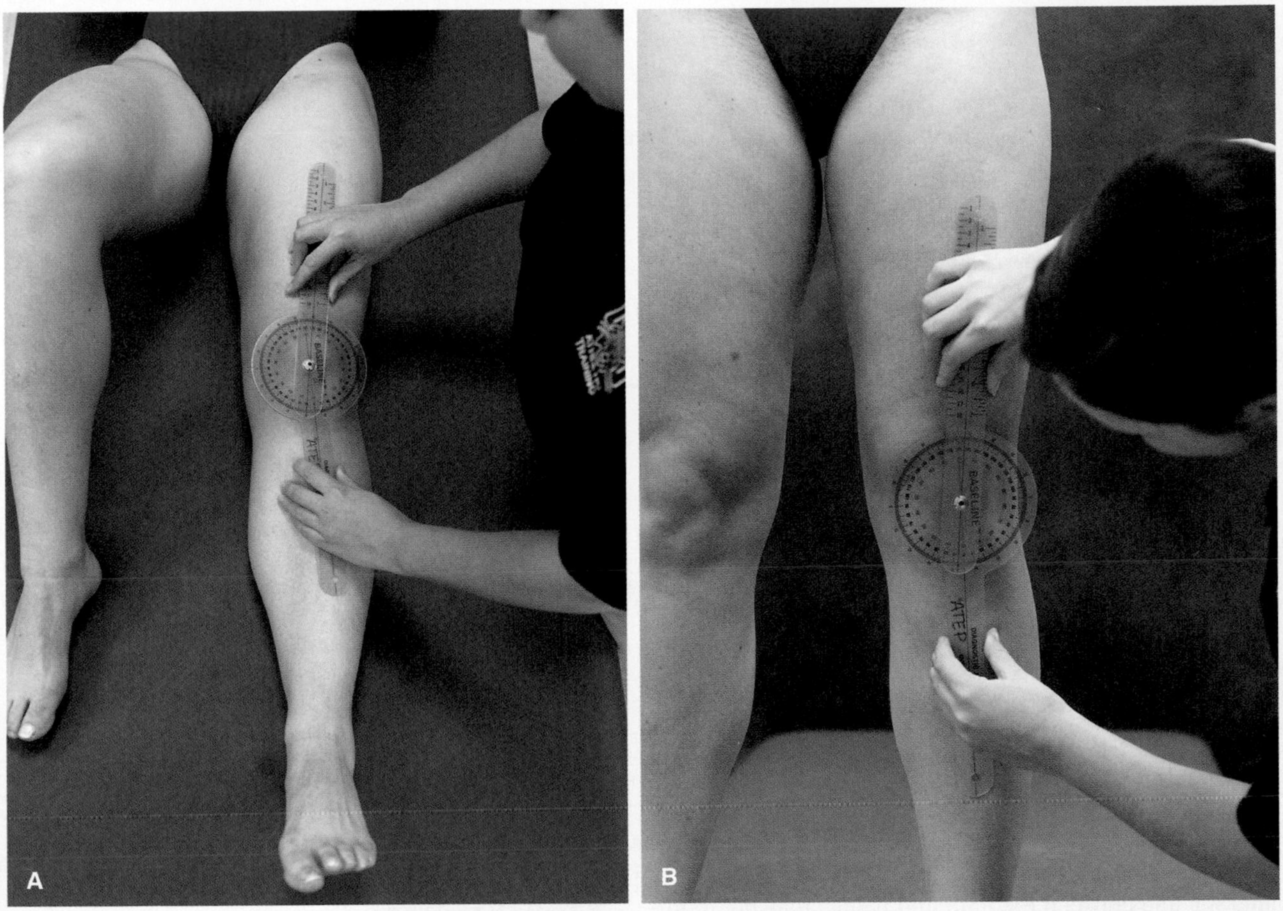

Measurement of the Q-angle with the knee extended in (A) a non–weight-bearing position and (B) weight bearing; the anatomic landmarks of the ASIS, center of the patella, and the tibial tuberosity are used to align the goniometer. Q-angle measurements are most meaningful when they are obtained with the patient weight bearing.

Patient Position	**(A)** Lying supine with the knee fully extended, the ankle in neutral, and the toes pointing up, replicating the standing position. Standardized foot position improves the reliability of this assessment.[46] **(B)** Standing with the feet shoulder-width apart
Position of Examiner	Standing on the side of the limb to be measured
Evaluative Procedure	The examiner identifies and marks the ASIS, the midpoint of the patella, and the tibial tuberosity. A goniometer is placed so that the axis is located over the patellar midpoint, the center of the stationary arm is over the line from the ASIS to the patella, and the moving arm is placed over the line from the patella to the tibial tuberosity.
Positive Test	A Q-angle greater than 13° in men or 18° in women
Implications	Increased lateral forces leading to a laterally tracking patella
Modification	Remeasure the Q-angle with the quadriceps isometrically contracted. Differences between the two measures may provide insight to patellar tracking abnormalities.[47] The Q-angle may be measured with the knee in 30° of flexion, centering the patella within the femoral trochlea.

Continued

Selective Tissue Test 11-1
Q-Angle Measurement—cont'd

Comments	Measurement of the Q-angle with the patient standing better replicates the functional alignment of the lower extremity.[45] The Q-angle measured with the patient short-sitting should be smaller than measures obtained with the patient standing or long-sitting. When correlated with radiographic Q-angle measurements, clinical measurements routinely overestimate the angle.[48] Q-angle should be measured bilaterally, as asymmetry may increase the risk of running injury.[25]
Evidence	*Supine*

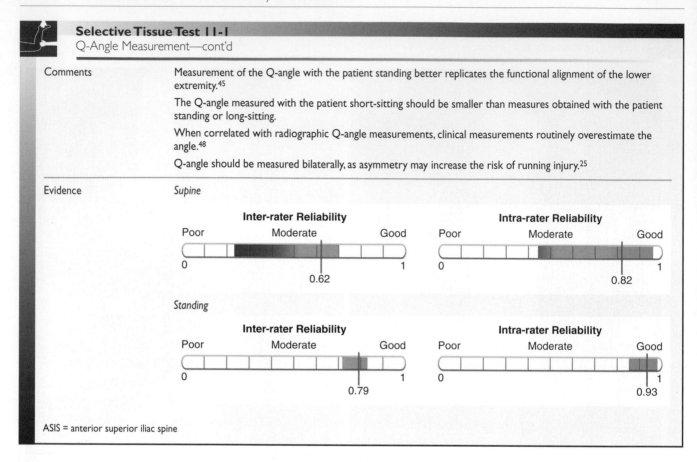

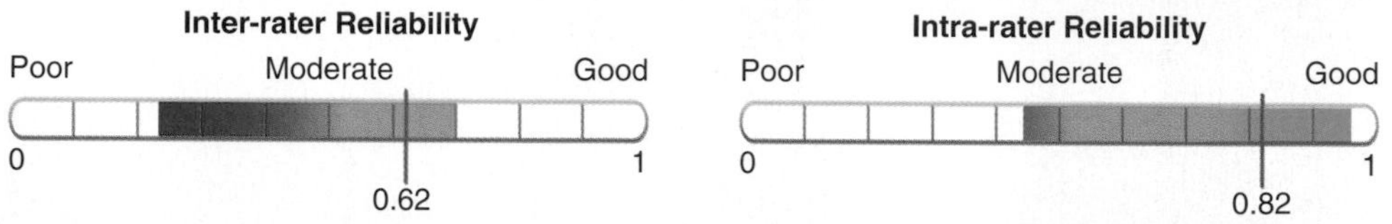

Standing

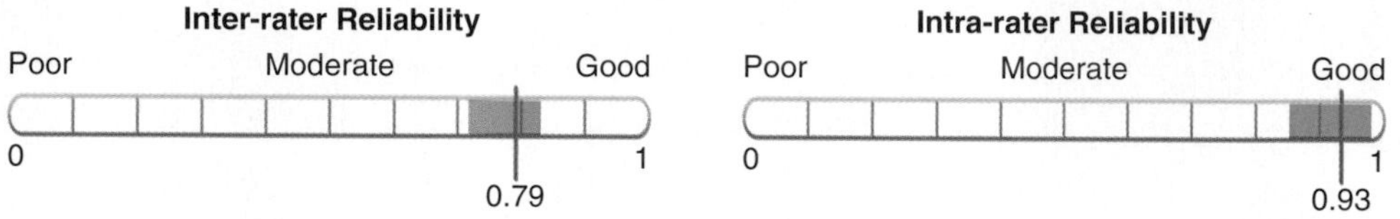

ASIS = anterior superior iliac spine

joint. The line between the ASIS and patella may not represent the line of pull of the quadriceps due to variations in timing and strength imbalances. A patella that is laterally positioned due to tight lateral structures may result in a Q-angle measurement that is within normal limits.

✱ Practical Evidence

A bilateral difference in Q-angle of more than 4 degrees predisposes runners to lower leg injury. A Q-angle of more than 20 degrees also results in a greater risk of injury.[25]

- **Patellar tendon:** Inspect the length of the patellar tendon, noting for signs of inflammation or other defects. An inflamed infrapatellar fat pad may cause bulging from beneath either side of the tendon.
- **Tubercle sulcus angle:** With the patient short sitting, observe the relationship between the tibial tuberosity and the inferior patellar pole. If the tuberosity is more than 10 degrees lateral to the inferior pole, the patient is predisposed to lateral patellar tracking (Fig. 11-11). Note that this alignment will also result in an increased Q-angle.
- **Leg-length difference:** Structural or functional leg-length differences can affect the extensor mechanism and influence patellar tracking. Refer to Chapter 6 for methods of determining the presence of structural and functional leg-length differences.

✱ Practical Evidence

Instrumented measurement demonstrating unequal heights of the anterior superior iliac spine is 83% accurate in predicting patients who will demonstrate patellofemoral pain from those who will not and is more reliable than leg-length discrepancies identified using a tape measure.[52]

- **Foot posture:** Observe the position of the foot. While the patient is weight bearing, the foot should maintain a neutral or slightly pronated position. Excessive pronation results in internal tibial rotation, and excessive supination results in external tibial rotation. Pronation of one foot and supination of the other indicates a leg-length discrepancy, with the supinated foot representing the shorter leg. A standing leg-length difference can be confirmed if supinating the pronated foot brings the anterior superior iliac spine (ASIS) to an equal level (see Fig. 6.10).
- **Areas of scars, skin disruption, or skin discoloration:** Examine for any scars from previous injury such as lacerations or abrasions or prior knee surgeries. These areas may develop a keloid (see Fig. 1.4) or result in the formation of a neuroma, either of which may be the source of the pain. Because of its superficial location, the prepatellar bursa is predisposed to infections from abrasions or other wounds.

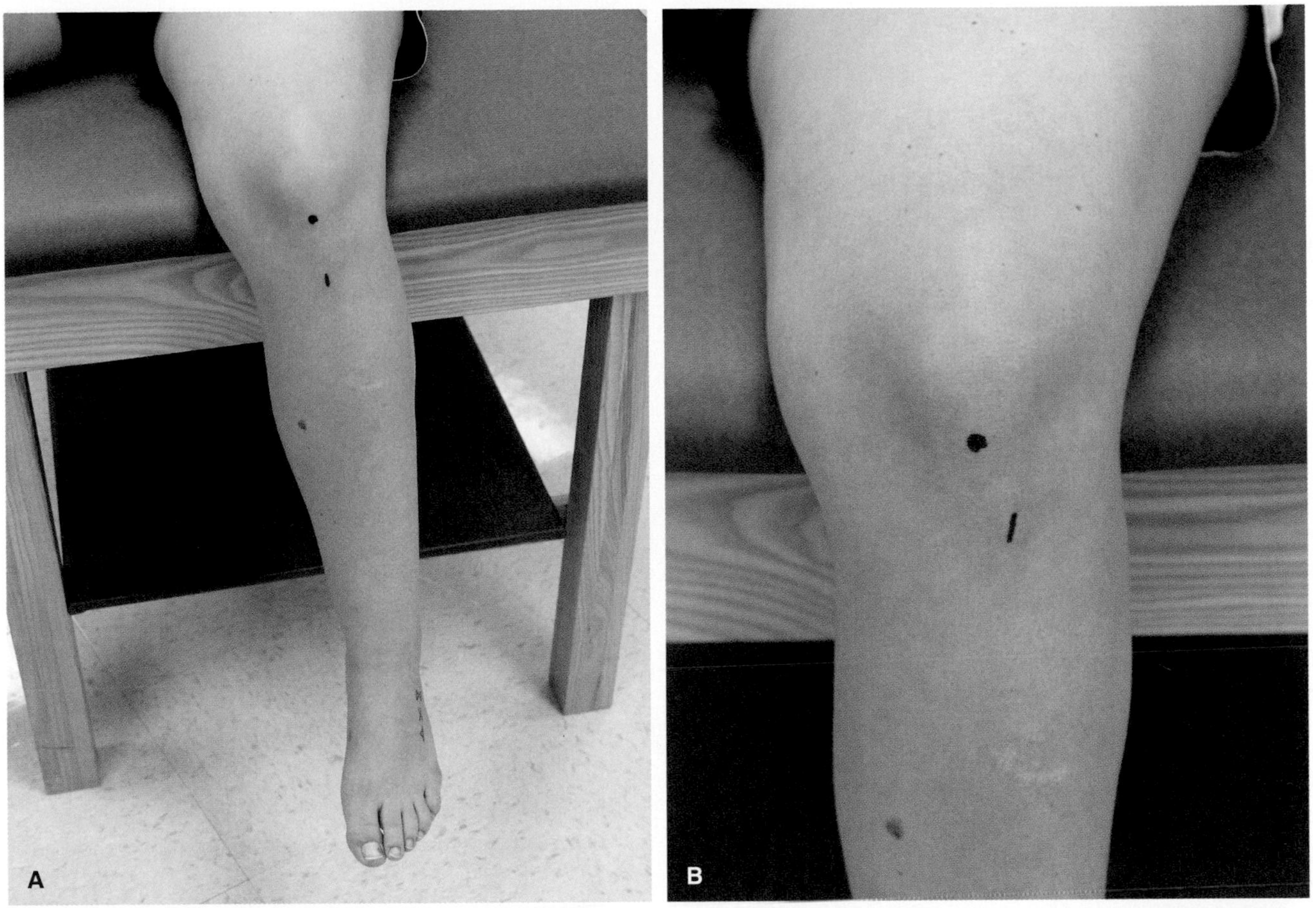

FIGURE 11-11 ■ Tubercle sulcus angle. (A) The tibial tuberosity is positioned inferior to the inferior pole of the patella, demonstrating normal alignment. (B) Laterally positioned tibial tuberosity, increasing lateral tracking of the patella.

PALPATION

Caution is necessary when moving the patella, especially laterally. Patients who have a history of patellar dislocations or subluxations may become fearful or apprehensive about the patella being displaced as it is moved during the examination process. The complete palpation of the patellofemoral articulation must also include the tibiofemoral articulation.

This section describes palpation of the knee and patella only as it relates to patellar dysfunction.

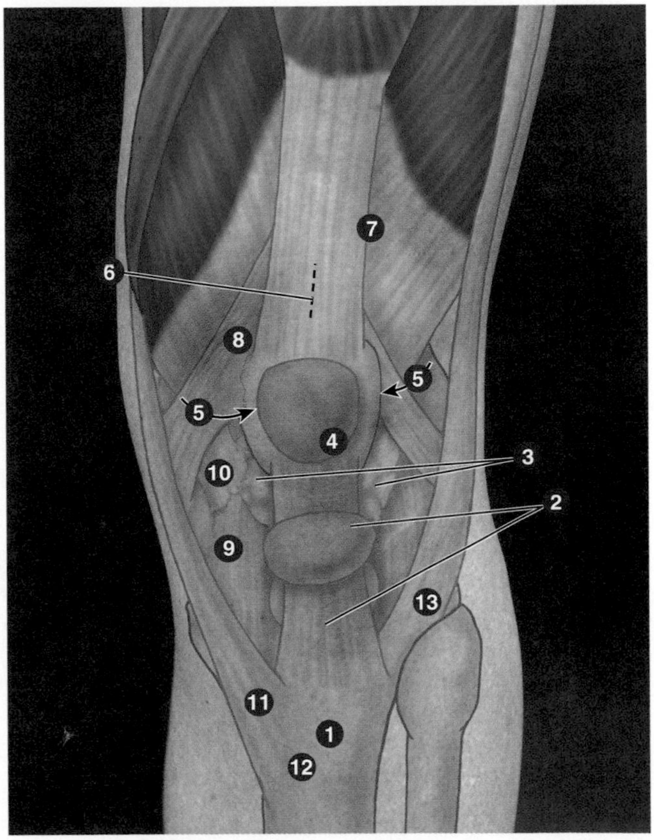

1 Tibial tuberosity: Palpate the tibial tuberosity, identified by the insertion of the patellar tendon. The tibial tuberosity can become tender secondary to patellar tendinopathy or a contusion. Tenderness and enlargement of the tuberosity in adolescent patients may indicate Osgood-Schlatter disease (OSD).

2 Patellar tendon and bursae: Palpate the tendon at the level of the infrapatellar pole, moving distally to the tendon's midsubstance to its insertion at the tibial tuberosity. Pain or thickening detected at the infrapatellar pole through the midsubstance may indicate patellar tendinopathy; pain localized in the midsubstance may reflect tendon pathology. Palpate the **subcutaneous infrapatellar bursa** and **deep infrapatellar bursa** for tenderness, swelling, and the skin's ability to glide freely over the tibial tuberosity.

3 Fat pads: Place the knee in extension to squeeze the fat pads beneath the patellar tendon out to either side, masking the deep infrapatellar bursa from palpation. Palpate these fat pads for signs of inflammation as they exit from behind, medially, and laterally to the patellar tendon, spanning the area from the inferior patellar pole to the tibial tuberosity.[24] Because these structures are highly innervated, they are prone to hypersensitivity during inflammatory conditions; and these symptoms may mimic patellar tendinopathy.

4 Patella and bursae: During palpation of the patella, be alert for pain arising from the bone itself to distinguish it from pain arising from the soft tissue. Palpate the patellar body to rule out the presence of fracture, indicated by pain, roughening, discontinuity, or crepitus. Continue to palpate along the periphery of the four borders, attempting to elicit tenderness secondary to inflammatory conditions. If pain is present at the superior border, palpate up the length of the quadriceps group, noting the point at which the pain disappears. A bipartite patella, although not always identified through palpation, may be present either from previous trauma or a congenital defect (Fig. 11-12).

The **prepatellar bursa** overlies the patella. Ensure that the skin over the patella moves freely and is not painful. The prepatellar bursa may become irritated and inflamed from overuse; from a contusing force to the anterior patella; or from prolonged periods of kneeling, as is seen with wrestlers. This bursa is also a common site of bacterial (e.g., staphylococcal) infection.

5 Patellar articulating surface: With the knee extended, move the patella laterally to expose the outer portion of the lateral articular facet and medially to expose the odd facet. The exposed facets are palpated for signs of tenderness. Exercise caution when moving the patella laterally, as this motion duplicates the mechanism for patellar dislocations and can create patient apprehension.

6 Femoral trochlea: In the patella's resting position on an extended knee, palpate the medial and lateral femoral trochlear borders for tenderness, keeping in mind that the lateral border is more exposed than the medial border is. Moving the patella medially and laterally exposes more of the femoral articular surface.

Compressing the patella and moving it against the femur may produce a grinding sensation. Because this is present in symptomatic and asymptomatic knees, its relevance is limited.

7 Suprapatellar bursa: Locate the suprapatellar bursa under the quadriceps group approximately 3 inches (four-finger breadth) above the patella. With the exception of puncture wounds, the suprapatellar bursa is rarely injured by direct trauma. It may, however, become inflamed or enlarged secondary to effusion of the knee joint capsule.

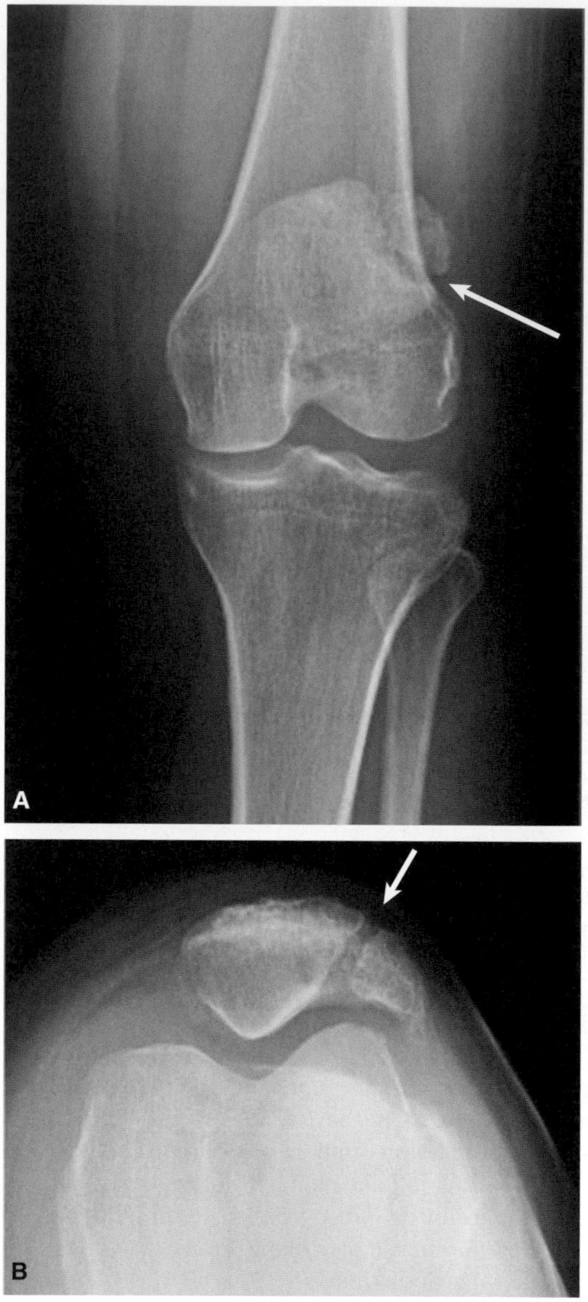

FIGURE 11-12 ■ (A) Anterior view of a bipartite patella of the left knee. (B) Merchant view of the patella. Note the discrepancy in the continuity of the left and right patellae. Image courtesy of Akira Murakami, MD. Boston Medical Center.

8 Medial patellofemoral ligament: Palpate the length of the MPFL from the femur's adductor tubercle and MCL to the superomedial aspect of the patella. This structure will become tender after acute dislocation of the patella.

9 Retinacular and capsular structures: Palpate the medial and lateral retinacula, patellofemoral ligaments, and capsule for pain. The retinaculum and the associated structures may become painful with patellar hypermobility.

10 Synovial plica: Palpate the anteromedial and anterolateral joint capsule for bands of thickened or folded tissue, denoting a synovial plica. These areas may become irritated and inflamed from being rubbed across bony structures or other tissues.

11-13 Related structures: The **(11) pes anserine muscle group** and its associated bursae in the area of the medial tibial flare are common sites of inflammation. Hypersensitivity of one or more nerves can result in pain radiating through the knee and lower extremity. A neuroma, most commonly occurring from laceration of nerves during surgery involving the **(12) infrapatellar branch of the saphenous nerve**, may be confirmed via a test for Tinel's sign over the medial aspect of the knee. Determine the extensibility of the **(13) IT band** because tightness of this structure serves to increase the amount of lateral patellar tracking. Trigger points can be found in the IT band, causing tightness along its entire length.

Joint and Muscle Function Assessment

Unrestricted movement of the patella is required for the lower leg to achieve its full ROM. Pain at the patella during movement may indicate a malalignment, resulting in soft tissue stretch as well as compressive forces on the articular facets, more so on the medial side. The extent to which discernible malalignment is associated with the development of pathology is debatable.[10] The normal and abnormal movement of the patella as the knee moves from flexion to extension is discussed here. The complete ROM testing of the knee joint is described in Chapter 10, and the hip is presented in Chapter 12.

Active Range of Motion

As the knee moves from flexion into extension, the patella normally glides superiorly and tracks somewhat laterally, creating the **J sign**. Tightness of the lateral structures and hamstrings accentuates the lateral glide and tilt of the patella.[5] During flexion, the patella glides inferiorly and medially as it situates itself in the femoral trochlea. The **reverse J sign** occurs when tight medial restraints pull the patella medially during terminal extension.

Manual Muscle Testing

Strength assessment of the quadriceps and hamstrings at the knee joint is described in Chapter 10. Weakness of the hip extensors, abductors, and external rotators such as gluteus maximus and medius is frequently implicated in patellofemoral pathology, as these muscles eccentrically control the internal rotation and adduction of the lower extremity that occurs during the stance phase of gait.[35,54] Weakness of these muscles could result in excessive internal rotation and adduction that causes increased lateral forces at the patellofemoral joint.[4,10]

Strength and ROM deficits do not necessarily translate to altered functional biomechanics, and it is unclear if altered patellofemoral biomechanics are the result of hip muscle weakness or vice versa.[54] Improving hip abductor and external rotator function decreases patient-reported symptoms of patellofemoral pain syndrome.[55]

Manual muscle tests of the hip are described in Chapter 12.

Passive Range of Motion

Passively assess motion at the hip, knee, and ankle for joint restrictions. Assess the muscle length of the hamstrings, quadriceps, and triceps surae (see Chapter 6). A limitation in knee flexion with the hip in neutral indicates tightness of the rectus femoris. A limitation in hip flexion with the knee extended indicates insufficient hamstring length, and a limitation in ankle dorsiflexion with the knee fully extended or flexed may indicate tightness in the triceps surae. Decreased gastrocnemius and soleus length, particularly when coupled with decreased strength of the hip abductors, is associated with patellofemoral pain.[56,57] Decreased hamstring flexibility results in increased joint reaction forces at the patellofemoral joint secondary to the added force generated by the quadriceps group.[37]

Joint Stability Tests

The ligamentous and capsular stability of the patella is assessed using patellar tilt and glide. Glide tests are performed to assess the laxity or tightness of the retinacula by assessing how far the patella can be moved passively from its resting position in the trochlea.

Stress Testing

Evaluate all major knee ligaments for normal integrity, as described in Chapter 10. Laxity of the knee joint can result in abnormal patellar tracking secondary to uniplanar or rotatory shifting of the tibia or femur, causing patellofemoral pain.

Joint Play Assessment

The following descriptions of the assessment of patellar glide and tilt have been adapted from the American Academy of Orthopaedic Surgeons' guidelines.[53]

- **Resting position:** Before determining the extent of mobility, the resting position of the patella must be assessed (see Box 11-1).
- **Patellar glide:** To determine the amount of glide, visualize the patella as having four quadrants. Place the knee on a bolster so that it is flexed to 30 degrees. The patient must be fully reclined to relax the quadriceps muscles (Fig. 11-13). To ensure accuracy during the measurements, avoid tilting the patella as it is glided medially and laterally (Joint Play 11-1).
- **Patellar tilt:** The amount of patellar tilt, the rotation of the patella about its longitudinal axis, evaluates the tension within the lateral retinaculum, lateral capsule, IT band, and lateral portion of the quadriceps tendon. Patella tilt is described by the direction that the medial

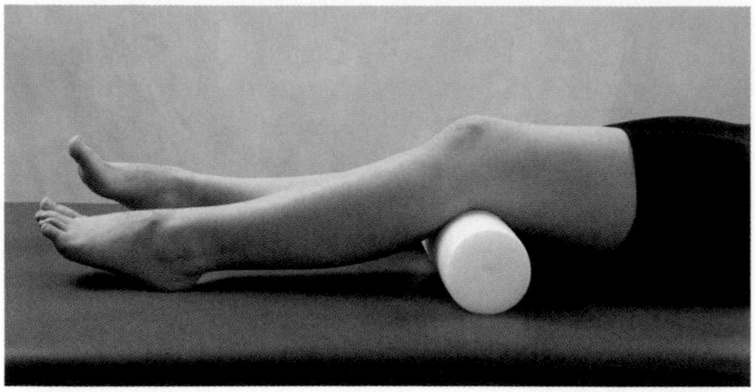

FIGURE 11-13 ■ Positioning of the patient during patellar glide tests. Positioning of the patient during patellar glide tests. The knee is flexed to 30° and the individual is encouraged to keep the quadriceps musculature relaxed.

and lateral borders are positioned. The evaluation is performed with the patient lying supine with the knee extended and the femoral condyles parallel to the table (Joint Play 11-2).

Practical Evidence

A hypomobile medial glide in the presence of a restricted lateral tilt result tends to respond favorably to conservative treatment. A normal patellar tilt test result combined with a hypomobile medial glide may require the surgical release of the lateral retinacular structures to permit proper glide within the trochlea. A negative preoperative patellar tilt result has been positively correlated with a successful outcome of the release of the lateral structures.[53]

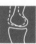

Joint Play 11-1
Medial and Lateral Patellar Glide

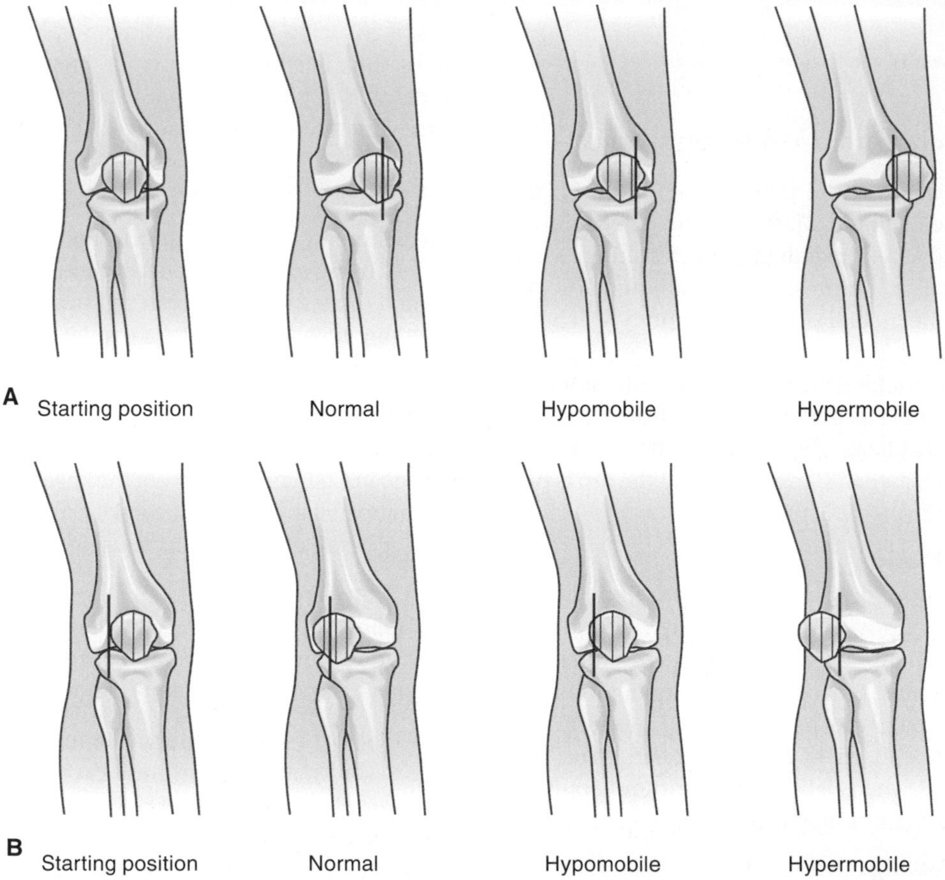

During (A) medial and (B) lateral patellar glide tests, the patella is viewed as having four quadrants. The amount of glide is based on the movement relative to the quadrants.

Patient Position	Supine with a bolster placed under the knee so that it is flexed to 30°
Position of Examiner	Standing lateral to the patient
Evaluative Procedure	**(A)** Medial glide: Move the patella medially, placing stress on the lateral retinaculum and other soft tissue restraints. **(B)** Lateral glide: Move the patella laterally, placing stress on the medial retinaculum, VMO, and medial capsule.

Joint Play 11-1
Medial and Lateral Patellar Glide—cont'd

Positive Test

Medial glide: The patella should glide one to two quadrants (approximately half its width) medially. Movement of less than one quadrant is considered hypomobile. Movement of more than two quadrants is hypermobile medial glide.

Lateral glide: Normal lateral motion is 0.5–2.0 quadrants of glide. Less than that is hypomobile lateral glide; greater than two quadrants is hypermobile lateral glide.

Implications

Medial glide:
Hypomobile glide: Tightness of the lateral retinaculum or IT band
Hypermobile glide: Laxity of the lateral restraints

Lateral glide:
Hypomobile glide: Tightness of the medial restraints, specifically the medial patellofemoral ligament[15]
Hypermobile glide: Laxity of the medial restraints

Comments

The patient may be apprehensive during lateral glide tests, fearful that the motion could result in a patellar dislocation or subluxation.

Hypermobile lateral glide creates a predisposition to patellar dislocations.

Hypomobile medial glide is more common than hypermobile medial glide.

Evidence

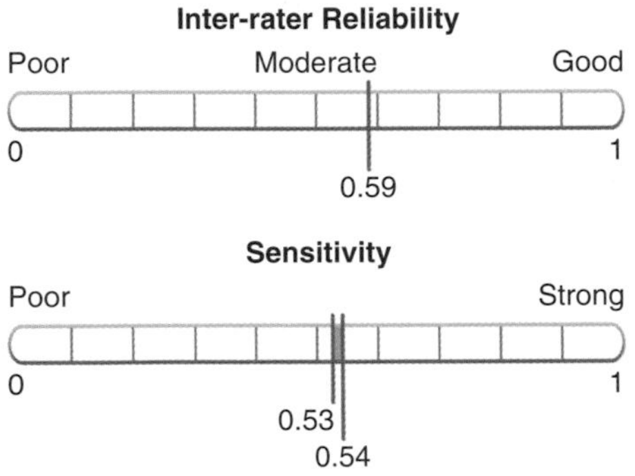

LR+: 1.74–1.96

IT = iliotibial; VMO = vastus medialis oblique

Selective Tissue Tests

IT band tightness is associated with increased lateral tracking secondary to its attachment on the lateral retinaculum. The tension of the IT band can be assessed via the Ober test (Chapter 12). The navicular drop test (Chapter 8) is used to identify excessive pronation. Foot structure, including an assessment of rearfoot and forefoot position (Chapter 8) statically and during gait, is routinely determined with patellofemoral conditions of gradual onset.

Neurological and Vascular Testing

The assessment of the sensory, motor, and reflex function and vascular testing for the patellofemoral joint is the same as described for the knee in Chapter 10.

Hip pathology such as **Legg-Calvé-Perthes disease** or a **slipped capital femoral epiphysis** may refer pain to the knee. A childhood history of these conditions warrants an examination of the hip.

Region-Specific Pathologies and Selective Tissue Tests

The interrelated nature of patellofemoral pathologies makes classification difficult, at best. The nonspecific terms "patellofemoral dysfunction" and "patellofemoral pain syndrome" describe a wide range of knee and patella symptoms, but they do little to reveal the underlying cause of the symptoms.[37] Symptoms range from dull to sharp pain arising from anterior (prepatellar) or posterior (retropatellar) portions of the patella or borders. The working diagnosis of patellofemoral dysfunction is often made for cases of unexplained pain when other more serious soft tissue and bony pathologies have been ruled out.[29,58]

Pain and dysfunction arising from the patellofemoral complex often mimic the symptoms of meniscal injury. Table 11-2 presents subjective findings that are used to differentiate between injuries of the two structures.

Joint Play 11-2
Patellar Tilt Assessment

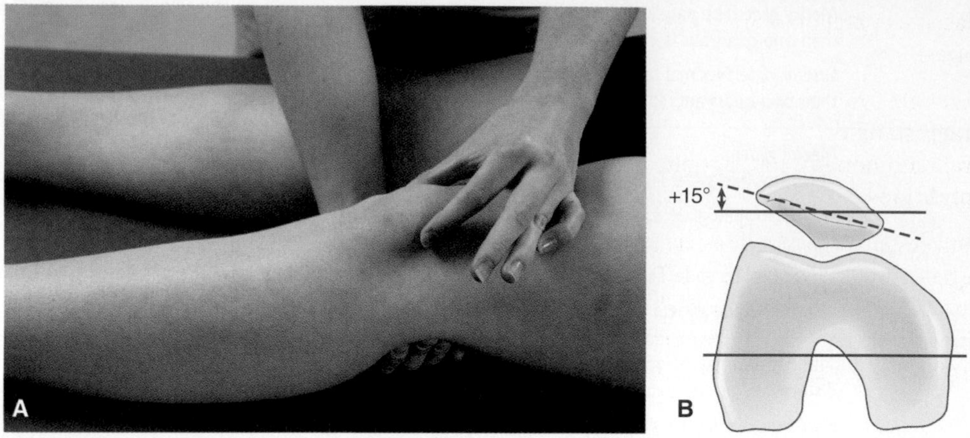

The patellar tilt test evaluates rotation of the patella around its midsagittal axis.

Patient Position	Supine with the knee extended and the femoral condyles parallel to the table
Position of Examiner	Standing lateral to the patient
Evaluative Procedure	Grasp the patella with the forefinger and thumb, elevating the lateral border and depressing the medial border.
Positive Test	A normal result is the lateral border raising between 0° and 15°. More than 15° is a hypermobile lateral tilt; less than 0° is a hypomobile lateral tilt.
Implications	A tilt of less than 0° indicates tightness of the lateral restraints and often occurs in the presence of a hypomobile medial glide. A tilt of more than 15° may predispose the individual to anterior knee pain.
Evidence	

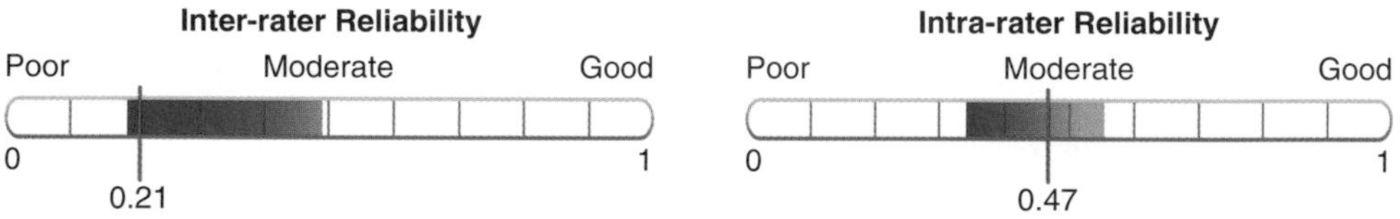

Table 11-2 Differential Diagnosis Between Meniscal and Patellar Pathology

History	Meniscus	Patella
Onset	Usually acute twisting injury; may occur secondary to degenerative changes	Occasionally direct anterior knee blow but usually insidious related to overuse and training errors
Symptom Site	Localized medial or lateral joint line	Diffuse, most commonly anterior
Locking	Frank transient locking episodes with the knee unable to fully terminally extend	Catching without locking, stiffness after immobility
Weight Bearing	Pain sharp and simultaneous with loaded weight bearing	Pain possibly coming on during weight bearing but often continuing into the evening and night
Cutting Sports	Pain with loaded twisting maneuvers	Some pain possible but not sharp or clearly related to cutting
Squatting	Pain at full squat; inability to "duck walk"	Pain when extensors used to descend or rise from a squat
Kneeling	Not painful because meniscus is not weight loaded	Pain from patellar compression
Jumping	Loaded without torque or twist tolerated	Extensors heavily stressed, causing pain on descent impact
Stairs or Hills	Pain often going upstairs with loaded knee flexion, causing compression	More patellar loading and pain going downstairs because gravity-assisted impact increases patellofemoral stress
Sitting	No pain	Stiffness and pain from lack of the distraction-compression effect on abnormal articular cartilage

Patellofemoral pain may also be the result of osteochondral defects of the femur or patellar articulating surface (see Chapters 4 and 10).

This section classifies patellofemoral joint pathology in four major categories:

- Patellofemoral pain syndrome (PPS)
- Patellofemoral instability
- Patellofemoral tendinopathy and apophysitis
- Traumatic conditions

This classification system organizes the examination findings and forms the basis for developing the optimal intervention strategy. For example, treatment for patellofemoral instability must emphasize restoration of dynamic control of the hip and foot to avoid forces that force the patella laterally.

Patellofemoral Pain Syndrome

Patellofemoral pain syndrome (PPS) is a diagnosis of exclusion in patients with anterior knee pain.[58] While the diagnostic criteria for this condition vary widely, there is consensus that development of the condition is multifactorial, with proximal, distal, and local influences contributing to the dysfunction (Fig. 11-14).[10] Locally, patellar tracking is primarily influenced by the geometry of the femur, with abnormal femoral motion altering patellofemoral mechanics. Proximally, insufficient dynamic control of hip adduction and internal rotation results in excessive knee valgus—and subsequent lateral tracking of the patella—during functional tasks. Distally, excessive pronation results in internal rotation of the tibia and creates additional knee valgus.

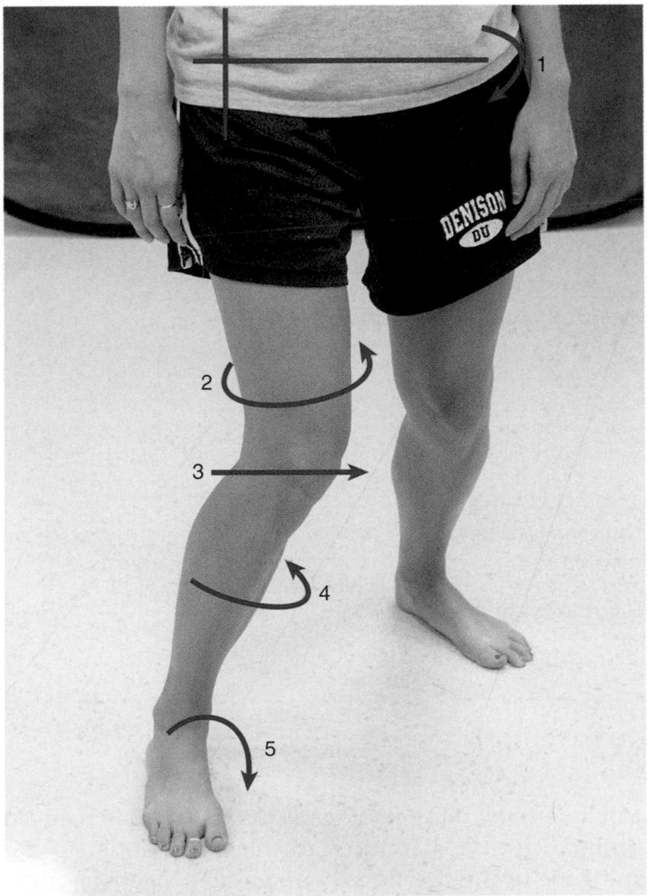

FIGURE 11-14 ■ Contributors of lower extremity segments to abnormal alignment: (1) contralateral pelvic drop, (2) internal rotation of the femur, (3) valgus knee alignment, (4) internal rotation of the tibia, and (5) foot pronation.

Soft tissue adaptations may also influence the development of or result from PPS. For example, a tight IT band creates lateral tension on the patella, influencing its tracking. Effective intervention for PPS is particularly important, as recent evidence suggests that PPS at a younger age is associated with the development of patellofemoral OA later in life.[10]

Many of the predisposing factors for patellofemoral pain syndrome are congenital (see Table 11-1). However, injury to the patella or knee may cause a change in one of the variables. For example, a lateral dislocation of the patella results in tearing of the medial restraints, causing increased laxity and increased lateral migration of the patella during knee extension. Likewise, an injury to the knee can cause atrophy of the VMO, increasing the amount of lateral patellar glide with subsequent shortening of the lateral restraints. Other variables affecting the equation are increased body weight and gait mechanics.[59]

In healthy individuals, the VMO contracts simultaneously with or before vastus lateralis contraction. This contractile pattern results in normal patellar tracking. When the knee is effused, a fluid buildup of 20 to 30 mL of excess fluid neurologically inhibits the VMO. With an effusion of 50 to 60 mL, the rest of the extensor mechanism is inhibited. When the VMO is inhibited, the relatively unopposed pull from the VL can cause excessive lateral tracking and increase compressive forces on the lateral facet.[60] Activation of the VMO is delayed in patients demonstrating the signs and symptoms of patellofemoral pain syndrome and a group of patients who are symptom free.[18]

Patients suffering from patellofemoral pain syndrome describe a gradual onset with symptoms related to an increase or change in activity. Complaints of pain are usually associated with descending stairs, sitting for long periods of time, and other activities in which the knee is flexed for prolonged periods. Occurring more frequently in females, patients may describe "popping" and "clicking," and palpation during active motion will reveal that this is occurring at the patellofemoral articulation. Mild swelling in the peripatellar region may be present (Examination Findings 11-1).

The functional examination may reveal increased and prolonged pronation and an inability to control medial rotation and adduction of the hip when accepting weight during the stance phase of gait. This aberration may become more apparent with fatigue, which associates with increased complaints of pain with a longer duration of activity. Lower extremity internal rotation is also demonstrated when the excessive valgus occurs when stepping

Examination Findings 11-1
Patellofemoral Pain Syndrome

Examination Segment	Clinical Findings
History of Current Condition	*Onset:* Gradual, with typical description of abrupt change in surface, activity level, or activity intensity *Pain characteristics:* Pain arising from the peripatellar area, frequently at lateral facet and lateral trochlea secondary to increased compressive forces *Other symptoms:* The patient may describe symptoms such as "clicking" or the knee "giving out." *Mechanism:* A discrete mechanism of injury is typically not reported. *Predisposing conditions:* Increased Q-angle, shallow trochlear groove, patella alta, patella baja, increased angle of inclination[35] Females are more than twice as likely to be affected as males.[61] A change in footwear may also be implicated.
Functional Assessment	Increased pain with sitting, descending and ascending stairs, and squatting;[38] inadequate proximal hip control may result in a contralateral drop of the pelvis (Trendelenburg) or a shifting weight over the involved side to compensate for weak abductors.[4]
Inspection	Increased Q-angle, patella alta, patella baja, femoral anteversion, excessive tibial torsion, or pronated foot may be noted.
Palpation	Pain at medial retinaculum, odd medial facet, lateral facet, lateral femoral condyle
Joint and Muscle Function Assessment	*AROM:* Knee extension may increase symptoms. *MMT:* Quadriceps pain and weakness Weakness of the hip abductors, extensors, and external rotators is commonly noted (see Chapter 12). *PROM:* End-range of knee flexion may increase symptoms due to compression of the patella. Shortened quadriceps, hamstrings, or triceps surae
Joint Stability Tests	*Stress tests:* A full examination of the knee may be warranted to rule out chronic tibiofemoral instability. *Joint play:* Lateral patellar glide may be increased. Medial patellar glide may be decreased.
Selective Tissue Tests	Ober test for IT band tightness (Chapter 12) Navicular drop test for excessive foot pronation/internal tibial rotation (Chapter 8)
Neurological Screening	Within normal limits
Vascular Screening	Within normal limits
Imaging Techniques	Skyline view radiograph
Differential Diagnosis	Meniscal tear, patellar instability, synovial plica, patellar tendinopathy
Comments	Patellofemoral problems are often related to poor neuromuscular control of the hip, which is worsened by fatigue and which increases valgus forces at the knee.

AROM = active range of motion; IT = iliotibial; MMT = manual muscle test; PROM = passive range of motion

down, such as descending stairs.[6] Both of these functional deviations result in increased lateral tracking of the patella.

Physical examination of the joint may reveal patella baja or alta, both of which contribute to atypical joint function. Patella baja increases joint compressive forces and subsequent stiffness;[1] patella alta leads to decreased patellofemoral joint stability as the patella has reduced contact with the stabilizing trochlea. At rest, lateral tilt and glide of the patella may be present, signifying tight lateral restraints and/or lax medial restraints. During joint play, lateral glide may be excessive, with medial glide restricted. Tightness of the lateral retinaculum may increase the tightness of the IT band and biceps femoris, also contributing to excessive lateral forces (see Joint Play 11-1).[62]

Examination of the ankle, foot, and hip is needed to understand fully the contributions to PPS. An assessment of the foot and ankle in subtalar joint neutral (see p. 198) frequently reveals a forefoot varus alignment, the cause of the increased and prolonged pronation. Reduced passive extension of the great toe in a relaxed stance also signifies a pronated foot and is predictive of patellofemoral pathology.[63] Strength and endurance of the hip external rotators and abductors is frequently diminished (Fig. 11-15).

Pain increases with active and resisted extension of the knee and during the end-range of passive flexion. **Clarke's sign**, where the patient contracts the quadriceps while the clinician applies an inferior force, produces an unreliably high rate of false-positive results, causing pain in otherwise-healthy individuals, and its use is NOT recommended.[58,64]

Patellofemoral Pain Syndrome Intervention Strategies

Because of its multifactorial nature, PPS must be treated with an individualized approach. Interventions include the use of orthotics,[65] change of footwear, alteration of gait patterns,[66] restoration of normal neuromuscular control and strength of the hip muscles,[4] stretching, patellar taping,[65] anti-inflammatory medications, weight loss, lumbopelvic manipulation,[67] and modification of activity. Because the scope of treatment is so broad, it is necessary to delineate subgroups of patients who might benefit from specific treatments. Clinical prediction rules to identify these subgroups have been identified for taping,[65] orthotic use,[63] and lumbopelvic manipulation.[67]

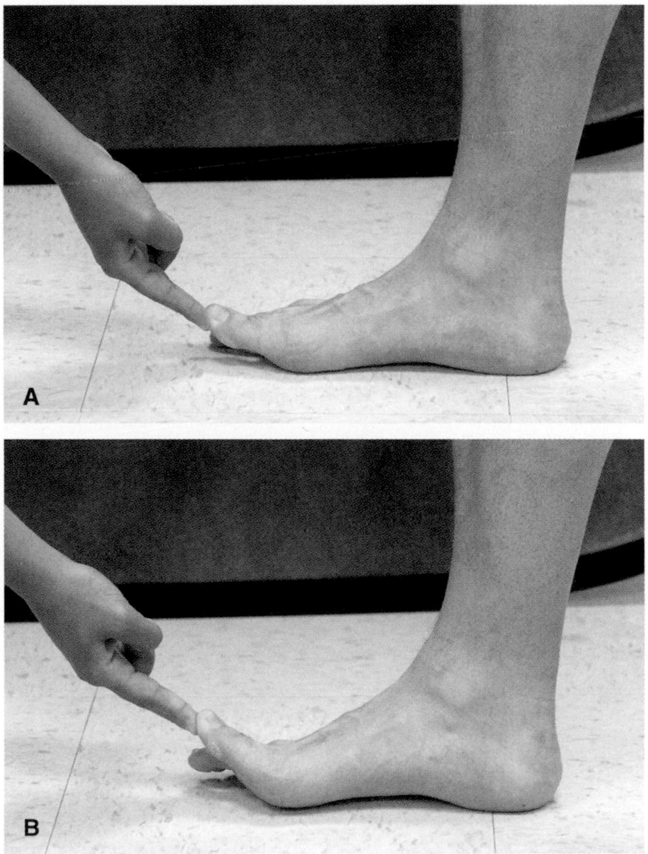

FIGURE 11-15 ■ The influence of foot position on toe extension. (A) Note the limited great toe extension in relaxed stance. (B) With the patient positioned in subtalar joint neutral, the flexor hallucis longus is no longer on stretch, allowing full motion into extension.

✱ Practical Evidence

In patients with patellofemoral pain syndrome, a positive patellar tilt test or tibial varum greater than 5 degrees is associated with a favorable response to patellar taping.[65]

Patellofemoral Instability

Patellofemoral instability can be subtle, resulting in subluxations, or dramatic, resulting in a dislocation. Resulting from laxity of the static restraints such as the medial and lateral retinacula, the patellofemoral articulation is typically unstable in the lateral direction due to the slight valgus arrangement of the knee. Medial instability is rare.

True (frank) dislocation of the patella causes it to shift laterally and lock out of place, resulting in obvious gross deformity and spasm of the quadriceps group as it guards the injury (see Acute Patellar Dislocation). Acute, chronic, or congenital laxity of the medial patellar restraints or abnormal tightness of the lateral retinaculum causes an increased lateral glide of the patella. Subtle patellar subluxations may occur without the patient's interpretation as such, producing symptoms described as the knee "giving out" during weight bearing (Examination Findings 11-2). Patients suffering from chronic patellar instability also produce a positive **apprehension test,** which should be performed before conducting a valgus stress test (Selective Tissue Test 11-2).

The patella is most apt to dislocate or subluxate when the maximum tensile strain is placed on the lateral patellar restraints, normally within the range of 20 to 30 degrees of knee flexion, pulling the patella laterally,[69] or after a valgus blow to the knee. Dislocations caused by blunt trauma may also result in a fracture of the patella.[70] Noncontact dislocations may result in osteochondral damage, patellar bone bruises, or osteochondritis dissecans.[71,72] Multiple dislocations or subluxations may cause erosion of the articular cartilage. However, the incidence of true OA is reduced in this population relative to those having normal tension in the patellar restraints.[73]

Several factors predispose an individual to patellar subluxations and dislocations. Those with patellar subluxations exhibit lateral displacement of the patella in weight bearing and non–weight bearing. In weight bearing, the internal femoral rotation is increased compared with non–weight bearing, suggesting that the femur is moving under the patella. Those with hypomobile medial glide have an increased tendency for subluxations compared with persons with hypermobile lateral glide.[74] The tightness of the lateral restraints serves to pull the patella laterally

Examination Findings 11-2
Patellofemoral Instability: Subluxation

Examination Segment	Clinical Findings
History of Current Condition	*Onset:* Recurrent *Pain characteristics:* Medial joint capsule, indicating trauma to the medial patellar restraints The patient may describe pain beneath the patella. *Other symptoms:* Reports of the knee "giving out," especially with change-of-direction maneuvers *Mechanism:* During extension of the knee, change of direction, or an eccentric contraction of the quadriceps group within the last 30° of the ROM *Predisposing conditions:* Lateral patellar tracking; increased Q-angle; tight lateral restraints; lax medial restraints; family history of patellar dislocation/subluxation
Functional Assessment	Symptoms (pain and "giving out") described with eccentric loading of the knee, such as when descending stairs. Observation of knee flexion in standing may reveal medial rotation of the lower extremity. The patient may demonstrate a significant difference (greater than 15% deficit) during the single-legged hop test (see p. 168) and/or during isokinetic testing.[37]
Inspection	Increased Q-angle Patella alta
Palpation	Pain is produced over the medial retinaculum and lateral articular facet.
Joint and Muscle Function Assessment	The following assume the patella has reduced and no obvious deformity exists: *AROM:* Pain occurring during the first 30° of flexion or terminal extension *MMT:* Hip abductors and external rotators may be weak, especially with repeated testing (see Chapter 12). The quadriceps are weak, and contraction may produce patellofemoral pain. Strength decreases during extension when the knee is positioned between 0° and 30°. *PROM:* Pain may arise secondary to stretching of the retinaculum, especially as the knee enters into flexion.
Joint Stability Tests	*Stress tests:* Unremarkable unless prior history of acute knee injury *Joint play:* Hypermobile lateral glide usually associated with a positive patellar tilt test result; hypomobile medial glide
Selective Tissue Tests	Positive patellar apprehension test
Neurological Screening	Within normal limits
Vascular Screening	Within normal limits
Imaging Techniques	AP (standing and/or supine), lateral, Merchant axial views
Differential Diagnosis	Meniscal tear, synovial plica, patellar pain syndrome
Comments	Repeated subluxations of the patella may result in osteochondral fractures to the lateral femoral condyle or posterior surface of the patella.

AP = anteroposterior; AROM = active range of motion; MCL = medial collateral ligament; PROM = passive range of motion; VMO = vastus medialis oblique

Selective Tissue Test 11-2
Apprehension Test for Patellar Instability

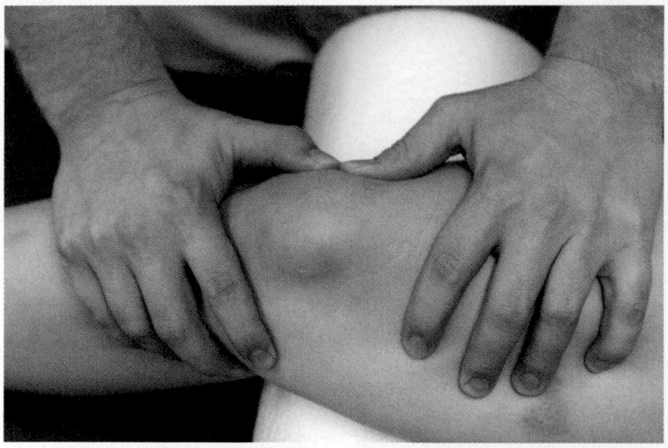

The apprehension test for patellar instability on a left knee. The examiner glides the patella laterally. A positive test is indicated by the patient's contracting the muscle or showing apprehension (anticipation) of an impending subluxation or dislocation.

Patient Position	Lying supine with the knee extended
Position of Examiner	Standing to the patient's side
Evaluative Procedure	The examiner attempts to move the patella as far laterally as possible, taking care not to cause it to actually dislocate.
Positive Test	Forcible contraction of the quadriceps by the patient to guard against dislocation of the patella. The patient may also demonstrate apprehension verbally or through facial expression.
Implications	Laxity of the medial patellar retinaculum, predisposing the patient to patellar subluxations or dislocations
Modification	To improve the specificity of the test by isolating the medial patellofemoral ligament, move the patella distally and laterally.[13] The **Fairbanks apprehension test** is performed with the patient's knee passively flexed to 30°. A lateral gliding force is placed on the patella while the knee is passively extended to the point where the patient experiences pain or apprehension.[68]
Evidence	

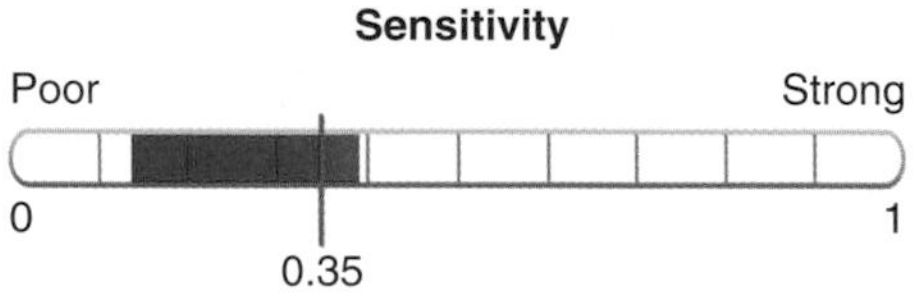

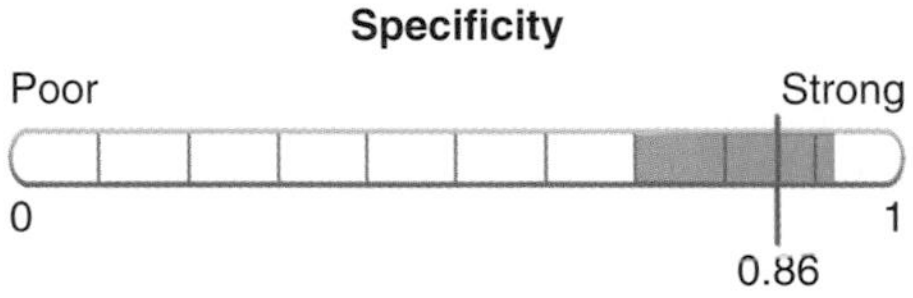

LR+: 0.90–1.20–2.90

LR−: 0.79–0.90–1.01

during knee extension. A shallow trochlea or flattened posterior (articulating) patellar surface increases the likelihood of spontaneous (non–contact-related) patellar dislocation.[75] Factors such as external tibial rotation and excessive pronation increase the Q-angle, causing the patella to track laterally.[76] A family history of patellar dislocations or subluxations also increases the risk of patellofemoral instability.[77]

Acute Patellar Dislocation

Acute patellar dislocations result in large, bloody effusions within 24 hours after the onset of the injury (Fig. 11-16). A complete dislocation seldom occurs without tearing of the VMO from the patella or from its origin near the adductor tubercle or the adjacent intermuscular septum.[78,79] The insertion of the medial patellar retinaculum is often avulsed from the patella, and the MPFL is often torn.[78,79] Palpation

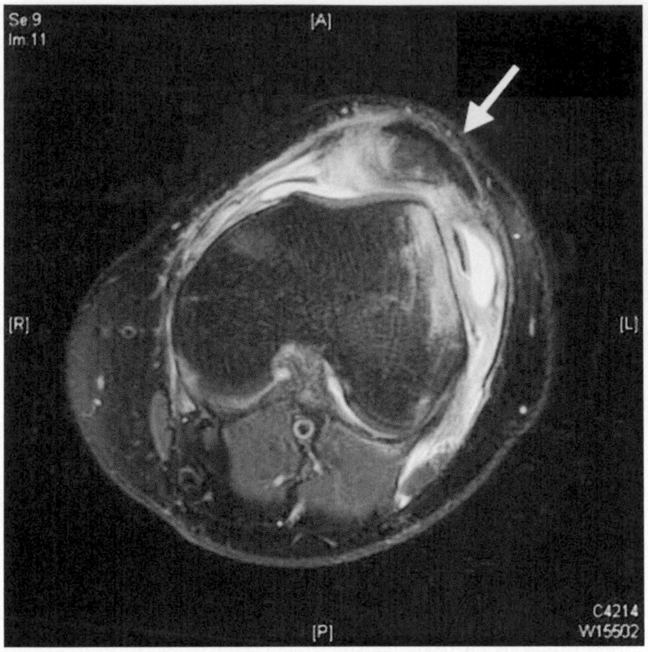

FIGURE 11-16 ■ MRI of a laterally dislocated patella. This view, obtained in the transverse plane, demonstrates the patella resting on the lateral femoral condyle.

of the medial patellar retinaculum, MPFL, and/or the VMO at either its origin or insertion produces pain (Examination Findings 11-3). Radiographic examination should be conducted for all dislocations or subluxations to rule out osteochondral fractures of the patella and femur. The mechanism for patellar dislocations and subluxations is similar to that of an MCL sprain, and the possibility of this injury must be ruled out.

✱ Practical Evidence

The patella most easily dislocates or subluxates when the knee is in 20° to 30° of flexion.[15]

Patellar Instability Intervention Strategies

The use of prophylactic or rehabilitative braces has little effect on preventing the recurrence of patellar dislocations or subluxations.[80] Treatment of subtle patellar instability emphasizes restoration of proximal hip control to minimize valgus forces, stretching tight lateral structures (e.g., IT band, lateral retinaculum) and decreasing pronation during gait.

First-time patellar dislocations are often treated conservatively, with early restoration of straight-ahead gait and strengthening of the quadriceps and hip musculature. With a large hemarthrosis, joint aspiration may be indicated to reduce quadriceps inhibition and pain. Recurrence of dislocations is fairly common.[78,79] Surgical procedures for frank dislocations, which are not recommended for children and adolescents, include repair of the MPFL and/or a release of tight lateral structures.[78,79]

Patellofemoral Tendinopathies

Much like patellofemoral pain syndrome, patellofemoral tendinopathies have multifactorial causes. Apophysitis, an outgrowth of bone at the tendon insertion, occurs in children and adolescents.

Patellofemoral Tendinopathy

Common in individuals participating in jumping activities, running sports, and weight lifting, patellar tendinopathies most often have an insidious onset. Repetitive motions on a biomechanically malaligned extensor mechanism can result in unequal loads on the extensor tendon.[81,82] Anatomic or biomechanical abnormalities are not present in many patients suffering from patellofemoral pain, and the onset of symptoms cannot be associated with a specific activity.[37]

Acute tendinopathy, characterized by an inflammatory response, can occur as the result of a blow to the tendon or a sudden increase in intensity or duration of activity. Tendinosis, a degenerative condition associated with collagen disorganization, is far more prevalent than tendinitis.

Histologic examination of tissue removed during surgery for patellar tendinopathies confirms that tendinosis is a more accurate descriptor of the chronic pathology than is tendinitis. Microtearing of the fibers results in the formation of excess connective tissues and endothelial cells, increased vascularity, and the alteration of the tendon's normal cellular structure.[82,84] The proximal portion of the posterior middle and the central third of the patellar tendon is the most frequently involved portions of the tendon.[82,84] Prolonged patellar tendon irritation can result in an elongation of the inferior patellar pole[84] and **morphologic** changes in the medial patellar retinaculum.[85]

The inferior pole of the patella is the common site of pain associated with patellar tendinopathy. Pain may also be described at the superior pole in the case of quadriceps tendinopathy (jumper's knee), in the midsubstance of the tendon, or at the tendon's attachment to the tibial tuberosity (Examination Findings 11-4). Moderate and severe pain with palpation is more predictive of patellar tendinopathy as confirmed by ultrasound than is mild pain, which is frequent in those with and without symptoms of patellar tendinopathy.[86] Resisted knee extension increases pain with a resulting decrease in strength. The end-range of passive knee flexion, performed with the patient in the prone position, elicits pain in the patellar tendon and may reveal decreased quadriceps flexibility when compared with passive knee flexion when the hip is flexed. Crepitus can be palpated in tendons during active or resisted movements. MRI is useful in identifying the presence of patellar tendinopathy.[82,84,87]

Pain that is elicited from either side of the patellar tendon may be caused by infrapatellar fat pad inflammation

Morphologic Changes in form and structure with regard to function

Examination Findings 11-3
Patellar Dislocation

Examination Segment	Clinical Findings
History of Current Condition	*Onset:* Acute *Pain characteristics:* Medial joint capsule, indicating trauma to the medial patellar restraints Pain in the vastus medialis, especially the oblique fibers Pain beneath the patella may be reported. *Mechanism:* Valgus blow to the knee; rapid change of direction with the foot fixed *Predisposing conditions:* Patella alta, history of previous dislocations or patellofemoral instability Low Q-angles may lead to patellar dislocation.[50]
Functional Assessment	The patient is unable to actively extend the knee or bear weight while the patella is still dislocated. Immediately after reduction, pain and soft tissue disruption limit strength and ROM. Significant gait alterations arise.
Inspection	Obvious deformity, with patella positioned laterally and knee flexed If examined postreduction, a large effusion will be present. If the capsule is torn, the fluid may extravasate distally.
Palpation	Obvious deformity of displaced patella Pain at the origin of the VMO at the adductor tubercle or intermuscular septum or at its insertion on the patella Tenderness over the medial patellofemoral ligament
Joint and Muscle Function Assessment	*AROM:* Not performed in the presence of dislocation If examined post-reduction, extension may be limited, or the patient may exhibit apprehension when approaching full extension. *MMT:* Not performed in the presence of a dislocation Following reduction, quadriceps strength will be decreased secondary to pain and, possibly, swelling. *PROM:* Not performed in the presence of a dislocation After reduction, ROM may be limited going into flexion.
Joint Stability Tests	*Stress tests:* Not performed in the presence of a dislocation If examined post-reduction, the major ligaments of the knee should be stressed to rule out concomitant injury, especially of the MCL. *Joint play:* Not performed in the presence of a dislocation
Selective Tissue Tests	Positive apprehension test post-reduction. This test should not be performed if a dislocation was known to occur.
Neurological Screening	Within normal limits
Vascular Screening	Within normal limits
Imaging Techniques	AP, PA, and skyline view radiographs; ultrasound (soft tissue damage)
Differential Diagnosis	Patellar tendon rupture, fracture of posterior aspect of patella or lateral femoral condyle
Comments	With an acutely dislocated patella, passive knee extension will often reduce the dislocation. The sooner the dislocation is reduced, the less damage there is to soft tissue restraints.

AP = anteroposterior; AROM = active range of motion; MCL = medial collateral ligament; MMT = manual muscle test; PA = posteroanterior; PROM = passive range of motion

Examination Findings 11-4
Patellar Tendinopathy

Examination Segment	Clinical Findings
History of Current Condition	*Onset:* Onset is insidious in most cases, but inflammation is possible secondary to contusive forces to the tendon. *Pain characteristics:* Inferior patellar poles, midsubstance of the tendon, or the tendon's point of insertion on the tibial tuberosity *Other symptoms:* The patient may complain of crepitus. *Mechanism:* Repeated activity involving resisted knee extension (e.g., jumping) or secondary to contusive forces on the patella Tendinitis may result from a rapid increase in activity level. *Predisposing conditions:* Patellar maltracking; overuse; rapid increase in training volume[88]
Functional Assessment	Increased pain with eccentric loading of the tendon, such as when landing from a jump or descending stairs
Inspection	Swelling may be localized around the patellar tendon and inferior patellar pole.
Palpation	Tenderness of the patellar tendon, especially at its insertion on the infrapatellar pole Thickening of the tendon and/or crepitus may be noted.
Joint and Muscle Function Assessment	*AROM:* Pain during active knee extension *MMT:* Quadriceps: Pain and weakness *PROM:* Pain at the end-range of knee flexion that may limit motion
Joint Stability Tests	*Stress tests:* Not applicable *Joint play:* Not applicable
Selective Tissue Tests	Not applicable
Neurological Screening	Within normal limits
Vascular Screening	Within normal limits
Imaging Techniques	Osteophytes and calcification within the tendon can be identified on AP and lateral radiographs. MRI can identify tendon lesions and bone edema within the tibial tuberosity.[89] MRI has a sensitivity of 0.78 and a specificity of 0.86.[90] Scar tissue and necrosis may be identified using diagnostic ultrasound.[89] Diagnostic ultrasound has a sensitivity of 0.58 and specificity of 0.94 for identifying thickening and calcification of the tendon. This procedure is better at ruling in tendinopathy than ruling it out.[90]
Differential Diagnosis	Fat pad impingement, meniscal tear, patellofemoral maltracking
Comments	There may be an associated tightness of the quadriceps musculature.

AP = anteroposterior; AROM = active range of motion; MMT = manual muscle test; MRI = magnetic resonance imaging; PROM = passive range of motion

(Hoffa's disease). This condition is marked by pain caused during knee extension that impinges the posterior (synovial) surface of the fat pad between the anterior portion of the femur and tibia and the posteroinferior part of the patella. Inflammation of the fat pad may trigger sympathetic spasm of the hamstring muscles, limiting knee ROM to reduce compression of the infrapatellar fat pad from the patellar tendon.[24] MRI may be required for the differential diagnosis between patellofemoral bursitis, tendinopathy, and fat pad inflammation.

Apophysitis

In adolescents, pain in the patellar tendon region can be associated with apophysitis, termed Osgood-Schlatter disease (OSD) or Sinding-Larsen-Johansson disease (SLJD) depending on the location of the pathology.

Osgood-Schlatter disease. The onset of OSD, which occurs at the insertion of the patellar tendon on the tibial tuberosity, is traced to repeated avulsion fractures of the tendon from its attachment and is caused by rapid growth, increased strength of the quadriceps, or both. These forces result in osteochondritis of the tubercle (Fig. 11-17). The symptoms of OSD are similar to those of patellar tendinopathies. However, differentiation is made by the patient's age (i.e., in adolescents) and the pain being localized to the tibial tuberosity and distal portion of the patellar tendon (Examination Findings 11-5). A history of OSD may lead to residual enlargement of the tibial tuberosity

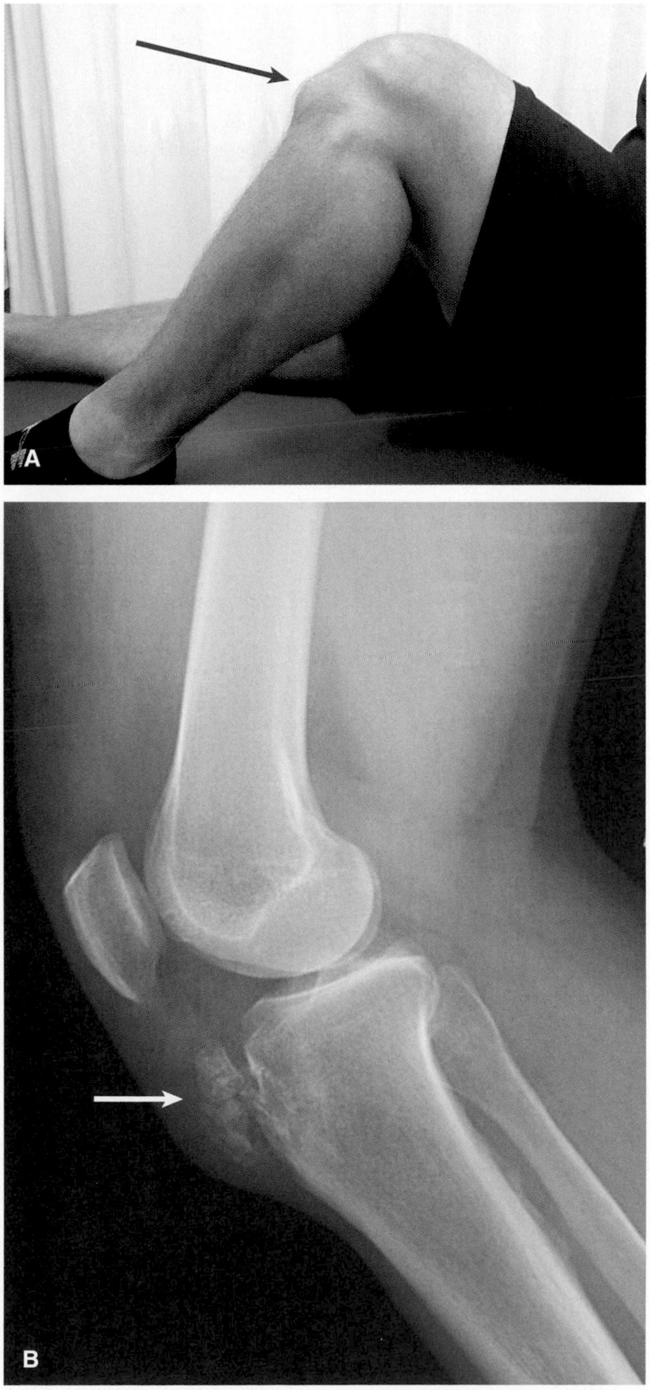

FIGURE 11-17 ■ Radiograph of Osgood-Schlatter disease showing the bony outgrowth. Image courtesy of Akira Murakami, MD. Boston Medical Center.

and mild exacerbation of symptoms with strenuous activity during adulthood.[91]

Sinding-Larsen-Johansson disease. SLJD is found at the attachment of the patellar tendon into the inferior patellar pole or, less commonly, at the quadriceps tendon attachment at the proximal pole of the patella.[93,94] As with OSD, SLJD is caused by a stress fracture or avulsion because of the repetitive forces associated with running and jumping. Continued traction forces on the growth areas of the patella lead to the disruption of the epiphysis.

SLJD affects males more often than females and is most common in the 11- to 14-year age group.[95] Complaints of pain and swelling at the affected pole of the patella are usually accompanied by an antalgic gait. Physical examination reveals point tenderness at the lesion site, pain with quadriceps stretching, and pain with active and resisted quadriceps function. Radiographs typically reveal the fragmentation at the superior or inferior pole of the patella. As with OSD, the fragmentation of SLJD may cause a visible or palpable deformity at the lesion site (see Examination Findings 11-5).

Patellar Tendinopathies and Apophysitis Intervention Strategies

The treatment of patellar tendinopathy should focus on finding the patient's envelope of function and working within that range, expanding it as the patient improves.[37,88] The rehabilitation program should also focus on postural control with emphasis on the trunk and pelvis. A program emphasizing eccentric quadriceps exercise and transverse friction massage across the tendon may be beneficial.[88] On rare occasions, surgical debridement of the tendon may be required if the patient fails to improve.[83]

OSD and SLJD are managed conservatively, with patients allowed to be as active as symptoms will allow. Quadriceps stretching is emphasized, along with **palliative** treatments such as ice and nonsteroidal anti-inflammatory medication. As physical development continues, symptoms may periodically reemerge until the patient's skeleton matures.

Patellofemoral Bursitis

The extensor mechanism's bursa may be inflamed secondary to a single traumatic force, repeated low-intensity blows, overuse, or infection (e.g., with ***Staphylococcus***). The superficial prepatellar bursa and the subcutaneous infrapatellar bursa are most often injured secondary to direct trauma, resulting in localized swelling (Fig. 11-18). The suprapatellar and deep infrapatellar bursae become inflamed secondary to overuse. Pain caused by bursitis usually remains localized, and the infrapatellar fat pads often become sympathetically tender (Examination Findings 11-6). Conditions with a sudden onset, associated redness and warmth about the knee, and no history of trauma or overuse require referral to a

Palliative Serving to relieve or reduce symptoms without curing

Examination Findings 11-5
Osgood-Schlatter Disease/Sinding-Larsen-Johansson Disease

Examination Segment	Clinical Findings
History of Current Condition	*Onset:* SLJD and OSD are insidious and affect a younger population. *Pain characteristics:* OSD: Radiating up the distal one-third of the patellar tendon; SLJD: Superior or inferior patellar pole point tenderness, beginning as activity-related pain and progressing to pain at all times *Mechanism:* Stress placed on the growth plate of the tibial tuberosity by forceful contraction or passive tension of the extensor mechanism; onset is often associated with a rapid growth spurt or overtraining. *Predisposing conditions:* Rapid bone growth during adolescence
Functional Assessment	Increased pain with going up or down stairs, single leg squats, and/or jumping The patient may describe increased pain and associated antalgic gait with increased activity.
Inspection	OSD: Swelling or deformity of the tibial tuberosity SLJD: Swelling at inferior patellar pole
Palpation	OSD: Tenderness and perhaps crepitus over the tibial tuberosity and patellar tendon SLJD: Pain and possible mass over the tendon's bony insertion
Joint and Muscle Function Assessment	*AROM:* Pain possibly experienced over the tibial tuberosity during active knee extension, especially when bearing weight *MMT:* Pain and weakness during quadriceps testing *PROM:* Pain over the tibial tuberosity or distal patellar pole during the end-range of knee flexion secondary to strain placed on the patellar tendon and associated pain
Joint Stability Tests	*Stress tests:* Not applicable *Joint play:* Not applicable
Selective Tissue Tests	Not applicable
Neurological Screening	Within normal limits
Vascular Screening	Within normal limits
Imaging Techniques	Standing or supine AP, lateral, and Merchant or sunrise views In children, the diagnosis is often made based on the clinical findings without the use of radiographs.[92]
Differential Diagnosis	Patellar tendinopathy, bipartite patella, patellar bursitis
Comments	The signs and symptoms of OSD may mimic those of patellar tendinopathy, but the symptoms are localized to the tibial tuberosity. These findings in postadolescent patients may indicate a history of apophysitis. SLJD may remain periodically symptomatic until the patient's skeleton matures.

AP = anteroposterior; AROM = active range of motion; MMT = manual muscle test; OSD = Osgood-Schlatter disease; PROM = passive range of motion; SLJD = Sinding-Larsen-Johansson disease

physician to rule out infection. Treatment of patellar bursitis consists of modifying activity to reduce painful stresses, padding to limit reinjury, and controlling inflammation.

Synovial Plica

Formed during the embryonic stage of development, synovial plicae are normal folds of the fibrous membrane that project into the joint cavity.[96] During maturation, these folds are absorbed into the joint capsule; however, in the majority of the population, either a thickened area or a crease within the membrane remains.[97] Four plicae are found in the knee and are named relative to the patella: suprapatellar, medial patellar, infrapatellar (ligamentum mucosum), and lateral patellar.[96]

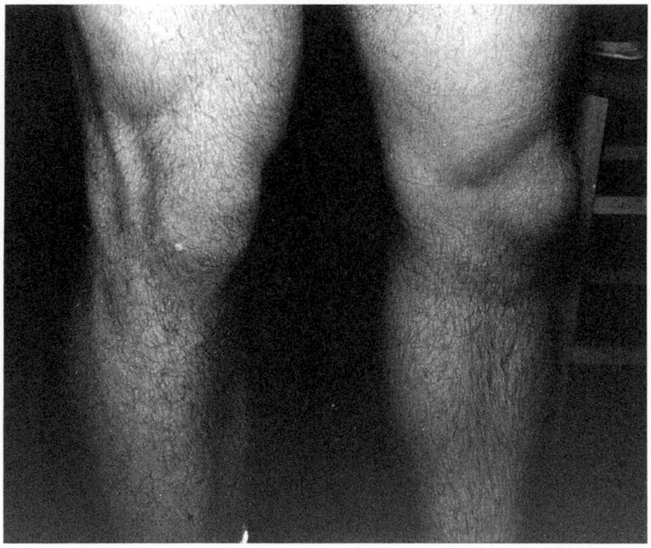

FIGURE 11-18 ■ Visibly swollen prepartellar bursa of the left knee.

A synovial plica will remain asymptomatic until the area is traumatized by a direct blow to the capsule, becomes inflamed secondary to stretching and friction caused by the plica bow-stringing across the femoral condyle during flexion, or develops inflammation secondary to OA.[98,99] Symptomatic plicae lose their normal elastic properties and, with time, become fibrotic, resulting in two reservoirs for synovial fluid: a suprapatellar reservoir and the cavity of the knee joint itself.[96,99,100] Although the onset of symptoms occurs most commonly in adolescents, plical syndromes may afflict patients of all ages at all stages of developmental maturity.[101] Synovial plica syndrome most commonly involves the medial joint capsule, but it can also involve the lateral capsule.[102]

When the plica becomes symptomatic, it loses its elastic qualities and alters the biomechanics of the patellar gliding mechanism. Prolonged inflammation of the plica leads to fibrosis and chronic disturbances within the knee.

Examination Findings 11-6
Patellofemoral Bursitis

Examination Segment	Clinical Findings
History of Current Condition	*Onset:* Acute or chronic *Pain characteristics:* Localized to a specific bursa and possibly the infrapatellar fat pads *Mechanism:* Direct trauma to the bursa or overuse *Predisposing conditions:* Other local inflammatory conditions (e.g., patellar tendinitis); weight bearing on the knees (e.g., wrestling)
Functional Assessment	Pain increases with activities that compress the bursa.
Inspection	Localized extra-articular swelling
Palpation	Point tenderness when directly palpating the bursa or the area over the bursa; tenderness over the infrapatellar fat pads may also be described.
Joint and Muscle Function Assessment	*AROM:* In chronic or severe cases, the patient may describe pain within a specified range *MMT:* Quadriceps: Pain and weakness *PROM:* The patient experiences pain at a specific point in the ROM, illustrating irritation of the bursa.
Joint Stability Tests	*Stress tests:* Not applicable *Joint play:* Unremarkable
Selective Tissue Tests	Not applicable
Neurological Screening	Within normal limits
Vascular Screening	Within normal limits
Imaging Techniques	Magnetic resonance imaging
Differential Diagnosis	Patellar tendinopathy; synovial plica; osteoarthritis; infection
Comments	The specific bursa involved is based on the location of pain. Patients with no relevant history for the onset of bursitis or who have superficial wounds over the bursa should be referred to a physician to rule out the possibility of infection.

AROM = active range of motion; MMT = manual muscle test; PROM = passive range of motion; ROM = range of motion

The symptoms presented by synovial plica syndrome may mimic those of meniscal tears, patellar subluxation, and patellar maltracking syndromes (Examination Findings 11-7).[100,103] Longitudinal tears of the plica can result in pseudolocking of the knee.[100] The suspicion of medial plica syndrome may be supported based on a positive finding on the **test for medial plica syndrome** (Selective Tissue Test 11-3) or the **stutter test** (Selective Tissue Test 11-4). A medial synovial plica can be confirmed via MRI.

Initial management of a symptomatic synovial plica includes modifying activity to reduce the irritating stresses and controlling the inflammatory response. Strengthening the VMO may lessen the symptoms by reducing the tensile forces placed on the plica.[100]

Examination Findings 11-7
Synovial Plica Syndrome

Examination Segment	Clinical Findings
History of Current Condition	*Onset:* Insidious *Pain characteristics:* Pain is located in the anterior portion of the knee; the patient may describe clicking, popping, or pseudolocking of the knee. The patient often describes symptoms as being worse in the morning, with a gradual decrease as the day progresses. *Other symptoms:* The patient may describe symptoms of the knee giving way. *Mechanism:* Friction caused by the plica rubbing across a femoral condyle *Predisposing conditions:* Congenitally large or thickened plica; OA[98]; the likelihood of onset decreases with increasing age.
Functional Assessment	Weight-bearing activities, including gait, can be disrupted when the knee is within the ROM that irritates the plica.
Inspection	Joint effusion or swelling over the involved plica may be noted.[96]
Palpation	Symptomatic plica possibly felt as a thickened, bandlike structure that is tender to the touch Plicae affect the anteromedial capsule more than the anterolateral capsule. Swelling possibly noted during palpation
Joint and Muscle Function Assessment	*AROM:* Pain experienced as the plica crosses the femoral condyle, with possible clicking or "catching" described by the patient; a snapping heard by the examiner and felt by palpating the joint capsule *MMT:* Quadriceps weakness secondary to pain *PROM:* A clicking or pseudolocking as the knee is flexed and extended over the point at which the plica rubs or catches on the femoral condyle. A flexion contracture of 5°–10° may be noted.
Joint Stability Tests	*Stress tests:* Not applicable *Joint play:* Lateral patellar glide may be decreased.
Selective Tissue Tests	Positive medial synovial plica test or stutter test result
Neurological Screening	Within normal limits
Vascular Screening	Within normal limits
Imaging Techniques	MRI
Differential Diagnosis	Meniscal tear, patellar subluxation, patellar maltracking, fat pad impingement
Comments	The symptoms of synovial plica may mimic those of a meniscal tear, subluxating patella, or other biomechanical dysfunction that has been caused by biomechanical changes in the knee. Longitudinal tears within the plica can result in pseudolocking of the knee.

AROM = active range of motion; MMT = manual muscle test; MRI = magnetic resonance imaging; OA = osteoarthritis; PROM = passive range of motion; ROM = range of motion

Traumatic Conditions

A laterally directed blow to the patella, a valgus stress, or other acute force can cause patellar dislocation. Refer to page 405 for a discussion of this condition.

Patellar Fractures

Patellar fractures can result from a direct blow, by an eccentric contraction of the quadriceps that places a tensile force on the bone, or as the result of a compressive force combined with a tensile force (Examination Findings 11-8).[3] The subsequent fracture line(s) are the result of the combined forces placed on the patella at the time of the fracture (Fig. 11-19). In some cases, the fracture may be readily apparent (Fig. 11-20). A rupture of the prepatellar bursa may cause immediate swelling and obscure the findings. Palpation may reveal crepitus over the body of the patella and one or more false joints.

Selective Tissue Test 11-3
Test for Medial Synovial Plica

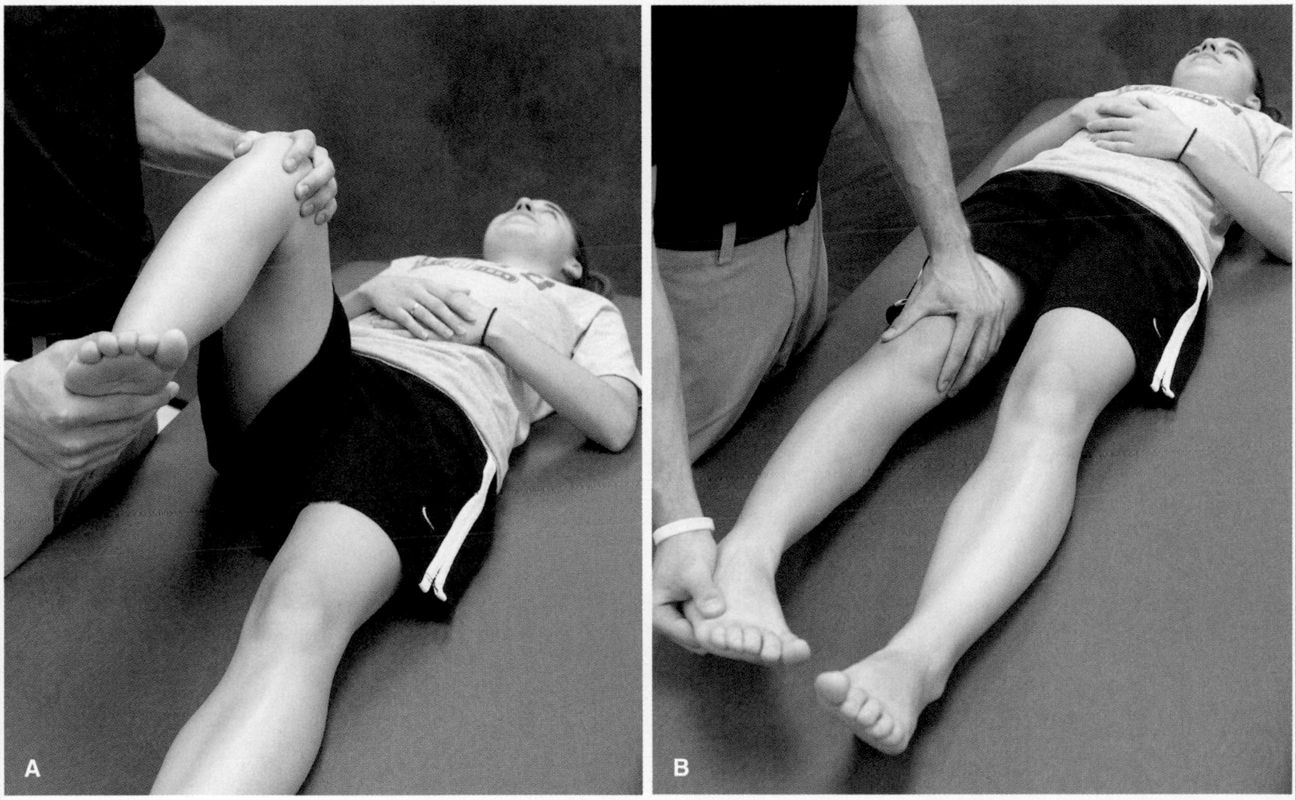

A positive test reproduces the patient's symptoms; the examiner may feel the plica as it crosses the medial femoral condyle.

Patient Position	Seated or lying supine with the knee flexed
Position of Examiner	Standing on the side being tested
Evaluative Procedure	**(A)** With the patient's knee flexed to 90° and the tibia internally rotated, the examiner passively moves the patella medially while palpating the anteromedial capsule. **(B)** The knee is then extended and flexed from 90° to 0° while the tibia is internally rotated.
Positive Test	The patient describes reproduction of the symptoms. The clinician may feel the plica as it crosses the medial femoral condyle, especially in the range of 60°–45° of flexion.
Implications	Symptomatic medial synovial plica
Evidence	Absent or inconclusive in the literature

Selective Tissue Test 11-4
Stutter Test for a Medial Synovial Plica

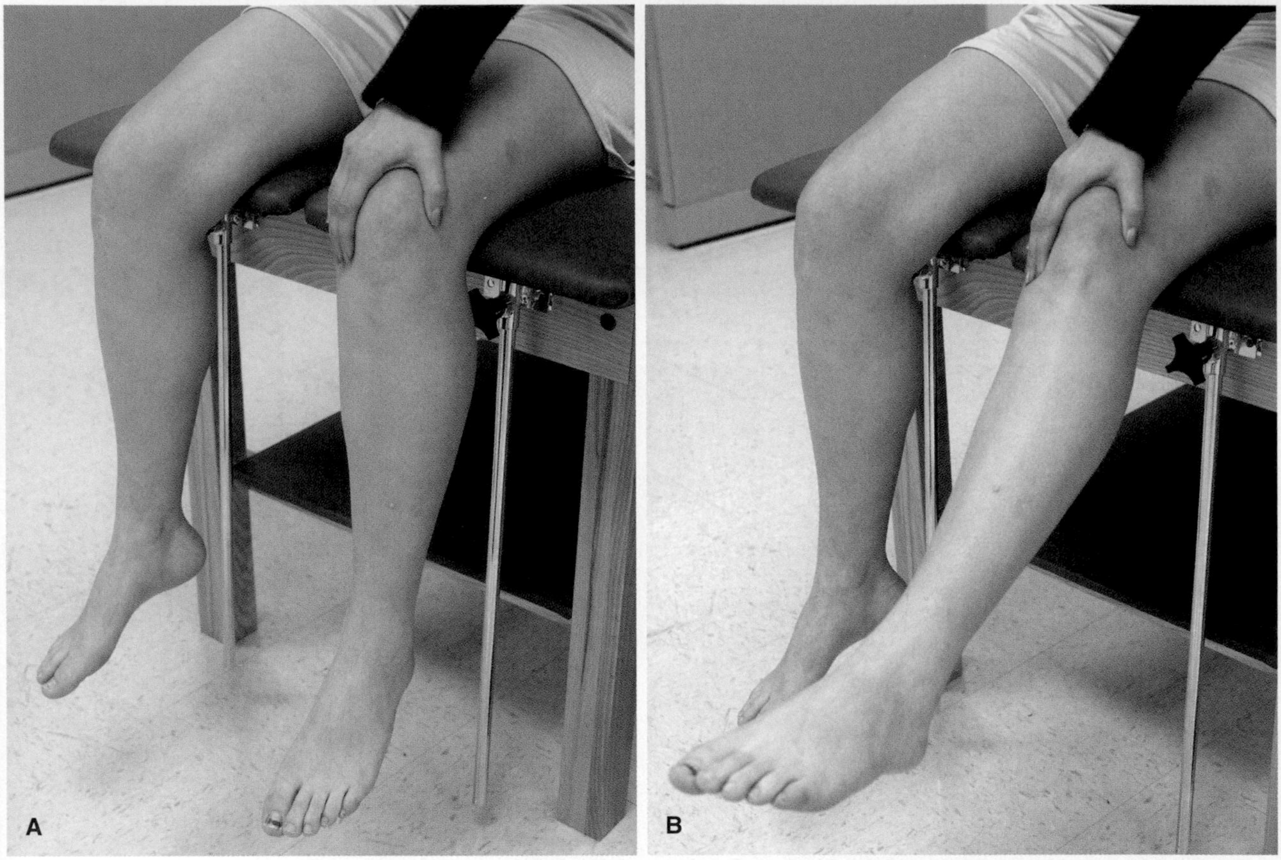

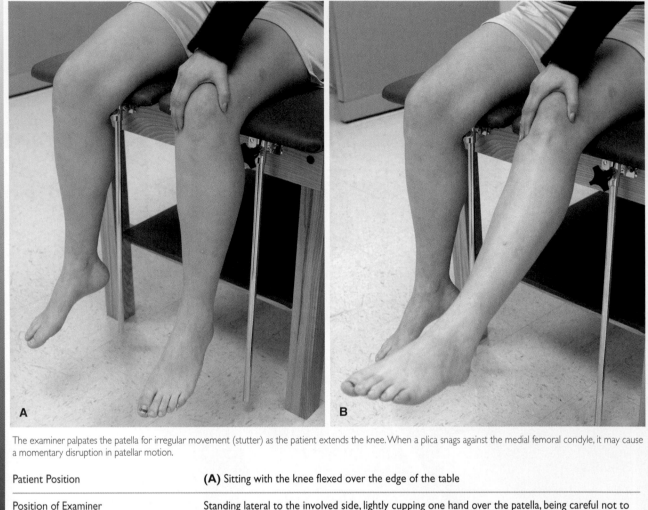

The examiner palpates the patella for irregular movement (stutter) as the patient extends the knee. When a plica snags against the medial femoral condyle, it may cause a momentary disruption in patellar motion.

Patient Position	**(A)** Sitting with the knee flexed over the edge of the table
Position of Examiner	Standing lateral to the involved side, lightly cupping one hand over the patella, being careful not to compress the articular surfaces
Evaluative Procedure	**(B)** The patient slowly extends the knee.
Positive Test	Irregular motion or stuttering between 40° and 60° as the plica passes over the medial condyle
Implications	Medial synovial plica
Evidence	Absent or inconclusive in the literature

Active knee extension (if possible) and passive knee flexion produce severe pain. Manual muscle testing cannot be performed because of pain secondary to the pressures placed on the fracture site. Avulsion fractures (sleeve fractures) can occur at the superior or inferior pole and may mimic a patellar tendon rupture.[62]

The risk of patellar fracture is increased following bone–patellar tendon–bone autograft ACL reconstruction.[104,105] Children are at a decreased risk of sustaining a patellar fracture because the patella is primarily cartilaginous and has increased mobility relative to that of adults.[62]

Patellar Tendon Rupture

Sudden overloading of the extensor mechanism can result in a rupture of the patellar tendon in its midsubstance or an avulsion from its attachment on the patella's inferior pole or the tibial tuberosity. The quadriceps' attachment on the patella's superior pole is another possible site of rupture. This muscular load most commonly occurs secondary to

Examination Findings 11-8
Patellar Fracture

Examination Segment	Clinical Findings
History of Current Condition	*Onset:* Acute *Pain characteristics:* Pain arising from the patella *Mechanism:* A direct blow to the patella; rapid hyperflexion A history of a strong eccentric quadriceps contraction at the time of impact may increase the likelihood of a patellar fracture. *Predisposing conditions:* Patellar stress fractures
Functional Assessment	The patient is often unable to bear weight on the affected limb.
Inspection	Swelling over and around the patella Other deformity may be noted.
Palpation	Pain over the fracture site; a false joint may be noted.
Joint and Muscle Function Assessment	*Do not perform if a fracture has not been ruled out.* *AROM:* Extension lag of 10°–30° *MMT:* Decreased quadriceps strength *PROM:* Flexion is limited by pain.
Joint Stability Tests	*Stress tests:* Not applicable *Joint play:* Not applicable
Selective Tissue Tests	Not applicable
Neurological Screening	Not applicable
Vascular Screening	Within normal limits
Imaging Techniques	AP and lateral radiographs
Differential Diagnosis	Patellar tendon rupture, quadriceps tendon rupture, patellar dislocation
Comments	The femoral articular surfaces may be fractured concurrently with the patella.

AP = anteroposterior; AROM = active range of motion; MMT = manual muscle test; PROM = passive range of motion

hyperflexion of the knee or a powerful quadriceps contraction from a weight-bearing position.[106]

Mechanical failure of the patellar tendon is uncommon in otherwise healthy individuals. Diseases such as rheumatoid arthritis, diabetes, **lupus**, chronic renal disease, or gout as well as chronic irritation of the patellar tendon or the use of corticosteroid medications may predispose patients to patellar tendon ruptures.[107-109]

Patellar tendon ruptures cause immediate gross deformity as the patella is displaced proximally on the femur, exposing the condyles (Fig. 11-21). During palpation, a depression is noted in the infrapatellar region.[106] Because of the severity of the trauma, gross swelling rapidly accumulates. The ability to actively extend the knee is lost, and the individual is unable to perform a straight leg raise on the affected side. However, the patient is still able to contract the quadriceps (Examination Findings 11-9). Although the ligaments of the involved knee may have been compromised at the time of injury, no ligamentous stability tests are performed before a physician examines the patient.

Lupus A systemic disease affecting the internal organs, skin, and musculoskeletal system

Patellar Tendon Rupture Intervention Strategies

Patients suffering from patellar tendon ruptures require immediate immobilization and transportation to the hospital (see the On-Field Management of Patellar Tendon Ruptures section). Surgical intervention within 7 to 10 days of the injury and appropriate rehabilitation can fully restore

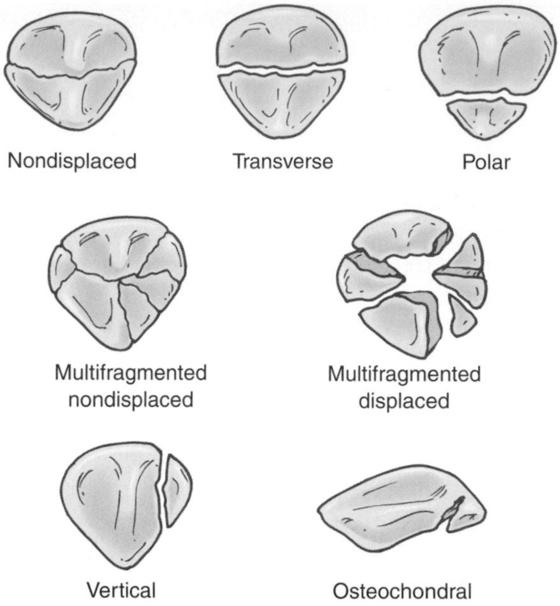

FIGURE 11-19 ■ Classification of patellar fractures.

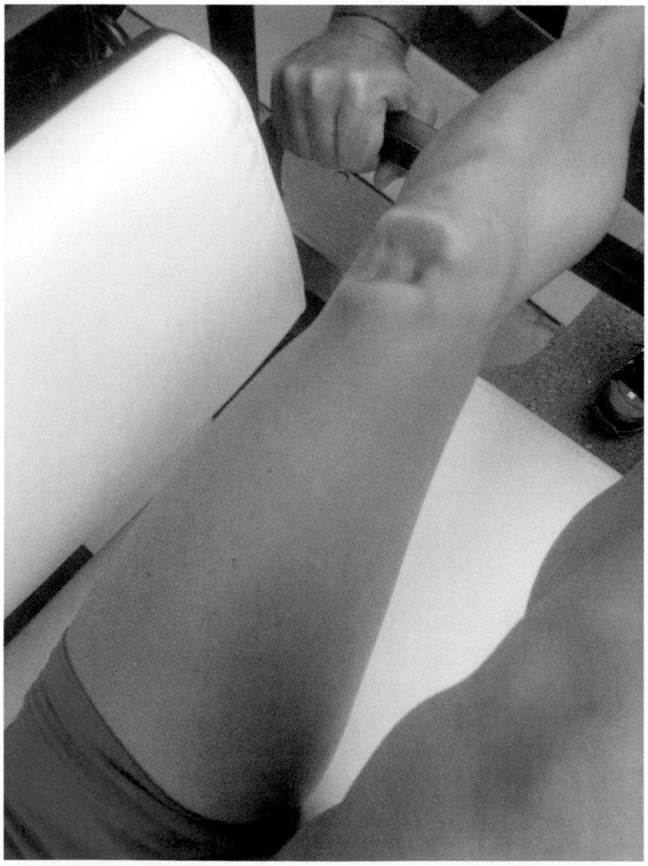

FIGURE 11-20 ■ Transverse fracture of the patella. Spasm of the quadriceps femoris (and slight knee flexion) displace the fractured segments, creating an obvious void over the femoral trochlea.

function to the knee. Most patients are able to progress to a full return to activity approximately 12 months after surgery.[112] Delaying surgery significantly decreases the functional outcome.[106]

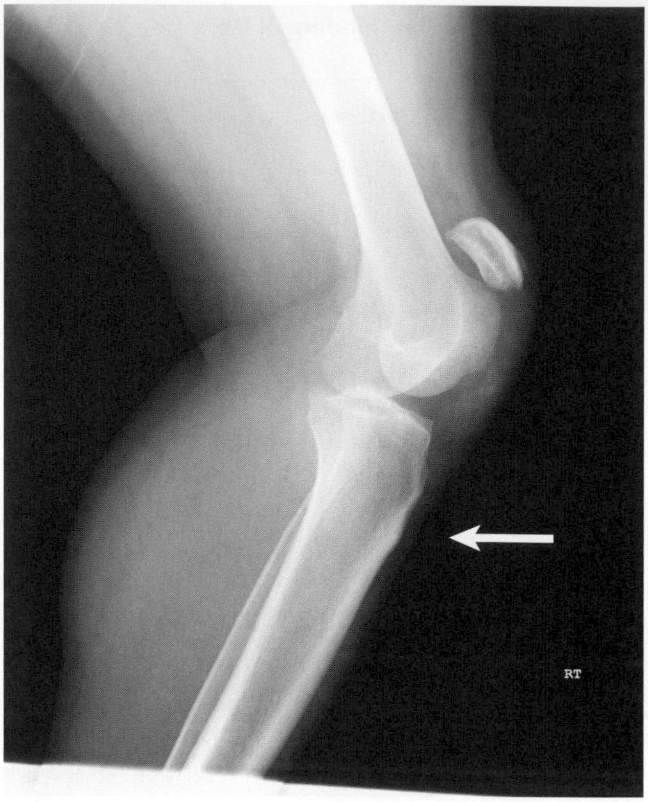

FIGURE 11-21 ■ Radiograph of a patellar tendon rupture showing patellar displacement associated with a patellar tendon rupture.

On-Field Evaluation of Patellofemoral Injuries

Acute traumatic injuries of the patellofemoral articulation mainly involve the patellar tendon, tracking of the patella within the femoral trochlea, and, on rare occasions, the bone itself. This type of trauma tends to produce gross deformity and loss of knee function.

Equipment Considerations

Refer to Chapter 10 for a discussion of the removal of equipment surrounding the knee.

On-Field History

Unless the nature of the athlete's condition is obviously apparent, the location of pain, mechanism of injury, and any associated sounds or other descriptors of the injury must be established. Initially, it may be difficult to differentiate trauma to the patellofemoral joint from tibiofemoral injury.

Inspect the patella to ensure that it assumes its normal position on the femur and has a normal shape. The patellar tendon should be visible as it runs from the tibial tuberosity to the infrapatellar pole. Rupture of this tendon results in violent spasm of the quadriceps muscle,

Examination Findings 11-9
Patellar Tendon Rupture

Examination Segment	Clinical Findings
History of Current Condition	*Onset:* Acute *Pain characteristics:* Patellar tendon, patella, and quadriceps muscle group *Mechanism:* Dynamic overload of the extensor mechanism secondary to extending the knee against resistance or a forceful eccentric contraction of the quadriceps muscle *Predisposing conditions:* Recurrent microtrauma, tendon degeneration, repeated corticosteroid injections, metabolic disease such as diabetes mellitus, gout, rheumatic disease[110]
Functional Assessment	Unwillingness to move or bear weight on the injured limb
Inspection	Patellar tendon rupture: Patella alta may be observed in the affected knee. Quadriceps tendon rupture: Patella baja is sometimes observed in the affected knee.[1] Obvious anterior soft tissue swelling, possibly masking the underlying deformity
Palpation	A palpable defect may be identified in the patellar tendon or superior to the patella's superior pole. The anterior surfaces of the femoral condyles may be palpable. Point tenderness will be noted over the defect. Swelling can mask the tendon defect during palpation.
Joint and Muscle Function Assessment	*AROM:* The patient is able to contract the quadriceps but is unable to extend the knee against gravity. *MMT:* Not advised because further damage to the extensor mechanism may result *PROM:* Pain moving into flexion An empty end-feel during flexion or a soft end-feel owing to the approximation of the hamstrings and gastrocnemius; PROM not performed acutely in the presence of an obvious tendon rupture
Joint Stability Tests	*Stress tests:* Not performed during the initial evaluation and management of a suspected tendon rupture, although damage to the knee ligaments is suspected *Joint play:* Not performed during the initial evaluation of a suspected tendon rupture
Selective Tissue Tests	Not applicable
Neurological Screening	Examine the lower-extremity dermatomes to rule out secondary trauma to the peroneal or tibial nerve.
Vascular Screening	Within normal limits
Imaging Techniques	MRI, diagnostic ultrasound[110]
Differential Diagnosis	Tibial tuberosity avulsion fracture
Comments	Patellar tendon ruptures tend to occur in men younger than age 40, although any segment of the population is susceptible. Harvesting of the central one-third of the patellar tendon for use as an autograft in ACL repair may increase the possibility of tendon rupture.[111]

ACL = anterior cruciate ligament; AROM = active range of motion; MMT = manual muscle test; MRI = magnetic resonance imaging; PROM = passive range of motion causing it to "ball up" on the femur. In the event of an obvious injury, a secondary screen must be performed to rule out any less obvious injury. Confirm any suspicions of injury obtained during the history-taking or inspection process through palpation. Any indication of a patellar dislocation, fracture, or patellar tendon rupture warrants immediate immobilization and referral for further medical evaluation.

On-Field Palpation

Begin by palpating the patellar tendon for tenderness, indicating possible tearing or aggravation of existing inflammation, from the tibial tuberosity to its insertion on the infrapatellar pole. Continue to palpate up the quadriceps muscles, paying close attention to the tone of muscle and tenderness over the VMO. Spasm of the quadriceps muscle may indicate a patellar dislocation, especially if the knee remains flexed. Tenderness may be elicited over the VMO secondary to tearing of the fibers during lateral dislocation of the patella.

From the VMO, palpate inferiorly to locate the medial joint capsule, which is tender after a lateral patellar dislocation. Palpate the lateral joint capsule for tenderness, indicating possible medial displacement of the patella.

On-Field Functional Assessment

After the possibility of major disruption to the patellofemoral joint has been ruled out, an assessment of functional status may begin. Some of these movements may have been voluntarily performed by the patient earlier in the examination.

- **Willingness to move the involved limb:** Ask the athlete to fully flex and extend the involved limb. An unwillingness or inability to complete this task is a sign that the athlete must be assisted off the field or court. If the athlete is able to complete the full ROM, break pressure may be applied with the knee near full extension and again in partial flexion to obtain a gross determination of muscular strength.
- **Willingness to bear weight:** If the preceding tests show normal or near-normal results, assist the athlete to the standing position and let him or her bear weight on the uninvolved limb. The athletic trainer then assumes a position under the involved side to help support the athlete's body weight, if needed.

Initial Management of On-Field Injuries

The primary concerns for the on-field management of patients with patellofemoral injuries involve the rupture of the patellar tendon, fractures of the patella, or an unreduced patellar dislocation. The following protocol is suggested for the initial management of patients with these conditions.

Patellar Tendon Rupture and Patellar Fracture

The management of patellar fractures and patellar tendon ruptures is essentially the same. Splint the knee in extension and immediately seek further medical attention for the athlete.

Patellar Dislocation

Gross dislocation of the patella is marked by obvious deformity caused by the laterally displaced patella. Spontaneous reductions may occur if the quadriceps are relaxed and gravity causes the knee to extend or if the patient attempts to actively extend the knee. All cases of acute or traumatic patellar dislocation require referral to a physician so that fractures to the articulating surfaces of the patella and femur may be ruled out.

Reduced patellar subluxations or dislocations are splinted with the knee fully extended or slightly flexed. Patellar dislocations are generally reducible by assisting the athlete with passive knee extension. An unreduced dislocation must be splinted in the position in which the knee was found. This can be accomplished using a long moldable aluminum splint, bending one end to serve as a truss between the femur and lower leg, or by using a vacuum splint.

REFERENCES

1. Tecklenburg, K, et al: Bony and cartilaginous anatomy of the patellofemoral joint. *Knee Surg Sports Traumatol Arthrosc*, 14:235, 2006.
2. Moore, KL, and Daily, AF: *Clinically Oriented Anatomy*, ed 5. Philadelphia, PA: Lippincott Williams & Wilkins, 2006.
3. Melvin, JS, and Mehta, S: Patellar fractures in adults. *J Am Acad Orthop Surg*, 19:198, 2011.
4. Powers, CM: The influence of abnormal hip mechanics on knee injury: a biomechanical perspective. *J Orthop Sports Phys Ther*, 40:42, 2010.
5. Elias, JJ, et al: Hamstrings loading contributes to lateral patellofemoral malalignment and elevated cartilage pressures: an in vitro study. *Clin Biomech (Bristol, Avon)*, 26:841, 2011.
6. Powers, CM: The influence of altered lower-extremity kinematics on patellofemoral joint dysfunction: a theoretical perspective. *J Orthop Sports Phys Ther*, 33:639, 2003.
7. Lee, TQ, Morris, G, and Csintalan, RP: The influence of tibial and femoral rotation on patellofemoral contact area and pressure. *J Orthop Sports Phys Ther*, 33:686, 2003.
8. Powers, CM: Patellar kinematics, part II: the influence of the depth of the trochlear groove in subjects with and without patellofemoral pain. *Phys Ther*, 80:965, 2000.
9. Cohen, ZA, et al: Patellofemoral stresses during open and closed kinetic chain exercises. *Am J Sports Med*, 29:480, 2001.
10. Davis, IS, and Powers, C: Patellofemoral pain syndrome: proximal, distal, and local factors: an international research retreat. *J Orthop Sports Phys Ther*, 40:A1, 2010.
11. Reese, NB, and Bandy, WD: Use of an inclinometer to measure flexibility of the iliotibial band using the Ober test and modified Ober test: differences in the magnitude and reliability of measurements. *J Orthop Sports Phys Ther*, 33:326, 2003.

12. Waryasz, GR, and McDermott, AY: Patellofemoral pain syndrome (PFPS): a systematic review of anatomy and potential risk factors. *Dyn Med*, 7:9, 2008.
13. Tanner, SM, et al: A modified test for patellar instability: the biomechanical basis. *Clin J Sport Med*, 13:327, 2003.
14. Nomura, E, Inoue, M, and Osada, N: Anatomical analysis of the medial patellofemoral ligament of the knee, especially the femoral attachment. *Knee Surg Sports Traumatol Arthrosc*, 13:510, 2005.
15. Bicos, J, Fulkerson, JP, and Amis, A: Current concepts review: the medial patellofemoral ligament. *Am J Sports Med*. 35:484, 2007.
16. Philippot, R, et al: Medial patellofemoral ligament anatomy: implications for its surgical reconstruction. *Knee Surg Sports Traumatol Arthrosc*, 17:475, 2009.
17. Peeler, J, et al: Structural parameters of the vastus medialis muscle. *Clin Anat*, 18:281, 2005.
18. Pal, S, et al: Patellar maltracking correlates with vastus medialis activation delay in patellofemoral pain patients. *Am J Sports Med*, 39:590, 2011.
19. Brownstein, BA, Lamb, RL, and Mangine, RE: Quadriceps torque and integrated electromyography. *J Orthop Sport Phys Ther*, 6:309, 1985.
20. Hanten, WP, and Schultheis, SS: Exercise effect on electromyographic activity of the vastus medialis oblique and vastus lateralis muscles. *Phys Ther*, 70:561, 1990.
21. Devan, MR, et al: A prospective study of overuse knee injuries among female athletes with muscle imbalances and structural abnormalities. *J Athl Train*, 39:263, 2004.
22. Witvrouw, E, et al: Intrinsic risk factors for the development of anterior knee pain in an athletic population: a two-year prospective study. *Am J Sport Med*, 28:480, 2000.
23. Elias, JJ, et al: In vitro characterization of the relationship between the Q-angle and the lateral component of the quadriceps force. Proc *Inst Mech Engrs*, 218:63, 2004.
24. Gallagher, J, et al: The infrapatellar fat pad: anatomy and clinical correlations. *Knee Surg Sports Traumatol Arthrosc*, 13:268, 2005.
25. Rauh, MT, et al: Quadriceps angle and risk of injury among high school cross-country runners. *J Orthop Sports Phys Ther*, 37:725, 2007.
26. Christoforakis, JJ, and Strachan, RK: Internal derangements of the knee associated with patellofemoral joint degeneration. *Knee Surg Sports Traumatol Arthrosc*, 13:581, 2005.
27. Saffagnini, S, et al: Single-bundle tendon versus non-anatomical double-bundle hamstrings ACL reconstruction: a prospective randomized study at 8-year minimum follow-up. *Knee Surg Sports Traumatol Arthrosc*, 19: 390, 2011.
28. Kettunen, JA, et al: Primary cartilage lesions and outcome among subjects with patellofemoral pain syndrome. *Knee Surg Sports Traumatol Arthrosc*, 13:131, 2005.
29. Näslund, J, et al: Comparison of symptoms and clinical findings of subgroups of individuals with patellofemoral pain. *Physiother Theor Pract*, 22:105, 2006.
30. Mouzopoulos, G, Borbon, C, and Siebold, R: Patellar chondral defects: a review of a challenging entity. *Knee Surg Sports Traumatol Arthrosc*, 19:1990, 2011.
31. Atanda, A Jr, et al: Approach to the active patient with chronic anterior knee pain. *Phys Sportsmed*, 40:41, 2012.
32. Pihlajamäki, HK, et al: Reliability of clinical findings and magnetic resonance imaging for the diagnosis of chondromalacia patellae. *J Bone Surg*, 92:927, 2010.
33. Brechter, JH, and Powers, CM: Patellofemoral joint stress during stair ascent and descent in persons with and without patellofemoral pain. *Gait Posture*, 16:115, 2002.
34. Thompson, LR, et al: The knee pain map: reliability of a method to identify knee pain location and pattern. *Arthritis Rheum*, 61:725, 2009.
35. Souza, RB, and Powers, CM: Predictors of hip internal rotation during running: an evaluation of hip strength and femoral structure in women with and without patellofemoral pain. *Am J Sports Med*, 37:579, 2009.
36. Bennett, G, and Stauber, W: Evaluation and treatment of anterior knee pain using eccentric exercise. *Med Sci Sports Exerc*, 18:526, 1986.
37. Witvrouw, E, et al: Clinical classification of patellofemoral pain syndrome: guidelines for non-operative treatment. *Knee Surg Sports Traumatol Arthrosc*, 13:122, 2005.
38. MacIntyre, NJ, et al: Patellofemoral joint kinematics in individuals with and without patellofemoral pain syndrome. *J Bone Joint Surg*, 88-A: 2596, 2006.
39. Fitzgerald, GK, and McClure, PW: Reliability of measurements obtained with four tests for patellofemoral alignment. *Phys Ther*, 75:84, 1995.
40. Nicolaas, L, Tigchelarr, S, and Koëter, S: Patellofemoral evaluation with magnetic resonance imaging in 51 knees of asymptomatic subjects. *Knee Surg Sports Traumatol Arthrosc*, 19:1735, 2011.
41. Harilainen, A, et al: Patellofemoral relationships and cartilage breakdown. *Knee Surg Sports Traumatol Arthrosc*, 13:142, 2005.
42. Powers, CM, et al: Criterion-related validity of a clinical measurement to determine the medial/lateral component of patellar orientation. *J Orthop Sports Phys Ther*, 29:386, 1999.
43. Ingersoll, CD: Clinical and radiological assessment of patellar position. *Athl Ther Today*, 5:19, 2000.
44. Snyder-Mackler, L, and Lewek, M: The knee. In Levangie, PK, and Norkin, CC: *Joint Structure and Function: A Comprehensive Analysis*, ed 4. Philadelphia, PA: FA Davis, 2005.
45. Smith, TO, Hunt, NJ, and Donell, ST: The reliability and validity of the Q-angle: a systematic review. *Knee Surg Sports Trumatol Arthrosc*, 16:1068, 2008.
46. Livingston, LA, and Spaulding, SJ: OPTOTRAK measurement of the quadriceps angle using standardized foot positions. *J Athl Train*, 37:252, 2002.
47. Guerra, JP, Arnold, MJ, and Gajdosik, RL: Q angle: effects of isometric quadriceps contraction and body position. *J Orthop Sport Phys Ther*, 19:200, 1992.
48. Greene, CC, et al: Reliability of the quadriceps angle measurement. *Am J Knee Surg*, 14:97, 2001.
49. Grelsamer, RP, Dubey, A, and Weinstein, CH: Men and women have similar Q angles: a clinical and trigonometric evaluation. *J Bone Joint Surg*, 87(B):1498, 2005.
50. Sandridsson, J, et al: Femorotibial rotation and the Q-angle related to the dislocating patella. *Acta Radiol*, 42:218, 2001.
51. Binder, D, et al: Peak torque, total work and power values when comparing individuals with Q-angle differences. *Isokinet Exer Sci*, 9:27, 2001.
52. Clarkson, M, and Wilkerson, J: Are differences in leg length predictive of patella-femoral pain? *Physiother Res Int*, 12:29, 2007.
53. Elkousy, H: Complications in brief: arthroscopic lateral release. *Clin Orthop Relat Res*, 470:2949, 2012.
54. Bolgla, LA, et al: Hip strength and hip and knee kinematics during stair descent in females with and without patellofemoral pain syndrome. *J Orthop Sports Phys Ther*, 38:12, 2008.
55. Nakagawa, TH, Muniz, TB, and de Marche Baldon, R: The effect of additional strengthening of hip abductor and lateral rotator muscles in patellofemoral pain syndrome: a randomized controlled pilot study. *Clin Rehabil*, 22:1051, 2008.
56. Piva, SR, Goodnite, EA, and Childs, JD: Strength around the hip and flexibility of soft tissues in individuals with and without patellofemoral pain syndrome. *J Orthop Sports Phys Ther*, 35:793, 2005.
57. Backman, LJ, and Danielson, P: Low range of ankle dorsiflexion predisposes for patellar tendinopathy in junior elite basketball players. *Am J Sports Med*, 39:2626, 2011.

58. Cook, C, et al: Diagnostic accuracy and association to disability of clinical test findings associated with patellofemoral pain syndrome. *Physiother Can*, 62:17, 2010.
59. Khayambashi, K, Mohammadkhani, Z, and Ghaznavi, K: The effects of isolated hip abductor and external rotator muscle strengthening on pain, health status, and hip strength in females with patellofemoral pain: a randomized controlled trial. *J Orthop Sports Phys Ther*, 42:22, 2012.
60. Hopkins, JT: Knee joint effusion and cryotherapy alter lower chain kinetics and muscle activity. *J Athl Train*, 41:177, 2006.
61. Boling, M, et al: Gender differences in the incidence and prevalence of patellofemoral pain syndrome. *Scand J Med Sci Sports*, 20:725, 2010.
62. Kumar, K, and Knight, DJ: Sleeve fracture of the superior pole of the patella: a case report. *Knee Surg Sports Traumatol Arthrosc*, 13:229, 2005.
63. Sutlive, TG, et al: Identification of individuals with patellofemoral pain whose symptoms improved after a combined program of foot orthosis use and modified activity: a preliminary investigation. *Phys Ther*, 84:49, 2004.
64. Doberstein, ST, Romeyn, RL, and Reineke, DM: The diagnostic value of the Clarke Sign in assessing chondromalacia patella. *J Athl Train*, 43:190, 2008.
65. Lesher, JD, et al: Development of a clinical prediction rule for classifying patients with patellofemoral pain syndrome who respond to patellar taping. *J Orthop Sports Phys Ther*, 36:854, 2006.
66. Noehren, B, and Davis, I: Effect of gait retraining on hip mechanics, pain and function in runners with patellofemoral pain syndrome. *PFPS Retreat*. Baltimore, MD, 2009.
67. Iverson, CA, et al: Lumbopelvic manipulation for the treatment of patients with patellofemoral pain syndrome: development of a clinical prediction rule. *J Orthop Sports Phys Ther*, 38:297, 2008.
68. Nijs, J, et al: Diagnostic value of five clinical tests in patellofemoral pain syndrome. *Man Ther*, 11:69, 2006.
69. Luo, ZP, et al: Tensile stress of the lateral patellofemoral ligament during knee motion. *Am J Knee Surg*, 10:139, 1997.
70. Willis, RB, and Firth, G: Traumatic patellar dislocation: loose bodies and the MPFL. *J Pediatr Orthop*, 32:S47, 2012.
71. Stanitski, CL, and Paletta, GA: Articular cartilage injury with acute patellar dislocation in adolescents: arthroscopic and radiographic correlation. *Am J Sports Med*, 26:52, 1998.
72. Hsiao, M, Owens, BD, and Burks, R: Incidence of acute traumatic patellar dislocation among active-duty United States military service members. *Am J Sports Med*, 38:1997, 2010.
73. Maenpaa, H, and Lehto, MU: Patellofemoral osteoarthritis after patellar dislocation. *Clin Orthop*, 339:156, 1997.
74. Stanitski, CL: Articular hypermobility and chondral injury in patients with acute patellar dislocation. *Am J Sports Med*, 23:146, 1995.
75. Maenpaa, H, Huhtala, H, and Lehto, MU: Recurrence after patellar dislocation: redislocation in 37/75 patients followed for 6–24 years. *Acta Orthop Scand*, 68:424, 1997.
76. Cameron, JC, and Saha, S: External tibial torsion: an underrecognized cause of recurrent patellar dislocation. *Clin Orthop*, 328:177, 1996.
77. Rebolledo, BJ, et al: Familial association of femoral trochlear dysplasia with recurrent bilateral patellar dislocation. *Orthopedics*, 35:e574, 2012.
78. Nietosvaara, Y, et al: Acute patellar dislocation in children and adolescents. *J Bone Joint Surg*, 91(A):S139, 2009.
79. Sillanpää, PJ, et al: Treatment with and without initial stabilizing surgery for primary traumatic patellar dislocation. *J Bone Joint Surg Am*, 91:263, 2009.
80. Muhle, C, et al: Effect of a patellar realignment brace on patients with patellar subluxation and dislocation: evaluation with kinematic magnetic resonance imaging. *Am J Sports Med*, 27:350, 1999.
81. Verheyden, F, Geens, G, and Nelen, G: Jumper's knee: results of surgical treatment. *Acta Orthop Belg*, 63:102, 1997.
82. Yu, JS, et al: Correlation of MR imaging and pathologic findings in athletes undergoing surgery for chronic patellar tendinitis. *Am J Roentgenol*, 165:115, 1995.
83. Griffiths, GP, and Selesnick, FH: Operative treatment and arthroscopic findings in chronic patellar tenditis. *Arthroscopy*, 14:836, 1998.
84. McLoughlin, RF, et al: Patellar tendinitis: MR imaging features, with suggested pathogenesis and proposed classification. *Radiology*, 197:843, 1995.
85. Grossfeld, SL, and Engebresten, L: Patellar tendinitis—a case report of elongation and ossification of the inferior pole of the patella. *Scand J Med Sci Sports*, 5:308, 1995.
86. Cook, JL, et al: Reproducibility and clinical utility of tendon palpation to detect patellar tendinopathy in young basketball players. *Br J Sports Med*, 35:65, 2001.
87. Popp, JE, Yu, JS, and Kaeding, CC: Recalcitrant patellar tendinitis: magnetic resonance imaging, histologic evaluation, and surgical treatment. *Am J Sports Med*, 25:218, 1997.
88. Rutland, M, et al: Evidence-supported rehabilitation of patellar tendinopathy. *N Am J Sports Phys Ther*, 5:166, 2010.
89. Sarimo, J, et al: Distal patellar tendinosis: an unusual form of jumper's knee. *Knee Surg Sports Traumatol Arthrosc*, 15:54, 2007.
90. Wilson, JJ, and Best, TM: Common overuse tendon problems: a review and recommendations for treatment. *Am Fam Physician*, 72:811, 2005.
91. Ross, MD, and Villard, D: Disability levels of college-aged men with a history of Osgood-Schlatter disease. *J Strength Cond Res*, 17:659, 2003.
92. Sarwark, JF, and Shore, RM (section eds): Pediatric orthopaedics. In Johnson, TR, and Steinbach, LS (eds): *Essentials of Musculoskeletal Imaging*. Rosemont, IL: American Academy of Orthopaedic Surgeons, 2004, p 760.
93. Duri, ZA, Patel, DV, and Aichroth, PM: The immature athlete. *Clin Sports Med*, 21:461, 2002.
94. Freednab, DM, Kono, M, and Johnson, EE: Pathologic patellar fracture at the site of an old Sinding-Larsen-Johansson lesion: a case report of a 33-year-old male. *J Orthop Trauma*, 19:582, 2005.
95. Ogden, JA: *Sinding-Larsen-Johansson Disease in Skeletal Injury in the Child*. Philadelphia, PA: WB Saunders, 1990, pp 765-768.
96. Demirag, B, Ozturk, C, and Karakayali, M: Symptomatic infrapatellar plica. *Knee Surg Sports Traumatol Arthrosc*, 14:156, 2006.
97. Bellary, SS, B, et al: Medial synovial plica syndrome: a review of the literature. *Clin Anat*, 25:423, 2012.
98. Lyu, SR, and Hsu, CC: Medial plicae and degeneration of the medial femoral condyle. *Arthroscopy*, 22:17, 2006.
99. Lyu, S, Chiang, J, and Tseng, C: Medial plica in patients with knee osteoarthritis: a histomorphological study. *Knee Surg Sports Traumatol Arthrosc*. 18:769, 2010.
100. Gerbino, PG II, and Micheli, LJ: Bucket-handle tear of the medial plica. *Clin J Sport Med*, 6:265, 1996.
101. Kim, SJ, Min, BH, and Kim, HK: Arthroscopic anatomy of the infrapatellar plica. *Arthroscopy*, 12:561, 1996.
102. Kurosaka, M, et al: Lateral synovial plica syndrome: a case report. *Am J Sports Med*, 20:92, 1992.
103. Blok, A, et al: Medial synovial plica. *Orthop Traumatol Rehabil*, 30:397, 2005.
104. Tjoumakaris, FP, Herz-Brown, AL, and Bowers, AL: Complications in brief: anterior cruciate ligament reconstruction. *Clin Orthop Relat Res*, 470:630, 2012.
105. Viola, R, and Vianello, R: Three cases of patella fracture in 1,320 anterior cruciate ligament reconstructions with bone-patellar tendon-bone autograft. *Arthroscopy*, 15:93, 1999.
106. Levine, RJ: Patellar tendon rupture: the importance of timely recognition and repair. *Postgrad Med*, 100:241, 1996.

107. Podesta, L, Sherman, MF, and Bonamo, JR: Bilateral simultaneous rupture of the infrapatellar tendon in a recreational athlete: a case report. *Am J Sports Med*, 19:325, 1991.
108. Rosenberg, JM, and Whitaker, JH: Bilateral infrapatellar tendon rupture in a patient with jumper's knee. *Am J Sports Med*, 19:94, 1991.
109. Chen, SK, et al: Patellar tendon ruptures in weight lifters after local steroid injections. *Arch Orthop Trauma Surg*, 129:369, 2009.
110. Heyde, CE, et al: Ultrasonography as a reliable diagnostic tool in old quadriceps tendon ruptures: a prospective multicentre study. *Knee Surg Sports Traumatol Arthrosc*, 13:564, 2005.
111. Mickelsen, PL, et al: Patellar tendon rupture 3 years after anterior cruciate ligament reconstruction with a central one third bone-patellar tendon-bone graft. *Arthroscopy*, 17:648, 2001.
112. Enad, JG: Patellar tendon ruptures. *South Med J*, 92:563, 1999.

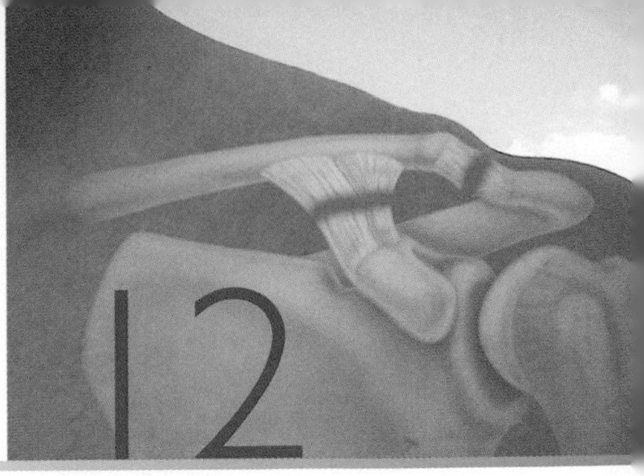

CHAPTER 12

Pelvis and Thigh Pathologies

The pelvic girdle forms the structural base of support between the lower extremities and the trunk. A relatively immobile structure, the pelvis is formed by pairs of three fused bones joined anteriorly by the pubic symphysis. The posterior portion of the pelvis is formed by the sacrum's wedging itself between the two halves of the pelvis. The hip articulation, formed by the femoral head and the acetabulum, is the strongest and most stable of the body's joints. However, this benefit is gained at the expense of range of motion (ROM).

The hip is subject to large forces. When standing on one leg, three to four times the body weight is transmitted through the hip,[1] and, when jogging, up to eight times the body weight is transmitted through each joint.[2] Tolerating these forces is possible because of the sturdy bony alignment and ligamentous arrangement of the pelvis coupled with its encompassing dynamic support.

Clinical Anatomy

The anterior and lateral portion of the pelvis is formed by two **innominate bones**, each consisting of the ilium, the ischium, and the pubis (Fig. 12-1). These bones fuse during the teenage years, but their two primary bony prominences, the ischial tuberosity and anterior superior iliac spine (ASIS), may not fuse until the third decade of life.[2] The posterior junction of the pelvic girdle is formed by its articulation with the **sacrum**, a broad, thick bone that fixates the spinal column to the pelvis. The sacrum is responsible for stabilizing the pelvic girdle.

On the lateral aspect of the pelvis, the **acetabulum**, a downwardly and outwardly directed depression, accepts the femoral head within its fossa. The superior wall of the acetabulum is formed by the ilium, the inferior wall by the ischium, and the internal (medial) wall by the pubis. There is a discontinuity inferiorly. This space is spanned by the transverse ligament.[3] A depression for the **ligamentum teres** is centered within the fossa. The **labrum**, a thick ring of fibrocartilage, lines the outer rim of the acetabulum and deepens the acetabulum by approximately 21%.[4] The labrum is thicker and stronger superiorly than inferiorly (Fig. 12-2).

The **femoral head** is globular, with an articular surface that is slightly over a 180-degree arc in diameter. Its articulating surface is thickly covered with hyaline cartilage except for a central depression that accepts the ligamentum teres. Connected to the femur's shaft by the **femoral neck**, the head is angled at approximately 125 degrees in the frontal plane (Fig. 12-3). This relationship, known as the **angle of inclination**, changes as an individual grows and develops, starting at a high angle at birth and then decreasing when weight bearing.[5] The angle of inclination is slightly decreased in women. In the transverse plane, the relationship between the femoral head and femoral shaft is the **angle of torsion**, normally an angle of 15 to 20 degrees (Fig. 12.4).[6] The angle of torsion describes the amount of twist in the femur.

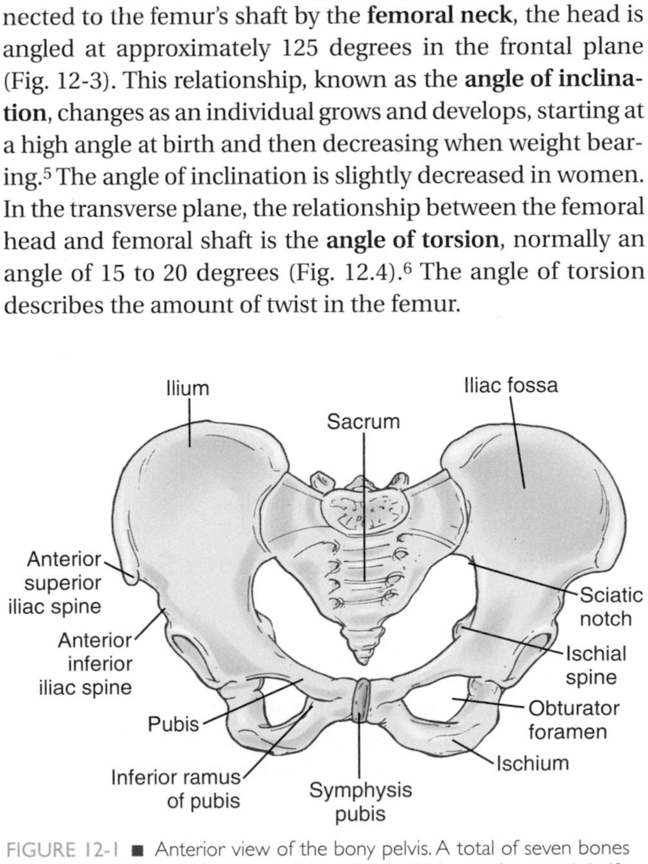

FIGURE 12-1 ■ Anterior view of the bony pelvis. A total of seven bones form the pelvis: Two ischial, two pubic, and two ilial bones form each half, and the posterior border is formed by the sacrum.

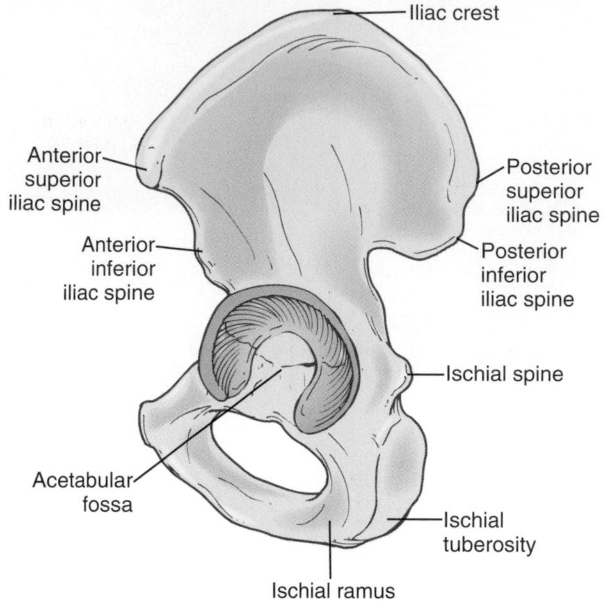

FIGURE 12-2 ■ Lateral view of the pelvis showing the acetabulum. The acetabular fossa is bordered by the fibrocartilaginous glenoid labrum.

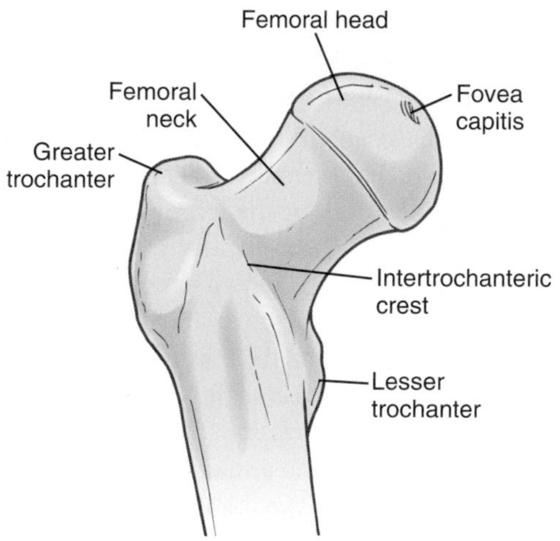

FIGURE 12-3 ■ Femoral neck and head.

On the proximal portion of the femoral shaft, the **greater trochanter** projects laterally, and the **lesser trochanter** projects medially. The trochanters are the attachment sites for many of the pelvic and hip muscles.

Articulations and Ligamentous Support

The pelvic bones articulate anteriorly at a relatively immobile joint, the **pubic symphysis** (see Fig. 12-1). Completed by the fibrocartilaginous interpubic disk, a small degree of spreading (distraction), compression, and rotation between the two halves of the pelvic girdle occurs here.

Posteriorly, each ilium articulates with the sacrum at the **sacroiliac (SI) joints**. A combination of synovial and syndesmotic joints, the SI joints vary considerably in their shapes and sizes. The surfaces of each bone are a collection of concave and convex areas with the concavities of one bone corresponding to convexities of the opposing bone. The resulting articulation is very sturdy with limited mobility.

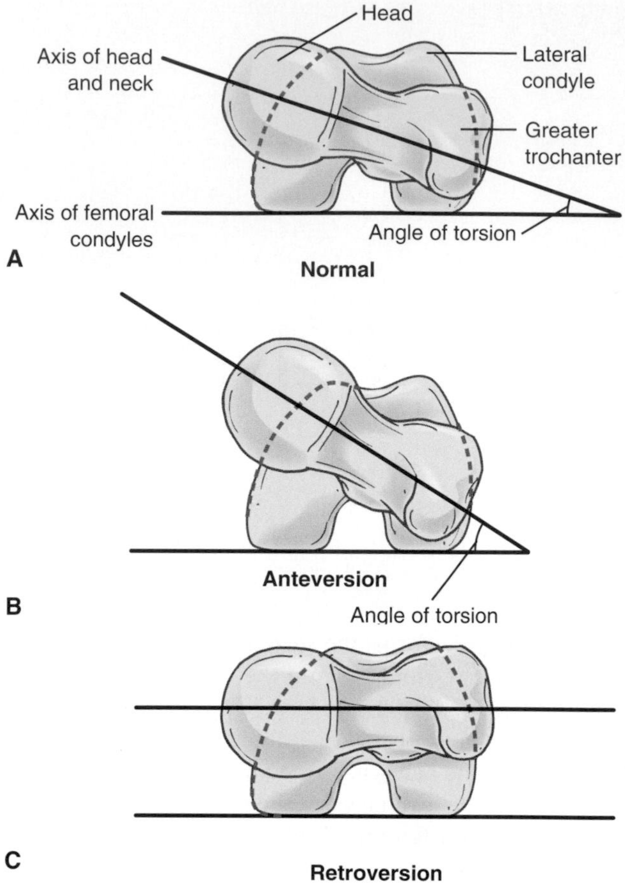

FIGURE 12-4 ■ Deviations of the hip in the transverse plane. (A) Normal hip angulation, 15 to 20°; (B) an increased angle, anteversion; (C) A more parallel alignment of the femoral condyles and femoral head and neck, retroversion.

The hip articulation, the **coxofemoral joint**, is a ball-and-socket joint possessing three degrees of freedom of movement: flexion and extension, abduction and adduction, and internal and external rotation. The depth of the acetabulum, the relative strength of the ligaments, and the strong muscular support limit the hip's ROM in all planes (Table 12-1).

Surrounding the joint, a strong, dense synovial capsule arises from the acetabular rim and runs to the distal aspect of the femoral neck. Accessory bands, or ligaments, associated with the capsule assist in reinforcing the joint (Fig. 12-5).

The Y-shaped **iliofemoral ligament** (also referred to as the "inverted Y ligament of Bigelow") originates from the anterior inferior iliac spine (AIIS). Its central fibers split, with one band inserting on the distal aspect of the anterior intertrochanteric line and the other band inserting on the proximal aspect of the anterior intertrochanteric line and the femoral neck. This strong structure reinforces the anterior portion of the joint capsule, thus limiting extension. Its superior fibers limit adduction, and its inferior fibers limit abduction. The fibrous arrangement of the iliofemoral ligament allows us to stand upright with a minimal amount of muscular activity.

Table 12-1 Ligaments Acting on the Hip

Ligament	Motion Restricted
Iliofemoral Ligament	Reinforces the anterior joint capsule Anterior fibers: Hyperextension Superior fibers: Adduction Inferior fibers: Abduction Allows standing with minimal muscular effort
Pubofemoral Ligament	Abduction Hyperextension
Ischiofemoral Ligament	Extension, extreme flexion

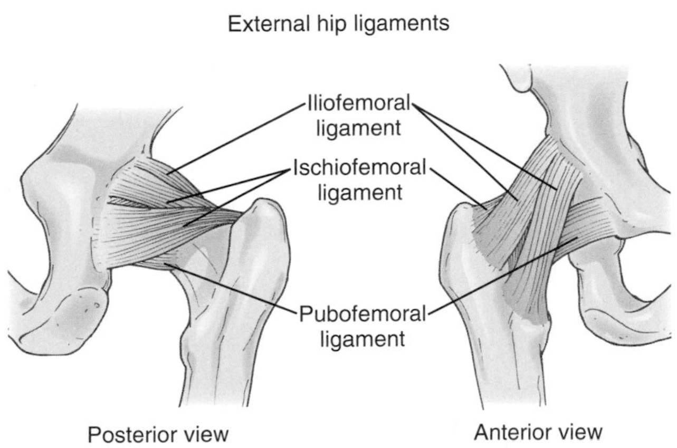

FIGURE 12-5 ■ External hip ligaments.

Also reinforcing the anterior capsule is the **pubofemoral ligament**. Emerging from the pubic **ramus** and inserting on the anterior aspect of the intertrochanteric fossa, this ligament limits abduction and hyperextension of the hip.

Posteriorly, the hip joint is augmented by the **ischiofemoral ligament**. This triangular ligament has an origin spanning from the posterior acetabular rim with upwardly twisting fibers attaching to the joint capsule and the inner surface of the greater trochanter. The spiraling nature of this ligament results in it limiting hip extension.

Within the hip joint, the **ligamentum teres** (also referred to as the "ligament of the head of the femur") serves as a conduit for the artery of the ligamentum teres, which provides little nutrition to the femoral head in adults.[7] Historically thought to have little contribution to hip pathology, the ligamentum teres is now believed to contribute to hip pain when injured (Fig. 12-6).[7]

The inguinal ligament originates off the ASIS and inserts at the pubic symphysis. This ligament serves to contain the soft tissues as they course anteriorly from the trunk to the lower extremities. This structure demarcates the superior border of the femoral triangle. More detailed anatomy of the sacroiliac joint is presented in Chapter 13.

Ramus A division of a forked structure

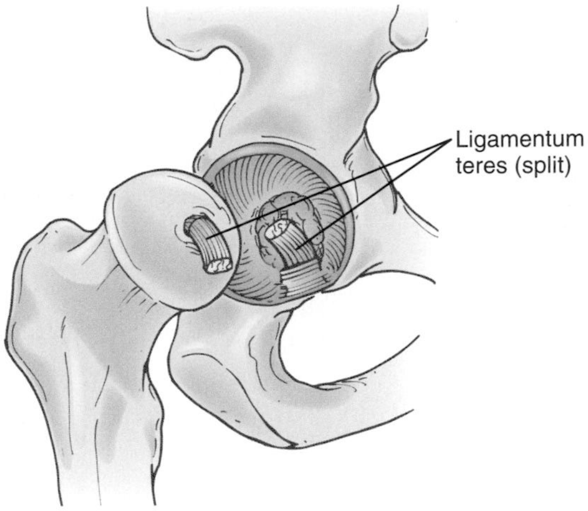

FIGURE 12-6 ■ Ligamentum teres. This structure serves little, if any, role in supporting the hip. It serves primarily as a conduit for the passage of the artery of the ligamentum teres.

Muscular Anatomy

Movements of the hip joint are controlled by groups of large extrinsic and small intrinsic muscles. The large muscle groups act primarily to flex, extend, and internally rotate the hip. The smaller intrinsic hip muscles serve to externally rotate it. During activities such as running and cutting, the hip abductors and adductors act to stabilize the hip rather than generate mechanical power.[8] During walking and running, the rectus femoris and iliopsoas muscles are active to accelerate the limb during the swing phase, and the hamstring muscles extend the hip and decelerate knee extension. Most anterior propulsion when running is derived from hip flexion and knee extension rather than from ankle plantarflexion.[2] The muscles acting on the hip, along with their origins, insertions, and innervations, are presented in Table 12-2.

Anterior Musculature

Crossing the anterior portion of both the knee joint and the hip, the **rectus femoris**, part of the **quadriceps femoris group**, is a powerful flexor of the hip, providing the greatest contribution to hip flexion when the knee is also flexed. The **sartorius**, in addition to flexing the knee, contributes to flexion, abduction, and external rotation of the hip. The psoas major, psoas minor, and iliacus, collectively known as the **iliopsoas group**, are the primary hip flexors (Fig. 12-7).

When the leg is fixed, the rectus femoris, sartorius, and iliacus all anteriorly rotate the pelvis on the sacrum as they contract. Tightness in these muscles can cause increased stress on the SI joint, also causing the pelvis to rotate anteriorly on the sacrum.

Medial Musculature

The medial hip muscles adduct and internally rotate the femur. The bulk of the inner thigh is formed by the **adductor group**, consisting of the adductor longus, adductor magnus, and adductor brevis. This muscle group's action is supplemented by the pectineus (Fig. 12-8). One additional adductor, the **gracilis**, is described in Chapter 10.

Table 12-2 Muscles Acting on the Hip

Muscle	Action	Origin	Insertion	Innervation	Root
Adductor Brevis	Hip adduction Hip internal rotation	Pubic ramus	Pectineal line Medial lip of linea aspera	Obturator	L2, L3, L4
Adductor Longus	Hip adduction Hip internal rotation	Pubic symphysis	Middle one-third of medial linea aspera	Obturator	L2, L3, L4
Adductor Magnus	Hip adduction Hip internal rotation	Inferior pubic ramus Ramus of ischium Ischial tuberosity	Line spanning from the gluteal tuberosity to the adductor tubercle of the medial femoral condyle	Obturator Sciatic	L2, L3, L4 L5, S1
Biceps Femoris	Hip extension Hip external rotation Knee flexion External rotation of the tibia	Long head • Ischial tuberosity • Sacrotuberous ligament Short head • Lateral lip of the linea aspera • Upper two-thirds of the supracondylar line	Lateral fibular head Lateral tibial condyle	Long head • Tibial Short head • Common peroneal	Long head • S1, S2, S3 Short head • L4, L5, S1
Gemellus Inferior	Hip external rotation	Tuberosity of ischium	Greater trochanter of femur via the obturator internus tendon	Sacral plexus	L4, L5, S1
Gemellus Superior	Hip external rotation	Spine of ischium	Greater trochanter of femur via the obturator internus tendon	Sacral plexus	L4, L5, S1
Gluteus Maximus	Hip extension Hip external rotation Hip adduction (lower fibers) Hip adduction (upper fibers)	Posterior gluteal line of ilium Posterior sacrum Posterior coccyx	Gluteal tuberosity of femur Through a fibrous band to the iliotibial tract	Inferior gluteal	L5, S1, S2
Gluteus Medius	Hip abduction Anterior fibers Hip flexion Hip internal rotation Posterior fibers Hip extension Hip external rotation	External surface of superior ilium Anterior gluteal line Gluteal aponeurosis	Greater trochanter of femur	Superior gluteal	L4, L5, S1
Gluteus Minimus	Hip abduction Hip internal rotation Hip flexion	Lower portion of ilium Margin of greater sciatic notch	Greater trochanter of femur	Superior gluteal	L4, L5, S1
Gracilis	Hip adduction Knee flexion	Symphysis pubis Inferior pubic ramus	Medial tibial flare	Obturator	L3, L4

Iliacus	Hip flexion	Superior surface of the iliac fossa Internal iliac crest Ala of sacrum	Lateral to the psoas major, distal to the lesser trochanter	Lumbar plexus	L1, L2, L3, L4
Obturator Externus	Hip external rotation	Pubic ramus	Trochanteric fossa of femur	Obturator	L3, L4
Obturator Internus	Hip external rotation	Obturator membrane Margin of obturator foramen Pelvic surface of ischium	Greater trochanter of femur	Sacral plexus	L5, S1, S2
Pectineus	Hip adduction	Superior pubis symphysis	Pectineal line of femur	Obturator	L3, L4
Piriformis	Hip external rotation	Pelvic surface of sacrum Rim of greater sciatic foramen	Greater trochanter of femur	Sacral plexus	S1, S2
Psoas Major and Minor	Hip flexion	Transverse process of T12 and all lumbar vertebrae	Lesser trochanter of femur	Lumbar plexus	L1, L2, L3, L4
Quadratus Femoris	Hip external rotation	Tuberosity of ischium	Intertrochanteric crest of femur	Sacral plexus	L4, L5, S1
Rectus Femoris	Hip flexion Knee extension	AIIS Groove located superior to the acetabulum	To the tibial tuberosity via the patella and patellar ligament	Femoral	L2, L3, L4
Sartorius	Hip flexion Hip abduction Hip external rotation Knee flexion Internal tibial rotation	ASIS	Proximal portion of the anteromedial tibial flare	Femoral	L2, L3
Semimembranosus	Hip extension Hip internal rotation Knee flexion Internal tibial rotation	Ischial tuberosity	Posteromedial portion of the medial condyle of the tibia	Tibial	L5, S1
Semitendinosus	Hip extension Hip internal rotation Knee flexion Internal tibial rotation	Ischial tuberosity	Medial portion of the tibial flare	Tibial	L5, S1, S2
Tensor Fasciae Latae	Hip flexion Hip internal rotation Hip abduction	ASIS External lip of the iliac crest	Iliotibial tract	Superior gluteal	L4, L5, S1

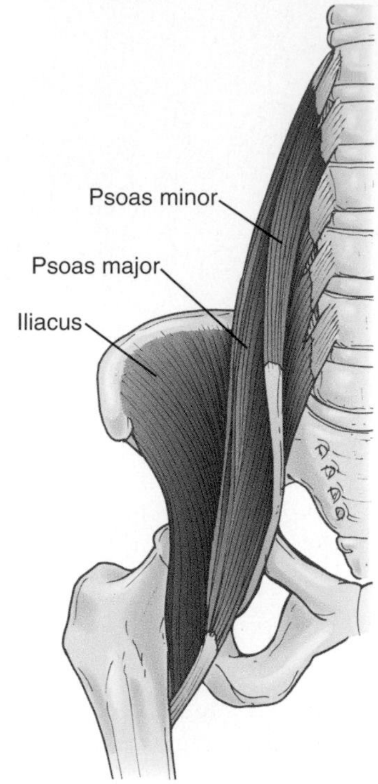

FIGURE 12-7 ■ Iliopsoas group formed by the iliacus, psoas major, and psoas minor muscles.

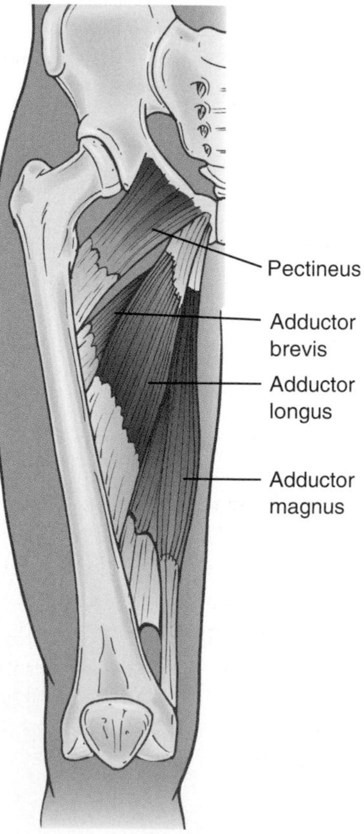

FIGURE 12-8 ■ Adductors of the hip. The only muscle of this group that is uniquely identifiable is the adductor longus, which becomes visible during resisted adduction.

Lateral Musculature

The most superficial of the lateral muscles are the **gluteus medius** and the **tensor fasciae latae (TFL)** (Fig. 12-9). A prime abductor of the hip joint, the gluteus medius is also important in maintaining the horizontal position of the pelvis and the torso's upright posture during gait. For example, weakness of the right gluteus medius causes the pelvis to lower on the left side when the left leg is not bearing weight. The torso compensates for the unequal position of the pelvis by leaning to the right. This compensating movement is termed **Trendelenburg gait pattern**. Through its insertion on the iliotibial (IT) band, the TFL is an abductor and internal rotator of the hip.

Although not contractile tissue, the IT band exerts biomechanical influences on the hip and provides an indirect insertion of several muscles onto the femur. The TFL attaches directly to the anterior portion of the IT band, and the gluteus maximus attaches directly to the IT band on its posterior aspect. The gluteus medius attaches to the IT tract via an overlying aponeurosis. Depending on the position of the hip, these muscles exert a force on the IT band, pulling it anteriorly or posteriorly and keeping it taut as the hip moves from flexion to extension.[9] Inflammation or tightness of the IT band can cause irritation as it moves over the greater trochanter.

Six intrinsic muscles form a posterolateral cuff around the femoral head (Fig. 12-10). The primary function of the piriformis, quadratus femoris, obturator internus, obturator externus, gemellus superior, and gemellus inferior is to

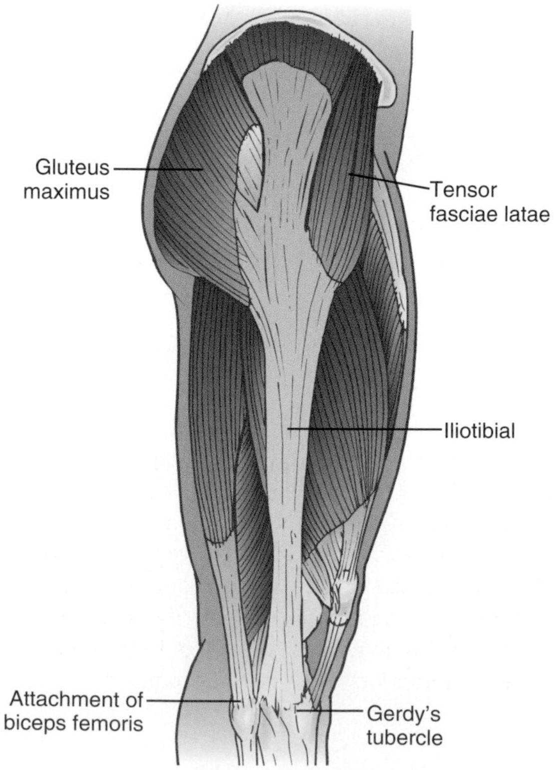

FIGURE 12-9 ■ Superficial lateral and posterior hip muscles. The tensor fasciae latae muscle attaches to Gerdy's tubercle via the iliotibial band.

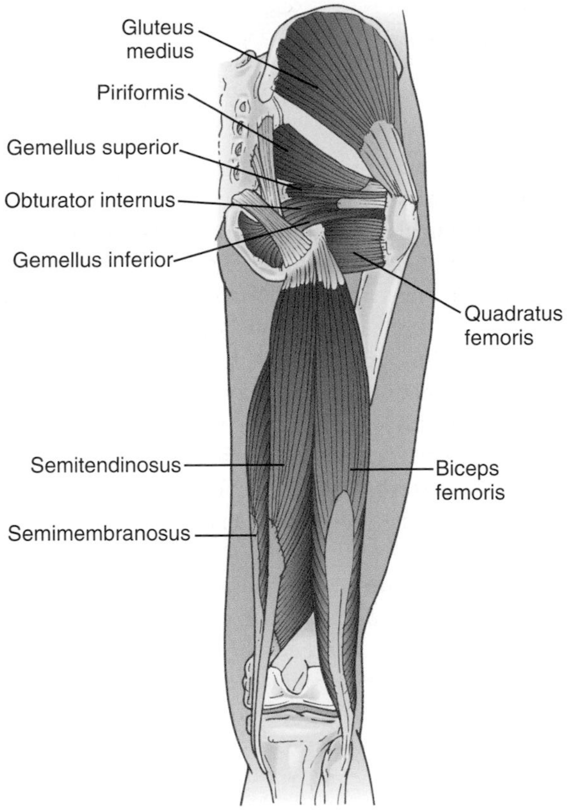

FIGURE 12-10 ■ Intrinsic hip muscles. Functionally, the intrinsic muscles serve primarily to control hip internal rotation during gait.

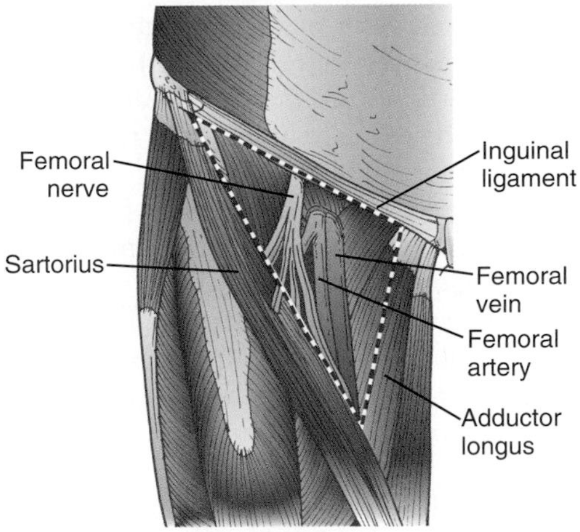

FIGURE 12-11 ■ Femoral triangle. This anatomical area is formed by the sartorius muscle laterally, the adductor longus medially, and the inguinal ligament superiorly. The femoral neurovascular bundle passes through this area.

externally rotate the hip in an open chain. During walking and running, these muscles serve a critical function to control hip internal rotation during the loading response and midstance phases of gait.

Posterior Musculature

The mass of the buttocks is formed by the **gluteus maximus**, a powerful extensor of the hip, especially when the knee is flexed (see Fig. 12-9). When the knee is extended, the **hamstring muscle group** also acts as a hip extensor. In addition, the hamstring group is responsible for decelerating knee extension and hip flexion during running through an eccentric contraction. When the leg is fixed, the contraction of the hamstrings causes posterior rotation of the pelvis on the sacrum from their attachment on the ischial tuberosity.

Femoral Triangle

Formed by the inguinal ligament superiorly, the sartorius laterally, and the adductor longus medially, the femoral triangle represents a clinically significant landmark (Fig. 12-11). The **femoral nerve, femoral artery,** and **femoral vein** pass through this area. The femoral pulse is palpable as it crosses the crease between the thigh and abdomen. Likewise, the triangle contains lymph nodes that may become enlarged with an infection or active inflammation in the lower extremities.

Bursae

Four primary bursae are found in the hip and pelvic region, each serving to decrease friction between the gluteus maximus and its adjacent bony structures. The trochanteric bursa lubricates the site at which the gluteus maximus passes over the greater trochanter. The gluteofemoral bursa separates the gluteus maximus from the origin of the vastus lateralis. The ischial bursa serves as a weight-bearing structure when an individual is seated, cushioning the ischial tuberosity where it passes under the gluteus maximus. The iliopsoas bursa is the largest synovial bursa in the body, measuring up to 7 cm long and 4 cm wide, covering the area from the iliopectineal line, AIIS, iliac fossa, and the lesser trochanter. The iliopsoas bursa frequently communicates with the hip joint.[9]

Neurological Anatomy

The femoral and obturator nerves arise from the lumbar plexus, comprised of nerve roots from T12–L4. The motor branch of the femoral nerve innervates the hip flexors and knee extensors. The sensory distribution of the femoral nerve includes the anterior-medial thigh and the lower leg (via the saphenous nerve). The motor branches of the obturator nerve innervate the hip adductor muscles and the obturator externus, with a sensory distribution to the medial thigh.

Nerves emanating from the sacral plexus (L4–S4) converge and pass through the pelvis as the sciatic nerve via the greater sciatic foramen. Small nerves, including the nerve to the piriformis, the nerve to the obturator internus and gemellus superior, and the nerve to the quadratus femoris and gemellus inferior, innervate the muscles as named. The superior gluteal nerve innervates the gluteus medius and minimus and TFL, with the inferior gluteal nerve innervating the gluteus maximus.

Vascular Anatomy

The blood supply of the hip joint, including the femoral head and neck, arises from the medial and lateral femoral circumflex arteries, both of which originate at the deep femoral artery from the femoral artery. The medial femoral circumflex artery runs deep to the femoral triangle and under the neck of the femur to become the primary source of blood for the femoral head.[10]

The lateral circumflex femoral artery provides the primary blood supply to the inferior femoral neck and trochanteric region. The obturator artery, originating from the internal iliac artery, sends a slip through the ligamentum teres, providing limited blood to the femoral head. Trauma to the ligamentum teres via axial compression of the femoral head or dislocation of the joint may result in disruption of this artery.

In general, the labrum has a poor blood supply. Its vascularization mimics that of the knee meniscus, with the sections closer to the bone attachment more richly vascularized.[11]

The extent of vascular damage and potential for avascular necrosis associated with hip fractures depends on the location of the fracture.

Clinical Examination of the Pelvis and Thigh

Serving as the anatomic and mechanical interface between the lower extremities and spinal column, the pelvis influences and is influenced by these areas. A complete evaluation of the pelvis and thigh may also include a thorough evaluation of the lower extremities, spine, and posture.

To permit the complete examination of these areas, the patient typically is dressed in shorts and a T-shirt. Use discretion when evaluating areas around the genitalia. Always do the examination in the presence of a witness.

History

The majority of pelvic girdle and hip injuries in active individuals tend to be of a chronic or overuse origin, increasing the importance of a complete and accurate history of the injury (Table 12-3).

Past Medical History

- **Prior medical conditions:** Congenital or childhood abnormalities of the hip can result in altered biomechanics of the hip, knee, or ankle during adulthood. **Legg-Calvé-Perthes** disease can lead to residual flattening of the proximal femoral epiphysis, resulting in decreased hip internal rotation and abduction.[12] A **slipped capital femoral epiphysis** can lead to excessive external rotation of the hip and restricted or painful internal rotation.[13]
- **History of steroid use or alcohol abuse:** Both of these increase the risk for osteonecrosis, or avascular necrosis, of the hip.
- **Menstrual history:** Irregular or absent menses can decrease bone density, thereby increasing the risk of stress fractures. The Female Athlete Triad, describes a cycle whereby low energy availability (often resulting from an eating disorder) causes amenorrhea, which ultimately results in decreased bone mineral density.

Legg-Calvé-Perthes Avascular necrosis occurring in children aged 3 to 12, causing osteochondritis of the proximal femoral epiphysis and potentially decreasing the range of hip motion in adult life

Slipped capital femoral epiphysis Displacement of the femoral shaft relative to the femoral head; common in children aged 10 to 15 and especially prevalent in boys

Table 12-3 Differential Diagnosis Based on the Location of Pain*

Location of Pain	Medial	Anterior	Lateral	Posterior
Soft Tissue	Adductor tear Gracilis tear	Rectus femoris tear Iliopsoas tear Sartorius tear Symphysis pubis instability Rectus femoris or iliopsoas tendinopathy Hip sprain Labral tear Iliofemoral bursitis Lymphatic edema/infection	Trochanteric bursitis Gluteus medius tear Gluteus minimus tear Nerve compression	Ischial bursitis Hamstring tear Gluteus maximus tear Nerve compression
Bony	Adductor avulsion fracture Stress fracture	Pubic bone fracture Osteoarthritis Stress fracture	Iliac crest contusion Hip joint dysfunction Stress fracture	Sacroiliac pathology Stress fracture

*Excluding gross injury.

Examination Map

HISTORY

Past Medical History

History of the Present Condition

Mechanism of Injury

FUNCTIONAL ASSESSMENT

Gait evaluation

INSPECTION

Hip Angulations
- Angle of inclination
- Angle of torsion

Inspection of the Anterior Structures
- Hip flexors

Inspection of the Medial Structures
- Adductor group

Inspection of the Lateral Structures
- Iliac crest
- Nélaton's line

Inspection of the Posterior Structures
- Posterior superior iliac spine
- Gluteus maximus
- Hamstring muscle group
- Median sacral crests

Leg-Length Discrepancy

PALPATION

Palpation of the Medial Structures
- Gracilis
- Adductor longus
- Adductor magnus
- Adductor brevis

Palpation of the Anterior Structures
- Pubic bone
- Inguinal ligament
- Anterior superior iliac spine
- Anterior inferior iliac spine
- Sartorius
- Rectus femoris

Palpation of the Lateral Structures
- Iliac crest
- Tensor fasciae latae
- Gluteus medius
- Iliotibial band
- Greater trochanter
- Trochanteric bursa

Palpation of the Posterior Structures
- Median sacral crests
- Posterior superior iliac spine
- Gluteus maximus
- Ischial tuberosity
- Ischial bursa
- Sciatic nerve
- Hamstring muscles

JOINT AND MUSCLE FUNCTION ASSESSMENT

Goniometry
- Flexion
- Extension
- Abduction
- Adduction
- Internal rotation
- External rotation

Active Range of Motion
- Flexion
- Extension
- Abduction
- Adduction
- Internal rotation
- External rotation

Manual Muscle Tests
- Hip flexion (iliopsoas)
- Knee extension (rectus femoris)
- Hip extension
- Abduction
- Adduction
- Internal rotation
- External rotation

Passive Range of Motion
- Flexion
  - Thomas test
  - Hip flexion contracture test
  - Ely's test
- Extension
- Abduction
- Adduction
- Internal rotation
- External rotation

JOINT STABILITY TESTS

Stress Testing
- Not applicable

Joint Play Assessment
- Passive range of motion

NEUROLOGICAL EXAMINATION

Lower Quarter Screen

Sciatic Nerve

Femoral Nerve

VASCULAR EXAMINATION

Distal capillary refill

Distal pulse
- Posterior tibial artery
- Dorsal pedal artery

REGION-SPECIFIC PATHOLOGIES AND SELECTIVE TISSUE TESTS

Iliac Crest Contusions

Muscle Strains
- Hamstring tear

Quadriceps Contusion

Slipped Capital Femoral Epiphysis

Iliotibial Band Friction Syndrome

Legg-Calvé-Perthes Disease

Femoral Neck Stress Fracture

Degenerative Hip Changes

Labral Tears
- Hip subluxation

Athletic Pubalgia

Osteitis Pubis

Piriformis Syndrome

Snapping Hip Syndrome
- Internal cause
- External cause
- Intra-articular cause

Bursitis
- Trochanteric bursitis
- Ischial bursitis

History of the Present Condition

- **Location of symptoms:** Deep hip joint pain can originate in the coxofemoral joint or be referred from the lumbar spine, sacroiliac joint, or both. Pathology in the coxofemoral joint can refer pain into the lumbar spine, adductor group, buttocks, and lateral knee. In females, the pain can resemble that of dysmenorrhea.[14]

A tear to the hip adductors or hip flexors causes pain in the pubic region or anterior hip, respectively. Lateral hip pain is commonly associated with greater trochanteric bursitis and tendinopathy of the gluteus medius and minimus.[15] Pain and paresthesia in the upper lateral thigh, called **meralgia paresthetica**, is indicative of neuropathy of the lateral femoral cutaneous nerve.

- **Onset:** Most pelvic girdle and hip pathologies tend to be chronic or caused by overuse. The date of onset of the patient's symptoms must be correlated with any changes in training techniques such as a different running surface, changes in footwear, or alterations in training techniques or intensity.
- **Aggravating activities:** Question the patient regarding any increased pain with bowel movements or coughing. Anterior pain in the inguinal region coupled with pain during bowel movements or coughing may indicate the presence of a hernia. An increase in symptoms with sitting is consistent with femoral acetabular impingement.[16]
- **Training techniques:** Recent changes in training techniques can lead to overuse injuries, including greater trochanteric bursitis or hip flexor tendinopathy, especially if the patient's running regimen includes training on a banked surface or the addition of hills. Development of stress fractures may be related to recent increases in training intensity, frequency, or duration.
- **Mechanism of injury:** A direct blow to the iliac crest may lead to a contusion (**hip pointer**). Blows to the buttocks, such as from a fall, can lead to a contusion of the coccyx or ischium or to sacroiliac pathology. A sudden pain, especially during an eccentric contraction of a muscle, usually indicates a tear of that muscle. Pain that gradually builds over time may indicate a stress fracture or tendinopathy.

The history-taking process may be expanded based on the patient's responses in the preceding categories.

Functional Assessment

- Ask the patient to demonstrate the functional tasks that exacerbate the symptoms. Frequently, these are walking or running. As described in Chapter 7, observation of gait patterns can provide diagnostic information. For example, a shortened swing phase of gait is associated with a hamstring tear. Lateral hip pain coupled with a pain during the loading response and midstance of gait may indicate gluteus medius involvement. Posterior pain with pushing off during a sprint start implicates the gluteus maximus and/or hamstring.

*** Practical Evidence**

Posterior hip pain elicited with squatting is highly associated with hip osteoarthritis (OA).[17]

Inspection

Inspection of most acute injuries is difficult because of the bony, muscular, and ligamentous arrangement of the hip and pelvis. With the exception of contusions to the iliac crest and hip dislocations, most trauma to this area does not leave visible signs. Therefore, the focus of the inspection phase is to identify secondary indications of pathology, such as muscle atrophy, or to determine the presence of conditions that may alter the biomechanics of the hip and lower extremities, predisposing the patient to injury. Patients who have inflammation of the hip joint may posture the hip in its loose-packed position of flexion, abduction, and external rotation, known as **Bonnet's position**, to reduce pain.

Inspection of Hip Angulations

- **Angle of inclination:** The angular relationship of the femoral head and the femoral shaft may be roughly determined by observing the relationship between the femur and tibia (see Inspection Findings 10-1). Abnormalities at the epiphysis, trochanteric, or subtrochanteric regions can result in significant deviations in the angle of inclination, especially when the deformity develops during childhood (Fig. 12-12).[18,19] An

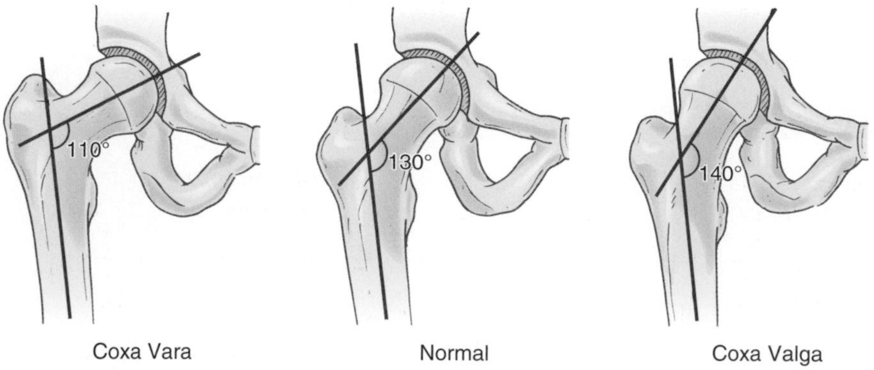

FIGURE 12-12 ■ Deviations in the angle of inclination.

increase in the angle of inclination, coxa valga, may be manifested through either genu varum or a laterally positioned patella. Decreases in this angle, coxa vara, may lead to genu valgum or a medially positioned "squinting" patella. In each case, the mechanical advantage of the gluteus medius is reduced by altering its line of pull on the femur. Radiographic examination is necessary to definitively determine the angle of inclination.

- **Angle of torsion:** Just like the angle of inclination, the angle of torsion must be definitively measured by using radiographs. However, the accuracy of this method is questionable.[20,21] Selective Tissue Test 12-1

Selective Tissue Tests 12-1
Clinical Determination of the Angle of Torsion

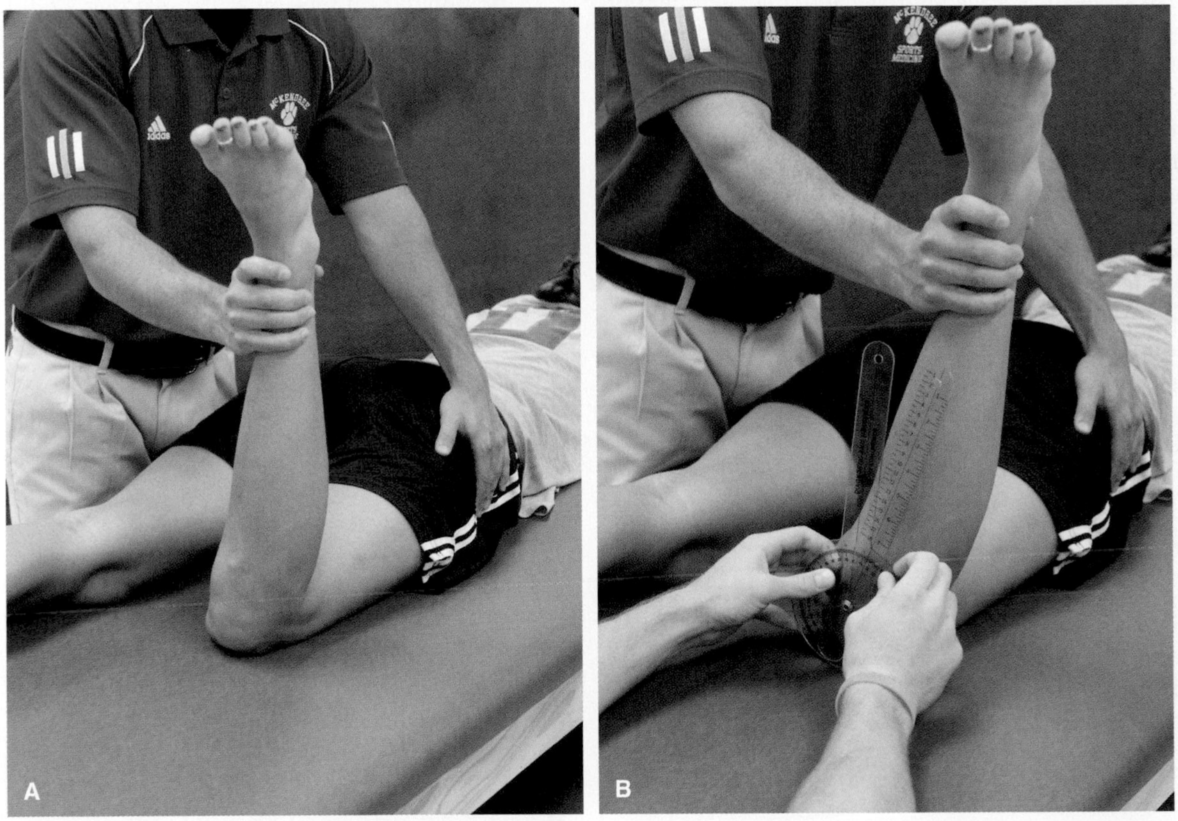

This procedure is most easily performed by two clinicians: one to maneuver the leg and the other to goniometrically measure the angle of the lower leg perpendicular to the table.

Patient Position	Prone with the knee of the leg being evaluated flexed to 90°
Position of Examiner	Examiner 1: On the contralateral side to that being tested; one hand palpates the greater trochanter, and the other hand manipulates the lower extremity. Examiner 2: Holding a goniometer distal to the flexed knee with the stationary arm perpendicular to the tabletop
Evaluative Procedure	**(A)** Examiner 1 internally rotates the femur by moving the lower leg inward and outward until the greater trochanter is maximally prominent. This represents the point at which the femoral head is parallel with the tabletop. **(B)** Examiner 2 then measures the angle formed by the lower leg while the knee remains flexed to 90°.
Positive Test	Angles less than 15° represent femoral retroversion; angles greater than 20° represent anteversion.[6]
Implications	As described in Positive Test above
Evidence	

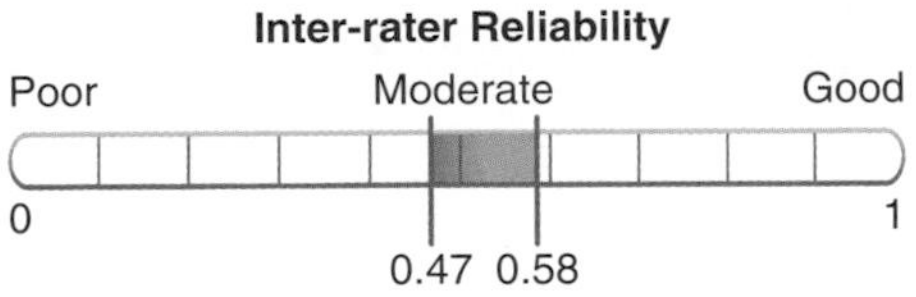

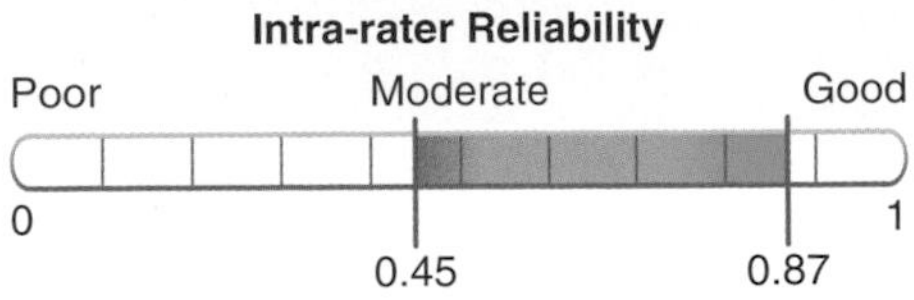

presents a method for clinically estimating the angle of torsion.

- **Anteverted femur:** Increases greater than 20 degrees in the angle of torsion, called anteversion, result in internal femoral rotation, squinting patellae, and a toe-in (pigeon-toed) gait. Compensatory external tibial rotation often occurs.[6] Patients with anteverted femurs typically display a limitation in external rotation coupled with greater-than-normal internal rotation.
- **Retroverted femur:** When the angle of torsion is less than 15 degrees, called retroversion, the alignment of the femoral neck and condyles approaches parallel, resulting in a toe-out (duck-footed) position of the feet. The patella is laterally positioned with a decrease in hip internal rotation and an increase in external rotation. The amount of retroversion demonstrated in early adolescence tends to diminish with age.[22]

Inspection of the Medial Structures

- **Adductor group:** Observe the area overlying the adductor muscle group for signs of swelling or ecchymosis, indicating a tear of these structures or a contusion to the area.

Inspection of the Anterior Structures

- **Hip flexors:** Observe the area of the hip flexors distal to the ASIS for swelling or herniation of these muscles, indicating a tear.

Inspection of the Lateral Structures

- **Iliac crest:** Inspect the iliac crest, located immediately beneath the skin. This area is vulnerable to contusions that initiate a very active inflammatory process. These contusions, or hip pointers, result in pain, swelling, and discoloration (Fig. 12-13).

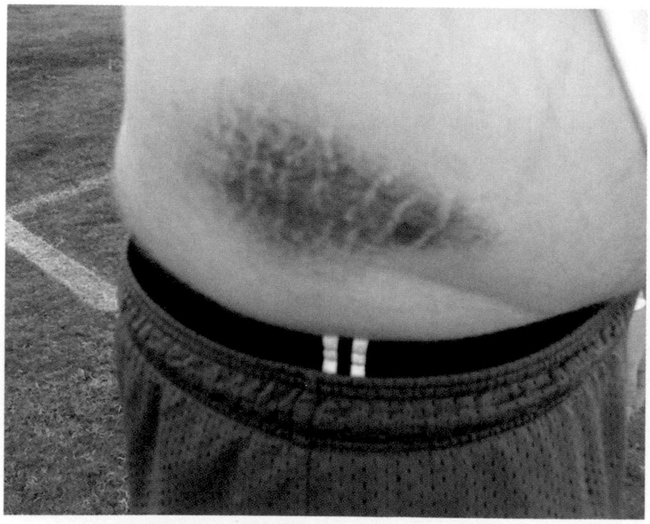

FIGURE 12-13 ■ Contusion to the iliac crest. This injury, the so-called "hip pointer," results in gross discoloration, swelling, pain, and loss of function.

Inspection of the Posterior Structures

- **Posterior superior iliac spine:** If visible, compare the skin indentations bilaterally for symmetry. This should include height of the posterior superior iliac spine (PSIS) from the floor and identification of localized swelling.
- **Gluteus maximus:** Inspect the gluteals for bilateral symmetry. Atrophy of the muscle group could indicate an L5–S1 nerve root pathology.
- **Hamstring muscle group:** Inspect the length of the hamstring muscles to look for deformity or discoloration indicating a muscular tear (Fig. 12-14).
- **Median sacral crests:** Observe the sacral area. Although injury to this area is rare, a **pilonidal cyst**, an infection over the posterior aspect of the **median** sacral crests, causes severe pain and disability. As the cyst matures, it protrudes from the gluteal crease and appears violently red. Patients suspected of suffering from a pilonidal cyst require an immediate referral to a physician.

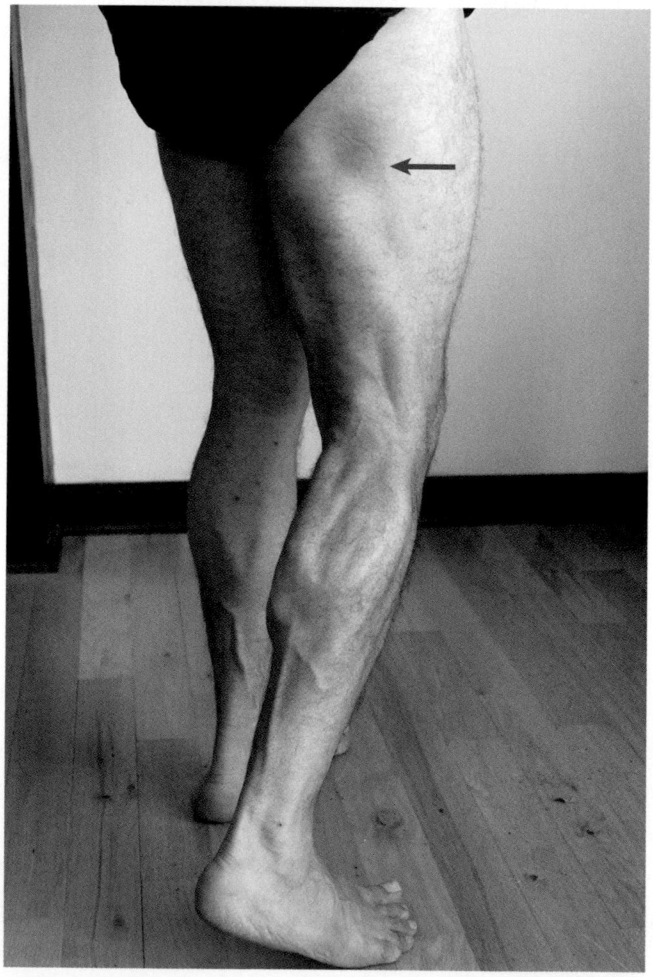

FIGURE 12-14 ■ A tear of the biceps femoris muscle. Note the indentation on the proximal portion of the posterolateral thigh.

Median Along the body's midline

Inspection of Leg-Length Discrepancy

Pain emanating from the foot, lower leg, knee, hip, or spine or deficits in gait may be related to leg-length differences greater than 2 cm.[23] Refer to Chapter 6 for information on the various methods of determining leg-length differences.

PALPATION

The hip and thigh are characterized by areas of subcutaneous bone and other areas of large muscle mass. When performing palpation, use discretion and communicate with the patient.

Palpation of the Medial Structures

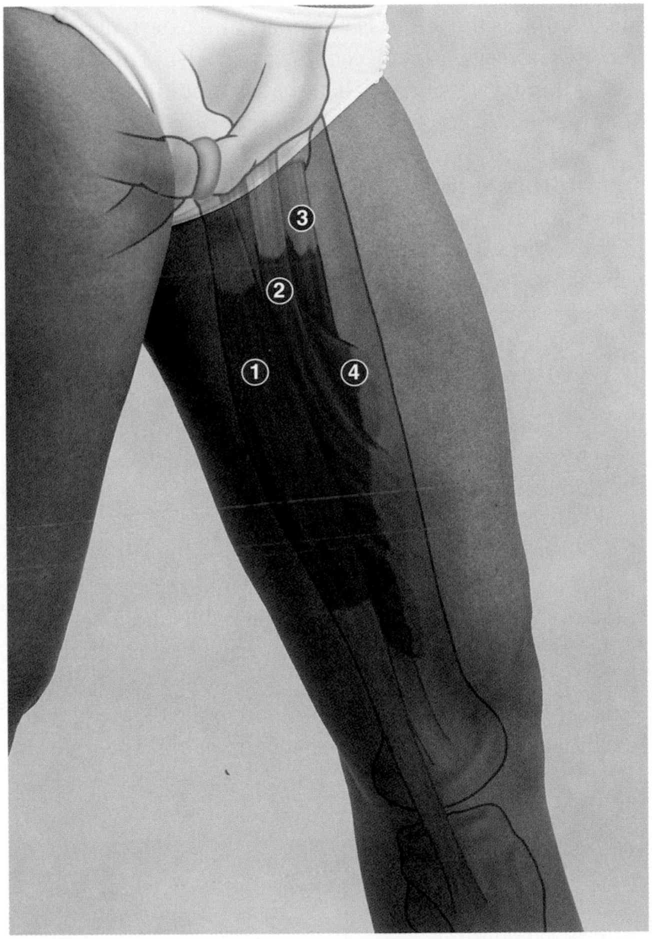

1 Gracilis: Abduct the hip to place the adductor muscles on stretch, making the adductor longus muscle visibly prominent at the point that it arises from the symphysis pubis. Palpate the gracilis proximally from its insertion on the medial tibial flare.

2 Adductor longus: Using discretion, palpate close to the origin of the adductor group for any tenderness or defect indicating an avulsion fracture.

3 Adductor magnus: Locate the adductor magnus superior and lateral to the adductor longus. This muscle makes up the bulk of the inner thigh.

4 Adductor brevis: Locate the bulk of the adductor brevis under the quadriceps muscle. Continue to palpate superiorly to locate the **pectineus**.

Palpation of the Anterior Structures

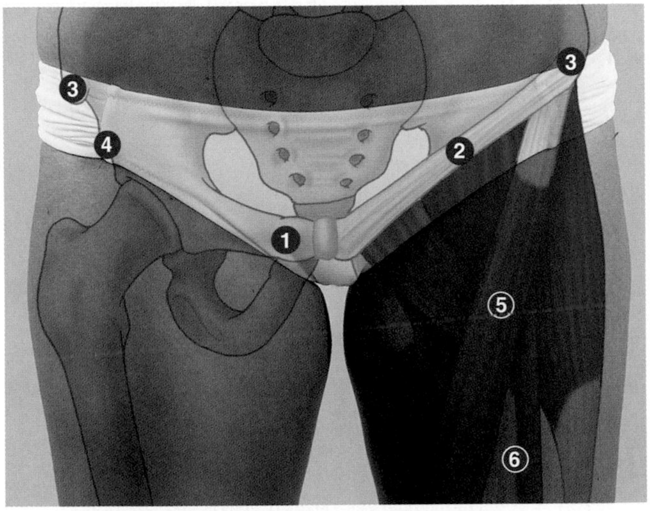

1 Pubic bone: Use discretion palpating this area. Follow the femoral creases downward toward the pubic bone, located under the pubic fat pad (mons pubis) superior to the genitalia. These bones, as well as the symphysis pubis, may be injured secondary to a blunt force such as when a gymnast strikes his or her pubic bone against the horse, balance beam, or bars. The pubic symphysis can become inflamed secondary to overuse injuries and sheer forces, leading to **osteitis pubis**.

2 Inguinal ligament: Palpate the inguinal ligament along its length from the ASIS to the pubic tubercle. Note any abnormal masses or tenderness that may be indicative of a hernia.

3 Anterior superior iliac spine: Follow the iliac crest anteriorly to locate the ASIS. This structure is easily palpable in thin patients but may become obscured in muscular or obese individuals. With the patient standing, palpate the ASIS bilaterally. These structures should be of equal height; any difference indicates a functional or true leg-length discrepancy.

4 Anterior inferior iliac spine: From the ASIS, continue to palpate downward to locate the AIIS. This structure is not always identifiable.

5 Sartorius: Palpate the sartorius from its insertion on the ASIS to where it crosses the femoral crease. In some patients, the sartorius may be palpable along its entire length.

6 Rectus femoris: Keep in mind that both heads of the rectus femoris lie under the sartorius and therefore are not palpable. However, when the knee is flexed and the hip forced into extension, the resulting tension may cause a tear of the rectus femoris or an avulsion of its origin. The length of the muscle belly becomes palpable just distal and lateral to the sartorius and should be palpated to its insertion on the patella.

Palpation of the Lateral Structures

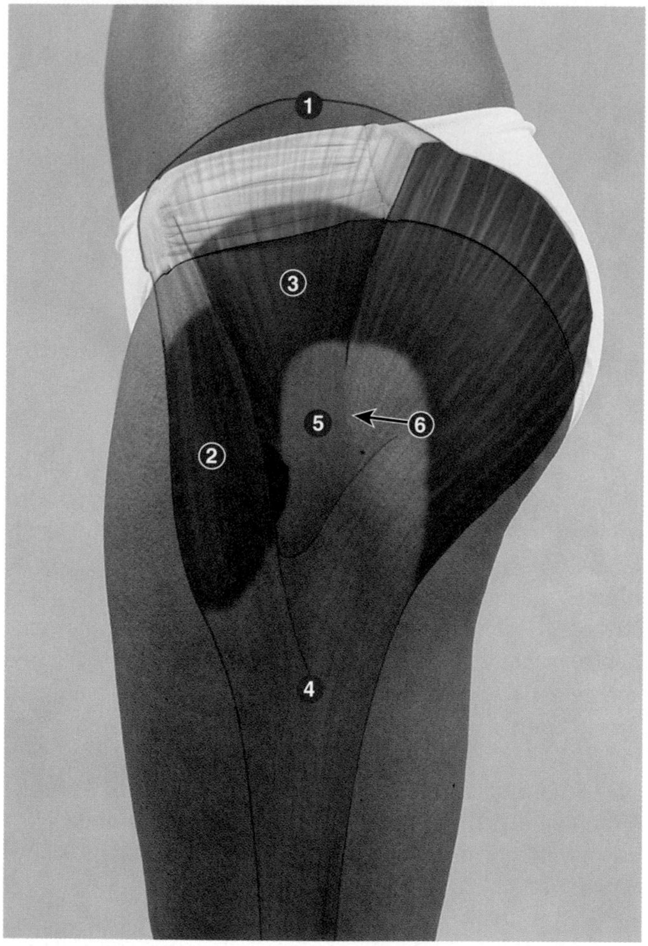

1 Iliac crest: Find the iliac crest, usually easily located on most patients, and palpate along its length from the ASIS to the PSIS. After a contusion, the iliac crest becomes swollen and tender to the touch.

2 Tensor fasciae latae: Locate this area below the anterior third of the iliac crest. The TFL is not easily distinguished from the gluteus medius.

3 Gluteus medius: To isolate the gluteus medius, position the patient in a side-lying position with the upper hip actively abducted 10 to 15 degrees. The length of the muscle is palpable from its origin just inferior to the iliac crest to its insertion on the superior portion of the greater trochanter (Fig. 12-15). The inability to maintain this position during the examination may indicate gluteus medius weakness, which is then confirmed through the **Trendelenburg test**.

4 IT band: Palpate the length of the IT band from its origin from the TFL to its insertion on Gerdy's tubercle. The IT band is a common site of trigger points and may become adhered to the underlying tissues.

5 Greater trochanter: Locate the greater trochanter at approximately the midline on the lateral thigh 6 to 8 inches below the iliac crest. The greater trochanter becomes more identifiable as the femur is internally and externally rotated and its posterior aspect becomes exposed. This area becomes tender secondary to bursitis, tendinopathy of the gluteus medius, or IT band tightness.

6 Trochanteric bursa: Overlying the posterior aspect of the greater trochanter, the trochanteric bursa is not directly palpable unless it is inflamed. Inflammation of this bursa causes it to feel thick and elicits pain at the posterior aspect of the greater trochanter.

Palpation of the Posterior Structures

1 Median sacral crests: Palpate the fused remnants of the sacral spinous processes from below the L5 vertebra to the midportion of the gluteal crease.

2 Posterior superior iliac spine: Locate the PSIS at the inferior portion of the gluteal dimples. Under normal circumstances, these bony landmarks are palpable and align at the same level. Tenderness may indicate sacroiliac pathology.

3 Gluteus maximus: Palpate the bulk of the gluteus maximus. This structure is easily palpable and may be

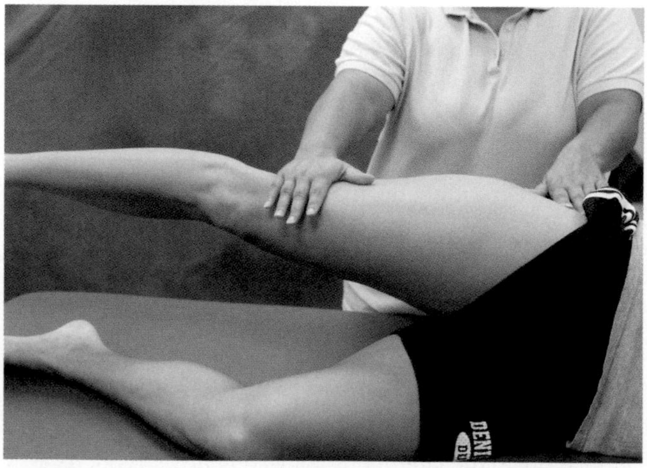

FIGURE 12-15 ■ Positioning of the patient to isolate the gluteus medius during palpation. The gluteus medius is more palpable if the patient slightly abducts the hip.

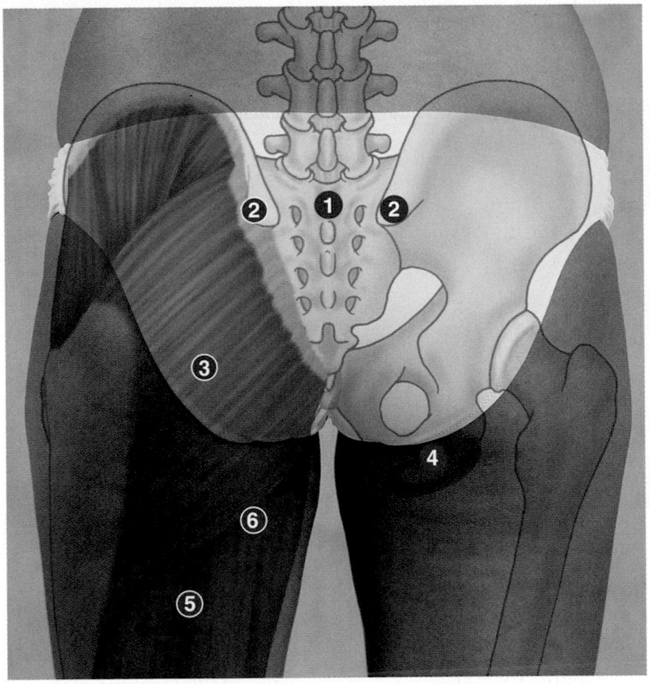

made more identifiable by having the patient squeeze the buttocks together or extend the hip.

4 Ischial tuberosity and bursa: Position the patient in a side-lying position with the upper hip flexed. Identify the ischial tuberosity by locating the gluteal fold and palpating deeply at approximately the midline of the gluteal fold. Tenderness at this site may indicate an avulsion fracture or hamstring tendinopathy. Similar to the trochanteric bursa, the ischial bursa cannot be identified unless it is inflamed, at which time it is tender to the touch.

5 Sciatic nerve: Although the sciatic nerve is not directly palpable, attempt to palpate its approximate course for tenderness. Begin palpation of this structure by locating the ischial tuberosity and the greater trochanter. The sciatic nerve is found as a cord midway between these two structures. An irritated sciatic nerve is exquisitely tender when compared with the contralateral side.

6 Hamstring muscles: Position the patient prone with the knee flexed between 45 and 90 degrees. Locate the common origin of the hamstring group on the ischial tuberosity, a common site of avulsion fractures. With the exception of the short head of the biceps femoris, the hamstring tendons originate as a single mass. Approximately 5 to 10 cm distal to the tuberosity, the muscles begin to diverge, with the semimembranosus the first muscle to become prominent.[24] Palpate the semitendinosus and semimembranosus down the medial side of the posterior femur. Also palpate the biceps femoris down the lateral border, noting any spasm, defects, or pain.

Joint and Muscle Function Assessment

The ROM available to the hip joint is limited by its bony and soft tissue restraints. The position of the knee also can further limit the hip's ROM, and assessment of hip motion should occur with the knee flexed and extended. A fully flexed knee can limit the amount of extension at the hip because the rectus femoris is stretched to its limits. An extended knee with stretched hamstrings can limit the amount of hip flexion available. Goniometric evaluation of hip ROM is presented in Goniometry 12-1 to 12-3. The muscles acting on the hip in each of its motions are presented in Table 12-4.

Active Range of Motion

With three degrees of freedom, the hip has a range of motion second only to the shoulder and the carpometacarpal joint of the thumb. There is no true active range of motion (AROM) at the sacroiliac joints or the pubis symphysis. Motion in these joints is accessory in nature.

- **Flexion and extension:** The arc of motion available to the hip with the knee flexed ranges from 130 to 150 degrees. The majority of this motion (120 degrees to 130 degrees) occurs during flexion. Hamstring muscle length is assessed by flexing the hip with the knee extended. Length of the rectus femoris is assessed by extending the hip while maintaining knee flexion.
- **Adduction and abduction:** AROM for abduction of the hip is approximately 45 degrees from the neutral position and for adduction 20 to 30 degrees after the opposite limb is cleared from the movement.
- **Internal and external rotation:** With the hip in the flexed position, such as when a patient is sitting with legs bent at the end of a table, external rotation ranges from 40 to 50 degrees from the neutral position. Internal rotation is slightly less, approximately 45 degrees from the neutral position. Anteversion and retroversion of the femur influence the available range in rotation. Extending the hip reduces the ROM available in each direction.

Manual Muscle Testing

The iliopsoas muscle group is the primary flexor of the hip. The rectus femoris, a two-joint muscle crossing the hip and knee, contributes to hip flexion, especially when combined with knee extension such as when kicking a ball. Several approaches attempt to differentiate the contribution of the iliopsoas and rectus femoris to hip flexion (e.g., knee flexed, knee extended). It is recommended to first test hip flexion as described in Manual Muscle Test 12-1 and then to test knee extension (see Manual Muscle Test 10-1). Testing of the sartorius, another two-joint muscle that acts on the hip and the knee, is described in Manual Muscle Test 10-3.

Manual muscle tests for the other hip muscles are presented in Manual Muscle Tests 12-2 through 12-4. In addition to the standard testing of the hip muscles, the postural muscles of the pelvic girdle are assessed during gait. Patients suffering from weakness of the gluteus medius tilt the pelvis to the side opposite the insufficiency, which is noted during the **Trendelenburg test** (Selective Tissue Test 12-2). Trendelenburg gait is discussed in detail in Chapter 7.

Goniometry 12-1
Flexion and Extension

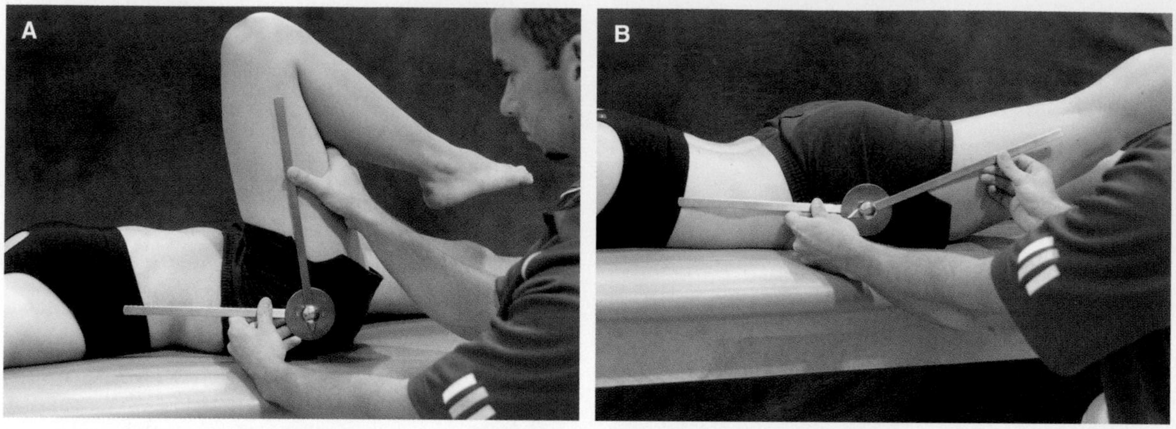

	Flexion 0°–120°	Extension 0°–30°
Patient Position	Supine	Prone

Goniometer Alignment

Fulcrum	The axis is aligned over the greater trochanter.
Proximal Arm	The stationary arm is aligned with the midline of the trunk.
Distal Arm	The movement arm is aligned with the long axis of the femur, using the lateral epicondyle as the distal reference point.
Comments	Allow the knee to flex during the hip flexion measurement. The hip flexion measurement can also be taken with the knee extended to determine the influence of hamstring length. When measuring hip extension, stabilize the pelvis to avoid trunk extension. This may require help from someone. The hip extension measurement can also be taken with the knee flexed to determine the influence of rectus femoris length.
Evidence	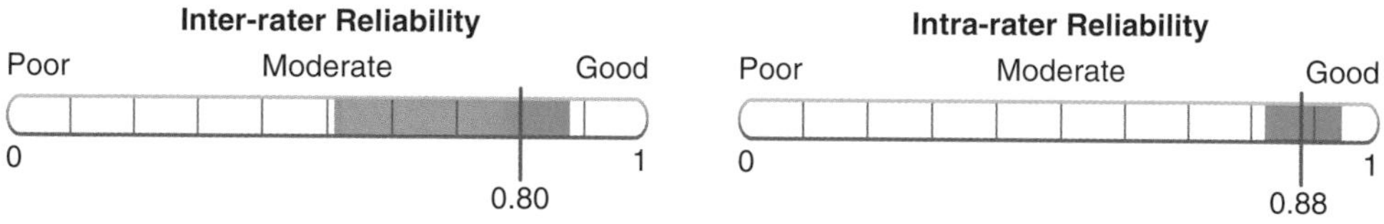

✱ Practical Evidence

Hip abduction strength is often reduced in the presence of chronic ankle instability and recurrent ankle sprains.[25]

Passive Range of Motion

Hip passive range of motion (PROM) most frequently results in a firm end-feel resulting from soft tissue stretch or soft tissue approximation (Table 12-5).

- **Flexion and extension:** To measure passive flexion of the hip, the patient is in the supine position. The distal hand is at the posterior thigh, just above the knee. The proximal hand is under the lumbar spine to detect pelvic rotation, which will occur at the end-range of hip flexion. As the hip is flexed, the knee is allowed to flex from tension placed on the hamstring muscles and gravity. With pressure applied proximal to the knee joint (i.e., without forcing knee extension), the normal end-feel for hip flexion is soft owing to the approximation of the quadriceps group with the abdomen. When the knee is forced to remain in extension during hip flexion, the end-feel is firm because of the stretching of the hamstring muscle groups (Fig. 12-16).

Tightness of the hip flexors can result in an increased lordotic curvature of the lumbar spine. The Thomas test is used to differentiate between tightness of the iliopsoas muscle group and tightness of the rectus femoris muscle (Selective Tissue Test 12-3). Tightness of the hip flexors can also be identified using Ely's test (Selective Tissue Test 12-4).

Goniometry 12-2
Hip Abduction and Adduction

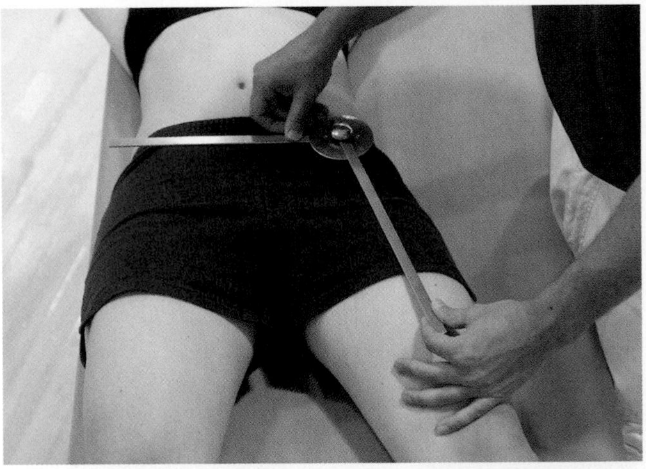

	Abduction 0°– 45°	Adduction 0°–30°
Patient Position	Supine	Supine; the opposite leg is abducted.

Goniometer Alignment

Fulcrum	The axis is aligned over the ASIS.
Proximal Arm	The stationary arm is placed over the opposite ASIS.
Distal Arm	The movement arm is positioned over the long axis of the femur, using the middle of the patella as the distal reference.
Comments	Note that the start position of the goniometer is 90°, which is the baseline. Measurements are made relative to that position. The end of hip adduction is reached when the pelvis begins to laterally tilt.
Evidence	

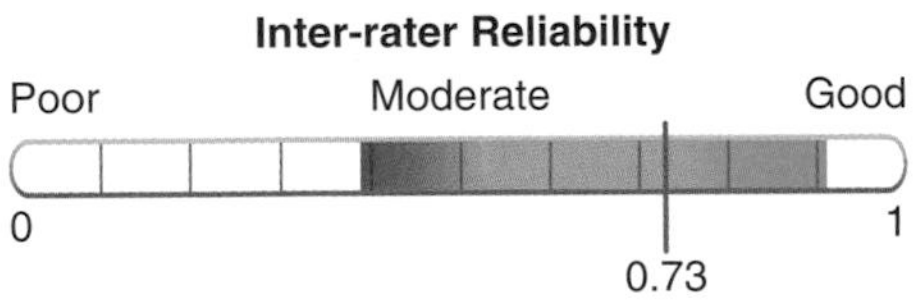

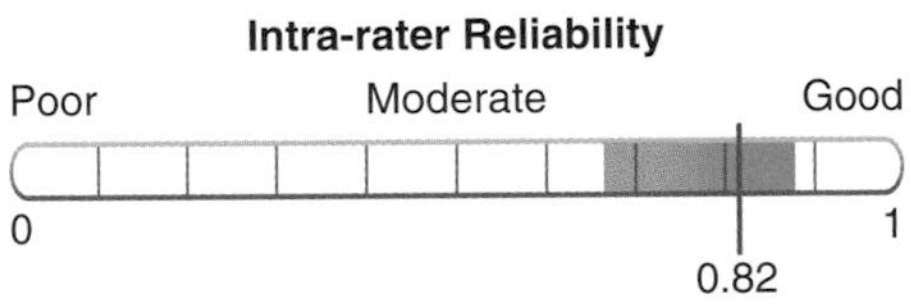

ASIS = anterior superior iliac spine

IT band tightness can be identified by the Ober test (Selective Tissue Test 12-5).

During passive hip extension ROM measurements, the patient is prone, and the knee is kept extended. The pelvis is stabilized to prevent it from being lifted off the table. The normal end-feel for hip extension is firm because of the stretching of the anterior joint capsule and the iliofemoral, ischiofemoral, and pubofemoral ligaments. If extension is assessed with the knee flexed, a firm end-feel is obtained from tension within the rectus femoris muscle (Fig. 12-17).

- **Adduction and abduction:** The patient is in the supine position with the knee extended for the measurement of both passive adduction and abduction. The leg opposite that being tested is abducted to permit unrestricted adduction of the extremity being tested. To isolate the hip joint, the pelvis is stabilized to prevent lateral tilting during the motion. The normal end-feel during adduction is firm owing to tension produced in the lateral joint capsule, the IT band, and the gluteus medius muscle. During abduction, a firm end-feel is obtained because of the tightness in the medial joint capsule and in the pubofemoral, ischiofemoral, and iliofemoral ligaments.
- **Internal and external rotation:** The patient is supine with the hip and knee flexed to 90 degrees for a rough estimate of range and end-feel. Stabilize the distal femur with one hand and maneuver the distal lower leg to rotate the femur. Measure joint motion with the patient seated.

Goniometry 12-3

Hip Internal and External Rotation

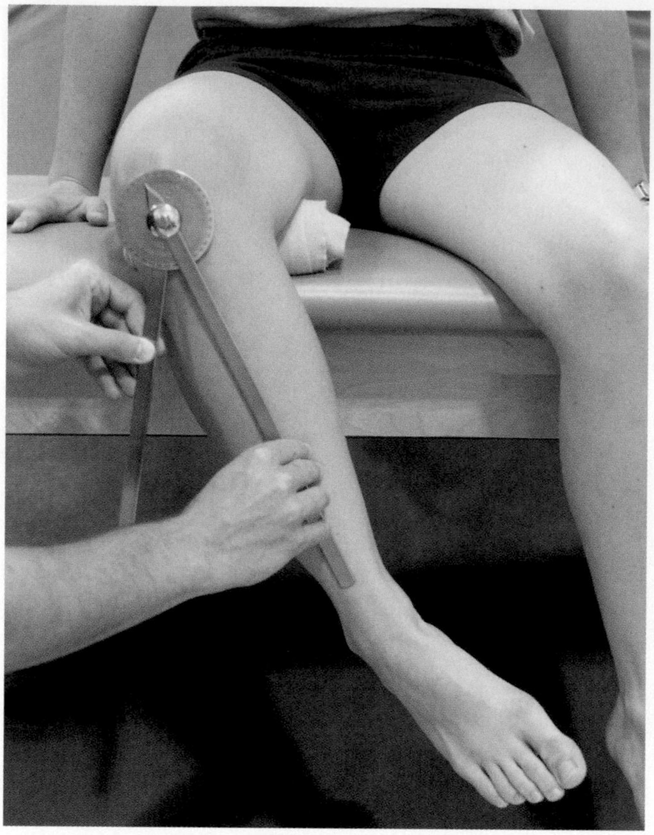

Internal Rotation 0°– 45° External Rotation 0°– 45°

Patient Position	Seated Place a bolster under the distal femur to keep it parallel with the tabletop.

Goniometer Alignment

Fulcrum	The axis is aligned over the center of the patella.
Proximal Arm	The stationary arm is held perpendicular to the floor.
Distal Arm	The movement arm is positioned with the long axis of the tibia, using the center of the talocrural joint as the distal reference.

Evidence

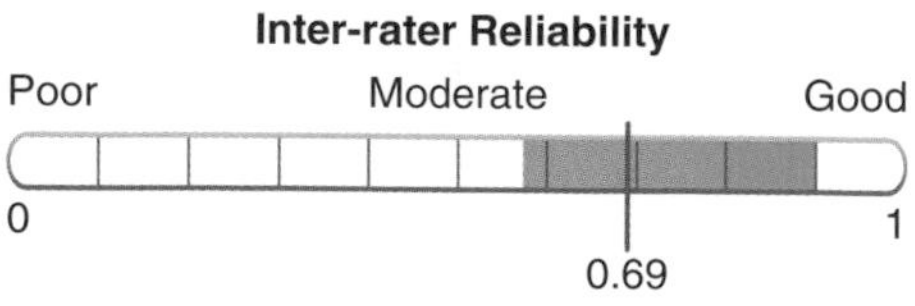

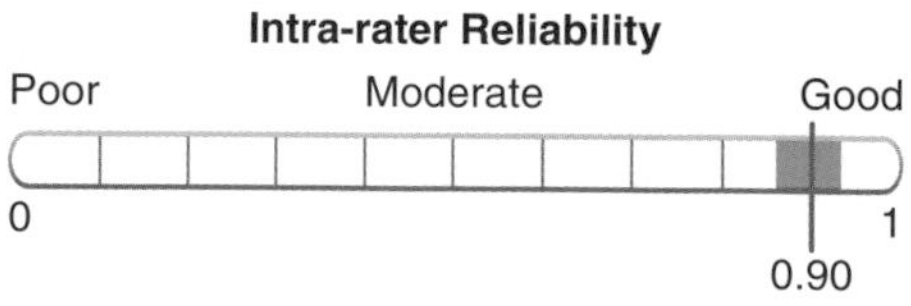

Manual Muscle Test 12-1
Hip Flexion

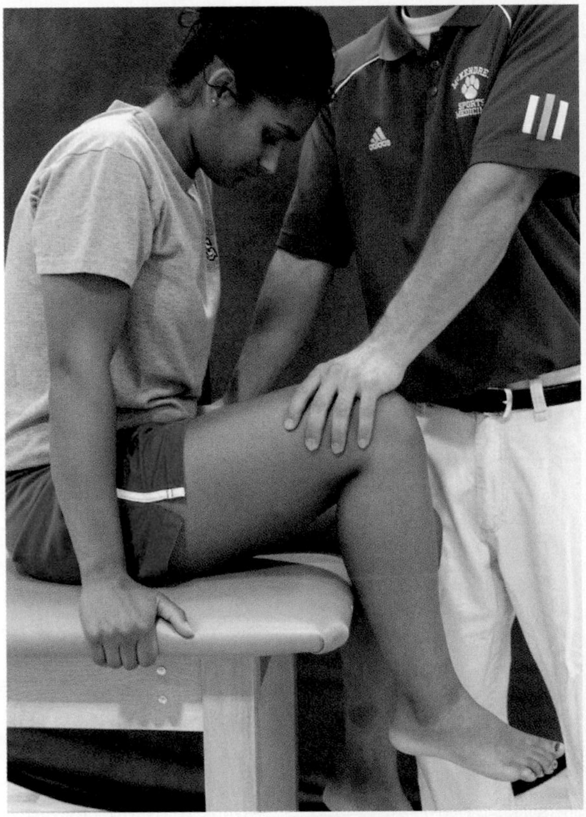

Patient Position	Seated, leaning slightly forward The patient should lightly grip the table.
Test Position	The knee is flexed over the edge of the table with the hip in slight flexion.
Stabilization	Over the anterior superior iliac spine
Resistance	Anterior aspect of the distal femur just proximal to the knee
Primary Movers (Innervation)	Iliopsoas (L1, L2, L3, L4)
Secondary Movers (Innervation)	Rectus femoris (L2, L3, L4) Sartorius (L2, L3)
Substitution	The patient may attempt to lean backwards to maximize the contribution of the rectus femoris.
Comments	There is no agreement on the optimal position for testing the hip flexors.

Table 12-4 Muscles Acting on the Hip According to Motion

Flexion	Abduction	Internal Rotation
Gluteus medius (anterior fibers)	Gluteus maximus (lower fibers)	Adductor brevis
Gluteus minimus	Gluteus medius	Adductor longus
Iliacus	Gluteus minimus	Adductor magnus
Psoas major	Sartorius	Gluteus medius (anterior fibers)
Psoas minor		Gluteus minimus
Rectus femoris		
Sartorius		
Extension	**Adduction**	**External Rotation**
Biceps femoris	Adductor brevis	Gemellus inferior
Gluteus maximus	Adductor longus	Gemellus superior
Gluteus medius (posterior fibers)	Adductor magnus	Gluteus medius (posterior fibers)
Gluteus maximus	Gluteus maximus (upper fibers)	Obturator extremis
Semimembranosus	Gracilis	Obturator internus
Semitendinosus	Pectineus	Piriformis
		Quadratus femoris
		Sartorius

When the knees are flexed, the lower leg rotates in the direction opposite that of the femur (e.g., when the femur is internally rotated, the lower leg rotates outwardly). The end-feel is firm in both directions. Internal femoral rotation is limited by tension in the posterior joint capsule and the intrinsic external hip rotators. External femoral rotation is limited by the anterior joint capsule and the iliofemoral and pubofemoral ligaments. Internal rotation may be increased in patients who have anteverted femurs and decreased in the presence of retroverted femurs. External rotation may be increased in individuals with retroverted femurs and decreased in those with anteverted femurs.

Joint Stability Tests

Stress Testing

There are no specific tests to determine the integrity of the hip ligaments. Pathology of the ligaments is determined through testing the passive movement of the joint. Extension of the hip places the iliofemoral, pubofemoral, and ischiofemoral ligaments on stretch. Adducting the hip stresses the ligamentum teres and the superior fibers of the iliofemoral ligament, while abducting the hip places a strain on the pubofemoral ligament and the lower fibers of the iliofemoral ligament (see Table 12-1). The FABER test stresses the anterior joint capsule (see Stress Test 13-15).

Joint Play

Assessment of joint play at the hip is not commonly performed. The large amount of soft tissue around the hip makes it difficult to maneuver the joint and to detect subtle joint motion; however, joint mobilization at the hip is a common intervention to optimize arthrokinematics. Restriction in joint PROM may identify hypomobility. For example, a restriction in hip flexion may result from decreased posterior mobility.

Neurological Testing

Pain, paresthesia, and inhibition of muscular innervation may be referred to the hip from low-back involvement. Radicular symptoms into the hip and lower extremity may result from impingement of the lumbar or sacral plexus or their associated nerve roots. A complete lower quarter screen should be performed for pathology involving the femoral or sciatic nerve (see Box 1-5). Impingement of the sciatic nerve from spasm of the piriformis muscle, **piriformis syndrome**, is discussed in the Region-Specific Pathologies section of this chapter.

Region-Specific Pathologies and Selective Tissue Tests

Most often, trauma to the hip and pelvis and the related muscles results in contusions or tears. Chronic conditions often result from improper biomechanics stemming from poor posture, leg-length discrepancies, or overuse. The amount of force needed to traumatize the hip acutely makes any injury to it a potential medical emergency.

Because of the magnitude of the injury and the subsequent emergent management, frank femoral fractures and hip dislocations and subluxations are presented in the On-Field Management section of this chapter.

Iliac Crest Contusion

The iliac crest is rich with multiple muscle attachments, blood vessels, and nerves. The major trunk muscles, the internal oblique, external oblique, latissimus dorsi, paraspinals, and many of the hip muscles, including the gluteus medius, gluteus minimus, the fascia of the gluteus maximus, and TFL attach to the iliac crest. Contusions to the iliac crest ("hip pointers") result in a seemingly disproportionate amount of pain, swelling, discoloration, and subsequent loss of function (see Fig. 12-13). After injury, any trunk and/or hip motions stress these muscle attachments, causing pain. The formation of a hematoma can produce pressure on the nerves, especially the femoral or lateral femoral cutaneous nerve.[2] Once the diagnosis is made (Examination Findings 12-1), the key to reducing the amount of time lost because of this injury lies in its immediate management.

Manual Muscle Test 12-2
Hip Extension

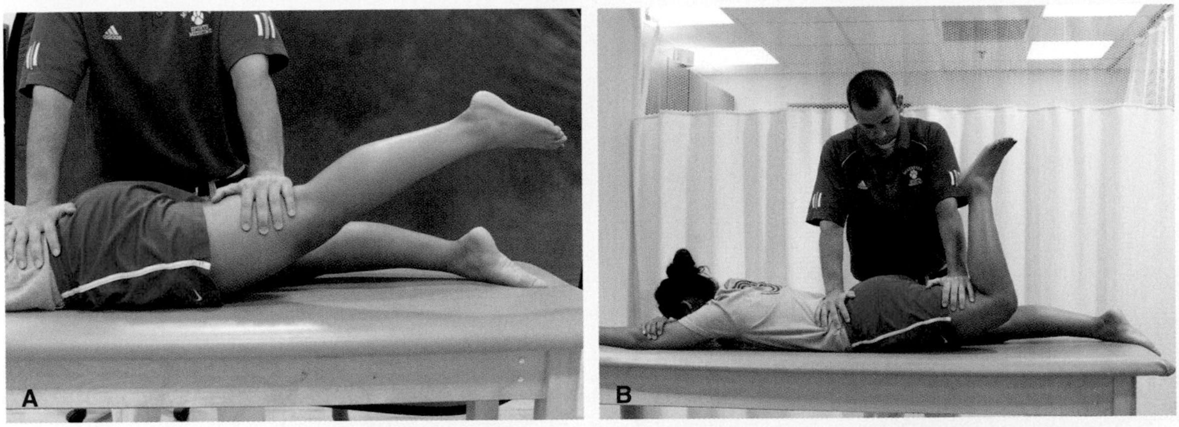

	Hamstrings and Gluteus Maximus (A)	Gluteus Maximus (B)
Patient Position	Prone	Prone
Test Position	The knee and hip are extended.	The knee is flexed to 90°, and the hip is extended.
Stabilization	Posterior pelvis	Posterior pelvis
Resistance	Posterior aspect of the distal femur	Posterior aspect of the distal femur
Primary Movers (Innervation)	Hamstrings (L4, L5, S1, S2, S3) Gluteus maximus (L5, S1, S2)	Gluteus maximus (L5, S1, S2)
Secondary Movers (Innervation)	Not applicable	Hamstrings (L4, L5, S1, S2, S3)
Substitution	Trunk extension	Trunk extension
Comments	Pain with the knee extended that decreases with the knee flexed implicates the hamstrings. This can be confirmed by resisting knee flexion.	Not applicable

Iliac Crest Contusion Intervention Strategies

Individuals with iliac crest contusions require immediate removal from competition or other potential stress, treatment with ice packs, and placement on crutches to avoid weight-bearing stresses. Stretching of the affected muscles should be initiated as tolerated. Radiographs may be warranted to rule out iliac fracture.

If the injury is minor and occurs during a game situation, the athlete may be allowed to return to competition, provided that full lower extremity and torso function is demonstrated. In this case, the injured area is padded to protect against further injury, with treatment following the competition.

Muscle Tears

Tears of the iliopsoas, quadriceps, adductors, or hamstrings frequently occur secondary to a dynamic overload during an eccentric muscle contraction or overstretching of the muscle fibers. Many times, these injuries are typified by pain at the muscular insertion into the bone or at the musculotendinous junction. Table 12-6 presents an overview of the mechanisms and ROM deficits common to muscular tears of the hip and thigh (also see Table 4-1 for the current classification of muscle injury).

In skeletally immature patients or patients with osteoporosis, eccentric muscle contractions can result in avulsion and apophyseal injuries. Clinically resembling muscle tears, these injuries tend to have pain localized to the muscle attachment. The defect can often be identified on radiographs.

In general, muscle tears present with pain during activities (or avoidance of those activities) during which the muscle is most active. For example, a quadriceps tear would result in increased pain during the loading response phase of gait, during which the quadriceps muscle is eccentrically controlling knee flexion.

Manual Muscle Test 12-3
Hip Adduction and Abduction

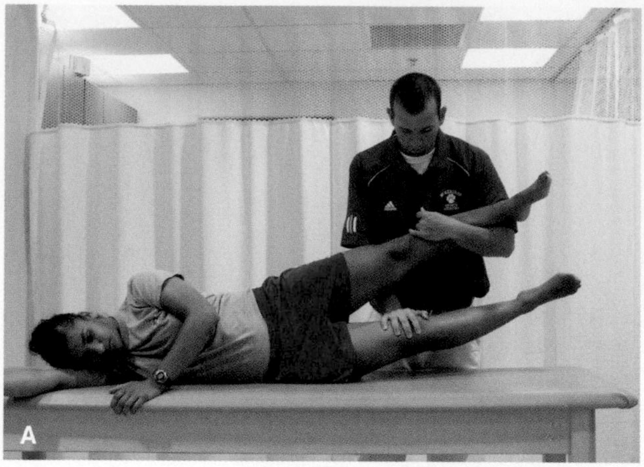

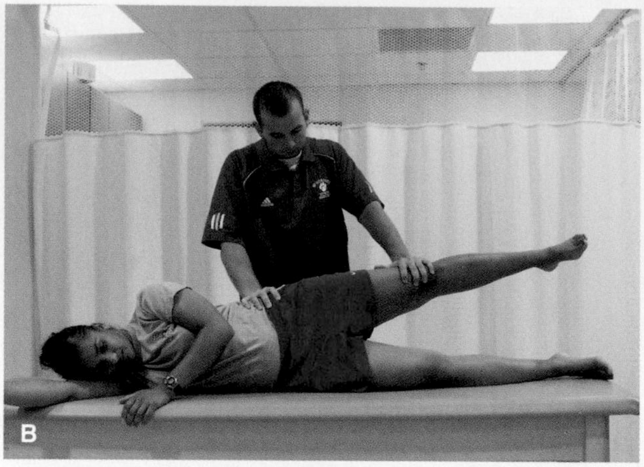

	Adduction (A)	Abduction (B)
Patient Position	Side-lying on the side being tested	Side-lying on the opposite side being tested
Test Position	The knee is extended. The opposite (nontested) leg is supported by the examiner, and the test leg position is in slight adduction.	The knee is flexed slightly with the hip abducted to midrange.
Stabilization	The pelvis and torso are stabilized by the patient.	The pelvis and torso are actively stabilized by the patient.
Resistance	Over the medial femur, proximal to the knee	Over the lateral femoral condyle
Primary Movers (Innervation)	Adductor magnus (L2, L3, L4, L5, S1) Adductor longus (L2, L3, L4) Adductor brevis (L2, L3, L4) Gracilis	Gluteus medius (L4, L5, S1) Gluteus minimus (L4, L5, S1)
Secondary Movers (Innervation)	Gluteus maximus (lower fibers) (L5, S1, S2) Pectineus (L3, L4)	Tensor fasciae latae (L4, L5, S1) Sartorius (L2, L3)
Substitution	Not applicable	Hip flexion
Comments		The tensor fascia latae is more active during abduction with slight hip flexion. The gluteus medius is more active with the hip in the anatomical position.

Hamstring Tears

Hamstring tears are common in many explosive activities. Tears of the biceps femoris, the most common, typically occur during sprinting with resulting injury in the intramuscular region.[31] Activities that incorporate simultaneous hip flexion and knee extension, such as kicking, increase risk to the semimembranosus and the semitendinosus and generally involve the proximal tendon and/or musculotendinous junction. Because tears in the intramuscular region are associated with a faster recovery and different rehabilitation needs than tears in the proximal region, the location of injury and the involved muscle must be determined during the examination process. Risk factors for hamstring tears include age, a prior history of hamstring injury, hamstring weakness and fatigue, imbalance between the quadriceps and hamstrings, and decreased quadriceps flexibility.[31] Hamstring injuries tend to recur if the strength deficits are not corrected, and chance of reinjury increases proportionally to the size of the original injury.[32]

Patients suffering hamstring tears typically report a distinct "popping" or "snapping" sensation when initially contracting the muscle or quickly increasing running speed. In most cases, the individual cannot continue the activity. Palpation performed immediately after the injury may reveal a divot in the muscle, depending on the extent of the injury. Any defects are soon obscured by the collection of edema at

Manual Muscle Test 12-4
Hip Internal and External Rotation

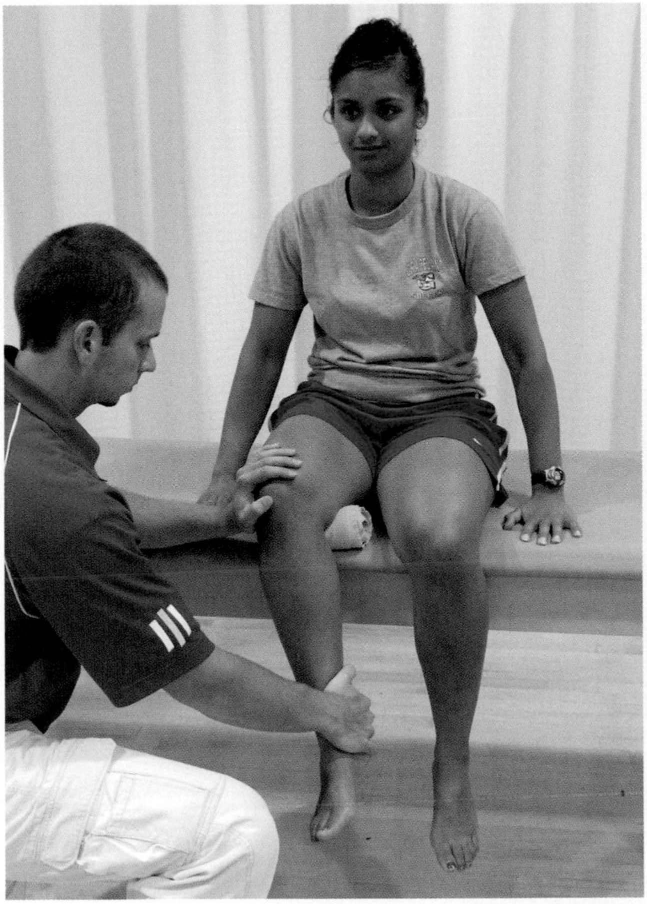

	Internal Rotation	External Rotation (shown)
Patient Position	Seated with the knees flexed over the edge of the table A bolster is placed under the distal femur to keep it parallel with the tabletop.	Seated with the knees flexed over the edge of the table A bolster is placed under the distal femur to keep it parallel with the tabletop.
Test Position	The hip is internally rotated 45°.	The hip is externally rotated 45°.
Stabilization	The patient's arms support the torso on the table.	The patient's arms support the torso on the table.
Resistance	On the lateral aspect of the distal lower leg	On the medial aspect of the distal lower leg
Primary Movers (Innervation)	Gluteus minimus (L4, L5, S1) Tensor fascia latae (L4, L5, S1) Gluteus medius (anterior fibers) (L4, L5, S1) Adductor longus (L2, L3, L4) Adductor magnus (L2, L3, L4, L5, S1)	Obturator internus (L5, S1, S2) Obturator externus (L3, L4) Quadratus femoris (L4, L5, S1) Piriformis (S1, S2) Gemellus inferior and superior (L4, L5, S1) Gluteus maximus (L5, S1, S2)
Secondary Movers (Innervation)	Adductor brevis (L2, L3, L4) Semimembranosus (L5, S1) Semitendinosus (L5, S1, S2)	Sartorius (L2, L3) Biceps femoris (long head) (S1, S2, S3) Psoas major (L1, L2, L3, L4)
Substitution	Trunk lateral flexion	Knee flexion

Selective Tissue Tests 12-2
Trendelenburg Test for Gluteus Medius Weakness

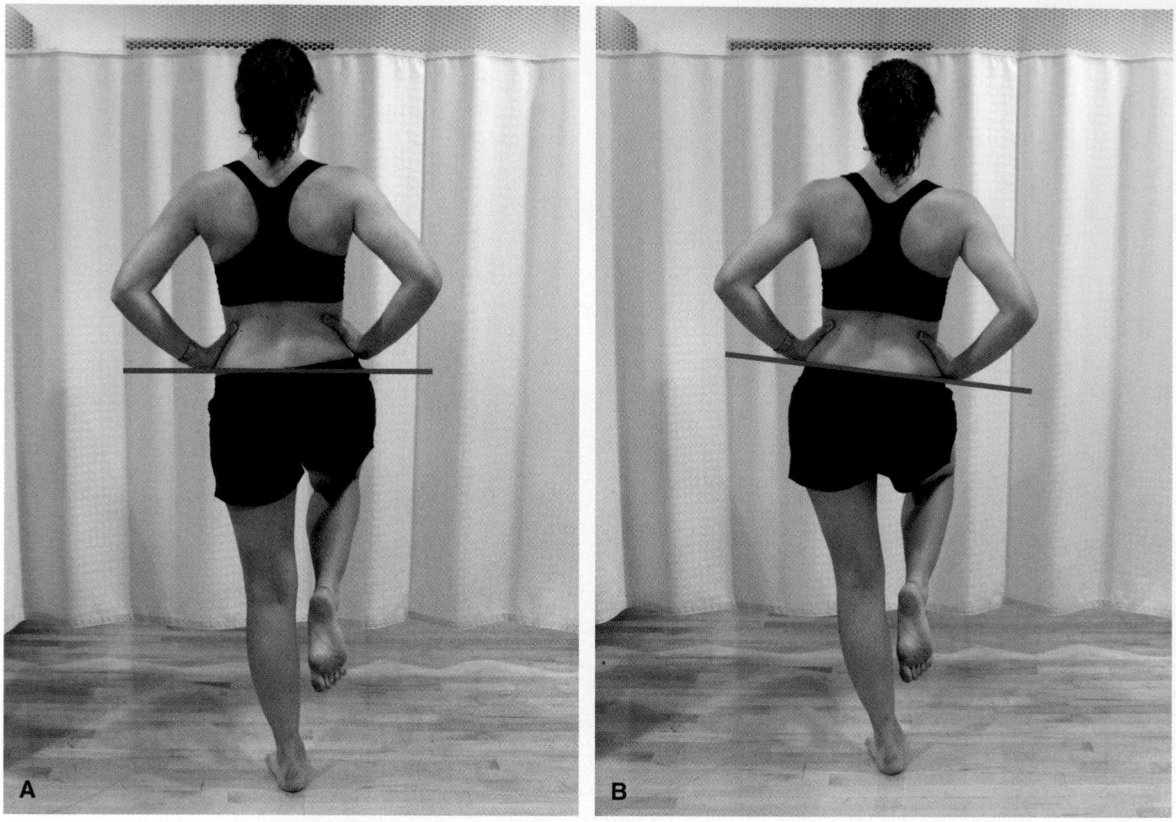

The patient is asked to stand on the affected leg (A). In the presence of gluteus medius weakness, the pelvis lowers on the opposite side of the affected leg (B).

Patient Position	Standing with the weight evenly distributed between both feet The iliac crests or posterior superior iliac spines should be visible.
Position of Examiner	Behind the patient
Evaluative Procedure	The patient lifts the leg opposite the side being tested.
Positive Test	The pelvis lowers on the non–weight-bearing side.
Implications	Insufficiency of the gluteus medius to support the torso in an erect position, indicating weakness in the muscle
Modification	Repeated testing may be necessary, as fatigue can magnify this weakness.
Comments	Muscle weakness can result from nerve root impingement or damage to the superior gluteal nerve.
Evidence	

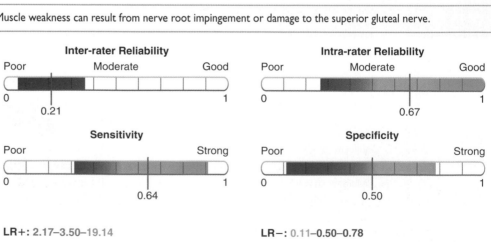

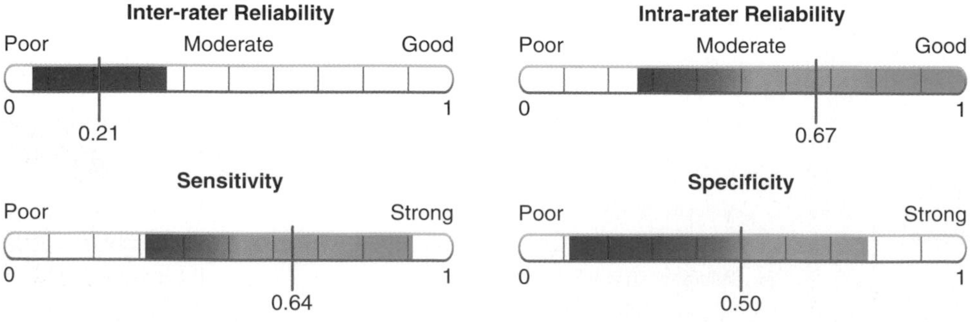

LR+: 2.17–3.50–19.14

LR−: 0.11–0.50–0.78

Table 12-5 Hip Capsular Pattern and End-Feels

Capsular Pattern: Internal rotation, abduction, flexion, extension	
End-Feels:	
Flexion	Firm or soft: Soft tissue approximation or hamstring tension
Abduction	Firm: Stretch of the adductors
Adduction	Firm: Stretch of the abductors and joint capsule
Internal rotation	Firm: Stretch of the external rotators
External rotation	Firm: Stretch of the internal rotators
Extension	Firm: Stretch of the iliopsoas and joint capsule

the injury site. The patient will experience pain with resisted knee flexion and passive hip flexion combined with knee extension. Resisting knee flexion with the tibia internally and externally rotated may help differentiate between the biceps femoris and the medial hamstrings. Ecchymosis may develop. The patient will display an antalgic gait with a shortened swing phase. Avulsion fractures should be considered if the pain is located at or close to the ischial tuberosity and the patient is not skeletally mature (an adolescent). Plain radiographs will detect avulsion fractures, but MRIs are needed to detect the extent of soft tissue injury. Other causes of posterior thigh pain should also be considered. In patients who describe a history of multiple hamstring injuries, the sciatic nerve may become scarred and lose mobility following repeated hamstring injury and may be a source of radicular pain to the posterior thigh.[31]

*** Practical Evidence**

Palpating hamstring tears yields useful information. The more proximal the point tenderness—the closer to the origin—the longer the time needed to return to the preinjury level of activity.[31,33]

Muscle Tear Intervention Strategies

Muscles tears are generally treated by avoiding painful movements during functional tasks without creating harmful movement patterns during compensation. For example, if the patient cannot walk without a limp following a quadriceps strain, then partial weight bearing using crutches is indicated. Other palliative treatments following acute injury include ice and gentle stretching. Once normal gait is restored, a gradual return to activity, including a progression from slow to fast activities, is warranted.

Hamstring tears normally require only surgical repair when the muscle's tendon has been avulsed and there is a significant amount of separation between the bone and tendon. Otherwise, rehabilitation that emphasizes agility and stabilization is more successful at preventing reinjury than rehabilitation that emphasizes stretching and strengthening.[34]

Quadriceps Contusion

Even mild contusive forces transmitted to the quadriceps group can result in the death of muscle fibers. As the severity of the impact increases, so does the proportion of muscle fiber death that occurs. Contusions to the quadriceps group result in decreased force during knee extension. Associated pain and spasm limit the amount of flexion available to the joint. The thigh is often discolored and painful to the touch. Intramuscular hematoma gives the muscle a hardened feel in the area and increases the girth of the muscle. Over time, the contour of the quadriceps group is lost secondary to atrophy. The risk of heterotopic ossification increases with effusion of the knee joint (Fig. 12-18).

Quadriceps Contusion Intervention Strategies

Athletes who display functional limitations during gait, who describe pain during active knee or hip flexion, or who have weakness during manual muscle testing of the involved muscles are to be removed from competition for immediate management of their injury.

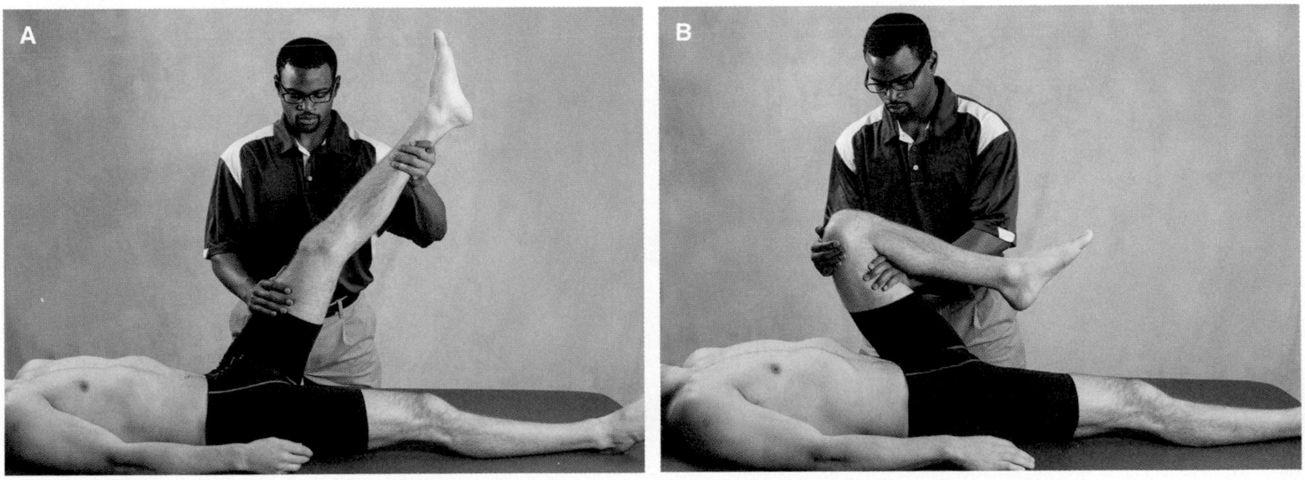

FIGURE 12-16 ■ Passive hip flexion: (A) knee extended; (B) knee flexed. The motion should also be replicated by adding pressure to the posterior distal femur. Note that hip flexion with the knee extended (shown in A) is the provocative phase of the straight-leg raise test and may produce sciatic nerve symptoms (see Chapter 13).

Selective Tissue Tests 12-3

Thomas Test for Hip Flexor Tightness Rectus Femoris Contracture

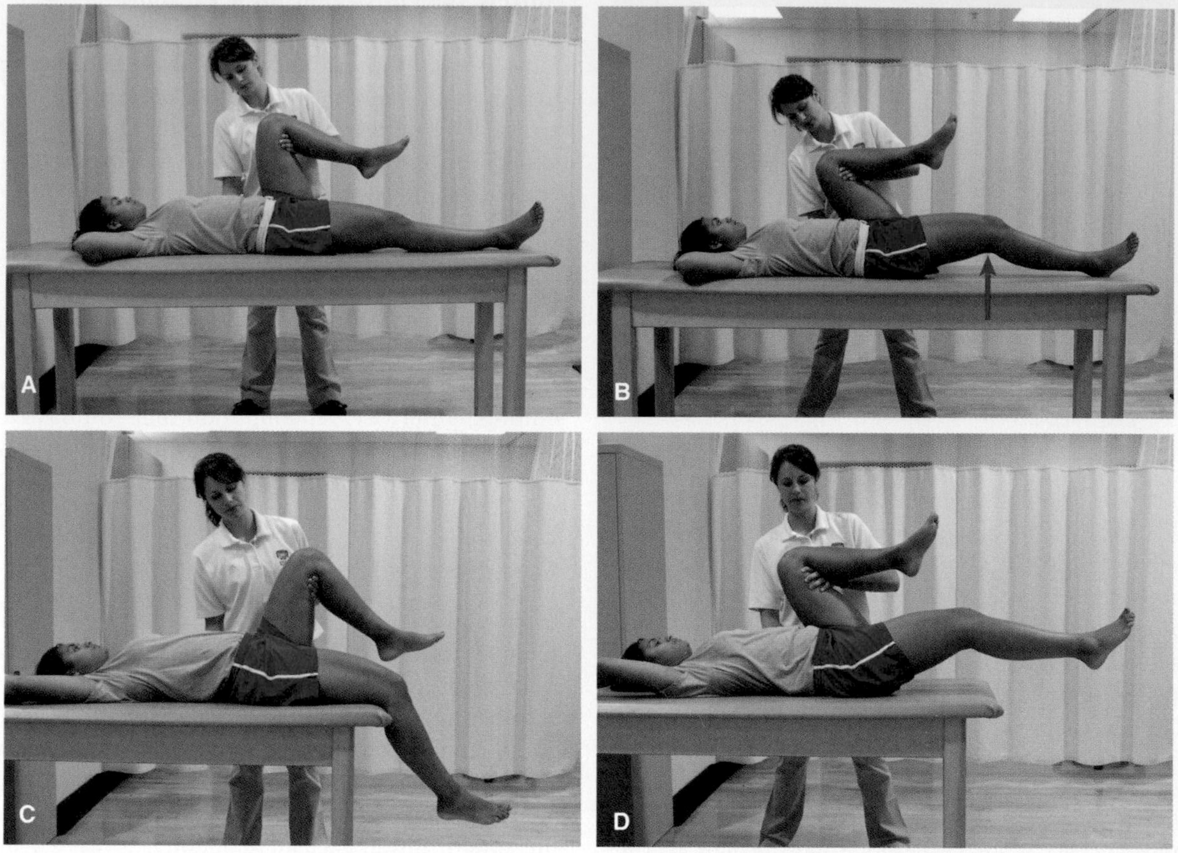

Thomas test for hip flexor tightness. The patient's right (forward) leg is tested. (A) Starting position; (B) Tightness of the right iliopsoas group; (C) Rectus femoris contracture test (a modification of the homas test). The patient is positioned so that the knee of the test leg is off the table. (D) Tightness of the rectus femoris and iliopsoas results in the opposite knee extending and the hip flexing.

Patient Position	TT: Lying prone on the table RFCT: Lying supine with the knees bent at the end of the table
Position of Examiner	Standing beside the patient
Evaluative Procedure	The examiner places one hand between the lumbar lordotic curve and the tabletop. One leg is passively flexed to the patient's chest, allowing the knee to flex during the movement. The opposite leg (the leg being tested) rests flat on the table.
Positive Test	TT: The involved leg rises off the table. RFCT: The knee moves into extension.
Implications	Tightness of the iliopsoas muscle group Tightness of the rectus femoris
Modification	The hip position may be measured goniometrically.
Comments	The patient may passively flex the hip and knee by using the arms to pull the leg to the chest.[26] Tightness of the hip flexors may also result in lumbar extension.
Evidence	

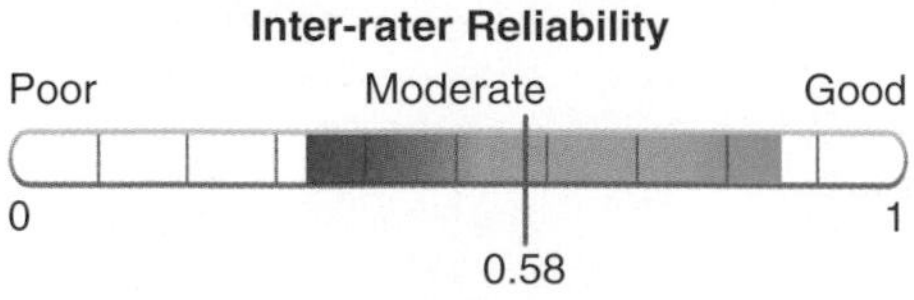

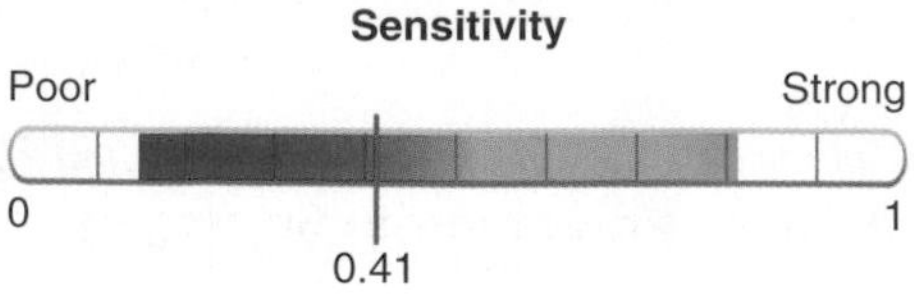

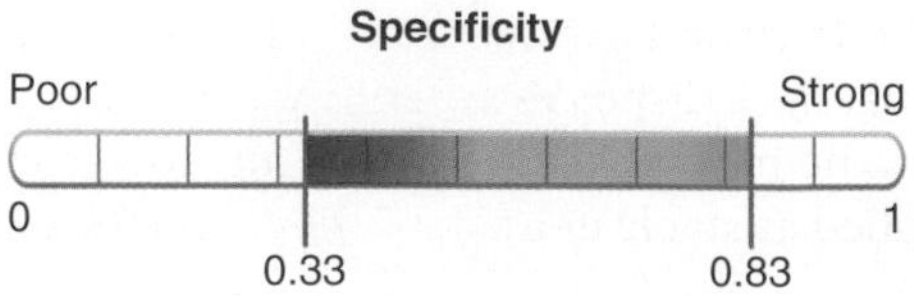

LR+: 0.16–3.35

LR−: 0.12–0.52

RFCT = rectus femoris contracture test; TT = Thomas test

Selective Tissue Tests 12-4
Ely's Test

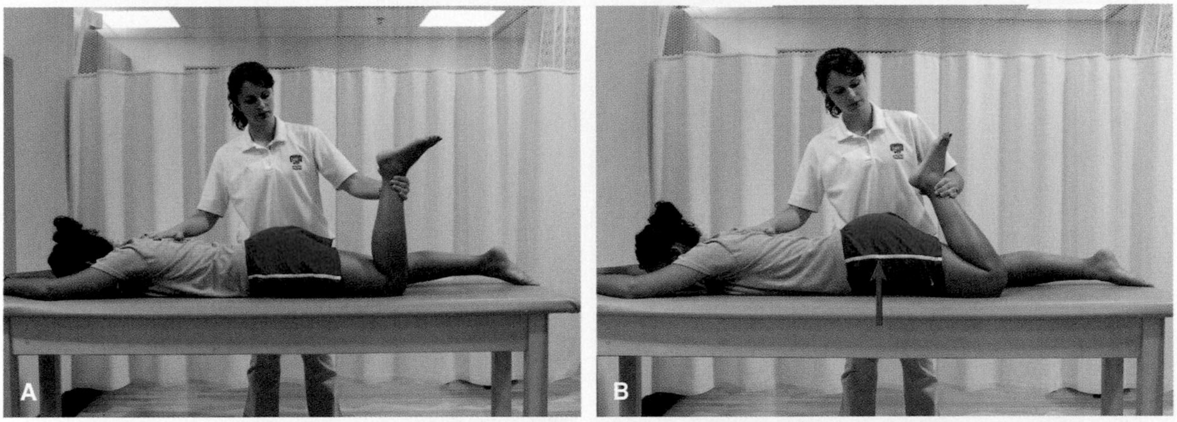

Ely's test for hip flexor tightness (A). Passive flexion of the knee results in hip flexion, causing it to rise off the table (B).

Patient Position	Lying prone
Position of Examiner	Standing beside the patient
Evaluative Procedure	The knee is passively flexed.
Positive Test	The hip on the side being tested flexes, causing it to rise from the table.
Implications	Tightness of the rectus femoris
Evidence	Absent or inconclusive in the literature

After the determination of the injury has been made, ice packs are applied to the area, and flexion of the knee joint, as much as pain allows, is encouraged. Immobilization in 120 degrees of flexion for 24 hours has been associated with a faster return to play.[35] As the treated area becomes numb, the amount of knee flexion is gradually increased to tolerance (Fig. 12-19). Maintaining the knee's ROM decreases the possibility of heterotopic ossification. Weight bearing is restricted until control of the quadriceps muscle is regained and the patient has 90 degrees of pain-free knee ROM.

Slipped Capital Femoral Epiphysis

Describing displacement of the femoral head relative to the femoral neck, slipped capital femoral epiphysis (SCFE) is the most common hip disorder in adolescents and more commonly affects boys than girls. The risk of acquiring a slipped capital femoral epiphysis is increased in children who are overweight and experiencing a growth spurt.[34] This condition occurs bilaterally in 18% to 50% of the cases.[36]

The femoral head remains in the acetabulum, and the femoral neck displaces anteriorly, causing the proximal femur to be retroverted and a resulting toeing out. SCFEs are classified as stable or unstable based on the patient's ability to bear weight.[36] Stable SCFEs, where patients can bear weight with or without crutches, account for about 90% of all cases. Depending on the extent of the slip, a stable SCFE can result in a permanent retroverted deformity as the bone remodels with increased bone growth posteriorly. This retroversion results in a gait marked by external femoral rotation and toeing out. Unstable SCFEs, characterized by a patient's inability to bear weight, have a much worse prognosis, with 20% to 50% developing osteonecrosis.[36]

The onset of symptoms may be chronic (gradual onset of symptoms over a 3-week period), acute-on-chronic where pain has existed for several weeks or more but is suddenly increased by a single episode that precludes walking, or, rarely, due to trauma.[37] SCFE is characterized by a limitation in internal rotation and a gait pattern with the involved extremity in external rotation. Describing poorly localized pain in the hip region, patients may also complain of referred knee pain secondary to irritation of the obturator nerve (Examination Findings 12-2).

Anteroposterior radiographs will reveal an irregular physis that is wider than normal. The epiphysis falls posterior to the anteriorly displaced femoral neck. On bilateral radiographic comparison, the affected epiphysis is lower than the contralateral epiphysis.[36]

Slipped Capital Femoral Epiphysis Intervention Strategies

If a SCFE is suspected, the patient should be non–weight bearing and immediately referred to a physician. To prevent further displacement, a stable SCFE is usually managed

Selective Tissue Tests 12-5

Ober Test for Iliotibial Band Tightness

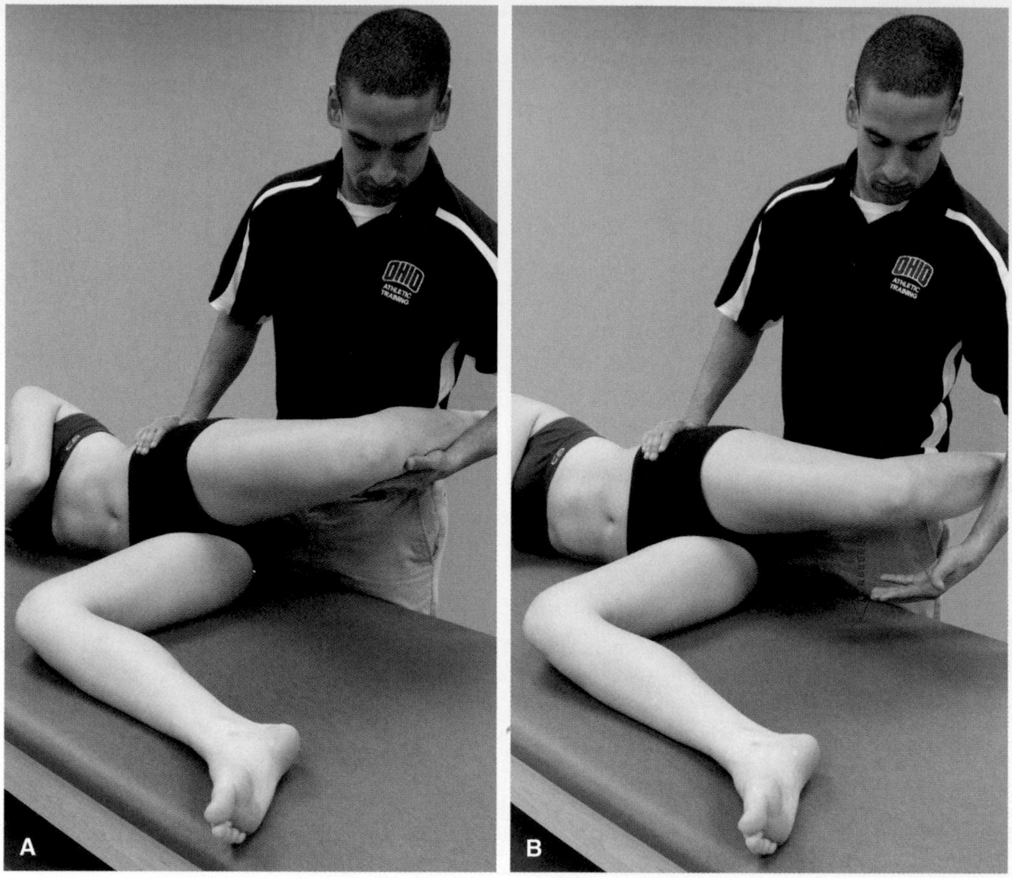

The original Ober test. To eliminate false-positive test results, the tensor fasciae latae must first clear the greater trochanter. A positive test result occurs when the knee does not adduct past horizontal.

Patient Position	Lying on the side opposite that being tested The knee flexed to 90° and the opposite hip (the bottom leg) is flexed to 45° to stabilize the torso and pelvis. The knee of the involved leg is flexed to 90°. *Modified Ober Test:* The knee of the involved leg is extended.[27]
Position of Examiner	Standing behind the patient One hand stabilizes the patient's pelvis. The opposite hand supports the leg being tested along the medial aspect of the distal tibia.
Evaluative Procedure	**(A)** Passively abduct and extend the patient's hip to allow the tensor fasciae latae to clear the greater trochanter. **(B)** The hip is then allowed to passively adduct to the table.
Positive Test	Normal: The femur adducts past horizontal. Minimal tightness: The femur adducts to horizontal. Maximal tightness: The leg is unable to adduct to horizontal.
Implications	Tightness of the IT band, predisposing the individual to IT band friction syndrome and/or lateral patellar alignment
Modification	A goniometer can be used to quantify the results. The proximal arm is aligned with both ASISs, and the distal arm is aligned with the midline of the thigh. An inclinometer can be placed over the lateral femoral condyle. If the leg remains in abduction relative to 0°, it is recorded as a negative value. If the leg adducts past 0°, it is recorded as a positive value.[27,28]
Comments	Flexing the knee to 90° can place tension on the femoral nerve (see Femoral Nerve Stretch Test in Chapter 13) and on the medial structures of the knee. Adequate pelvic stabilization (limiting trunk lateral flexion) is important to avoid false-negative results. The modified Ober test produces less adduction; therefore, both tests should be performed.[29] Deviations in pelvic position may create a bony block to hip adduction, thereby yielding a false-positive result.[30]
Evidence	

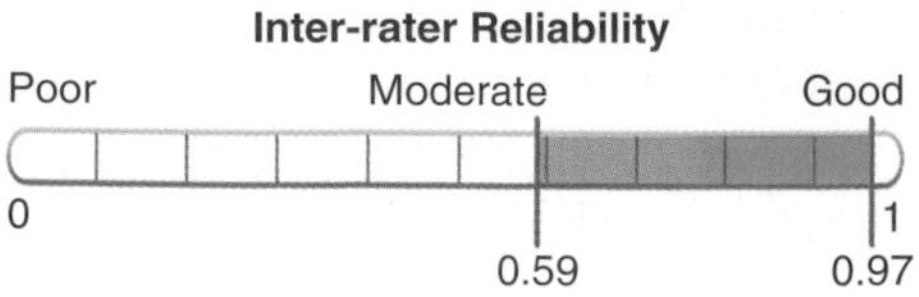

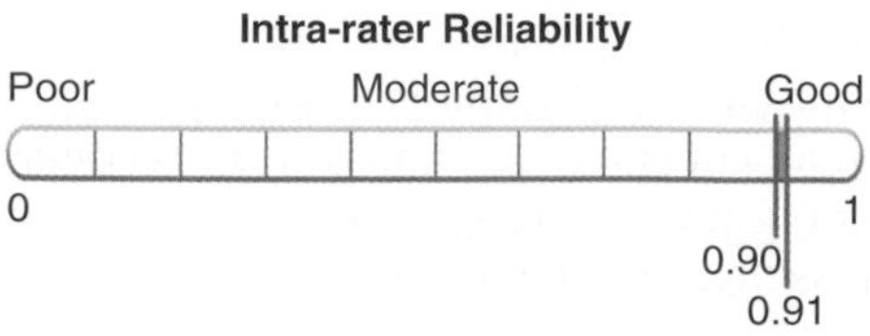

ASIS = anterior inferior iliac spine; IT = iliotibial

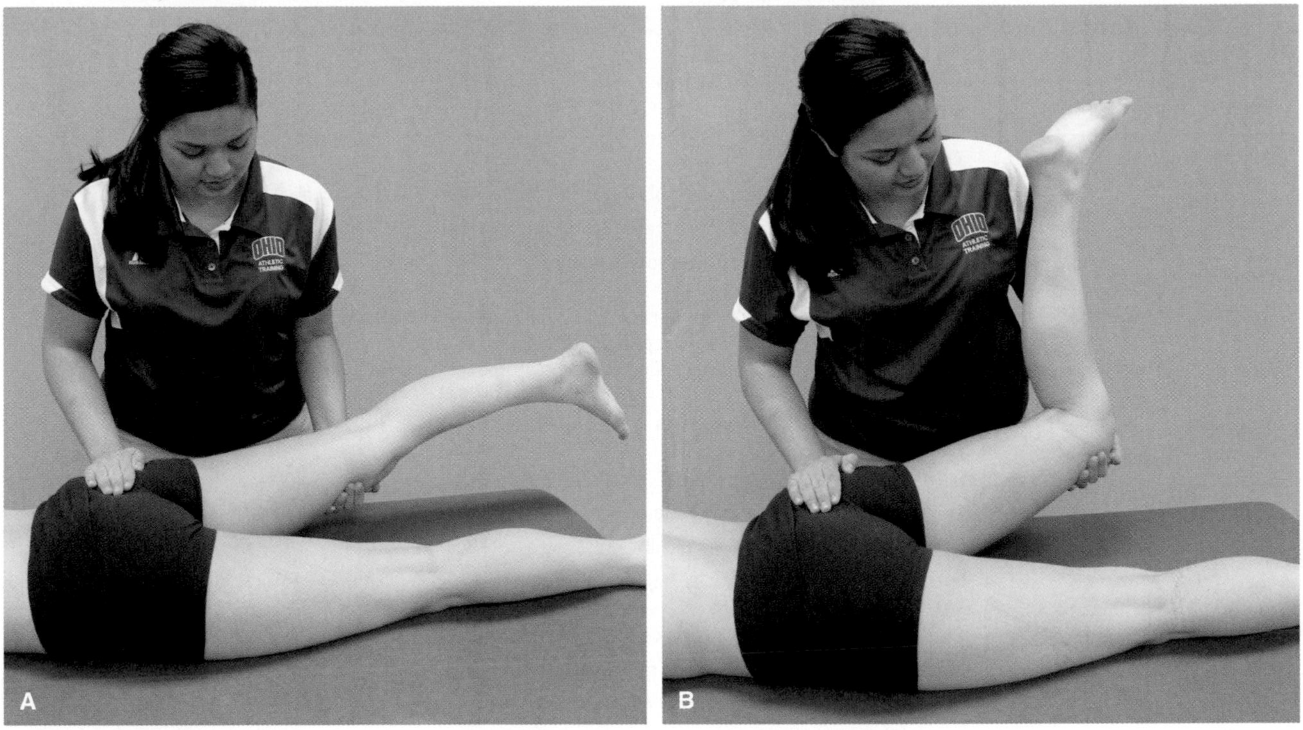

FIGURE 12-17 ■ Passive hip extension: (A) knee extended; (B) knee flexed.

surgically soon after it is identified, and outcomes are generally good, especially with mild to moderate displacement. Standard surgical repair for stable SCFEs uses single-screw fixation **in situ** followed by a gradual return to activity. Unstable SCFEs are also managed operatively, but outcomes are worse with a higher number of associated complications including avascular necrosis and chondrolysis.[34]

Legg-Calvé-Perthes Disease

Legg-Calvé-Perthes disease is an ischemic lesion of the femoral head that develops during the first decade of life. The degenerative process is marked by ischemia that results in resorption, collapse, and repair of the femoral head. Permanent damage to the femoral head can result in a marked decrease in hip abduction and internal rotation. The disease develops bilaterally in 10% to 20% of the cases, but each side may degenerate at different rates. If untreated, childhood Legg-Calvé-Perthes disease will lead to disabling hip arthritis by the sixth decade of life in half of the people affected.[38]

Although a necrotic process, the triggering events for Legg-Calvé-Perthes disease are not fully understood. Genetic and environmental factors are both thought to contribute.[39] Possible causes of the condition include single traumatic or multiple chronic events that disrupt the blood supply, maternal smoking or exposure to secondhand smoke, and blood-borne clotting factor and/or endocrine disorders such as thyroid disease.[38,39]

Legg-Calvé-Perthes disease tends to develop between the ages of 2 and 14 and is more frequent in boys than in girls. Pain may be referred to the medial thigh (obturator nerve), buttock (sciatic nerve), or suprapatellar region (femoral nerve). The child often has a painless antalgic gait and/or gluteus medius lurch. Abduction and internal hip rotation, especially when the hip is extended, are limited. Early in the degenerative process, ROM is limited secondary to muscle spasm and synovitis. As the disease progresses, ROM is limited by bony degeneration.[38]

Clinically, the affected leg may appear shorter than the unaffected leg secondary to a contracture, but actual bony leg-length differences rarely occur. The Trendelenburg test is often positive (see Selective Tissue Test 12-2). Radiographic studies are used to confirm the presence of Legg-Calvé-Perthes disease.[38] Poor long-term prognosis is predicted when at least two of the following signs are visible on radiographs: a radiolucent "V" on the lateral epiphysis, calcification of the lateral epiphysis, lateral subluxation of the femoral head, a horizontal physis, metaphyseal cysts, **coxa magna**, or a decreased joint space in later life.[38]

The long-term functional consequence of Legg-Calvé-Perthes disease is a flattening of the femoral head, resulting in the permanent loss of abduction and rotation. The less congruent the shape of the femoral head and the acetabulum, the more severe the dysfunction and the more likely that arthritis will develop.[38]

in situ In the original position or place

Coxa magna The femoral head is at least 10% larger than normal.

Examination Findings 12-1
Iliac Crest Contusion (Hip Pointer)

Examination Segment	Clinical Findings
History of Current Condition	*Onset:* Acute *Pain characteristics:* Iliac crest, possibly radiating into the internal and external oblique muscles *Other symptoms:* Paresthesia over the anterolateral thigh *Mechanism:* Direct blow to an unprotected ilium
Functional Assessment	All muscles having an origin or insertion along the iliac crest may be affected by this injury. In most cases, the internal and external obliques elicit pain when the trunk is flexed away from the involved side. In more severe instances, hip flexion and abduction and movement of the trunk in any direction also cause pain.
Inspection	Rapid onset of swelling and redness Ecchymosis develops over time.
Palpation	Crepitus felt during palpation of the iliac crest Point tenderness elicited along the iliac crest and associated muscles Spasm of the associated muscles may also be present.
Joint and Muscle Function Assessment	*AROM:* Pain during hip flexion, trunk rotation, trunk flexion *MMT:* Painful according to involved muscles *PROM:* Pain with stretch of involved muscles
Joint Stability Tests	*Stress tests:* Not applicable *Joint play:* Not applicable
Selective Tissue Tests	Not applicable
Neurological Screening	A complete sensory check of the involved lower leg is necessary to rule out trauma to the nerves about the hip. The lateral femoral cutaneous nerve, supplying sensation to the anterolateral thigh, is most commonly involved.
Vascular Screening	Within normal limits
Imaging Techniques	Radiographs can rule out fracture of the ilium.
Differential Diagnosis	Ilium fracture, muscle tear (gluteus medius, gluteus minimus, internal oblique, external oblique), avulsion fracture, bursitis
Comments	With more severe contusions, swelling can appear in the lower extremity or testicular region.

AROM = active range of motion; MMT = manual muscle test; PROM = passive range of motion

Legg-Calvé-Perthes Disease Intervention Strategies

Treatment for Legg-Calvé-Perthes centers around maintaining good hip ROM and containing the femoral head in the acetabulum so that the femoral head ossifies in a rounded shape.[39] The effectiveness of bisphosphonate therapy, now used to restore bone density in cases of osteoporosis, is also being investigated. Surgical intervention including a femoral osteotomy is effective in some groups of patients.[39]

Femoral Stress Fractures

Femoral shaft and neck stress fractures account for 8% to 11% of stress fractures in military personnel and athletes. Like all stress fractures, femoral stress fractures occur more often in women than in men and are most prevalent in women with infrequent or absent menstruation.[40,41] Repetitive activities such as running combined with rapid increase in volume (frequency and/or intensity) that do not provide sufficient recovery periods predispose the development of fatigue stress fractures. **Insufficiency stress fractures** are associated with normal stresses in bone that lacks expected bone density. In the femoral neck, weight-bearing or muscle-tension forces create either tension-side or compression-side stress fractures on the superior or inferior surface of the neck respectively. Tension-side fractures tend to be more unstable than compression-side fractures and have a poorer prognosis.[40]

Table 12-6 Characteristics of Muscular Tears of the Hip and Thigh

		Pain or Deficit Elicited During Range of Motion Testing	
Muscle	Injuring Force	Active	Passive
Rectus Femoris	Hyperextension of the hip and flexion of the knee Dynamic overload; isometric contraction	Hip flexion, knee extension	Hip extension, knee flexion
Iliopsoas	Hyperextension of the hip Resisted hip flexion	Hip flexion	Hip extension
Quadriceps (other than rectus femoris)	Hyperflexion of the knee Dynamic overload; resisted knee extension	Knee extension with a flexed hip	Knee flexion
Hamstring	Dynamic overload; eccentric contraction Tensile force; overstretching the muscle	Knee flexion Hip extension with an extended knee	Knee extension Hip flexion
Gluteus Maximus	Dynamic overload; eccentric contraction; isometric contraction	Hip extension with a flexed knee	Hip flexion with a flexed knee
Adductor Group	Tensile; overstretching the muscle Dynamic overload; eccentric contraction; isometric contraction	Hip adduction	Hip abduction

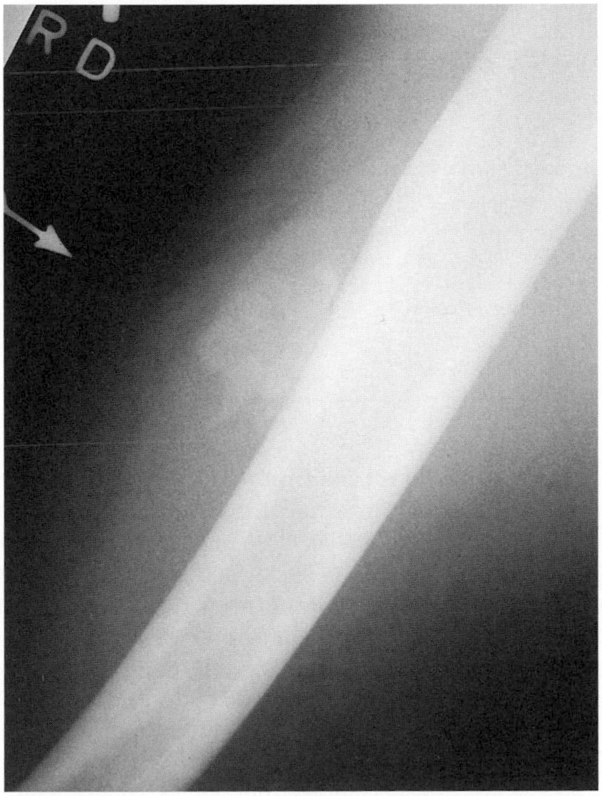

FIGURE 12-18 ■ Femoral heterotopic ossification resulting from a quadriceps contusion.

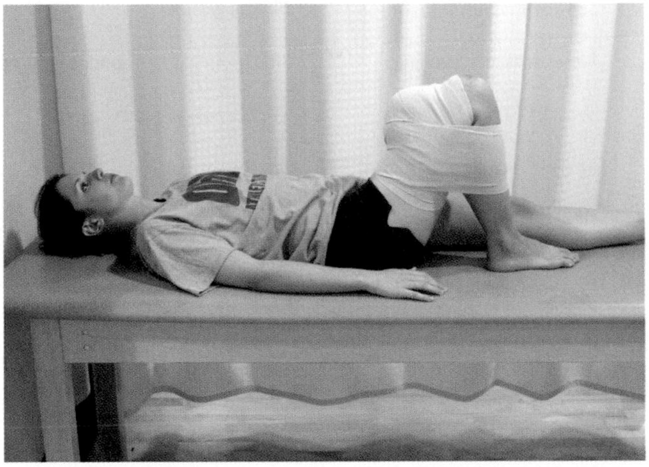

FIGURE 12-19 ■ Method of managing a quadriceps contusion. The quadriceps is flexed to the point that pain is experienced and then extended to the point that the pain disappears. Ice is applied and the process is repeated when the patient reports numbness.

The patient will complain of a deep aching pain arising from the thigh, hip, or adductor region that increases with the duration and intensity of activity. Night pain is often reported, especially when the patient log rolls on the involved side.[42] Symptoms of femoral shaft stress fractures mimic those of chronic quadriceps injury, potentially delaying diagnosis of a stress fracture. Mature stress fractures will elicit pain when the involved region is palpated. ROM is limited and painful near the end-ranges; strength may also be decreased. Axial loading of the hip joint or shear forces placed

Examination Findings 12-2
Slipped Capital Femoral Epiphysis

Examination Segment	Clinical Findings
History of Current Condition	*Onset:* Acute, chronic, acute-on-chronic *Pain characteristics:* Stable: Pain in the adductor group or hip increases with walking. Pain may be referred to the anterior distal quadriceps (femoral nerve), adductor area (obturator nerve), and/or buttocks and hamstrings (sciatic nerve). Unstable: Pain intense enough to prevent walking *Mechanism:* Gradual onset or abrupt maneuver *Predisposing conditions:* Obesity, skeletal immaturity, male, growth spurt
Functional Assessment	Stable: The patient demonstrates an antalgic gait with hip externally rotated. Unstable: The patient is unable to bear weight, and walking is not possible, even with crutches.
Inspection	A leg-length difference may be noted.
Palpation	Tenderness over the femoral head and neck
Joint and Muscle Function Assessment	*AROM:* Possible decrease in internal rotation, hip flexion, and/or abduction *MMT:* Weak internal rotation In advanced cases, weakness will be noted for all hip muscles. *PROM:* Decreased internal rotation, decreased hip flexion, and abduction may also be noted.
Joint Stability Tests	*Stress tests:* Not applicable *Joint play:* Not applicable
Selective Tissue Tests	Not applicable
Neurological Screening	Unexplained knee and hip pain in children should raise the suspicion of a slipped capital femoral epiphysis.
Vascular Screening	Within normal limits
Imaging Techniques	Anteroposterior and "frog-leg" pelvic radiographs are usually diagnostic. "Pistol-grip" deformity may be noted if OA has developed.
Differential Diagnosis	Muscle injury, avulsion fracture
Comments	Long-term consequences include chronic pain and osteoarthritis.

AROM = active range of motion; MMT = manual muscle test; OA = osteoarthritis; PROM = passive range of motion

on the femoral neck, such as when standing on one leg, may cause pain (Examination Findings 12-3).

Pain may be referred to the hip from the lumbar or sacral plexus or be referred proximally from the lower extremity. Concurrent examination of the lower extremities, spine, sacrum, and gait may be required to obtain a definitive clinical diagnosis.

Only 10% of patients will demonstrate positive findings on plain radiographs taken within the first week of symptoms, and fewer than 55% of patients with femoral neck stress fractures will ever have radiographic evidence of the condition.[43] Although bone scans provide a high sensitivity in detecting stress fractures, their low specificity combined with a relatively high dose of radiation make magnetic resonance imaging (MRI) the modality of choice in detecting stress fractures.[40]

Femoral Stress Fracture Intervention Strategies

Treatment of femoral stress fractures depends on their location. Stress fractures in the shaft are treated symptomatically with restriction of any pain-causing activities and a progressive return to activity following resolution of symptoms. Stable compression-side femoral neck stress fractures are frequently managed conservatively, too. Tension-side stress fractures are assessed and monitored closely for displacement and commonly require surgical fixation.[40]

Intra-Articular Pathology

Femoral Acetabular Impingement

Femoral acetabular impingement (FAI) is a common source of hip pain in young and middle-aged athletic individuals.

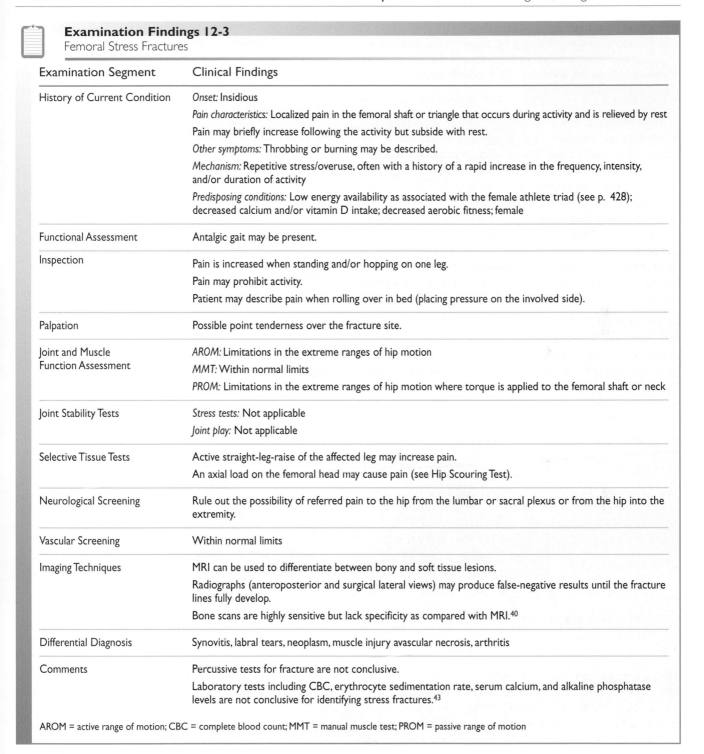

Examination Findings 12-3
Femoral Stress Fractures

Examination Segment	Clinical Findings
History of Current Condition	*Onset:* Insidious *Pain characteristics:* Localized pain in the femoral shaft or triangle that occurs during activity and is relieved by rest Pain may briefly increase following the activity but subside with rest. *Other symptoms:* Throbbing or burning may be described. *Mechanism:* Repetitive stress/overuse, often with a history of a rapid increase in the frequency, intensity, and/or duration of activity *Predisposing conditions:* Low energy availability as associated with the female athlete triad (see p. 428); decreased calcium and/or vitamin D intake; decreased aerobic fitness; female
Functional Assessment	Antalgic gait may be present.
Inspection	Pain is increased when standing and/or hopping on one leg. Pain may prohibit activity. Patient may describe pain when rolling over in bed (placing pressure on the involved side).
Palpation	Possible point tenderness over the fracture site.
Joint and Muscle Function Assessment	*AROM:* Limitations in the extreme ranges of hip motion *MMT:* Within normal limits *PROM:* Limitations in the extreme ranges of hip motion where torque is applied to the femoral shaft or neck
Joint Stability Tests	*Stress tests:* Not applicable *Joint play:* Not applicable
Selective Tissue Tests	Active straight-leg-raise of the affected leg may increase pain. An axial load on the femoral head may cause pain (see Hip Scouring Test).
Neurological Screening	Rule out the possibility of referred pain to the hip from the lumbar or sacral plexus or from the hip into the extremity.
Vascular Screening	Within normal limits
Imaging Techniques	MRI can be used to differentiate between bony and soft tissue lesions. Radiographs (anteroposterior and surgical lateral views) may produce false-negative results until the fracture lines fully develop. Bone scans are highly sensitive but lack specificity as compared with MRI.[40]
Differential Diagnosis	Synovitis, labral tears, neoplasm, muscle injury avascular necrosis, arthritis
Comments	Percussive tests for fracture are not conclusive. Laboratory tests including CBC, erythrocyte sedimentation rate, serum calcium, and alkaline phosphatase levels are not conclusive for identifying stress fractures.[43]

AROM = active range of motion; CBC = complete blood count; MMT = manual muscle test; PROM = passive range of motion

Resulting from altered morphology of the femoral head and/or acetabulum, FAI creates abnormal stresses on the surrounding soft tissue and bone, resulting in labral tears, chondral degeneration, and, ultimately, OA.

Two types of FAI deformities exist. **Cam lesions** are located on the femoral head and result from an abnormally shaped femoral head repeatedly contacting the acetabulum and surrounding labrum. Occurring most often in young, athletic males, cam lesions are thought to develop in response to extensive sports participation during the high-growth period of adolescence.[44,45] **Pincer lesions**, more common in middle-aged, active females, result when the acetabulum is overly covering the femoral head, resulting in compression between the acetabular rim and femoral head-neck function, especially during hip flexion.[16] A combination of pincer and cam lesions may also develop (Fig. 12-20).

✱ Practical Evidence

Diagnostic images are indicated for patients who demonstrate pain, motion restriction, and other symptoms that are produced with the hip flexed, adducted, and internally rotated and who have a positive FABER test.[14]

The individual with FAI will complain of groin pain that is sporadic at first and then progresses to constant. The pain may extend to the lateral thigh.[46] Athletic activities, walking, and prolonged sitting may provoke symptoms. The physical examination will reveal limited internal rotation with the hip in 90 degrees of flexion. Adding adduction to this position (hip flexion, internal rotation, and adduction) describes the anterior impingement test (see Selective Tissue Test 12-6), which also often reproduces symptoms (Examination Findings 12-4).[16] Diagnosis of FAI is made via radiographs and MRI, which determines any resulting chondral or labral damage.[16]

Femoral Acetabular Impingement Intervention Strategies

Initial treatment is generally conservative, consisting of avoiding aggravating activities and altering movement patterns to avoid excessive internal rotation and adduction.[47] Because of the active population affected and the bony nature of the problem, surgery may be needed to correct the interface between the femur and the acetabulum and address any resulting pathologies such as labral tears (see Labral Tear Intervention Strategies). Short-term and midterm outcomes of surgical management of FAI reveal good outcomes related to returning to activity.[16,48,49]

Labral Tears

Improved imaging techniques have increased the number of labral tears diagnosed. Once thought to occur only as the result of major trauma such as hip dislocations, we now understand that labral tears can be the result of femoral acetabular impingement, hypermobility, **dysplasia**, or degeneration.[16,47,50]

Patients may describe a localized dull groin pain with sporadic episodes of sharp pain. Pain may extend to the lateral hip or buttock, and night pain and pain with prolonged

Dysplasic (dysplasia) Abnormal tissue development

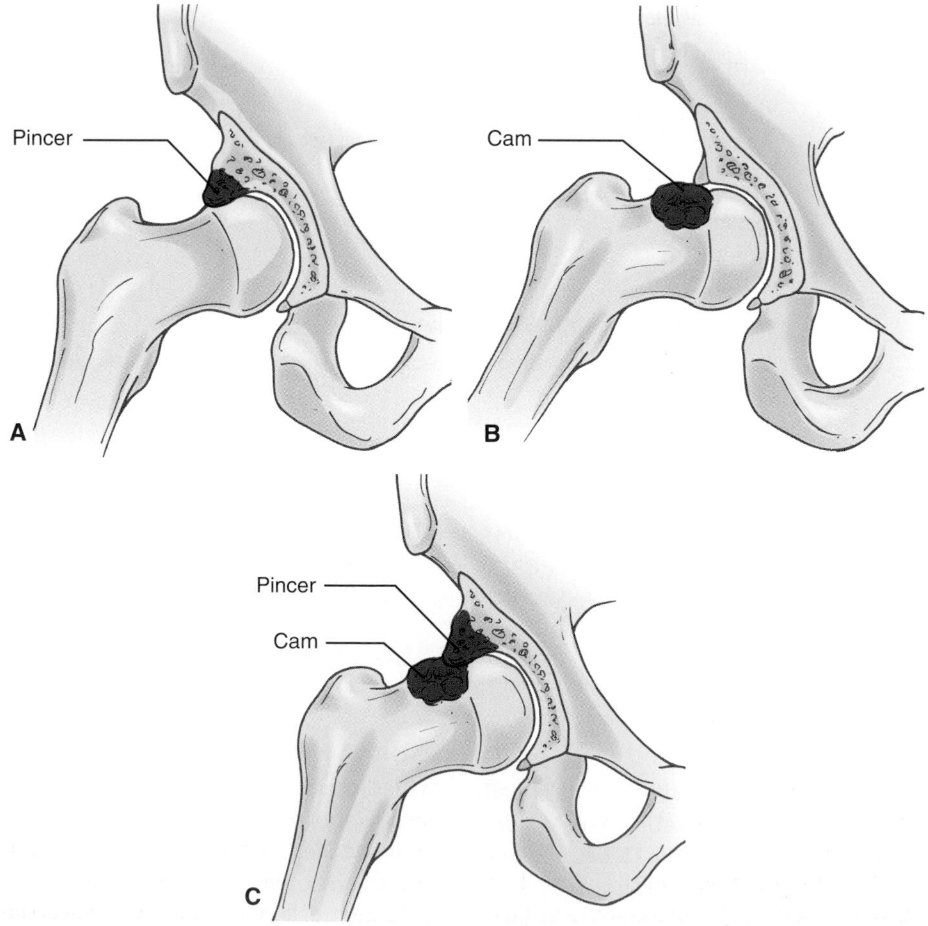

FIGURE 12-20 ■ Causes of femoral acetabular impingement. Outgrowths from the acetabulum and/or femoral neck can entrap the associated soft tissue. (A) A pincer lesion, a bony outgrowth of the acetabulum, (B) a cam lesion, a bony outgrowth of the femoral neck, (C) a mixed cause involving the concurrent formation of pincer and cam lesions.

Examination Findings 12-4
Femoral Acetabular Impingement

Examination Segment	Clinical Findings
History of Current Condition	*Onset:* Gradual *Pain characteristics:* Groin pain that may extend to the lateral thigh; initially sporadic and progressing to constant; exacerbated by activity or prolonged flexed postures such as sitting *Mechanism:* Repeated compressive forces from an abnormally shaped femoral head (cam lesion) or acetabulum (pincer lesion) or both *Predisposing conditions:* Acetabular dysplasia, slipped capital femoral epiphysis, Legg-Calvé-Perthes disease
Functional Assessment	Activities requiring hip flexion (e.g., squatting down, rowing, stair climbing) may reproduce symptoms. Antalgic gait secondary to pain Poor hip control with squatting (increased internal rotation and adduction)
Inspection	Unremarkable
Palpation	Deep pain in the anterior hip region
Joint and Muscle Function Assessment	*AROM:* Internal rotation and adduction may be limited, especially with the hip flexed to 90°. *MMT:* Weak hip external rotators *PROM:* Decreased hip internal rotation when hip is flexed to 90°; increased pain with hip flexion
Joint Stability Tests	*Stress tests:* Not applicable *Joint play:* Not applicable
Selective Tissue Tests	Positive FABER test with underlying labral pathology Positive anterior impingement test (hip flexed to 90° and passively internally rotated and adducted)
Neurological Screening	Within normal limits
Vascular Screening	Within normal limits
Imaging Techniques	Radiographs MRI to detect resulting soft tissue pathology
Differential Diagnosis	Labral tear, hip flexor tear, inguinal hernia, OA, greater trochanteric bursitis

AROM = active range of motion; MMT = manual muscle test; MRI = magnetic resonance imaging; OA = osteoarthritis; PROM = passive range of motion

sitting is common. Patients most commonly also describe clicking, with some describing catching, locking, or giving way.[50,51] Medically, the location of the tear is described using a clock face (e.g., tear extends from the 1 o'clock to 3 o'clock position).[52] Anterior tears produce pain and catching when the hip is moved into flexion, internal rotation, and adduction (**the anterior impingement test, see** Selective Tissue Test 12-6). Posterior labral tears are marked by pain during passive hip flexion and internal rotation while a posterior load is being applied.[2] Pain tends to increase with activity, especially weight-bearing hip internal and external rotation (Examination Findings 12-5).[53] Hip scouring and FABER tests may be positive (see Selective Tissue Tests 12-7 and 13-5).

A diagnosis of a labral tear may be made by injecting a local anesthetic into the joint. If pain relief is obtained after the injection and arthrographic findings are normal, then an intra-articular defect should be assumed. MRI, especially high-resolution MRI, and magnetic resonance arthrography have improved the accuracy and specificity of identifying labral lesions and are used to rule out other possible pathologies.[50-52]

Labral Tear Intervention Strategies

Initial treatment of labral tears focuses on relative rest and restoration of normal movement patterns. Conservative treatment is often ineffective, with patients reporting a return of symptoms as soon as activity is increased.[50] Surgical treatment of labral tears is controversial, with a movement towards repair as opposed to resection, especially if the tear is in the vascular zone close to the acetabular rim. While excision provides symptomatic relief, residual instability may

Selective Tissue Tests 12-6
Anterior Impingement Test

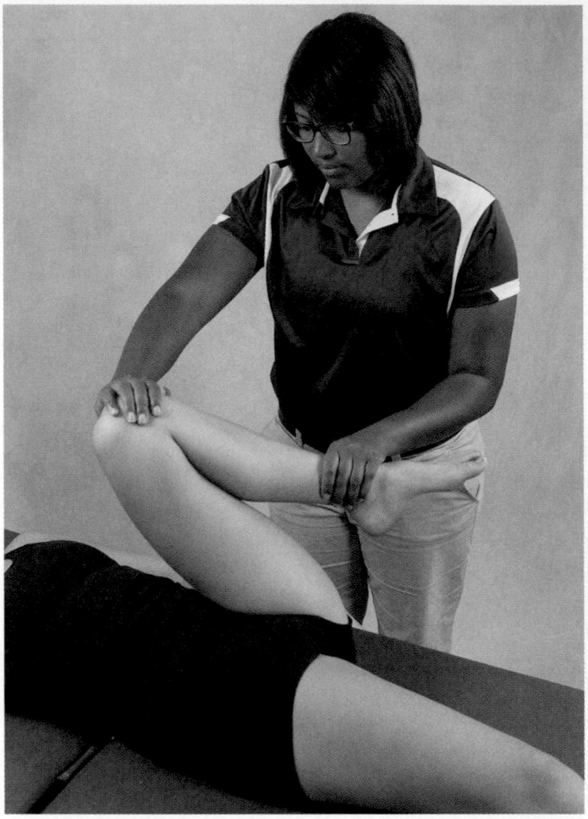

This test positions the femoral head to entrap the labrum, thereby reproducing symptoms of femoral acetabular impingement (FAI) and/or a labral tear.

Patient Position	Supine
Position of Examiner	At the side of the patient
Evaluative Procedure	The examiner flexes, internally rotates, and adducts the hip.
Positive Test	Pain or symptoms in the hip are reproduced.
Implications	Femoral acetabular impingement Labral tear
Evidence	

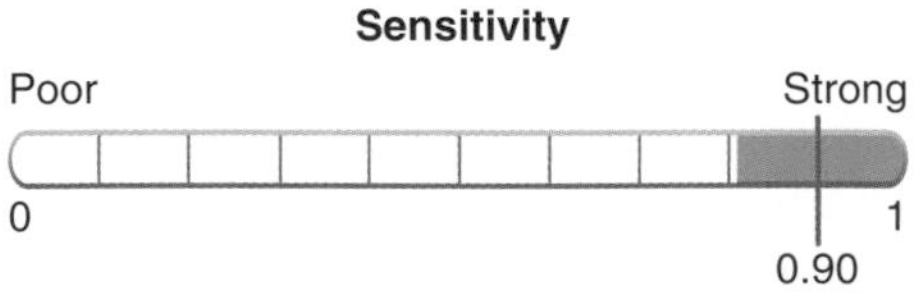

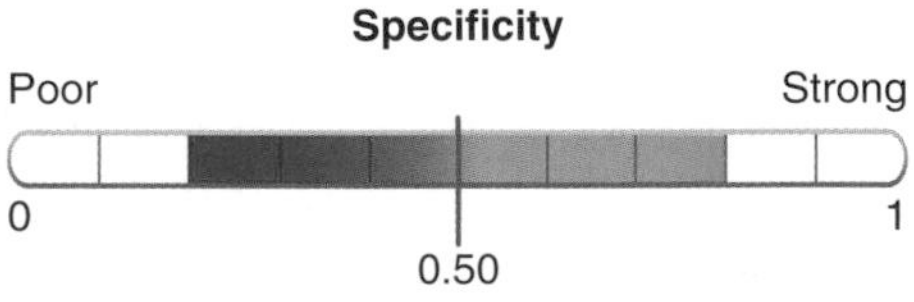

LR+: 1.01–1.32–2.42

LR−: 0.05–0.20–0.58

Examination Findings 12-5
Labral Tears

Examination Segment	Clinical Findings
History of Current Condition	*Onset:* Acute or degenerative *Pain characteristics:* Pain most commonly presents in the anterior or medial hip; posterior or lateral pain is reported less frequently. Night pain is common. *Other symptoms:* Clicking, catching, or locking may be described. *Mechanism:* Acute: Hip dislocation or subluxation Insidious: Repeated subtle subluxations, impingement of the anterior capsule; repeated weight-bearing internal or external rotation, hyperabduction, or hyperextension[4] *Predisposing conditions:* Femoral acetabular impingement, hip dysplasia, slipped capital femoral epiphysis
Functional Assessment	Increased symptoms with activities requiring hip flexion, including sitting A limp or shortened stance phase on the involved leg may be noted. Walking/running distance is often limited.
Inspection	Unremarkable
Palpation	Often unremarkable; anterior tears may yield tenderness over the anterior joint capsule. Clicking or popping may be noted during joint motion.
Joint and Muscle Function Assessment	*AROM:* May be limited secondary to pain at end-range of adduction, flexion, internal or external rotation *MMT:* Within normal limits *PROM:* Anterior tear: Pain and/or catching when the hip is moved from flexion, internal rotation, and adduction Posterior tear: Pain during passive hip flexion and internal rotation while a posterior load is applied
Joint Stability Tests	*Stress tests:* Not applicable *Joint play:* Not applicable
Selective Tissue Tests	Hip scouring test may be positive. Positive anterior impingement test The use of the Thomas test has been suggested to identify labral tears, but the sensitivity and specificity of this procedure are poor in detecting this condition.[51] The Trendelenburg test may be positive.[53]
Neurological Screening	Within normal limits
Vascular Screening	Within normal limits
Imaging Techniques	Radiographs are used to rule out bony trauma and identify underlying bony deformity. Magnetic resonance arthrography is more accurate in diagnosing a labral tear than MRI.[50,51]
Differential Diagnosis	Hernia, athletic pubalgia, osteitis pubis, OA, bursitis, referred pain from lumbosacral region, adductor strain, snapping hip syndrome, osteochondral defect, femoral acetabular impingement, hip dysplasia, avascular necrosis of the femoral head[50]

AROM = active range of motion; MMT = manual muscle test; MRI = magnetic resonance imaging; OA = osteoarthritis; PROM = passive range of motion result.[54] Patients report better outcomes following repair as compared with resection.[55]

Hip Osteoarthritis

Age, repetitive trauma, acute trauma, or dysplasia of the hip can lead to degeneration of the articular surfaces of the femur and acetabulum. In athletes, these conditions most commonly include arthritis, osteochondritis dissecans, acetabular labrum tears, femoroacetabular impingement, and avascular necrosis. All share the common characteristic of further degeneration if left undetected and untreated. Chronic hip degeneration occurs with age, commonly affecting people older than age 50 (Table 12-7). Younger patients may develop degenerative hip changes secondary to acute trauma.

Osteoarthritis of the coxofemoral joint involves the degeneration of the articular cartilage, fibrocartilage, bone, and synovium. **Primary osteoarthritis** results from decreased blood supply (osteonecrosis), infection (sepsis), or rheumatoid arthritis. Primary OA is often a diagnosis of exclusion. The presence of congenital hip disease, slipped capital femoral epiphysis, or other existing anatomical abnormalities can lead to **secondary osteoarthritis**, the most common form of hip arthritis.[1]

The primary complaint associated with the early stages of hip degeneration is pain only during weight bearing. As the degeneration continues, the pain becomes more constant. The location of this pain may lead to the suspicion of lumbar spine or sacroiliac pathology because pain may be referred to the low back and distally into the anterior thigh, knee, or adductor group.

Physical evaluation reveals a loss of motion in all of the hip's planes, with rotational motions being lost first, followed by abduction. Strength assessment with manual muscle testing may be inconclusive secondary to pain. **Hip scouring** causes the two articular surfaces to compress and rub over one another, resulting in pain (Selective Tissue Test 12-7). Radiographic evaluation may provide conclusive evidence of deterioration of the hip's articular surfaces and the resulting diminished joint space.

Table 12-7 Etiological Factors Contributing to the Development of Hip Osteoarthritis

Factor	Increased Rate of Osteoarthritis
Body Weight	Increased body weight (obesity) Heavier individuals may be less active, thereby decreasing the rate of OA progression.
Occupation	Lifting heavy loads Participation in track, field, racket sports, and soccer, especially if the patient is genetically predisposed to hip OA
Anatomy	Developmental hip dysplasia Acetabular abnormalities Femoral anteversion (inconclusive)
Genetics	Family history of hip OA

OA = osteoarthritis

Hip Osteoarthritis Intervention Strategies

Initial treatment of hip OA includes modifying risk factors via weight loss and changes in activity. Pharmacologic interventions begin with acetaminophen and, if this is not effective, progresses to nonsteroidal antiinflammatory medications (e.g., ibuprofen). Glucosamine and chondroitin are often prescribed, but evidence suggests that they are ineffective in reducing pain.[56] Arthroplasty is indicated for those individuals with significant participation restrictions following conservative treatment.

Hip Subluxation

Hip subluxations often have a subtle presentation and occur as the result of a fall onto a flexed knee with the hip adducted, or a jump-stop or pivot, that forces the femoral head posteriorly in the acetabulum. Subluxations are characterized by the femoral head being forced into, but not over, the posterior acetabulum, allowing the joint to spontaneously reduce.[2] In addition to stressing the joint capsule and ligaments, which may lead to chronic instability and recurrent subluxations, the mechanisms associated with hip subluxations may result in a tear of the ligamentum teres, fractures or contusions of the femoral head, or an osteochondral defect of the articular surface. The involved structures are identified via MRI.

Hip Subluxation Intervention Strategy

Hip subluxations are managed by the patient non–weight bearing for up to 6 weeks. Serial MRIs are obtained to monitor possible osseous changes.

Athletic Pubalgia

Athletic pubalgia—also known as a sports hernia—is the result of increased muscular loads placed on the pubis from repetitive, high-volume twisting, cutting, running, and kicking activities.[56-58] Athletic pubalgia results from unbalanced tension between the upward pull of the rectus abdominis and the downward and lateral pull of the adductor muscle group, and its onset is usually insidious. This high-tensile load weakens the posterior inguinal wall, a finding generally identified only during surgery. Unlike an inguinal hernia where the defect is palpable, no palpable defect is present with a sports hernia.

Some patients describe an acute episode with resulting disability, but this often follows a period of low-grade symptoms.[57,58] The actual source of pain may be the **transversalis fascia**, conjoined tendons of the adductor group, the insertion of the rectus abdominis, the external oblique aponeurosis, or the avulsion of the internal oblique from the pubic tubercle (Fig. 12-21).[57,58]

Selective Tissue Tests 12-7
Hip Scouring Test (Hip Quadrant Test)

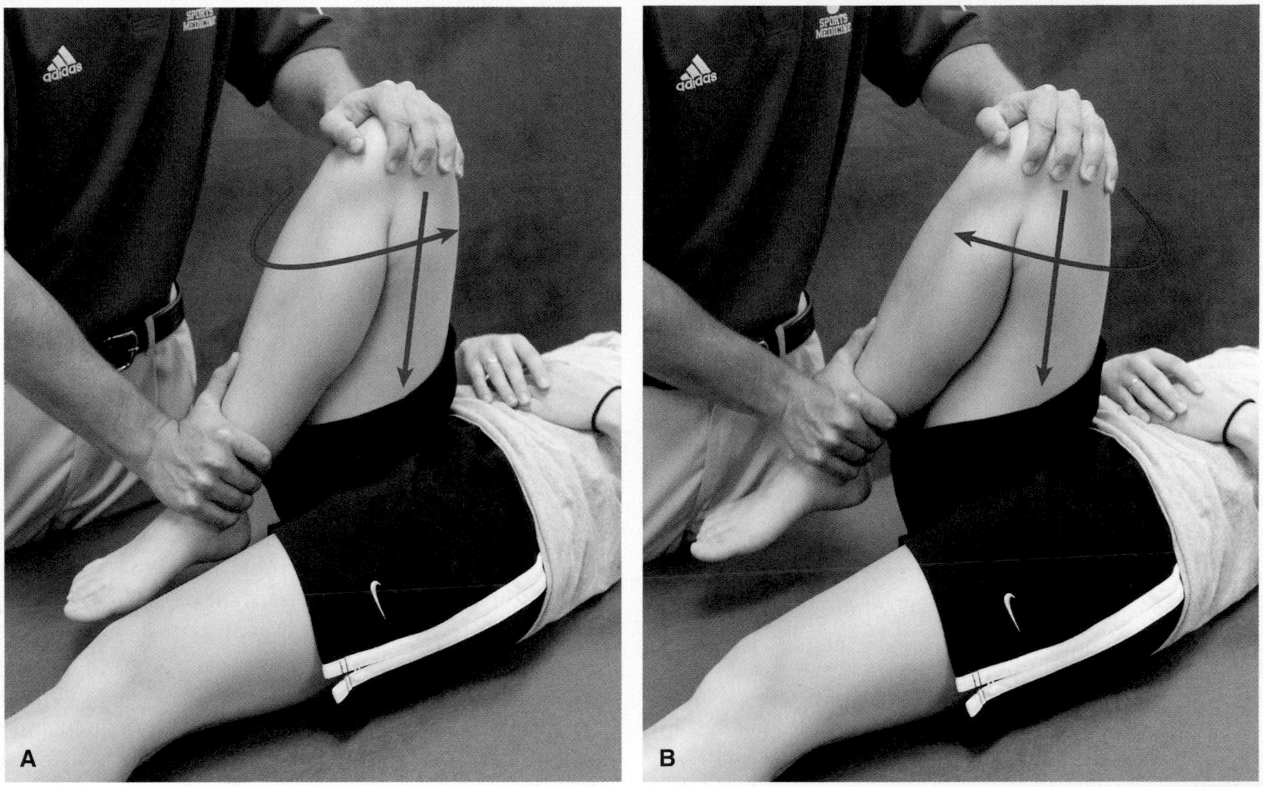

This procedure moves the hip through its ROM while an axial load is placed on the femur. Pain within a specific location may indicate a defect of the articular surface or labral tear.

Patient Position	Supine
Position of Examiner	At the side of the patient, fully flexing the patient's hip and knee
Evaluative Procedure	The examiner applies pressure downward along the shaft of the femur to compress the joint surfaces. The femur is **(A)** internally and **(B)** externally rotated with the hip in multiple angles of flexion.
Positive Test	Pain or symptoms in the hip are reproduced.
Implications	A possible defect in the articular cartilage of the femur or acetabulum (e.g., osteochondral defects, arthritis) Labral tear
Evidence	

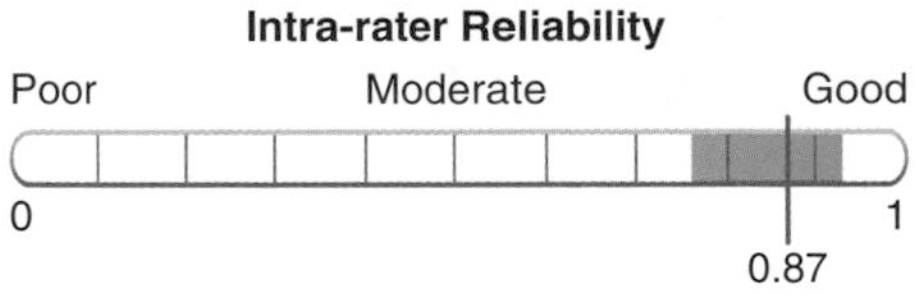

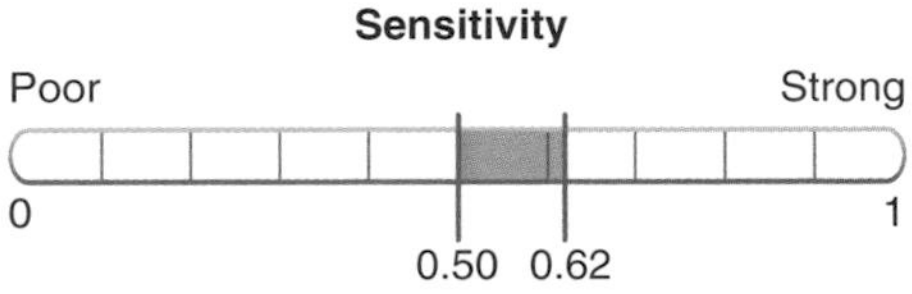

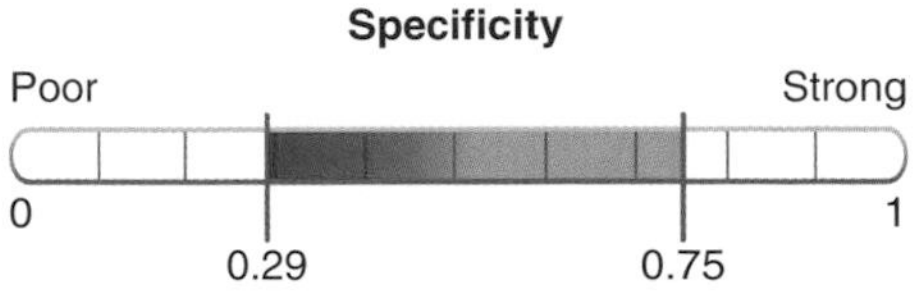

LR+: 0.70–2.48

LR−: 0.51–1.72

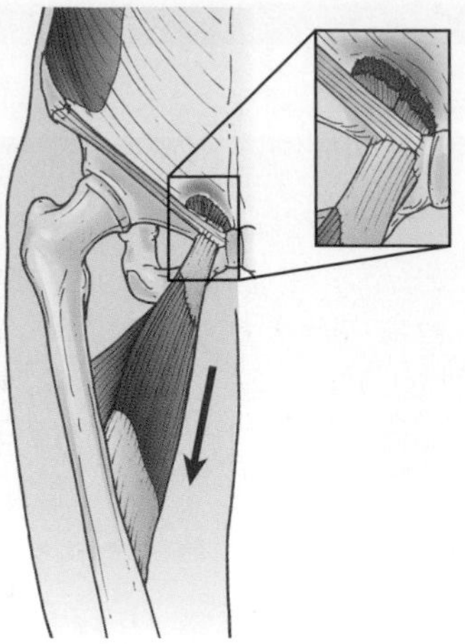

FIGURE 12-21 ■ Muscles contributing to athletic pubalgia. A muscle imbalance exists between the strong pull of the adductor group (arrow) and the weak abdominal stabilizers, resulting in a stretching or avulsion of the pelvic floor.

Clinically, the patient will describe deep lower abdominal or groin pain that is present with activity and abates when activity stops. Classically, symptoms return soon after resuming activity after a period of rest.[57,58] Males may complain of testicular pain.[58] Physical examination reveals pain with palpation at the pubic ramus, proximal adductor region, and insertion of the rectus abdominis. Adding resistance to hip adduction and a sit-up will also reproduce pain. Plain film radiographs may be ordered to rule out other underlying bony trauma; MRI is useful in identifying defects in the surrounding muscle or fascia (Examination Findings 12-6).

Athletic Pubalgia Intervention Strategies

Conservative treatment including soft tissue and joint mobilization, stretching, and exercise may be indicated for those athletes who describe a gradual onset of symptoms and who can tolerate a prolonged rehabilitation process.[58] Those for whom conservative treatment has failed or high-level competitive athletes with an acute diagnosis of athletic pubalgia may be candidates for corrective surgery, which is associated with a good outcome. Multiple surgical techniques have been recommended, including imbedding reinforcing mesh over the weakened area (**herniorrhaphy**), repair of the rectus abdominis insertion, and releasing the adductor tendon.[59]

Osteitis Pubis

Osteitis pubis—an inflammation of the pubis symphysis and subsequent stress reaction of the surrounding bone—is caused by rotational, tension, or shear forces placed on the symphysis.[60] Although osteitis pubis may be caused by acute injury such as fracture, in the physically active population, long-term activities such as running, the kicking motion in soccer, or vigorous ice skating may also lead to the development of this condition. A leg-length difference may further predispose an individual to osteitis pubis.[61]

Patients complain of pain centered over the symphysis pubis, lower abdominal muscles, and adductor muscles. Spasm of the adductor muscles may also occur.[62,63] Aggravating activities typically include running, cutting, and any activities that load the rectus abdominis. Resisted hip adduction and trunk flexion are painful. MRI is used to identify the condition. As described in the section on athletic pubalgia, many conditions can present with similar symptoms.

Osteitis Pubis Intervention Strategies

Initial intervention is usually conservative, consisting of rest from aggravating activities and possibly a corticosteroid injection. Recalcitrant cases may require surgery.[60]

Piriformis Syndrome

The sciatic nerve passes under or through the piriformis muscle as the nerve travels across the posterior pelvis. Spasm or hypertrophy of the piriformis places pressure on the sciatic nerve, mimicking the signs and symptoms of lumbar nerve root compression or sciatica in the buttock and posterior leg.[64] The resulting symptoms, piriformis syndrome, are more common in women than in men.[65] Improved diagnostic tests for lumbar nerve root impingement and intervertebral disk disease have decreased the frequency with which piriformis syndrome is diagnosed.[66]

Although the signs and symptoms of piriformis syndrome are similar to those caused by other lumbopelvic conditions, piriformis syndrome remains relatively undefined and confusing.[67] Complaints include burning, pain, numbness, or paresthesia that are increased with contraction of the piriformis or during palpation or prolonged sitting.[64] Symptoms may be heightened by the straight-leg-raise test on the involved side, passive hip internal rotation, and resisted external rotation with the patient seated (Examination Findings 12-7). Resisted hip abduction with the patient seated may also increase the symptoms (Fig. 12-22). These symptoms may also be caused by entrapment of the sciatic nerve by the hamstring muscles, termed **hamstring syndrome**.[68]

Piriformis Syndrome Intervention Strategies

Treatment of piriformis syndrome includes stretching, strengthening, and possible steroid or botulinum toxin injection into the piriformis muscle. Surgical release of the piriformis muscle may be indicated in cases that do not respond to conservative care.[69]

Snapping Hip Syndrome (Coxa Saltans)

Snapping hip syndrome, or coxa saltans, is characterized by a palpable and audible "snapping" within the hip as the joint flexes and extends. Although the physical sensation of snapping may be the patient's only complaint, pain may arise from the anterior or lateral aspect of the hip, especially when there is concurrent bursal inflammation (Examination Findings 12-8). Although there are many possible causes for this condition, snapping hip syndrome can be classified as having an internal or external origin.[9,70-72] Labral tears may present with symptoms similar to snapping hip syndrome.

Examination Findings 12-6
Athletic Pubalgia

Examination Segment	Clinical Findings
History of Current Condition	*Onset:* Usually insidious, although the patient may describe a single episode that results in severe localized pain *Pain characteristics:* Pain is localized to the pubic ramus, pubic symphysis, lower abdominal and/or adductor muscles, and/or testicles. Pain is exacerbated with activity and generally resolves when activity stops. Coughing or sneezing may also cause pain. *Mechanism:* A tensile force caused by the pull of the adductor muscle group and the lower abdominal muscles *Predisposing conditions:* Weak abdominal muscles; repetitive kicking, running, or cutting maneuvers
Functional Assessment	Explosive athletic activities create symptoms. Increased pain with resisted sit-ups Patients may describe pain when coughing.
Inspection	No visible abnormality
Palpation	Pain over the adductor tendon, pubic ramus, midinguinal region. A tender, dilated superficial inguinal ring may also be reported.
Joint and Muscle Function Assessment	*AROM:* Pain may be experienced during hip adduction. Any motion in which the involved muscles place tension on the pubis may cause pain. *MMT:* Adductor muscle group Trunk flexion *PROM:* Abduction causes pain by causing tension in the adductors.
Joint Stability Tests	*Stress tests:* Not applicable *Joint play:* Not applicable
Selective Tissue Tests	Pain may be reported during the Valsalva maneuver (see p. 502).
Neurological Screening	Within normal limits
Vascular Screening	Within normal limits
Imaging Techniques	Radiographs are used to rule out concomitant bony injury. MRI can be diagnostic of muscular lesions or surrounding soft tissue.
Differential Diagnosis	Osteitis pubis, adductor tears, iliopsoas tendinopathy, arthritis, tumor, inguinal hernia, OA, femoral acetabular impingement, nerve root impingement, urinary tract infection, epididymitis, endometriosis, ovarian cysts[58]
Comments	The diagnosis of athletic pubalgia can be complicated by the presence of multiple conditions and symptoms.

AROM = active range of motion; MMT = manual muscle test; MRI = magnetic resonance imaging; OA = osteoarthritis; PROM = passive range of motion

Internal Cause

The iliopsoas tendon is held in position by the inguinal ligament. When the hip is flexed, abducted, and externally rotated, the tendon is positioned laterally; when the hip is extended, adducted, and internally rotated, the tendon is medially positioned. Internal snapping hip syndrome is attributed to the iliopsoas passing over the femoral head, iliopectineal ridge, iliopsoas bursa, or bony outgrowth on the lesser trochanter as the hip moves from flexion to extension and back (Fig. 12-23).[9,72]

Clinically, internal snapping hip syndrome can be replicated by having a supine patient move the femur from a flexed, abducted, and externally rotated position into extension, adduction, and internal rotation and back. The snapping can be reduced by applying manual pressure on the iliopsoas tendon where it crosses the hip.[9]

External Cause

External causes of snapping hip syndrome are associated with the IT band sliding over the greater trochanter. When the hip is extended, the IT tract is posterior to the greater trochanter. During hip flexion, the band "snaps" over the trochanter. The symptoms are worsened when the posterior portion of the IT tract and/or the anterior fibers of the

Examination Findings 12-7
Piriformis Syndrome

Examination Segment	Clinical Findings
History of Current Condition	*Onset:* Acute: Rapid onset of symptoms may be associated with spasm of the piriformis muscle resulting from hyperinternal rotation of the hip or a blow to the buttock. Insidious: Gradual, progressive onset that occurs secondary to hypertrophy of the piriformis muscle or biomechanical changes in the hip, pelvis, or sacrum; in most cases, the time of onset is not discernible. *Pain characteristics:* Pain deep in the posterior aspect of the hip, radiating into the buttock and down the posterior aspect of the leg; increases on standing and often decreases with the patient lying supine and the knees flexed *Mechanism:* May result from a rapid increase in activity *Predisposing conditions:* Anatomic deviation in which the sciatic nerve passes through the piriformis muscle; females have an increased risk of acquiring piriformis syndrome.
Functional Assessment	The patient may present with an antalgic gait, with increased pain during the loading response and midstance phases.
Inspection	In chronic conditions, atrophy of the gluteus maximus may be noted.
Palpation	Tenderness during palpation of the sciatic notch. Palpation may also cause an increase in symptoms reported.
Joint and Muscle Function Assessment	*AROM:* Pain may be experienced during external rotation owing to the piriformis muscle's contracting and placing pressure on the sciatic nerve. *MMT:* Pain elicited or symptoms increased during resisted hip abduction with the patient in the seated position (see Fig. 12-22); pain is also possible during hip abduction. *PROM:* Increased symptoms with internal rotation of the hip while patient is supine; symptoms reduced with external rotation
Joint Stability Tests	*Stress tests:* Not applicable *Joint play:* Not applicable
Selective Tissue Tests	Positive straight-leg-raise test result
Neurological Screening	The L2–L4 dermatomes require evaluation for numbness or paresthesia.
Vascular Screening	Within normal limits
Imaging Techniques	MRI is used to rule out other bony or soft tissue abnormality. Hypertrophy of the piriformis may be noted.
Differential Diagnosis	Nerve root compression and many others
Comments	The signs and symptoms of piriformis syndrome closely replicate those of other lumbopelvic disorders.

AROM = active range of motion; MMT = manual muscle test; MRI = magnetic resonance imaging; PROM = passive range of motion

gluteus maximus are inflamed and thickened.[9] The maximum amount of pressure is placed on the greater trochanter when the hip is adducted with the knee extended.[2]

With the patient either lying on the unaffected side or standing, the IT band can often be felt snapping over the greater trochanter. Applying manual pressure over the trochanter and reducing the snapping sensation helps confirm the clinical diagnosis of external snapping hip syndrome.

Snapping Hip Syndrome Intervention Strategies

Most cases of internal and external snapping hip syndrome are managed conservatively, focusing on reducing inflammation, correcting biomechanical predispositions, stretching shortened tissues, and avoiding activities that cause the symptoms. Oral or injectable anti-inflammatory medications may be prescribed.[71]

On rare occasions, surgery may be required to relieve the symptoms. These procedures include excising the offending bursa, lengthening the IT band, and/or reducing the size of bony prominences that are impinging on the soft tissue structures.[9,71,72]

Bursitis

Resulting from increased friction between a muscle or tendon and bone, bursitis in the hip region usually is isolated

Examination Findings 12-8
Snapping Hip Syndrome

Examination Segment	Clinical Findings
History of Current Condition	*Onset:* Insidious *Pain characteristics:* Pain and discomfort associated with the snapping tend to be localized over the greater trochanter (external type) or the anterior hip (internal type). Pain is usually secondary to bursitis. *Mechanism:* Internal snapping represents the iliopsoas tendon contacting the femoral head or other structure. External snapping is caused by the IT band catching on the greater trochanter. The motion of hip flexion and extension produces the snapping. *Predisposing conditions:* Athletes, especially dancers, in their late teens or early 20s are at an increased risk.[9] External type: Greater trochanteric bursitis; IT band inflammation and/or tightness; reduced femoral neck angle Anterolateral knee instability (secondary to gait changes)[9] May be the result of total hip arthroplasty
Functional Assessment	Pain and snapping may be experienced during running, jumping, and carioca-type cross-stepping activities.[70]
Inspection	Gross inspection is unremarkable. The patient may voluntarily demonstrate the motions that produce the snapping.
Palpation	The patient may feel the mechanical snapping of the tendon over the anterior hip for the internal type or over the greater trochanter for the external type.
Joint and Muscle Function Assessment	*AROM:* Snapping may be replicated when the hip moves from flexion to extension and back.[70] The internal type has more pronounced findings when the hip is moved from a flexed, abducted, and externally rotated position into extension, adduction, and internal rotation and back. *MMT:* Unremarkable *PROM:* In some cases, the symptoms can be reproduced during passive hip flexion and extension.
Joint Stability Tests	*Stress tests:* Not applicable *Joint play:* Not applicable
Selective Tissue Tests	None
Neurological Screening	Within normal limits
Vascular Screening	Within normal limits
Imaging Techniques	Radiographs and MRI may be used to rule out intra-articular lesions and identify hip angulations that may cause structural impingement. **Bursography** can be used to image the size and shape of the bursae, especially the iliopsoas bursa, to identify structural involvement.
Differential Diagnosis	Labral tear, trochanteric bursitis, iliopsoas bursitis, intra-articular lesion, chronic positional subluxation of the hip joint
Comments	A loose body within the articular space will present with symptoms similar to snapping hip syndrome.

AROM = active range of motion; IT = iliotibial; MMT = manual muscle test; MRI = magnetic resonance imaging; PROM = passive range of motion

Bursography Imaging technique that highlights the bursae

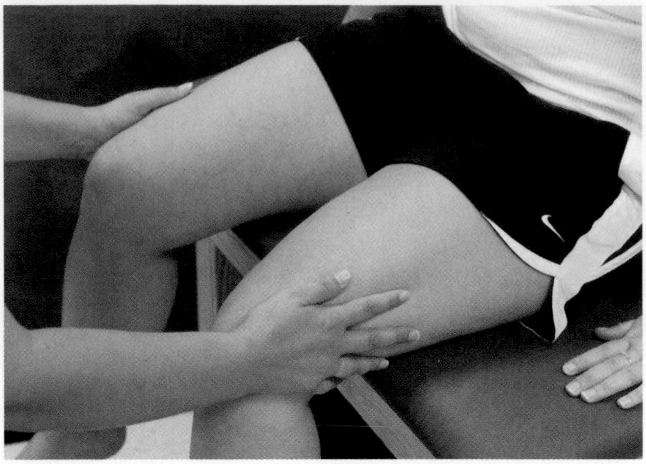

FIGURE 12-22 ■ Resisted hip abduction with the patient seated to duplicate pain caused by piriformis syndrome.

to the greater trochanteric, ischial, or iliopsoas bursae. The onset of these conditions may be related to biomechanical factors, congenital influences, or environmental conditions such as prolonged periods of sitting. Septic infection has also been cited as a cause of inflammation of the hip bursae.[73] A definitive diagnosis of these conditions can be made via ultrasonic imaging, CT scans, or MRI.[73]

Trochanteric Bursitis

Irritation of the trochanteric bursa may result from a single blow. However, more commonly, it may be caused by friction from the IT band as it crosses over this structure during the movements of flexion, extension, internal rotation, and external rotation. A history of a rapid increase in the frequency, intensity, or duration of training is often associated with this condition. Women may be predisposed to this condition because of an increased Q-angle (Examination Findings 12-9).

Chronic inflammation of the trochanteric bursa is one of the possible causes of external **snapping hip syndrome**, in which an audible snap occurs as the IT band passes over the greater trochanter (see p. 460). Greater trochanteric bursitis commonly results in reduced hip ROM, especially in flexion and extension and internal and external rotation secondary to pain located directly posterior to the greater trochanter. Trochanteric bursitis can mimic or mask the signs and symptoms of a femoral neck stress fracture.[74]

Ischial Bursitis

Movement of the buttocks while the patient is weight bearing in the seated position, such as the rocking motion associated with rowing or biking, can cause friction to irritate the ischial bursa. This structure can also be traumatized secondary to a direct blow, such as a fall. Ischial bursitis can be further irritated by prolonged periods of sitting, as occurs during bus or airplane trips. Point tenderness at the ischial tuberosity is characteristic of ischial bursitis. A careful history is necessary to rule out the possibility of a hamstring tear or an avulsion of its attachment, both of which have signs and symptoms similar to those of ischial bursitis (Examination Findings 12-10). Use of an inflatable doughnut pad for sitting during prolonged periods to lessen the weight-bearing forces placed on these structures may be helpful.

Iliopsoas Bursitis

Inflammation of the iliopsoas bursa, seldom occurring as an isolated event, may be associated with rheumatoid arthritis or OA of the hip.[75] Pain in the anterior hip is often the only symptom of iliopsoas bursitis. However, a mass may be palpated in the inguinal region and femoral fold.[75,76] The condition has also been implicated as another cause of snapping hip syndrome.[73,77-79]

Bursitis Intervention Strategies

The initial management of bursitis is conservative, with the patient advised to avoid the offending activity and stretch soft tissue that may lead to bursal inflammation. For example, adequate length of the iliotibial tract and the attached gluteus medius is necessary to reduce irritation of the greater trochanteric bursa. Patients with ischial bursitis may get symptomatic relief by sitting on a donut pad. Equipment changes (such as changing the bike seat) may be indicated to prevent recurrence.

On-Field Evaluation of Pelvis and Thigh Injuries

Trauma to the coxofemoral joint is rare in sports. The bony and muscular anatomy is normally well padded in collision sports, such as football and ice hockey, which mandate the use of protective padding over the anterior thigh, ilium, and sacrum. However, when trauma does occur, it is usually severe. More commonly, acute injuries to this region involve muscular tears, contusions, and sprains of the SI joint.

On arriving at the scene, note whether the athlete is moving the involved leg. If the femur is moving, a gross dislocation of the hip or fracture of the femur is less probable. However, a subluxation of the hip must still be considered. A fixed, immobile, awkwardly positioned, or noticeably shortened leg may indicate a dislocation of the hip joint or a fracture of the femoral neck. Inspect the shaft of the femur for normal contour.

The mechanism of injury and other factors surrounding the onset of the injury must be ascertained as soon as possible in the history-taking process. Relevant questions include determining the injurious force, associated sounds and sensations, and any pertinent history of injury.

After a hip dislocation or subluxation and femoral fracture have been ruled out, AROM of both the knee and the hip is initiated. This is easily performed by having the athlete flex the thigh to the chest and straightening the leg back out again. If the athlete is unable to fully bear weight, a decision needs to be made on how to remove that individual from the playing arena. These techniques are described in Chapter 1.

Examination Findings 12-9
Trochanteric Bursitis

Examination Segment	Clinical Findings
History of Current Condition	*Onset:* Acute or insidious *Pain characteristics:* Over the greater trochanter, radiating posteriorly to the buttock; increased pain when the patient climbs stairs *Other symptoms:* Increased pain or inability to sleep on involved side *Mechanism:* Acute: Direct blow to the greater trochanter Chronic: Irritation from the IT band passing over the bursa *Predisposing conditions:* Increased Q-angles (above the norm for the patient's gender) possibly predisposing him or her to overuse forces being placed on the trochanteric bursa; leg-length discrepancy
Functional Assessment	Increased pain during loading response and midstance phase of gait
Inspection	The area over the greater trochanter is usually unremarkable.
Palpation	Palpation reveals tenderness over the trochanteric bursa. Crepitus may also be noted during active movement of the hip.
Joint and Muscle Function Assessment	*AROM:* Flexion and extension and internal and external rotation cause pain as the IT band passes over the greater trochanter, resulting in decreased ROM. *MMT:* Hip extension and abduction weak secondary to pain Hip adduction weak secondary to pain *PROM:* Flexion and extension and internal and external rotation cause pain as the IT band passes over the greater trochanter, resulting in decreased ROM.
Joint Stability Tests	*Stress tests:* Not applicable *Joint play:* Not applicable
Selective Tissue Tests	Ober test for IT band tightness
Neurological Screening	Within normal limits
Vascular Screening	Within normal limits
Imaging Techniques	MRI Diagnostic ultrasound
Differential Diagnosis	Tendinopathy, femoral neck stress fracture, contusion, gluteus medius tear, tensor fascia latae tear
Comments	Chronic trochanteric bursitis may result in external "snapping hip" syndrome. The signs and symptoms of trochanteric bursitis may mimic those of a femoral neck stress fracture. Pain may be referred from the sacroiliac joint or low back.

AROM = active range of motion; IT = iliotibial; MMT = manual muscle test; MRI = magnetic resonance imaging; PROM = passive range of motion; ROM = range of motion

Examination Findings 12-10
Ischial Bursitis

Examination Segment	Clinical Findings
History of Current Condition	*Onset:* Acute or insidious *Pain characteristics:* Over the ischial tuberosity in the vicinity of the gluteal fold *Mechanism:* Acute: Direct blow to the ischial tuberosity, such as falling on it Chronic: Repeated shifting and moving while weight bearing in the seated position (e.g., rowing) *Predisposing conditions:* Tightness of the hamstring muscle group, prolonged sitting and rocking, especially on a hard surface (i.e., bike seat, scull seat)
Functional Assessment	Prolonged periods of sitting may cause an increase in symptoms.
Inspection	Unremarkable
Palpation	Tenderness over the ischial tuberosity; the bursa feels thick.
Joint and Muscle Function Assessment	*AROM:* Pain during active hip flexion *MMT:* Pain during resisted hip extension with the knee flexed to isolate the gluteus maximus *PROM:* Pain at the end of passive hip flexion, especially with knee extended
Joint Stability Tests	*Stress tests:* Not applicable *Joint play:* Not applicable
Selective Tissue Tests	Not applicable
Neurological Screening	Prolonged irritation of the ischial bursa possibly placing pressure on the sciatic nerve, requiring the evaluation of the sensory and motor nerves of the posterior lower leg
Vascular Screening	Within normal limits
Imaging Techniques	MRI Diagnostic ultrasound
Differential Diagnosis	Hamstring avulsion fracture

AROM = active range of motion; MMT = manual muscle test; MRI = magnetic resonance imaging; PROM = passive range of motion

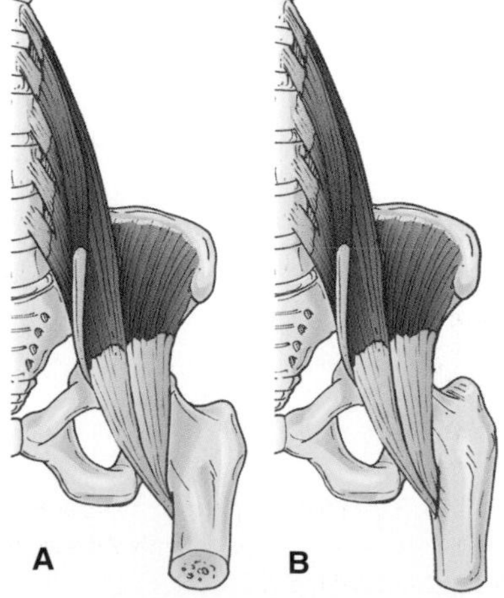

FIGURE 12-23 ■ Internal snapping hip syndrome. (A) During hip flexion the iliopsoas tendon shifts laterally, catching on a femoral bony prominence. (B) During hip extension the tendon moves medially.

Initial Evaluation and Management of On-Field Injuries

Contusions or muscle strains are the typical pelvis and thigh injuries that necessitate on-field evaluation of the athlete. However, hip dislocations and femur fractures represent medical emergencies requiring astute management to limit the scope of trauma and increase the athlete's chances for a full recovery.

Hip Dislocation

Because of the hip's strong ligamentous and bony arrangement, dislocations are rare. However, their occurrence represents a medical emergency requiring immediate care. The majority of hip dislocations involve posterior displacement of the femoral head.[80] Fractures to the femoral neck or the acetabulum (or both) may also result. Most dislocations occur when the hip is in flexion and adduction and an axial force is delivered to the femur, displacing it posteriorly and causing the head to be driven through the posterior capsule.[81]

Athletes suffering from a hip dislocation complain of immediate, intense pain within the joint and buttock, possibly describing the sensation of the hip's "going out." The femur and lower leg are often positioned in flexion, internal rotation, and adduction so that the involved knee rests against the knee of the opposite side (Fig. 12-24).[2] AROM is impossible or results in severe pain. Although no attempt is made to reduce the dislocation on the field, the examiner must perform a sensory and vascular check of the involved extremity. Integrity of the motor nerves can be determined by asking the athlete to extend and flex the toes. These results are documented for reference by the emergency room staff. Immediate transport to an emergency facility is necessary to allow rapid reduction of the dislocation.[80]

Closed reduction of the dislocation can often be performed with the patient sedated or anesthetized. More complex dislocations or dislocations that involve a concomitant fracture may require open reduction and/or internal fixation.

Femoral Fracture

Resulting from a torsional or shear force to the shaft, femoral fractures are relatively rare in athletes. This fact is based on the "weak link" principle, in which these forces are more likely to result in trauma to the ankle, lower leg, or knee. Because they result in immediate loss of function, pain, and deformity, complete fractures of the femur are easily recognizable (Fig. 12-25). Suspected femoral fractures also constitute a medical emergency. Distal pulses and neurological function should be assessed, with the results reported to emergency personnel. The athlete's leg will be immobilized prior to transport. Femoral fractures, especially in adults, generally require surgical intervention.

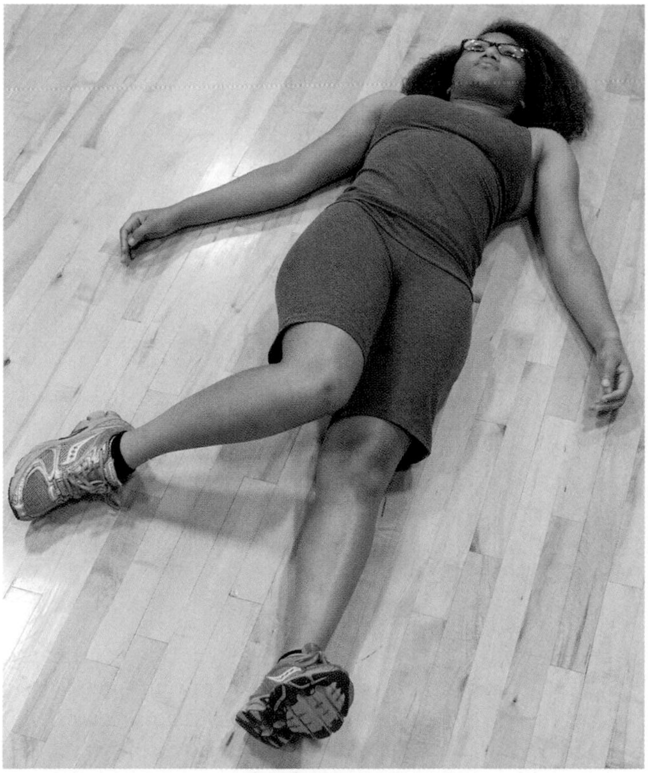

FIGURE 12-24 ■ Position of the lower leg following a posterior hip dislocation: adduction and internal rotation of the hip.

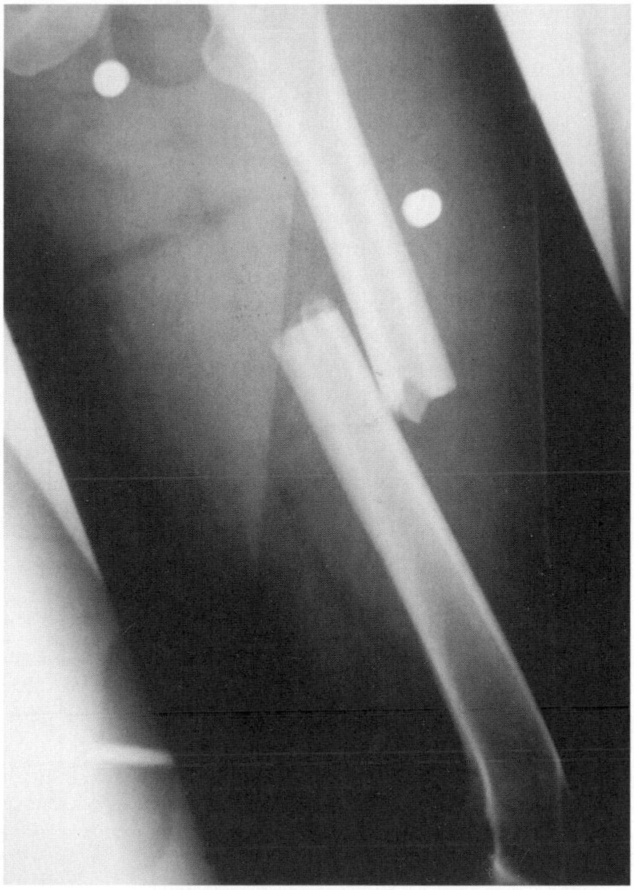

FIGURE 12-25 ■ Radiograph of a complete fracture of the femoral shaft. This type of injury results in obvious deformity of the thigh.

REFERENCES

1. Hoaglund, FT, and Steinbach, LS: Primary osteoarthritis of the hip: etiology and epidemiology. *J Am Acad Orthop Surg*, 9:320, 2001.
2. Anderson, K, Strickland, SM, and Warren, R: Hip and groin injuries in athletes. *Am J Sports Med*, 29:521, 2001.
3. Hong, RJ, et al: Magnetic resonance imaging of the hip. *J Magn Reson Imaging*, 27:435, 2008.
4. Lewis, CL, and Sahrmann, SA: Acetabular labral tears. *Phys Ther*, 86: 110, 2006.
5. Martin, RL, and Kivlan, B: The hip complex. In Levangie, PK, and Norkin, CC (eds): *Joint Structure and Function: A Comprehensive Analysis*, ed 5. Philadelphia, PA: FA Davis, 2011, p 359.
6. Tonnis, D, and Heinecke, A: Current concepts review – acetabular and femoral anteversion: relationship with osteoarthritis of the hip. *J Bone Joint Surg Am*, 81:1747, 1999.

7. Bardakos, NV, and Villar, RN: The ligamentum teres of the adult hip. *J Bone Joint Surg*, 91(B):8, 2009.
8. Neptune, RR, Wright, IC, and van den Bogert, AJ: Muscle coordination and function during cutting movements. *Med Sci Sports Exerc*, 31:294, 1999.
9. Deslandes, M, et al: The snapping iliopsoas tendon: new mechanisms using dynamic sonography. *AJR Roentgenol*, 190:576, 2008.
10. Zlotorowicz, M, et al: Anatomy of the medial femoral circumflex artery with respect to the vascularity of the femoral head. *J Bone Joint Surg*, 93(Br):1471, 2011.
11. Kelly, BT, et al: Vascularity of the hip labrum: a cadaveric investigation. *Arthroscopy*, 21:3, 2005.
12. Carney, BT, and Minter, C: Nonsurgical treatment to regain hip abduction motion in Perthes disease: a retrospective review. *South Med J*, 97:485, 2004.
13. Loder, RT, Starnes, T, and Dikos, G: Atypical and typical (idiopathic) slipped capital femoral epiphysis: reconfirmation of the age-weight test and description of the height and age-height tests. *J Bone Joint Surg*, 88(A):1574, 2006.
14. Mitchell, B, et al: Hip joint pathology: clinical presentation and correlation between magnetic resonance arthrography, ultrasound, and arthroscopic findings in 25 consecutive cases. *Clin J Sport Med*, 13:152, 2003.
15. Woodley, SJ, et al: Lateral hip pain: findings from magnetic resonance imaging and clinical examination. *J Orthop Sports Phys Ther*, 38:313, 2008.
16. Imam, S, and Khanduja, V: Current concepts in the diagnosis and management of femoroacetabular impingement. *Int Orthop*, 35:1427, 2011.
17. Sutlive, TG, et al: Development of a clinical prediction rule for diagnosing hip osteoarthritis in individuals with unilateral hip pain. *J Orthop Sports Phys Ther*, 38:542, 2008.
18. Stief, F, et al: Dynamic loading of the knee and hip joint and compensatory strategies in children and adolescents with varus malalignment. *Gait Posture*, 33:490, 2011.
19. Sabharwal, S, and Zhao, C: The hip-knee-ankle angle in children: reference values based on a full-length standing radiograph. *J Bone Joint Surg*, 91(A):2461, 2009.
20. Sugano, N, Noble, PC, and Kamaric, E: A comparison of alternative methods of measuring femoral anteversion. *J Comput Assist Tomogr*, 22:610, 1998.
21. Liodakis, E, et al: The neck-malleolar angle: an alternative method for measuring total lower limb torsion that considers the knee joint rotation angle. *Skeletal Radiol*, 40:617, 2011.
22. Matovinovic, D, et al: Comparison in regression of femoral neck anteversion in children with normal, intoeing and outtoeing gait: prospective study. *Coll Antropol*, 22:525, 1998.
23. Brand, RA, and Yack, HJ: Effects of leg length discrepancies on the forces at the hip joint. *Clin Orthop Relat Res*, 333:172, 1996.
24. Dallinga, JM, Benjaminse, A, and Lemmink, KA: Which screening tools can predict injury to the lower extremities in team sports? A systematic review. *Sports Med*, 42:791, 2012.
25. Friel, K, et al: Ipsilateral hip abductor weakness after inversion ankle sprain. *J Athl Train*, 41:74, 2006.
26. Winters, MV, et al: Passive versus active stretching of hip flexor muscles in subjects with limited hip extension: a randomized clinical trial. *Phys Ther*, 84:800, 2004.
27. Herrington, L, Rivett, N, and Munro, S: The relationship between patella position and length of the iliotibial band as assessed using Ober's test. *Man Ther*, 11:182, 2006.
28. Reese, NB, and Bandy, WD: Use of an inclinometer to measure flexibility of the iliotibial band using the Ober test and modified Ober test: differences in the magnitude and reliability of measurements. *J Orthop Sports Phys Ther*, 33:326, 2003.
29. Gajdosik, RL, Sandler, MM, and Marr, HL: Influence of knee positions and gender on the Ober test for length of the iliotibial band. *Clin Biomech (Bristol, Avon)*, 18:77, 2003.
30. Boyle, KL, and Demske, JR: Management of a female with chronic sciatica and low back pain: a case report. *Physiother Theory Pract*, 25:44, 2009.
31. Heiderscheit, BC, et al: Hamstring strain injuries: recommendations for diagnosis, rehabilitation, and injury prevention. *J Orthop Sports Phys Ther*, 40:67, 2010.
32. Verrall, GM, et al: Assessment of physical examination and magnetic resonance imaging findings of hamstring injury as predictors for recurrent injury. *J Orthop Sports Phys Ther*, 36:215, 2006.
33. Askling, CM, et al: Acute first-time hamstring strains during high speed running: a longitudinal study including clinical and magnetic resonance imaging findings. *Am J Sports Med*, 35:197, 2007.
34. de Visser, HM, et al: Risk factors of recurrent hamstring injuries: a systematic review. *Br J Sports Med*, 46:124, 2012.
35. Aronen, JG, et al: Quadriceps contusions: clinical results of immediate immobilization in 120 degrees of knee flexion. *Clin J Sports Med*, 16:383, 2006.
36. Peck, D: Slipped capital femoral epiphysis: diagnosis and management. *Am Fam Physician*, 82:258, 2010.
37. Golve, PA, Cameron, DB, and Millis, MB: Slipped capital femoral epiphysis update. *Curr Opin Pediatr*, 21:39, 2009.
38. Larson, AN, et al: A prospective multicultural study of Legg-Calvé-Perthes disease: functional and radiographic outcomes of nonoperative treatment at a mean follow-up of twenty years. *J Bone Joint Surg*, 94:584, 2012.
39. Kim, HKW: Pathophysiology and new strategies for the treatment of Legg-Calvé-Perthes disease. *J Bone Joint Surg Am*, 94:659, 2012.
40. Pegrum, J, Crisp, T, and Padhiar, N: Diagnosis and management of bone stress injuries of the lower limb in athletes. *BMJ*, 344:e2511, 2012.
41. Shaffer, RA, et al: Predictors of stress fracture susceptibility in young female recruits. *Am J Sports Med*, 34:108, 2006.
42. Gurney, B, Boissonnault, WG, and Andrews, R: Differential diagnosis of a femoral neck/head stress fracture. *J Orthop Sports Phys Ther*, 36:80, 2006.
43. Shin, AY, and Gillingham, BL: Fatigue fractures of the femoral neck in athletes. *J Am Acad Orthop Surg*, 4:293, 1997.
44. Agricola, R, et al: The development of cam-type deformity in adolescent and young male soccer players. *Am J Sports Med*, 40:1099, 2012.
45. Johnson, AC, Shaman, MA, and Ryan, TG: Femoroacetabular impingement in former high-level youth soccer players. *Am J Sports Med*, 40:1342, 2012.
46. Audenaert, EA, et al: Hip morphological characteristics and range of internal rotation in femoroacetabular impingement. *Am J Sports Med*, 40:1329, 2012.
47. Austin, AB, et al: Identification of abnormal hip motion associated with acetabular labral pathology. *J Orthop Sports Phys Ther*, 38:558, 2008.
48. Cohen, SB, et al: Treatment of femoroacetabular impingement in athletes using a mini-direct anterior approach. *Am J Sports Med*, 40:1620, 2012.
49. Nho, SJ, et al: Outcomes after the arthroscopic treatment of femoroacetabular impingement in a mixed group of high-level athletes. *Am J Sports Med*, 39 Suppl:14S, 2011.
50. Groh, MM, and Herrera, J: A comprehensive review of hip labral tears. *Curr Rev Musculoskelet Med*, 2:105, 2009.
51. Narvani, AA, et al: A preliminary report on prevalence of acetabular labrum tears in sports patients with groin pain. *Knee Surg Sports Traumatol Arthrosc*, 11:403, 2003.
52. Blankenbaker, DG, et al: Classification and localization of acetabular labral tears. *Skelet Radiol*, 36:391, 2007.
53. Burnett, SJ, et al: Clinical presentation of patients with tears of the acetabular labrum. *J Bone Joint Surg*, 88(A):1448, 2006.
54. Petersen, W, Petersen, F, and Tillmann, B: Structure and vascularization of the acetabular labrum with regard to the pathogenesis and healing of labral lesions. *Arch Orthop Trauma Surg*, 123:283, 2003.
55. Larson, CM, Giveans, MR, and Stone, RM: Arthroscopic debridement versus refixation of the acetabular labrum associated with femoroacetabular impingement. *Am J Sports Med*, 40:1015, 2012.

56. Wandel, S, et al: Effects of glucosamine, chondroitin, or placebo in patients with osteoarthritis of hip or knee: network meta-analysis. *BMJ*, 16:341, 2010.
57. Preskitt, JT: Sports hernia: the experience of Baylor University Medical Center at Dallas. *Proc (Bayl Univ Med Cent)*, 24:89, 2011.
58. Kachingwe, AF, and Grech, S: Proposed algorithm for the management of athletes with athletic pubalgia (sports hernia): a case series. *J Orthop Sports Phys Ther*, 38:768, 2008.
59. Litwin, DE, et al: Athletic pubalgia (sports hernia). *Clin Sports Med*, 30: 417, 2011.
60. Hiti, CJ, et al: Athletic osteitis pubis. *Sports Med*, 41:361, 2011.
61. Morelli, V, and Smith, V: Groin injuries in athletes. *Am Fam Physician*, 64:283, 2001.
62. LeBlanc, KE, and LeBlanc, KA: Groin pain in athletes. *Hernia*, 7:68, 2003.
63. Mehin R, et al: Surgery for osteitis pubis. *Can J Surg*, 49:170, 2006.
64. Parziale, JR, Hudgins, TH, and Fishman, LM: The piriformis syndrome. *Am J Orthop*, 25:819, 1996.
65. McCrory, P, and Bell, S: Nerve entrapment syndromes as a cause of pain in the hip, groin, and buttock. *Sports Med*, 27:261, 1999.
66. Hughes, SS, et al: Extrapelvic compression of the sciatic nerve: an unusual cause of pain about the hip: report of five cases. *J Bone Joint Surg Am*, 74:1553, 1992.
67. Silver, JK, and Leadbetter, WB: Piriformis syndrome: assessment of current practice and literature review. *Orthopedics*, 21:1133, 1998.
68. Bresler, M, Mar, W, and Toman, J: Diagnostic imaging in the evaluation of leg pain in athletes. *Clin Sports Med*, 31:217, 2012.
69. Hanania, M, and Kitain, E: Perisciatic injection of steroid for the treatment of sciatica due to piriformis syndrome. *Reg Anesth Pain Med*, 23:223, 1998.
70. Keskula, DR, Lott, J, and Duncan, JB: Snapping iliopsoas tendon in a recreational athlete: a case report. *J Athl Train*, 34:382, 1999.
71. Dobbs, MB, et al: Surgical correction of the snapping iliopsoas tendon in adolescents. *J Bone Joint Surg*, 84(A):420, 2002.
72. Gruen, GS, Scioscia, TN, and Lowenstein, JE: The surgical treatment of internal snapping hip. *Am J Sports Med*, 30:607, 2002.
73. Ginesty, E, et al: Iliopsoas bursopathies: a review of twelve cases. *Rev Rhum Engl Ed*, 65:181, 1998.
74. Jones, DL, and Erhard, RE: Diagnosis of trochanteric bursitis versus femoral neck stress fracture. *Phys Ther*, 77:58, 1997.
75. Parziale, JR, O'Donnell, CJ, and Sandman, DN: Iliopsoas bursitis. *Am J Phys Med*, 88:690, 2009.
76. McCormick, JJ, Demos, TC, and Lomasney, LM: Radiologic case study: iliopsoas bursitis. *Orthopedics*, 26:1106, 2003.
77. Blankenbaker, DG, and Tuite, MJ: Iliopsoas musculotendinous unit. *Semin Musculoskelet Radiol*, 12:13, 2008.
78. Vaccaro, JP, Sauser, DD, and Beals, RK: Iliopsoas bursa imaging: efficacy in depicting abnormal iliopsoas tendon motion in patients with internal snapping hip syndrome. *Radiology*, 197:853, 1995.
79. Janzen, DL, et al: The snapping hip: clinical and imaging findings in transient subluxation of the iliopsoas tendon. *Can Assoc Radiol J*, 47:202, 1996.
80. Berkes, MB, et al: Traumatic posterior hip instability and femoroacetabular impingement in athletes. *Am J Orthop*, 41:166, 2012.
81. Stiris, MG: MR imaging after sports-induced hip dislocations: report of three cases. *Acta Radiol*, 41:300, 2000.

SECTION 3

Torso Examination

Patient-Reported Outcome Measures

The multifactorial nature of low back pain, combined with the difficulty in identifying a structural culprit, means that the use of outcome measures is important in understanding the impact of the pain on the patient's life.[1] The Oswestry Disability Index and the Roland-Morris Disability Questionnaire, both commonly used for patients with low back pain, may suffer from ceiling effects when used with highly active patients who have transient conditions. Generic measures, described in the section opener at the beginning of this text, are also often used. Additionally, because low back pain is often associated with fear avoidance beliefs and symptoms of depression, different scales are often used to determine their influence.[1]

Oswestry Disability Index (ODI)

The ODI is the most commonly used outcome measure in patients with low back pain. The ODI includes the following 10 sections, each with six statements from which the patient can choose: pain intensity, personal care, lifting, walking, sitting, standing, sleeping, sex life, social life, and traveling. The modified ODI has slightly different sections. Each selection is scored from 0 to 5, with 5 representing worse symptoms. The total score is then doubled and reported from 0 to 100, with a higher score representing greater disability.[2]

Minimal Detectable Change: 15–19[3]
Minimally Clinically Important Difference: 10-point change from baseline

Roland-Morris Disability Questionnaire (RDQ)

Consisting of 24 yes/no items, the RDQ assesses the impact of pain on the patient's perceived disability over the past 24 hours. Scores range from 0 to 24, with higher scores representing greater disability. The RDQ may be more discriminatory in patients with mild or moderate disability than in those with severe disability.

Minimum Detectable Change: 2–7, depending on time interval, treatment type, and baseline scores[4]
Minimum Clinically Important Difference: 2–7 in patients with baseline scores <10; 5.5–13.8 in patients with baseline scores > 15[5]

Beck Depression Inventory (BDI)

Symptoms of depression are a frequent comorbidity in patients with low back pain. The 21-item BDI is used to screen for the presence and severity of depression. For each item, the patient selects one of four options. Scores range from 0 to 63 and are interpreted as follows:

1–10: Normal ups and downs
11–16: Mild mood disturbance
17–20: Borderline clinical depression
21–30: Moderate depression
31–40: Severe depression
>40: Extreme depression[2]

Fear Avoidance Beliefs Questionnaire (FABQ)

The FABQ is used to assess the patient's fear and the extent to which the patient is avoiding activity in response to low back pain. Because a high FABQ is associated with worse clinical outcomes if not addressed, measuring this psychosocial component is warranted as part of the examination process to determine treatment options.[6,7] The questionnaire is composed of two subscales measuring work (11 items) and activity (5 items). Patients are asked to circle a number from 0 to 6, with higher numbers associated with higher avoidance. Certain items are not used in scoring. The scores for activity range from 0 to 24, and the scores for work range from 0 to 42.

The FABQ is generally not used to measure treatment success, so Minimum Detectable Change and Minimum Clinically Important Differences are not reported.[1]

REFERENCES

1. Vela, LI, Haladay, DE, and Denegar, C: Clinical assessment of low-back-pain treatment outcomes in athletes. *J Sport Rehabil*, 20:74, 2011.
2. Chapman, JR: Evaluating common outcomes for measuring treatment success for chronic low back pain. *Spine*, 36(21 Suppl):S54, 2011.

3. Davidson, M, and Keating, JL: A comparison of five low back disability questionnaires: reliability and responsiveness. *Phys Ther*, 82:8, 2002.
4. Ostelo, RW, et al: Interpreting pain and functional status in low back pain: towards international consensus regarding minimal important change. *Spine*, 33:90, 2008.
5. Smeets, R, et al: Measures of function in low back pain/disorders. *Arthritis Care Res*, 63(Suppl 11):S158, 2011.
6. Grotle, M, Vollestad, NK, and Brox, JI: Clinical course and impact of fear-avoidance beliefs in low back pain. *Spine*, 31:1038, 2006.
7. DeLitto, A, et al: Low back pain: clinical practice guidelines linked to the International Classification of Functioning, Disability, and Health from the Orthopaedic Section of the American Physical Therapy Association. *J Orthop Sports Phys Ther*, 42:A1, 2012.

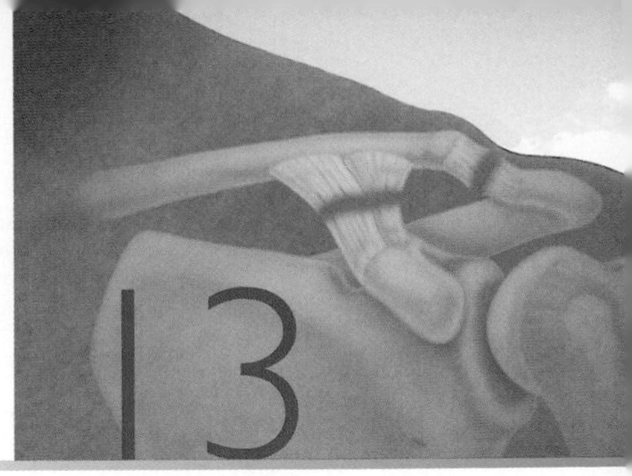

CHAPTER 13

Lumbosacral Pathologies

Formed by 33 vertebral segments and divided into four distinct portions, the spinal column and its associated muscles provide postural control to the torso and skull, while also protecting the spinal cord. The conflicting needs for range of motion (ROM) versus protection of the spinal cord are met in varying degrees throughout the spine (Fig. 13-1).

The cervical spine provides the greatest ROM, but here the spinal cord is the most vulnerable. The thoracic spine provides the greatest protection of the spinal cord but does so at the expense of ROM. The lumbar spine provides a more equal balance between protection of the spinal cord and available ROM. The sacrum and coccyx are composed of fused bones. The sacrum affixes the spinal column to the pelvis and serves as a site for muscle attachment. At this level, the spinal cord has exited the column.

Spine-related pain is a prevalent condition. During any given year, up to 36% of adults will experience low back pain for the first time, with recurrence of symptoms a common phenomenon.[1] The prevalence of back pain in adolescents mimics that in adults, with reports of up to 70% to 80% of the population affected.[2,3] The high prevalence, the significant association of back pain to mental illnesses such as depression, and the resulting demands on the healthcare system make the cost of back pain exorbitant. Acute injury to the spine during athletic competition accounts for an estimated 10% to 15% of all spinal injuries, and each injury carries the risk of traumatizing the spinal cord or spinal nerve.[4] This chapter discusses conditions affecting the lumbar and sacral regions. Conditions affecting the cervical and thoracic regions are presented in Chapter 14. Traumatic (emergent) spinal injuries are discussed in Chapter 20.

Clinical Anatomy

Figure 13-2 compares the relative sizes of the cervical ($n = 7$), thoracic ($n = 12$), and lumbar ($n = 5$) vertebrae and identifies the bony landmarks. The body's weight is transmitted primarily along the spinal column via the vertebral body, whose size is related to the amount of force it transmits. Carrying only the weight of the head, the vertebral bodies of

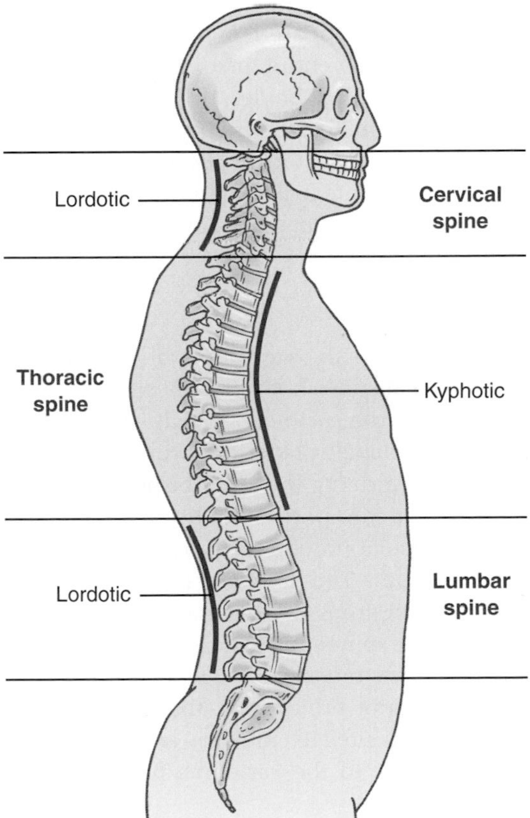

FIGURE 13-1 ■ The three segments of the mobile spinal column with their normal curvature noted.

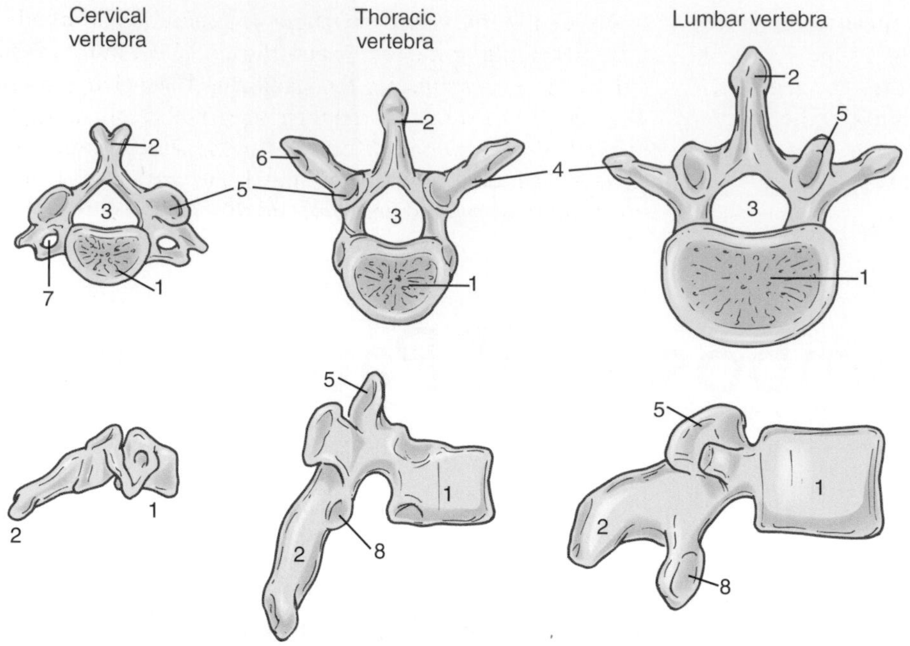

FIGURE 13-2 ■ Comparative anatomy of the cervical, thoracic, and lumbar spine. (1) Vertebral body, (2) spinous process, (3) vertebral foramen, (4) transverse process, (5) superior articular facet, (6) costotransverse facet, (7) transverse foramen, (8) inferior articular facet.

the cervical vertebrae are much smaller than those of the lumbar vertebrae, which are required to transmit and absorb the weight of the entire torso. A segment, comprised of two adjacent vertebral bodies, the intervening disc, and the soft tissue that holds the vertebrae together, represents the smallest functional unit of the spine. The vertebrae of the cervical spine are included in this section for a basis of comparison. Refer to Chapter 14 for further description of the cervical spine.

Bony Anatomy

Each vertebra, with the exception of the first cervical vertebra, has a distinct body that is situated anteriorly and comprises the primary weight-bearing surface. Projecting immediately posteriorly from the body are the sturdy pedicles, forming the anterior portion of the neural arch. The posterior portion of the arch is composed of the lamina, articular processes, transverse processes, and spinous processes. The laterally projecting **transverse processes**, arising from the laminae, provide an attachment site for the spine's intrinsic ligaments and muscles and increase the muscles' mechanical leverage. The prominent posterior projections, the **spinous processes**, act as attachment sites for muscles and ligaments. Their angulation relative to the vertebrae below limits extension of the spine.

The **neural arch**, forming the posterior element of the spinal canal, serves as the protective tunnel through which the spinal cord passes. Lined with a continuation of the cerebral meninges (see Chapter 20), the spinal cord is normally buffered from the walls of the spinal canal by cerebrospinal fluid. Narrowing of the canal, stenosis, due to an acute, acquired, or congenital development of soft tissue or bone, leads to an increased possibility of pressure being placed on the spinal cord that results in radicular symptoms.[5]

Two sets of articular processes arise from the superior and inferior surfaces of the laminae. The superior facets of the vertebrae articulate with the inferior facets of the vertebrae immediately above, forming synovial **facet joints** (zygapophyseal joints), which transmit 20% of the weight-bearing forces through the spine in healthy individuals and up to 47% in patients with disc degeneration.[6] The bony arrangement of these joints is such that the lateral portion of the superior facet articulates with the medial portion of the inferior facet. The orientation and resulting direction of motion change throughout the spine. In the rotating upper cervical region, the facet joints have a more horizontal orientation. In the lower cervical and thoracic regions, the more frontal plane orientation allows lateral flexion but restricts rotation. In the lumbar region, the sagittal plane orientation favors flexion and extension.[7] The extension of the laminae between the superior and inferior facets of a vertebra is called the **pars interarticularis**, a common site of stress fractures in the lumbar spine.

The anterior portions of each pedicle contain vertebral notches, concave depressions along the inferior surfaces and superior portions of the bone. The vertebral notch on the inferior portion of one pedicle is matched with the vertebral notch on the superior portion of the pedicle below,

Facet joints An articulation of the facets between each contiguous part of vertebrae in the spinal column forming the **intervertebral foramen**, the space where spinal nerve roots exit the vertebral column (Fig. 13-3).

The relative sizes of the vertebral bodies and the transverse and spinous processes vary according to their function at each of the spinal levels (Table 13-1). The cervical spine, the most mobile of the vertebral segments, has the smallest vertebral bodies.

Molded by five fused vertebrae, the sacrum is a broad, thick, triangular bone that fixates the spinal column to the pelvis and is responsible for stabilizing the pelvic girdle (Fig. 13-4). The weight of the torso and skull is transmitted through the **sacroiliac (SI) joints** to the lower extremity. Ground reaction forces from the lower extremities are transmitted through the SI joints up the spinal column.

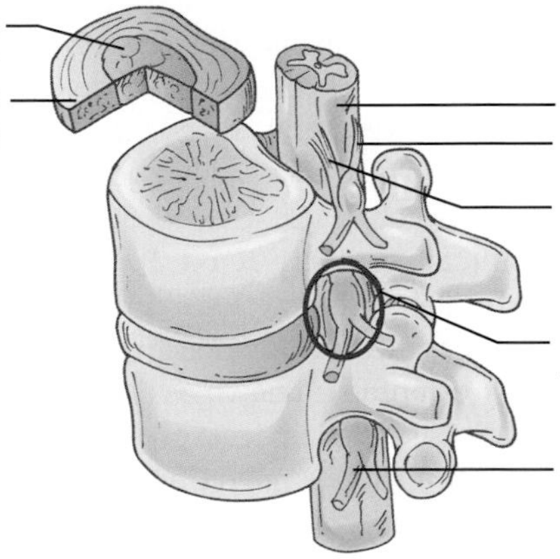

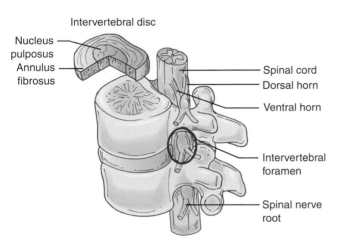

FIGURE 13-3 ■ Nerve roots exiting between the vertebrae. The pedicles of the superior and inferior vertebrae align to form the intervertebral foramen, allowing the spinal nerves to exit the vertebral column.

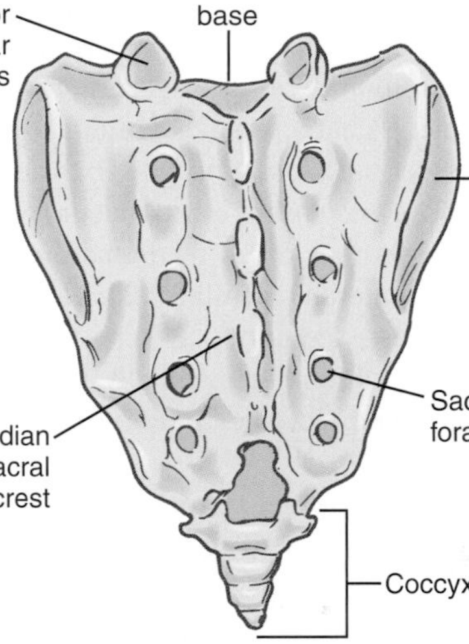

FIGURE 13-4 ■ Posterior view of the sacrum and coccyx.

Table 13-1 Structural Adaptations of Vertebral Anatomy at the Different Spinal Levels

	Bony Anatomy			
Level	Vertebral Body	Transverse Process	Spinous Process	Facet Joints
Cervical	Small; view in the frontal plane is wider than in the sagittal plane Vertebral body is absent in C1; C2 body has vertical projection called the dens; the remaining bodies progressively increase in size.	Short; processes contain the transverse foramen for passage of the vertebral artery.	Small and short, except for C7, which has characteristics of a thoracic vertebra.	C0 and C1: Ellipsoid joint C1 and C2: Positioned in the transverse plane C3–C7: Approximately 45° from transverse plane in the frontal plane
Thoracic	Diameter and thickness increase as the spine continues inferiorly. Demifacets are present to accept the head of the ribs.	Solid configuration allows for the attachment of muscles and costovertebral ligaments. The processes of T1–T12 have articular surfaces for the ribs.	Long and slender; their downward projections result in an overlap of spinous process of the vertebra below; the spinous processes of the lower thoracic vertebrae gradually thicken and straighten to resemble those of the lumbar vertebrae.	Oblique, but lying primarily in the frontal plane
Lumbar	Vertebral bodies are broad in both the frontal and sagittal planes.	Long for leverage; thin in the cross section	The superior borders are posteriorly projected with a large inferior flare.	The facet joints of L1–L3 are located in the sagittal plane; the facets of L4 and L5 are frontally oriented.

The laterally projecting articular surfaces of the sacrum have an irregular shape that, when matched to the iliac facets, form the very stable SI joint. Its anterior and posterior surfaces are roughened to permit firm attachment of muscles acting on the femur and pelvis. Four pairs of foramina perforate the bone to permit the passage of the dorsal and ventral primary divisions of the nerves of the sacral plexus from their posterior origin into the pelvic cavity. Once adulthood is reached, the amount of movement at the sacroiliac joint is minimal, and it continues to decrease with age.[7]

Lumbarization occurs when the first sacral vertebra fails to unite with the remainder of the sacrum, forming a separate vertebra having characteristics similar to those of the lumbar spine, essentially becoming a sixth lumbar vertebra. **Sacralization**, on the other hand, occurs when the fifth lumbar vertebra becomes fused to the sacrum (Fig. 13-5). This may occur unilaterally or bilaterally, resulting in complete fusion of these segments. Except for radiographic diagnosis, these conditions are virtually undetectable and typically asymptomatic. However, patients may demonstrate decreased lumbar ROM.

The distal end of the spinal column is formed by the **coccyx**. Formed by the fusion of three or four rudimentary bony pieces, the coccyx provides an attachment site for some of the muscles of the pelvic floor and, sometimes, portions of the gluteus maximus.

Intervertebral Discs

Found in varying thicknesses between the cervical, thoracic, and lumbar vertebrae, intervertebral discs act to increase the total ROM available to the spinal column. The discs also serve as shock absorbers of longitudinal and rotational stresses placed on the column through compression. Each disc is formed by a tough, dense outer layer, the **annulus fibrosus**, surrounding a flexible inner layer, the **nucleus pulposus** (Fig. 13-6).

Twenty-three intervertebral discs are found along the spinal column. No disc is found between the skull and the first cervical vertebra (C0–C1) or between the first and second cervical vertebrae (C1–C2). Individual discs are referenced by the vertebrae between which they are found. For instance, the disc located between the fourth and fifth lumbar vertebrae is known as the L4–L5 intervertebral disc. The discs in the cervical spine are thinner than the discs in the lumbar spine, reflecting the differing load-bearing demands.

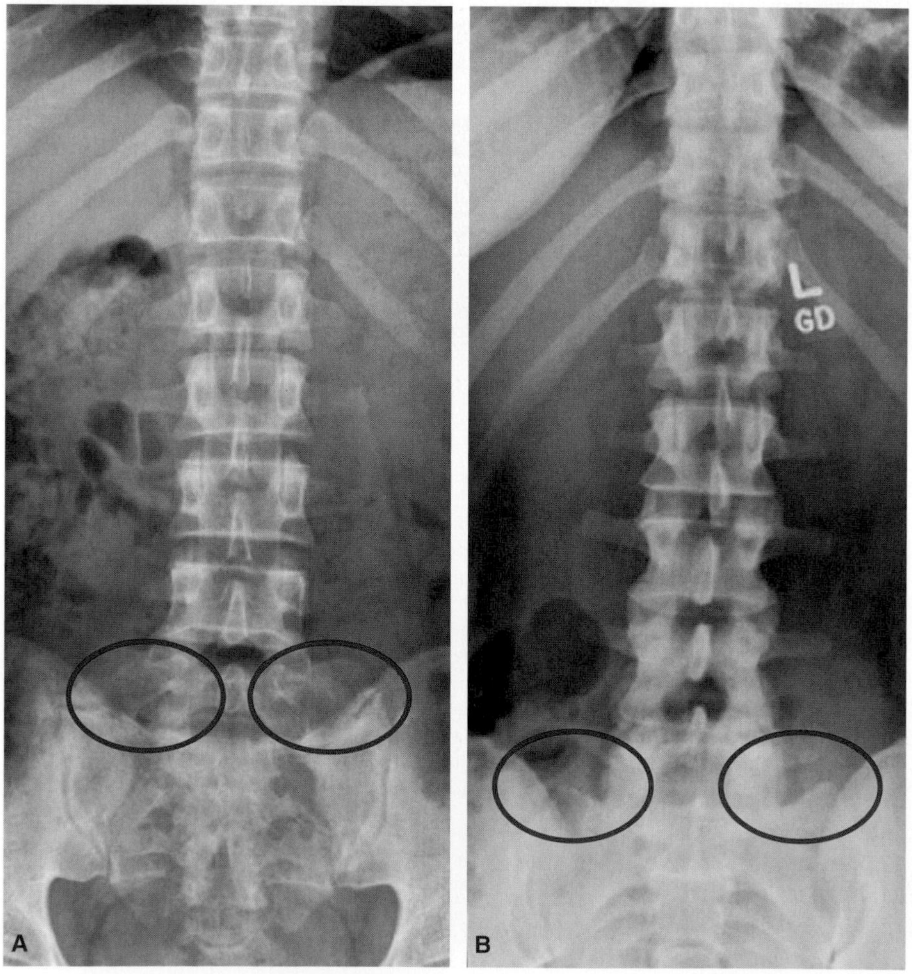

FIGURE 13-5 ■ Sacralized L5 vertebrae. (A) The L5 and S1 vertebra are fused together. (B) Radiograph of a normal L5/S1 junction. *(Image courtesy of Akira Murakami, MD. Boston Medical Center.)*

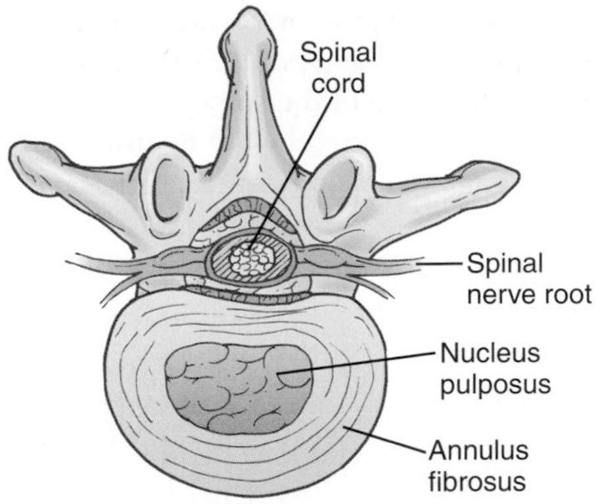

FIGURE 13-6 ■ Illustration of an intervertebral disc. The firm, outer annulus fibrosus surrounds the pliable nucleus pulposus.

The annulus fibrosus consists of multilayered fibers that cross from opposite directions, forming an X pattern. This arrangement leaves some portion of the disc taut regardless of the position of the vertebral column and increases the overall strength of the tissue. When viewed in cross section, the annulus fibrosus is thinner posteriorly than anteriorly. A vertebral endplate, an expanse of fibrocartilage from the annulus fibrosus, inserts on the vertebra above and below to secure the disc to the spinal column.

The core of the disc, the nucleus pulposus, is a highly elastic, semigelatinous substance that is 60% to 70% water.[8] The high water content makes the nucleus pulposus resistant to compression while allowing it to be deformable. During the course of the day, the nucleus pulposus becomes dehydrated from the body weight placed on it, compressing water out of its core. During sleep or other long periods of reclining, the compressive forces placed on the discs are eliminated, allowing the nucleus pulposus to become rehydrated. Physical activity such as running compresses the intervertebral discs between T7–L1 and L5–S1, resulting in a decreased ROM in the lumbar spine after activity.[9]

Permanent dehydration also occurs through the aging process. Until the age of approximately 40 years, the disc is fully hydrated. After this age, dehydration begins. By age 60, the discs have reached their maximum state of dehydration, resulting in decreased ROM and a slight narrowing of the intervertebral foramen.[6]

The annulus fibrosus and the posterior longitudinal ligament (PLL) are richly innervated by sensory nerves.[10] This nerve supply can account for much of the pain associated with disc degeneration or herniation. This type of pain is referred to as **discogenic pain**.

The amount of stress placed on the lumbar intervertebral discs is influenced by the position of the trunk. In the supine position, the disc is under a load of approximately 75 kg of pressure. When an individual stands up, the load increases to 100 kg. When sitting and leaning forward, the total load increases to 275 kg.[11] Lateral bending, flexion, lateral shear, and compression place the largest shear loads on the disc.[12]

Articulations, Ligamentous and Fascial Anatomy

The spinal column allows for three degrees of freedom of movement: (1) flexion and extension, (2) rotation, and (3) tilting, resulting in lateral bending. The accessory motions occurring at the facet joints allowing these physiologic motions to occur include (1) anterior and posterior glide, or flexion; (2) lateral glide, or extension; and (3) compression and distraction, or sidebending and rotation (Fig. 13-7). The articulation between each pair of vertebrae is formed by cartilaginous and synovial joints. The union between an intervertebral disc and the superior and inferior vertebrae forms the **cartilaginous joint**, and the facet joints represent the synovial articulations. The exception to this is the joint formed between the first and second cervical vertebrae. The end-range of motion is limited by the supporting ligaments (Table 13-2).

The motion at the spine occurs as an interdependent function of the interbody articulations and the facet joints. The *amount* of movement is largely determined by the size of the discs, while the facet joints largely influence the *direction* of movement.[7] The amount of movement between any two vertebrae is rather limited, but the sum of these motions provides a large amount of ROM for the spinal column as a whole. **Coupled motions** occur because of the varied orientations of the facet joints. For example, lateral flexion occurs concurrently with rotation and vice versa: neither is a pure, single-plane movement.

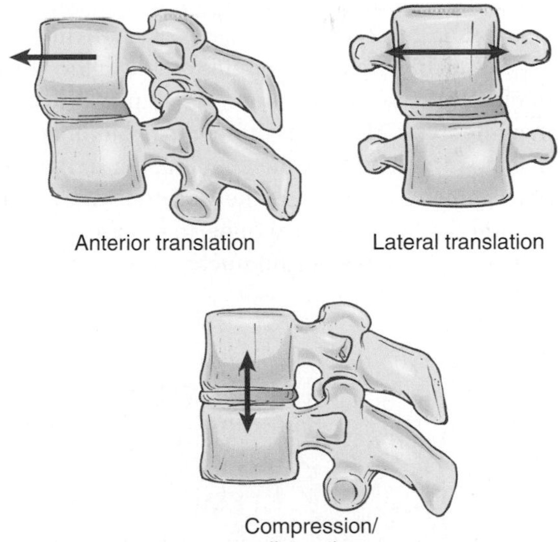

FIGURE 13-7 ■ Accessory vertebral motions. In addition to the cardinal spinal movements of flexion and extension, rotation, and lateral bending, the facet joints allow for anterior and posterior translation, lateral translation, and compression and distraction of contiguous vertebrae.

Cartilaginous joint A relatively immobile joint in which two bones are fused by cartilage

Coupled motion The concurrent and necessary association of a motion around one axis with a different motion around another axis

Table 13-2 Spinal Ligaments Stressed During the End-Range of Passive Range of Motion Assessment

Motion	Ligaments Stressed
Flexion	Posterior longitudinal ligament
	Supraspinous ligament (thoracic and lumbar spine)
	Interspinous ligament
	Ligamentum flavum
Extension	Anterior longitudinal ligament
Rotation	Interspinous ligament
	Ligamentum flavum
*Lateral Bending**	Interspinous ligament
	Ligamentum flavum

*Assessing these motions is usually inconclusive.

The entire length of the spinal column is reinforced by the **anterior and posterior longitudinal ligaments** (Fig. 13-8). The broader, thicker anterior longitudinal ligament (ALL) spans the length of the vertebral column from the occiput to the sacrum, attaching to both the vertebral bodies and the intervertebral discs. The fibrous arrangement of this ligament strengthens the anterior portion of the intervertebral discs and vertebrae, functioning to limit extension of the spine. The ALL is well developed in the lumbar spine.[7]

The PLL originates from the occiput as a thick structure but gradually thins as it progresses down the vertebral column. Lining the anterior portion of the vertebral canal, the PLL fans out and thickens as it passes over the intervertebral discs, attaching to their margins only to allow the passage of blood vessels. This ligament serves primarily to limit flexion of the spine. The PLL is thinner in the lumbar region.

Traversing the length of the spinal column, the **supraspinous ligament** attaches to the posterior apex of each spinous process. In the cervical spine, the supraspinous ligament becomes the **ligamentum nuchae**. Two ligaments are intrinsic to the adjoining vertebrae. Filling the space formed between the spinous processes, the **interspinous ligaments** limit flexion and rotation of the spine. The posterior margin of the vertebral canal is lined by the **ligamentum flavum**, a pair of elastic ligaments connecting the lamina of one vertebra to the lamina of the vertebra above it. The ligamentum flavum reinforces the facet joints, and its unusual elastic property assists the trunk in returning from flexion to the neutral position without getting pinched.

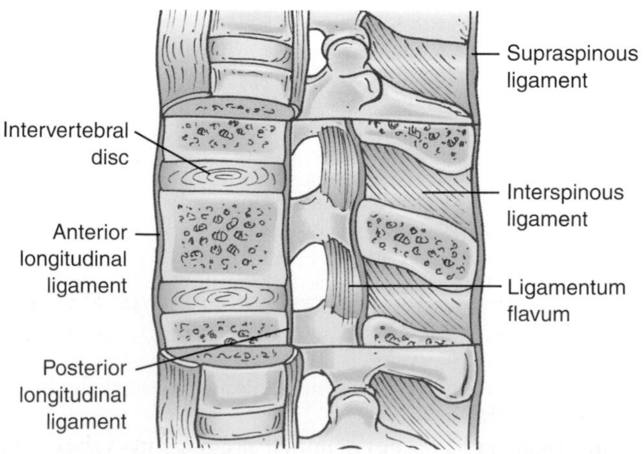

FIGURE 13-8 ■ Cross-sectional view of the ligaments of the vertebral column.

Thoracolumbar Fascia

Surrounding the middle and lower trunk, the thoracolumbar fascia helps transfer forces between the spine and the trunk and abdominal muscles.[7] The thoracolumbar fascia, comprised of anterior, middle, and posterior layers, separates muscles with different directions of pull, allowing them to slide past each other.[13] The fascia surrounds the erector spinae and multifidus muscles and serves as an origin for the latissimus dorsi, the gluteus maximus, the internal and external abdominal obliques, and the transversus abdominis. The fascia may be a source of pain in those with pathology in the lumbar region.

Sacroiliac Joint

A series of ligaments serve to bind the sacrum to the pelvis. The **interosseous sacroiliac** ligaments are formed by strong fibers spanning the anterior portion of the ilium and the posterior portion of the sacrum, filling the void behind the articular surfaces of these bones (Fig. 13-9). The anterior and posterior surfaces of the articulation are strengthened by the **dorsal and ventral sacroiliac ligaments**. The dorsal SI ligament is made of fibers that run transversely to join the ilium to the upper portion of the sacrum and vertical fibers connecting the lower sacrum to the posterior superior iliac spine (PSIS). Lining the anterior portion of the pelvic cavity, the ventral SI ligaments attach to the anterior portion of the sacrum. Two accessory ligaments assist in

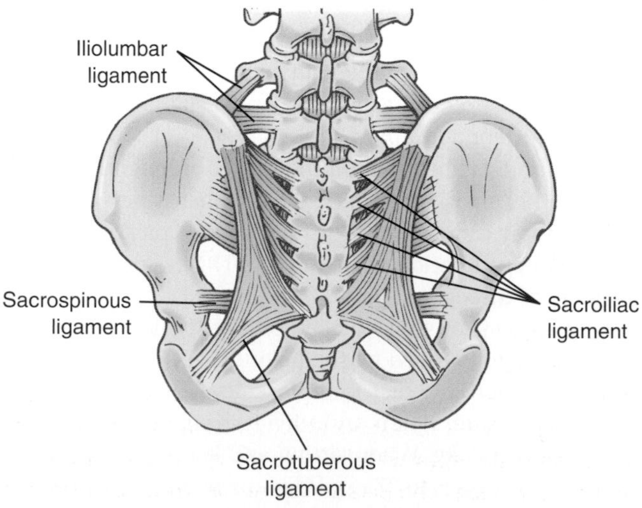

FIGURE 13-9 ■ Posterior sacroiliac ligaments. The strong ligamentous configuration of the sacroiliac joint permits only slight movement.

maintaining the stability of the SI joint. The **sacrotuberous ligament** arises from the ischial tuberosity to blend with the inferior fibers of the dorsal SI ligaments. Indirectly supporting the sacrum, the **sacrospinous ligament** originates from the sacrum's ischial spine and attaches to the coccyx.

The SI joints are more mobile in young individuals and become less mobile with age. In **postpartum** females, the stresses of athletics can injure the structurally weakened SI joints. During pregnancy and at the time of birth, the hormone relaxin is released into the mother's system. Relaxin increases the extensibility of the ligamentous structures in and around the birth canal.[14] These hormones affect the ligaments of the SI joint and pubic symphysis, resulting in increased pelvic motion and increasing the risk of pathology at the pelvic ring.

Neurological Anatomy

A nerve plexus is a network formed by a consecutive series of spinal nerves. These systems are formed by both **convergent** and **divergent** pathways, causing an intermixing of sensory and motor impulses. Although the root of a plexus may be supplied by one spinal nerve, the nerves exiting the plexus contain fibers from more than one spinal nerve root.

Thirty-one pairs of nerve roots exit the spinal column (Fig. 13-10). The thoracic and lumbar regions have a pair of nerves exiting below the corresponding vertebra (e.g., the T1 nerve root exits below the body of the first thoracic vertebra). There are 12 pairs of thoracic nerves and five pairs of lumbar nerves. Although there are seven cervical vertebrae, eight pairs of nerve roots exit in this area. The first seven cervical nerves exit above the vertebrae. The "odd" cervical nerve, C8, exits below the seventh cervical vertebra (between the seventh cervical and first thoracic vertebrae).

Several pairs of nerve plexuses are formed by the sacral, lumbar, thoracic, cervical, and cranial nerve roots. This chapter addresses the lumbar plexus and sacral plexus. The brachial plexus is described in Chapter 14, and the cranial plexus is presented in Chapter 20. Note that few resources agree on the actual nerve roots forming each plexus.

Lumbar Plexus

Formed by the 12th thoracic nerve root and the L1–L5 nerve roots, the lumbar plexus innervates the anterior and medial muscles of the thigh and the dermatomes of the medial leg and foot. The posterior branches of the L2, L3, and L4 nerve roots converge to form the **femoral nerve**, and their anterior branches merge to form the obturator nerve (Fig. 13-11).

Sacral Plexus

A portion of the L4 nerve root, the L5 nerve root, and the lumbosacral trunk courses downward to form the superior portion of the sacral plexus (Fig. 13-12). This plexus supplies the muscles of the buttocks and, via the sciatic nerve, innervates the muscles of the posterior upper leg and the entire lower leg. The sciatic nerve has three distinct sections: (1) the **tibial nerve**, formed by the anterior branches of the upper five nerve roots; (2) the **common peroneal nerve**, formed by the posterior branches of the upper four nerve roots; and (3) a slip of the tibial nerve that innervates the hamstring muscles.

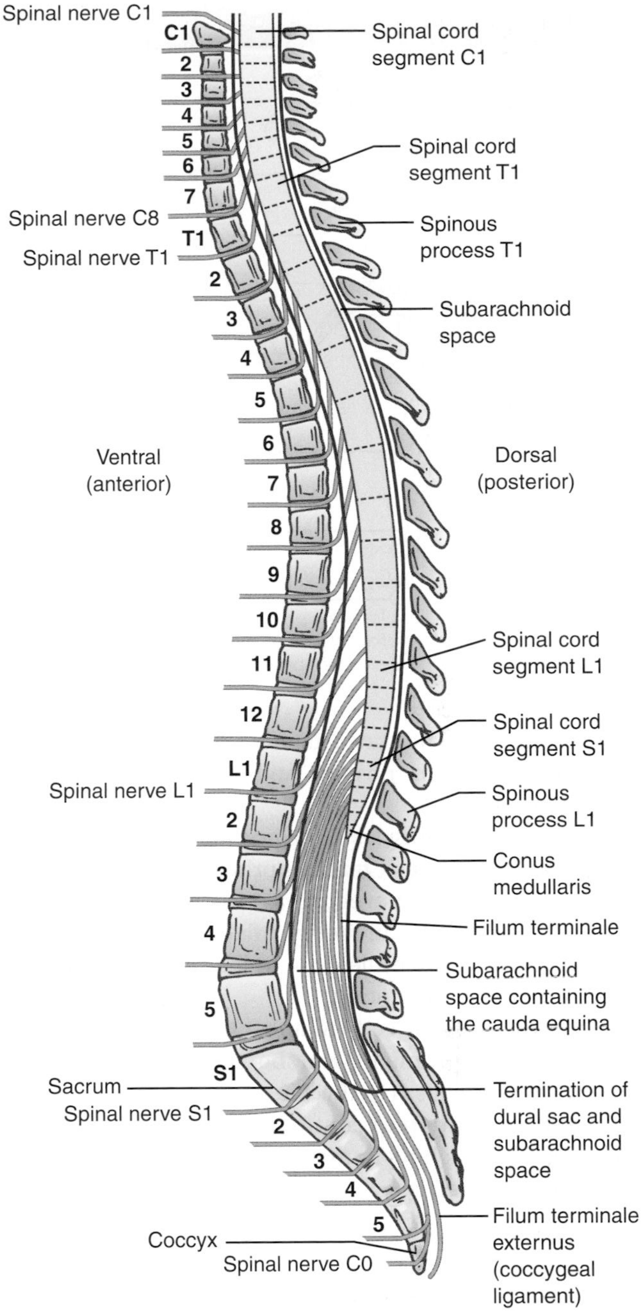

FIGURE 13-10 ■ Relationship between the vertebrae and spinal nerve roots.

Muscular Anatomy

A complex network of muscles acts on the spinal column. These muscles, interwoven with the fibers of other muscles,

---

Postpartum After childbirth
Convergent Two nerves combining together to form a single nerve
Divergent One nerve splitting to form two individual nerves

Table 13-4 Motions Produced by the Internal and External Oblique Muscles—cont'd

Muscle	Bilateral Contraction	Unilateral Contraction
External Oblique	Flexion of the lumbar spine Posterior pelvic rotation Compression of the abdominal viscera Depression of the thorax Assistance in respiration	Contralateral rotation of the trunk Ipsilateral lateral flexion of the trunk Rotation of the pelvis
Internal Oblique	Flexion of the lumbar spine Compression of the abdominal viscera Depression of the thorax Assistance in respiration	Ipsilateral rotation of the trunk Ipsilateral lateral flexion of the trunk

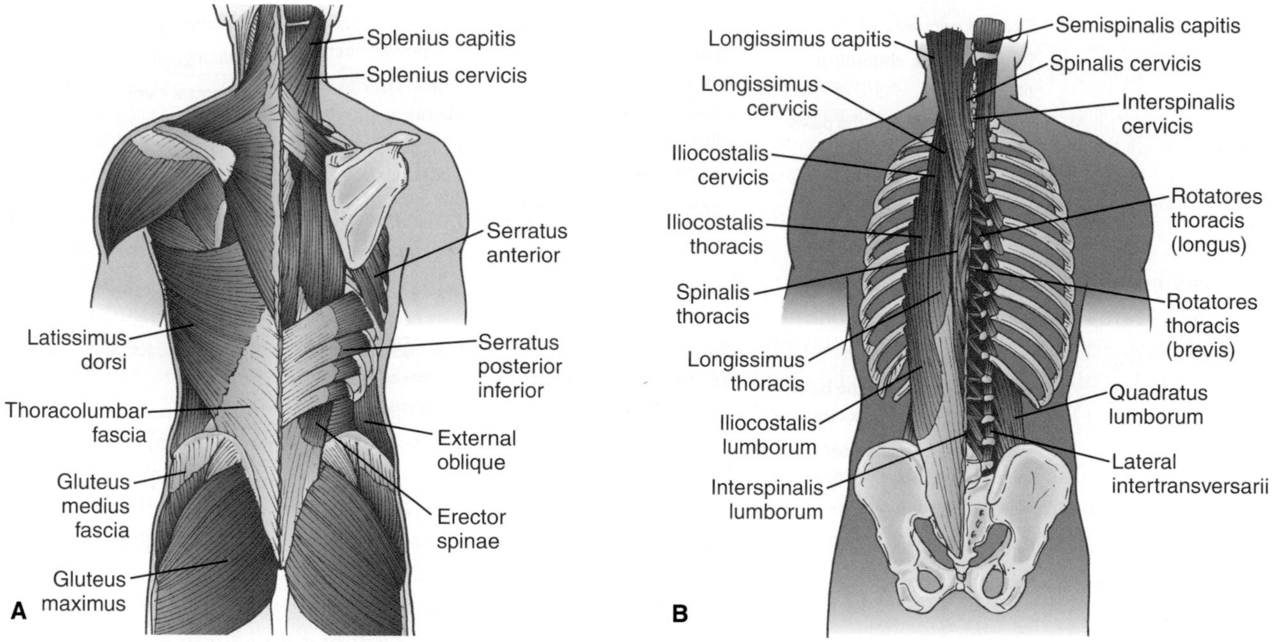

FIGURE 13-13 ■ Muscles of the spinal column: (A) superficial muscles, (B) deep muscles.

The deep intrinsic layer is collectively known as **transversospinal** muscles because the fibers run from one transverse process to the spinous process superior to them. Individually, this group is formed by the **semispinalis, multifidus**, and **rotatores** muscles. The multifidii muscles play an important role in the dynamic, segmental stabilization of the lumbar spine and are active in concert with the transversus abdominis during lifting and rotational maneuvers.[16,17] The multifidii show atrophy, weakness, and decreased activation in individuals who experience low back pain.[16,18]

The semispinalis muscle is divided into the thoracis, cervicis, and capitis segments. These muscles act primarily to contralaterally rotate the spinal column, especially above the lumbar level. They also contribute slightly to spinal extension and ipsilateral lateral flexion.

Clinical Examination of the Lumbar Spine

Because of the important role of the vertebrae in protecting the spinal cord and spinal nerve roots, vertebral injuries can have catastrophic results. In acute trauma, the primary role of the initial evaluation is to rule out the presence of trauma that has jeopardized, or can jeopardize, the integrity of the spinal cord or nerve roots. Chapter 20 discusses these evaluative procedures. The techniques presented in this chapter assume that significant vertebral fractures or dislocations have been ruled out.

Low back pain is multidimensional, with psychological and physiological influences. Identification of specific structures that are pathologically involved is difficult, leading to the widespread diagnosis of nonspecific low back

Table 13-5 Intrinsic Muscles Acting on the Spinal Column

Muscle	Action	Origin	Insertion	Innervation	Root
Iliocostalis Lumborum	Bilateral contraction: Extension of spinal column Unilateral contraction: Lateral bending of spinal column to the same side	Posterior aspect of the iliac crest	Inferior angles of ribs 6–12	Posterior primary divisions of the spinal nerves	Multiple roots, segmentally along the length of the muscle
Iliocostalis Thoracis	Bilateral contraction: Extension of spinal column Unilateral contraction: Lateral bending of spinal column to the same side	Ribs 6–12	Ribs 1–6 Transverse process of C7	Posterior primary divisions of the spinal nerves	Multiple roots, segmentally along the length of the muscle
Longissimus Thoracis	Bilateral contraction: Extension of spinal column Unilateral contraction: Lateral bending of spinal column	Common erector spinae tendon	Transverse process of T3–T21 Ribs 3–12	Posterior primary divisions of the spinal nerves	Multiple roots, segmentally along the length of the muscle
Spinalis Thoracis	Bilateral contraction: Extension of the spine Unilateral contraction: Lateral bending of the spine to the same side	Common erector spinae tendon	Spinous processes of upper thoracic spine	Posterior primary divisions of the spinal nerves	Multiple roots, segmentally along the length of the muscle
Semispinalis Thoracis	Bilateral contraction: Extension of thoracic and cervical spine Unilateral contraction: Rotation to the opposite side	Transverse process	Travel upwardly and medially to attach to a spinous process 5 or 8 vertebrae above the origin	Posterior primary divisions of the spinal nerves	Multiple roots, segmentally along the length of the muscle
Multifidus (or multifidii)	Bilateral contraction Stabilization of vertebral column Unilateral contraction: Rotation of spine to the opposite side	Lumbar region • Superior aspect of sacrum • Thoracic region • Transverse processes • Cervical region • Articular processes	Spinous process	Posterior primary divisions of the spinal nerves	Multiple roots, segmentally along the length of the muscle
Quadratus lumborum		Inferior portion of the 12th rib Transverse process of L1-L4	Iliac crest Iliolumbar ligament	Posterior primary divisions of the spinal nerves	T12, L1-L4
Rotatores	Bilateral contraction: Extension of spine Stabilization of vertebral column Unilateral contraction: Rotation of spine	Transverse process	Spinous process of the vertebra immediately above the origin	Posterior primary divisions of the spinal nerves	Multiple roots, segmentally along the length of the muscle

pain. Many spinal pain syndromes are associated with or complicated by improper foot mechanics, muscular tightness of the lower extremity, and imbalances of the pelvic and abdominal muscles (see Chapter 6).

History

Pain produced during activities of daily living (ADLs) provides valuable information about the cause of the pain and other activities that may reproduce or decrease the pain (refer to Table 13-6). These patient-described activities serve as the foundation for the functional assessment portion of the exam. Pain that occurs during certain times of the day can indicate a postural position that irritates the involved nerve root (or roots) or other soft tissue structures.

Past Medical History

- **History of spinal injury:** Any pertinent history that may lead to structural degeneration or predispose the

Examination Map

HISTORY

Past Medical History

Mental health status

History of the Present Condition

Location of pain

Radicular symptoms

Onset and severity of symptoms

FUNCTIONAL ASSESSMENT

Gait Observation

General movement

Posture

INSPECTION

Gait

Movement

Posture

General Inspection

Frontal curvature

Sagittal curvature

Skin markings

Inspection of the Lumbar Spine

Lordotic curve

Standing posture

Erector muscle tone

Faun's beard

PALPATION

Palpation of the Lumbar Spine

Spinous processes

- Step-off deformity

Paravertebral muscles

Palpation of the Sacrum and Pelvis

Median sacral crests

Iliac crests

Posterior superior iliac spine

Gluteals

Ischial tuberosity

Greater trochanter

Sciatic nerve

Pubic symphysis

JOINT AND MUSCLE FUNCTION ASSESSMENT

Goniometry

Flexion

Extension

Lateral bending

Rotation

Active Range of Motion

Flexion

Extension

Lateral bending

Rotation

Manual Muscle Tests

Flexion

Extension

Rotation

Pelvic elevation

Passive Range of Motion

Flexion

Extension

Rotation

Side gliding

JOINT STABILITY TESTS

Joint Play Assessment

Spring test

SELECTIVE TISSUE TESTS

Test for Nerve Root Impingement

Valsalva

Milgram

Kernig

Straight leg raise

Well straight leg raise

Slump test

Quadrant test

NEUROLOGICAL EXAMINATION

Lower quarter screen

REGION-SPECIFIC PATHOLOGIES AND RELATED SELECTIVE TISSUE TESTS

Spinal Stenosis

Intervertebral Disc Lesions

Femoral nerve stretch test

Tension sign

Segmental Instability

Erector spinae tear

Facet joint dysfunction

Spondylopathies

Spondylolysis

Spondylolisthesis

- Single-leg stance test

Sacroiliac Dysfunction

FABER sign

Patrick's test

Gaenslen's test

Long sit test

Table 13-6 Ramifications of Spinal Pain Exhibited During the Activities of Daily Living

Activity	Ramifications
Bending	Pain may be initially worsened with flexion exercises.
Sitting	Pain may be initially worsened with flexion exercises.
Rising From Sitting	This motion causes changes in the forces within the disc. Sharp pain suggests derangement of the disc.
Standing	The spine is placed in extension. Pain may be initially experienced with extension exercises.
Walking	The amount of spinal extension increases as the speed of gait increases.
Lying Prone	The spine is placed in or near full extension.
Lying Supine	When lying supine on a hard surface, the amount of extension is maintained. When lying on a soft surface, the spine falls into flexion.

patient to chronic problems is important. The current symptoms may be the result of the formation of scar tissue that is impinging or restricting other structures. Following an episode of acute low back pain, approximately 25% of people will experience a recurring episode.[19] Low back pain as an adolescent is a significant predictor of low back pain as an adult.[20]

- **General health and lifestyle:** Infection of the kidney, urinary tract, or reproductive organs may cause back pain. A history of cancer is a red flag for a potential recurrence. Obesity and smoking both increase the risk of developing low back pain.[3]
- **Occupation:** While certain repetitive tasks may put the low back at risk, systematic review findings have not identified that occupations that require walking, standing, lifting, sitting, or carrying independently cause back pain.[3] Understanding the impact of symptoms on the individual's ability to work is important.

- **Changes in activity:** Changes in the level, intensity, or duration of activity or changes in running surfaces, footwear, sleeping mattress, and so on can redistribute the forces transmitted to the spinal column. (Refer to Chapters 6 and 8 for more information on how these changes can affect posture and cause pain.)
- **Mental health status:** The association between mental health status and onset, chronicity, and disability associated with low back pain has been studied extensively. Emotional distress, negative expectation about recovery, fear-avoidance behaviors, and depressed moods are all associated with an increased risk, prolonged duration, and increased severity of low back pain.[20-24]

✻ Practical Evidence

Multidimensional in nature, the pain and disability associated with low back pain relates to psychological variables such as depression, anxiety, and distress.[20] Depression coupled with low back pain is associated with a worse outcome than low back pain alone. A positive response to either or both of the questions (1) "During the past month, have you often been bothered by feeling down, depressed, or hopeless?" or (2) "During the past month, have you often been bothered by little interest or pleasure in doing things?" warrants referral of the patient for evaluation for depression.[25]

History of the Present Condition

- **Location of the pain and referred or radicular symptoms:** Pain radiating into the extremity or peripheral paresthesia or numbness is the result of impingement or pressure on the spinal cord itself, a nerve root exiting the intervertebral foramen, or dural irritation proximal to the site of pain. In addition, leg or buttock pain may be referred from structures in the low back and not related to nerve root compression. Unlike pain in other anatomical areas, the exact location and underlying cause of low back pain are often ambiguous.[26] Sacroiliac pathology usually causes pain around the PSIS of the affected side or radiating into the hip and groin. Spasm of the piriformis muscle can cause symptoms of sciatic nerve dysfunction. Having the patient complete a pain drawing by placing symbols on the body representing pain locations may provide insight as to pathology. For example, the patient might indicate symptoms along a dermatomal distribution, describing impingement of a specific nerve. Pain in the buttock and pelvis area but not in the lumbar region is consistent with sacroiliac joint pathology.[27]
- **Onset of the pain:** The patient's description of the onset of the pain, such as a description of acute, chronic, or insidious onset of pain, along with other symptoms is important. Although patients may describe a single incident that acutely initiated the pain, the injury often results from an accumulation of repetitive stresses and macrotrauma developed during the episode described.
- **Severity of pain:** Several reliable pain severity scales can be used to quantify the patient's pain (see Box 1-3).
- **Mechanism of injury:** Any known mechanism of injury (e.g., flexion, extension, lateral bending, or rotation) can be used to possibly identify the involved structures. A direct blow to the lumbar or thoracic area may cause a contusion of the involved structures, the kidneys, or other internal organs. Sports (e.g., gymnastics, blocking in football, cheerleading) in which the spine is regularly hyperextended place increased compressive stress on the pars interarticularis and other posterior spinal structures. Offensive linemen in football place enormous compressive and shear forces on the lumbar spine and therefore are particularly predisposed to injury.[28] Frequently, patients are unable to identify a specific episode of injury.
- **Consistency of the pain:** The frequency and consistency of the patient's pain can serve as an indication of the type of pathology that is involved.
    - **Constant pain:** Pain that is unyielding and does not increase or subside based on the position of the patient's spine is indicative of chemically induced pain, such as that resulting from inflammation of the dural sheath. Unremitting pain or pain that cannot be modified by change of position can also be a signal of another space-occupying lesion such as a tumor and warrants referral.
    - **Intermittent pain:** Symptoms that increase or decrease based on the position of the spine (e.g., flexion, extension, lateral bending) indicate pain of a mechanical origin. Placing the body in one position may cause compression or stretching of the tissues. Likewise, relief (or a decrease in symptoms) can be obtained by moving the spine into a specific position that lessens the pressure on the involved structure, a posture that the patient will try to maintain.
- **Bowel or bladder control:** Reports of changes in bowel or bladder control, **incontinence**, urinary retention, or slow-healing wounds may indicate central stenosis, lower nerve root lesions (e.g., cauda equina syndrome) or spinal cord injury warranting immediate referral to a physician.[29]
- **Disability associated with low back pain:** Many region-specific measures, such as the Oswestry Disability Index (ODI), attempt to measure perceived disability attributed to low back pain. Given the nonspecific nature of low back pain and the difficulty in identifying a specific structure as the source of pain, these measures of the multiple facets of disability are particularly helpful. The ODI has demonstrated reliability and detects clinically significant changes in patient-reported disability in the general adult population; however, it has not been validated in an athletic population (see p. 475).[30,31]

Incontinence A loss of bowel or bladder control

- **Sleeping pattern:** Disrupted sleep or difficulty falling asleep is commonly associated with low back pain. Question the patient regarding the most comfortable sleeping position: lying on the stomach positions the trunk in extension while lying supine causes the spine to assume a relatively flexed position.

Nonorganic Origin of Pain

Nonorganic contributors to low back pain, where no structural or physiological source can be identified, can impact the course of treatment. **Waddell signs** are physical findings such as pain with axial loading, widespread tenderness, and an excessive show of emotion that may be present in patients with greater behavioral influences on their pain. Patients who display Waddell signs have worse outcomes than patients who do not.[32] Unlike in malingering patients, nonorganic low back pain is not generally associated with potential secondary gain such as receiving workman's compensation or validation of not playing in the case of an athlete.[33]

By their very nature, lumbopelvic disorders are difficult to evaluate objectively, forcing the clinician to rely on subjective information gained from the history of the condition. On occasion, a person may intentionally describe or produce symptoms for secondary gain, such as prolonging the absence from work or activity. Malingering is extremely difficult to diagnose and the label of "malingerer" should be used only in the presence of conclusive evidence. Warning signs of malingering include persistent noncompliance, inconsistency between the physical exam and stated symptoms, and referral from an insurance company or attorney.[34] The **Hoover test** (Selective Tissue Test 13-1) is a classic procedure used to determine whether the individual is malingering during the performance of functional and selective tissue tests.[35-37]

Functional Assessment

Observing the patient performing activities or assuming positions that aggravate or alleviate the symptoms provides compelling evidence about the involved structures and possible treatment strategies. Difficulty in standing and reaching may reflect a reluctance to extend the spine. A preference for standing (as opposed to sitting) implicates lumbar flexion as a causative factor (Table 13-6).

- **Gait observation:** Note the patient's gait. Spinal pain may grossly influence walking and running gait. Common gait deviations resulting from spinal pain include a slouched, shuffling, or shortened gait. Chapter 7 provides detailed discussion regarding gait analysis. In addition, a patient's unwillingness to move the body as a whole after injury to the spinal region may become evident during walking.
- **General movement and posture:** Observe the patient for poor postural movement habits such as improper standing or sitting postures and improper lifting mechanics (e.g., bending instead of squatting to lift objects). When the patient is standing, observe for the **mannequin posture**, where the involved-side leg is flexed at the hip and knee with the pelvis tilted to the involved side. This posture is associated with a disc herniation.[38]

Inspection

A general inspection of the entire spinal column is necessary to determine the alignment in the sagittal and frontal planes. The muscles of the spinal column and torso require inspection to determine the presence of spasm or atrophy, each indicating a possible irritation of one or more spinal nerve roots. Last, finite inspection at the level of each spinal segment may provide an indication of a malalignment of one vertebra relative to the ones above and below it. The patient's general posture, as described in Chapter 6, also must be assessed.

General Inspection

- **Frontal curvature:** Inspect the alignment of the lumbar, thoracic, and cervical vertebrae with the patient standing. Normally, this alignment should be relatively straight. Lateral curvature of the spinal column, scoliosis, generally afflicts the thoracic or lumbar spine (or both) and is visible in the frontal plane (Fig. 13-14). Most scoliosis in children is idiopathic, although it may be congenital or representative of neuromuscular dysfunction or connective-tissue diseases. Routine scoliosis screening often includes observing the shoulders and spine with the individual standing and while forward flexed (Selective Tissue Test 13-2); however, this technique is associated with a high rate of false positives given that trunk asymmetry is common in adolescents.[39] In those with functional scoliosis, a curve observed in standing will disappear with forward flexion. With structural scoliosis, the curve remains in both positions. Adolescents who have not reached skeletal maturity and are diagnosed with scoliosis require monitoring on a regular basis for increases in the amount of curvature. Individuals who are suspected of having previously undiagnosed scoliosis need to be referred to a physician for further evaluation, although scoliosis is a common finding in adults who do not suffer any back pain.[39]

* Practical Evidence

With the exception of general back pain and cosmetic concerns, patients with late-onset idiopathic scoliosis who do not receive treatment fair as well as those patients who do receive treatment.[40]

- **Sagittal curvature:** From the side, observe the patient's cervical, thoracic, lumbar, and sacral curvature. Changes in any of these curves may be cause the symptoms or result from pathology. In either event, these changes produce abnormal stresses on spinal structures, leading to pain and dysfunction. Muscular spasm, as seen in patients with acute injuries, usually serves to flatten these curves.
- **Skin markings:** Note the presence of any darkened areas of skin pigmentation. **Café-au-lait spots** may

be normally occurring skin discolorations or may represent collagen disease or **neurofibromatosis**.[41,42]

Inspection of the Lumbar Spine

- **Lordotic curve:** Note the patient's lumbar lordotic curve. The lordotic curve can be either accentuated or reduced in patients suffering from low back pain or trauma. Reduction of the lordotic curve may be attributed to acute pain, muscle spasm, or tightness of the hamstring muscle group. Increased lordosis may be traced to tightness in the hip flexor muscle groups or weakness in the abdominal musculature.
- **Standing posture:** While observing the patient from behind, look for a lateral shift in the trunk and pelvis, indicating possible impingement of a nerve root. In this case, the patient instinctively shifts the upper trunk to reduce the amount of pressure on the nerve (Fig. 13-15).

Neurofibromatosis Increased cell growth of neural tissues; normally a benign condition; pain possible secondary to pressure on the local nerves

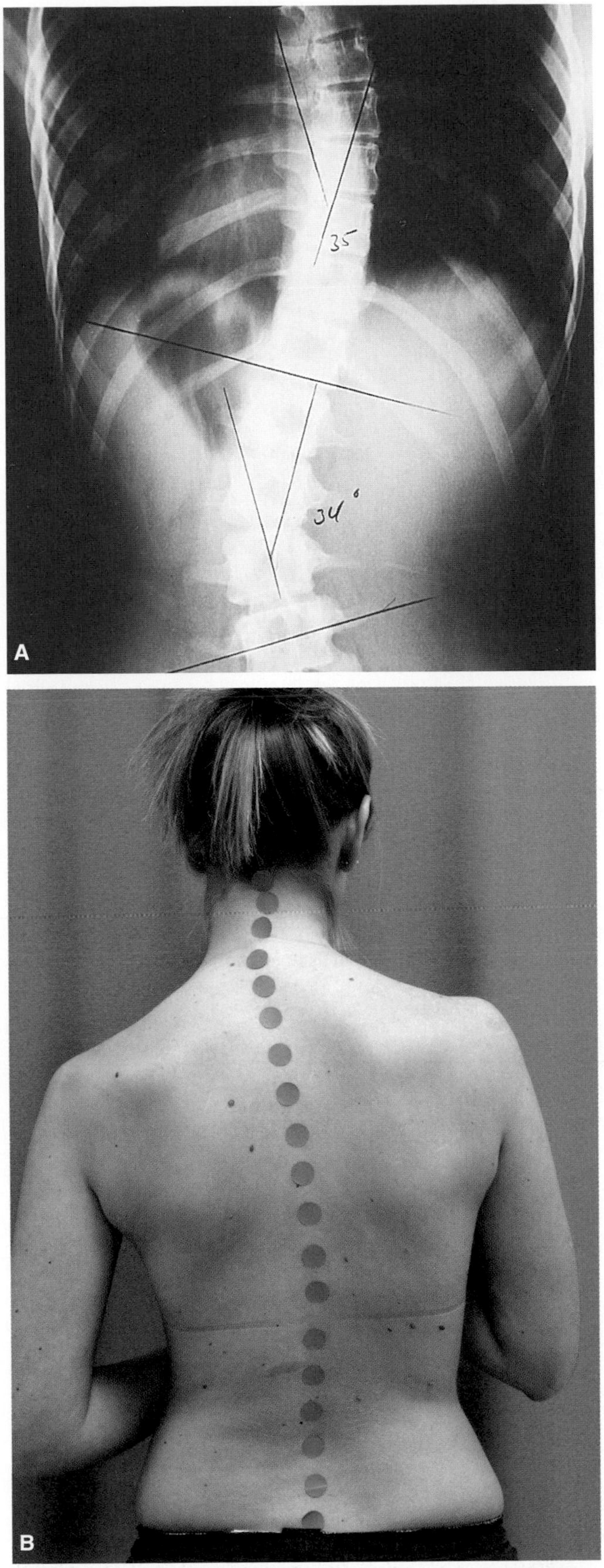

FIGURE 13-14 ■ Scoliosis, lateral bending of the spinal column in the frontal plane. (A) A radiograph of moderate to severe scoliosis. (B) Dots have been placed over the spinous processes.

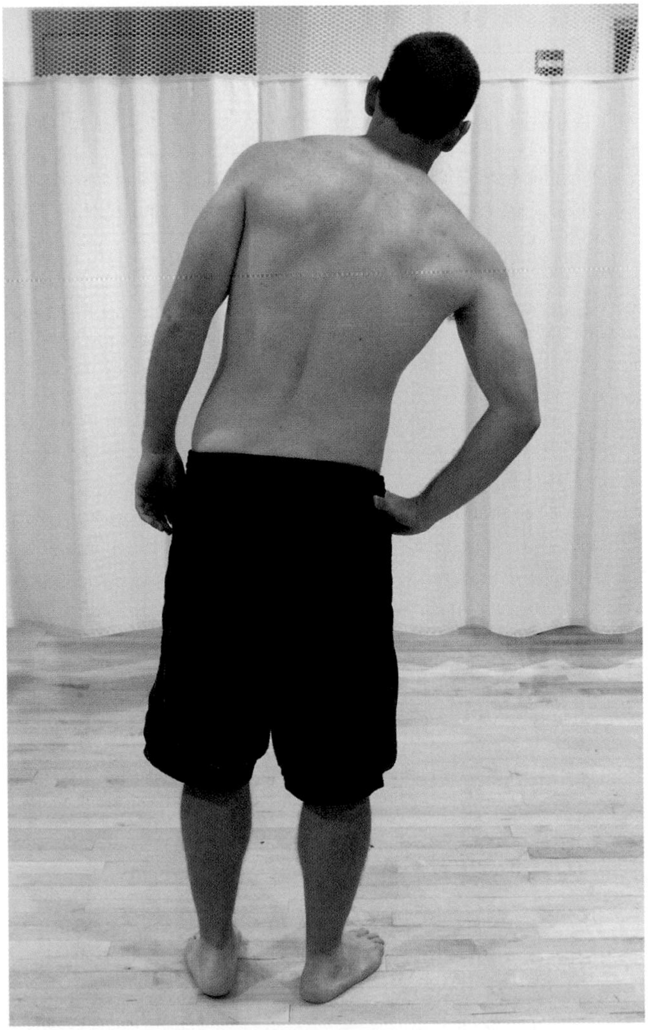

FIGURE 13-15 ■ Compensatory posture for nerve root impingement. The patient will naturally shift the body to lessen the pressure on the nerve root. The posture is categorized based on the affected side of the patient's body. This would be a right compensatory posture.

Selective Tissue Test 13-1
Hoover Test

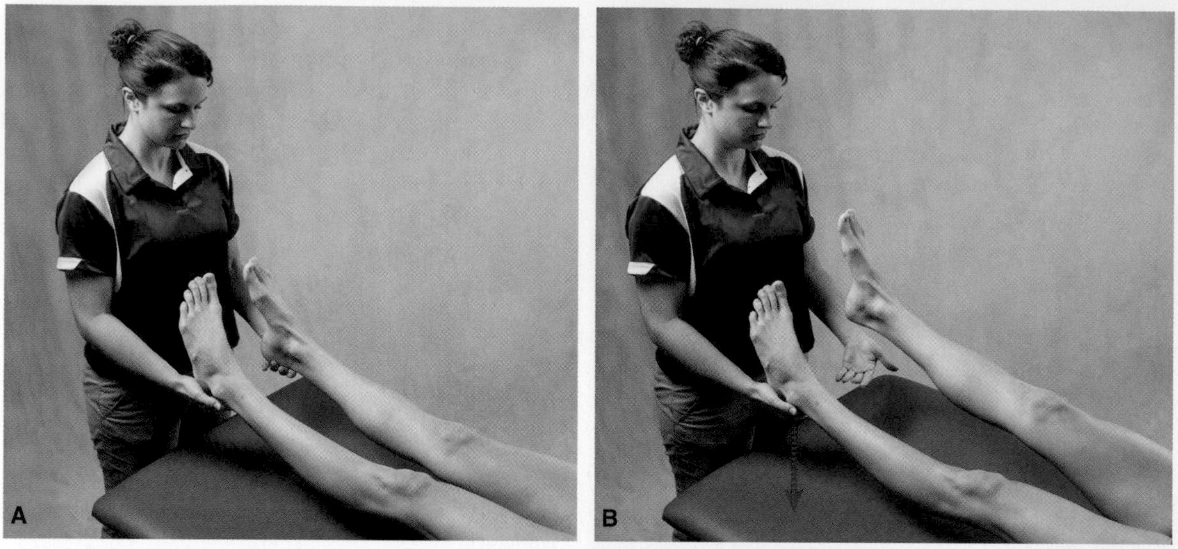

The Hoover Test is used to identify if a patient is actually exerting effort during the testing procedure. A positive test suggests that the patient is malingering.

Patient Position	Supine
Position of Examiner	At the feet of the patient with the evaluator's hands cupping the calcaneus of each leg (A).
Evaluative Procedure	The patient attempts an active straight leg raise (SLR) on the involved side.
Positive Test	The patient does not attempt to lift the leg, and the examiner does not sense pressure from the uninvolved leg pressing down on the hand as should instinctively happen (B).
Implications	The patient is not attempting to perform the test (i.e., malingering).
Comments	Although the contemporary clinical use of the Hoover Test is to identify patients who may be malingering, its original purpose was to diagnose mild cases of hemiparesis. Patients with unilateral weakness would yield a positive test but would not be malingering.[37]
Evidence	Absent or inconclusive in the literature

The shift is named for the direction the upper trunk moves relative to the patient.

- **Erector muscle tone:** Inspect the paraspinal muscles for equal tone. A unilaterally hypertrophied or atrophied muscle could indicate instability or poor or abnormal posture.
- **Faun's beard:** Observe the sacrum and lower lumbar spine for a tuft of hair, **Faun's beard**, possibly indicating **spina bifida occulta.**

PALPATION

Table 13-7 presents a list of landmarks used to orient the location of specific spinal structures. The ease of palpation of these structures depends on the patient's body

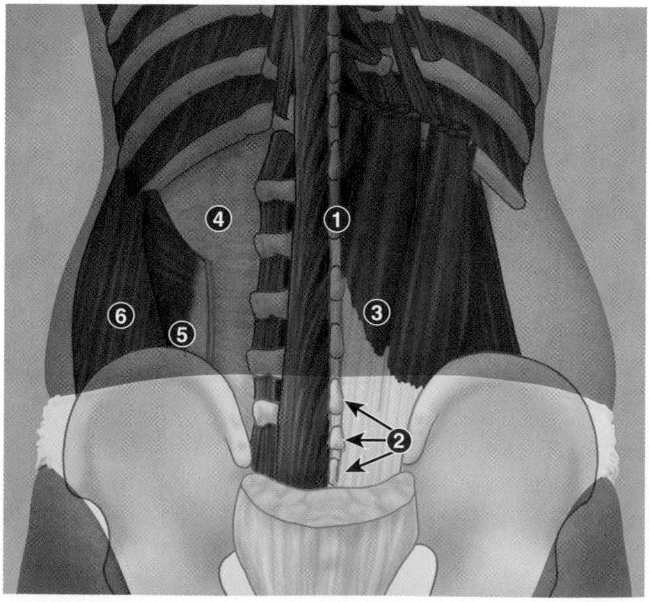

Palpation of the Lumbar Spine

Spina bifida occulta Incomplete closure of the spinal vertebrae

Selective Tissue Test 13-2
Test for Scoliosis (Adams Forward Bend Test)

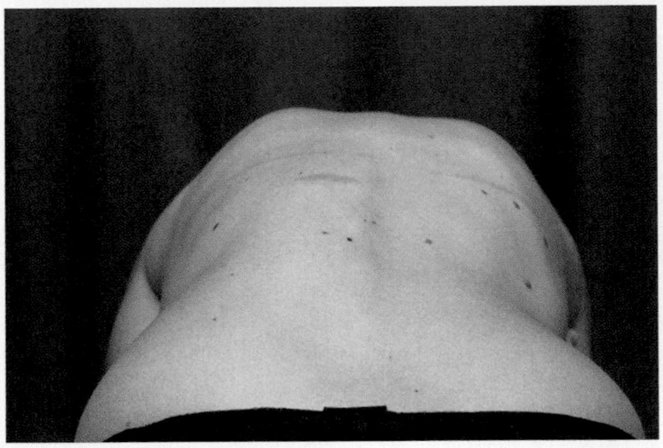

Posterior view of the spinal column while the patient flexes the spine; note the presence of a hump over the left thoracic spine, suggesting scoliosis.

Patient Position	Standing with hands held in front with the arms straight
Position of Examiner	Seated in front of or behind the patient
Evaluative Procedure	The patient bends forward, sliding the hands down the front of each leg.
Positive Test	An asymmetrical hump is observed along the lateral aspect of the thoracolumbar spine and rib cage.
Implications	If scoliosis is present but disappears during flexion, then functional scoliosis is suggested. Scoliosis that is present while the patient is standing upright and while forwardly flexed indicates structural scoliosis. A leg-length discrepancy may create a false positive. Positive findings in those who are skeletally immature warrant referral to a physician for further evaluation.

Evidence

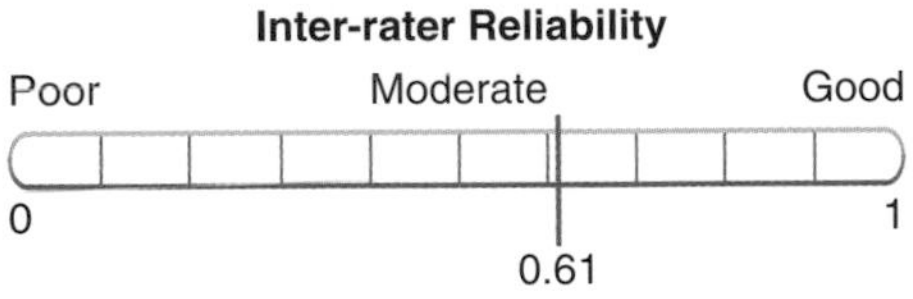

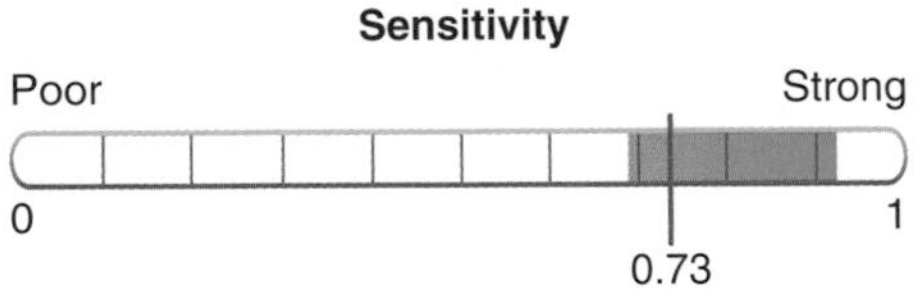

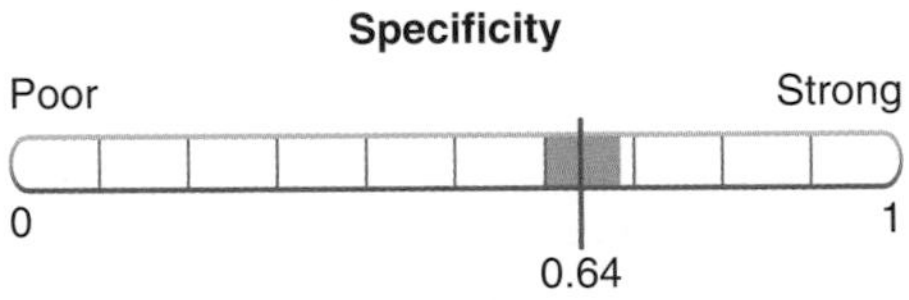

LR+: 2.28–2.29–2.30

LR−: 0.13–0.27–0.40

Table 13-7 Bony Lumbar Landmarks During Palpation	
Structure	Landmark
Lumbar Spinal Bodies	Upper portion of the spinous processes overlying the inferior half of the same vertebra
L3 Vertebra	In normal body build, posterior from the umbilicus
L4 Vertebra	Level with the iliac crest
L5 Vertebra	Typically demarcated by bilateral dimples, but variable from person to person
S2	At the level of the posterior superior iliac spine

mass. Identification of landmarks, including vertebral level (e.g., L4 or L5) has poor interrater reliability, making the validity of techniques that require known landmarks questionable from the start.[43]

Palpation of the Lumbar Spine

1 Spinous processes: Palpate the spinous processes along the entire length of the lumbar spine, with the L4 process at approximately the same level as the iliac crests. The L5 spinous process is relatively smaller and rounder than the other spinous processes and normally disappears when the hip is passively extended.

2 **Step-off deformity:** During palpation of the lumbar spinous process, note whether one process is located more anteriorly than the one below it. **Step-off deformities** indicate **spondylolisthesis**, which most commonly occurs between the L4 and L5 or L5 and S1 vertebrae.

3 **Paravertebral muscles:** From the thoracic spine, continue to palpate the length of the erector spinae muscles along the lumbar spine. Tightness of these muscles increases the amount of lordosis in the lumbar spine.

4 **Latissimus dorsi:** Palpate the large **latissimus dorsi** muscles from their origin at the thoracolumbar fascia along their length through the axilla and terminating on the humerus.

5-6 **Oblique muscles:** A portion of the (5) **internal oblique** muscle can be palpated from its insertion on the medial iliac crest. Moving laterally, palpate the (6) **external oblique** as it arises from the lateral portion of the iliac crests.

Palpation of the Sacrum and Pelvis

1 **Median sacral crests:** Attempt to palpate the fused remnants of the sacral spinous processes from below the L5 vertebra to the midportion of the gluteal crease.

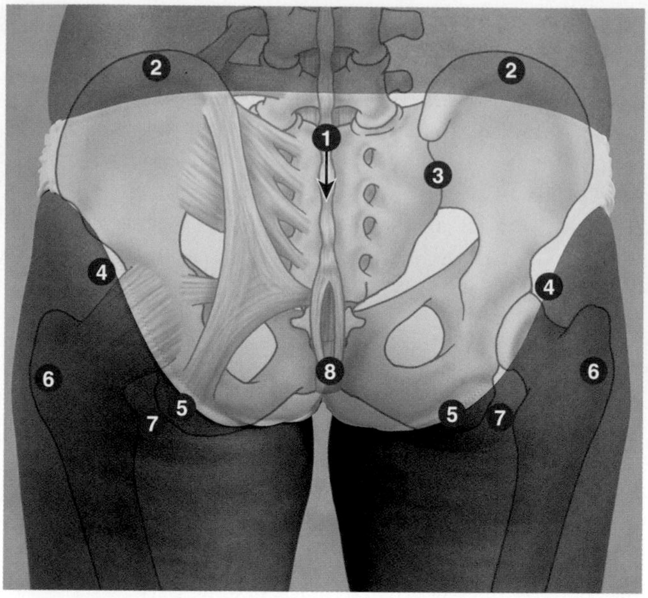

Palpation of the Sacrum and Pelvis

2 **Iliac crests:** Palpate laterally from the PSIS to find the **iliac crests** and anteriorly to locate the anterior superior iliac spine (ASIS) and check for level and symmetry (see Fig. 3.9).

3 **Posterior superior iliac spine:** Locate the **PSIS** near the inferior portion of the gluteal dimples (Fig. 13-16). Under normal circumstances, these bony landmarks are palpable and align at the same level (see Fig. 6-12). Tenderness may indicate sacroiliac pathology.

4 **Gluteals:** Posteriorly, locate the gluteus maximus, the most prominent muscle mass. From this point, palpate laterally to identify the gluteus medius as it emerges from beneath the iliac crest. Atrophy of the gluteals can indicate nerve pathology.

5 **Ischial tuberosity:** Locate the **ischial tuberosity** at the proximal aspect of the hamstrings. The ischial tuberosity

Spondylolisthesis The forward slippage of a vertebra on the one below it

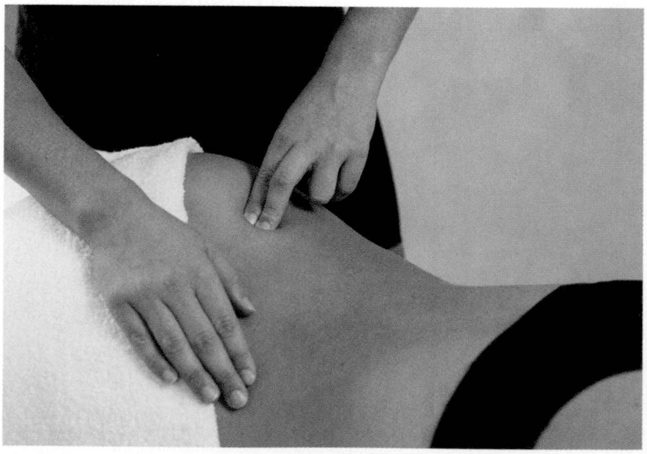

FIGURE 13-16 ■ Location of the posterior superior iliac spine.

may become irritated secondary to proximal hamstring tears, ischial bursitis, or contusive forces.

6 **Greater trochanter:** Palpate the lateral femur to locate the **greater trochanter**. During active or passive internal and external hip rotation, the greater trochanter can be felt as it rolls beneath the fingers. Localized pain may be caused by inflammation of the gluteus medius attachment or by greater trochanteric bursitis or referred spinal pain.

7 **Sciatic nerve:** Palpate the **sciatic nerve** by placing the thumb on the ischial tuberosity and the middle finger on the PSIS. The second finger will fall into the sciatic notch. The nerve is at its most superficial point as it passes by the ischial tuberosity. Tenderness on one tuberosity and not on the other may indicate sciatic nerve inflammation.

8 **Pubic symphysis (anterior):** Locate the **symphysis pubis** on the anterior portion of the pelvis, just superior to the genitalia at the midline of the body. This structure may become irritated secondary to a hard jarring injury such as a fall. Use good communication and appropriate draping when palpating this area.

Joint and Muscle Function Assessment

Although various forms of goniometers and protractors are available to assess the ROM available in the spine, in actual practice, gross observation of the ROM is typically used, and the grade is expressed as a percentage of the total possible normal ROM. Similar to what occurs with the body's other joints, spinal ROM is graded quantitatively as well as qualitatively, noting any pain produced during or at the end of the movement. ROM fluctuates throughout the day, even in those with chronic low back pain. Reliability will be improved if measurements are taken at the same time each day.[44]

A set of 10 repetitions of any particular motion can be used to determine the effect of repeated movement on the quantity and location of pain. In general, repeated movements in one direction that result in pain radiating distally are to be avoided during the rehabilitation program.

The total motion produced by the hips and the thoracic and lumbar spines is difficult to isolate into its individual segments. In addition, it is difficult to isolate passive motion in a gravity-dependent position, so active and passive ROM testing often occurs concurrently when the techniques described in the Active Range of Motion section are used.

Tape measures, inclinometers, goniometers, and specially designed devices have been used to quantify spinal ROM measurement. Goniometry 13-1 describes the use of an inclinometer to assess trunk flexion and extension. Goniometry 13-2 describes the use of an inclinometer to quantify lateral bending and rotation.

Active Range of Motion

Active range of motion (AROM) is assessed with the patient standing. ROM assessment, as described in this section, is contraindicated for patients with acute injuries until the possibility of a vertebral fracture or dislocation has been ruled out.

- **Flexion and extension:** While the patient is flexing and returning to a neutral position, note any pain, catches, or deviations from a straight sagittal plane movement or pushing on the anterior thighs to extend the trunk. Any of these findings may indicate instability or decreased motor control.[24] Gravity-assisted flexion is a more accurate indication of available motion than trunk flexion from the **hook-lying position**. Testing in the hook-lying position is the initial step to assess the strength of the abdominal muscles as they overcome the weight of the trunk. To avoid motion initiating at the hips and ensure that spinal flexion is being observed, forward flexion is begun by bending the patient's chin to the chest and then rolling the flexion down the vertebral column until hip flexion is seen or felt (Fig. 13-17).

Assess extension with the patient standing, feet shoulder-width apart and hands on the hips. The end-range occurs when the hips begin to extend (see Fig. 13-17).

- **Lateral bending:** The patient stands with the feet shoulder-width apart and the hand opposite the direction of the movement resting on the ilium. The patient then bends the trunk laterally, attempting to touch the fingertips to the ground as the clinician stabilizes the pelvis to prevent lateral tilt. The distance between the ground and the fingertips can be compared bilaterally, measured, and recorded (Fig. 13-18).
- **Rotation:** Because of the orientation of the facet joints, there is limited rotation in the lumbar spine. Most motion occurs in the thoracic and cervical spines (Chapter 14).

Manual Muscle Tests

Because of their essential function in trunk control and postural endurance, assess the trunk muscles for their ability to maintain a contraction for a longer duration (Manual Muscle Tests 13-1 through 13-5). Typical isometric trunk strength appears to have limited relationship to back pain.[46] Assessment should also include the extent to which the patient can volitionally control muscles such as the transversus abdominis and multifidii because weakness and subsequent lack of control of these stabilizing muscles is associated with low back pain. Assessment of transversus abdominis control is done with the patient supine and the examiner's fingers medially and inferiorly to the iliac spine but avoiding the more superficial rectus abdominis. The patient is instructed to draw in the stomach without any movement of the pelvis or lumbar spine. Activation of the transversus abdominis is noted via palpation.[47]

Hook-lying position Lying supine with the hips and knees flexed and the feet flat on the table

Goniometry 13-2
Lateral Bending (Inclinometer)

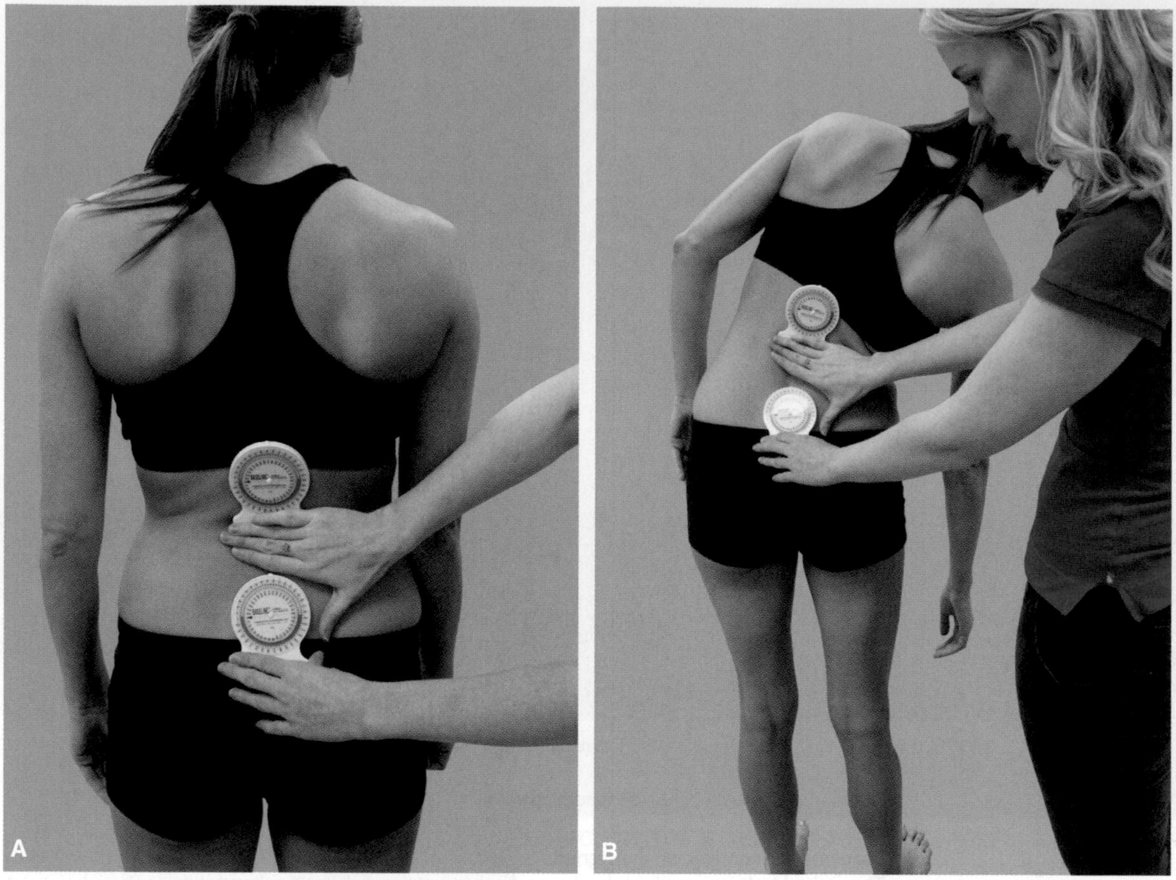

Patient Position	Standing with the feet shoulder-width apart
Procedure	Place one inclinometer on the sacrum. The second inclinometer is at the thoracolumbar junction. Set both inclinometers at 0°.
Motion	The patient laterally flexes while the clinician holds the inclinometers.
Final Measurement	Lateral flexion ROM is recorded as superior inclinometer reading minus the reading obtained from the inferior inclinometer.
Evidence	Absent or inconclusive in the literature

Joint Stability Tests

There are no tests to check the integrity of single isolated ligaments. However, these results may easily be confused with pain caused by intervertebral disc lesions or pathology to the nerve roots or peripheral nerves.

Sprains to the spinal ligaments usually occur more frequently in the cervical spine because of its increased ROM. The conclusion of a ligamentous sprain is generally derived by excluding the possibility of other pathologies. The history of a mechanism that would stress the spinal ligaments, pain along the spinal column and at the end of range of motion, and static pain when the muscles are relatively relaxed and the ligaments are acting as the only static stabilizers can lead to the conclusion of a sprain. This assumes that all other possible pathologies have been ruled out.

Joint Play Tests

The total ROM available to the spinal column is equal to the sum of the motions between any two contiguous vertebrae.

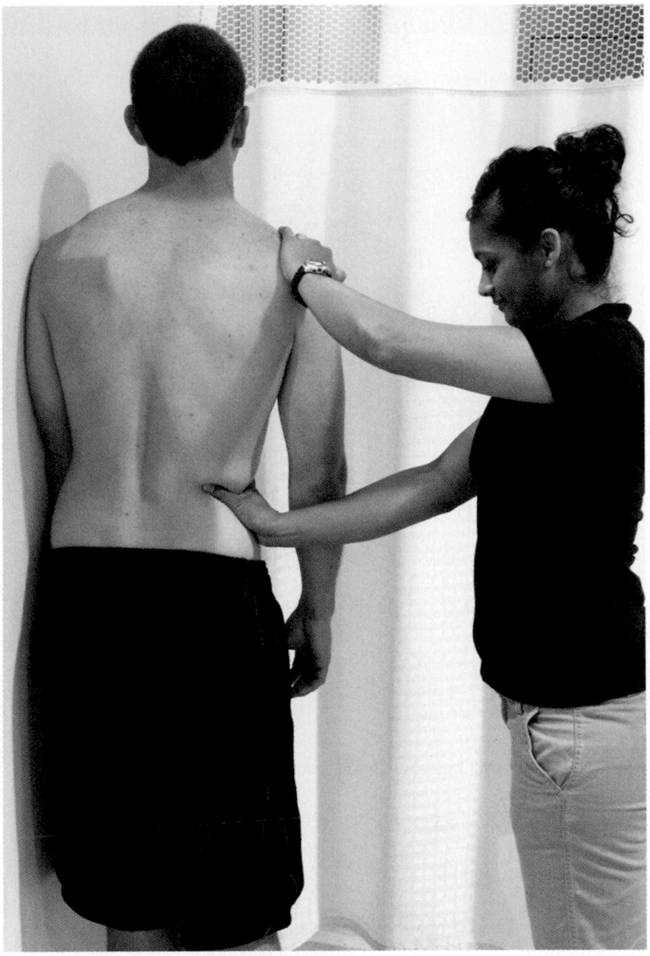

FIGURE 13-19 ■ Passive lateral glide of the trunk. The patient's shoulder is stabilized against the wall while the examiner forces the pelvis laterally.

Although it is difficult to quantify the amount of motion that occurs at each individual spinal segment, the accessory movement of the segment can be grossly determined. Passive intervertebral motion testing is used to assess segmental mobility. Posterior-to-anterior (P–A) joint play (Joint Play 13-1) and palpating for segmental motion by moving the hips and trunk with the patient side-lying may detect hypomobility, hypermobility and/or pain at a vertebral segment. Causative factors include facet joint pathologies, degenerative changes, or spondylotic defects. Reliability of P–A joint play is affected by the surface on which the patient is lying, so repeat testing should be performed on the same surface.[55]

Selective Tissue Tests

Several selective tissue tests (STT) are commonly incorporated into all spinal evaluations. They are presented in this section, and the remaining tests are described in their appropriate locations in the Region-Specific Pathologies section of this chapter.

Test for Nerve Root Impingement

Impingement of spinal nerve roots may result from a narrowing of the intervertebral foramen caused by stenosis, facet joint degeneration, herniated intervertebral discs, or other space-occupying lesions. Increased **intrathecal** pressure can increase the patient's symptoms by forcing the annulus pulposus outward, compressing the nerve root and causing radicular pain. The **Valsalva test** (Selective Tissue Test 13-3) is used clinically to identify the effect of increased intrathecal pressure, but equally persuasive findings are self-reported increase in symptoms while bearing down during a bowel movement, sneezing, or while lifting weights.

Practical Evidence

A dermatomal distribution of pain, pain worse in the leg than in the back, pain that worsens with coughing and sneezing, and a cold sensation in the leg are all associated with nerve root compression.[25]

Several tests are designed to place tension on peripheral nerves, nerve roots, and the dura mater. Each of these tests involves provoking and then relieving symptoms. A positive SLR test (Selective Tissue Test 13-4) indicates either sciatic nerve irritation or a herniated intervertebral disc that is irritating the nerve root. A positive SLR is associated with patients who have disc herniations with root compression requiring surgery.[57] The well or cross SLR, a modification of the SLR test, can be used to discriminate between symptoms caused by sciatic neuropathy or disc herniations.[58-60] The slump test (Selective Tissue Test 13-5), another test that assesses the effect of increasing nerve tension, can be used to identify possible compression of the lumbar nerve roots from spinal stenosis, disc herniation, or distal entrapment of a nerve. Because many patients report radicular symptoms while sitting, the slump test may be better than the SLR test in reproducing symptoms.[61]

Practical Evidence

The clinical results of the SLR are rarely conclusive, and the results are more accurate in a younger population.[62]

The **quadrant test** (Selective Tissue Test 13-6) is used to determine dural irritation and facet joint compression.

Neurological Testing

Because of the close involvement of the spinal column with the spinal cord and its nerve roots, many of the maladies affecting the spine may result in decreased neurological function in the extremities as well as the trunk. Impingement of the lower spinal cord, including disc disease, stenosis, or the lumbar or sacral nerve roots is likely to result in radicular pain to the extremity.[67] Clinically, this involvement can be determined through the use of manual muscle tests, deep tendon reflexes, and sensory testing. Chapter 20 discusses the management of acute spinal injuries.

Intrathecal Within the spinal canal

Manual Muscle Test 13-1
Trunk Flexors

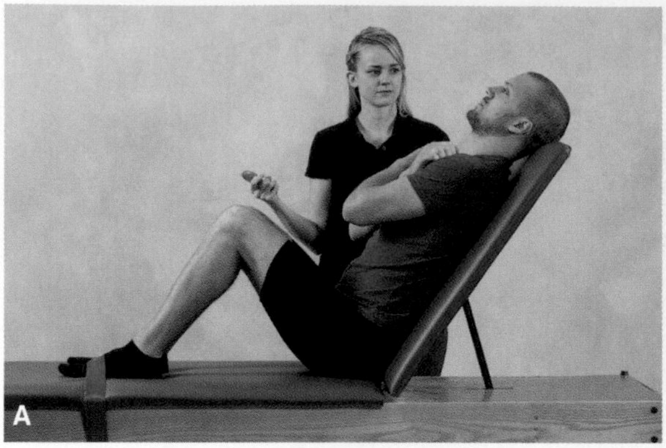

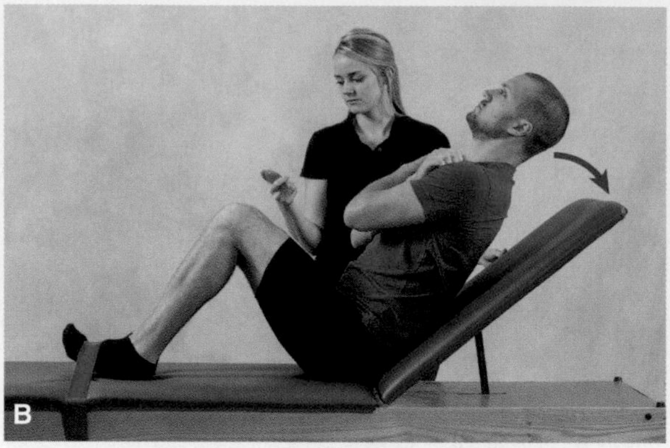

Patient Position Test Position

Patient Position	The patient is reclined with the trunk supported at a 60-degree angle from the table either by a split table or by the examiner. Both hips and knees are in 90 degrees of flexion. The feet are stabilized with straps or by another examiner. The arms are crossed over the chest.
Test Procedure	The examiner lowers the supporting table (or removes the support). The duration that the patient can maintain the position is timed.
Interpretation/Normative Data	**Young healthy males average 144±76 seconds, and young healthy females average 149±99 seconds, with duration decreasing as age increases.[48]** **In a different study, young, healthy adults averaged 340±215 seconds.[49]**
Muscles Assessed	Rectus abdominis, hip flexors, internal and external obliques
Evidence	A ratio of flexion to extension endurance >1.0 suggests an imbalance (see Manual Muscle Test 13-2). This test has excellent repeat reliability, regardless of whether the stabilization is provided by a human or by straps.[48,49]

Manual Muscle Test 13-2
Extension Endurance

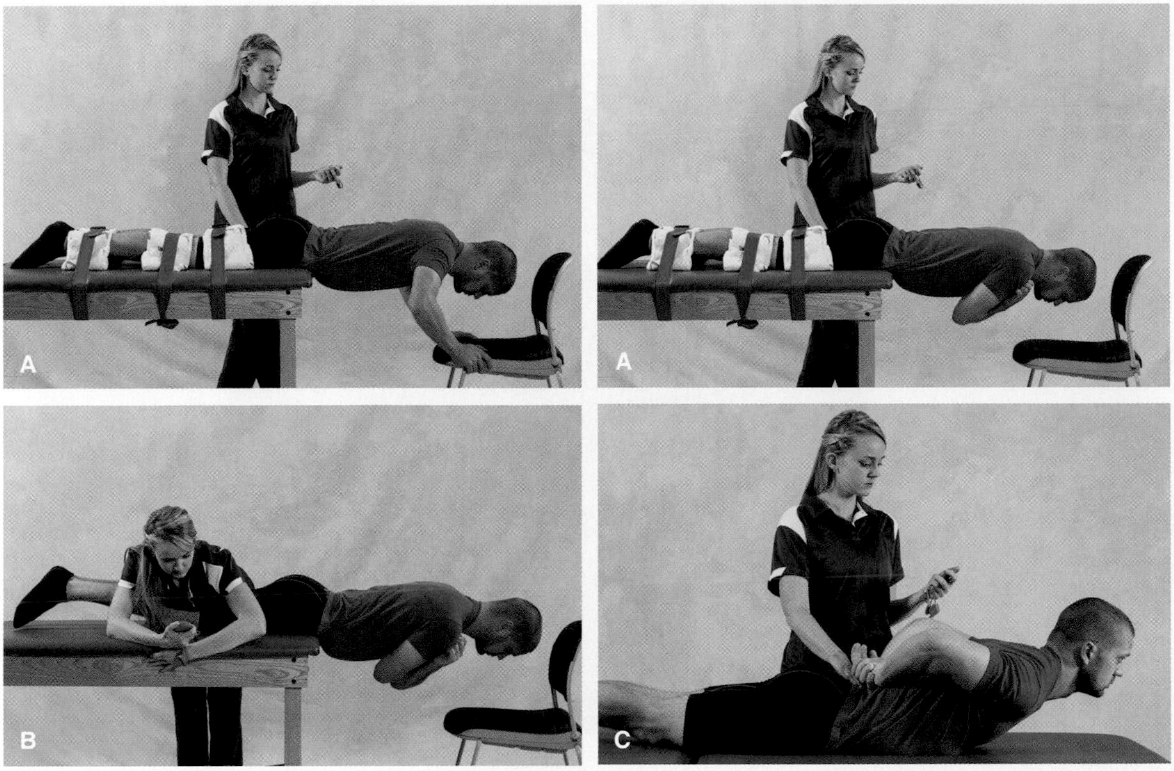

(A)The Sorensen test. (B) A modification of the Sorensen test. (C)The extension endurance test.

Patient Position	**(A)** In the **Sorensen test**, the patient is positioned with the torso off the table with the upper border of the iliac crests aligned with the edge of the table. The patient's hips and legs are stabilized with straps.
Test Procedure	With the arms crossed over the chest, the patient is asked to maintain the upper body in a horizontal position. The examiner times the duration that the patient can hold the position.
Interpretation/Normative Data	Decreased back extensor endurance is associated with development and persistence of low back pain.[50,51] The average duration for young, adult men and women is 146±51 seconds and 189±60 seconds, respectively.[48] In another study with a broader age range, the average endurance time was 113±46 seconds, with decreasing endurance with increasing age.[52]
Muscles Assessed	Iliocostalis lumborum, iliocostalis thoracis, longissimus thoracis, spinalis thoracis, semispinalis thoracis, multifidus, rotatores, latissimus dorsi, quadratus lumborum
Substitution	Hip extension
Modification	**(C)** For a modification of this test, the patient is prone, with the hands behind the back or by the sides. The patient is instructed to raise the chest off the table by extending the lumbar spine to approximately 30 degrees and holding the position.
Comments	Individuals with a higher body mass index fatigue more quickly.[53] Males with chronic low back pain demonstrate shorter durations, indicating faster time to fatigue than healthy individuals.[53] Good test–retest reliability for the Sorensen has been demonstrated in asymptomatic patients (0.77) and patients with nonspecific low back pain (0.80).
Evidence	

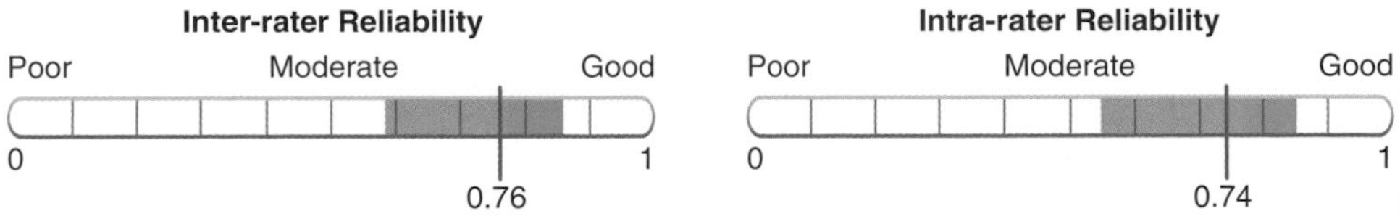

Manual Muscle Test 13-3
Transversus Abdominis

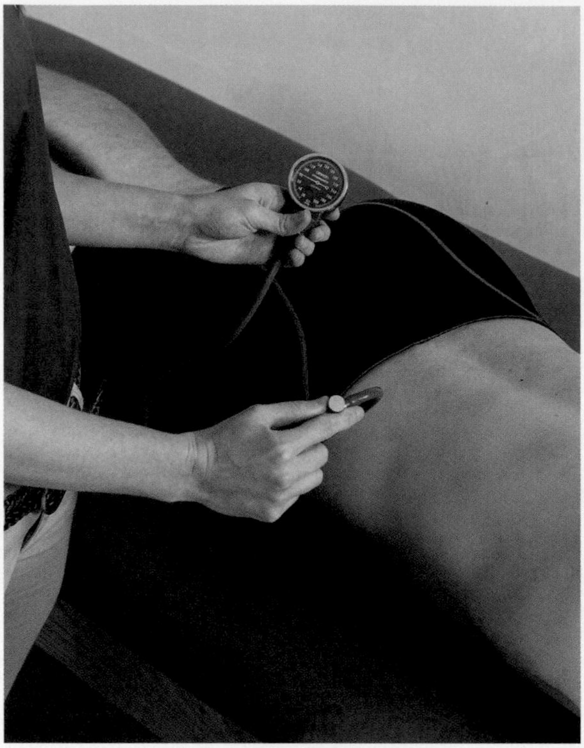

Patient Position	The patient is prone with a pressure biofeedback unit or blood pressure cuff under the abdomen. The pressure unit is inflated to 70 mm Hg.
Test Procedure	The patient draws in the abdomen without moving the pelvis for 10 seconds. The decrease in pressure is noted.
Interpretation	4 mm decrease = normal; inability to decrease by 2 mm associated with incidence of low back pain
Muscles Assessed	Transversus abdominis
Substitution	Allowing pelvic motion indicates increased activity from the surrounding musculature.
Comments	Poor ability to recruit the transversus abdominis is associated with chronic low back pain.[54]
Evidence	The studies found moderate to good reproducibility (intra-class correlation coefficients from 0.47 to 0.82) and acceptable construct validity (intra-class correlation coefficients from 0.48 to 0.90).

Manual Muscle Test 13-4
Lateral Abdominals Endurance

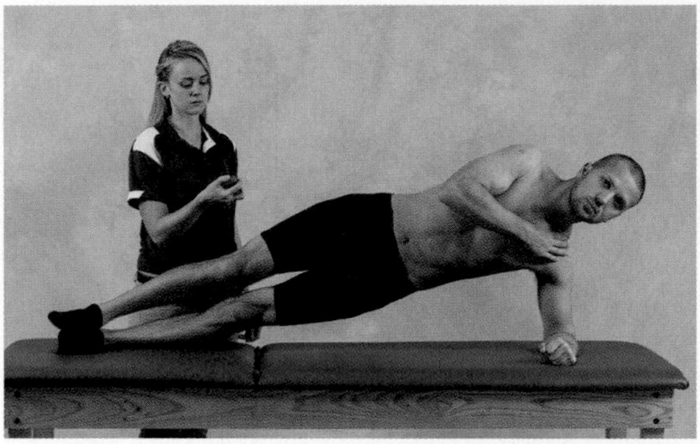

Patient Position	The patient is side-lying with the legs straight and the body resting on the flexed elbow. Alternatively, the patient's knees are flexed.
Test Procedure	The patient lifts the pelvis off the table while maintaining the spine in a neutral (neither flexed nor extended) position—a side bridge. The hand of the uninvolved arm crosses the chest to the opposite shoulder. The examiner times the duration that the patient can maintain the position. Repeat the test on the opposite side.
Interpretation	A right-to-left difference of greater than 5% suggests an imbalance. On average, healthy males can maintain the position for approximately 94±34 [R] and 97±35 [L] seconds, and females can maintain the position for 72±31 [R] and 77±35 [L] seconds.[48]
Muscles Assessed	Internal oblique, external oblique, quadratus lumborum
Substitution	Hip extension
Evidence	Test–retest reliability (intra-subject): 0.96–0.99[48]

Manual Muscle Test 13-5
Pelvic Elevation

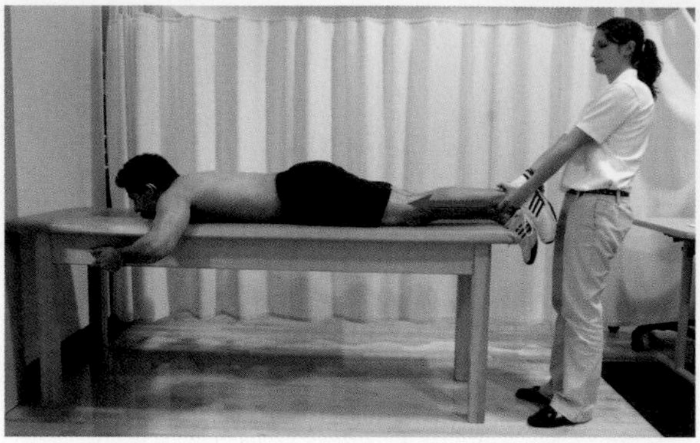

Patient Position	Supine or prone
Starting Position	The examiner grasps the patient's leg just proximal to the ankle.
Stabilization	The patient holds the edges of the table to maintain stabilization.
Resistance	The examiner distracts the leg by applying longitudinal resistance. The patient is then instructed to "hike" the pelvis, attempting to move the pelvis on the side being tested toward the rib cage.
Primary Movers (Innervation)	Quadratus lumborum External oblique (T1 - T12) Internal oblique (T7-T12)
Secondary Movers (Innervation)	Latissimus dorsi (with the patient's shoulder flexed) Iliocostalis lumborum (multiple roots; segmentally)
Substitution	Hip flexion Trunk lateral flexion (abdominals) Pulling with the arms
Comments	The test may also be performed with the patient standing on a raised platform and hiking the opposite leg.

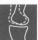

Joint Play 13-1
Posterior–Anterior Vertebral Joint Play (Passive Accessory Intervertebral Motion)

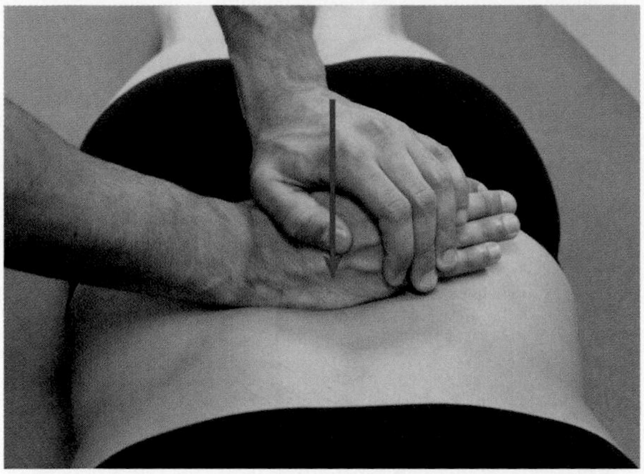

Posterior–anterior joint play is used to assess segmental mobility.

Patient Position	Prone
Position of Examiner	Standing over the patient with the hypothenar eminence of one hand placed over the spinous process to be tested
Evaluative Procedure	The examiner carefully applies an anterior force on the spinous process, feeling for the extent of the vertebral translation.
Positive Test	The vertebra does not move ("spring"), or moves excessively.
Implications	Lumbar segmental hypomobility or hypermobility
Evidence	

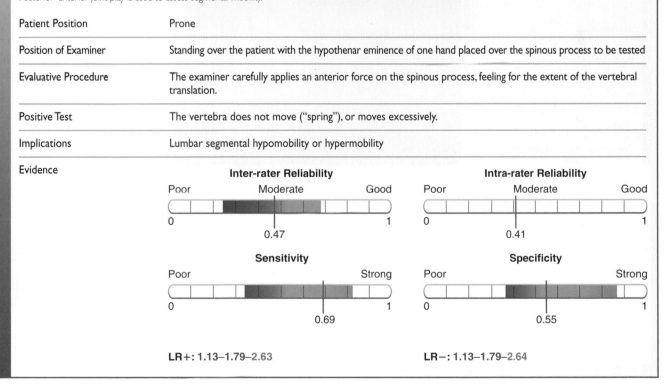

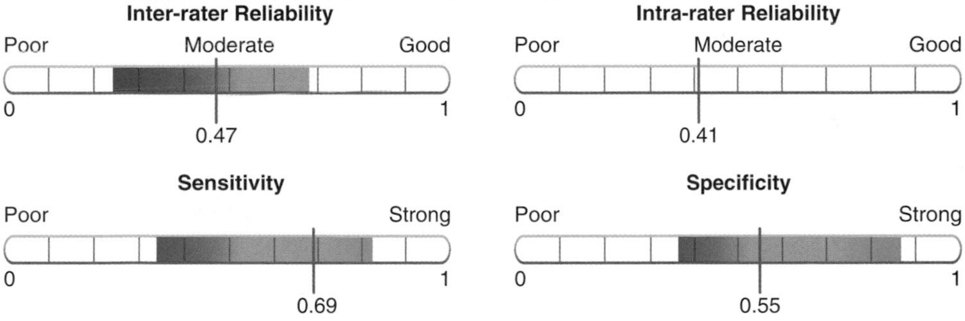

LR+: 1.13–1.79–2.63

LR−: 1.13–1.79–2.64

Selective Tissue Test 13-3
Valsalva Test

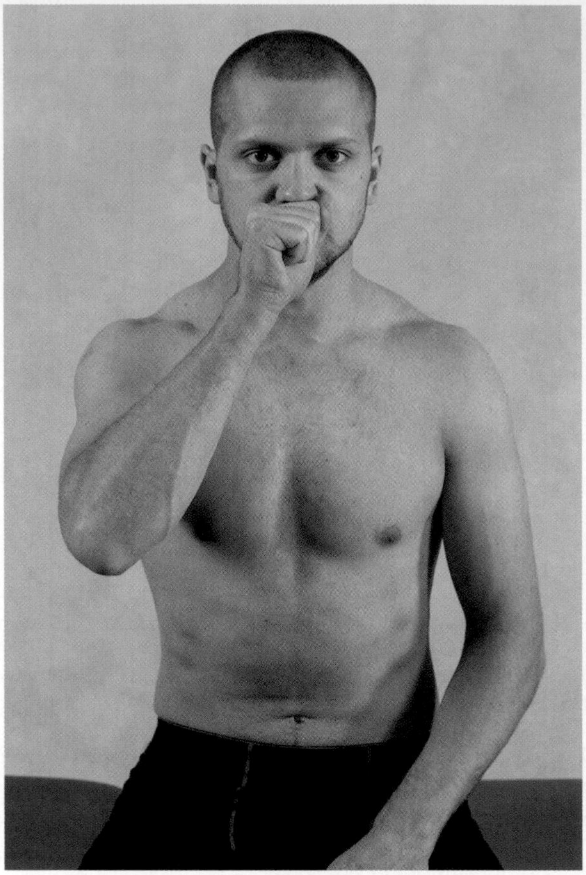

The Valsalva test attempts to increase intrathecal pressure, duplicating nerve-root pain that may be elicited while coughing or with bowel movements. The patient often self-reports these findings rather than being identified clinically.

Patient Position	Sitting
Position of Examiner	Standing within arms' reach in front of the patient
Evaluative Procedure	The patient takes and holds a deep breath while bearing down similar to performing a bowel movement.
Positive Test	Increased spinal or radicular pain
Implications	Increase in intrathecal pressure causes pain secondary to a space-occupying lesion such as a herniated disc, tumor, or osteophyte anywhere along the spinal column.
Modification	The Valsalva maneuver is performed with the patient standing and the lumbar spine flexed to 35° to 75° (Cecin's sign). The patient stands and leans forward until pain or paraesthesia is experienced. This position is held, and the patient is asked to cough. The test is positive if symptoms worsen. If pain is not experienced at this point, the spine is flexed to approximately 35° and the test repeated.[56]
Comments	If the patient is embarrassed or apprehensive about simulating a bowel movement, he or she may be instructed to blow into a closed fist as if inflating a balloon. The test increases intrathecal pressure throughout the spinal column, resulting in a slowing of the pulse, decreased venous return, and increased venous pressure, all of which may cause fainting.

Evidence

Cecin's sign

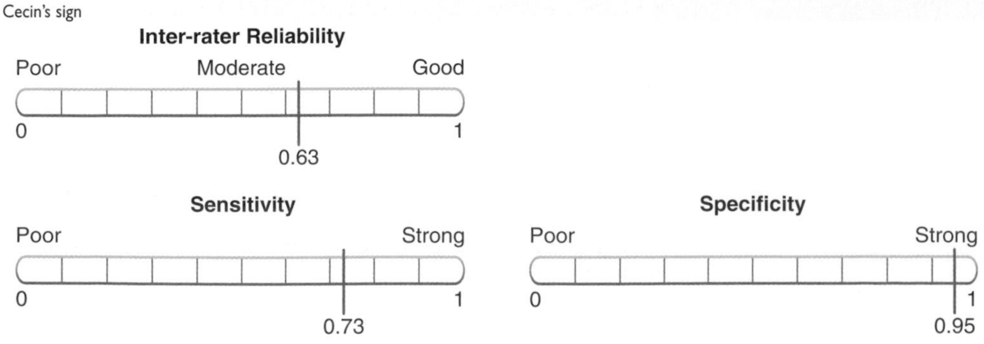

LR+: 14.60

LR−: 0.28

Selective Tissue Test 13-4

Straight Leg Raise Test (Test of Lasègue)/Well (Cross) Straight Leg Test

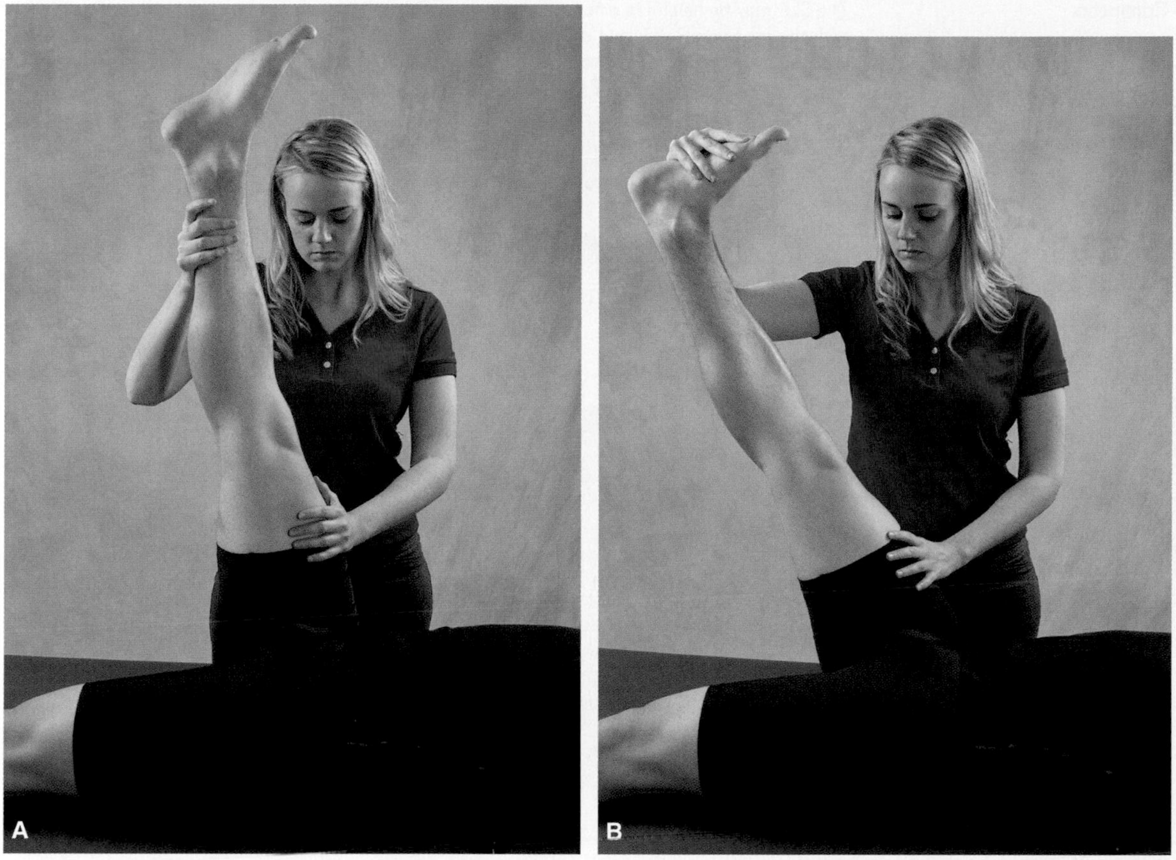

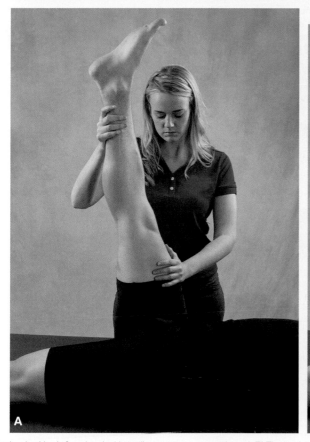

(A) The involved leg is flexed at the hip until symptoms are experienced. (B) The involved leg is lowered approximately 10° (until symptoms subside), and the ankle is then passively dorsiflexed. A return of the symptoms indicates a stretching of the dural sheath. The well SLR test differs from the SLR test in that the leg on the unaffected side is raised.

Patient Position	Supine
Position of Examiner	At the side to be tested; one hand grasps under the heel, while the other is placed on the anterior knee to keep it in full extension during the examination.
Evaluative Procedure	While keeping the knee in extension, the examiner raises the leg by flexing the hip until discomfort is experienced or the full ROM is obtained.
Positive Test	**SLR:** The patient complains of pain or reproduction of symptoms before the end of the normal ROM (70°). The pain may be described as radiating distally along the tested leg, usually in the posterior thigh, radiating into the calf and perhaps the foot. The findings are highly significant if they are elicited at less than 30° of hip flexion.[28] **Well SLR:** Pain or reproduction of symptoms is experienced on the side opposite that being raised.
Implications	**SLR:** Sciatic nerve irritation/compression Pain described before the hip reaches 70° of flexion may indicate disc involvement.[63] The sensitivity and specificity of the SLR is significantly improved for L5 and S1 nerve root levels than for the L2–L4 levels.[64] **Well SLR:** A large space-occupying lesion such as a herniated disc
Modification	After pain is experienced, the leg is lowered to the point at which the pain stops. The examiner passively dorsiflexes the ankle and/or has the patient flex the cervical spine. Serving to stretch the dural sheath, this flexion recreates the symptoms. If the patient's prior pain was caused by tight hamstrings, this modification does not elicit pain. Although the SLR can be performed with the patient seated, this position reduces the sensitivity of the findings.[65]

Continued

Selective Tissue Test 13-4

Straight Leg Raise Test (Test of Lasègue)/Well (Cross) Straight Leg Test—cont'd

Comments

The SLR may be helpful in differentiating between tarsal tunnel syndrome and plantar fasciitis. Beginning with the foot dorsiflexed and everted additionally stresses the tibial nerve. The SLR is then performed. An increase in symptoms points to tibial nerve entrapment because strain on the plantar fascia would not further increase.[66] (See p. 218 for a description of tarsal tunnel syndrome.)

Evidence

Straight Leg Raise

Inter-rater Reliability

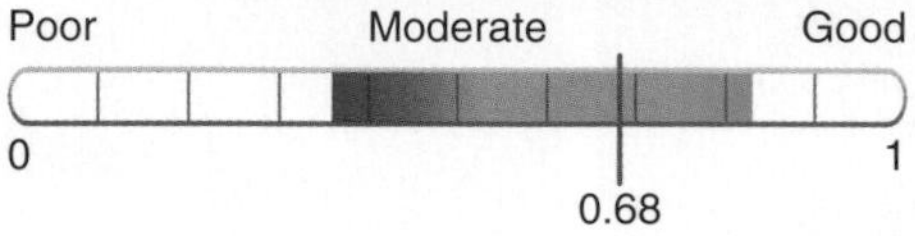

No data

Sensitivity

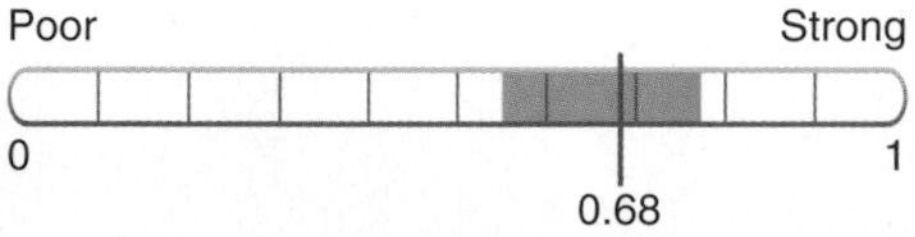

Specificity

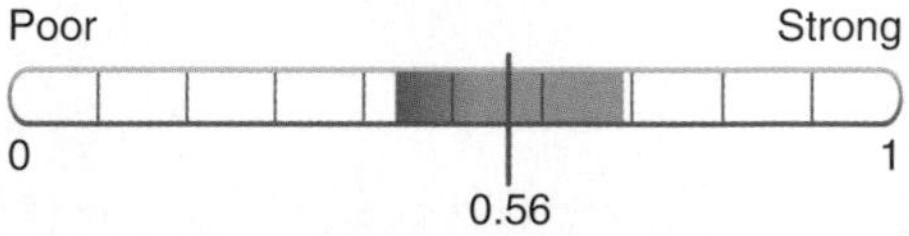

LR+: 0.72–4.68–8.63

LR−: 0.41–0.61–0.81

Well Straight Leg Raise

Sensitivity

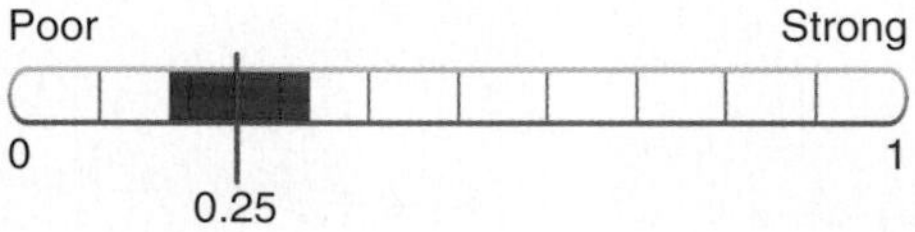

Specificity

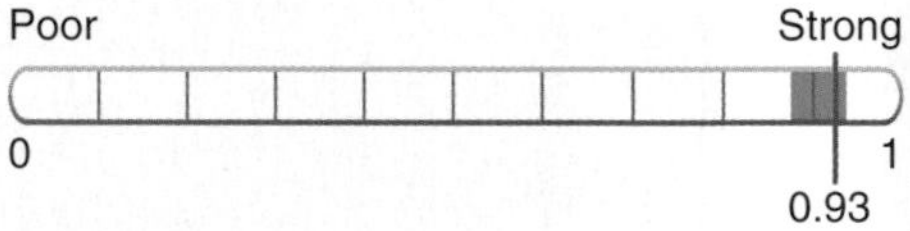

LR+: 1.83–2.33–3.36

LR−: 0.76–0.83–0.90

ROM = range of motion; SLR = straight leg raise

Selective Tissue Test 13-5
Slump Test

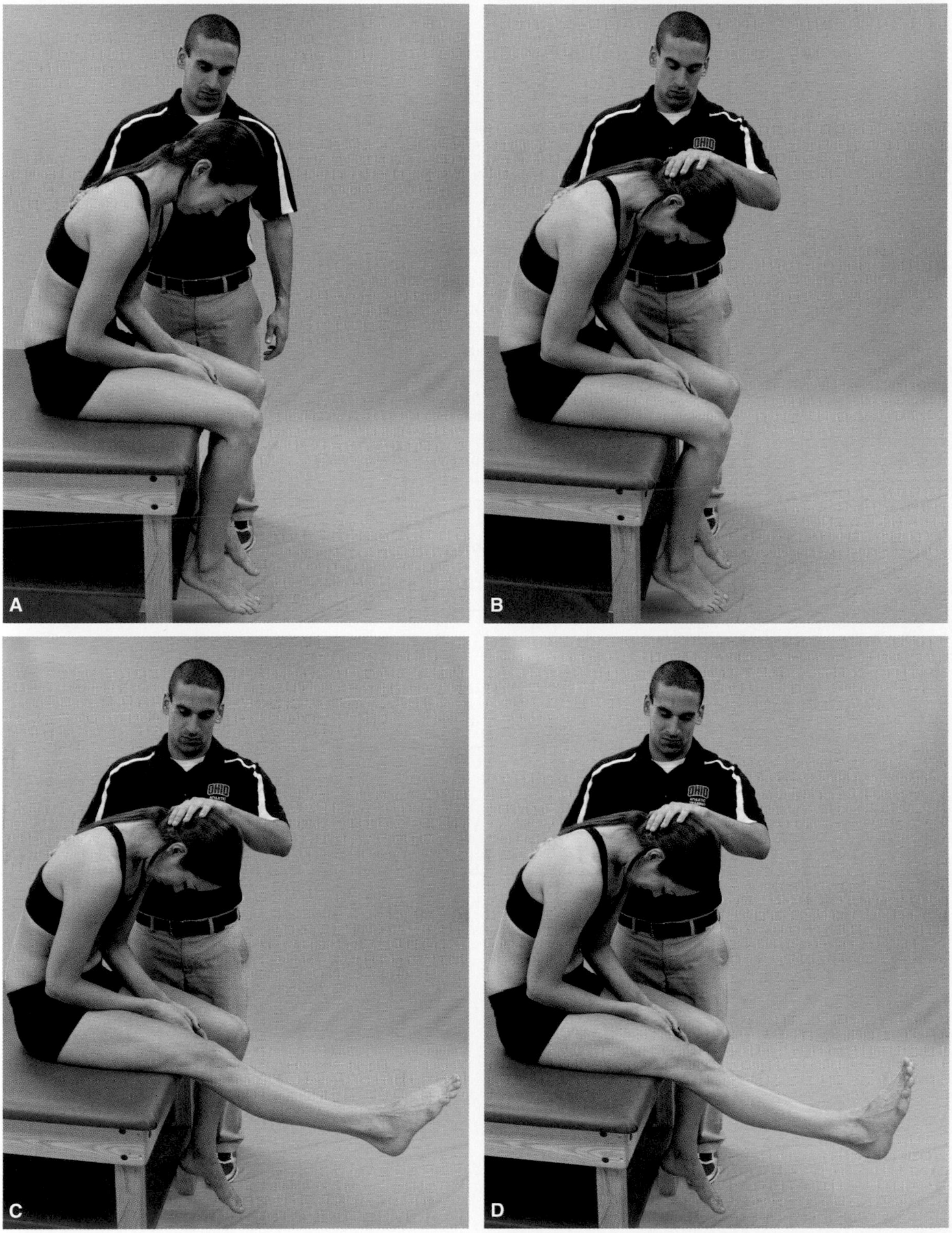

The slump test is designed to place progressively more tension on the nerve and nerve roots by systematically positioning the patient to provoke and subsequently alleviate symptoms.

Continued

Selective Tissue Test 13-5
Slump Test—cont'd

Patient Position
Sitting upright

Position of Examiner
At the side of the patient

Evaluative Procedure
The following sequence is followed until symptoms are provoked:

1. The patient slumps forward along the thoracolumbar spine, rounding the shoulders while keeping the cervical spine in neutral **(A)**. Overpressure to trunk flexion is then applied.
2. The patient flexes the cervical spine by bringing the chin to the chest. The clinician then holds the patient in this position **(B)**.
3. The knee is actively extended **(C)**.
4. The ankle is actively dorsiflexed **(D)**.
5. Repeat steps 2 to 4 on the opposite side.
6. Alleviation maneuver: At any step that symptoms are elicited, the provoking position is slightly relieved and tension is reduced at the other end of the nervous system. For example, if knee extension reproduces symptoms, slightly flex the patient's knee and extend the cervical spine. Extend the patient's knee again. In this example, if the symptoms reappear, the cause is nerve tension as opposed to hamstring pathology.

Positive Test
Sciatic pain or reproduction of other neurological symptoms

Implications
Impingement of the dural lining, spinal cord, or nerve roots

Modification
Many modifications have been proposed, most of which describe different sequences of motions.

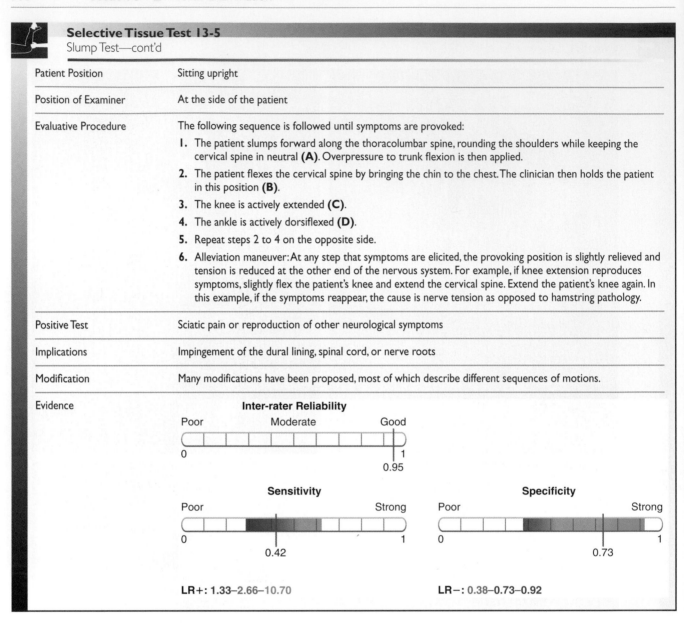

Evidence

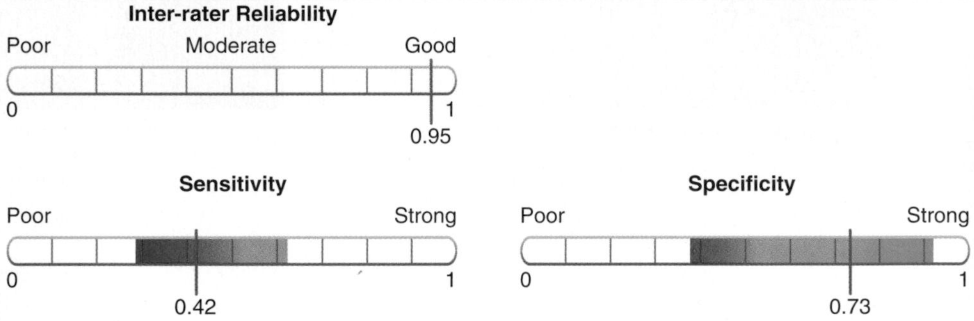

LR+: 1.33–2.66–10.70

LR−: 0.38–0.73–0.92

Selective Tissue Test 13-6
Quadrant Test

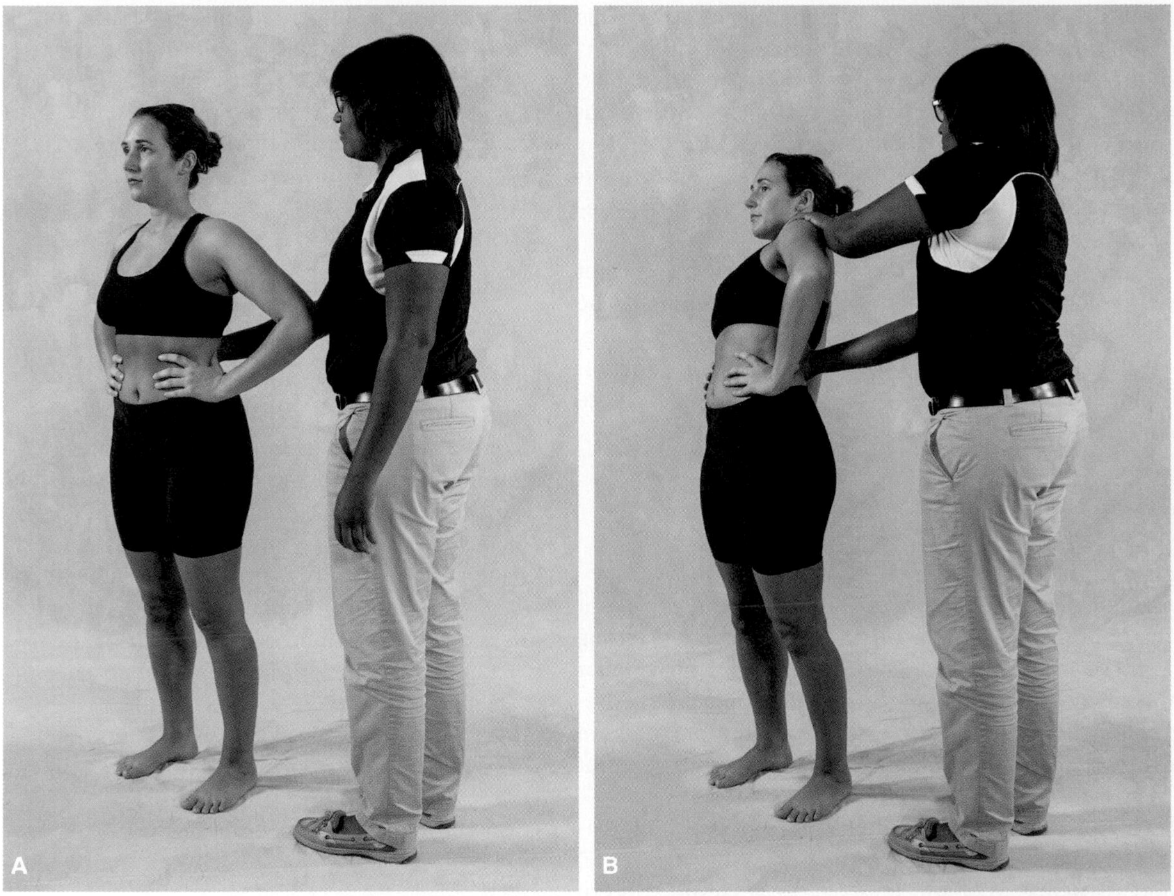

The patient moves into extension, followed by sidebending and rotation to the same side. The examiner provides overpressure to emphasize the position.

Patient Position	Standing with the feet shoulder-width apart
Position of Examiner	Standing behind the patient, grasping the patient's shoulders
Evaluative Procedure	The patient extends the spine as far as possible, then sidebends and rotates to the affected side. The examiner provides overpressure through the shoulders, supporting the patient as needed.
Positive Test	Reproduction of the patient's symptoms
Implications	Radicular symptoms indicate compression of the intervertebral foramina that impinges on the lumbar nerve roots. Local (nonradiating) pain indicates facet joint pathology. Symptoms isolated to the area of the PSIS; may also indicate SI joint dysfunction
Evidence	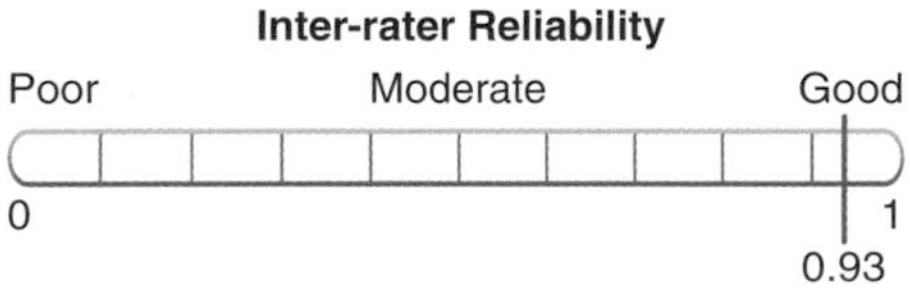

PSIS = posterior superior iliac spine; SI = sacroiliac

Tests for Lower Motor Neuron Lesions

Lower motor neuron involvement of the spinal nerve roots or the peripheral nervous system results in **hyporeflexia**, flaccidity of the muscles, and denervation atrophy. This condition most often results from compression or stretching of the nerves. Temporary hyporeflexia, sensory deficit, or muscle weakness or paralysis may indicate nerve root impingement or transient quadriplegia (see Chapter 20).

Lower motor neuron injuries include neurapraxia, axonotmesis, and neurotmesis. Refer to Chapter 1 for a description of upper motor neuron lesions.

The upper and lower quarter screens provide an efficient evaluation for neurological function in the extremities. The screens use manual muscle testing, sensory testing, and deep tendon reflexes to assess neurological function (Neurological Screening 13-1). Upper quarter screens are presented in Chapter 14.

Region-Specific Pathologies and Selective Tissue Tests

The structure and function of the spinal column exposes it and its supportive structures to almost constant stress during ADLs. These stresses are increased further during heavy labor or athletic competition. In addition to the contact forces related to athletic competition, movement of the torso results in shear forces across the column. Sitting or standing upright places an axial load on these structures.

Regardless, the spinal column displays an enormous capability to adapt to the forces placed on it. When the spinal column is unable to adapt, injury occurs. Dysfunction of the SI joint can occur acutely secondary to a dynamic overload or insidiously from an unknown cause.

The evaluation of back injuries relies on a thorough, accurate history to provide the examiner with, minimally, an understanding of the positions and movements that aggravate and alleviate the symptoms and, possibly, identification of the involved structure. Identification of the specific pathology is often difficult with chronic low back pain, leading to a general classification of nonspecific low back pain. Chronic low back pain is often idiopathic, with the patient unable to describe any instigating factor. The correlation between imaging studies such as MRI and low back pain is poor.[68]

The idiopathic and inconsistent behavior of low back pain makes identifying the underlying involved structures difficult and likely unnecessary. Treatment-based classification systems have been developed that categorize the findings from the low back examination into clusters (Fig. 13-20).[21,69-72] Each cluster of signs and symptoms is associated with an improved responsiveness to a certain intervention. With this strategy, specific identification of the involved structures isn't necessary, and the emphasis is on identifying a treatment plan. For example, patients who demonstrate pain during flexion and pain relief during extension are grouped into the specific exercise category, and extension is emphasized during the initial rehabilitation and education protocol. An understanding of the treatment-based classification system helps the examiner determine what information to gather during the examination. While the clinical presentation of discrete structure pathology is included for organizational purposes, the clinical examination should eliminate red flags that indicate the need for immediate referral and build the foundation for the appropriate intervention.

Spinal Stenosis

Spinal stenosis, narrowing of the spinal canal or intervertebral foramen, most often results from degeneration associated with aging and collapse of the disc space, which results in increased stress to the facet joints and subsequent degeneration and osteophyte formation.[5] These changes narrow the space available in the spinal canal and compress the contents within and exiting the canal. While narrowing may be evident with imaging, the extent of narrowing correlates poorly with symptoms, and, conversely, narrowing may be apparent in asymptomatic individuals.[73] Stenosis can also result from congenital factors. Degenerative stenosis is most common in 50- to 60-year-old people.[74]

Bilateral buttock or leg pain, the absence of pain when seated, the improvement of symptoms when bending forward, and a wide-based gait are common clinical indicators of lumbar spinal stenosis.[73] Patients describe a decreased tolerance for standing and walking, with walking improved by assuming a forward flexed posture.[5]

Spinal Stenosis Intervention Strategies

Initial treatment often includes nonsteroidal anti-inflammatory medications and core-strengthening exercises. The role of epidural steroid injections is equivocal. When symptoms significantly affect quality of life, surgical intervention to decompress the canal and stabilize segments as necessary.[5]

Intervertebral Disc Lesions

The degeneration of intervertebral discs involves the loss of water from the nucleus pulposus, decreasing the protein content and altering the chemical structure. Biochemical changes associated with the aging process further extenuate the loss of water, causing an increased stress load to be placed on the annulus fibrosus and leading to the bulging of the nucleus pulposus (Fig. 13-21). Tears of the annulus in early adulthood are likely to lead to eventual disc degeneration and herniation.[12]

Disc herniation is the extrusion of the nucleus pulposus through a weakened region in the annulus fibrosus with subsequent impingement on one or more lumbar nerve roots, with L5 and S1 nerve roots most commonly affected.[75] A complete herniation typically results in pressure of the nerve root exiting below the affected disc (Fig. 13-22). For example, a herniation of the L4–L5 disc places pressure on the L5 nerve root. The lesion can involve any protrusion of the nuclear material into the annulus, even if it has not

Part 1

Does the patient have a DP?
A DP is established if certain postures or repeated end-range movements in 1 direction (e.g., flexion) cause the symptoms to improve or centralize (pain moves from a distal to a proximal area), and in the opposite direction (e.g., extension) cause the symptoms to worsen or peripheralize (pain moves from a proximal to a distal area).

→ Yes → Direction-specific exercises

↓ No

Does the patient meet the following 4 criteria:
(1) No symptoms distal to the knee
(2) Low v score (<19)
(3) ≥ 1 hypomobile segment on lumbar segmental mobility testing
(4) Hip internal rotation ROM (>35° for at least 1 hip)

→ Yes → Spinal manipulation

↓ Or

Does the patient have at least 3 of the following?
(1) Greater general flexibility (average SLR ROM >91° or postpartum or high BLLS (≥4 of 9)
(2) Positive prone instability test
(3) Positive aberrant movements
(4) Age <40 yr

For postpartum patients (no cutoff value defined):
Positive thigh thrust test, positive ASLR, positive modified Trendelenburg, pain, provocation with palpation of the long dorsal sacroiliac ligament, or pubis symphysis.

→ Yes → Stabilization

↓ No

Part 2

Which subgroup does the patient fit best into?

Spinal Manipulation	Stabilization		Direction-Specific Exercises	
Factors against	Factors favoring	Factors against	Factors favoring	Factors against
• Symptoms below the knee • Increasing episode frequency • No pain with mobility testing • No hypomobility • Less discrepancy in left-to-right hip internal rotation (<10°) • Negative Gaenslen's sign • Peripheralization with motion testing	• Hypermobility with spring testing • Increasing episode frequency • 3 or more prior episodes • Previous severe low back/pelvis incident	• Discrepancy in SLR ROM (>10°) Does the patient have at least 3 of the following? • FABQPA score <9 • Negative prone instability test • Absence of aberrant movements • Absence of lumbar hypermobility	• Strong preference for sitting or walking or cycling • Peripheralization in direction opposite to centralization Flexion DP: • >50 yr of age • Imaging evidence of lumbar spinal stenosis Lateral DP: • Visible lateral shift	• LBP only

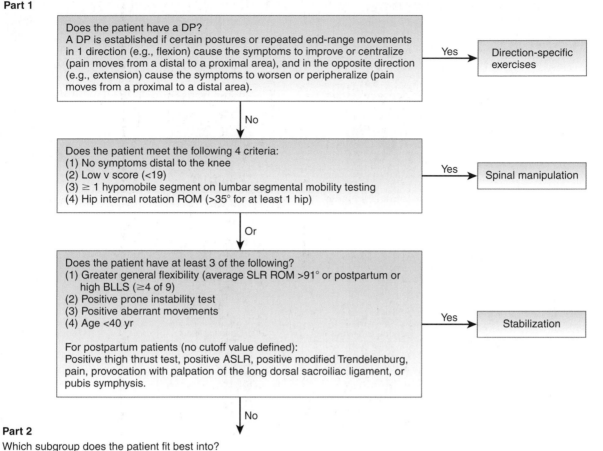

FIGURE 13-20 ■ Classification Categories of Low Back Injury Based on the Treatment Approach. ASLR = Active Straight Leg Raise; BLSS = Beighton Ligamentous Laxity Scale; DP = Directional Preference; FABQ = Fear-avoidance Beliefs Questionnaire; ROM = Range of Motion; SLR = Straight Leg Raise *(Appledorn, A, Ostelo, R, van Helvoirt, H, et al: A Randomized Controlled Trial on the Effectiveness of a Classification-Based System for Subacute and Chronic Low Back Pain. Spine, 37(16):1347-1356, 2012.)*

herniated through the entire structure. Note that many disc protrusions remain asymptomatic.[76]

The signs and symptoms of an intervertebral disc herniation are primarily those of nerve root compression that results in pain in the lumbar spine and radicular pain aggravated by activity (Examination Findings 13-1).[63] The patient typically describes an insidious onset, but the pain may be related to a single specific episode. Often, the breakdown of the disc is related to repetitive stress, but the episode resulting in the symptoms reflects the final failure in the annulus fibrosus to contain the nucleus pulposus. Changes in body position (e.g., sitting to standing or standing to lying) are

Neurological Screening 13-1
Lower Quarter Neurologic Screening

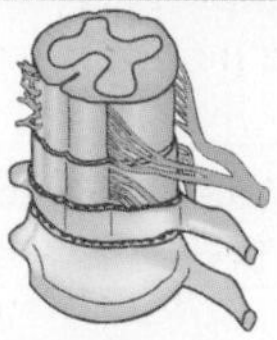 Nerve Root Level	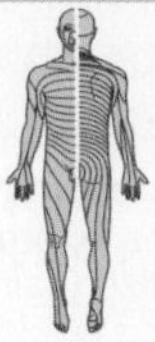 Sensory Testing	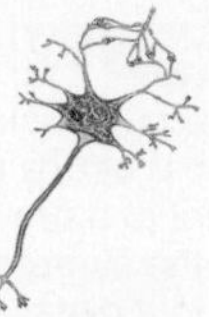 Motor Testing	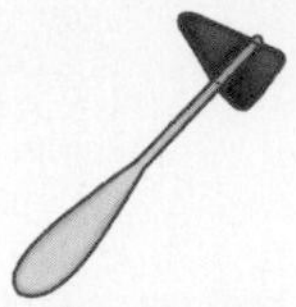 Reflex Testing
L1	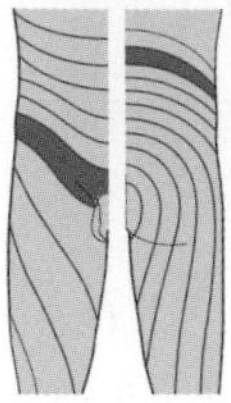 Femoral cutaneous n.	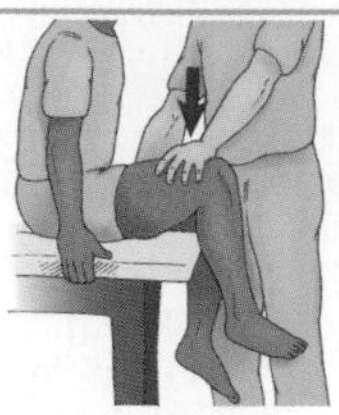 Lumbar plexus	 None
L2	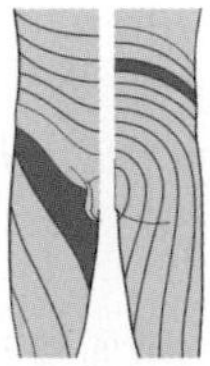 Femoral cutaneous n.	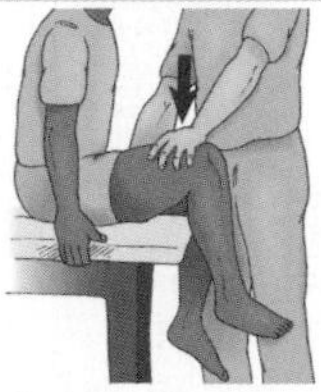 Lumbar plexus	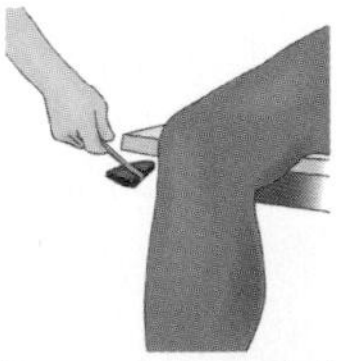 Femoral n. (partial)
L3	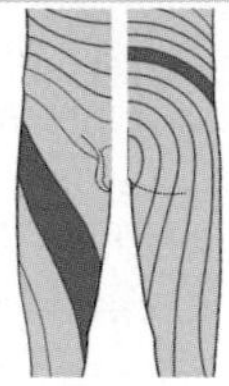 Femoral cutaneous n.	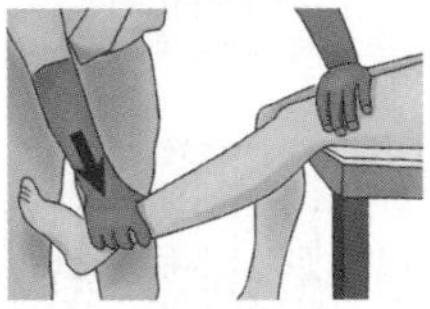 Femoral n.	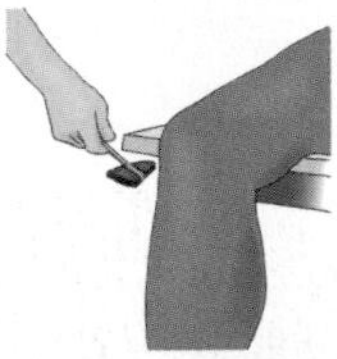 Femoral n. (partial)
L4	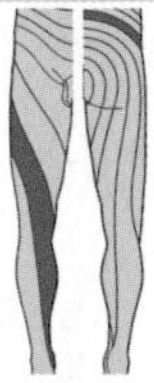 Saphenous n.	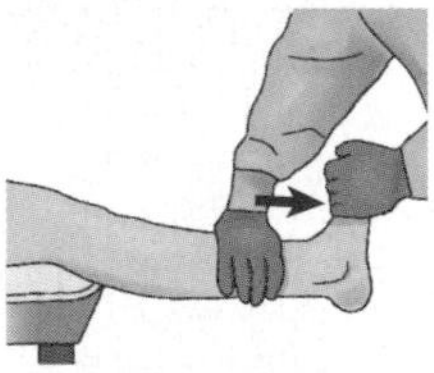 Deep peroneal n.	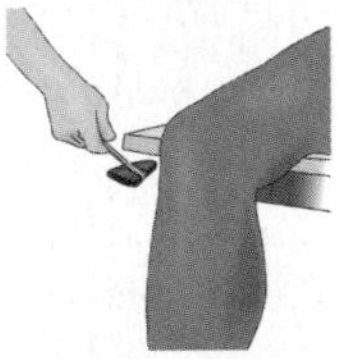 Femoral n. (partial)
L5	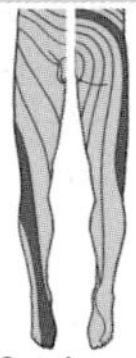 Superficial peroneal n.	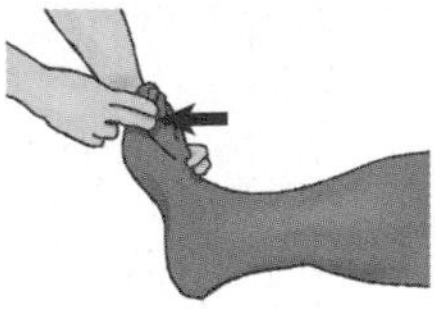 Deep peroneal n.	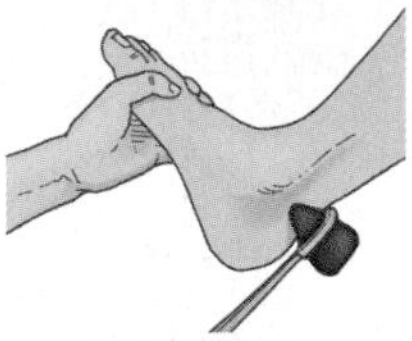 Tibial n. (medial hamstring or tibialis posterior)
S1	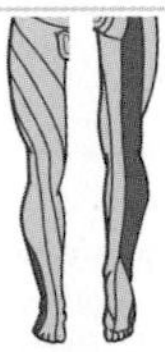 Posterior femoral cutaneous n. and sural n.	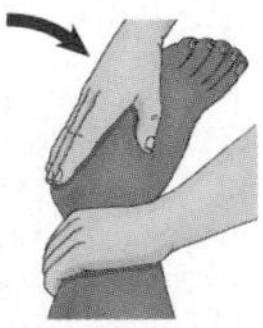 Superficial peroneal n.	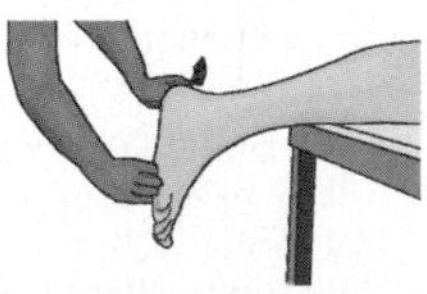 Tibial n. (Achilles)
S2	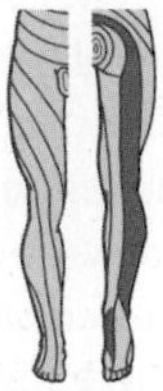 Posterior femoral cutaneous n.	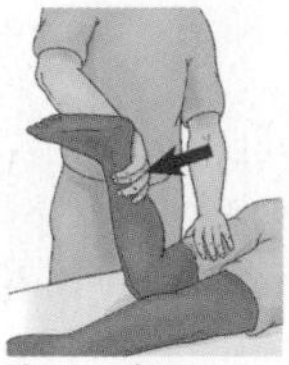 Tibial n. and common peroneal n.	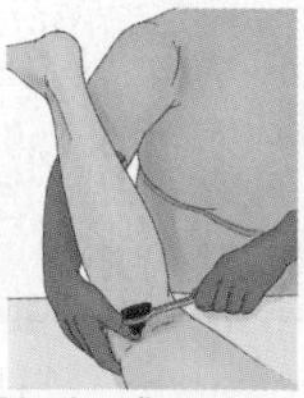 Tibial n. (hamstring)

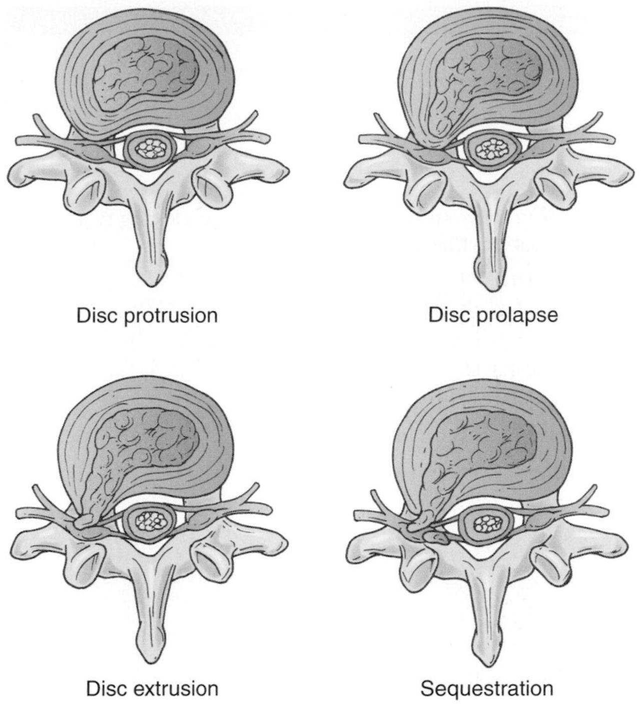

FIGURE 13-21 ■ Classification of intervertebral disc lesions.

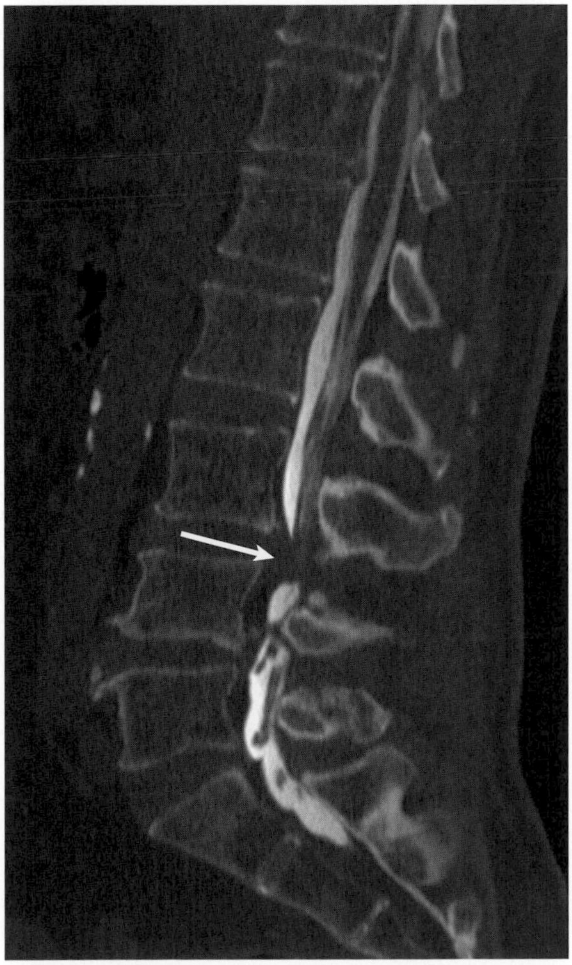

FIGURE 13-22 ■ Myelogram of a disc herniation. Notice the narrowing of the spinal canal.

painful as the changes in disc pressure increase pressure on the structures. On inspection, the patient may be noted as having a slow, deliberate gait and, in the acute and subacute stages, a decreased lumbar lordosis. In an attempt to decrease the pressure on the nerve root, the patient may stand with a lateral shift, usually away from the side of the leg pain. If the patient demonstrates a leg-length discrepancy, the pain usually occurs on the side of the body with the shorter leg.[77]

Question the patient to determine the exact location (or locations) of pain. Typically, the pain is in the low back, buttocks, and posterior thigh. However, herniations impinging on the midlumbar nerve roots (L2, L3, or L4) can present with pain in the groin or anterior thigh and into the calf, ankle, or foot (Box 13-1).[81] The pain patterns stemming from disc lesions may be inconsistent, with changes in the position of the lumbar spine reducing the pressure on the nerve root, causing a decrease in symptoms. Because lying down allows the disc to rehydrate, symptoms are usually improved in the morning and worsen as the day progresses. A precise neurological evaluation is needed to determine the spinal levels that are involved. A lower quarter neurological screen is used to evaluate strength, deep tendon reflexes, and sensation. Findings of bilateral leg pain, absent deep tendon reflexes, or changes in bowel and bladder function warrant immediate referral for evaluation of stenosis or **cauda equina syndrome**.

Selective tissue tests are used to confirm the findings identified during the history, inspection, and neurological screening portions of the evaluation. The Valsalva test (see Selective Tissue Test 13-3), SLR and the well SLR (see Selective Tissue Test 13-4), the **femoral nerve stretch test** (Selective Tissue Test 13-7), the **tension sign** (Selective Tissue Test 13-8), and the **Milgram test** (Selective Tissue Test 13-9) are commonly used to identify intervertebral disc lesions or resulting radiculopathy. **Kernig's test** and its modification the Brudzinski test are also used to identify disc pathology, but they present positive results in the presence of inflammation of the nerve or its dural sheath; most references implicate positive findings as a sign of meningitis (Fig. 13-23).[90,91]

Standard radiographic examinations are effective only in measuring secondary changes associated with disc degeneration (i.e., a narrowing of the intervertebral space). The evaluation of disc changes through diagnostic imaging is

Box 13-1
Sciatica: "Shin Splints" of the Spine

Sciatica, a nondescript general term for any inflammation involving the sciatic nerve, does not describe the actual condition that is insulting the nerve and causing the inflammation. Whenever possible, this term should be avoided in favor of a more definitive diagnosis and/or treatment plan. Causes of sciatica include lumbar disc herniation, SI joint dysfunction, piriformis muscle spasm, scar tissue formation around the nerve root, nerve root inflammation, spinal stenosis, synovial cysts, cancerous or noncancerous tumors, and other disease states.[82-89]

Examination Findings 13-1
Lumbar Disc Pathology

Examination Segment	Clinical Findings
History of Current Condition	*Onset:* Insidious: Degeneration Acute: Rupture *Pain characteristics:* Pain localized to the affected segment; compression of the spinal nerve root leading to pain in the low back and buttocks possibly radiating into the thigh, calf, heel, and foot *Other symptoms:* Paresthesia along the affected dermatome *Mechanism:* Repetitive loading of the intervertebral disc over time *Risk factors:* History of lumbar spine trauma
Functional Assessment	Identify movement patterns that increase or decrease the symptoms. Motion that decreases symptoms is useful in determining the appropriate intervention. The single-leg sit-to-stand provides a functional assessment of knee extensor strength. Slow gait Changes in position are guarded and painful.
Inspection	Flattened lumbar spine
Palpation	Spasm of the musculature possible
Joint and Muscle Function Assessment	*AROM:* Limited by pain in all directions *MMT:* Weakness of the abdominal muscles may be noted. The patient may be unable to maintain a neutral spine. *PROM:* Hip flexion may be limited.
Joint Stability Tests	*Stress tests:* Not applicable *Joint play:* Initially, increased P–A mobility is demonstrated. As the condition worsens, the amount of play decreases.
Selective Tissue Tests	Straight leg raising, slump, well straight leg raising, Milgram test, sciatic and femoral nerve tension tests, bowstring sign
Neurological Screening	Lower quarter screen
Vascular Screening	Within normal limits
Imaging Techniques	Discography MRI can visualize the annulus fibrosus, nucleus pulposus, spinal cord, spinal nerve roots, and vertebrae and represents the reference standard for diagnosis of nerve root impingement; however, degenerative changes to the disc as assessed via MRI are often present in asymptomatic people.[78,79] Standard lumbar spine radiographs are reliable for making a definitive diagnosis of lumbar disc degeneration. All discs tend to begin degenerating by the fourth decade of life and may be a concurrent finding with other spine pathology.
Differential Diagnosis	Spondylolytic change, facet joint dysfunction, spinal stenosis, piriformis syndrome, peripheral nerve entrapment, tumor
Comments	Cases of lumbar disc degeneration are often first reported as complaints of a hamstring injury or knee pain.[80]

AROM = active range of motion; MMT = manual muscle test; P–A = posterior-to-anterior; PROM = passive range of motion

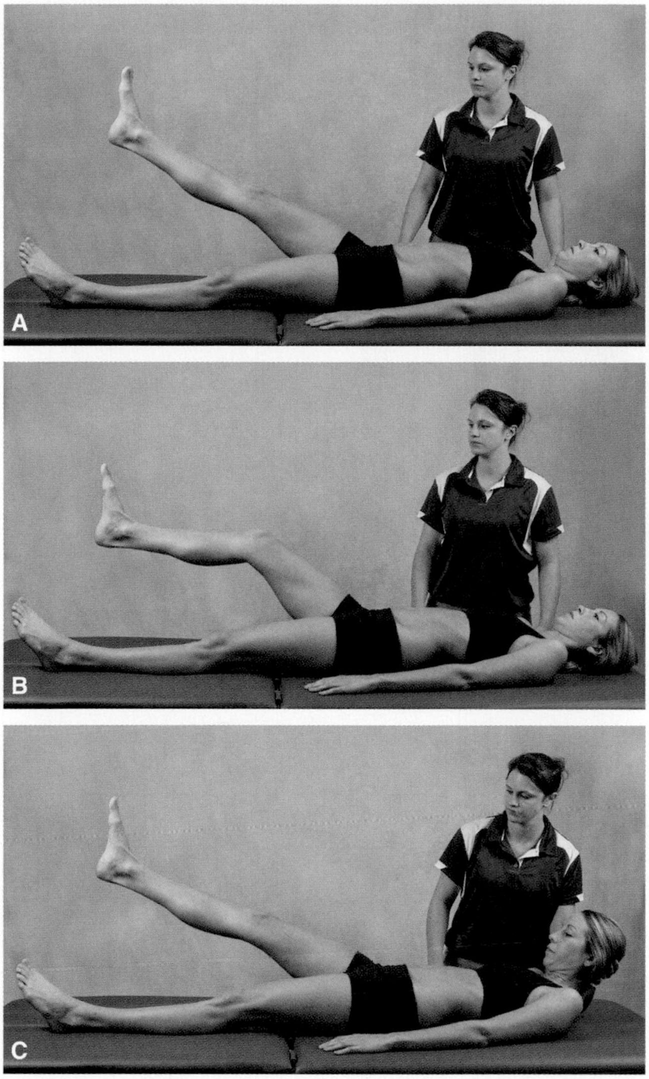

FIGURE 13-23 ■ Modifications of tension signs. (A & B) The Kernig test identifies nerve root entrapment caused by a bulging of an intervertebral disc or narrowing of the intervertebral foramen. The Brudzinski test (C) identifies symptoms caused by a stretching of the dural sheath. Both tests are also identified as meningeal signs, indicating a connection between positive findings and meningitis.

made more effective with MRI scans. MRI has a high sensitivity in detecting those who do not have disc herniation. A negative finding is good evidence that the patient does not have disc involvement. The high number of asymptomatic individuals with apparent disc degeneration makes the determination that the disc is contributing to symptoms more difficult, and MRI findings must be coupled with examination and history for a diagnosis.[93] Discography, a contrast dye injected into a disc to enhance the ensuing computed tomography (CT) images, is often considered to be the gold standard for diagnosing intervertebral disc lesions.

Disc Herniation Intervention Strategy

Often, patients with disc herniations fall into the specific exercise treatment classification system (See Fig. 13-20), whereby symptoms centralize using repeated movements in the same direction. Rehabilitation exercises consist of those motions, usually extension motions, and, ultimately, core stability and pelvic stabilization exercises. Physical activity is encouraged and has demonstrated a positive impact on recovery.[24] Disc pathology that does not respond to conservative care may require surgery to remove the involved section of the intervertebral disc and fuse the superior and inferior vertebrae.[10]

Segmental Instability

Stability of the spinal segment comes from active restraints (muscles), passive restraints (ligaments, facet joints, discs, vertebral bodies, and tension from musculotendinous units) and neural control.[17] Dysfunction in any of these can result in instability. For example, spondylolisthesis results in instability as a bony restraint is disrupted. Muscle weakness can result in a decreased ability to provide active stability.

Patients with segmental instability describe frequent recurrences of low back pain resulting from seemingly mild aggravating factors. They report increased pain with rolling over in bed and in the morning.[94] Rising from a seated position may also be painful. Returning to standing from a forward flexed position may reveal a "catch" or jerky movement, a compensatory response to a lack of stability. P–A joint play at the involved segment may demonstrate increased motion at that segment, with decreased joint play at the above and below segments, although this technique has widely variable reliability.[24] The **prone instability test** (Selective Tissue Test 13-10) examines the extent to which symptoms are reduced when stabilization is present.

Segmental Instability Intervention Strategy

Those with segmental instability generally benefit from stabilization exercises that emphasize postural control, core stability, and biomechanical education. Core stabilization exercises initially emphasize trunk control using the transversus abdominus and multifidii muscles and progress to exercises that require maintenance of that stabilization during increasingly complex movement patterns.

*** Practical Evidence**

Clusters of test findings may help identify appropriate treatments. Patients with a positive prone instability test, notable aberrant movement patterns, straight leg motion greater than 91 degrees, and who are under the age of 40 are more likely to benefit from stabilization exercises.[51]

Erector Spinae Muscle Tears

Acute injury of the spinal erector muscle group may be one of the most common orthopedic conditions seen for treatment.[95,96] Although injury to the lumbar musculature is common, it tends to be self-limiting conditions. Similar to sprains of the spinal ligaments, muscle tears are usually diagnosed after the exclusion of all other possible problems. Commonly, the patient presents with a history of heavy or

Selective Tissue Test 13-7
Femoral Nerve Stretch Test

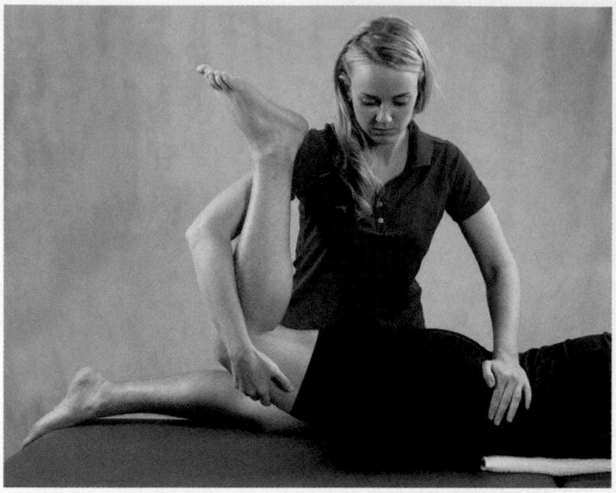

The tension placed on the femoral nerve (L2, L3, L4) is increased by passively flexing the patient's knee. The test can be modified by extending the hip.[92] Nerve root impingement will result in radicular pain in the anterior and/or lateral thigh.

Patient Position	Prone with a pillow under the abdomen
Position of Examiner	At the side of the patient
Evaluative Procedure	The examiner passively flexes the patient's knee.
Positive Test	Pain is elicited in the anterior and lateral thigh.
Implications	Nerve root impingement at the L2, L3, or L4 level
Modification	The femoral nerve may be further stressed by passively extending the patient's hip while maintaining knee flexion.[92] If the patient cannot lie prone, the test can be performed in side-lying with the pelvis stabilized.
Comments	This test is associated with a high number of false positives due to tight or injured quadriceps. The cross femoral stretch is positive when testing the opposite leg produces symptoms on the involved side.

Evidence

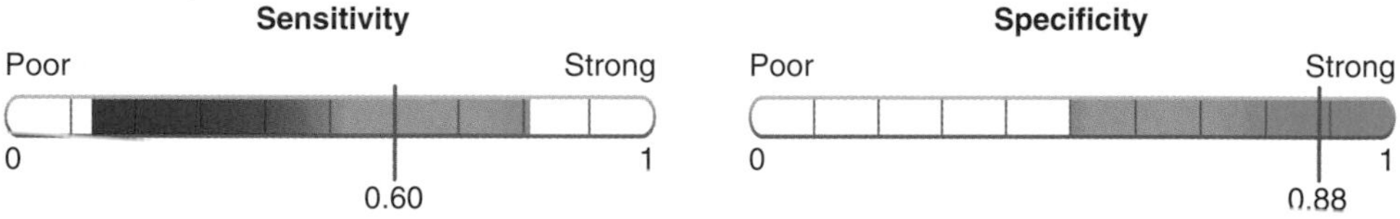

LR+: 0–5.83

LR−: 0.34–0.50–0.94

Selective Tissue Test 13-8
Tension Sign

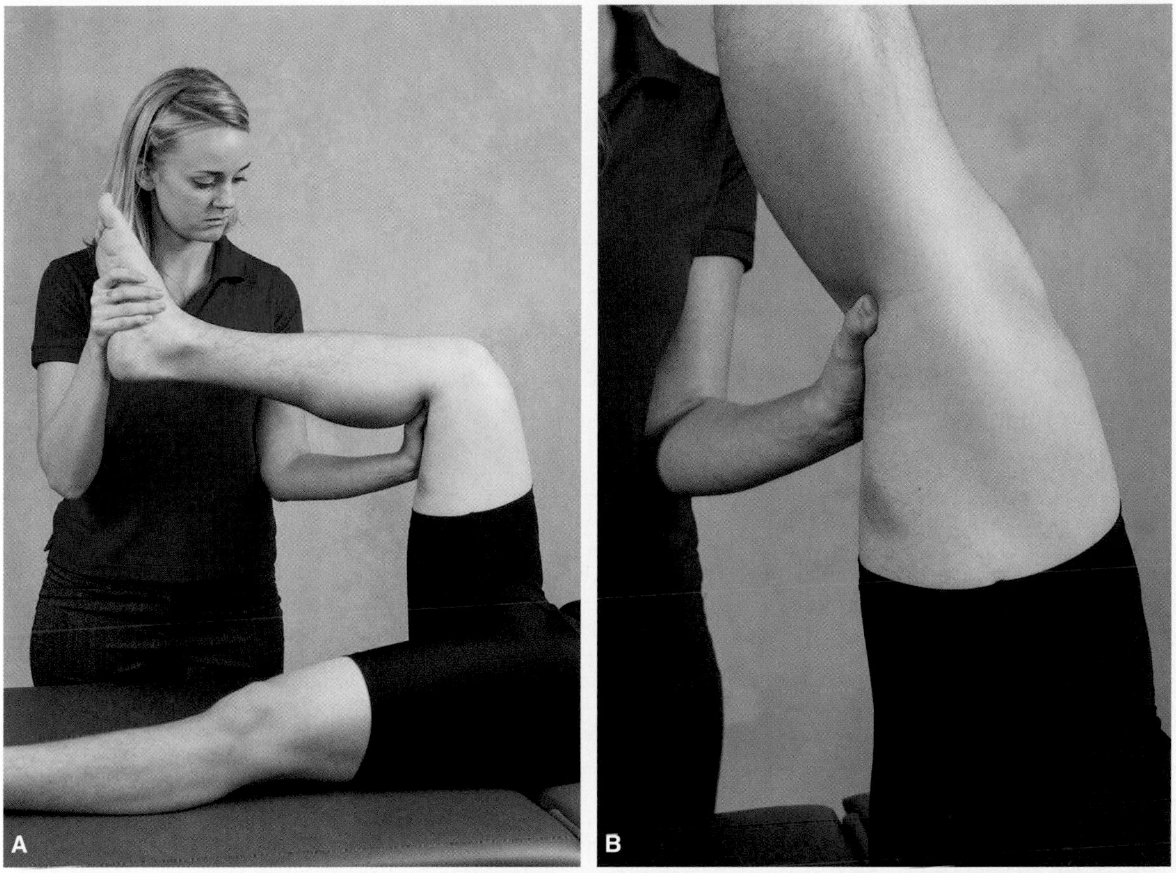

The sciatic nerve is stretched by extending the patient's knee with the hip flexed to 90° while palpating the nerve as it passes through the popliteal fossa.

Patient Position	Supine
Position of Examiner	At the patient's side that is to be tested; one hand grasps the heel, while the other grasps the thigh.
Evaluative Procedure	The hip is flexed to 90°, with the knee flexed to 90° (A). The knee is then extended as far as possible, with the examiner palpating the tibial portion of the sciatic nerve as it passes through the popliteal space (B).
Positive Test	Exquisite tenderness with possible duplication of sciatic symptoms, as compared with the opposite side
Implications	Sciatic nerve irritation
Modification	The bowstring test is a variation of this technique. The examiner extends the patient's knee until radiating symptoms are experienced. The knee is then flexed approximately 20° or until the symptoms are relieved. The examiner then pushes on the tibial portion of the sciatic nerve to reestablish the symptoms.
Evidence	Absent or inconclusive in the literature

Selective Tissue Test 13-9
Milgram Test

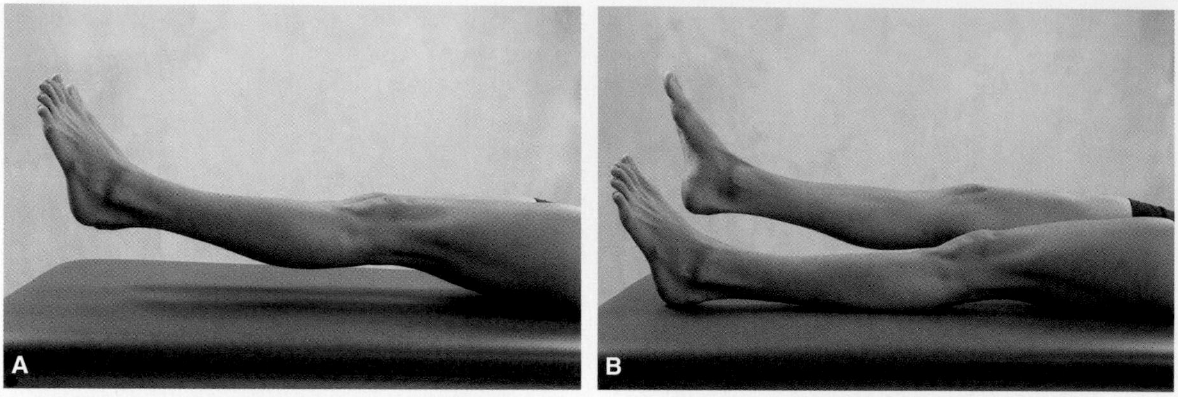

A bilateral SLR is used to increase pressure on the lumbar nerve roots. In the presence of a disc lesion, one or both legs will drop.

Patient Position	Supine
Position of Examiner	At the feet of the patient
Evaluative Procedure	**(A)** The patient performs a bilateral SLR to the height of 2–6 inches and is asked to hold the position for 30 seconds.
Positive Test	**(B)** The patient is unable to hold the position, cannot lift the leg, or experiences pain with the test.
Implications	Intrathecal or extrathecal pressure causing an intervertebral disc to place pressure on a lumbar nerve root
Evidence	Absent or inconclusive in the literature

repetitive lifting and complaints of aching pain centralized to the low back. Pain increases with passive and active flexion as well as resisted extension. Lower quarter screens show negative results.

Facet Joint Dysfunction

The lumbar facet joints give the spine rigidity and protect the intervertebral discs against rotational injury.[97,98] As with much lumbar spine pathology, facet joint pathology is closely linked to pathology in other spine components. For example, degenerative changes in the disc significantly increase load and subsequent degeneration of the facet joints.[99] Conversely, degenerative changes in the facet joint can alter load and ultimately damage the disc. Other associated pathologies, such as muscle spasm, may be protective in nature.

Facet joint pathology may involve subluxation of the facet or degeneration of the facet itself leading to hypermobility and osteophyte formation. A subluxed facet joint tends to "lock" the involved spinal segment, causing the involved segment to become hypomobile and the adjacent segments to become hypermobile over time (see Joint Play 13-1). The patient may report a history of extension, rotation, or lateral bending of the spine with pain that tends to be localized over the affected facet. Prolonged standing often provokes symptoms, as do motions that repeatedly load the joint such as extension, rotation, and side bending to the involved side (Examination Findings 13-2).[100]

Facet joint pathology often occurs from repetitive stress to the facet joint through movement or loading. Although pain is often localized to the region of the involved facets, radiating pain into the buttock, groin, or thigh that stops above the knee and accompanying hamstring tightness may also be present. Note that these are also symptoms associated with herniated discs.

Degeneration of the facet joint has an undefined history of injury. If the degeneration is significant, the size of the intervertebral foramen will decrease, potentially impinging the associated nerve root and causing radicular pain. Nerve entrapment can be reduced by the patient's assuming a posture that decreases pressure on the nerve root, usually caused by flexion reducing the size of the intervertebral foramen. A definitive diagnosis of facet joint degeneration is made using computed tomography or by relief of symptoms following injection of an anesthetic into the facet joint.[99,100]

Facet Joint Pathology Intervention Strategies

When facet joint pathology presents acutely and with no symptoms distal to the knee, the patient may benefit from manipulation (i.e., high-velocity thrust) performed by someone qualified in the technique. Other initial treatment of patients with facet joint pathologies involves the use of nonsteroidal anti-inflammatory drugs (NSAIDs) to decrease pain and facilitate movement. Instruct the patient to avoid postures and movements that irritate the facet and

Selective Tissue Test 13-10
Prone Instability Test

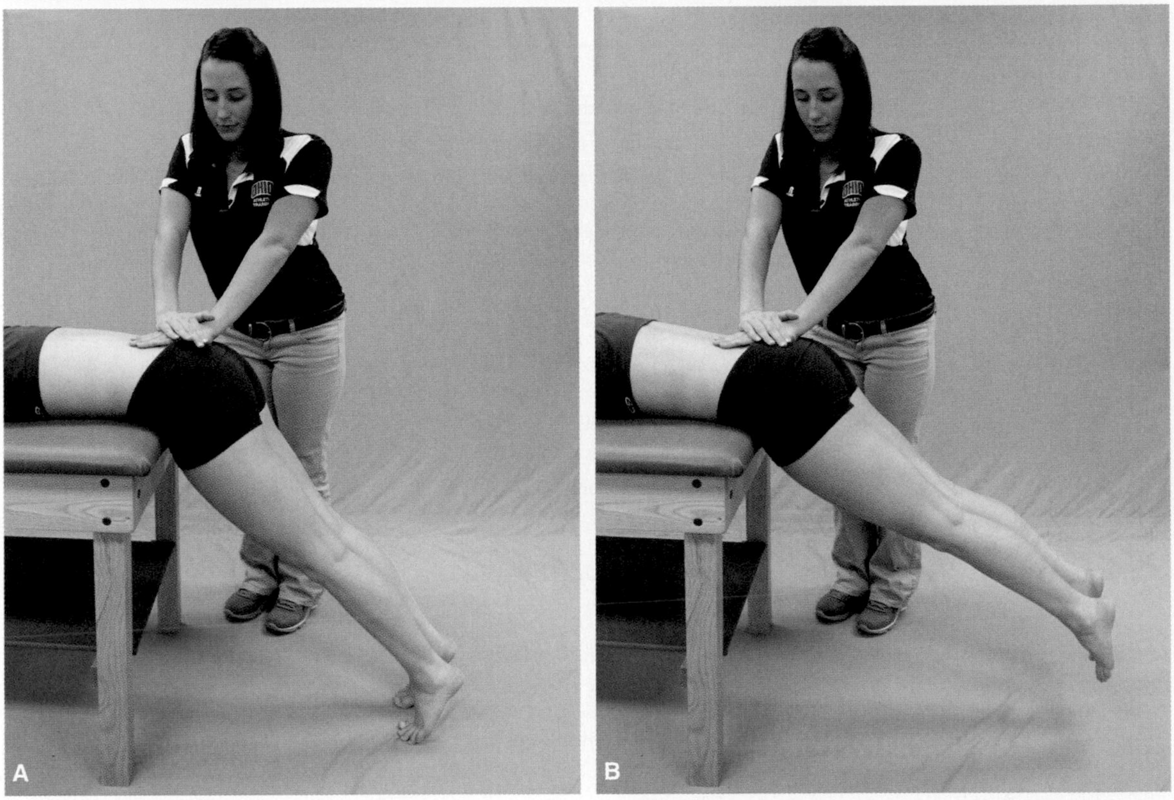

The prone instability test assesses the influence of dynamic stabilization. In the presence of segmental instability, the patient's symptoms will reduce when an external stabilizing force is applied. Patients with a reduction in symptoms tend to respond favorably to a spinal stabilization program.

Patient Position	The patient is prone with the trunk on the table, the pelvis off the table, and the feet on the floor.
Position of Examiner	At the side of the patient
Evaluative Procedure	The examiner applies P–A force on each spinous process of the lumbar spine, noting any provocation of pain and the involved level(s). The patient next lifts both feet off the floor, holding the table to maintain the position. The examiner then again applies the P–A force at the previously symptomatic level, noting any change in symptoms.
Positive Test	Symptoms that are provoked with unstabilized P–A glides are reduced when the trunk musculature is activated.
Implications	Active stabilization protects hypermobile segments, indicating that stabilization exercises may prove beneficial.
Modification	Perform the initial P–A glides with the patient fully supported on the table.
Evidence	

Inter-rater Reliability

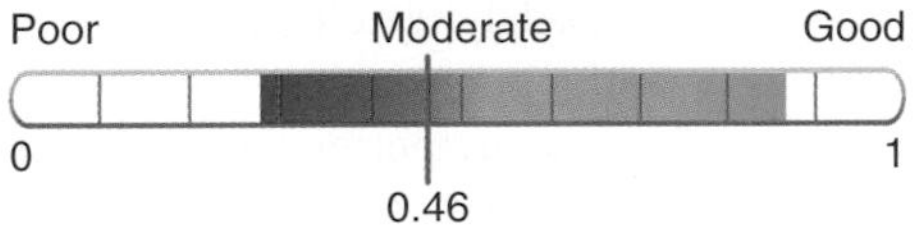

LR+: 1.70

LR−: 0.48

P–A = posterior-to-anterior

Examination Findings 13-2
Facet Joint Dysfunction

Examination Segment	Clinical Findings
History of Current Condition	*Onset:* Insidious or acute *Pain characteristics:* Localized over the involved facets and the surrounding musculature *Mechanism:* Extension, rotation, or lateral bending of the vertebrae *Risk factors:* Repeated motions of spinal extension, rotation, or lateral bending; lumbar disc pathology
Functional Assessment	Activities or motions that require extension, rotation, and/or lateral bending to the involved side all produce pain. Prolonged standing may exacerbate symptoms.
Inspection	The patient may assume a posture that decreases the pressure on the affected facets.
Palpation	Possible local muscle spasm is noted in the paravertebral muscles.
Joint and Muscle Function Assessment	*AROM:* Increased pain with extension and rotation, alleviation with flexion *MMT:* May have extensor weakness *PROM:* Increased pain with prone press-up
Joint Stability Tests	*Stress tests:* Not applicable *Joint play:* Spring test may cause pain or reveal hypo- or hypermobility.
Selective Tissue Tests	Quadrant test may be positive. Tests for concomitant intervertebral disc lesion may be positive.
Neurological Screening	Within normal limits unless secondary nerve root impingement occurs Secondary nerve root impingement warrants a lower quarter screen (see Neurological Screening 13-1).
Vascular Screening	Within normal limits
Imaging Techniques	CT scan is preferred over MRI for detecting osteophyte formation and osteoarthritis.[99]
Differential Diagnosis	Herniated disc, spondylotic defect
Comments	Continued degeneration of the facet joint may reduce the size of the intervertebral foramen and result in compression of the spinal nerve root. Diagnosis is definitively made via pain relief after injection of an anesthetic into the joint.[100]

AROM = active range of motion; CT = computed tomography; MMT = manual muscle test; PROM = passive range of motion

increase pain, especially sleeping in a prone position. Local therapeutic modalities such as moist heat, electrical stimulation, or ice may be helpful to decrease subsequent muscle spasm. Long-term treatment revolves around restoring normal arthrokinematics by mobilizing hypomobile segments and using stabilization exercises to control hypermobility. Facet joint injections may be helpful to reduce pain and spasm and allow sufficient strengthening and stabilization to occur.[100]

Spondylopathies

Bony disorders of the posterior elements of the spinal column, spondylopathies, are a common cause of persistent low back pain in young athletes[101] and tend to be more prevalent in those who repeatedly hyperextend and rotate, or rotate their torso against resistance during activity.[102] The development of spondylolysis is general attributed to repetitive microtrauma and/or a genetic predisposition to thinner, weakened, or elongated pars interarticularis.[102] Lumbar spondylytic defects are rarely caused by acute trauma. These defects are caused by repetitive forced hyperextension such as that experienced by football linemen, gymnasts, divers, and cheerleaders. Spondylopathies most commonly occur at the L5 level but may develop anywhere along the vertebral column.[102] Table 13-8 presents a description of terminology associated with common spondylopathies.

Spondylolysis

Spondylolysis is a defect in the pars interarticularis, the area of the vertebral arch between the inferior and superior articular facets, usually brought on by repetitive stress. It can occur bilaterally or unilaterally (Examination Findings 13-3). Bilateral defects in the pars interarticularis result in

Examination Findings 13-3
Spondylolysis and Spondylolisthesis

Examination Segment	Clinical Findings
History of Current Condition	*Onset:* Insidious; the pain begins as an ache and evolves to constant pain. *Pain characteristics:* Pain in the lumbar spine, possibly radiating into the buttocks and upper portion of the posterolateral thighs.[80] Pain may increase with activity and subside with rest. *Mechanism:* Repeated extension *Risk factors:* Adolescence, when pars is thinner; imbalances in trunk muscular strength, endurance, and flexibility; activities that repetitively place the lumbar spine into hyperextension; females have a higher incidence rate of spondylolisthesis than males.
Functional Assessment	Activities that require extension, such as reaching high overhead, may produce symptoms. The patient may walk with a stiff legged and/or short stride.
Inspection	Gross inspection of the spinal curvatures may reveal hyperlordosis in the lumbar spine.
Palpation	Spondylolisthesis: A palpable "step-off" deformity may be detected at the involved lumbar level. Possible spasm of the paraspinal muscles may be noted.
Joint and Muscle Function Assessment	*AROM:* ROM during trunk flexion is restricted but pain free. Pain is described, or a "catch" is experienced as the patient returns to an upright posture and during active extension of the spine. Pain may also be elicited during lumbar rotation and lateral rotation. *MMT:* Weakness of the spinal erector muscles *PROM:* Muscle length assessment reveals hamstring tightness.
Joint Stability Tests	*Stress tests:* Not applicable *Joint play:* Spring test may reveal pain and/or hypermobility at the involved segment.
Selective Tissue Tests	Single-leg stance; SLRs may produce a pain that is worse than that normally caused by tightness of the hamstring group.
Neurological Screening	Lower quarter screen is used to rule out involvement of one or more lumbar nerve roots. Results of this are typically negative, but the presence of positive neurological signs can indicate that the vertebrae is slipping, requiring immediate physician referral.
Vascular Screening	Within normal limits
Imaging Techniques	Radiographs are used to identify defects in the pars. A lateral view will reveal anterior slippage associated with spondylolisthesis. Spinal instability associated with spondylolisthesis can be diagnosed using flexion and extension radiographs.[102,106] CT scans have slightly higher sensitivity than bone scans with less radiation exposure.[106] MRI may be helpful to detect early spondylolysis that is not detectable on standard radiographs.[107]
Differential Diagnosis	Disc herniation, facet joint pathology
Comments	Tightness of the hamstrings or weakness of the abdominal muscles may be noted. Refer to Chapter 6 for muscle length assessment techniques.

AROM = active range of motion; CT = computed tomography; MRI = magnetic resonance imaging; PROM = passive range of motion; ROM = range of motion

Table 13-8 Classification of Spondylopathies

Term	Description
Spondylalgia	Pain arising from the vertebrae
Spondylitis	Inflammation of the vertebrae
Spondylolisthesis	Forward slippage of a vertebra on the one below it (may occur secondary to spondylolysis, in which the fracture of the pars interarticularis results in the anterior displacement of the vertebral body)
Spondylolysis	Degeneration of a vertebral structure secondary to repetitive stress, most commonly affecting the pars interarticularis but with no displacement of the vertebral body
Spondylopathy	Any disorder of the vertebrae
Spondylosis	Arthritis or osteoarthritis of the vertebrae; results in pressure being placed on the vertebral nerve roots

listhesis. The anterosuperior segment, consisting of the vertebral body, pedicles, and transverse processes, separates from the posteroinferior segment, consisting of the laminae, inferior articular processes, and spinous processes.[102] This defect, when seen on an oblique radiographic view, appears as a "collared Scotty dog" deformity, with the area of the stress fracture representing the dog's collar (Fig. 13-24). Defects in the pars are a common radiological finding in individuals with no symptoms, so CT scans are used to determine whether or not the fracture site is metabolically active.[103,104] Radiographs may show a flattening of the inferior facet on the vertebra above the affected site.[105]

The patient presents with localized low back pain that is increased during and after activity but decreases with rest. During observation, spinal alignment is usually normal. Those with spondylotic defects typically describe a pattern where extension (e.g., standing and walking) is aggravating and symptoms are alleviated with postures or activities that incorporate more flexion (e.g., sitting). Active ROM is normal for flexion, but pain restricts extension. Results of selective tissue tests and neurological tests are normal. The evaluative findings of advanced spondylolysis resemble those of spondylolisthesis.

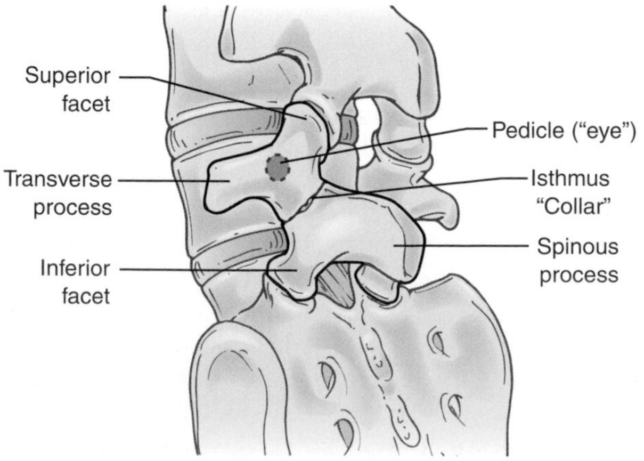

FIGURE 13-24 ■ "Collared Scotty dog" deformity. On an oblique radiograph, the presence of a collar on the Scotty dog indicates a nondisplaced stress fracture on the pars interarticularis, spondylolysis.

✻ Practical Evidence

Peak bone mineral density is realized between 20 and 30 years of age. Because of hormonal changes and decreased calcium intake, the risk of osteoporosis may be increased in endurance runners. Although this change is most common in females, males are also affected. After peak bone mass has been obtained, both males and females demonstrate decreased density with each cycle of remodeling. In females, this loss is accelerated in early menopause. Consequently, decreased bone mineral density increases the risk of stress fractures.[108]

Spondylolisthesis

Spondylolysis may progress to spondylolisthesis, in which the defects in both elements of the pars interarticularis result in the separation of the vertebrae into two uniquely identifiable structures and resulting spinal instability. The fixation between the affected vertebra and the one below it is lost, resulting in the superior vertebra's sliding anteriorly, and possibly inferiorly, on the one below it (Fig. 13-25). A

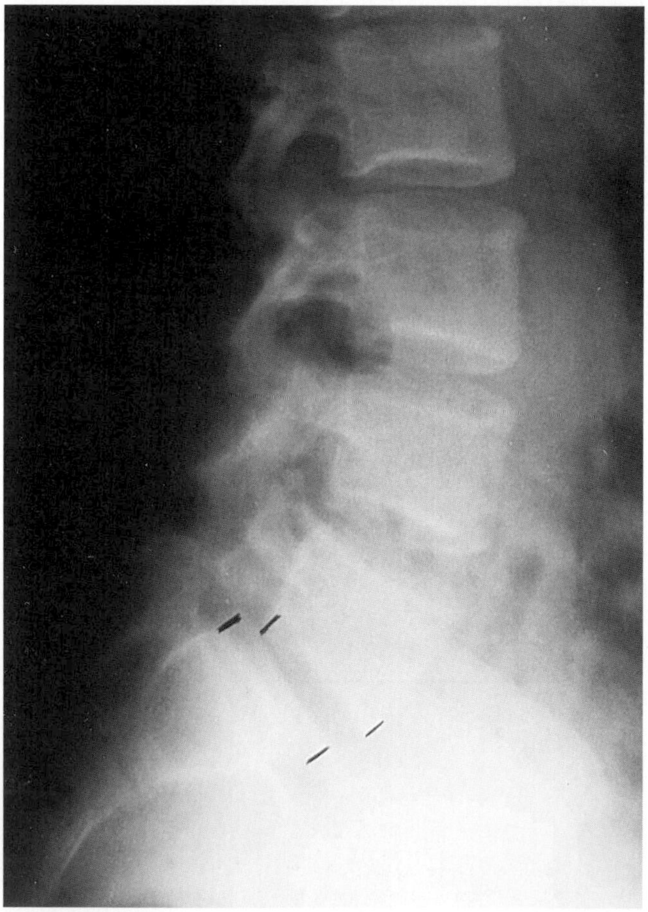

FIGURE 13-25 ■ Spondylolisthesis of the L5-S1 junction as seen on a lateral radiograph. Notice that the L5 vertebra is anteriorly displaced relative to S1.

radiographic examination of this condition reveals a "decapitated Scotty dog" deformity, in which the head of the dog, the anterior element of the vertebra, has become detached from the body, the posterior element (Fig. 13-26). The severity of the spondylolisthesis is determined by the relative amount of anterior displacement of the vertebra. After the fracture occurs, the displacement of the vertebra usually does not progress under the normal daily stresses.[109] However, the stresses of sports and other exertive activities may increase the amount of anterior displacement. True healing of the fracture site rarely occurs.[110]

Practical Evidence

Approximately half of the individuals diagnosed with spondylolisthesis will also demonstrate thoracic kyphosis, a slouching posture, anterior wedging of the vertebrae, and intravertebral disc herniation, or **Scheuermann's disease**.[80]

Spondylolisthesis is most prevalent in adolescents under the age of 16 and in women. Also, young gymnasts have an incidence of pars interarticularis defects four times higher than that of the average population.[111] Patients with spondylolisthesis have a history and physical presentation that is very similar to that of spondylolysis, with increased symptoms in postures that emphasize trunk extension. During AROM, the patient may reveal a "catch" when returning to upright from a flexed position.[112] The pain may be more intense and is likely to be more constant. On observation and with palpation of the spinous processes, an actual step-off deformity may be identified, as the normal continuity of the lumbar spine is lost when the vertebra shifts forward. Detecting anterior slippage via palpation has poor interrater reliability.[113] More severe cases of spondylolisthesis result in a flattening of the buttocks when viewed laterally and more severe limitations in ROM. As with intervertebral disc pathologies, pain may be described in the lumbar region when the patient returns to a standing posture.

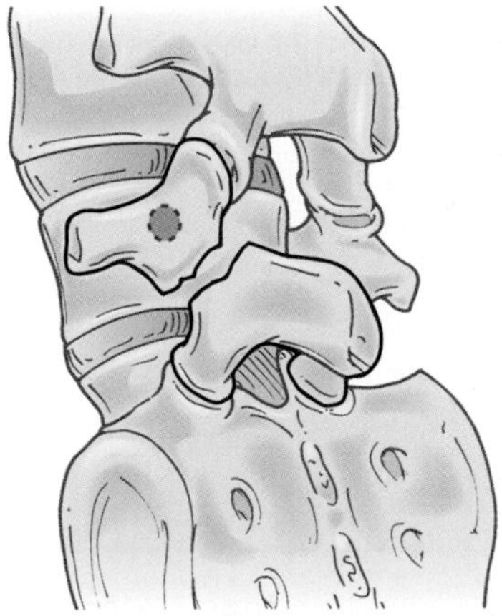

FIGURE 13-26 ■ "Decapitated Scotty dog" deformity. Further degeneration of the pars interarticularis can lead to a displaced fracture, spondylolisthesis. Here the "collared Scotty dog" loses its head as the superior vertebra slides anteriorly.

Results of selective tissue tests and neurological tests may become positive if the slippage of the vertebra is great enough to impinge on the neurological structures. Pain associated with spondylolysis and early stages of spondylolisthesis tends not to radiate.[109] Although its diagnostic utility is questionable, the **single-leg stance test** (Selective Tissue Test 13-11) may reinforce a suspicion of spondylolysis or spondylolisthesis.[101]

Spondylotic Pathology Intervention Strategies

The treatment of patients with spondylolysis and spondylolisthesis is primarily based on the patient's symptoms. Early detection of spondylolysis is associated with improved fracture healing.[101] Rehabilitation exercises should resolve muscular tightness and strength deficit problems, but extension exercises that place stress on the pars interarticularis are avoided in the early stages.[109,110] Posture awareness is emphasized. The patient is taught how to control pelvic position and instructed about ways to avoid placing the lumbar spine in extension. The most conservative form of treatment, the use of a lumbar brace, is attempted if other forms of rehabilitation fail to produce the desired results.

Sacroiliac Pathology

Although the SI joints are relatively immobile, a slight amount of accessory movement, rotation, or translation of the ilium on the sacrum occurs here. Although there are proponents of hypermobile and/or hypomobile SI joints as the cause of pain, evidence to support mechanical dysfunction of the joint is limited.[114] The SI joint is implicated as the source in approximately13% of patients with nonspecific low back pain.[115] Injury to or degeneration at the pubic symphysis—the anterior connection of the pelvic ring—can also lead to SI symptoms.[14] The resulting pain often resembles lumbar nerve root compression.

Patients with SI joint involvement often describe an acute mechanism such as falling on the buttocks or stepping into an unanticipated hole. Others describe pain of gradual onset. Palpation reveals pain over the PSIS and over the SI joint. Patients may also describe referred pain into the groin region. Functional assessment may reveal a decreased stride length, which decreases the forces transmitted up the leg following initial contact.[116]

Selective tissue tests for the SI joint either try to detect asymmetry or aberrant movement patterns or provoke symptoms by stressing the joint. Provocation tests, such as Gaenslen's test (or Patrick's test), sacral thrust, and thigh thrust are more reliable and valid than tests that attempt to detect differences in movement or position, such as the Gillet test. The amount of mobility at the SI joint is very small (2 mm or less), and individual variation in bony structure is very high, making it unlikely that displacements or changes in mobility can be detected.[27,114,117,118] In general, single tests for SI dysfunction are not reliable measures of the presence of pathology in this region

Selective Tissue Test 13-11
Single-Leg Stance Test

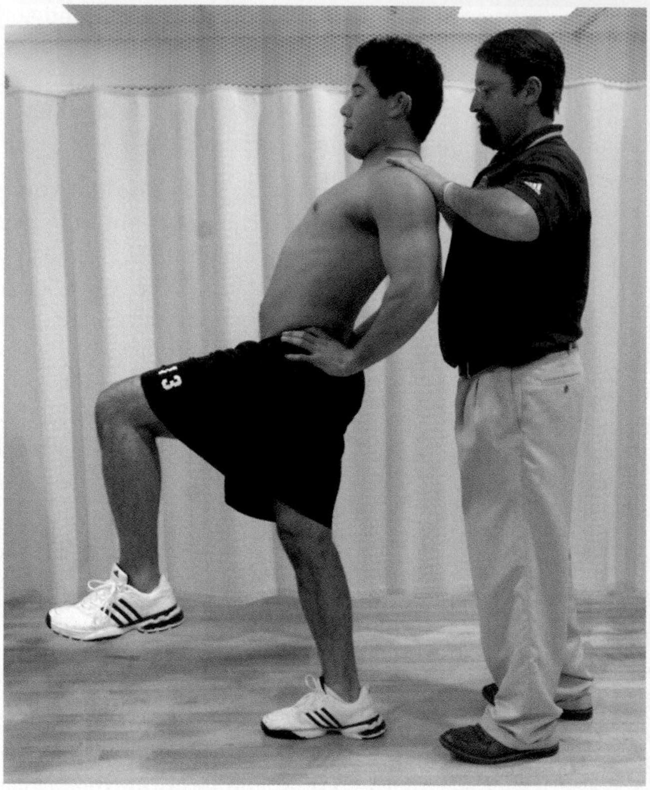

This test reproduces the positions that maximally stress the pars interarticularis by positioning the patient in extension and rotation.

Patient Position	Standing with the body weight evenly distributed between the two feet
Position of Examiner	Standing behind the patient, ready to provide support if the patient is unstable.
Evaluative Procedure	The patient lifts one leg, then places the trunk in hyperextension. The examiner may assist the patient during this motion. The procedure is then repeated for the opposite leg.
Positive Test	Pain is noted in the lumbar spine or SI area.
Implications	Shear forces are placed on the pars interarticularis by the iliopsoas pulling the vertebra anteriorly, resulting in pain.
Comments	When the lesion to the pars interarticularis is unilateral, pain is evoked when the opposite leg is raised. Bilateral pars fractures result in pain when either leg is lifted. This test may also result in pain specifically at the area of the PSIS secondary to SI joint irritation.
Evidence	

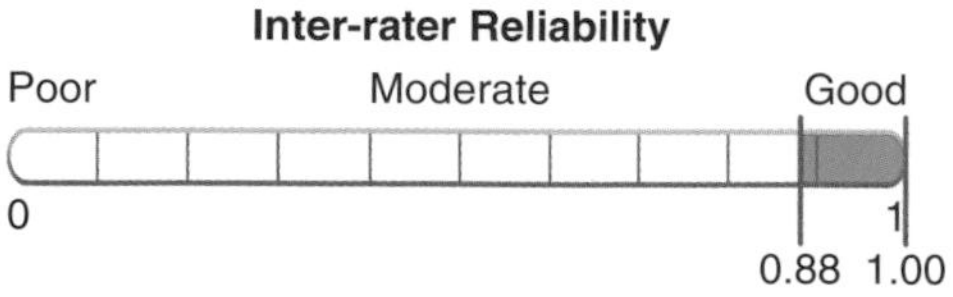

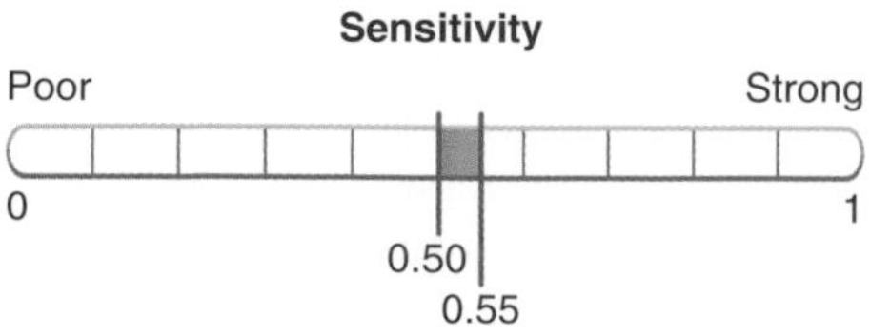

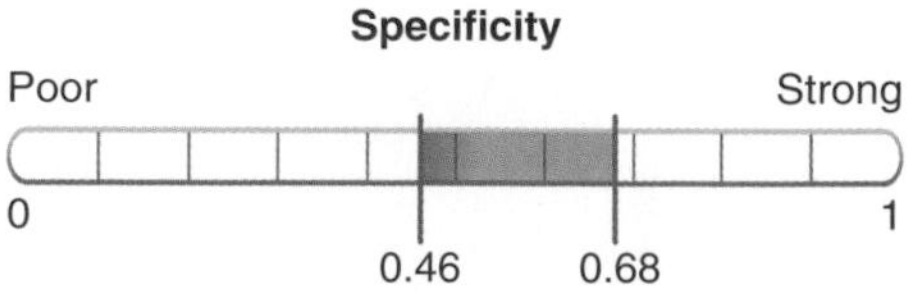

LR+: 1.02–1.56

LR−: 0.74–0.98

PSIS = posterior superior iliac spine; SI = sacroiliac

(Examination Findings 13-4).[27,114-117,119] Combining the results of a series of provocation tests, however, may improve diagnostic accuracy.[114,116] The validity of test clusters improves when a patient's symptoms do not centralize with repeated extension or flexion, that is, the pain is less likely to be of discogenic origin.[114]

Compression or distraction of the two halves of the pelvis creates tension at the SI joint, resulting in a duplication of the patient's symptoms if the joint is involved (Selective Tissue Test 13-12). The **FABER test** (Selective Tissue Test 13-13), or **Patrick's test**, is used to elicit pain in the SI joints and the hip. The term *FABER* is used as a mnemonic describing the position of the hip during testing: **F**lexion, **AB**duction, **E**xternal **R**otation, and Extension. **Gaenslen's test** (Selective Tissue Test 13-14) is used to place a rotatory stress on the SI joint by forcing one hip into hyperextension while the other hip is flexed. Applying a vertically oriented force through the femur on the patient's flexed hip, the **thigh thrust test** creates a posterior force on the ipsilateral SI joint (Selective Tissue Test 13-15). The sacral thrust test applies an anteriorly directed force at the midline of the sacrum at the apex of its curve, creating a posterior shearing force at the SI joint (Selective Tissue Test 13-16).

If a theory of mechanical dysfunction is supported, then differences in motion or position may be detectable. The **Gillet test**, whereby the movement of the PSIS is palpated while the patient flexes the hip, may reveal asymmetry (Fig. 13-27). Tightness of the hip flexors, tightness of the hamstrings, abdominal weakness, or leg-length differences may stress the ilium, causing abnormal rotation. Symptomatic relief following a guided injection of an anesthetic clearly implicates the SI joint as a source of pain.

Sacroiliac Joint Intervention Strategies

Conservative treatment is typical for those with SI joint pathology. Stabilization exercises for the lumbopelvic region are generally integrated into a treatment program and have demonstrated efficacy in postpartum women.[114] Manual therapy, including mobilization and manipulation, is often incorporated if a mechanical dysfunction is suspected. Guided corticosteroid injections may provide symptomatic relief.[114]

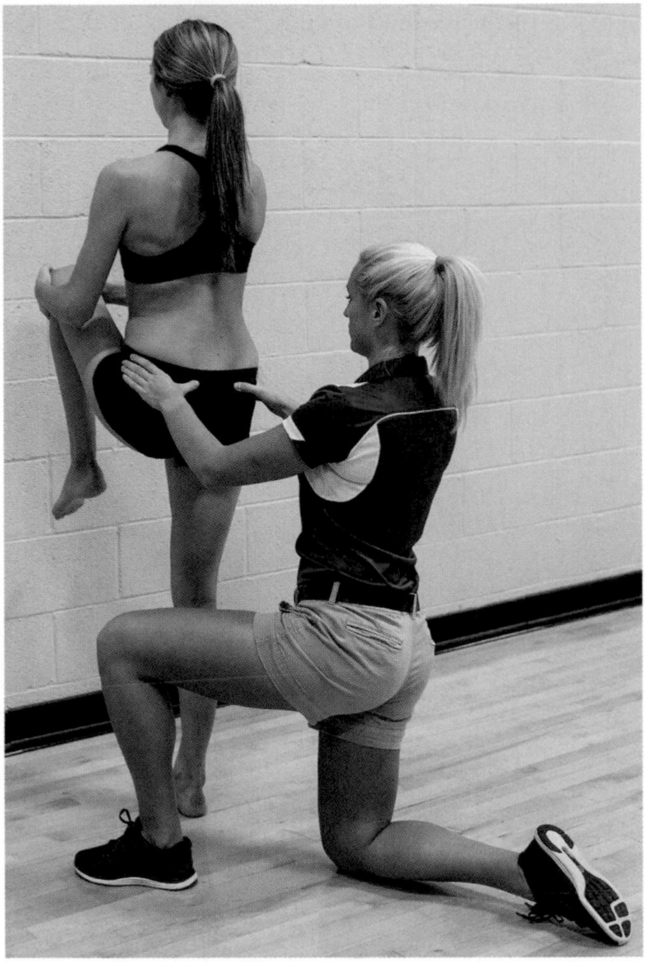

FIGURE 13-27 ■ The Gillet test. To assess for abnormal sacroiliac joint motion the thumbs are placed on each PSIS so that the two thumbs are aligned. The patient then flexes the hip on the side opposite of the palpation. The PSIS on the side of hip flexion should move slightly anteriorly. A positive test is marked by the PSIS on the tested side remaining stationary or moving downward. The test is performed on each side. SI tests that rely on palpation suffer from poor reliability.

Examination Findings 13-4
Sacroiliac Pathology

Examination Segment	Clinical Findings
History of Current Condition	*Onset:* Acute or insidious *Pain characteristics:* Over one or both SI joints; pain possibly radiating to the buttock, groin, or thigh. Pain does not generally go above the L5 level. The patient may complain of anterior pain at the pubis symphysis. *Other symptoms:* Not applicable *Mechanism:* No one mechanism leads to the onset of SI joint pathology, but it may be related to prolonged stresses placed across the SI joint by soft tissues. The patient may describe a fall on the buttocks as the instigating incident. *Risk factors:* Postpartum or pregnant women may be predisposed to SI joint pathology because relaxin released prior to and following birth increases the extensibility of the ligaments surrounding the SI joints. Hormonal changes before the menstrual period may increase the laxity of the SI ligaments, causing SI pain.
Functional Assessment	A shortened stride length may be apparent as the patient attempts to minimize ground reaction forces. Activities that require trunk flexion with the knees extended may cause sufficient movement of the sacrum on the ilia to cause pain.
Inspection	The levels of the iliac crests, ASIS, and PSIS are observed for symmetry.
Palpation	Tenderness may be elicited over the SI joint and the PSIS. Palpation for asymmetry such as unequal heights of the PSIS and ASIS
Joint and Muscle Function Assessment	*AROM:* Pain may be elicited at the extremes of trunk and hip motion. *MMT:* Hip abduction may increase symptoms. *PROM:* Hip flexion greater than 70° may produce symptoms. Restricted hip extension (tight hip flexors)
Joint Stability Tests	*Stress tests:* Not applicable *Joint play:* P–A joint play may provoke symptoms. Many selective tissue tests mimic joint play motions.
Selective Tissue Tests	SI compression and distraction; straight leg raising, FABER test; Gaenslen's test; quadrant test, sacral thrust, thigh thrust
Neurological Screening	A complete lower quarter screen of the sensory, motor, and reflex distributions to rule out lumbar nerve root involvement
Vascular Screening	Within normal limits
Imaging Techniques	Axial CT scans, MRI, and AP and lateral radiographs
Differential Diagnosis	Nerve root impingement, facet joint dysfunction, pelvic stress fracture
Comments	The pain distribution may mimic lumbar nerve root involvement. A combination of findings from multiple selective tissue tests is more reliable than the results of a single test. A diagnosis can be confirmed if an intra-articular injection of an anesthetic relieves symptoms.[114,120]

AP = anteroposterior; AROM = active range of motion; ASIS = anterior superior iliac spine; CT = computed tomography; MMT = manual muscle test; MRI = magnetic resonance imaging; PROM = passive range of motion; PSIS = posterior superior iliac spine; SI = sacroiliac; AROM = active range of motion; CT = computed tomography; MRI = magnetic resonance imaging; PROM = passive range of motion; ROM = range of motion

Selective Tissue Test 13-12
Sacroiliac Joint Compression and Distraction Tests

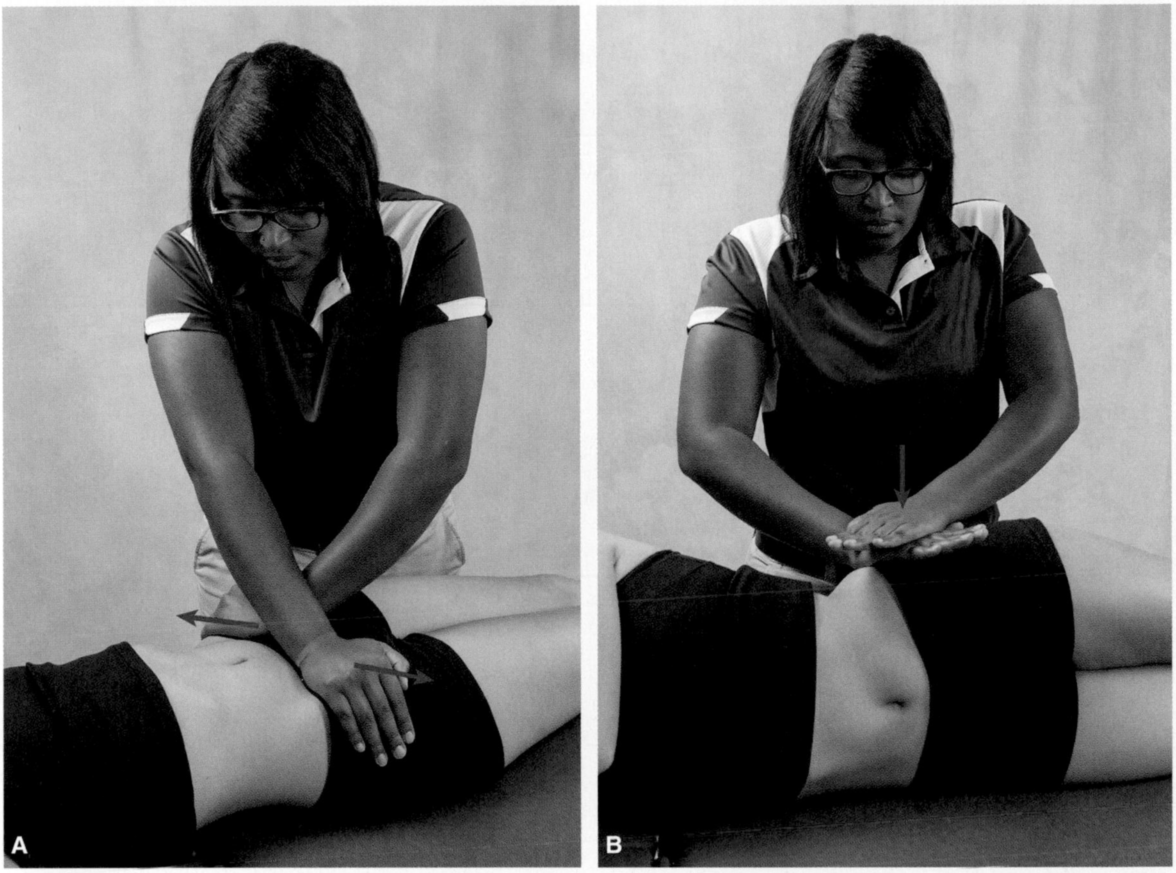

(A) Sacroiliac joint distraction test. (B) Sacroiliac joint compression test. The compression test should be performed on both sides.

Patient Position	***Compression:*** Side-lying, starting with the painful side up. Repeat the test with the painful side downward. ***Distraction:*** Supine
Position of Examiner	***Compression:*** Behind the patient with both hands over the lateral aspect of the pelvis ***Distraction:*** Standing next to the patient with each hand placed over the patient's corresponding ilial flare
Evaluative Procedure	***Compression:*** The examiner applies a downward force, thus compressing the posterior portions of the SI joints. ***Distraction:*** The examiner applies pressure down through the anterior portion of the ilium, spreading the anterior portions of the SI joints.
Positive Test	Pain arising from the SI joint
Implications	Sacroiliac pathology

Continued

Selective Tissue Test 13-12
Sacroiliac Joint Compression and Distraction Tests—cont'd

Evidence

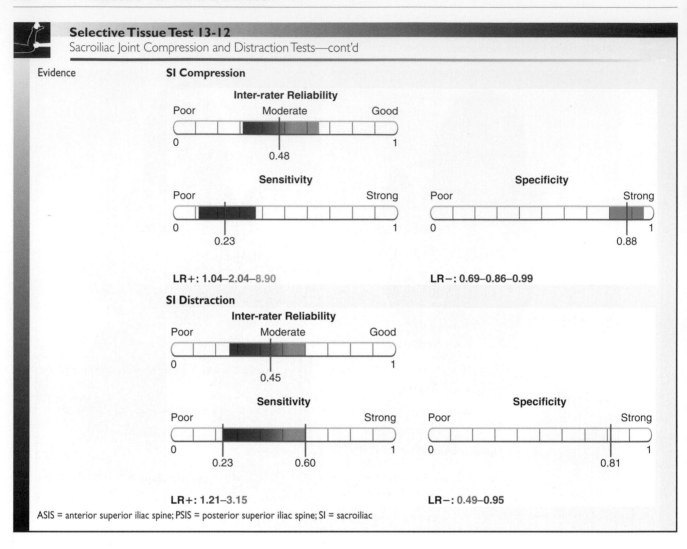

SI Compression

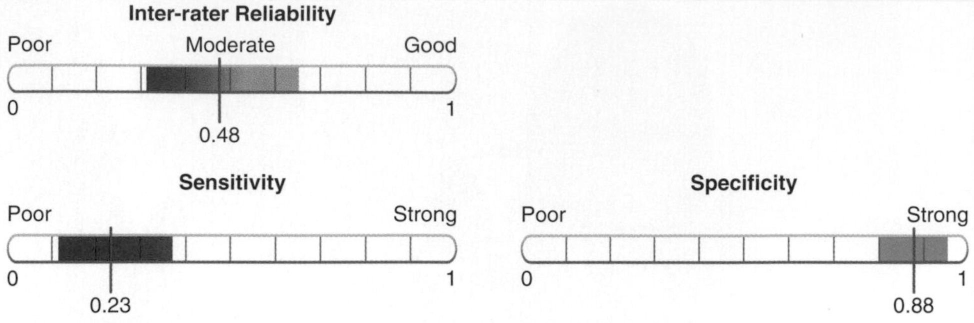

LR+: 1.04–2.04–8.90

LR−: 0.69–0.86–0.99

SI Distraction

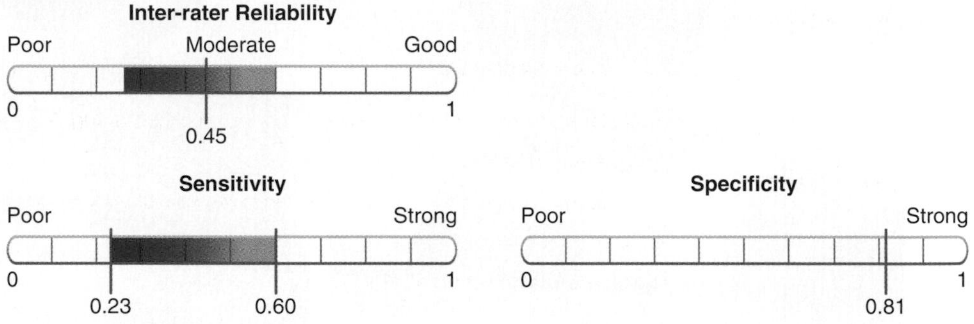

LR+: 1.21–3.15

LR−: 0.49–0.95

ASIS = anterior superior iliac spine; PSIS = posterior superior iliac spine; SI = sacroiliac

Selective Tissue Test 13-13
FABER (Patrick's) Test

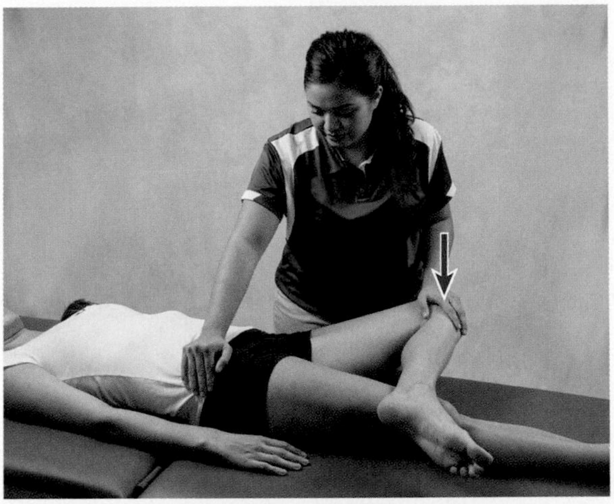

FABER (flexion, abduction, external rotation, and extension) test for hip or sacroiliac pathology.

Patient Position	Supine, with the foot of the involved side crossed over the opposite thigh
Position of Examiner	At the side of the patient to be tested with one hand on the opposite ASIS and the other on the medial aspect of the flexed knee
Evaluative Procedure	The extremity is allowed to rest into full external rotation followed by the examiner's applying overpressure at the knee and ASIS.
Positive Test	Reproduction of symptoms in the sacroiliac joint or hip
Implications	Pain in the inguinal area anterior to the hip may indicate hip pathology. Pain in the SI area during the application of overpressure may indicate SI joint pathology.

Evidence

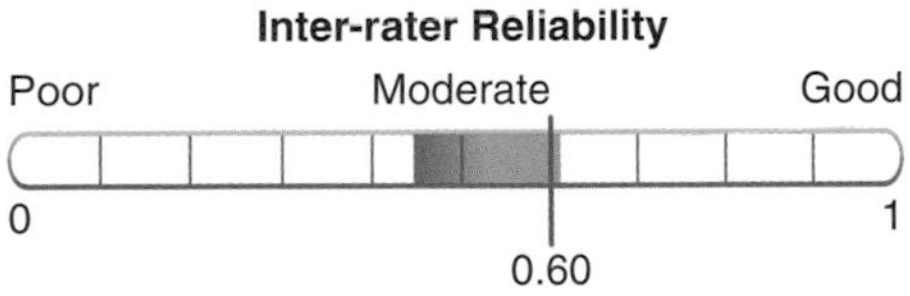

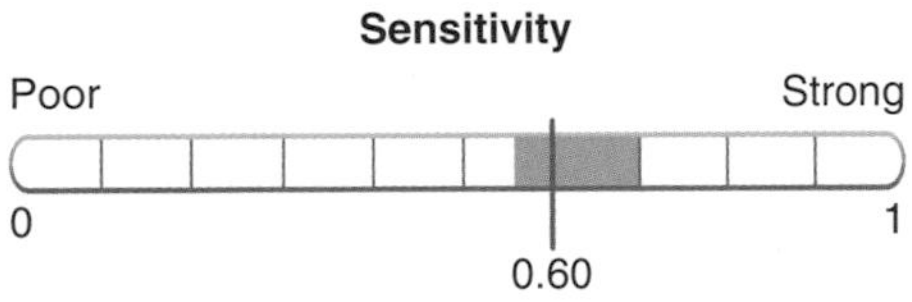

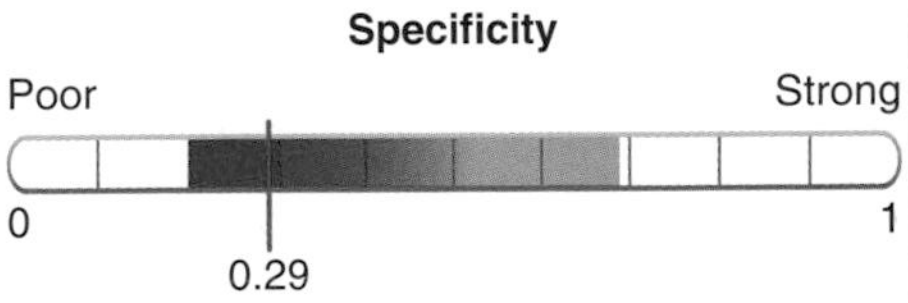

LR+: 0.82–1.08–1.53

LR−: 0.70–0.79–1.77

ASIS = anterior superior iliac spine; SI = sacroiliac

Selective Tissue Test 13-14
Gaenslen's Test

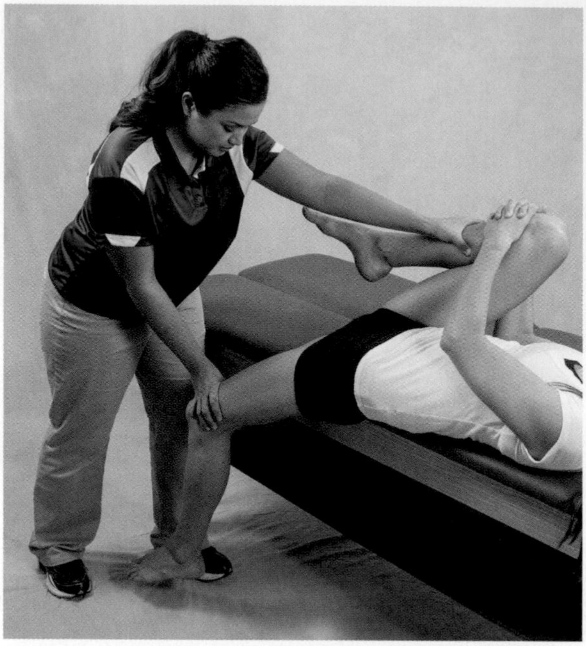

Gaenslen's test places a rotational force on the SI joints.

Patient Position	Supine, lying close to the side of the table
Position of Examiner	Standing at the side of the patient
Evaluative Procedure	The examiner slides the patient close to the edge of the table. The patient pulls the far knee up to the chest. The near leg is allowed to hang over the edge of the table. While stabilizing the patient, the examiner applies pressure to the near leg, forcing the hip into extension.
Positive Test	Pain in the SI region
Implications	SI joint pathology
Comments	The lumbar spine should not extend during this test.
Evidence	

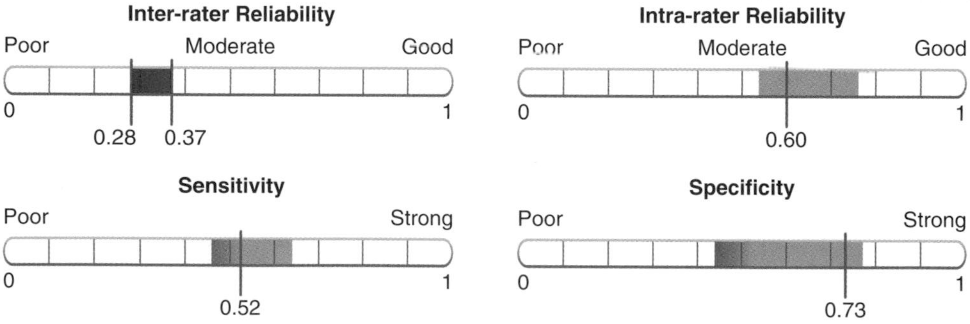

LR+: 1.13–1.78–2.20

LR−: 0.65–0.70–0.92

SI = sacroiliac

Selective Tissue Test 13-15
Thigh Thrust Test

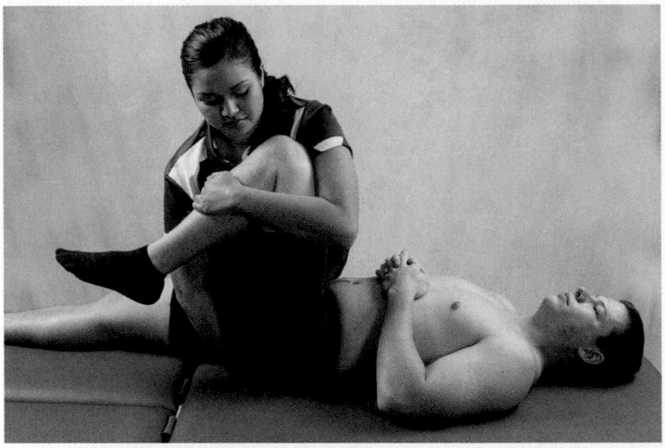

With one hand stabilizing the sacral base, the opposite arm places an axial load on the femur, creating a shear force on the SI joint.

Patient Position	Lying supine The patient's hip is flexed to 90 degrees, and the knee is fully flexed. Avoid adduction.
Position of Examiner	Standing next to the patient on the side opposite the one being tested, the examiner reaches one hand under the buttock and places it on the sacral base. The opposite hand is placed on the knee.
Evaluative Procedure	A downward force is placed through the femur, creating an axial load and torque over the SI joint.
Positive Test	Pain in the SI joint
Implications	SI joint dysfunction
Evidence	

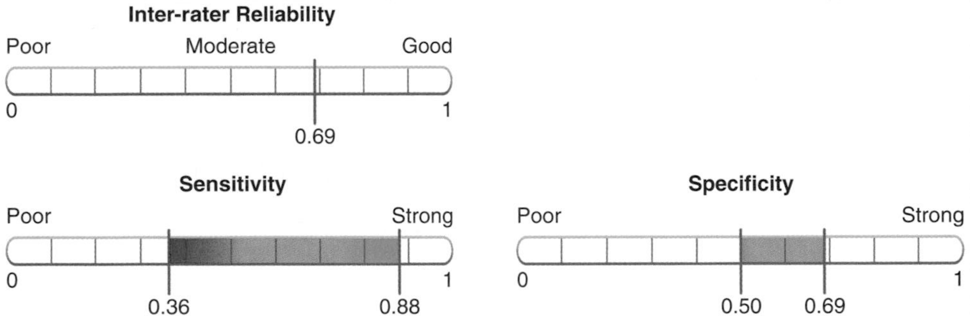

LR+: 0.72–2.84

LR−: 0.17–1.28

SI = sacroiliac

Selective Tissue Test 13-16
Sacral Thrust

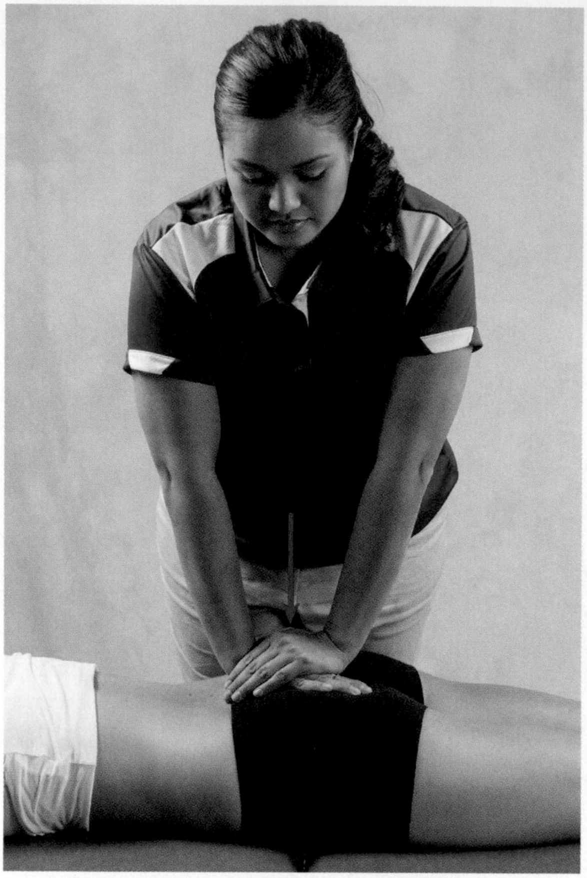

The sacral thrust test places an anterior force on the SI joint that results in pain in the presence of SI pathology.

Patient Position	Lying prone
Position of Examiner	Standing next to the patient The hands are placed one on top of the other over the sacrum.
Evaluative Procedure	An anterior force is placed through the sacrum.
Positive Test	Pain in the SI joint
Implications	SI joint dysfunction
Evidence	

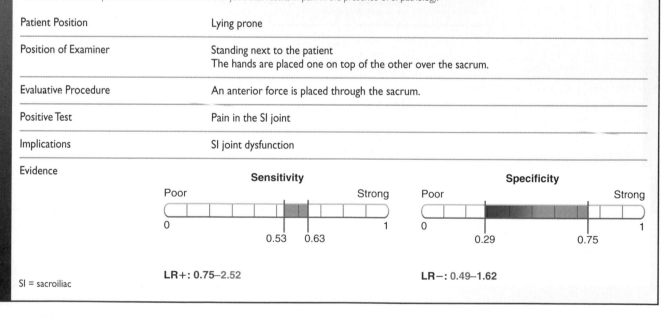

LR+: 0.75–2.52

LR−: 0.49–1.62

SI = sacroiliac

On-Field Examination of Lumbar Spine Injuries

All injuries to the spinal column requiring an on-field evaluation must be treated as being catastrophic in nature until determined otherwise. Bilateral symptoms in the upper extremities or symptoms in the lower extremities should alert the examiner to the potential of spinal cord involvement. The procedures described in this chapter assume that the potential of a catastrophic spinal cord injury has been ruled out. Chapter 20 discusses the evaluation and management of potentially catastrophic spinal cord injuries.

On-Field History

- **Location of pain:** Pain that is localized to the vertebral column can indicate a disc rupture, sprain, fracture, or facet pathology. Pain running parallel to the vertebral column may indicate spasm of the paravertebral muscles. Pain radiating into the extremities may indicate trauma to one or more spinal nerve roots.
- **Peripheral symptoms:** Pain, weakness, or numbness that radiates into the extremity is usually the result of nerve root impingement.
- **Mechanism of injury:** External forces that produce rotation of the spine may result in contusions, facet joint dislocation or subluxation, disc trauma, or ligamentous sprains. Eccentric contractions may result in a muscular tear.

On-Field Inspection

- **Position of the athlete:** Observe the athlete's position. Is the athlete prone or supine? If the athlete is supine and trauma to the vertebra, spinal cord, nerve roots, or spinal musculature is suspected, these structures cannot be palpated without moving the athlete.
- **Posture:** Note the presence of abnormal posture, including flexion or extension posturing of the extremities or flaccidity of the muscles, possibly indicating spinal cord involvement. The patient may also assume a posture that decreases the amount of pressure placed on the involved structure (e.g., disc, facet joints), or the posture may be influenced by muscle spasm.
- **Willingness to move:** Assume that a motionless athlete is unconscious until otherwise ruled out. Disc lesions, vertebral fractures, facet dislocations, or muscle spasm may cause the athlete to move in a guarded manner.[121]

On-Field Neurological Tests

If the athlete describes symptoms that radiate into the extremities, the following on-field neurological assessments are necessary. If these tests show positive results (or if there is reason to suspect a vertebral fracture or dislocation), then the athlete must be managed as described in Chapter 20.

- **Sensory tests:** Bilaterally check the anterior, posterior, medial, and lateral aspects of the extremities to assure equal sensory function within the dermatomes. Absent or diminished sensation in one or more extremity can indicate serious spinal cord trauma.
- **Motor tests:** Ask the athlete to wiggle the feet and hands and bend the knees and elbows. An inability to perform these tasks may indicate spinal cord trauma.

On-Field Palpation

If the athlete is in the prone position, the majority of the lumbar and thoracic spine can be easily palpated, although portions of the back may be covered by protective equipment.

- **Bony palpation:** Palpate the spinous processes of the lumbar and thoracic spine (typically easily palpable [refer to Tables 13-7 and 14-7 for the approximate location of the spinous processes]). The transverse processes may be masked by the paravertebral muscles, but their location can be palpated for tenderness.
- **Paraspinal muscles:** Palpate the paraspinal muscles to identify areas of spasm. If the trauma was caused secondary to a direct blow, the area may be tender to the touch.

On-Field Management of Lumbar Spine Injuries

This section describes the on-field management of lumbar spine injuries. Athletes suspected of having vertebral fractures or dislocations in this area of the spinal column should be spine boarded as described in Chapter 20.

Lumbar Spine

Catastrophic injury to the lumbar spine is relatively rare because of the decreased ROM of this area and the extremely high forces needed to cause this injury. However, this fact should not allow the athletic trainer or physician to become complacent during the evaluation process. As with all spinal injuries, the evaluation of the lumbar spine must be approached as if a catastrophic injury exists until it has been ruled out.

The athlete must be questioned for a history of symptoms, including pain and paresthesia. Pain localized over a spinous process may indicate a compression or burst fracture.[121] This alone is reason for immediate referral. Any symptoms suggesting neurological involvement must be investigated. An athlete reporting bilateral symptoms must be treated as having a spinal cord injury, immobilized on a spine board, and properly transported to a medical facility.

Direct blows to the lumbar or thoracic region may result in trauma to the kidneys, ribs, or other internal organs. The evaluation of these conditions is discussed in Chapter 14.

REFERENCES

1. Hoy, D, Brooks, P, Blyth, F, and Buchbinder, R: The epidemiology of low back pain. *Best Pract Res Clin Rheumatol*, 24:769, 2010.
2. Jones, GT, and Macfarlane, GJ: Epidemiology of low back pain in children and adolescents. *Arch Dis Child*, 90:312, 2005.
3. Balagué, F, et al: Non-specific low back pain. *Lancet*, 379:482, 2012.
4. Hall, NA, et al: Spine and axial skeleton injuries in the National Football League. *Am J Sports Med*, 40:1755, 2012.
5. Issack, PS, et al: Degenerative lumbar spinal stenosis: evaluation and management. *J Am Acad Orthop Surg*, 20:527, 2012.
6. Varlotta, GP, et al: The lumbar facet joint: a review of current knowledge: part 1: anatomy, biomechanics, and grading. *Skeletal Radiol*, 40:13, 2011.
7. Dalton, D: The vertebral column. In Levangie PK, and Norkin CC: *Joint Structure and Function*, ed 5. Philadelphia, PA: FA Davis, 2011.
8. Oegema, TR: Biochemistry of the intervertebral disc. *Clin Sports Med*, 12:419, 1993.
9. Carrigg, SY, and Hillemeyer, LE: The effect of running-induced intervertebral disc compression on thoracolumbar vertebral column mobility in young, healthy males. *J Orthop Sports Phys Ther*, 16:19, 1992.
10. Hanley, ED, and David, SM: Lumbar arthrodesis for the treatment of back pain. *J Bone Joint Surg*, 81(A):716, 1999.
11. Nachemson, A, and Morris, JM: In vivo measurements of intradiscal pressure. *J Bone Joint Surg*, 46(A):1077, 1964.
12. Costi, JJ, et al: Direct measurement of intervertebral disc maximum shear strain in six degrees of freedom: motions that place disc tissue at risk of injury. *J Biomech*, 40:2457, 2007.
13. Langevin HM, Fox JR, Koptiuch C, et al: Reduced thoracolumbar fascia shear strain in human chronic low back pain. *BMC Musculoskelet Disord*, 12:203, 2011.
14. Becker I, Woodley SJ, and Stringer MD: The adult human pubic symphysis: a systematic review. *J Anat*, 217:475, 2010.
15. Hodges, PW, and Richardson, CA: Inefficient muscular stabilization of the lumbar spine associated with low back pain: a motor control evaluation of transversus abdominis. *Spine*, 21:2640, 1996.
16. Hides, J, et al: The relationship of tranversus abddominis and lumbar multifidus clinical muscle tests in patients with chronic low back pain. *Man Ther*, 16:573, 2011.
17. Fritz, JM, Erhard, RE, and Hagen, BF: Segmental instability of the lumbar spine. *Phys Ther*, 78:889, 1998.
18. Kolber, MJ, and Beekhuizen, K: Lumbar stabilization: an evidence-based approach for the athlete with low back pain. *Strength Condit J*, 29:26, 2007.
19. Stanton, TR, et al: After an episode of acute low back pain, recurrence is unpredictable and not as common as previously thought. *Spine*, 33:2923, 2008.
20. Linton, SJ: A review of psychological risk factors in back and neck pain. *Spine*, 25:1148, 2000.
21. George, SZ, Bialosky, JE, and Donald, DA: The centralization phenomenon and fear-avoidance beliefs as prognostic factors for acute low back pain: a preliminary investigation involving patients classified for specific exercise. *J Orthop Sports Phys Ther*, 35:580, 2005.
22. Grotle, M, Vollestad, NK, and Brox, JI: Clinical course and impact of fear-avoidance beliefs in low back pain. *Spine*, 31:1038, 2006.
23. Hallegraeff, JN, et al: Expectations about recovery from acute non-specific low back pain predict absence from usual work due to chronic low back pain: a systematic review. *J Physiother*, 58:165, 2012.
24. DeLitto, A, et al: Low back pain: Clinical practice guidelines linked to the International Classification of Functioning, Disability, and Health from the Orthopaedic Section of the American Physical Therapy Association. *J Orthop Sports Phys Ther*, 42:A1, 2012.
25. Haggman, S, Maher, C, and Refshauge, KM: Screening for symptoms of depression by physical therapists managing low back pain. *Phys Ther*, 84:1157, 2004.
26. Boissonnault, W, and DiFabio, RP: Pain profile of patients with low back pain referred to physical therapy. *J Orthop Sport Phys Ther*, 24:180, 1996.
27. Potter, NA, and Rothstein, JM: Intertester reliability for selected clinical tests of the sacroiliac joint. *Phys Ther*, 65:1671, 1985.
28. Gatt, CJ, et al: Impact loading of the lumbar spine during football blocking. *Am J Sports Med*, 25:317, 1997.
29. Sizer, PS, Brismée, J, and Cook, C: Medical screening for red flags in the diagnosis and management of musculoskeletal spine pain. *Pain Pract*, 7:53, 2007.
30. Fairbank, JCT, and Pynsent, PB: The Oswestry Disability Index. *Spine*, 25:2940, 2000.
31. Davidson, M, and Keating, JL: A comparison of five low back disability questionnaires: reliability and responsiveness. *Phys Ther*, 82:8, 2002.
32. Fishbain DA, et al: A structured evidence-based review on the meaning of nonorganic physical signs: Waddell signs. *Pain Med*, 4:141, 2003.
33. Fishbain DA, et al. Is there a relationship between nonorganic physical findings (Waddell signs) and secondary gain/malingering? *Clin J Pain*, 20:399, 2004.
34. Greer, S, and Chambliss, L: What physical exam techniques are useful to detect malingering? *J Fam Pract*, 54:719, 2005.
35. Hoover, CF: A new sign for the detection of malingering and functional paresis of lower extremities. *JAMA*, 51:746, 1908.
36. Archibald, AC, and Wiechec, F: A reappraisal of Hoover's test. *Arch Phys Med Rehabil*, 51:234, 1970.
37. Arieff, AJ, et al: The Hoover sign: an objective sign of pain and/or weakness in the back or lower extremities. *Arch Neurol*, 5:673, 1961.
38. Westbrook, A, et al: The mannequin sign. *Spine*, 30:E115, 2005.
39. Hresko, MT: Idiopathic scoliosis in adolescents. *N Engl J Med*, 368:834, 2013.
40. Weinstein, SL, et al: Health and function of patients with untreated idiopathic scoliosis: a 50-year natural history study. *JAMA*, 289:599, 2003.
41. Landau, M, and Krafchik, BR: The diagnostic value of café-au-lait macules. *J Am Acad Dermatol*, 40:877, 1999.
42. Abeliovich, D, et al: Familial café-au-lait spots: a variant of neurofibromatosis type 1. *J Med Genet*, 32:985, 1995.
43. Binkley, J, Stratford, PW, and Gill, C: Interrater reliability of lumbar accessory motion mobility testing. *Phys Ther*, 75:786, 1995.
44. Ensink, F, et al: Lumbar range of motion: influence of time of day and individual factors on measurements. *Spine*, 21:1339, 1996.
45. Reese, NB, and Bandy, WD: *Joint Range of Motion and Muscle Length Testing*. Philadelphia, PA: W.B. Saunders, 2002.
46. Adams, MA, Mannion, AF, and Dolan, P: Personal risk factors for first-time low back pain. *Spine*, 24:23, 1999.
47. Barr, KP, Griggs, M, and Cadby, T: Lumbar stabilization: a review of core concepts and current literature, part 2. *Am J Phys Med Rehabil*, 86:72, 2007.
48. McGill, SM, et al: Endurance times for low back stabilization exercises: clinical targets for testing and training from a normal database. *Arch Phys Med Rehabil*, 80:941, 1999.
49. Reiman, MP, et al: Comparison of different trunk endurance testing methods in college-aged individuals. *Int J Sports Phys Ther*, 7:533, 2012.
50. Handrakis, JP, et al: Key characteristics of low back pain and disability in college-aged adults: a pilot study. *Arch Phys Med Rehabil*, 93:1217, 2012.
51. Demoulin, C, et al: Spinal muscle evaluation using the Sorensen test: a critical appraisal of the literature. *Joint Bone Spine*, 73:43, 2006.
52. Adedoyin, RA, et al: Endurance of low back musculature: normative data for adults. *J Back Musculoskelet Rehabil*, 24:101, 2011.
53. Süüden, E: Low back muscle fatigue during Sorensen endurance test in patients with chronic low back pain: relationship between electromyographic

spectral compression and anthropometric characteristics. *Electromyogr Clin Neurophysiol*, 48:185, 2008.
54. Ferriera, PH, et al: Changes in recruitment of transversus abdominis correlate with disability in people with chronic low back pain. *Br J Sports Med*, 44:1166, 2010.
55. Latimer, J, et al: Plinth padding and measures of posteroanterior lumbar stiffness. *J Manipulative Physiol Ther*, 20:315, 1997.
56. Cecin, HA: Cecin's Sign ("X" Sign): Improving the diagnosis of radicular compression by herniated lumbar discs. *Rev Bras Reumatol*, 50:44, 2010.
57. Majlesi, J, et al: The sensitivity and specificity of the slump and the straight leg raising tests in patients with lumbar disc herniation. *J Clin Rheumatol*, 14:87, 2008.
58. Scham, SM, and Taylor, TKF: Tension signs in lumbar disc prolapse. *Clin Orthop*, 75:195, 1971.
59. Hudgens, WR: The crossed-straight-leg-raising test. *N Engl J Med*, 297:1127, 1977.
60. Woodhall, R, and Hayes, GJ: The well-leg-raising test of Fajersztajn in the diagnosis of ruptured lumbar intervertebral disc. *J Bone Joint Surg Am*, 32:786, 1950.
61. Johnson, EK, and Chiarello, CM: The slump test: the effects of head and lower extremity position on knee extension. *J Orthop Sports Phys Ther*, 26:310, 1997.
62. Capra, F, et al: Validity of the straight-leg raise test for patients with sciatic pain with or without lumbar pain using magnetic resonance imaging results as a reference standard. *J Manipulative Physiol Ther*, 34:231, 2011.
63. Fritz, JM: Lumbar intervertebral disc injuries in athletes. *Athletic Ther Today*, March:27, 1999.
64. Suri, P, et al: The accuracy of the physical examination for the diagnosis of midlumbar and low lumber nerve root impingent. *Spine*, 36:63, 2011.
65. Rabin, A, et al: The sensitivity of the seated straight-leg raise test compared with the supine straight-leg raise test in patients presenting with magnetic resonance imaging evidence of lumbar nerve root compression. *Arch Phys Med Rehabil*, 88:840, 2007.
66. Coppieters, MW, et al: Strain and excursion of the sciatic, tibial, and plantar nerves during a modified straight leg raising test. *J Orthop Res*, 24:1883, 2006.
67. Beskin, JL: Nerve entrapment syndromes of the foot and ankle. *J Am Acad Orthop Surg*, 5:261, 1997.
68. Weiner, DK, et al: Chronic low back pain in older adults: prevalence, reliability, and validity of physical examination findings. *J Am Geriatr Soc*, 54:11, 2006.
69. Fritz, JM, Cleland, JA, and Childs, JD: Subgrouping patients with low back pain: evolution of a classification approach to physical therapy. *J Orthop Sports Phys Ther*, 37:296, 2007.
70. Delitto, A, Erhard, RE, and Bowling, RW: A treatment-based classification approach to low back syndrome: identifying and staging patients for conservative treatment. *Phys Ther*, 75:740, 1995.
71. Fritz, JM, Erhard, RE, and Vignovic, M: A nonsurgical treatment approach for patients with lumbar spinal stenosis. *Phys Ther*, 77:963, 1997.
72. Apeldoorn, AT, et al: A randomized controlled trial on the effectiveness of a classification-based system for subacute and chronic low back pain. *Spine*, 37:1347, 2012.
73. de Schepper EI, et al: Diagnosis of lumbar spinal stenosis: an updated systematic review of the accuracy of diagnostic tests. *Spine*, 38:E469, 2013.
74. de Graaf, I, et al: Diagnosis of lumbar spinal stenosis. *Spine*, 31:1168, 2006.
75. Lee-Robinson, A, and Lee, AT: Clinical and diagnostic findings in patients with lumbar radiculopathy and polyneuropathy. *Am J Clin Med*, 7:80, 2010.
76. Jensen, MC, et al: Magnetic imaging of the lumbar spine in people without back pain. *N Engl J Med*, 331:69, 1994.
77. ten Brinke, A, et al: Is leg length discrepancy associated with the side of radiating pain in patients with a lumbar herniated disc? *Spine*, 24:684, 1999.
78. Luoma, K, et al: Low back pain in relation to lumbar disc degeneration. *Spine*, 25:487, 2000.
79. van der Windt, DAWM, et al: Physical examination for lumbar radiculopathy due to disc herniation in patients with low-back pain (Review). *Cochrane Database Syst Rev*. 17:CD007431, 2010. doi: 10.1002/14651858.CD007431.pub2.
80. Ginsburg, GM, and Bassett, GS: Back pain in children and adolescents: evaluation and differential diagnosis. *J Am Acad Orthop Surg*, 5:67, 1997.
81. Suri, P, et al: The accuracy of the physical examination for the diagnosis of midlumbar and low lumbar nerve root impingement. *Spine*, 36:63, 2011.
82. Waddell, G: *The Back Pain Revolution*. Edinburgh: Churchill Livingstone, 2004, p 186.
83. Jonsson, B, and Stromqvist, B: Clinical characteristics of recurrent sciatica after lumbar discectomy. *Spine*, 21:500, 1996.
84. Benyahya, E, et al: Sciatica as the first manifestation of a leiomyosarcoma of the buttock. *Rev Rhum Engl Ed*, 64:135, 1997.
85. Amundsen, T, et al: Lumbar spinal stenosis: clinical and radiological features. *Spine*, 20:1178, 1995.
86. Maheshwaran, S, et al: Sciatica in degenerative spondylolisthesis of the lumbar spine. *Ann Rheum Dis*, 54:539, 1995.
87. Spencer, DL: The anatomical basis of sciatica secondary to herniated lumbar disc: a review. *Neurol Res*, 21(suppl 1):S33, 1999.
88. Zwart, JA, Sand, T, and Unsgaard, G: Warm and cold sensory thresholds in patients with unilateral sciatica: C fibers are more severely affected than A-delta fibers. *Acta Neurol Scand*, 97:41, 1998.
89. Tomaszewski, D: Vertebral osteomyelitis in a high school hockey player: a case report. *J Athl Train*, 34:29, 1999.
90. Curtis S, et al: Clinical features suggestive of meningitis in children: a systematic review of prospective data. *Pediatrics*, 126:952, 2010.
91. Thomas, KE, et al: The diagnostic accuracy of Kernig's sign, Brudzinski's sign, and nuchal rigidity in adults with suspected meningitis. *Clin Infect Dis*, 35:46, 2002.
92. Nadler, SF, et al: The crossed femoral nerve stretch test to improve diagnostic sensitivity for the high lumbar radiculopathy: 2 case reports. *Arch Phys Med Rehabil*, 82:522, 2001.
93. Revel, M, et al: Capacity of the clinical picture to characterize low back pain relieved by facet joint anesthesia: proposed criteria to identify patients with painful facet joints. *Spine*, 23:1972, 1998.
94. Alqarni, AM, Schneiders, AG, and Hendrick, PA: Clinical tests to diagnose lumbar segmental instability: a systematic review. *J Orthop Sports Phys Ther*, 41:130, 2011.
95. Starkey, C: Injuries and illnesses in the National Basketball Association: a 10-year perspective. *J Athl Train*, 35:161, 2000.
96. Deitch, JR, et al: Injury risk in professional basketball players: a comparison of Women's National Basketball Association and National Basketball Association athletes. *Am J Sport Med*, 34:1077, 2006.
97. Natarajan, RN, et al: Study on effect of graded facetectomy on change in lumbar motion segment torsional flexibility using three-dimensional continuum contact representation for facet joints. *J Biomech Eng*, 121:215, 1999.
98. Boden, SD, et al: Orientation of the lumbar facet joints: association with degenerative disc disease. *J Bone Joint Surg*, 78(A):403, 1996.
99. Varlotta, GP, et al: The lumbar facet joint: a review of current knowledge: part I: anatomy, biomechanics, and grading. *Skeletal Radiol*, 40:13, 2011.
100. Varlotta, GP, et al: The lumbar facet joint: a review of current knowledge: part II: diagnosis and management. *Skeletal Radiol*, 40:149, 2011.

101. Masci, L, et al: Use of the one-legged hyperextension test and magnetic resonance imaging in the diagnosis of active spondylolysis. *Br J Sports Med*, 40:940, 2006.
102. Hicks, GE, et al: Preliminary development of a clinical prediction rule for determining which patients with low back pain will respond to a stabilization exercise program. *Arch Phys Med Rehabil*, 86:1753, 2005.
103. Congeni, J, McCulloch, J, and Swanson, K: Lumbar spondylolysis: a study of natural progression in athletes. *Am J Sports Med*, 25:248, 1997.
104. Soler, T, and Calderón, C: The prevalence of spondylolysis in the Spanish elite athlete. *Am J Sports Med*, 28:57, 2000.
105. Moore, KL: The perineum and pelvis. In Moore, KL (ed): *Clinically Oriented Anatomy*, ed 5. Baltimore, MD: Williams & Wilkins, 2005, p 389.
106. Miller, R, et al: Imaging modalities for low back pain in children: a review of spondylolysis and undiagnosed mechanical back pain. *J Pediatr Orthop*, 33:282, 2013.
107. Kobayashi, A, et al: Diagnosis of radiographically occult lumbar spondylolysis in young athletes by magnetic resonance imaging. *Am J Sports Med*, 1:169, 2013.
108. Voss, LA, Fadale, PD, and Hylstyn, MJ: Exercise-induced loss of bone density in athletes. *J Am Acad Orthop Surg*, 6:349, 1998.
109. Pezzullo, DJ: Spondylolisthesis and spondylolysis in athletes. *Athletic Ther Today*, March:36, 1999.
110. Alfieri, A, et al: The current management of lumbar spondylolisthesis. *J Neurosurg Sci*, 57:103, 2013.
111. Tertti, M, et al: Disc degeneration in young gymnasts: a magnetic resonance imaging study. *Am J Sports Med*, 18:206, 1990.
112. Kasai, Y, et al: A new evaluation method for lumbar spinal instability: passive lumbar extension test. *Phys Ther*, 86:1, 2006.
113. Collaer, JW, McKeough, DM, and Boissonnault, WG: Lumbar isthmic spondylolisthesis detection with palpation: interrater reliability and concurrent criterion-related validity. *J Man Manip Ther*, 14:22, 2006.
114. Laslett, M: Evidence-based diagnosis and treatment of the painful sacroiliac joint. *J Man Manip Ther*, 16:142, 2008.
115. Maigne, JY, Aivaliklis, A, and Pfefer, F: Results of sacroiliac joint double block and value of sacroiliac pain provocation tests in 54 patients with low back pain. *Spine*, 21:1889, 1996.
116. Simopoulos, TT, et al: A systematic evaluation of prevalence and diagnostic accuracy of sacroiliac joint interventions. *Pain Physician*, 15:E305, 2012.
117. Laslett, M, and Williams, M: The reliability of selected pain provocation tests for sacroiliac joint pathology. *Spine*, 19:1243, 1994.
118. Robinson, HS, et al: The reliability of selected motion- and pain provocation tests for the sacroiliac joint. *Man Ther*, 12:72, 2009.
119. Potter, NA, and Rothstein, JM: Intertester reliability for selected clinical tests of the sacroiliac joint. *Phys Ther*, 65:1671, 1985.
120. Freburger, JK, and Riddle, DL: Using published evidence to guide the examination of the sacroiliac joint region. *Phys Ther*, 81:1135, 2001.
121. Gertzbein, SD, et al: Thoracic and lumbar fractures associated with skiing and snowboarding injuries according to the AO comprehensive classification. *Am J Sports Med*, 40:1750, 2012.

CHAPTER

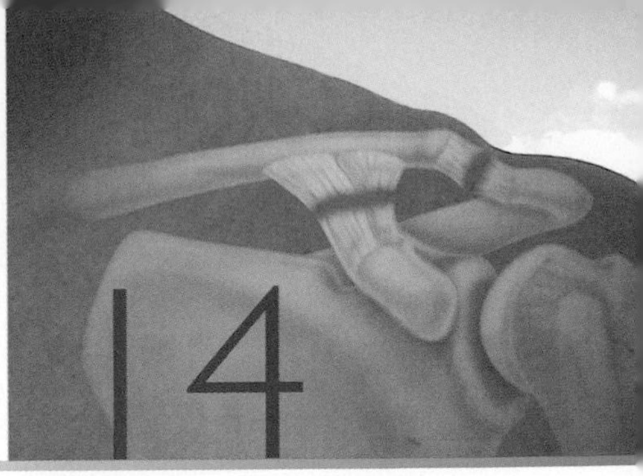

Cervical and Thoracic Spine and Thorax Pathologies

The cervical spine provides the greatest range of motion (ROM) among the segments of the spinal column. However, the spinal cord is the most vulnerable in this location of the spinal column. Because of the important role of the cervical vertebrae in protecting the spinal cord and spinal nerve roots, injury to this area can have catastrophic results. Noncatastrophic injury to the neck region can also impact daily life. Similar to low back pain, the origin of cervical spine pain is frequently nonspecific in that the involved structure cannot be identified. Because approximately one-third of the population will experience cervical pain during their lives, a systematic examination that leads to specific treatment options is required for proper patient care.[1] Serving as the posterior attachment site for the ribs, the thoracic spine provides exceptional protection of the spinal cord, but at the expense of ROM.

This chapter describes the clinical evaluation of cervical and thoracic spine and thorax pathology. Chapter 20 describes the on-field evaluation and management of patients with potentially catastrophic cervical spine trauma. The procedures described in this chapter assume that the possibility of spinal fracture and dislocation have been ruled out.

Clinical Anatomy

Cervical Spine

Carrying only the weight of the head, the vertebral bodies of the cervical vertebrae are much smaller than the other sections of the spinal column. The cervical transverse processes include a transverse foramen through which the vertebral artery and vein pass, a structure not found in the thoracic or lumbar vertebrae (Fig. 14-1). Each vertebra articulates with its adjacent vertebrae via an interbody articulation and superior and inferior facet (zygapophyseal) articulations that project from the pars interarticularis. The uncinate processes on the posteromedial margin of the body's endplates give the superior surface a concavity and increase the joint surface of the vertebral body. The uncinate processes on the inferior vertebrae articulate with the uncus process on the superior vertebrae to form the uncovertebral joints from C3 to C7.

The first two vertebrae of the cervical spine are unique. The first cervical vertebra, the atlas, has no vertebral body and supports the weight of the skull through two concave facet surfaces articulating with the occiput, forming the atlanto-occipital joint. The primary movement at the junction between the atlas and the skull (the C0–C1 articulation) is flexion and extension, such as when nodding the head "yes." A slight amount of lateral flexion also occurs at the

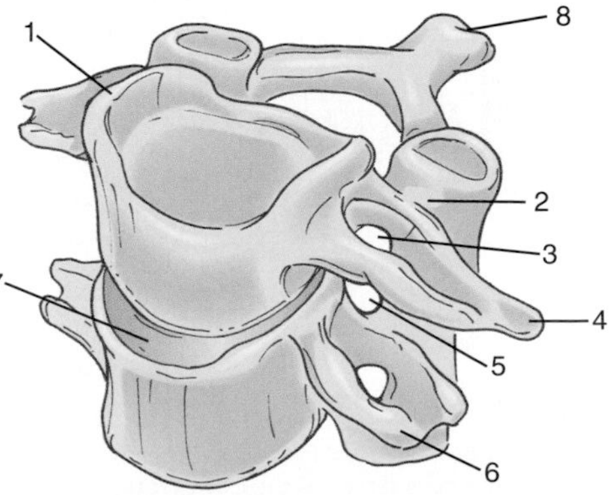

FIGURE 14-1 ■ C4 and C5 cervical vertebrae. 1, uncinate process; 2, intervertebral foramen (spinal nerve foramen); 3, superior intervertebral notch; 4, transverse foramen; 5, posterior tubercle of transverse process; 6, anterior tubercle of transverse process; 7, C4–C5 disc; 8, spinous process.

C0–C1 articulation. At the C1 vertebrae, the transverse processes are exceptionally long, and no true spinous process exists. The second cervical vertebra, the axis, has a small body with a superior projection, the dens. The articulation between the anterior arch of the atlas and the dens forms the atlanto-axial joint, providing the majority of cervical rotation, as when shaking the head "no" (Fig. 14-2). The C0–C1 and C1–C2 articulations are entirely synovial joints that are lacking the substantial bony facet joints found along the remainder of the vertebral column. These superior facet joints are oriented horizontally and lack the bony congruence found in the lower cervical region. The absence of a bony restraint increases the possibility of acute or congenital subluxations at these joints.[2]

Moving inferiorly along the remainder of the cervical vertebrae, the dimensions of the bone and intervertebral disc increase to provide the stability needed to support the increasing loads and larger muscle masses attaching at these levels. As with the lumbar spine, the facet joints of the cervical spine are formed by the lateral portion of the superior facet that articulates with the medial portion of the inferior facet. Refer to Chapter 13 for more information regarding facet joints. The facet joints in the cervical region are positioned approximately 45 degrees from the frontal and horizontal planes, an orientation that favors rotation. As occurs throughout the spine, the configuration of the muscles, ligaments, bones, and discs prevents single-plane motion from occurring in isolation at the segmental level. Between the C3 and C7 articulations, level rotation must be accompanied by the **coupled motion** of lateral bending.[2]

Spinal nerve roots pass through the intervertebral foramen. During youth, the spinal nerve root occupies approximately one-third of the foramen's space. Aging and degenerative changes decrease the free space within the foramen. This space also decreases when the cervical spine is extended, thereby increasing the potential of traumatic spinal nerve root impingement.[3]

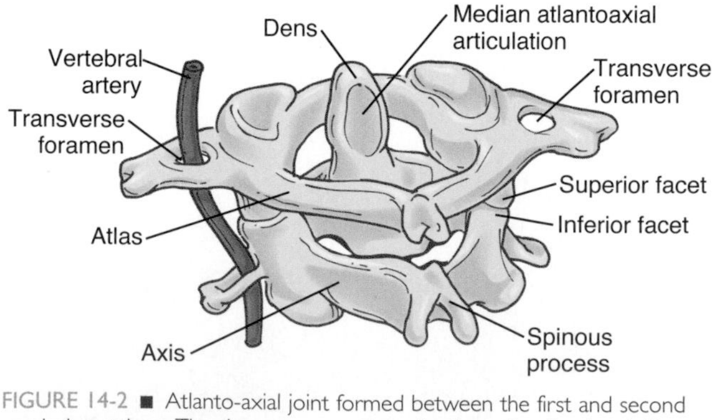

FIGURE 14-2 ■ Atlanto-axial joint formed between the first and second cervical vertebrae. The dens serves as the axis of rotation for the skull's movement on the vertebral column.

Coupled motion The association of one motion about an axis with another motion around a different axis

Thoracic Spine

In the thoracic region of the spinal column, the vertebral bodies begin to widen and thicken to assist in managing the weight of the torso. The spinous processes project downward to limit extension and provide a broad attachment site for the thoracic muscles and ligaments. The transverse processes thicken to articulate with the ribs, forming the **costotransverse joints** in ribs 1–10. Ribs 11 and 12 do not articulate with the transverse processes, so these joints do not exist at these levels. In addition to articulating with the transverse processes, a **costovertebral joint** is formed between each rib and the vertebral bodies. The joints formed on the T1 and T10–T12 vertebral levels articulate with a single rib on each side. The remaining ribs articulate with two vertebrae at the **superior costal** and **inferior costal facets** and the associated intervertebral disc on each side. Flexion and extension in the upper thoracic spine are limited secondary to rib attachments and the orientation of the facet joints in the frontal plane. Lateral rotation with its coupled motion of rotation occur in this region.[2,4]

Intervertebral Discs

The intervertebral discs in the cervical spine, as throughout the rest of the spine, are formed by the dense outer annulus fibrosus surrounding the flexible interdiscal tissue, the nucleus pulposus (see Chapter 13). Unlike the discs in the lumbar region, the annulus fibrosis does not completely encircle the nucleus pulposus. The anterior aspect of the disc is covered by a thick annulus that thins as it travels posteriorly. The lateral aspect of the disc is not covered, and the posterolateral portion of the disc receives some containment by the posterior longitudinal ligament. The posterior aspect of the disc is covered by a thin layer of annulus (Fig. 14-3).[5] In this region, the discs are smaller because they have less weight to support. Because of the unique anatomical features of the first two cervical vertebrae, intervertebral discs are not located at the C0–C1 and C1–C2 articulations.

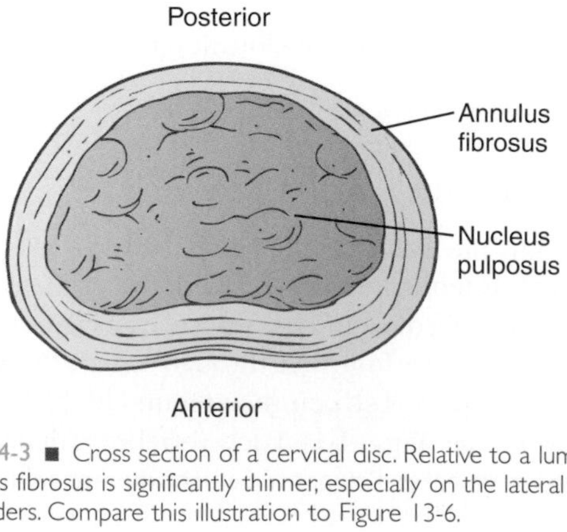

FIGURE 14-3 ■ Cross section of a cervical disc. Relative to a lumbar disc, the annulus fibrosus is significantly thinner, especially on the lateral and posterior borders. Compare this illustration to Figure 13-6.

Ligamentous Anatomy

Extending from the cervical spine to the lumbar spine, **anterior** and **posterior longitudinal ligaments** reinforce the spinal column (Fig. 14-4). The anterior longitudinal ligament runs from the sacrum to C2 and strengthens the anterior portion of the intervertebral discs and vertebrae, limiting extension of the spine. In the area between C2 and the skull, the anterior longitudinal ligament becomes the **anterior atlanto-axial** and the **atlanto-occipital** ligament.

Spanning the length of the vertebral column from the sacrum to C2, the posterior longitudinal ligament is most dense in the cervical spine, gradually thinning as it progresses down the anterior aspect of the vertebral canal. This ligament primarily limits flexion of the spine and reinforces the posterior aspect of the intervertebral disc. The posterior longitudinal ligament becomes the **tectorial membrane** as it runs from C2 to the skull.

In the cervical spine, the supraspinous ligament becomes the **ligamentum nuchae**, a triangular septum that serves as a broad area for muscle attachment. The ligamentum nuchae restricts flexion in the cervical spine (Fig. 14-5).

The **interspinous ligaments**, which occupy the space between the spinous processes, limit flexion and rotation of the spine. The posterior margin of the vertebral canal is formed by the **ligamentum flavum**, a pair of elastic ligaments connecting the lamina of one vertebra to the lamina of the vertebra above it. The ligamentum flavum limits flexion and rotation of the spine.

The transverse ligament and longitudinal bands, the atlantal cruciform ligament, maintains the position of the dens in the posterior aspect of the atlas and prevents displacement of C1 on C2.

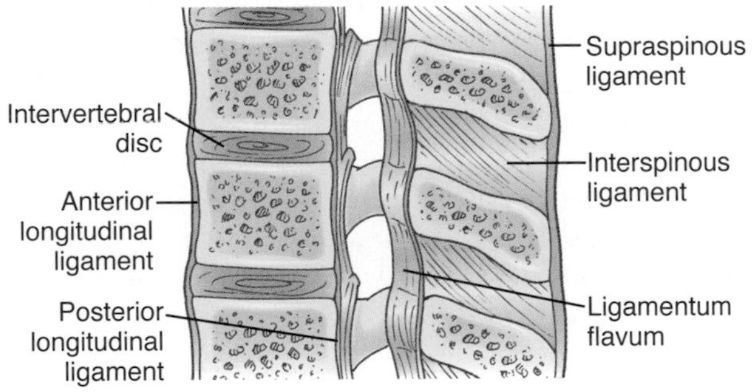

FIGURE 14-4 ■ Cross-sectional view of the ligaments of the cervical vertebral column.

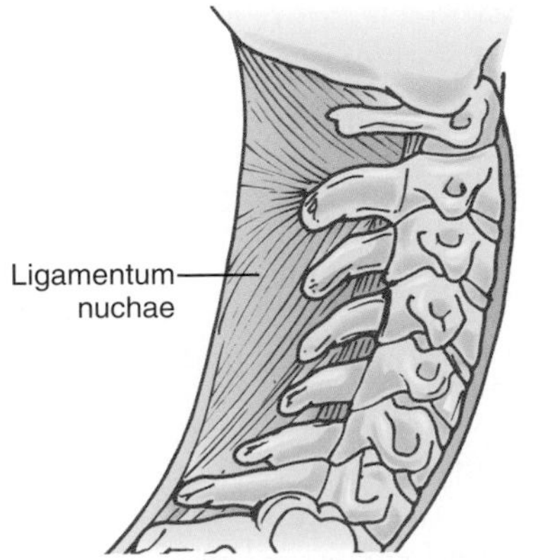

FIGURE 14-5 ■ In the cervical spine, the supraspinous ligament thickens to form the ligamentum nuchae.

Neurological Anatomy

The brain stem exits from the foramen magnum to become the spinal cord in the upper cervical region. The glossopharyngeal (IX), vagus (X), and accessory (XI) cranial nerves exit the skull via the jugular foramen. The cranial nerves are discussed in more detail in Chapter 20.

Eight pairs of spinal nerve roots exit between the seven cervical vertebrae. The first seven cervical nerves exit above the corresponding vertebrae. The "odd" cervical nerve, C8, exits below the seventh cervical vertebra (between the seventh cervical and first thoracic vertebrae) (Fig. 14-6). These spinal nerves, composed of anterior (ventral) roots and posterior (dorsal) roots that converge just outside of the intervertebral foramen, subsequently divide into two rami, a posterior (dorsal) **ramus** and an anterior (ventral) ramus, each carrying sensory and motor information (Fig. 14-7). The posterior rami innervate the facet joints of the spine, deep muscles of the back, and the overlying skin. The much larger anterior rami innervate the remaining trunk and upper extremities.[6] The accessory nerve provides motor input to the sternocleidomastoid (SCM) and trapezius (see Chapter 15).

Cervical Plexus

The cervical plexus is composed of the anterior rami of C1–C4. The cervical plexus provides sensory input to the occipital, supraclavicular, shoulder, and upper thoracic

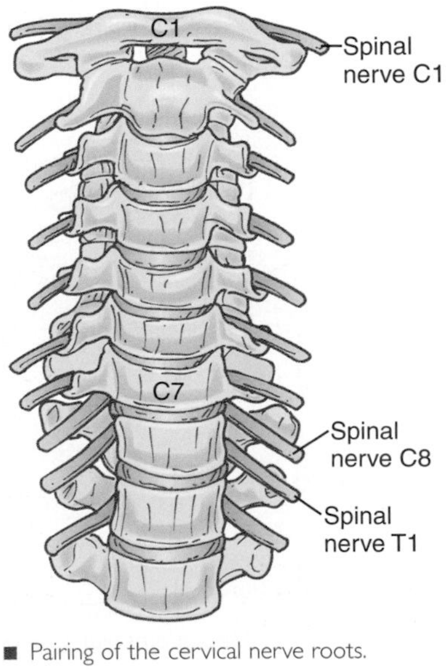

FIGURE 14-6 ■ Pairing of the cervical nerve roots.

Ramus (pl. rami) A branch of a nerve or blood vessel

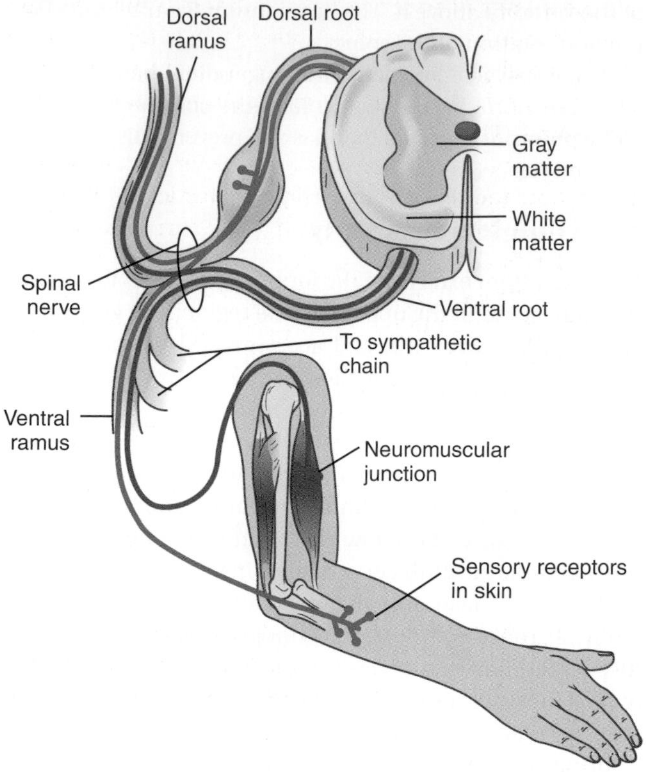

FIGURE 14-7 ■ Nerve root anatomy. The dorsal root, comprised of afferent sensory axons, and the ventral root, comprised of efferent motor axons, converge to form a single spinal nerve. This nerve then diverges into dorsal (posterior) and ventral (anterior) rami. The dorsal rami provide sensory and motor innervation to the facet joints, deep muscles and overlying skin. The ventral rami of C5–T1 form the brachial plexus.

region. The suboccipital nerve from the dorsal ramus of C1 innervates the deep cervical flexors.

Brachial Plexus

Supplying innervation to portions of the shoulder, the length of the arm, and the hand, the brachial plexus is formed by the C5 through C8 and the T1 nerve roots. The C4 or T2 nerve roots (or both) also may contribute (Fig. 14-8). The brachial plexus has five segmental areas: roots, trunks, divisions, cords, and branches. The ventral (anterior) portion of the cervical nerve roots contains the motor portion of the nerve; the dorsal (posterior) portion transmits sensory information.[3]

The C5 and C6 nerve roots converge to form the upper trunk. The C7 nerve root forms the middle trunk. The C8 and T1 nerve roots merge to form the lower trunk. Each trunk then diverges into anterior and posterior divisions. The posterior divisions of each trunk converge to form the posterior cord, the anterior divisions of the upper and middle trunks merge to form the lateral cord, and the anterior division of the lower cord forms the medial cord.

Each cord diverges to form the terminal branches of the brachial plexus. The lateral cord diverges into the lateral pectoral nerve and the musculocutaneous nerve and sends a branch that partially innervates the median nerve. The posterior cord splits into the axillary and radial nerves. One portion of the medial cord forms the ulnar nerve, and one portion converges with a division of the lateral cord to form the median nerve. These terminal branches innervate the arm, forearm, and hand. The nerves arising from the medial

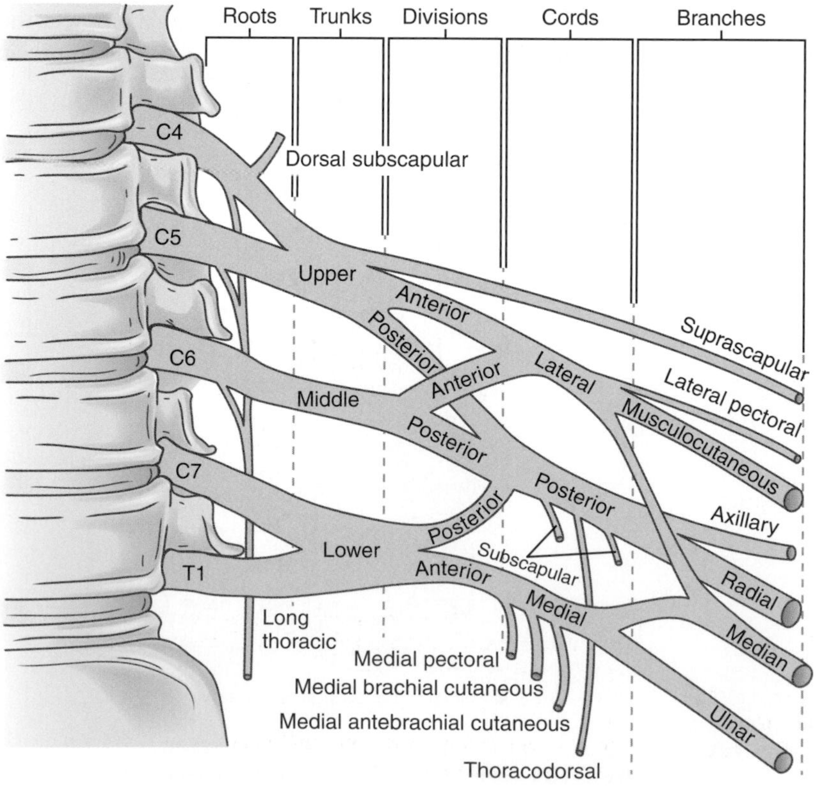

FIGURE 14-8 ■ Brachial plexus formed by the C5–C8 and T1 spinal nerve roots. Some references include the C4 and/or T2 nerve roots as a part of the brachial plexus.

and lateral cords are routed to the pectoral muscles and the flexor muscles originating on the anterior portion of the arm (relative to the anatomical position). The nerves emerging from the posterior cord innervate the muscles of the shoulder itself and the extensor muscles originating on the posterior aspect of the arm. In Figure 14-8, the other nerves that arise from the brachial plexus are identified.

Thoracic Nerves

Twelve pairs of nerve roots exit between T1 and T12. The thoracic nerves innervate muscles of the trunk and thorax and have dermatomal regions that approximate the ribs. As in the cervical region, the facet joints receive innervation from the lateral branch of the dorsal ramus of the corresponding spinal nerve. The costotransverse joints are innervated by the medial branch of the dorsal ramus.[7]

Thorax

With the sternum anteriorly, the vertebrae posteriorly, and the ribs connecting the two, the thorax forms a protective shell around the torso's upper internal organs (Fig. 14-9). The **sternum** consists of three sections: the **manubrium** superiorly, the central **body**, and the inferiorly projecting **xiphoid process**. The sternal body and the manubrium are connected by a fibrocartilaginous joint that fuses during adolescence to form a single, solid bone.

The upper seven ribs are classified as **true ribs** because they articulate with the sternum through their own **costal cartilages**. Ribs 8–10 articulate with the sternum through a conjoined costal cartilage. Thus, they are termed **false ribs**. Ribs 11 and 12, the **floating ribs**, do not have an anterior articulation. An anomalous **cervical rib** may project off the seventh cervical vertebra. Although this structure is often benign, it can be a source of compression on the brachial plexus, the subclavian artery, or the subclavian vein, predisposing the individual to **thoracic outlet syndrome (TOS)**.

The abdominal region has no anterior or lateral bony protection and receives only slight protection on its posterior surface from the thoracic and lumbar vertebrae and the floating ribs. The inferior portion of the abdomen is protected by the sacrum posteriorly and the ilium laterally.

Located within the thorax and abdomen are numerous internal organs. Many of the internal organs come in pairs. Reference to these organs is relative to the patient; thus, the right kidney is on the examiner's left side when facing the patient from the front (Fig. 14-10). Pain of **visceral** origin may be referred to the body's periphery (see Neurological Testing, p. 556).

Muscular Anatomy

Precise control of the cervical muscles is required for maintaining the head upright so that the eyes and ears can optimally function. Many of the muscles acting on the

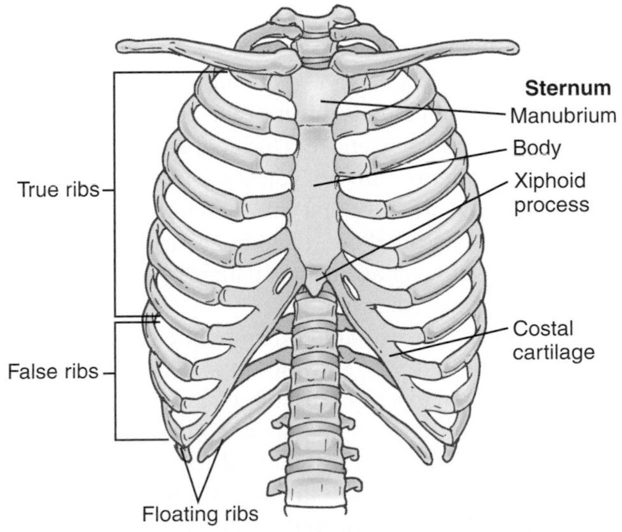

FIGURE 14-9 ■ The thorax. The rib cage formed by the true ribs (1–7), false ribs (8–10), and floating ribs (11 and 12); the sternum (manubrium, body, and xiphoid process); and the costal cartilage. The posterior margin of the thorax is formed by the thoracic vertebrae.

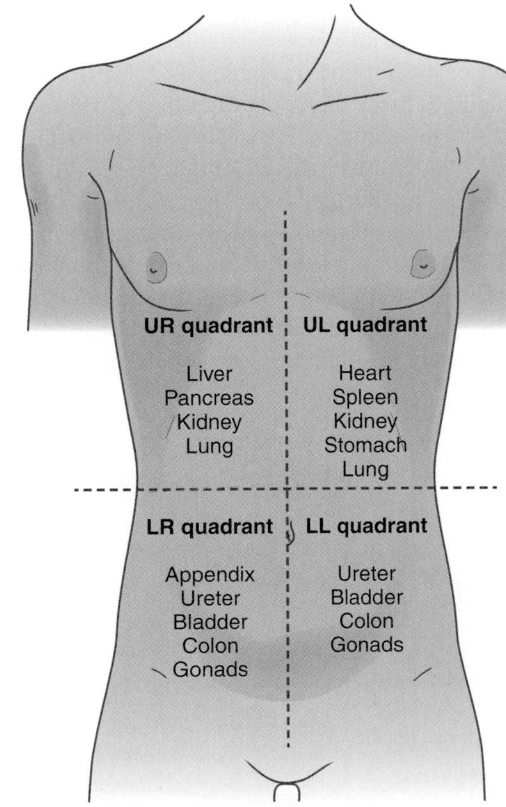

FIGURE 14-10 ■ Abdominal quadrant reference system. The sagittal quadrants are relative to the patient. Therefore, the right kidney is on the person's right-hand side.

Visceral Pertaining to the internal organs contained within the thorax and abdomen cervical spine are superficial and, depending on the fixation of the origin or insertion, act on the shoulder, cervical spine, or head. With bilateral contraction, the cervical spine muscles extend or flex the cervical spine and head. Unilateral contractions primarily result in lateral bending and contribute to cervical rotation. When coupled with the contractions of other muscles contralateral to themselves, these muscles work primarily to rotate the spine. The muscles acting on the thoracic spine are described in Chapter 13.

The superficial layer of the extensor cervical musculature is formed by the large, flat **splenius capitis** and **splenius cervicis** muscles. These muscles, when acting bilaterally, extend the head and neck. When acting alone, they laterally flex and rotate the head and cervical spine to the same side as the muscle (Fig. 14-11). Just deep to the splenius muscles are the rope-like **semispinalis capitis** and **semispinalis cervicis**, which traverse from the thoracic transverse processes to the spinous processes of the cervical spine. Deep and lateral to the semispinalis group are the **longissimus capitis** and **longissimus cervicis**, while the suboccipital group (spanning from C2 to the occiput) is the innermost muscle layer (Table 14-1).

The **longus capitis** and **longus colli** stabilize the cervical spine anteriorly. Injury to these muscles can occur with a high-velocity "whiplash" mechanism (Table 14-2).

The extrinsic muscles (those originating away from the spinal column) are presented in Table 14-3. When its insertion on the scapula is fixed, the upper one-third of the **trapezius** bilaterally acts to extend the cervical spine and skull. When the trapezius works unilaterally with other musculature, it laterally bends and rotates the cervical spine and skull.

The **sternocleidomastoid** (SCM) is responsible for rotating the skull to the opposite side and for lateral flexion of the cervical spine to the same side as the contracting muscle (Fig. 14-12). The angle of pull of the SCM extends the head on the cervical spine but acts as a flexor of the lower cervical spine. The anterior, middle, and posterior **scalene** muscles laterally flex the cervical spine. When the cervical spine is fixated, the scalenes elevate the rib cage to assist in inspiration. The scalene group is significant because the brachial plexus passes between its anterior and middle portions. Spasm or tightness of the scalenes can place pressure on the neurovascular structures of the upper extremities, resulting in thoracic outlet syndrome.

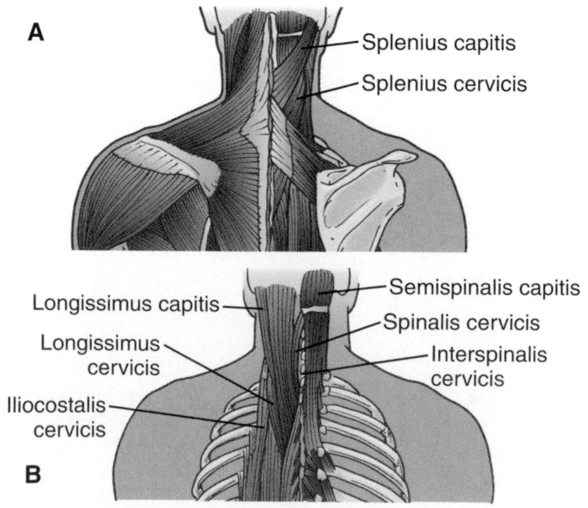

FIGURE 14-11 ■ Muscles of the spinal column: (A) superficial muscles, (B) deep muscles.

Muscles of Inspiration

The **diaphragm** is a muscular membrane that separates the thoracic cavity from the abdominal cavity. Innervated by the **phrenic nerve**, as the diaphragm contracts, it moves downward, creating a vacuum in the thorax and pulling air into the lungs. The diaphragm is interrupted at several points by portals through which the major vessels pass into the torso and lower legs.

The rib cage's intrinsic skeletal muscles are collectively referred to as the **intercostal muscles**. Spanning from rib to rib, these muscles assist in the respiratory process. Inspiration is also assisted by the scalene muscles that serve as secondary muscles of inspiration by elevating the first and second ribs. The SCM, trapezius, serratus anterior, pectoralis major and minor, and latissimus dorsi all function as secondary muscles of inspiration, used when breathing becomes difficult.

Muscles of Expiration

The abdominal muscles—the **rectus abdominis**, **internal oblique**, and **external oblique**—are supported across the abdomen by the **transverse abdominis**. In addition to flexing and rotating the lumbar and thoracic spine, the contraction of these muscles creates a positive pressure gradient across the diaphragm, resulting in the expiration of air. Testing of these muscles is described in Chapter 13.

Clinical Examination of the Cervical and Thoracic Spine and Thorax

The spinal cord and its nerve roots are vulnerable in the cervical spine. When the magnitude of the trauma is severe, catastrophic results may ensue. This chapter describes the evaluation of patients with noncatastrophic trauma to the cervical spine and assumes that vertebral fractures and dislocations have been ruled out. Chapter 20 describes the on-field evaluation and management of patients with potentially catastrophic cervical spine injuries.

The use of patient-centered outcome measures such as the Neck Disability Index provide important information in determining the extent of disability associated with the patient's symptoms. Examples of outcome measures are further described on p. 471. Repeated use of these functional scales helps assess the impact of intervention, provides a standard assessment tool, and determines whether the patient is getting worse or improving.[8]

As with the lumbar spine, identification of the anatomic cause of cervical and thoracic pain can be difficult and may

Table 14-1 Intrinsic Muscles That Extend the Cervical Spine and Head

Muscle	Action	Origin	Insertion	Innervation	Root
Iliocostalis Cervicis	Extension of spinal column Lateral bending of spinal column	Ribs 3–6	Transverse processes of C4–C6	Posterior rami of spinal nerves	C4–C8
Longissimus Capitis	Extension of skull and cervical spine Rotation of the face toward the same side	Articular processes of C5–C7	Mastoid process of skull	Posterior rami of spinal nerves	C4–C8
Longissimus Cervicis	Extension of spinal column Lateral bending of spinal column	Transverse processes of T1–T5	Transverse processes of C2–C6	Posterior rami of spinal nerves	C4–C8
Longissimus Thoracis	Extension of spinal column Lateral bending of spinal column	Common erector spinae tendon	Transverse process of T3–T12 Ribs 3–12	Posterior rami of spinal nerves	C4–C8
Multifidus (or Multifidi)	Rotation of spine to the opposite side Stabilization of vertebral column	Articular processes	Spinous process	Posterior rami of spinal nerves	C4–C8
Semispinalis Capitis	Extension of neck and head Rotation to the opposite side	Transverse process	Travel upwardly and medially to attach to a spinous process 5 or 8 vertebrae above the origin	Posterior rami of spinal nerves	C4–C8
Semispinalis Cervicis	Extension of thoracic and cervical spine	Transverse process	Travel upwardly and medially to attach to a spinous process 5 or 8 vertebrae above the origin	Posterior rami of spinal nerves	C4–C8
Semispinalis Thoracis	Extension of thoracic and cervical spine Rotation to the opposite side	Transverse process	Travel upwardly and medially to attach to a spinous process 5 or 8 vertebrae above the origin	Posterior rami of spinal nerves	C4–C8
Spinalis Capitis	Extension of the spine Lateral bending of the spine	Upper thoracic and lower cervical spinous processes	Ligamentum nuchae	Posterior rami of spinal nerves	C4–C8
Spinalis Cervicis	Extension of the spine Lateral bending of the spine	Upper thoracic and lower cervical spinous processes	Ligamentum nuchae	Posterior rami of spinal nerves	C4–C8
Splenius Capitis	Lateral bending of the cervical spine	Lower half of the ligamentum nuchae	Mastoid process of the temporal bone and adjacent occipital bone (capitis portion)	Posterior rami of middle cervical spinal nerves	C4–C8
Splenius Cervicis	Rotation of the head toward the same side Extension of the cervical spine	Spinous processes of C7–T6 vertebrae	Transverse processes of C2–C4 vertebrae (cervicis portion)	Posterior rami of spinal nerves	C4–C8

Table 14-2 Intrinsic Muscles Acting on the Head (atlanto-occipital flexion and extension)

Muscle	Action	Origin	Insertion	Innervation	Root
Longus Capitis	Flex head (atlanto-occipital motion)	Base of occiput	Anterior tubercles of C3–C6 transverse processes	Anterior rami of C1–C3 spinal nerves	C1, C2, C3
Longus Colli	Cervical flexion with rotation to opposite if unilateral	Anterior tubercle of C1; bodies of C1–C3 and transverse processes of C3–C6	Bodies of C5–T3 vertebrae; transverse processes of C3–C5 vertebrae	Anterior rami of spinal nerves	C2, C3, C4, C5, C6
Obliquus Capitis Inferior	Unilateral:ipsilateral rotation	Lateral surface of spinous process of axis	Inferior surface of transverse process of C1 (atlas)	Suboccipital nerve	C1
Obliquus Capitis Superior	Bilateral:extension of head on atlas Unilateral:ipsilateral rotation	Transverse process of atlas	Occipital bone	Suboccipital nerve	C1
Rectus Capitis Anterior	Flex head (atlanto-occipital motion)	Base of skull, anterior to occipital condyle	Anterior surface of lateral portion of C1 (atlas)	Branches from C1 and C2 spinal nerves	C1, C2
Rectus Capitis Lateralis	Flex and stabilize head (atlanto-occipital motion)	Jugular process of occiput	Transverse process of C1 (atlas)	Branches from C1 and C2 spinal nerves	C1, C2
Rectus Capitis Posterior Major	Bilateral: extension of head on atlas Unilateral: ipsilateral rotation	Posterior edge of spinous process of axis	Inferior nuchal line on occipital bone	Suboccipital nerve	C1
Rectus Capitis Posterior Minor	Bilateral: extension of head on atlas Unilateral: ipsilateral rotation	Posterior tubercle of axis	Inferior nuchal line on occipital bone (medial aspect)	Suboccipital nerve	C1

Table 14-3 Extrinsic Muscles Acting on the Cervical Spinal Column

Muscle	Action	Origin	Insertion	Innervation	Root
Trapezius (upper one-third)	Cervical extension Cervical side bending Elevation of scapula Upward rotation of scapula Rotation of the cervical spine to the opposite side	Occipital protuberance Nuchal line of the occipital bone Upper portion of the ligamentum nuchae	Lateral one-third of clavicle Acromion process	Spinal accessory	CN XI
Levator Scapulae	Elevation of the scapula Downward rotation of the scapula Extension of cervical spine	Spinous process of C7 Transverse processes of cervical vertebrae C1–C4	Superior medial border of scapula	Dorsal subscapular	C3, C4, C5
Sternocleidomastoid	Flexion of the cervical spine Rotation of the skull to the opposite side Lateral bending of the cervical spine Elevation of the clavicle and sternum	Medial clavicular head Superior sternum	Mastoid process of the skull	Spinal accessory	CN XI, C2, C3
Scalene, Anterior	Lateral bending of the cervical spine Elevation of the rib cage	Anterior portion of the transverse processes of C3–C6	Sternal attachment of the 1st rib	Cervical spinal nerves	C4, C5, C6
Scalene, Middle	Lateral bending of the cervical spine Elevation of the rib cage	Anterior portion of the transverse processes of C2–C7	Lateral to the insertion of the anterior scalene on the 1st rib	Anterior rami of cervical spinal nerves	C3, C4, C5, C6, C7, C8
Scalene, Posterior	Lateral bending of the cervical spine Elevation of the rib cage	Anterior portion of the transverse processes C5 and C6	Medial portion of the 2nd rib	Anterior rami of cervical spinal nerves	C7, C8

Examination Map

HISTORY

Past Medical History

Prior history of injury
Headaches/chest pain
Use of eyewear
Psychosocial factors

History of the Present Condition

Pain characteristics
Radicular symptoms
Mechanism of injury

FUNCTIONAL ASSESSMENT

Movement and posture

INSPECTION

Inspection of the Lateral Structures

Cervical and thoracic curvature
Posture

Inspection of the Anterior Structures

Level of the shoulders
Position of the head
Shape of the chest

Inspection of the Posterior Structures

Bilateral soft tissue comparison
Breathing patterns
Skin folds
Chest shape

PALPATION

Palpation of the Anterior Neck and Thorax

Hyoid
Thyroid cartilage
Cricoid cartilage
Carotid artery
Lymph nodes
Sternocleidomastoid
Scalenes

Sternum

Ribs and costal cartilage

Palpation of the Posterior Cervical and Thoracic Structures

Occiput and superior nuchal line
Transverse processes
Spinous processes
Supraspinous ligaments
Trapezius
Levator scapulae
Scapular muscles
Costovertebral junction
Paravertebral muscles

JOINT AND MUSCLE FUNCTION ASSESSMENT

Goniometry

Flexion
Extension
Lateral bending
Rotation

Active Range of Motion

Flexion
Extension
Lateral bending
Rotation

Manual Muscle Tests

Capital, Cervical, and Combined Capital and Cervical Flexion
Capital, Cervical, and Combined Capital and Cervical Extension
Lateral Flexion
Rotation and Flexion
Neck Flexor Endurance Test

Passive Range of Motion

Flexion
Extension
Lateral Bending
Rotation

JOINT STABILITY TESTS

Joint Play Assessment

Spring test
Mobility of the first rib

NEUROLOGICAL EXAMINATION

Upper Limb Nerve Tension Test
Upper Quarter Screen
Upper Motor Neuron Lesions
- Babinski test
- Oppenheim test
- Beevor's sign

REGION-SPECIFIC PATHOLOGIES

Cervical Radiculopathy

Cervical compression test
Spurling test
Cervical distraction test
Vertebral artery test

Intervertebral Disc Lesions

Shoulder abduction test
Valsalva maneuver (see Chapter 13)

Degenerative Joint and Disc Disease

Cervical Instability

Facet Joint Dysfunction

Brachial Plexus Pathology

Brachial plexus traction test

Thoracic Outlet Syndrome

Adson test
Allen test
Costoclavicular syndrome test
Roos test

Thoracic Spine Pathologies

Scheuermann's disease
Rib fracture
- Rib compression test

Costochondral injury

Thorax Pathologies

Splenic injury
Kidney trauma
Commotio cordis

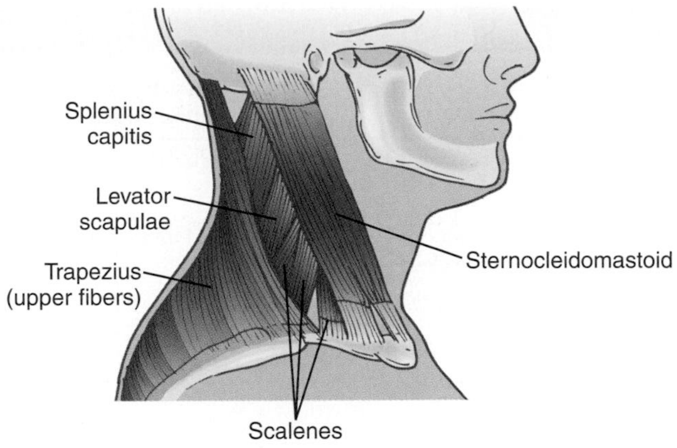

FIGURE 14-12 ■ Lateral cervical muscles.

not help determine an appropriate intervention. A treatment-based classification system whereby clusters of symptoms are matched with specific interventions has been proposed.[9,10]

History

Relevant Past History

- **History of spinal pathology:** Does the patient have a history of cervical or thoracic pain? Identify any pertinent history that may lead to structural degeneration or predispose the patient to chronic problems. The current symptoms may be the result of scar tissue formation's impinging or restricting other structures, a previously injured disc, or the formation of osteophytes within the intervertebral foramina.[11]
- **Recurrent brachial plexus trauma:** A prior history of injury to the brachial plexus makes the tissue more susceptible to reinjury. Repetitive injury may result in permanent impairment.
- **Chest/breast pain:** Angina-like chest pain or women with breast pain who have normal cardiac workups and who appear to be cancer free may be experiencing referred symptoms from the cervical or thoracic nerves.
- **Headaches or other head pain:** Neuropathy of the C2 or C3 nerve roots can produce complaints that include headaches, jaw and ear pain, pain in the occipital region, or superficial pain in the posterior cervical spine.[3] In addition, the greater occipital nerve pierces the semispinalis capitis, and spasm of this muscle can cause an occipital headache.
- **Eye examination:** Does the patient wear corrective lenses? If so, has the prescription recently changed? If not, when was the patient's last eye examination? Poor vision can result in postural changes that produce cervical headaches and neck pain.
- **Psychosocial factors:** Psychosocial behaviors such as **fear-avoidance** beliefs and depression are related to pain and disability associated with acute and chronic neck and back pain.[12,13] Patients who express high fear-avoidance beliefs avoid activities in the anticipation of pain, leading to further deconditioning and weakening of supporting and involved structures.

History of the Present Condition

The onset and identification of functional activities causing the symptoms assist in determining the appropriate intervention. Although usually mechanical in origin, cervical pain can arise from pathological sources such as tumors. A high index of suspicion of serious pathology is warranted if the patient describes unremitting pain, night pain, bowel and bladder dysfunction, or **hyperreflexia** (Table 14-4).[14]

- **Location of the pain:** Is the pain localized or does it radiate? Pain that is localized to the cervical spine may indicate a muscle injury, sprain, vertebral fracture or dislocation, or facet syndrome. Radicular symptoms are a strong indication of cervical nerve root or spinal cord involvement. Table 14-5 presents common symptoms relative to the involved nerve root.

  Musculoskeletal injuries to the ribs, costal cartilage, or abdominal muscles are usually tender at the site of the injury. Injury to the internal organs may result in a more diffuse pain at rest. However, these areas can be more specifically localized as the patient moves or the area is palpated. Blows to the low back may result in a kidney contusion, especially on the patient's right side. Pain in the thorax, abdomen, shoulder, or arm can be referred from the visceral organs. Pain in the upper left quadrant and shoulder, **Kehr's sign**, may indicate a ruptured spleen that is irritating the diaphragm.

  Cardiac dysfunction results in intense pain, tightness, or squeezing in the center of the chest. Another sign of cardiac tissue ischemia is referred pain into the left shoulder, arm, jaw, or epigastric area.

- **Mechanism and onset of injury:** Although patients can usually identify the specific mechanism of onset in acute pain, patients who report longer duration of symptoms or symptoms of a gradual onset should be questioned regarding postural or overuse causative factors. When an acute onset of injury is described, the mechanism of injury (MOI) can provide clues to the trauma (Table 14-6). When the patient reports an axial load being placed on the cervical spine, a possible vertebral fracture or dislocation must be considered until ruled out with radiographic examination. A whiplash mechanism, rapid extension followed by flexion, may be described following an automobile accident or fall.

  Injury to the thoracic and abdominal organs usually results from a direct blow to the area, such as being hit by a competitor, colliding with a piece of equipment, or falling.

Fear avoidance Refraining from tasks or movements because of the potential for pain or instability

Hyperreflexia Increased action of the reflexes

Table 14-4 Key Signs and Symptoms Associated With Serious Pathological Cervical Spine Conditions

Cervical Myelopathy	Neoplastic Conditions	Upper Cervical Ligamentous Instability	Vertebral Artery Insufficiency	Inflammatory or Systemic Disease
Sensory disturbance of the hands	Age older than 50	Occipital headache and numbness	Drop attacks	Temperature > 37°C
Muscle wasting of hand intrinsic muscles	Previous history of cancer	Severe limitation during neck active range of motion in all directions	Dizziness or lightheadedness related to neck movement	BP > 160/95 mm Hg
Unsteady gait	Unexplained weight loss	Signs of cervical **myelopathy**	**Dysphasia**	Resting pulse >100 bpm
Hyperreflexia	Constant pain; no relief with bed rest		**Dysarthria**	Fatigue
Bowel/bladder disturbance	Night pain		Double vision	
Multisegmental weakness and/or sensory changes			Positive cranial nerve signs	

Table 14-5 Overview of Cervical Spinal Nerve Root Dysfunction[3]

Cervical Nerve Root	Sensory Complaints	Motor/Functional Deficit
C2	Jaw Occipital headaches	None
C3	Headache Posterior cervical spine pain Occipital pain Ear pain/tinnitus	None
C4	Cervical spine pain Trapezius pain Superior/proximal shoulder	No skeletal muscle deficits Diaphragmatic dysfunction possible
C5	Superior aspect of the shoulder Lateral aspect of the upper arm	Deltoid muscle group weakness Biceps brachii weakness Impingement tests may be negative
C6	Cervical spine Area over the biceps brachii Dorsal hand between thumb and index fingers	Weak wrist extension Weak elbow extension Weak thumb extension
C7	Posterior aspect of arm Posterolateral forearm Middle finger	Triceps brachii weakness Wrist extensor weakness Finger extensor weakness Wrist pronator weakness
C8	Fourth or fifth finger	Weak interossei

- **Pain:** Establish the patient's current level of pain using a visual analogue scale. Is the pain constant or intermittent? Chemically induced pain, such as that relating to inflammation, is more constant with no change in symptoms as the spine changes position. Mechanical pain, caused by compression of a nerve root, tends to vary in intensity, and relief (or a decrease in symptoms) can be obtained by moving the spine into a specific position, such as tilting the head away from the involved side, which decreases the pressure on the involved structure. Question the patient regarding activities or postures that aggravate or alleviate symptoms.
- **Symptom location:** The location of symptoms by the patient may help identify a referred pain pattern and/or radicular symptoms. Pain drawings, whereby the patient shades the location of symptoms on an outline of a body, may be useful in identifying neurogenic pain.[15]
- **Other symptoms:** Complaints of visual disturbances, dizziness, lightheadedness, and headaches may be associated with decreased blood flow to the brain due to insufficiency of the vertebrobasilar artery.[16,17] Patients with these findings should be referred to a physician for further diagnostic testing. Often, patients who sustain flexion-extension, or whiplash, injuries may also experience dizziness due to altered proprioceptive input to the vestibular system.[18]

Functional Assessment

Ask the patient to describe or reproduce those motions and activities that increase the symptoms. Multiple repetitions of a task may be needed to determine the impact of fatigue.

Dysphasia Difficulty in generating speech caused by a brain lesion.

Dysarthria Speech impairment caused by dysfunction of the muscles and joints associated with speech

Table 14-6 Possible Pathology Based on the Mechanism of Injury

Mechanism	Pathology
Flexion	Compression of the anterior vertebral body and intervertebral disc
	Sprain of the supraspinous, interspinous, and posterior longitudinal ligaments and ligamentum flavum
	Sprain of the facet joints
	Tear of the posterior cervical musculature
Extension	Sprain of the anterior longitudinal ligament
	Compression of the posterior vertebral body and intervertebral disc
	Compression of the facet joints
	Fracture of the spinous processes
	Tear of the anterior cervical musculature
Lateral Bending	On the side toward the bending:
	Compression of the cervical nerve roots
	Compression of the vertebral bodies and intervertebral disc
	Compression of the facet joints
	On the side opposite the bending:
	Stretching of the cervical nerve roots
	Sprain of the lateral ligaments
	Sprain of the facet joints
	Tear of the cervical musculature
Rotation	Disc trauma
	Ligament sprain
	Facet sprain or dislocation
	Vertebral dislocation
Axial Load	Compression fracture of the vertebral body
	Compression of the intervertebral disc
Whiplash	Cervical instability
	Cervical muscle tear
	Facet joint dysfunction

Acute cervical spine pathology may dramatically limit active ROM, making such daily tasks as driving, sleeping, reaching up, and reading difficult and painful. Increased pain and peripheralization of symptoms with positions that require cervical flexion are often associated with cervical disc disease.

The patient's work or study environment may aggravate neck symptoms. Frequently, chronic cervical pain is associated with sustained positioning associated with working at a desk or a computer. Observe the patient's habitual work posture and position of the computer screen.

Observe the patient's breathing pattern and note any change in symptoms with deep or rapid breathing. Injury to the thoracic vertebrae, pressure on the thoracic nerve roots, or trauma to the ribs or costal cartilage may result in pain during respiration, resulting in irregular or shallow breathing patterns.

Inspection

A general inspection of the entire body is necessary to determine proper posture in the sagittal and frontal planes. Also see Inspection of the Lumbar Spine in Chapter 13 and Postural Evaluation in Chapter 6.

Inspection of the Lateral Structures

- **Cervical and thoracic curvature:** To keep the eyes level, the head is maintained in an upright and level position. The kyphotic curve of the thoracic spine is counterbalanced by the lordotic curve in the cervical spine to maintain this position. Pathology in the cervical or thoracic region can alter this relationship, resulting in increased or decreased curves. Observe the curves from the side. A flattening of the cervical curvature or lateral bending may indicate posturing to decrease pressure on the nerve roots (usually on the side away from the bend). An increased lordotic curve can lead to a forward head posture. Flattening of the lordotic curve or tilting to one side can indicate spasm of the cervical muscles.
- **Posture:** A forward head posture is characterized by excessive thoracic kyphosis combined with increased lordosis in the upper cervical region. This posture can result from adaptive tissue changes. Identify the cause and effect of muscle shortening, lengthening, and/or weakening (see Chapter 6).

Inspection of the Anterior Structures

- **Level of the shoulders:** Standing in front of the patient, observe the level of the patient's shoulders. The height of the acromioclavicular joints, the deltoid, and clavicles should be level; the dominant shoulder is often slightly depressed relative to the nondominant shoulder.
- **Position of the head on the shoulders:** The head should be seated symmetrically on the cervical spine with the shoulders held in an upright position. Unilateral spasm of the cervical muscles results in lateral flexion of the head toward the involved side. The rotation of the chin opposite the side of the tilt may indicate torticollis, a congenital or acquired spasm of the SCM muscle.
- **Shape of the chest:** The chest should be shaped symmetrically from side to side. An advanced scoliosis may cause a noticeable "rib hump" as the vertebrae rotate and side bend as the disease progresses. The vertebral rotation causes the ribs to become prominent in the posterior aspect of the spine.

Inspection of the Posterior Structures

Note that inspection of the posterior cervical and thoracic spine should also include inspection of the lumbar spine.

- **Bilateral soft tissue comparison:** Inspect the contour and tone of the trapezius and the other cervical musculature for equality of mass, tone, and texture. The trapezius of the dominant side may be hypertrophied relative to the opposite side. The posterior scapular muscles and the deltoids are inspected for normal muscle mass, tone, and texture. Atrophy of these muscles may result from impingement of a cervical nerve root or from brachial plexus trauma.

- **Bilateral comparison of skin folds:** The natural folds of the patient's torso are compared for symmetry. Unevenness or asymmetry of these folds could be caused by a bilateral muscle imbalance, increased or decreased kyphosis, scoliosis, or disease.

PALPATION

Table 14-7 presents a list of landmarks to assist in locating specific cervical and thoracic spine structures.

Table 14-7 Bony Landmarks for Palpation

Structure	Landmark
Cervical Vertebral Bodies	On the same level as the spinous processes
C1 Transverse Process	One finger breadth inferior to the mastoid process
C3–C4 Vertebrae	Posterior to the hyoid bone
C4–C5 Vertebrae	Posterior to the thyroid cartilage
C6 Vertebra	Posterior to the cricoid cartilage; movement during flexion and extension of the cervical spine
C7 Vertebra	Prominent posterior spinous process

Palpation of the Anterior Neck and Thorax

Refer to Chapter 15 for instructions on palpating the chest muscles.

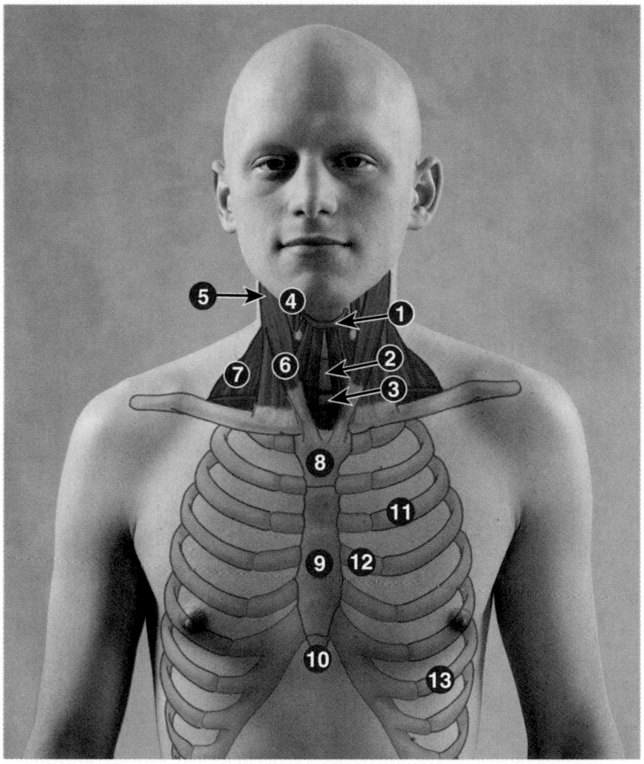

1 **Hyoid bone:** Located across from the C3 vertebra; palpate the **hyoid bone** for tenderness. While gently palpating this structure, request that the patient swallow, noting the superior and inferior movement of the hyoid bone.

2 **Thyroid cartilage:** Locate the **thyroid cartilage**, found at the level of the fourth and fifth cervical vertebrae. The thyroid cartilage is a fibrous shield protecting the anterior surface of the larynx. This structure gently shifts laterally and, similar to the hyoid bone, raises and lowers during the act of swallowing. Swelling in this region may be associated with thyroid gland enlargement.

3 **Cricoid cartilage:** Identify the **cricoid cartilage**, which lies at the level of the sixth cervical vertebra. The cricoid cartilage demarcates the location where the pharynx joins the esophagus and the larynx joins the trachea. The cartilage is identified by the thickened rings that can be palpated along its anterior surface.

4 **Carotid artery:** Palpate the **carotid pulse** between the thyroid cartilage and the SCM.

5 **Lymph nodes:** Near the upper trapezius and beneath the mandible, palpate the anterior cervical **lymph nodes** lying near the origin of the SCM. Lymph nodes become enlarged secondary to infection or illness.

6 **Sternocleidomastoid (SCM):** Palpate the cordlike **SCM** along its length from its origin on the mastoid process and superior nuchal line to its insertion on the sternum and clavicle. Rotating the head causes the SCM on the side opposite the movement to become more prominent.

7 **Scalenes:** Palpate the **scalene** muscles just posterior to the SCM muscle at about the C3 to C6 level. Tightness or spasm of this muscle group may cause abnormal cervical posture or lead to compression of the brachial plexus or subclavian blood vessels.

8–10 **Sternum:** Begin palpating the rib cage at the **(8) manubrium**, continuing inferiorly to include the **(9) sternal body** and **(10) xiphoid process** and noting for tenderness and deformity. Injury to the upper sternum may involve the sternoclavicular joint (see Chapter 11).

11–13 **Ribs and costal cartilage:** Palpate each **(11) rib**, **(12) costal cartilage**, and **(13) floating rib** from anterior to posterior, noting any pain, crepitus, and deformity. Stress fractures of the ribs result in focal point tenderness.

Palpation of the Posterior Cervical and Thoracic Structures

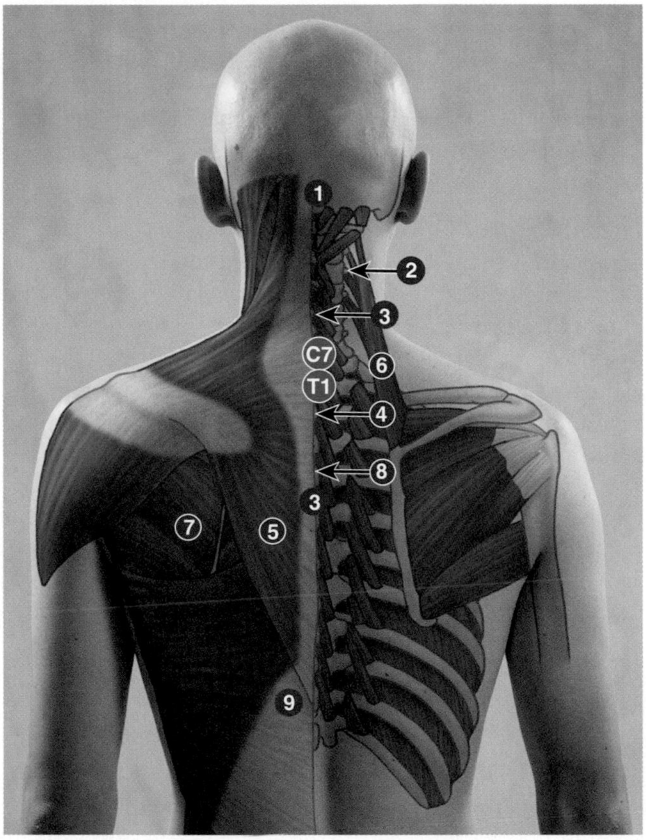

1 Occiput and superior nuchal line: The **occipital** bone, the most posterior aspect of the skull, is located at the apex of the cervical spine. Palpate this area for tenderness because it is the site of attachment for many cervical muscles. Identify the **supraspinous ligament** as it fills the space between the spinous processes. Other ligamentous structures of the spinal column can be palpated lateral to this structure.

2 Transverse processes: Located approximately one finger breadth inferior to the mastoid processes, the **transverse processes** of C1 are the only processes of the cervical spine that are palpable. The areas overlying the remaining transverse processes are palpated at the same level as the spinous processes for tenderness. The transverse processes of the thoracic spine are largely obscured by overlying muscle.

3 Spinous processes: The **spinous processes** are more easily palpated when the cervical spine is slightly flexed. Locate the area where the cervical and thoracic spines meet slightly above the superior angle of the scapula. Here two spinous processes are more prominent than the rest. The lower protrusion is the spinous process of **T1**, and the superior protrusion is the **C7** spinous process. From here, palpate the spinous processes of C6, C5, and, possibly, C4 and C3. Above the C5 level, the spinous processes begin to be masked by the soft tissue, but the area overlying the remaining processes should be palpated for tenderness. Each of these processes should be aligned immediately superior to the one below it. Continue to palpate the spinous processes along the length of the thoracic spine. The spinous process of T3 normally aligns with the medial border of the scapular spine, and T7 aligns with the inferior angle of the scapula. Use the "Rule of 3's" (Table 14-8) to help orient the spinous processes relative to the vertebral body.

4 Supraspinous ligaments: Identify the **supraspinous ligament** as it fills the space between the spinous processes. Other ligamentous structures of the spinal column can be palpated lateral to this structure.

5 Trapezius: Beginning at the occiput and superior nuchal line, the upper portion of the **trapezius** is palpated inferiorly to its insertion on the lateral clavicle, acromion process, and spine of the scapula. The thickness of this muscle is easily palpated as it spans from the cervical spine to the acromion process. Most of the remaining cervical musculature lies beneath the trapezius and is not directly palpable. The upper trapezius is a common site for trigger points.

6 Levator scapulae: Although deep to the trapezius, the **levator** may be discernible as a long, vertically oriented muscle at its origin on the medial superior scapula.

7 Scapular muscles: Palpate the muscles acting on the **scapula** to identify areas of tenderness, spasm, or atrophy. Precise palpation of these muscles is described in Chapter 15.

8 Costovertebral junction: The articulations between the ribs and thoracic vertebrae are not directly palpable

Table 14-8 Relative Alignment of the Thoracic Spinous Processes (Rule of 3's)

Level	Spinous Process Alignment
T1–T3	At the same level as the transverse processes and the vertebral body
T4–T6	Midway between the transverse processes of the originating vertebra and the transverse processes of the one below
T7–T9	At the same level as the transverse processes of the inferior vertebra
T10	At the level of the T11 vertebral body
T11	Halfway between T11 and T12
T12	At the same level as the T12 vertebral body

when they are covered by large paravertebral muscles but can be palpated on individuals with slender to normal builds.

9 Paravertebral muscles: Palpate the **paravertebral muscles** as they become prominent in the area of the scapula along their length to the pelvis (actual muscle group not shown in this figure).

Joint and Muscle Function Assessment

During ROM assessment, monitor the patient for symptoms such as **nystagmus**, dizziness, and lightheadedness, which may signal decreased blood supply to the brain. Should this occur, the patient should be referred for further diagnostic testing, and no further joint motions should be assessed. The vertebral artery test, described on page 574 should be performed following single-plane passive ROM assessment; however, the diagnostic accuracy of the vertebral artery test is questionable, and negative findings do not conclusively rule out vascular compromise.[19]

Cervical spine ROM decreases with age.[20] Active and passive ROM can be subjectively classified as "limited" or "not limited" or quantified with measurements using visual estimates, inclinometers, goniometers, or tape measures (Fig. 14-13 and Fig. 14-14). Goniometric and visual estimates of cervical ROM are highly inaccurate and have poor interrater reliability. Dual inclinometers are often used; however interrater reliability for some motions remains questionable (Goniometry 14-1, 14-2, and 14-3).[21]

Active Range of Motion

Active range of motion (AROM) is used to assess the upper and lower cervical regions. When the patient gets to the end of the voluntary range, apply slight passive pressure to assess for exacerbation of pain, tissue extensibility, and available range.[22] People who have sustained whiplash-type injuries may have significantly limited AROM in the acute and chronic stages.[23]

- **Cervical Flexion and Extension:** Assess flexion and extension while the patient is seated. Most of the flexion and extension motion that occurs in the cervical spine takes place at the atlanto-occipital joint (capital flexion

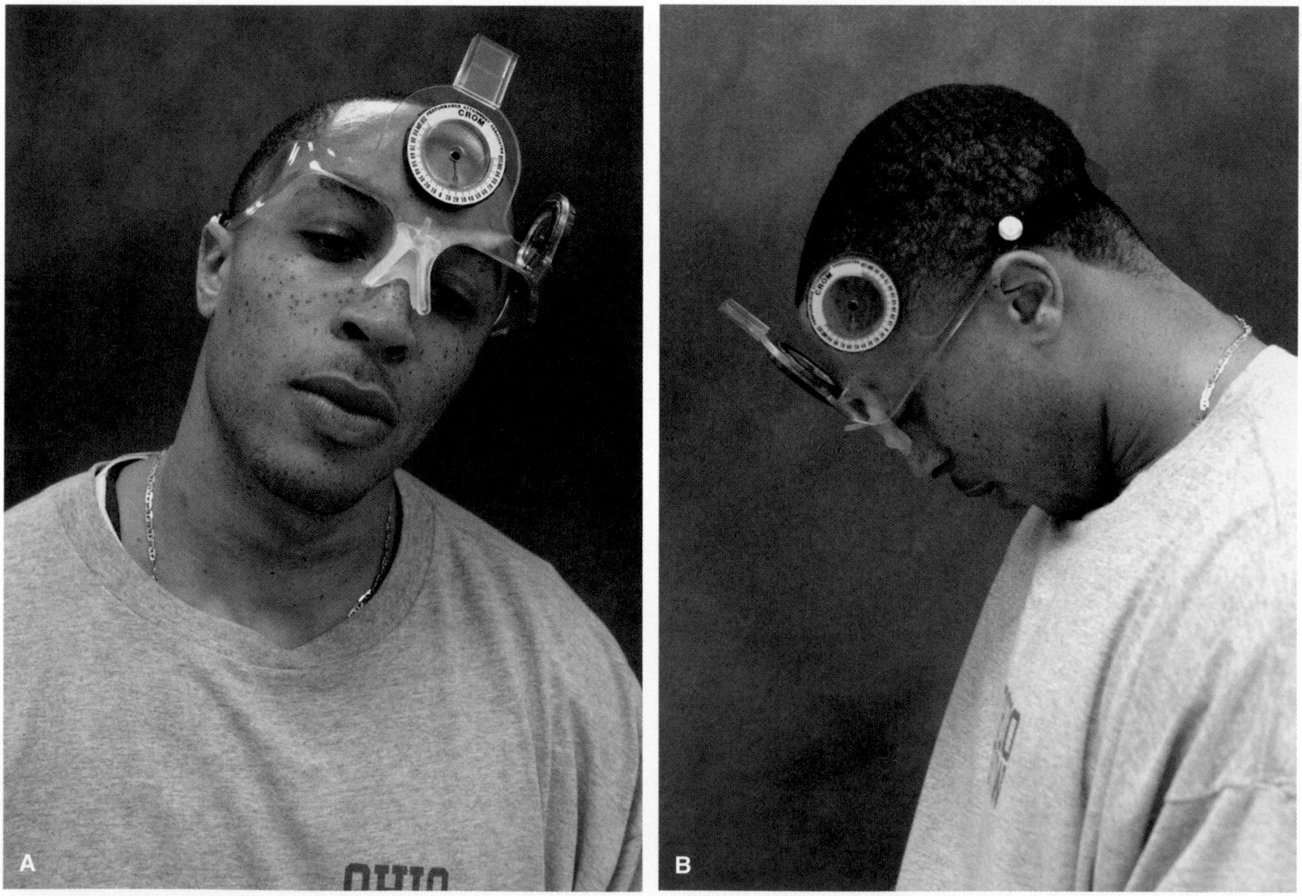

FIGURE 14-13 ■ A specialized cervical spine inclinometer such as the Cervical Range of Motion device can be used. These instruments yield more reliable results because there are fewer sources of measurement error, including not needing to use anatomical landmarks. (A) Lateral flexion; (B) Cervical flexion.

Nystagmus An uncontrolled side-to-side movement of the eyes

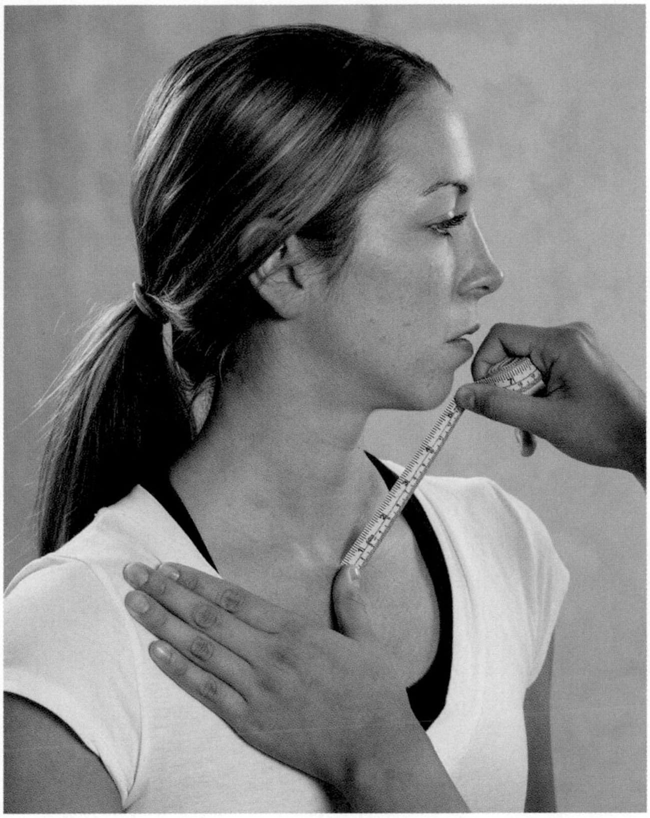

FIGURE 14-14 ■ Measuring cervical range of motion with a tape measure. The distance from the jugular notch on the sternum to the point of the chin is measured and recorded for each motion. Cervical rotation is demonstrated in this photograph.

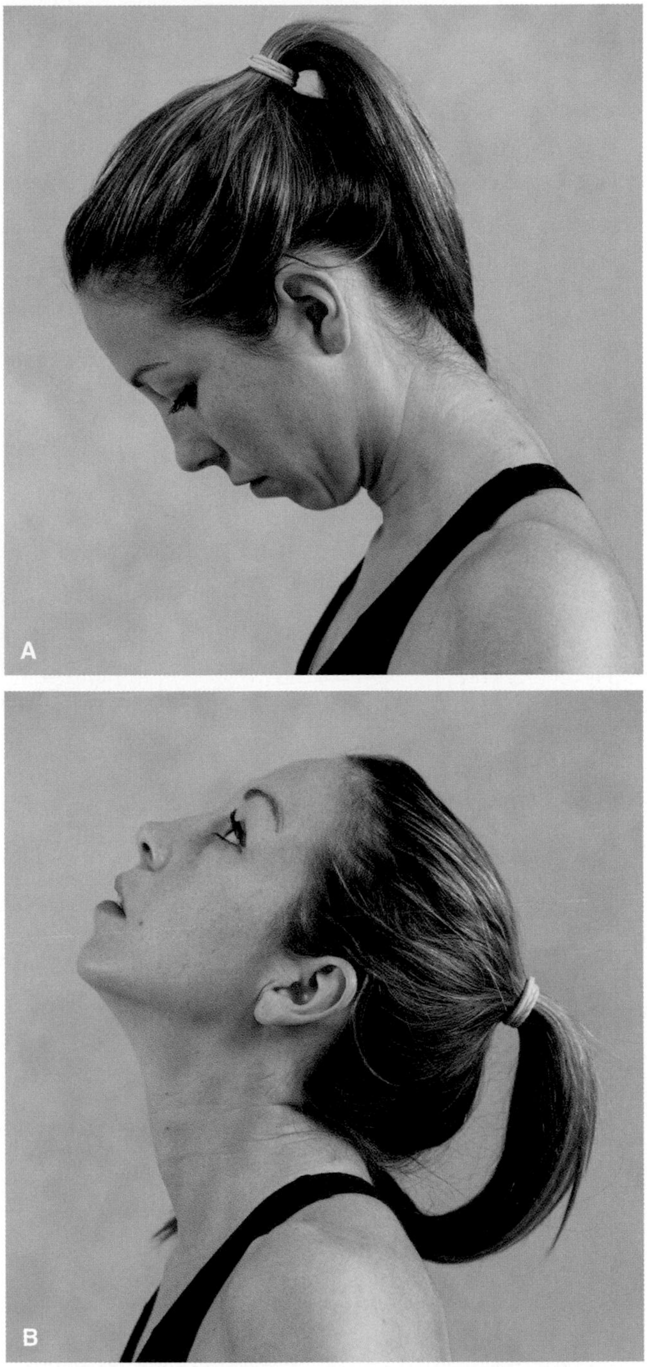

FIGURE 14-15 ■ Active (A) flexion and (B) extension of the cervical spine. The patient may attempt to compensate for a lack of cervical flexion by rounding the shoulders and compensate for a lack of extension by retracting the scapulae.

and extension) (Fig. 14-15A). Flexion of the head is achieved by asking the patient to "make a double chin." Cervical spine flexion is assessed by asking the patient to touch the chin to the chest, noting for rotation of the skull that indicates substitution by the SCM on the side opposite to the rotation. Extension is tested by having the patient look up toward the ceiling (Fig. 14-15B). When the patient reaches the end of the range, apply passive overpressure to assess for any increase in symptoms and the quality of the end-feel.

Limitations in cervical extension will result in compensatory trunk extension or knee flexion, while limitations in cervical flexion will result in compensation through trunk flexion. Compensation for limited or painful cervical rotation occurs through increased trunk rotation.

- **Cervical Lateral Flexion:** With the patient seated, determine if the ROM of the head toward each shoulder is equal and pain free. This motion occurs primarily in the upper vertebrae, producing approximately 45 degrees of motion in each direction. The patient may attempt to compensate for decreased cervical ROM by elevating the shoulder girdle.
- **Cervical Rotation:** With the patient seated and the head held upright and facing forward, observe for symmetry in the amount of rotation as the patient attempts to look over each shoulder. This motion, occurring primarily at the atlanto-axial joint, should be equal and pain free in each direction. The patient may compensate for a lack of cervical rotation by rotating the torso in the direction opposite that of the cervical movement.
- **Thoracic Spine Flexion and Extension:** With the patient seated and the hands laced behind the neck, the patient moves into flexion, keeping the elbows in

Goniometry 14-1
Cervical Flexion and Extension

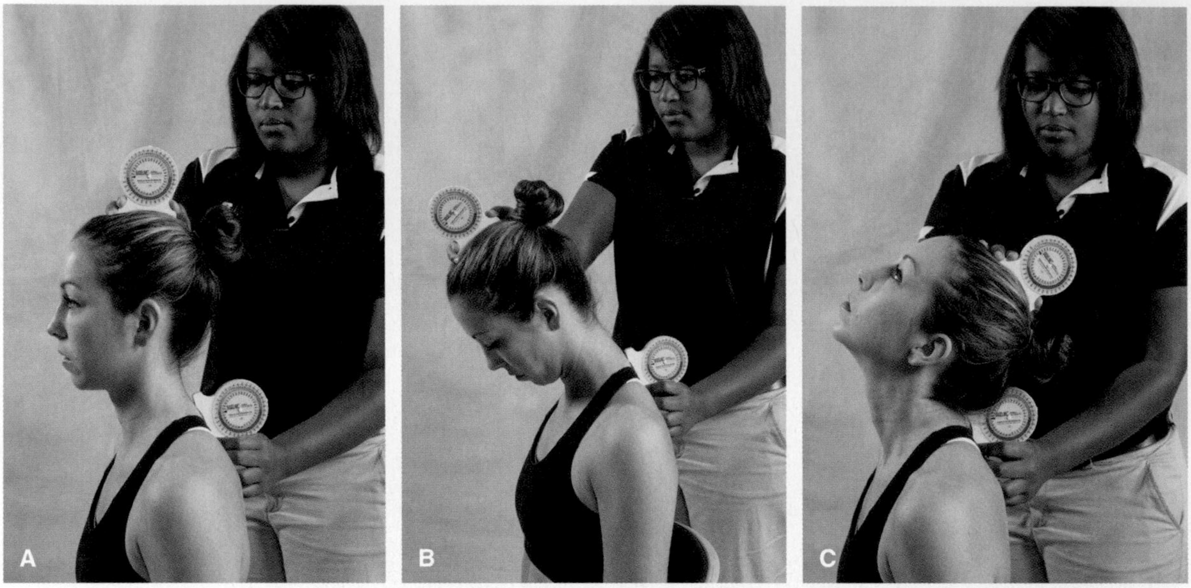

Total Excursion (flexion/extension): 50°–0°–60°

Patient Position	Seated
Procedure	Place one inclinometer over the T1 spinous process. Adjust the inclinometer to 0°. Place the second inclinometer on top of the patient's head. Adjust the inclinometer to 0°. **(A)** Have the patient bring the head and neck into flexion while keeping the trunk still. Note the degrees on each inclinometer. The difference between the values on the thoracic inclinometer and the second goniometer represents the flexion ROM. **(B)** Repeat the process with the patient moving into cervical extension. **(C)**
Comments	Cervical flexion and extension can also be assessed using a tape measure to measure the distance between the chin and the suprasternal notch. A goniometer can also be used.
Evidence	

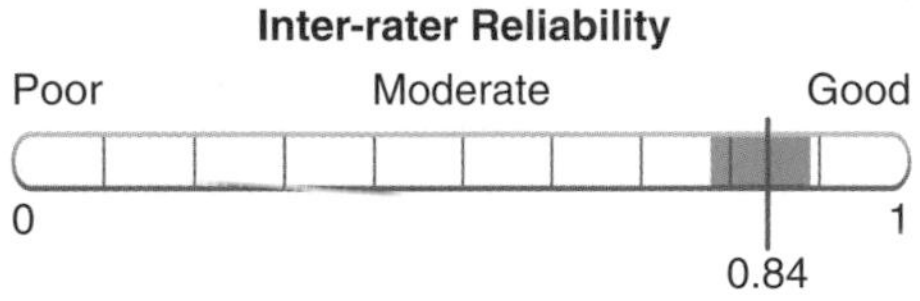

(Fig. 14-16A). For extension, instruct the patient to lift the elbows to the sky (Fig. 14-16B).[24] A restriction in physiological thoracic spine movement may be implicated in thoracic, shoulder, or cervical pain.

- **Thoracic Spine Rotation:** The patient is placed in the sitting position to stabilize the pelvis and lower extremity. The patient then rotates the shoulder girdles and spinal column as if looking behind the back (Fig. 14-16C). Rotation of the trunk occurs primarily in the thoracic spine. The amount of rotation should be equal in each direction. Overpressure can be applied at the end to assess end-feel.[24]

Manual Muscle Testing
Muscles in the cervical region require strength and endurance to maintain mechanical stability. Decreased strength and endurance in the cervical musculature is associated with neck pain, and reducing these impairments can be an important component of treatment.[25] Manual muscle testing and endurance assessment of the cervical muscles are presented in Manual Muscle Tests 14-1 to 14-5. The muscles of the shoulder girdle, especially those with attachment on the spine and scapula, may also be implicated in cervical and thoracic pain. Assessment of these muscles is presented in Chapter 15.

Goniometry 14-2
Cervical Rotation

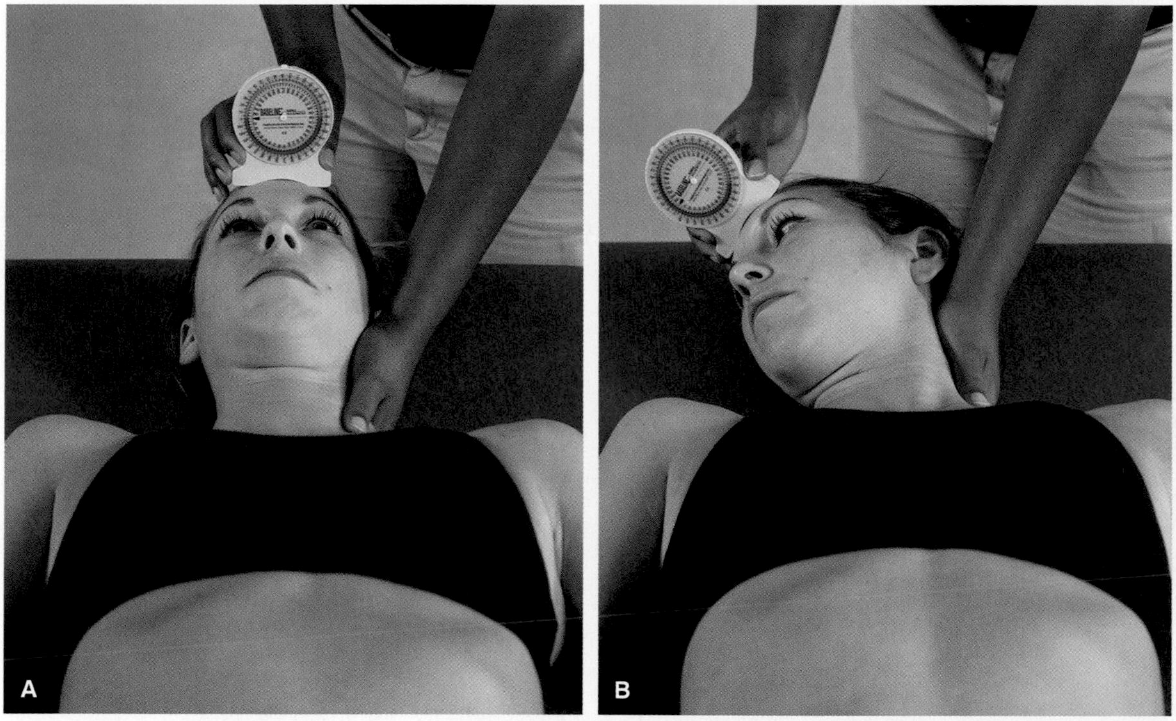

Rotation: 0–80° (each direction)

Patient Position	Supine
Procedures	Place an inclinometer in the middle of the patient's forehead. Adjust the inclinometer to 0°. **(A)** Ask the patient to rotate the head to one side, noting the inclinometer reading at the end of the range. Repeat the process, having the patient rotate to the other side. **(B)**
Evidence	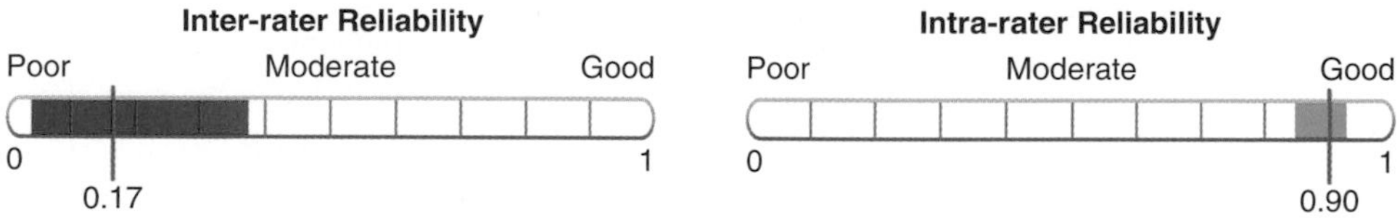

Passive Range of Motion

The available passive range of motion (PROM) and end-feel are assessed by applying over-pressure at the end of AROM. PROM is assessed with the patient supine and the head supported and moved by the examiner. If the patient describes symptoms associated with **cervical arterial dysfunction**, avoid end-range assessment of PROM—especially rotation from an extended position (see Vertebral Artery Test, p. 574).[30]

- **Flexion:** With the patient in the supine position and the head off the table to about the T2 level, grasp the patient's head under the occiput. First, assess motion at the upper cervical region by flexing only the head and bringing the chin to the chest. Next, repeat the motion, allowing the lower cervical spine to flex (Fig. 14-17A). The normal end-feel for this movement is firm owing to the chin striking the chest. Unilateral asymmetry may also be noted. Spasm in the posterior cervical muscles results in an early firm end-feel with complaints of "tightness"; mechanical blockage of the atlanto-occipital joint or the vertebrae causes a premature, hard end-feel.
- **Extension:** Assess PROM with the patient supine so that the head is off the end of the table and the neck is allowed to move into extension (Fig. 14-17B). First,

Goniometry 14-3
Cervical Lateral Flexion (Side bending)

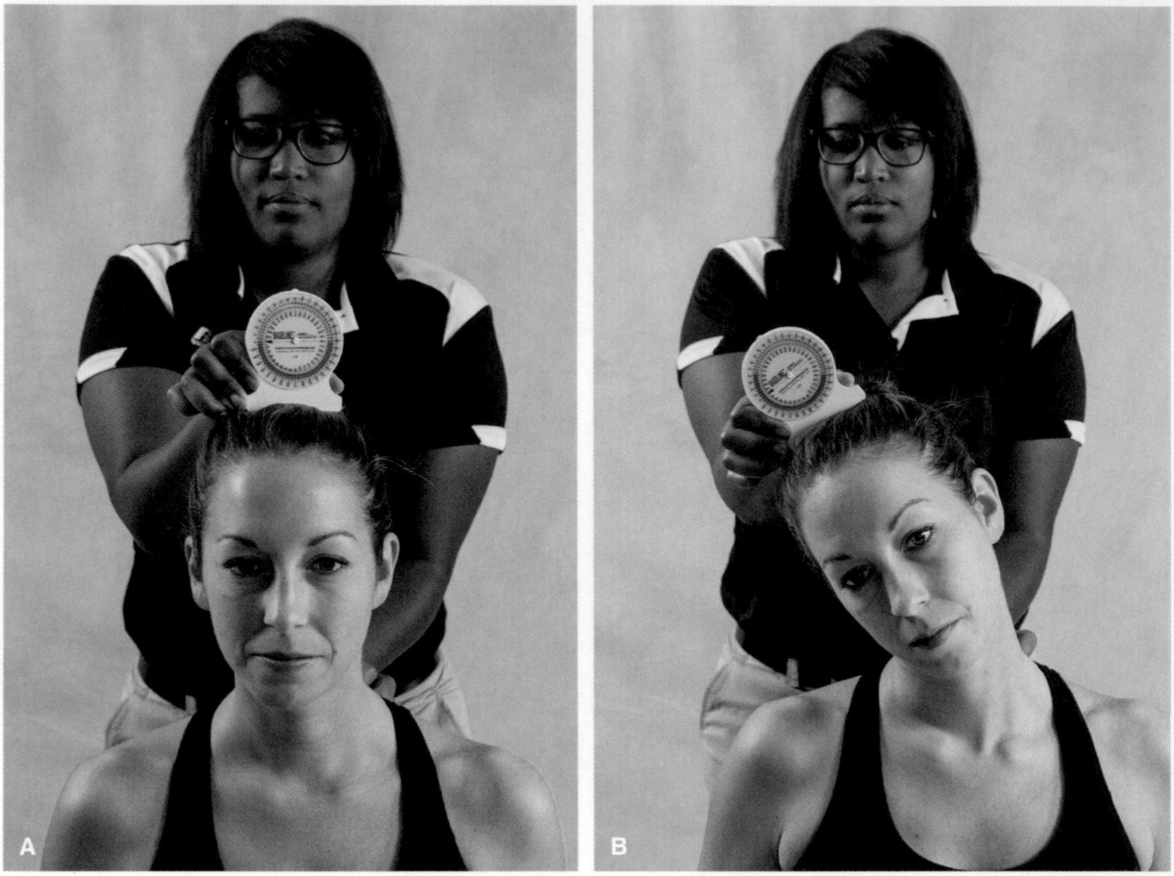

Lateral Flexion 45°–0°–45°

Patient Position

Seated with the trunk supported

Procedure

Place one inclinometer over the T1 spinous process in the frontal plane. Adjust the inclinometer to 0° [not shown].

Place the second inclinometer on top of the patient's head in the frontal plane. Adjust the inclinometer to 0°. **(A)**

Ask the patient to bring the head into lateral flexion while keeping the trunk still. The difference between the values on the thoracic inclinometer and the goniometer on the head represents the ROM. **(B)**

Repeat the process on the opposite side.

Evidence

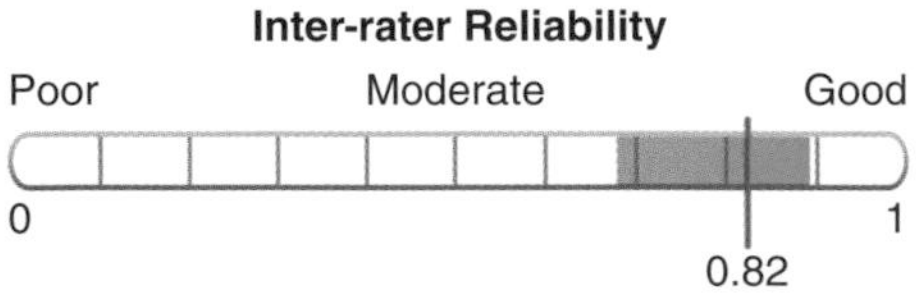

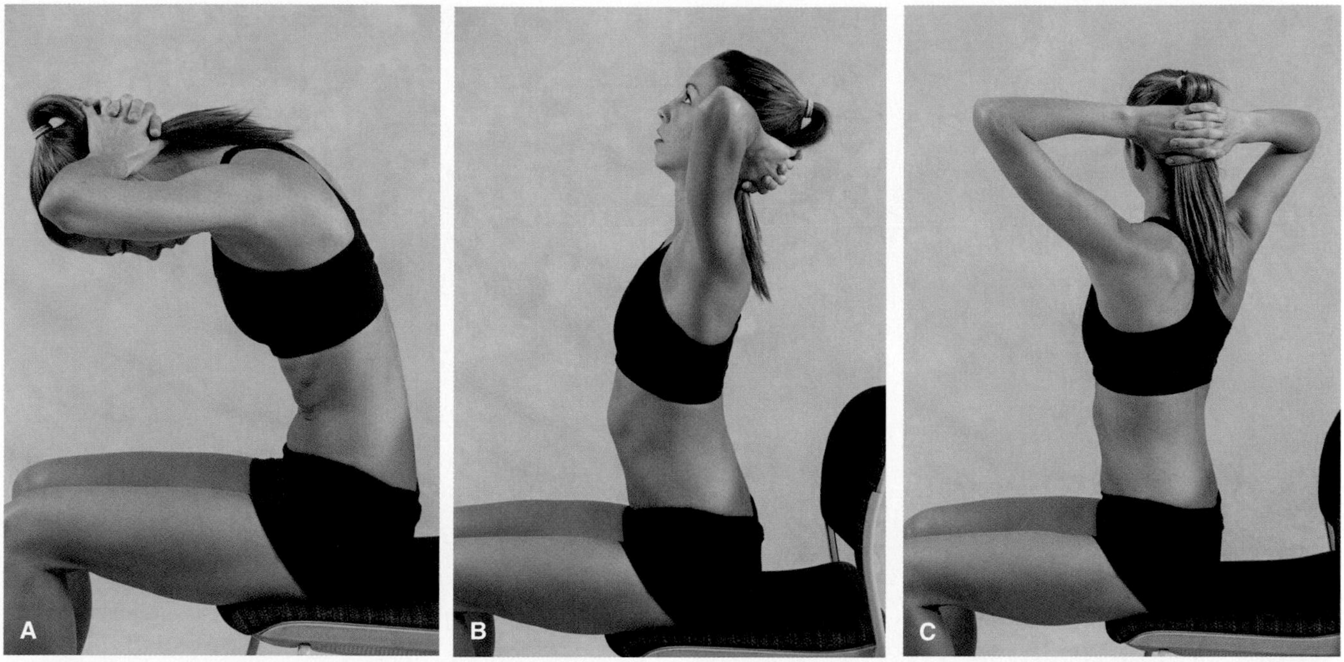

FIGURE 14-16 ■ Thoracic active range of motion. (A) Flexion, (B) Extension, (C) Rotation

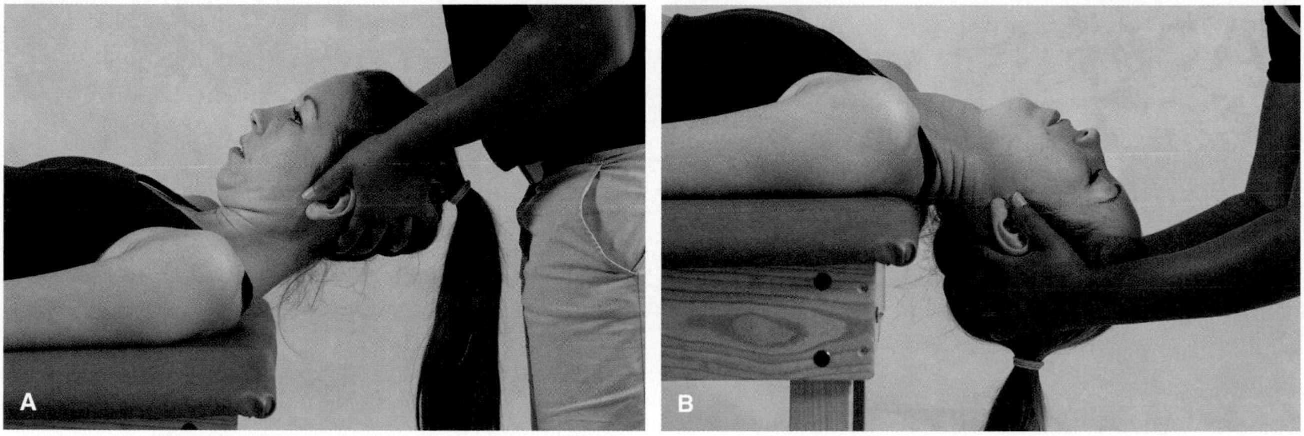

FIGURE 14-17 ■ Passive (A) flexion and (B) extension of the cervical spine. It is recommend that a table with a dropped face plate be used if the patient's head is off the table and supported by the clinician.

assess capitocervical extension by stabilizing the lower cervical spine and extending the head. Follow this with extension of the lower cervical spine, noting any unilateral asymmetry. The normal end-feel for this motion is hard as the occiput makes contact with the rest of the cervical spine. Avoid assessing passive extension in patients who describe dizziness or nystagmus, symptoms of impingement on the vertebrobasilar artery.

- **Lateral flexion:** Continuing in the supine position, keep the patient's cervical spine in the neutral position between flexion and extension. Sliding one hand under the occiput, tilt the head and neck to bring the ear toward the shoulder (Fig. 14-18). Stabilize the contralateral shoulder with the opposite hand if needed. The normal end-feel for lateral flexion is firm owing to soft tissue stretch.
- **Rotation:** With the patient supine, grasp the patient's forehead and occiput to maintain the cervical spine in its neutral position. Then apply pressure to rotate the skull and neck (Fig. 14-19). The skull and spine should be rotated together. A firm end-feel is expected from stretching of the SCM muscle and intrinsic neck ligaments. Fully flexing the neck before rotating the head better isolates the atlanto-axial joints by restricting motion in the lower cervical region.

Joint Stability Tests

Patient reports of dizziness, syncope, or nystagmus during vertebral joint stability tests warrant stopping the tests and further diagnostic testing by a physician.

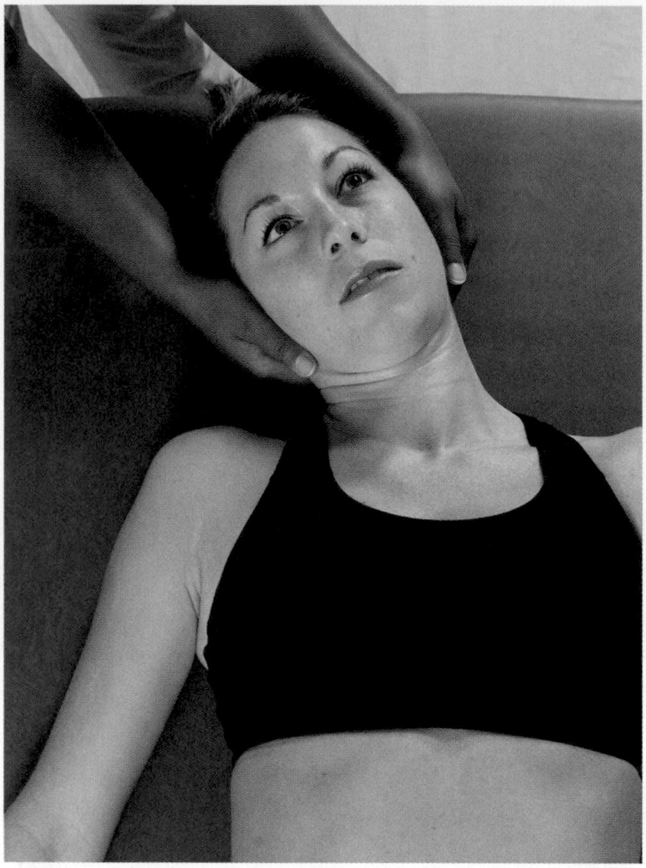

FIGURE 14-18 ■ Passive right lateral flexion of the cervical spine.

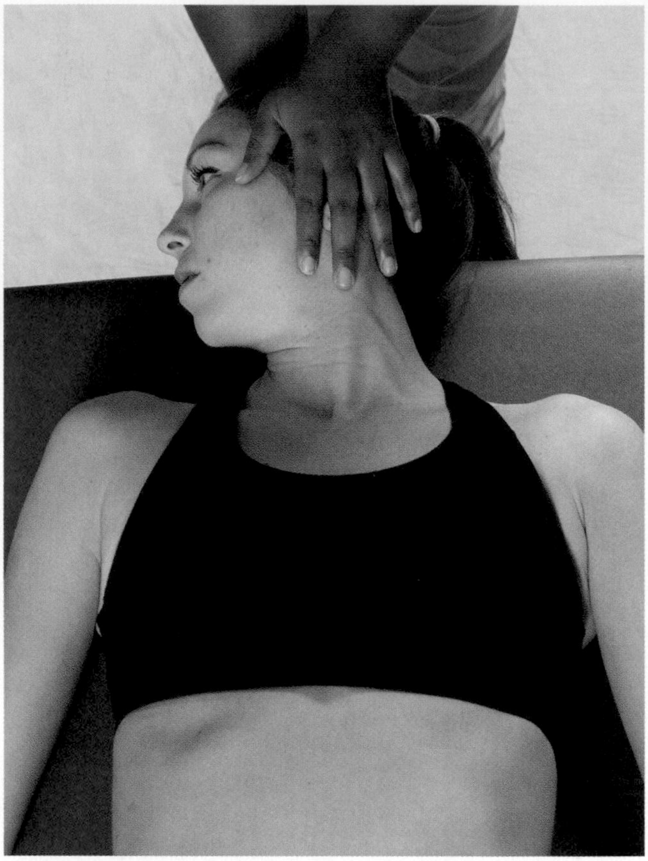

FIGURE 14-19 ■ Passive right rotation of the cervical spine.

Stress Testing

There are no specific ligamentous tests for the cervical spine. The end-range of PROM testing stresses the spinal ligaments, assuming the motion is not limited by muscular tightness or contractures (Table 14-9).

Joint Play

Accessory intervertebral motion and associated pain are assessed using joint play techniques (Joint Play 14-1). Theoretically, hypomobility at one segment may result in compensatory hypermobility at the segments above and below, although the small magnitude of the available range makes differences difficult to detect clinically. The interrater reliability of these techniques is low, likely because consistent identification of the same segment via palpation is problematic.[12] Hypomobility of the first rib can result in cervical pain (Joint Play 14-2).

Table 14-9 Cervical Spine Ligaments Stressed During Passive Range of Motion Testing

Motion	Ligaments Stressed
Flexion	Posterior longitudinal ligament Ligamentum nuchae Interspinous ligament Ligamentum flavum
Extension *Rotation*	Anterior longitudinal ligament Interspinous ligament Ligamentum flavum
*Lateral Bending**	Interspinous ligament Ligamentum flavum

*These assessments are usually inconclusive.

Neurological Testing

Because of the mobility and relative lack of protection of the cervical spine, lower motor neuron lesions in this area are common. An upper quarter neurological screen is used to determine pathology of the C5 through T1 nerve roots. The possibility of spinal cord involvement also requires a lower quarter screen (see Box 1-5). PROM may also provoke neurological symptoms such as aching, throbbing, or burning as the nerve root is compressed or placed on stretch.

Sometimes referred to as the "straight leg test of the upper extremity," the **upper limb nerve tension tests** (also known as the upper limb neurodynamic tests) assess the impact of changing nerve tension on provoking symptoms (Selective Tissue Test 14-1).[17,31] Similar to the straight leg raising test or the slump test in the lower extremity, the upper limb tension tests (ULTTs) involve placing the patient in sequential positions that gradually increase tension on a

Manual Muscle Test 14-1
Capital, Cervical, and Combined Capital and Cervical Flexion

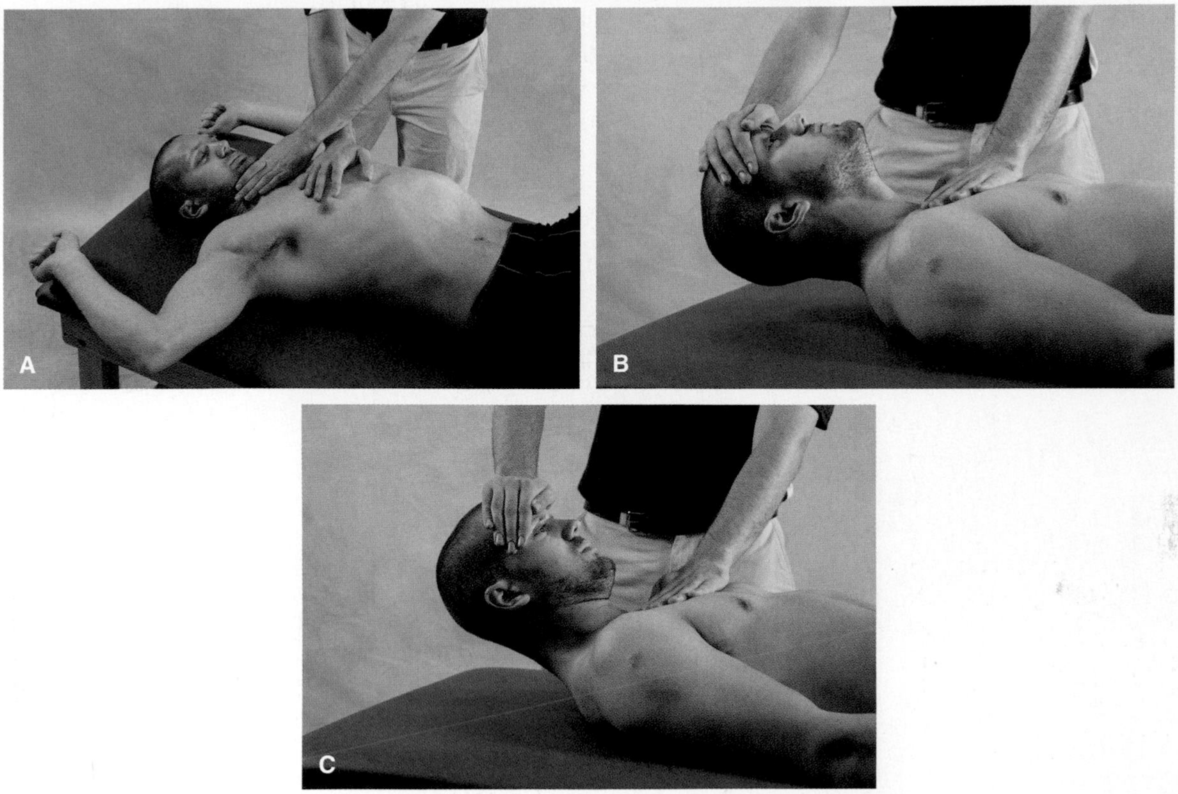

Patient Position	Supine with head supported on table and the cervical spine and head in a neutral position. The shoulders are abducted to 90° with the elbows flexed to 90°.
Test Position	*Capital flexion:* The patient's chin is tucked without lifting the head from the table as if nodding. **(A)** *Cervical flexion:* The patient's cervical spine is flexed without tucking the chin, looking at the ceiling. **(B)** *Combined capital and cervical flexion:* The patient's head and neck are flexed, with chin to chest. **(C)**
Stabilization	*Cervical and combined flexion:* Over the superior aspect of the sternum if the patient is unable to self-stabilize the trunk
Resistance	*Capital flexion:* Resistance is applied on the mandible, pulling the head up and backwards. *Cervical flexion:* Resistance is applied on the forehead. *Combined capital and cervical flexion:* Resistance is applied on the forehead.
Prime Movers (Innervation)	*Capital flexion:* Rectus capitis anterior (suboccipital nerve: C1) Rectus capitis lateralis Longus capitis (branches of CN C4, C5, C6, C7, C8) *Cervical flexion:* Sternocleidomastoid (spinal accessory: CN XI, C2, C3) Anterior scalene (dorsal rami: C4, C5, C6) Longus colli (anterior rami, C2, C3, C4, C5, C6)
Secondary Movers (Innervation)	*Capital flexion:* Suprahyoids (mylohyoid [CN III], digastric [CN III], stylohyoid [CN VII], geniohyoid [CN I–CN XII]) *Cervical flexion:* Middle scalene (dorsal rami: C3–C8) Posterior scalene (dorsal rami: C7, C8) Infrahyoids (sternothyroid, thyrohyoid, sternohyoid, omohyoid [CN I–CN III)
Substitution	Inability to keep the chin tucked during the combined movement signals weakness of the deep cervical flexors and overreliance on the sternocleidomastoid.[26]

Manual Muscle Test 14-2
Capital, Cervical, and Combined Capital and Cervical Extension

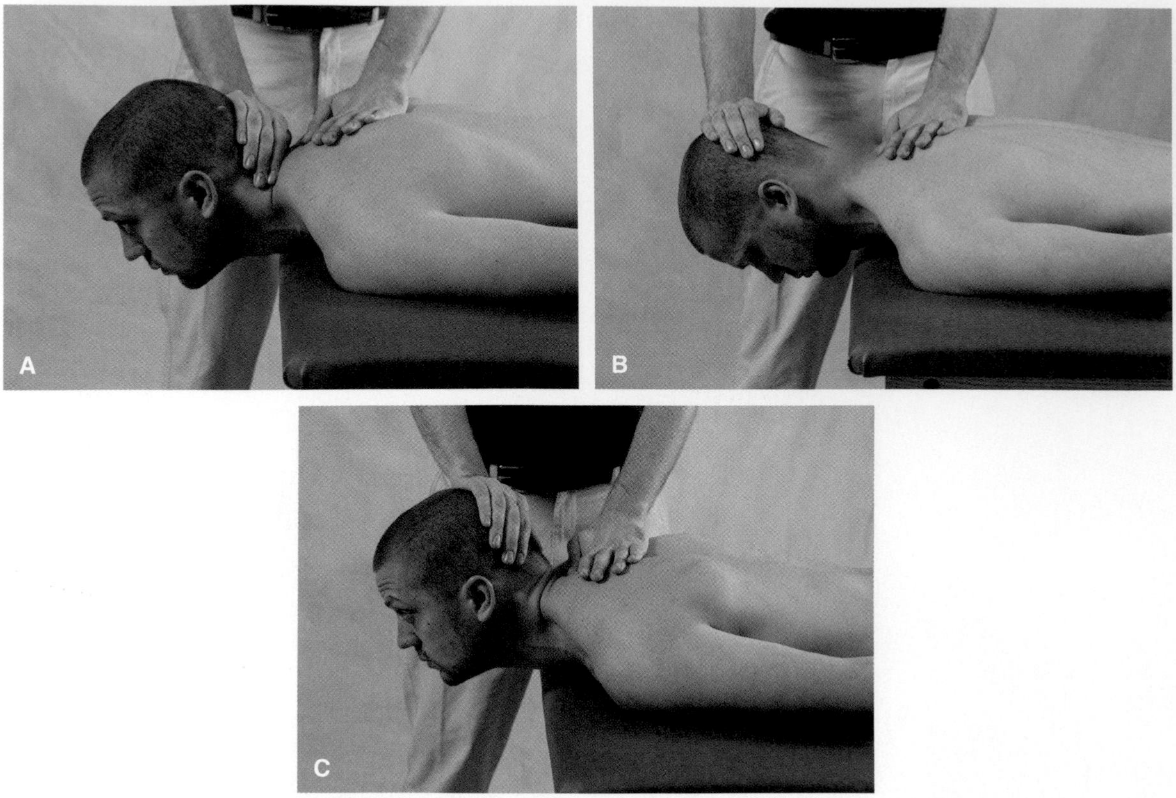

Patient Position	Prone with head off table The arms are at the side, or the shoulders are abducted to 90° and the elbows flexed to 90°.
Test Position	The cervical spine and head are in the neutral position. *Capital extension:* The patient's head is extended by tilting the chin upward ("Look at the wall."). **(A)** *Cervical extension:* The patient extends the head without tilting the chin upward ("Push up on my hand, but keep your chin down."). **(B)** *Capital and cervical extension:* The patient extends the head and then tilts the chin upward ("Look at the ceiling."). **(C)**
Stabilization	Superior aspect of the thoracic spine (e.g., T2–T9)
Resistance	*Capital extension:* At the base of the occiput *Cervical extension:* At the parietal-occipital area *Capital and cervical extension:* At the parietal-occipital area
Prime Movers (Innervation)	*Capital extension:* Capitus muscles (see Table 14-1) *Cervical extension:* Cervicis muscles (see Table 14-1) Upper trapezius (spinal accessory: CN XI) Levator scapulae (dorsal subscapular: C3, C4, C5) Multifidi
Secondary Movers (Innervation)	None
Substitution	Lumbar and thoracic paraspinals
Comments	It is recommend that a table with a dropped face plate be used if the patient's head is off the table and supported by the clinician.

Manual Muscle Test 14-3
Lateral Flexion

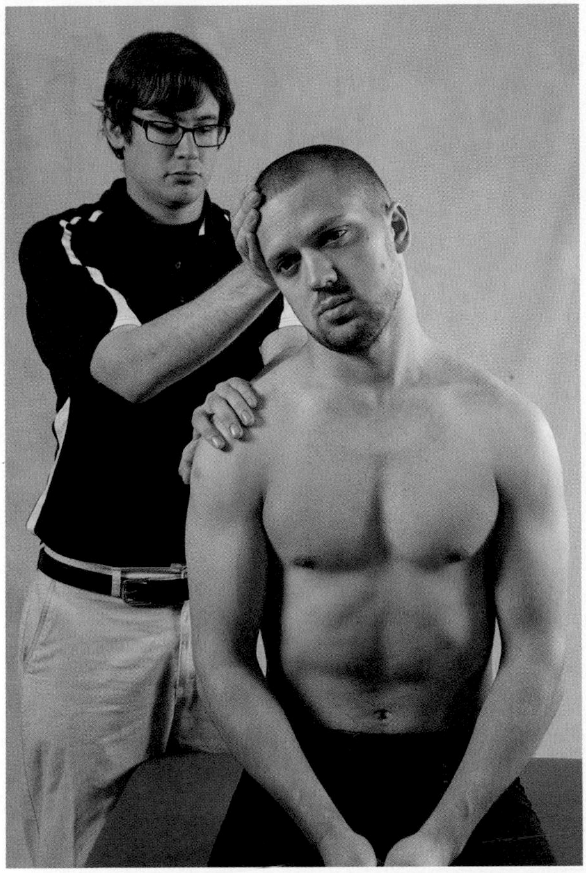

Patient Position	Seated with the cervical spine and head in the neutral position
Test Position	Slightly flexed on the side being tested
Stabilization	Over the acromioclavicular joint on the side toward the motion
Resistance	Over the temporal and parietal bones on the side toward the motion
Prime Movers (Innervation)	Sternocleidomastoid (spinal accessory: CN XI, C2, C3) Scalenes (dorsal rami: C3–C8) Paraspinal muscles on the side being tested
Secondary Movers (Innervation)	None
Substitution	Cervical flexors
Comments	The muscles tested during lateral flexion are redundant with those tested for cervical rotation, flexion, and extension.

Manual Muscle Test 14-4
Rotation and Flexion

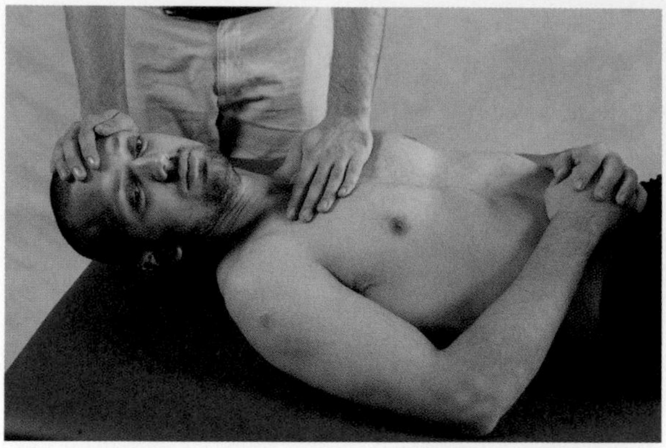

Patient Position	Supine with the shoulders abducted to 90° and the elbows flexed to 90°
Test Position	The head is rotated to the side opposite that being tested.
Stabilization	Over the sternum
Resistance	Over the temporal bone on the side toward the motion
Prime Movers (innervation)	Sternocleidomastoid (CN XI, C2, C3)
Secondary Movers (innervation)	Cervical flexors on same side
Substitutions	Uniplanar cervical flexion

specific peripheral nerve.[17,32] While tests that theoretically stretch the median, ulnar, and radial nerves have been described, research suggests that the ulnar and radial nerves are not selectively isolated and that only the ULTT for the median nerve demonstrates adequate specificity.[17] This ULTT commonly provokes responses such as pain or paresthesia in normal subjects as the nerve is progressively stretched, a so-called "normal positive."[31] Therefore, a positive response is considered reproduction of the patient's specified symptoms and motion limitation.[31,33] As with other nerve-tensioning techniques such as the slump test and straight leg raise (see Chapter 13), the response is confirmed when symptoms reduce when the exacerbating position is eliminated. Once a positive response is elicited, no further components are added to the test.

Upper Quarter Neurological Screen

Neurological Screening 14-1 presents the components of an upper quarter neurological screen.

Upper Motor Neuron Lesions

Trauma to the brain or spinal cord can result in hyperreflexia, spasticity, and hypertonicity of muscles; weakness of the muscles innervated distal to the lesion; loss of sensation; and ataxia. These findings are consistent with damage to the upper motor neurons, which connect the brain with the spinal cord and provide descending input to the muscles. Other findings of this condition include muscle tremor and uncontrollable involuntary movement. In addition, the loss of bowel and bladder control can be a sign of upper motor neuron lesions. The **Babinski test** (Selective Tissue Test 14-2) and the **Oppenheim test** (Selective Tissue Test 14-3) are used to evaluate for an upper motor neuron lesion and an associated disorder of the central nervous system.[34] Note that these tests are rarely needed with acute trauma: if an upper motor neuron lesion is present, other signs and symptoms will be readily apparent.

Normally, the abdominal muscles receive concurrent innervation from the T5–T12 nerve roots. **Beevor's sign** (Selective Tissue Test 14-4), a modified sit-up, can indicate pathology to the lower thoracic nerve roots.

Region-Specific Pathologies and Selective Tissue Tests

Acute injuries to the cervical spine occur in contact and collision sports when the spine is compressed (e.g., axial loading)

Manual Muscle Test 14-5
Neck Flexor Endurance Test

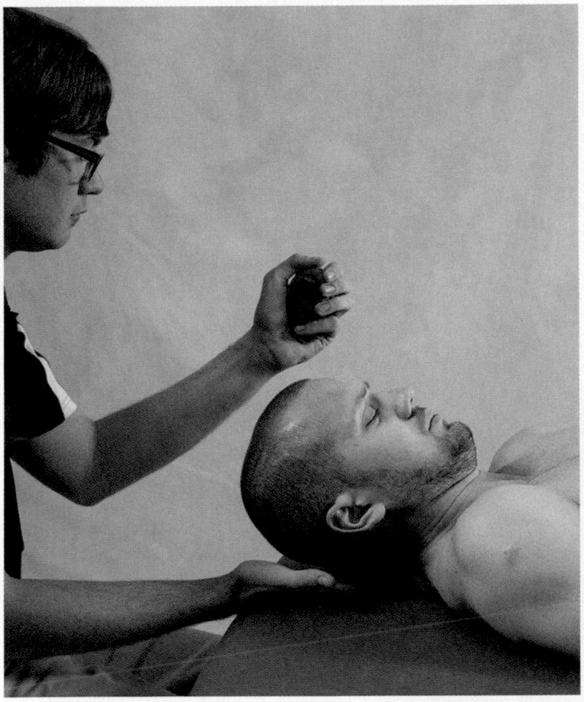

Patient Position	Supine, hook-lying
Test Position	The patient is asked to maximally tuck the chin and then lift the head approximately 1 inch (2.5 cm) from the table. The examiner slides a hand under the patient's head, just below the occiput, to note when the patient can no longer maintain the test position. The examiner times the duration that the patient can hold the position.
Prime Movers (Innervation)	Longus capitis (anterior rami C1 - C3) Longus colli (anterior rami C2 - C6) Rectus capitis anterior and lateralis (C1, C2)
Normative Data	Normative data in those without neck pain: 34.2 ± 17.7 sec [27]
Implications	Decreased control of the deep neck flexors is associated with increased cervical lordosis and may contribute to head and/or neck pain.[27,28] A review of published data on this test determined that its intrarater and interrater reliability have been adequately established.[29]

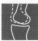

Joint Play 14-1
Cervical and Thoracic Vertebral Joint Play

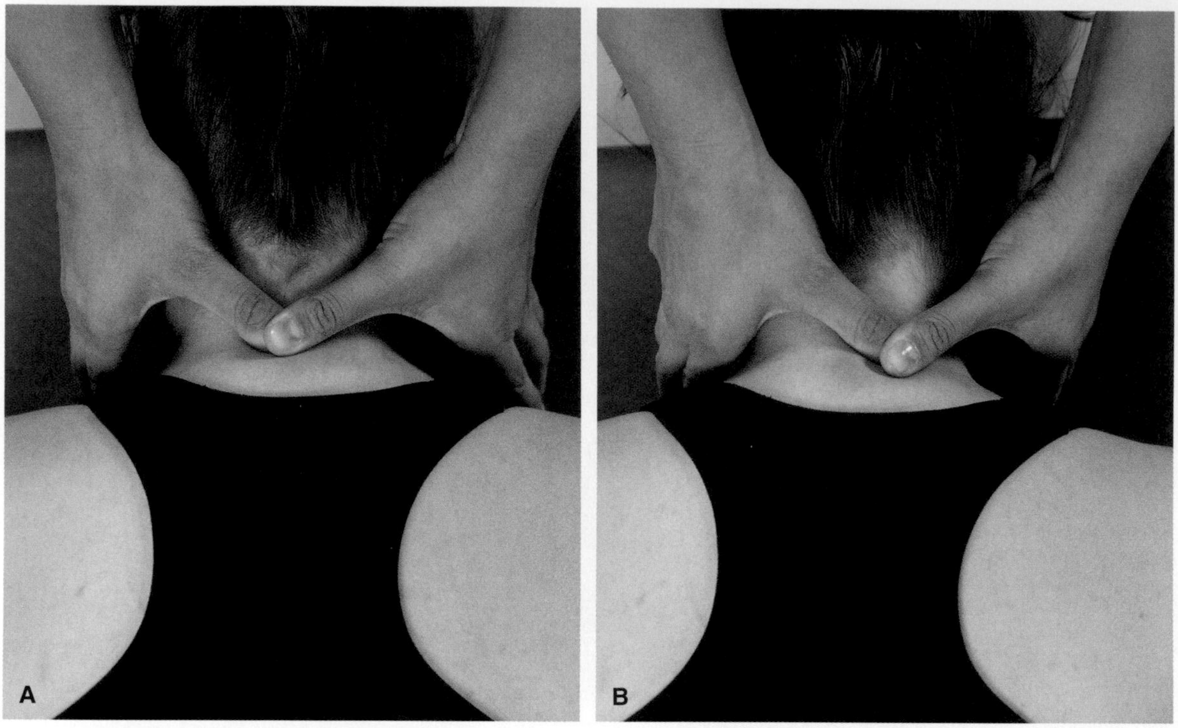

Joint play of the cervical spine. (A) Central posterior–anterior (CPA) and (B) unilateral posterior–anterior (UPA).

Patient Position	Prone; the head is in a neutral position.
Position of Examiner	Standing at the head of the patient
Evaluative Procedure	*CPA:* Palpate the target spinous process using the tips of the thumbs. Use the pisiform as a point of contact in the thoracic region. Apply a gradual anteriorly directed force until an end-feel is determined, noting any reproduction of pain. Repeat at each level, noting any differences. **(A)** Note that the degree of downward angulation of the spinous processes varies in the thoracic spine, so the moving segment may be one below the targeted spinous process. *UPA:* Palpate the target spinous process and move laterally approximately one thumb breadth to the raised area, the articular pillar. Apply an anteriorly directed force. Repeat at each level and then assess the opposite side. **(B)** In the thoracic spine, the facet joints are between the ribs and just lateral to the spinous process. To assess mobility at the costotransverse joint, apply a posterior anterior force at the junction, which is at the end of the transverse process approximately 1 inch lateral to the spinous process.
Positive Test	Hyper- or hypomobility compared with the segment above and below Pain provocation
Implications	*Hypermobility:* Insufficiency of the passive supporting structures (e.g., ligaments) *Hypomobility:* Restriction of the passive supporting structures
Evidence	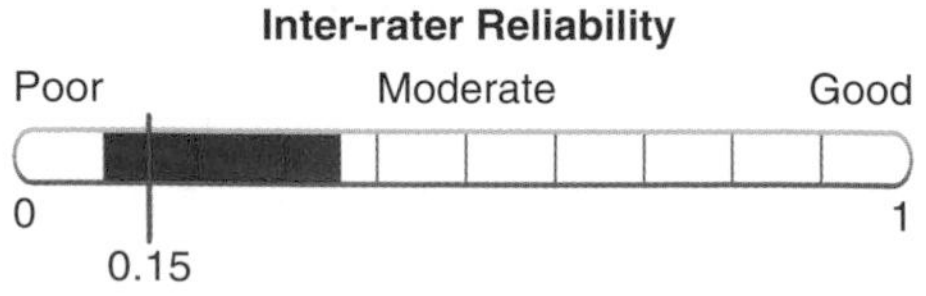

CPA = central posterior–anterior; UPA = unilateral posterior–anterior

Joint Play 14-2
Mobility of the First Rib

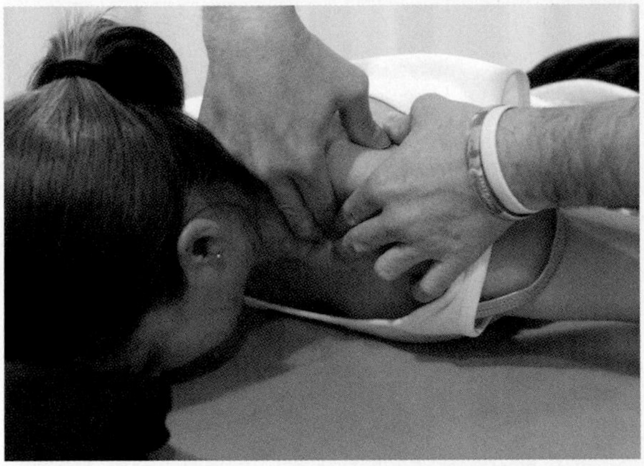

The first rib is mobilized to determine the amount of motion at the costovertebral junction.

Patient Position	Prone
Position of Examiner	Standing at the head of the patient
Evaluative Procedure	Palpate the posterior aspect of the first rib just anterior to the upper trapezius just above the vertebral border of the scapula. Provide an inferior gliding force to the rib.
Positive Test	Hypomobility and/or pain
Implications	Restricted mobility of the first costovertebral joint
Modification	There are several techniques for evaluating the mobility of the first rib.
Evidence	Absent or inconclusive in the literature

CPA = central posterior–anterior; UPA = unilateral posterior–anterior

or forced past its normal ROM. The "whiplash" type of injury occurs as the head is moving in one direction and the cervical muscles eccentrically contract to counter this motion. Chronic conditions develop from poor postural habits, repetitive movements, decreased flexibility, and dynamic insufficiency. These conditions worsen with time secondary to the adaptive shortening of tissues, resulting in increased pain and spasm. Certain disease states such as infections (e.g., meningitis), allergic reactions to medication, and other diseases may mimic the symptoms of injury to the cervical spine, especially if they create swelling and pain of surrounding lymph glands.[35]

Multiple structures are usually involved with acute and chronic neck pain. For example, degenerative joint disease is commonly associated with osteophyte formation and subsequent nerve root compression. Whiplash-associated disorder (WAD) incorporates the muscle and facet joint pathology that occurs following this mechanism.[23] Because of the close functional relationships among the structures of the spine, identifying one anatomical source is usually not possible.

The first step when evaluating cervical pathologies is to rule out the presence of any potentially catastrophic injuries. Evaluate the local cervical structures to determine any effect that the pathology may cause in distally signs and symptoms.

Cervical Radiculopathy

Pressure on one or more cervical nerve roots can result in radiculopathy, nerve-related symptoms in the neck and upper extremity. Impingement on the nerve root(s) can produce pain and paresthesia in the affected dermatome, muscular weakness, altered reflexes, and atrophy in the region supplied by the involved root (Examination Findings 14-1). Paresthesia in the upper extremity is a common symptom.[36] The mid and lower cervical nerve roots, and C7 in particular, are most commonly affected, likely because of the progressively smaller intervertebral foramen.[36]

Disc degeneration and herniations, and degenerative changes of the superior facet or uncovertebral joint can

Selective Tissue Tests 14-1
Upper Limb Tension Test (ULTT)

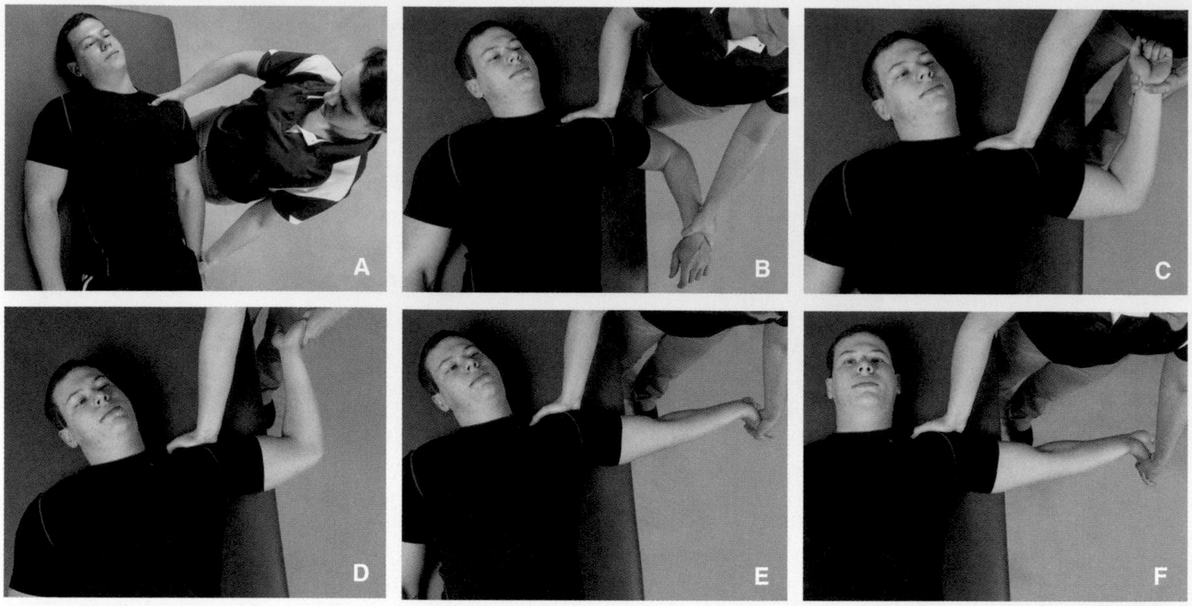

The patient's limb is sequentially positioned, pausing after each step to elicit symptoms.

Patient Position
Supine
The glenohumeral joint is at the side, the wrist and fingers are relaxed, the forearm is pronated, and the elbow is flexed.

Position of Examiner
On the test side

Evaluative Procedure
Hold each position for 6 seconds after the addition of each sequential position:
- **(A)** Passively lateral flex the cervical spine to the side not being tested and depress the shoulder girdle on the test side. Maintain this force throughout the remaining steps.
- **(B)** Abduct the glenohumeral joint to 90°.
- **(C)** Externally rotate the glenohumeral joint 90° with the elbow in 90° of flexion.
- **(D)** Supinate the forearm and extend the wrist and fingers.
- **(E)** Extend the elbow.
- **(F)** When symptoms are produced, return the patient's cervical spine to a neutral position and note any change in symptoms.

The test is discontinued at whatever position evokes positive findings.

Positive Test
Provocation of stated symptoms and restricted ROM

Implications
Hyperirritability of the peripheral nerve due to adaptive shortening, entrapment or impingement (e.g., cervical disc herniation)[33]

Modification
Positioning of the shoulder, elbow, and wrist can isolate specific peripheral nerves:[32]
Median n: Shoulder abducted to 110°, 60° external rotation, 10° extension; elbow is maintained at 0° extension and fully supinated; the wrist is extended to 70°.
Ulnar n: The shoulder is maximally abducted and externally rotated; the elbow is flexed to 120° and fully supinated; the wrist is extended to 70°.
Radial n: The shoulder is maximally abducted, extended, and internally rotated; the elbow is extended and maximally pronated. The wrist is flexed to 70°.

Comments
This procedure has a high false-positive rate, up to 88.1% in a healthy population. The diagnostic accuracy may be improved with a cutoff of 60° of elbow extension.[31]

Evidence

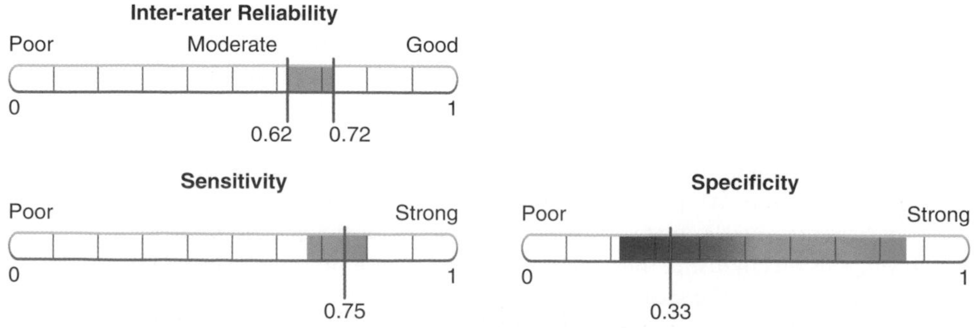

LR+: 0.91–1.24–4.79

LR−: 0.24–0.54–1.20

ROM = range of motion

Neurological Screening 14-1
Upper Quarter Neurologic Screen

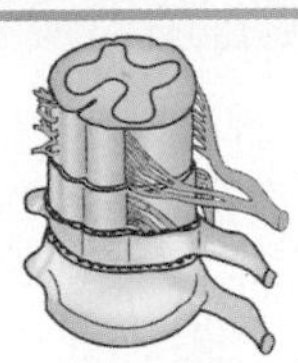 Nerve Root Level	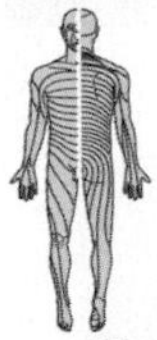 Sensory Testing	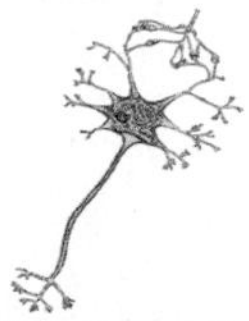 Motor Testing	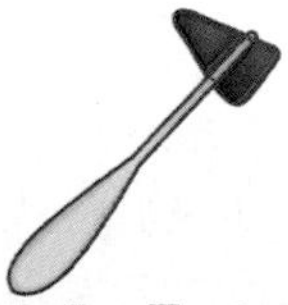 Reflex Testing
C4	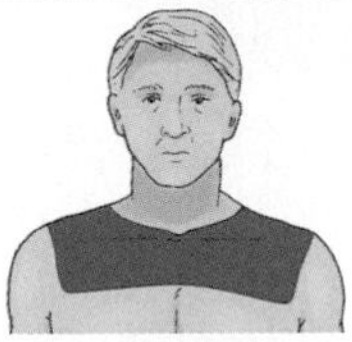 Supraclavicular n.	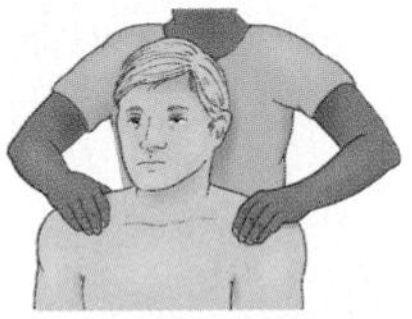 Shoulder shrug Dorsal scapular n.	None
C5	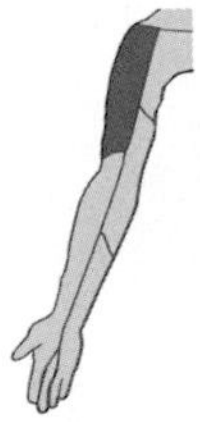 Proximal lateral brachial	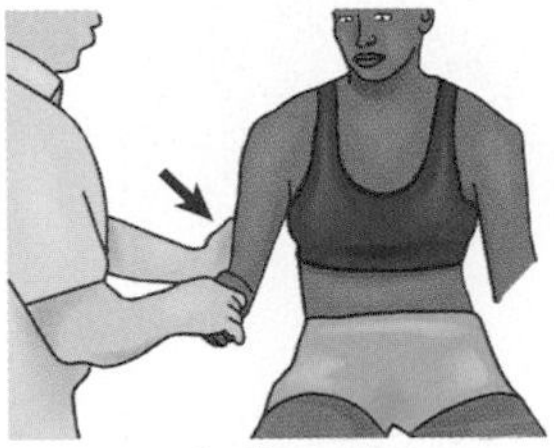 Axillary n.	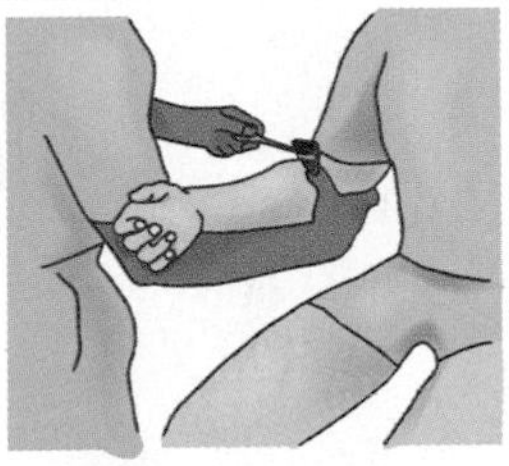 Musculocutaneous n.
C6	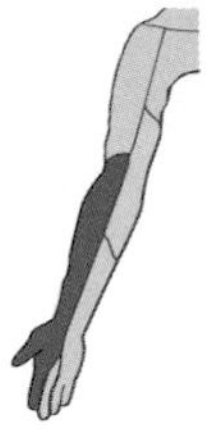 Lateral antebrachial Cutaneous n.	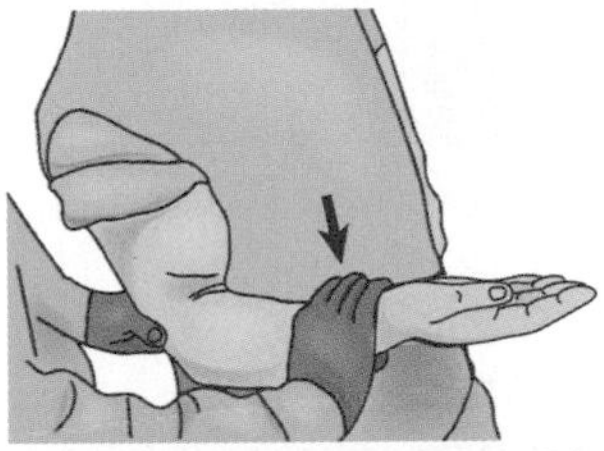 Musculocutaneous n. (C5 & C6)	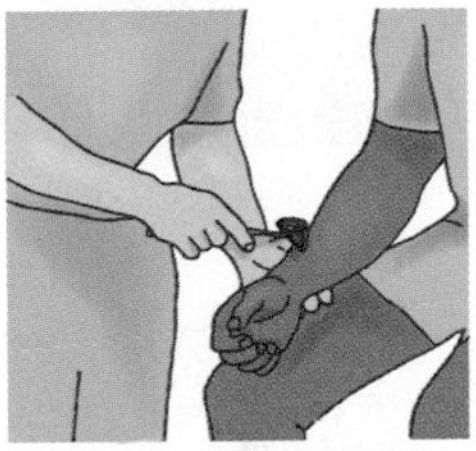 Musculocutaneous n.
C7	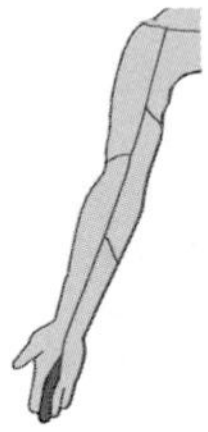 Radial n.	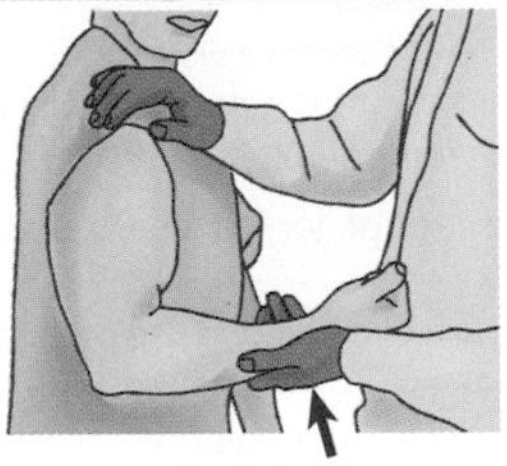 Radial n.	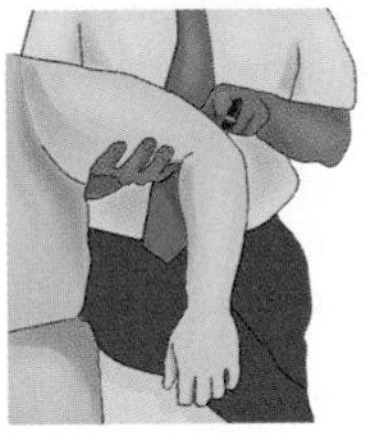 Radial n.
C8	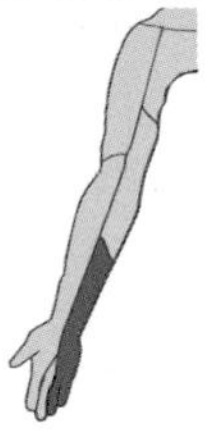 Ulnar n. (mixed)	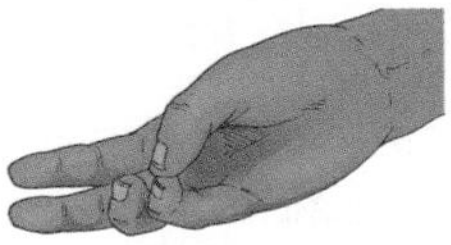 Median n.	None
T1	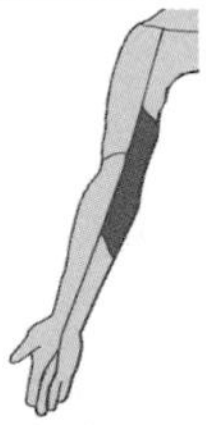 Med. brachial cutaneous n.	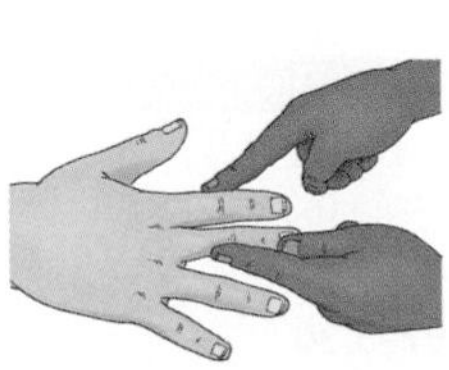 Med. brachial cutaneous n.	None

Selective Tissue Tests 14-2
Babinski Test for Upper Motor Neuron Lesions

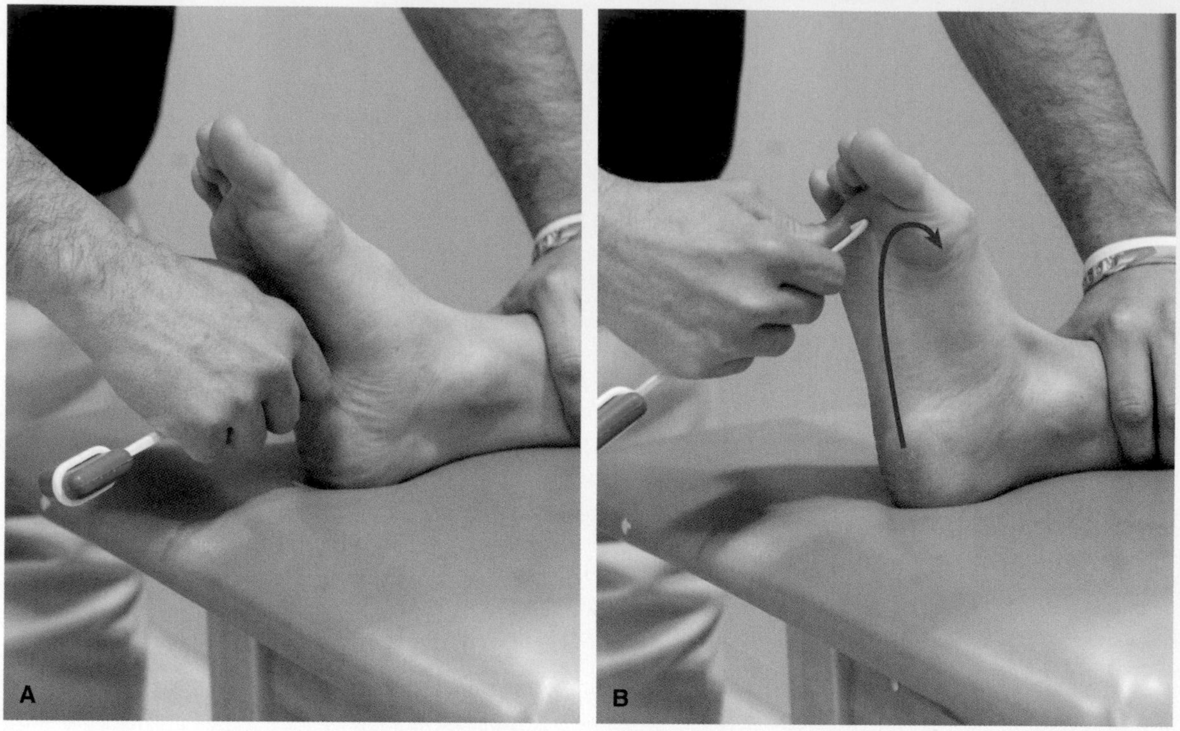

In adults, the Babinski test may be performed during the evaluation of an acute head or cervical spine injury to determine the presence of an upper motor neuron lesion.

Patient Position	Supine
Position of Examiner	At the foot of the patient; a blunt device, such as the handle of a reflex hammer or the handle of a pair of scissors, is needed.
Evaluative Procedure	The examiner runs the device up the plantar aspect of the foot, making an arc from the calcaneus medially to the ball of the great toe **(A)**. In the presence of normal innervation, the toes should curl **(B)**.
Positive Test	The great toe extends, and the other toes splay.
Implications	Upper motor neuron lesion, especially in the pyramidal tract, caused by brain or spinal cord trauma or pathology
Comments	The Babinski reflex occurs normally in newborns and should spontaneously disappear shortly after birth.
Evidence	

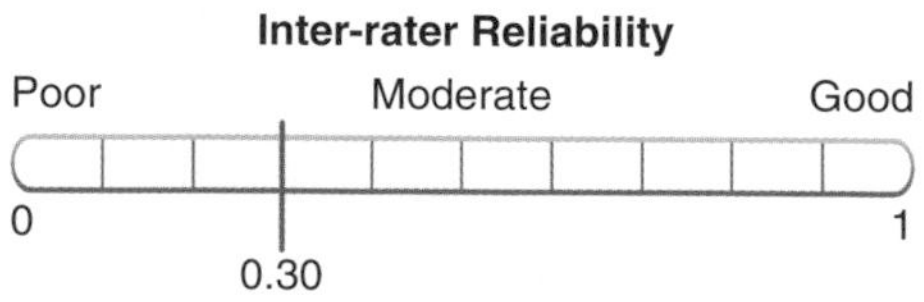

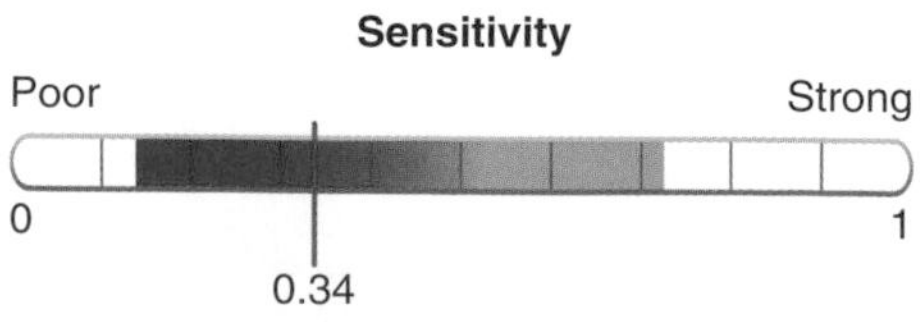

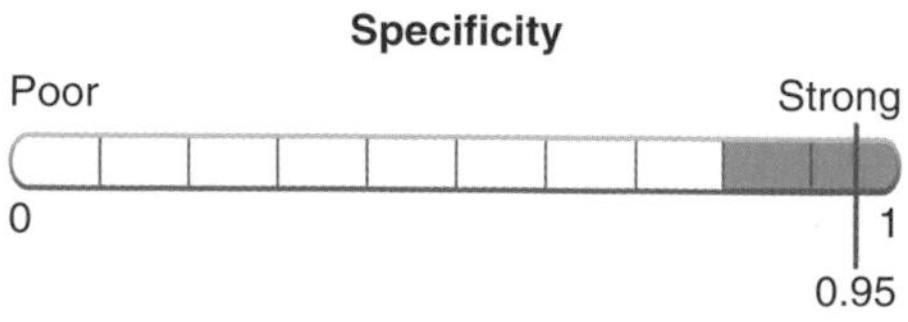

LR+: 1.52–3.30

LR–: 0.31–0.79–0.91

Selective Tissue Tests 14-3
Oppenheim Test for Upper Motor Neuron Lesions

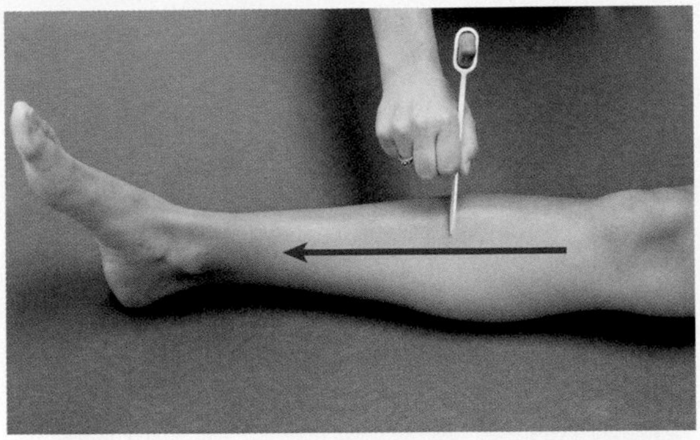

The Oppenheim test may be performed during the evaluation of a patient with suspected central nervous system pathology to determine the presence of an upper motor neuron lesion.

Patient Position	Supine
Position of Examiner	At the patient's side
Evaluative Procedure	A blunt object or the examiner's fingernail is run along the crest of the anteromedial tibia.
Positive Test	The great toe extends and the other toes splay, or the patient reports hypersensitivity to the test.
Implications	Upper motor neuron lesion caused by brain or spinal cord trauma or pathology
Evidence	Absent or inconclusive in the literature

impinge the nerve root (Fig. 14-20).[37] Degenerative causes are more common in older patients and discogenic causes more common in younger patients.[36,38]

The signs and symptoms of cervical nerve root impingement may closely mimic those of distal neuropathies such as radial tunnel or carpal tunnel syndrome. Neck pain may or may not be present, and often the patient will describe the upper extremity symptoms as more problematic than the cervical pain. An upper quarter neurological screen may be positive for altered sensation, decreased strength, and/or diminished reflexes. A diminished or absent biceps reflex is strongly suggestive of cervical radiculopathy.[17]

Narrowing of the intervertebral foramen secondary to exostosis of the vertebrae, enlargement or irritation of the dural sheath surrounding the cervical nerve root, and degeneration of the facet or uncovertebral joints may be confirmed with the **cervical compression test** (Selective Tissue Test 14-5). The **Spurling test** (Selective Tissue Test 14-6) is a modification of the cervical compression test that increases the compression of the cervical nerve root by unilaterally decreasing the size of the foramen.[39,40]

The **upper limb tension tests** (see Selective Tissue Test 14-1) may reproduce symptoms. Negative findings (reproduction of symptoms, involved/uninvolved differences in elbow motion or increased symptoms with contralateral neck side bending and/or decreased symptoms

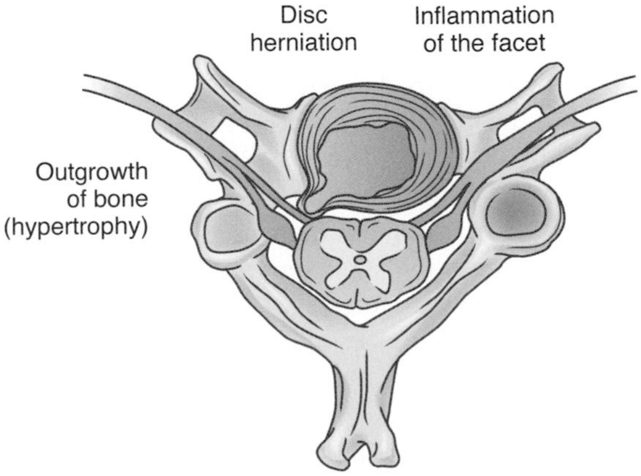

FIGURE 14-20 ■ Sources of cervical nerve root impingement.

Selective Tissue Tests 14-4
Beevor's Sign for Thoracic Nerve Inhibition

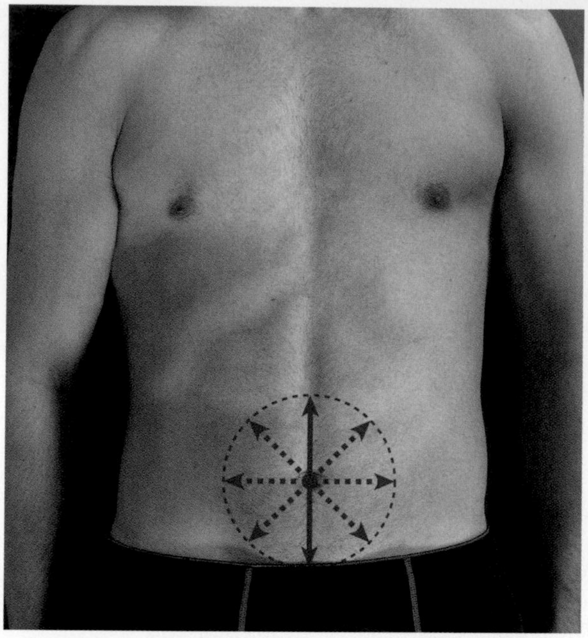

Lateral movement of the umbilicus can indicate inhibition of the thoracic nerves innervating the abdominal muscles.

Patient Position	Hook-lying
Position of Examiner	At the side of the patient
Evaluative Procedure	The patient performs an abdominal curl (partial sit-up).
Positive Test	The umbilicus moves up, down, or to one side.
Implications	Segmental involvement of the nerves innervating the rectus abdominis (T5–T12); this should draw suspicion to the paraspinal muscles innervated by the same nerve roots.
Comments	Normally, the umbilicus should not move at all during this test but will move toward the stronger muscle group in the presence of pathology.
Evidence	Absent or inconclusive in the literature

with side bending to the same side) with ULTT greatly reduce the probability that the patient has cervical radiculopathy.[17]

The **cervical distraction test** may help determine the underlying cause of pain (Selective Tissue Test 14-7). Manual traction to the skull separates the cervical vertebrae, reducing pressure on the nerve roots. This indicates that the pain is caused by mechanical pressure arising from entrapment of the nerve root or pressure caused by a disc herniation.

Cervical spine pathology such as instability or stenosis may also result in compromise of either the vertebrobasilar artery or internal carotid artery in the neck, collectively known as cervical arterial dysfunction (CAD). Patients who describe symptoms associated with CAD should be referred for additional testing. Cervical manipulation is contraindicated in patients who display these signs or symptoms (Table 14-10). A test for **patency** of the vertebral artery, the **vertebral artery test** (Selective Tissue Test 14-8), identifies potential for claudication and interruption of the blood flow to the brain; however, results should be interpreted

Patency Freely open

Examination Findings 14-1
Cervical Nerve Root Compression

Examination Segment	Clinical Findings
History of Current Condition	*Onset:* Acute or chronic *Pain characteristics:* May or may not have cervical pain; pain possibly radiating into the trapezius, scapula, shoulder, arm, wrist, and hand Increased symptoms as day progresses *Other symptoms:* Paresthesia along distribution of involved nerve root *Mechanism:* Compression or irritation of the associated nerve root (or roots) *Risk factors:* Disc pathology, stenosis of the intervertebral foramen, degenerative changes in the facet and/or uncovertebral joints, prior trauma to the cervical spine Disc pathology is more common in younger patients; degenerative pathology is more common in older patients.
Functional Assessment	The patient will often demonstrate limitations or compensations during those tasks that require full cervical rotation. Compensations generally include increased rotation of the trunk.
Inspection	The head and cervical spine are postured to relieve pressure on the involved nerve root.
Palpation	Point tenderness may be noted at the involved vertebral level.
Joint and Muscle Function Assessment	*AROM:* Pain experienced during extension, lateral bending toward the involved side, and rotation. Rotation to the involved side of less than 60 degrees is particularly suggestive of cervical radiculopathy.[17] *MMT:* Pain and weakness possible for all muscles tested *PROM:* Pain is experienced during extension, lateral bending toward the involved side, and rotation.
Joint Stability Tests	*Stress tests:* Not applicable *Joint play:* Segmental hypo- or hypermobility may be noted.
Selective Tissue Tests	Cervical compression test (increases symptoms), cervical distraction test (decreases symptoms), Spurling test, vertebral artery test, shoulder abduction test
Neurological Screening	Upper quarter screen may reveal muscle weakness, paresthesia, and diminished reflexes specific to the involved nerve root. C6 and C7 nerve roots are most commonly involved.[36]
Vascular Screening	Not applicable
Imaging Techniques	Radiographs are used to identify structural or degenerative changes to the vertebra and/or decreased intervertebral space caused by disc degeneration. T1- and T2-weighted MR images are used to image the spinal cord, cervical nerve roots, and intervertebral discs.
Differential Diagnosis	Cervical muscle tear, cervical spondylolysis, degenerative disc disease, facet joint dysfunction, disc herniation or rupture, TOS, clinical cervical instability, tumor, distal nerve entrapment, myelopathy, myocardial ischemia, regional pathology (e.g., rotator cuff disease)
Comments	The value of EMG in diagnosing radiculopathy is controversial, but this test may be helpful in the absence of other confirming tests.[36,37] Suspect a cervical fracture, dislocation, or sprain with acute symptoms following a traumatic force.

AROM = active range of motion; EMG = electromyography; MMT = manual muscle test; MR = magnetic resonance; PROM = passive range of motion; TOS = thoracic outlet syndrome

Herniation The protrusion of a tissue through the wall that normally contains it

Selective Tissue Tests 14-5
Cervical Compression Test

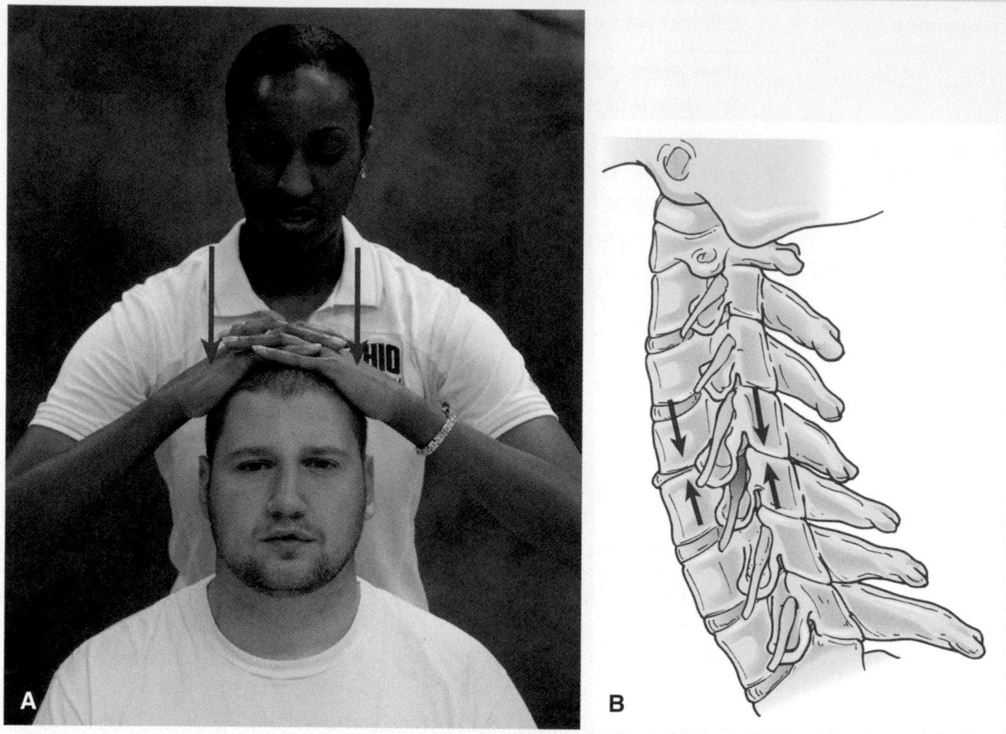

The cervical compression test attempts to duplicate the patient's symptoms by increasing pressure on the cervical nerve roots.

Patient Position	Sitting
Position of Examiner	Standing behind the patient with hands interlocked over the top of the patient's head
Evaluative Procedure	The examiner presses down on the crown of the patient's head.
Positive Test	The patient experiences pain or reproduction of symptoms in the upper cervical spine, upper extremity, or both.
Implications	Compression of the facet joints and narrowing of the intervertebral foramen resulting in pain
Comments	This test should not be performed until the possibility of a cervical fracture or instability has been ruled out. If compression reproduces symptoms, apply traction with the patient in the seated position to determine if symptoms are alleviated.

Evidence

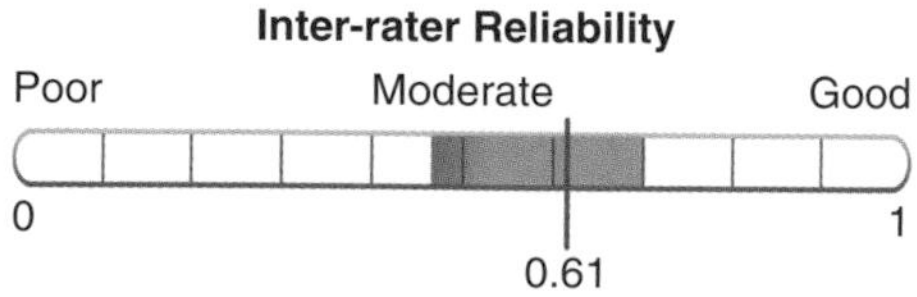

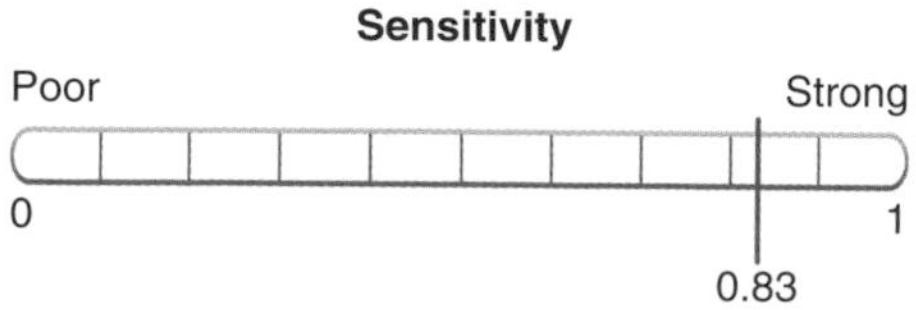

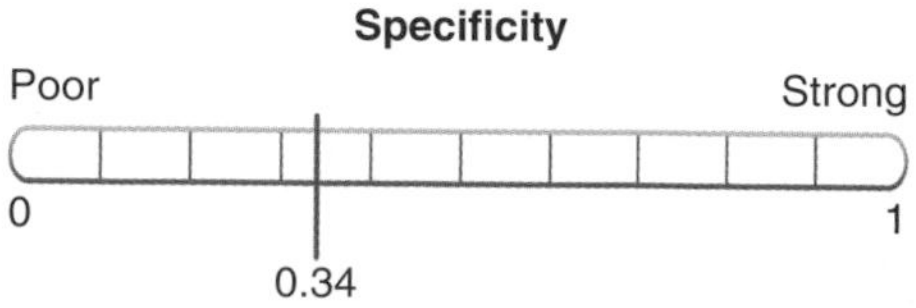

LR+: 1.66

LR−: 0.34

Selective Tissue Tests 14-6
Spurling Test

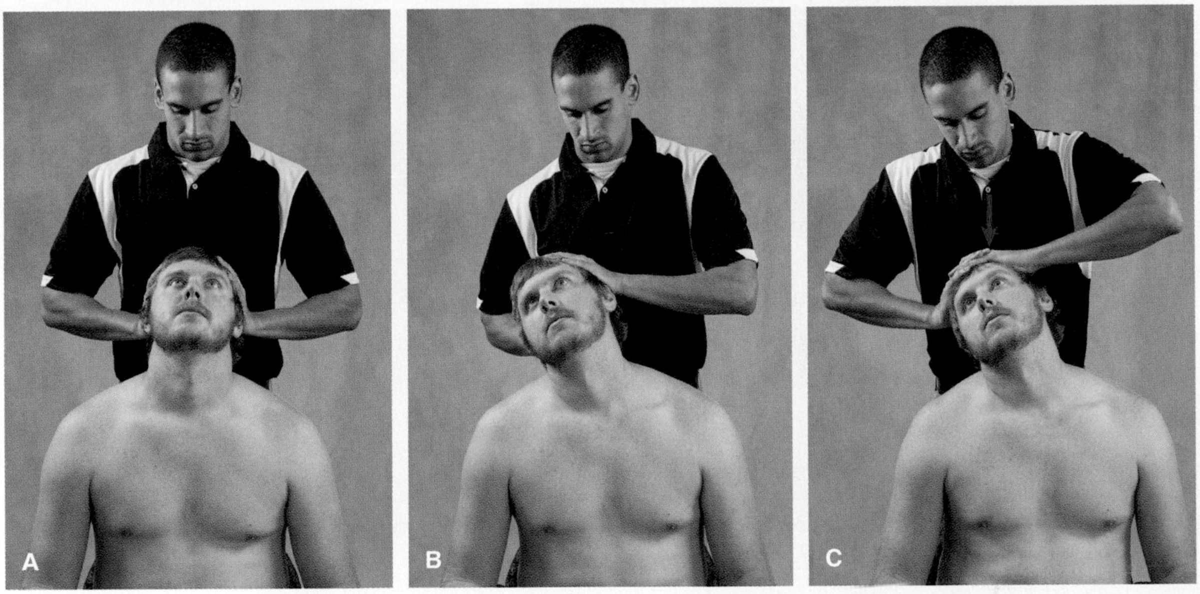

Similar to the cervical compression test, the Spurling test attempts to compress one of the cervical nerve roots.

Patient Position	Seated
Position of Examiner	Standing behind the patient with the hands interlocked over the crown of the patient's head
Evaluative Procedure	**(A)** The patient's head is passively moved into extension.[40] If no symptoms are produced: **(B)** Add lateral flexion. **(C)** Add axial compression to the cervical spine.
Positive Test	Pain or reproduction of symptoms radiating down the patient's arm
Implications	Nerve root impingement by narrowing of the neural foramina
Modification	Several modifications of this test have been proposed including various combinations of cervical compression, extension, and/or rotation.[17,40,41] The test may be performed supine, but the sensitivity and specificity decrease.[39]
Comments	This test should not be performed until the possibility of a cervical fracture or significant instability has been ruled out.
Evidence	

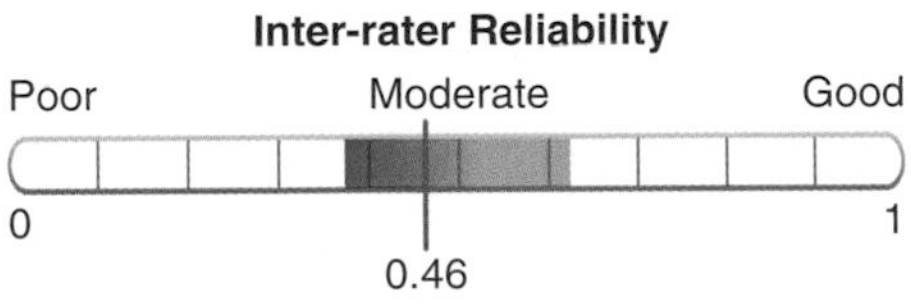

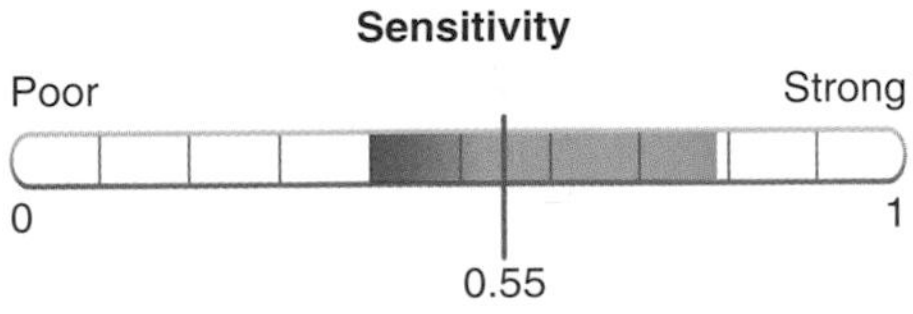

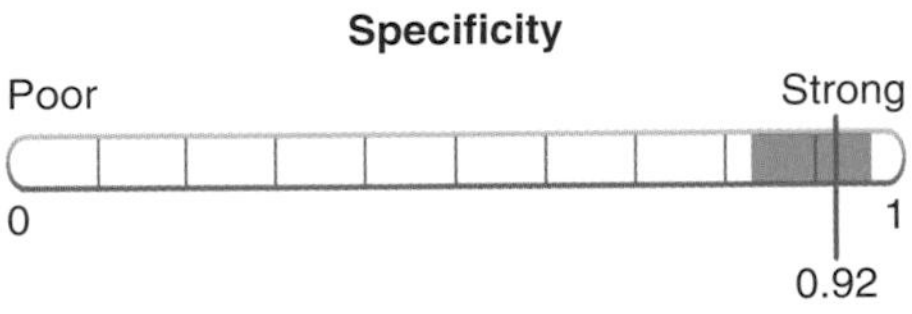

LR+: 2.33–4.64–8.47

LR−: 0.36–0.56–0.66

Selective Tissue Tests 14-7
Cervical Distraction Test

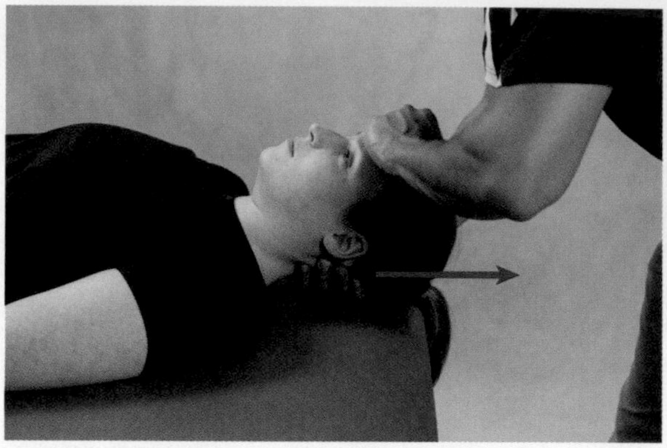

The cervical distraction test attempts to relieve the patient's symptoms by decreasing pressure on the cervical nerve roots.

Patient Position	Supine to relax the cervical spine postural muscles
Position of Examiner	At the head of the patient with one hand under the occiput and the other on top of the forehead, stabilizing the head
Evaluative Procedure	The examiner flexes the patient's cervical spine to a position of comfort.[17] A traction force is applied to the skull, producing distraction of the cervical spine.
Positive Test	The patient's symptoms are relieved or reduced.
Implications	Compression of the cervical facet joints and/or stenosis of the neural foramina
Modification	The distraction test may be performed with the patient seated. The advantage of this technique is that it places the patient in a functional position.
Comments	This test should not be performed until the possibility of a cervical fracture or significant instability has been ruled out.
Evidence	

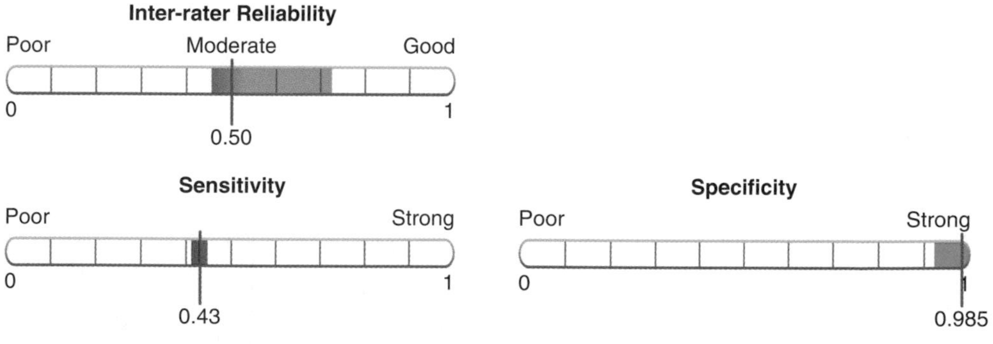

LR+: 4.40–13.30

LR−: 0.43–0.53–0.80

Table 14-10	Symptoms Associated With Cervical Arterial Dysfunction
Dizziness	
Drop attacks	
Diplopia	
Dysarthria	
Dysphagia	
Ataxia	
Nausea	
Numbness	
Nystagmus	

with caution. A negative test does not rule out vertebral artery involvement; a positive test warrants referral for further diagnostic testing.[19,30]

Diagnostic testing can help identify the source of radicular symptoms. Radiographs detect decreased disc space or spurs that may result from hypermobility. MRI is used to assess for stenosis and disc pathology. Electromyography may be necessary to differentiate symptoms of cervical radiculopathy from peripheral nerve entrapment.[42]

Disc Pathology

In the presence of disc herniations and vertebral impingement, pain is often influenced by the position of the patient's head and cervical spine. Because the annulus fibrosis is thin in the lateral region of the disc, pain arising from cervical disc pathology likely results from tension on the lateral aspect of the posterior longitudinal ligaments (Fig. 14-21).[5]

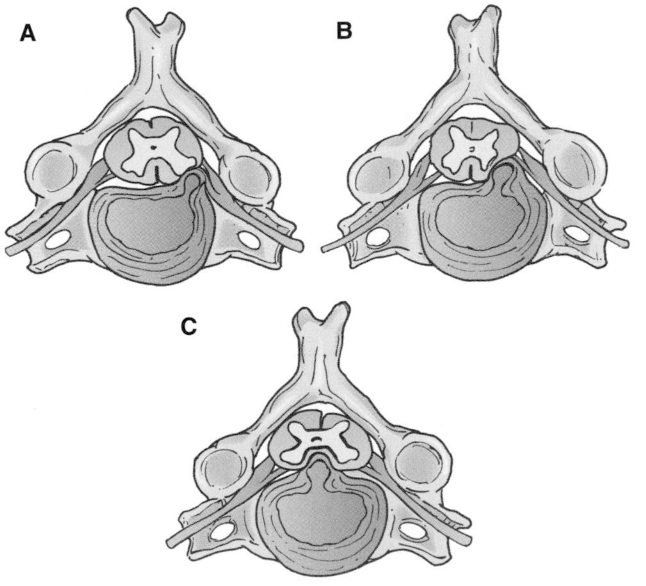

FIGURE 14-21 ■ Location of herniation influences the resulting dysfunction: (A) Intraforaminal—Radicular symptoms within a discrete dermatomal pattern. (B) Posterolateral—Motor deficits, atrophy. (C) Midline—Anterior spinal cord compression that may result in bowel and bladder changes, sexual dysfunction, gait disturbance, and decreased fine motor skills.

Unyielding pain may signify an intervertebral disc rupture or the presence of a tumor.[43] Pain that does not subside during treatment or has an unknown cause requires a physician's examination.

The majority of cervical disc herniations involve the C5–C6 or C6–C7 intervertebral discs and the C6 or C7 nerve roots.[2,44,45] The patient will experience increased symptoms when the cervical spine is placed in a position that forces the disc's nucleus pulposus toward the involved nerve root. The shoulder abduction test is a clinical test used to identify the presence of a herniated disc by alleviation of the symptoms (Selective Tissue Test 14-9). The patient may self-report assuming this position to reduce symptoms.[39,46] The patient may also describe pain during the Valsalva maneuver, such as when making a bowel movement, when sneezing, or during other activities that increase intrathecal pressure (see Valsalva Test, p. 502).

Degenerative Joint and Disc Disease

Degenerative joint and disc disease (cervical spondylosis) may be a normal consequence of aging that starts with disc degeneration or may be the result of repetitive stresses or trauma.[38] The collapse of the disc results in segmental hypermobility. Osteophyte formation and bony hypertrophy occur to compensate for this hypermobility. This cluster of pathologies can ultimately result in pressure on the spinal cord (**myelopathy**).[25] Myelopathy is characterized by bilateral symptoms, signs of upper motor neuron involvement such as hyperreflexia, and decreased manual dexterity.[25] Patients with examination findings suggesting myelopathy should be referred to a physician for further examination (Fig. 14-22).

Some age-related degeneration of the spine is expected and may not be symptomatic, even if there is radiologic evidence of degeneration such as osteophyte formation and decreased disc space. Likewise, patients may display signs

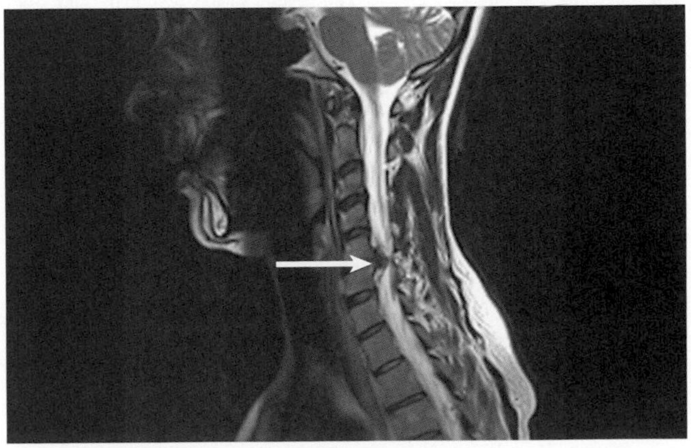

FIGURE 14-22 ■ MRI of a C4–C5 cervical disc herniation (arrow).

Myelopathy Diseases that affect the spinal cord

Selective Tissue Tests 14-8
Vertebral Artery Test

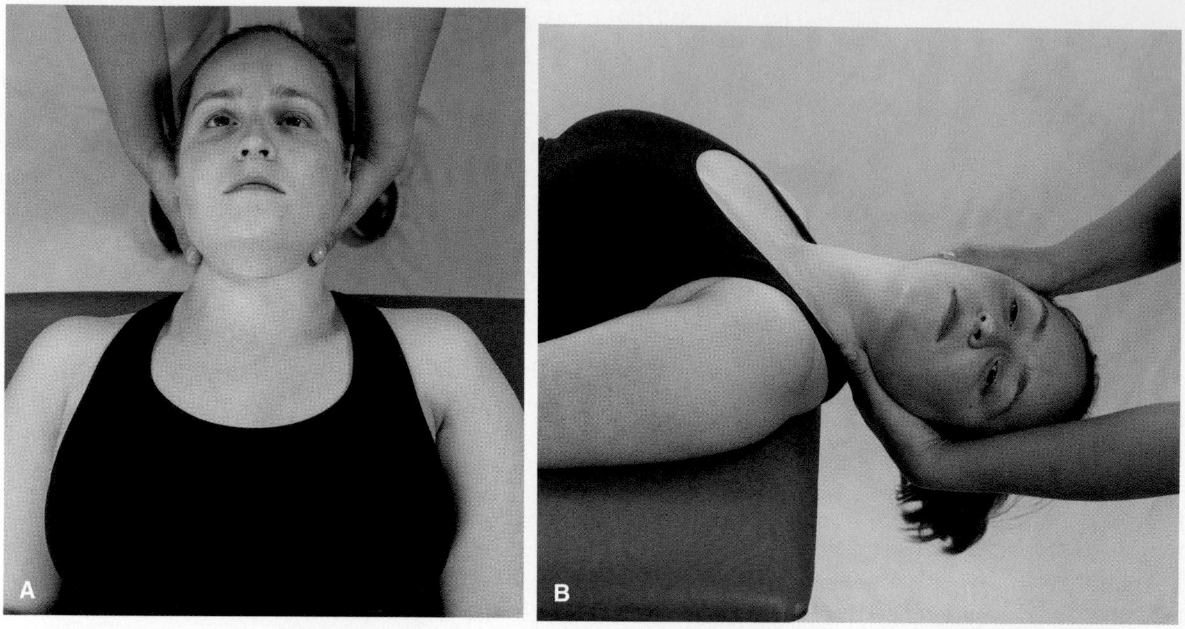

The vertebral artery test is performed to assess the competency of the vertebral artery before initiating treatment or rehabilitation techniques that may compromise a partially occluded artery. This test should not be performed until the presence of a cervical fracture, dislocation, or gross instability has been ruled out. It is recommend that a table with a dropped face plate be used if the patient's head is off the table and supported by the clinician.

Patient Position	Supine
Position of Examiner	Seated at the head of the patient with the hands placed under the occiput to stabilize the head
Evaluative Procedure	The examiner passively extends the cervical spine **(A)**. The head is then rotated to one side and held for 30 seconds **(B)**. Repeat the procedure for the opposite side. During this procedure, the examiner must monitor the patient's pupillary activity.
Positive Test	Dizziness, confusion, nystagmus, unilateral pupil changes, nausea
Implications	Occlusion of the cervical vertebral arteries
Comments	Patients with a positive test result should be referred to a physician before any other evaluative tests are performed or a rehabilitation plan is implemented and before being allowed to return to sport activity. The results of this test, especially the rotation component, may produce symptoms that occur following the procedure.[30]
Evidence	 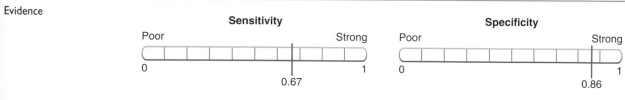 **LR+:** 4.79 **LR−:** 0.38

Selective Tissue Tests 14-9
Shoulder Abduction Test

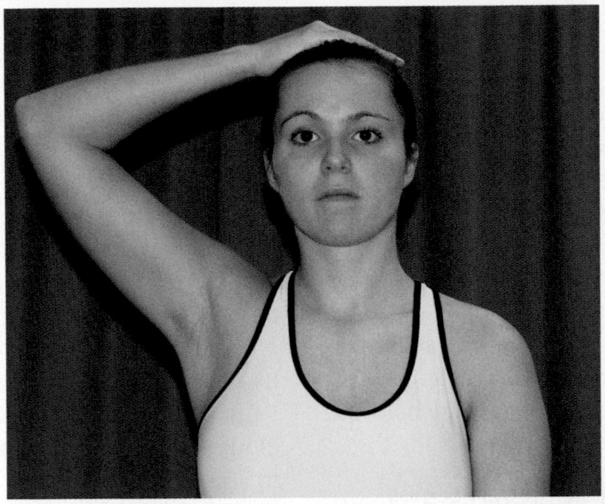

Because of its pain-relieving qualities, the patient may voluntarily assume this posture for comfort.

Patient Position	Seated or standing
Position of Examiner	Standing in front of the patient
Evaluative Procedure	The patient actively abducts the arm so that the hand is resting on top of the head and maintains this position for 30 seconds.
Positive Test	Decrease in the patient's symptoms secondary to decreased tension on the involved nerve root
Implications	Herniated disc or nerve root compression
Evidence	

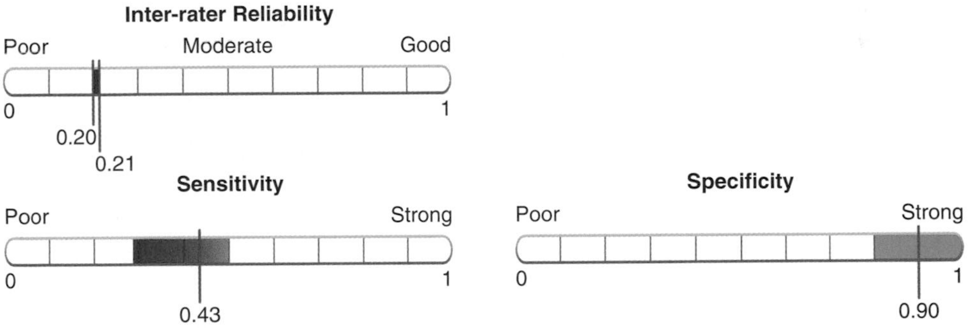

LR+: 2.13–2.15–2.44

LR−: 0.50–0.71–0.80

and symptoms of degenerative disease in the absence of radiographic evidence.

Patients with degenerative joint and disc disease describe a history of joint aggravation with episodes of joint pain and cervical stiffness. Questioning may reveal an acute neck injury or an occupation or activity that repetitively stresses the neck. Suboccipital pain and headaches may also occur. Radicular symptoms may occur as a result of encroachment on the nerve roots as the intervertebral foramen becomes narrowed. These most often involve the C6 and C7 nerve roots.

AROM and PROM may be limited secondary to pain and stiffness. Joint play may reveal hypomobility at one segment with compensatory hypermobility at the segments above and below. When radicular symptoms are present, palpation of affected muscles may detect atrophy before it becomes notable on inspection.

Cervical Radiculopathy Intervention Strategies

With a treatment goal of centralization of symptoms, conservative treatment consisting of patient education, strengthening exercises, and medication is effective in reducing symptoms in most patients.[10,42] Cervical traction may be beneficial for specific subgroups of patients. Medications used include anti-inflammatories and certain antidepressants, which may be helpful for neuropathic pain.[47] Steroid injections may also be needed to decrease nerve irritability.

Surgery is an option for patients who do not respond to conservative treatment. Degenerative disease may be treated with fusion and discectomy or, more recently, arthroplasty, in which a prosthetic disc replaces the diseased disc.[48] Cervical fusion above the C3 level or fusions that involve three or more spinal levels are absolute contraindications against participation in collision or contact sports.[2]

* Practical Evidence

Patients over the age of 55 who have peripheralization of symptoms with mobility testing of the lower cervical spine, who demonstrate positive shoulder abduction and upper limb tension tests, and who experience relief with distraction have a high probability of realizing positive results with traction interventions.[7]

Clinical Cervical Instability

Clinical cervical instability differs from gross instability caused by dislocations or acute fractures. Cervical stabilization is obtained through input from neurological, active, and passive structures. Alterations in neural input, muscle activity, or bony and ligamentous restraint can result in subtle cervical instability. In large joints, noticeable instability often occurs with damage to the passive restraints, such as ligaments. In the cervical spine, the passive restraints may be intact even when clinical cervical instability is present, representing dysfunction of the active and neurological stabilizers.[49]

Causes of clinical cervical instability include degenerative changes secondary to poor posture, repetitive movements, muscular weakness, and damage to the passive restraints such as occurs during acute trauma.

Patients with clinical cervical instability may describe symptom relief with external stabilization, such as a cervical collar or simply holding the neck with the hands. Pain or intolerance with sustained postures (e.g., working at a computer) is common, as are complaints of muscle tightness and referred pain to the shoulder and parascapular region. Occipital, frontal or retro-orbital headaches may also occur. Patients typically describe pain, weakness, or a "catching" sensation in the midrange of motion, consistent with disruption to the active and neurological stabilizers. Radiculopathy may or may not be present.

Poor control and uneven motion in the midrange of active movements are characteristic examination findings.[49,50] Palpation reveals general tenderness in the cervical region, along with notable increased paraspinal muscle density due to spasm. Findings from intervertebral joint play, although having poor reliability, may include hypermobility in the cervical region that is often coincident with hypomobility in the upper thoracic region.

Cervical Instability Intervention Strategies

Interventions for those with cervical instability with signs of nerve compression incorporate exercise for improved dynamic stability of the cervical spine.[10] These exercises generally require an ongoing commitment from the patient to avoid recurrence of symptoms.

In the event that clinical cervical spine instability degrades to result in gross instability, surgical correction is required. In most cases, fixation using plates, screws, and/or bone grafts is required to obtain stabilization.[51] Depending on the nature of the surgical procedure and the resulting loss of ROM, the patient may be excluded from participation in contact and collision sports.

Facet Joint Dysfunction

Facet joint dysfunction results from trauma or degenerative changes[52] and is characterized by posterior neck pain with motions that load the involved articulation. Traumatic mechanisms often include hyperextension, such as that associated with whiplash.

Examination findings include well-localized pain in the paraspinal region, just lateral to the spinous process of the involved segment. This pain may radiate into the shoulders or midback, likely the result of muscle spasm. Facet joint pathology is associated with a characteristic pattern of referred pain specific to the involved joint (Fig. 14-23).[52,53] PROM and AROM may provoke symptoms, especially with extension and rotation, and asymmetry of motion may be present. Not associated with radicular symptoms, the upper quarter screen and upper limb tension tests are typically normal. Central and unilateral posterior–anterior joint play (see Joint Play 14-1) may increase symptoms and reveal hypermobility or hypomobility. Radiographs are used to detect degenerative changes; however, these changes are

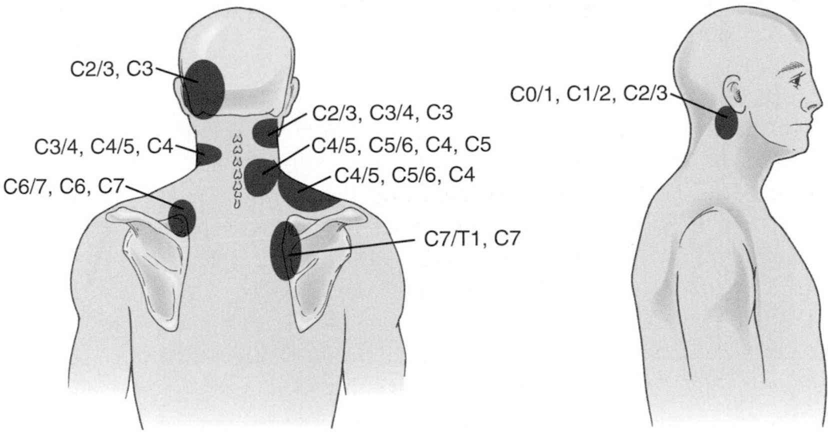

FIGURE 14-23 ■ Referred pain patterns from cervical facet joints.

a typical finding in adults without cervical pain.[52] The diagnosis of facet joint involvement may be confirmed when symptoms are relieved after an injection of anesthetic into the joint or the innervating branches of the dorsal rami.[54]

Facet Joint Dysfunction Intervention Strategies

Treatment of facet joint dysfunction depends on the underlying cause. Stabilization exercises may be indicated in the presence of hypermobility. Mobilization techniques are used to decrease pain and restore normal arthrokinematics. Corticosteroid injection into the joint is of questionable efficacy. Injection over the branches of the dorsal rami innervating the joint may be beneficial.[52]

Brachial Plexus Pathology

Acute trauma to the brachial plexus, often referred to as a "burner" or "stinger," is common in contact sports. The onset of this injury may be caused by a traction force placed on the brachial plexus (brachial plexus stretch) or an impingement of the cervical nerve roots (brachial plexus compression) through extension and lateral flexion to the same side. In football players, the brachial plexus can also be traumatized by compression of the brachial plexus between the shoulder pad and the superior medial scapula and is more common in defensive players.[55-57] This site, **Erb's point** (Fig. 14-24), is located 2 to 3 cm above the clavicle in front of the transverse process of the sixth cervical vertebra and represents the most superficial passage of the brachial plexus.

Stretching of the brachial plexus occurs when the head is forced laterally while the opposite shoulder is depressed, such as when tackling in football (Fig. 14-25). The resulting force places traction on the nerves on the side opposite the lateral bending of the neck. Any of the cervical nerve roots may be affected by a traction mechanism, but the lateral and posterior cords that are innervated by the C5 and C6 nerve roots (suprascapular, lateral pectoral, musculocutaneous, and axillary nerves) are most commonly involved when the mechanism involves side bending of the head and depression of the shoulder (see Fig. 14-8).[2,58,59] Forced abduction of the arm can involve the C8 and T1 nerve roots.

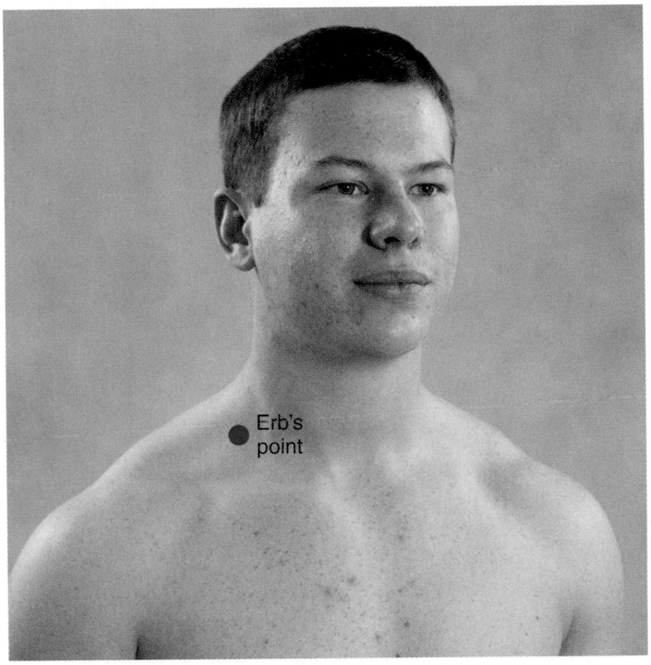

FIGURE 14-24 ■ Erb's point, representing the most superficial passage of the brachial plexus. Pressure to this area can result in pain and paresthesia radiating into the upper extremity.

Repeated low-intensity traction of the brachial plexus can hinder the local microcirculation of the plexus and cause ischemic changes in the nerves.[60] Cervical nerve root injury that quickly resolves without further consequence is associated with a traction mechanism. Recurrent and chronic nerve root injuries are associated with extension and ipsilateral side-bending mechanisms, functionally reproducing Spurling's sign. Individuals with chronic pathology are more likely to have degenerative changes in the cervical spine, disc disease, and spinal stenosis.[57,61]

Compression of the brachial plexus occurs on the side toward the bending of the neck when the nerve roots are impinged between the vertebrae. The likelihood of the impingement mechanism is increased by the narrowing of the intervertebral foramen (spinal stenosis).[38,57,62,63] A positive Spurling test (see Selective Tissue Test 14-6) is evidence of a

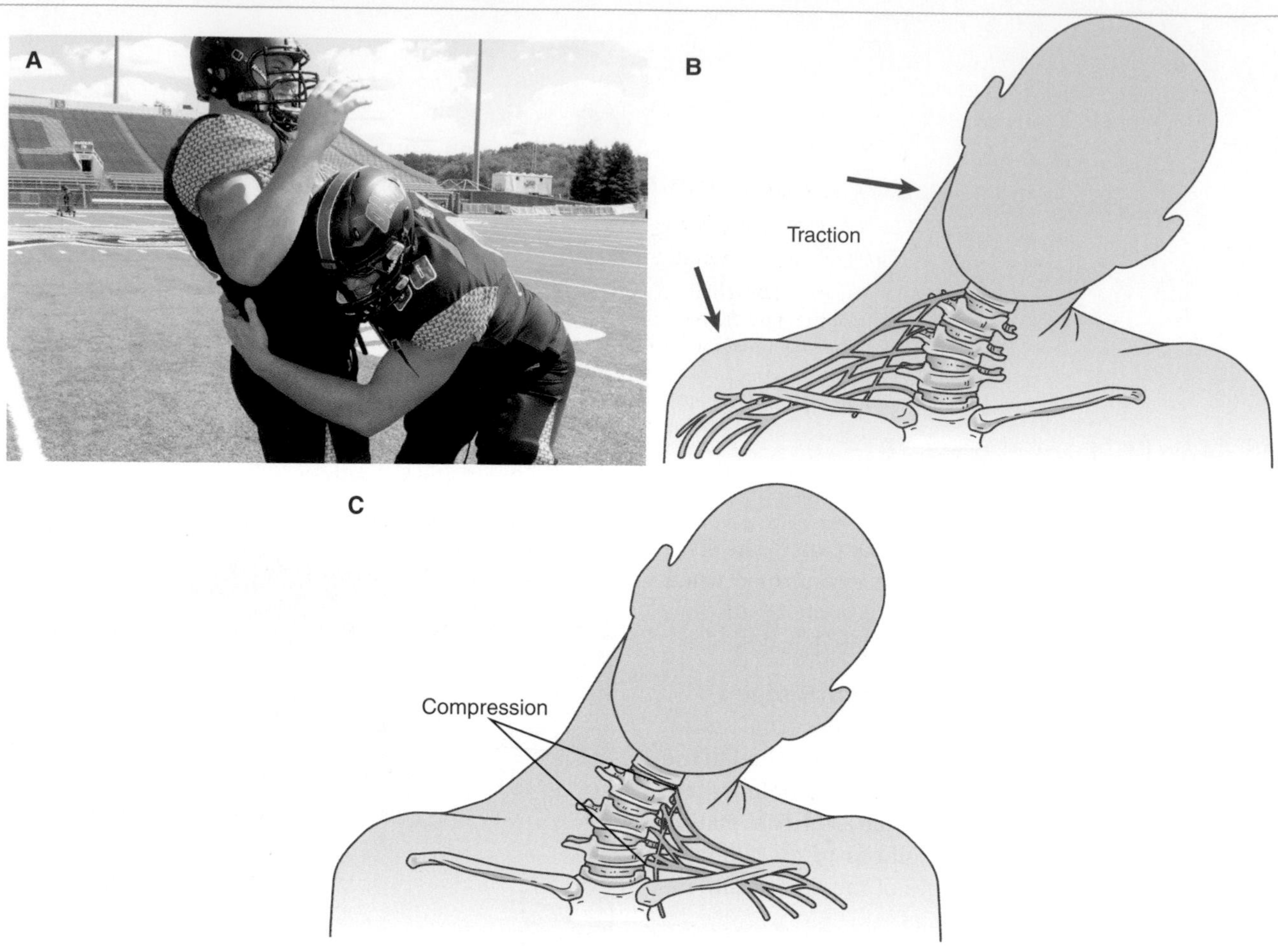

FIGURE 14-25 ■ Mechanism for a brachial plexus injury. (A) The cervical spine is forced laterally and the opposite shoulder is depressed, resulting in elongation of the trapezius and brachial plexus. (B) Elongation of the trapezius muscle with concurrent depression of the shoulder can result in a traction injury to the brachial plexus. (C) Compression (impingement) of the brachial plexus at the exiting nerve root can result on the side toward which the head is tilted.

mechanical narrowing of the intervertebral foramen by spinal stenosis, degenerative disc disease, or an asymmetric disc bulge (Examination Findings 14-2).[2,64]

The signs and symptoms of any type of brachial plexus pathology are similar. Immediate pain, often reported as "burning" or "an electrical shock" radiating through the upper extremity, is typically described, but the symptoms are not always limited to the involved dermatome(s).[3] During an acute examination, symptoms being limited to one side—rather than occurring in both arms—is a significant finding in the differential diagnosis between brachial plexus neuropathy and spinal cord involvement.[59]

Characteristically, the involved arm is found dangling limply at the side or the person may be shaking the hand and arm in an attempt to regain feeling. Neck pain is not typically associated with this condition.[55] Manual muscle testing often reveals decreased strength for the muscles innervated by the involved nerves with associated paresthesia. Upper quarter reflexes may be altered, especially in chronic cases.[3] These signs and symptoms normally subside within minutes, but prolonged symptoms can occur (Table 14-11).[2,57,58] Repeated or severe brachial plexus injuries may produce signs and symptoms that diminish much more slowly. Athletes suffering from chronic brachial plexus pathology display a dropped shoulder, atrophy of the shoulder and cervical musculature on the involved side, and note a decrease in bench press weight.[56,66]

Despite the presence of a common set of symptoms, examiners must not become complacent about the possibility of more severe cervical trauma. A thorough examination of the cervical spine is warranted to rule out the presence of a cervical fracture or dislocation. After these conditions have been ruled out, the **brachial plexus traction test**, which is fundamentally PROM with overpressure in side bending, may be used to duplicate the MOI and reproduce the patient's symptoms (Selective Tissue Test 14-10). Many of the selective tissue tests described in the cervical nerve root impingement section also produce positive results in the presence of brachial plexus pathology. Computed tomography (CT) scans, magnetic resonance imaging (MRI), and electromyographic (EMG) analysis can be used to identify local trauma to the nerves or nerve roots.[64]

Brachial Plexus Pathology Intervention Strategies

The immediate treatment and management of patients with brachial plexus trauma is discussed in the on-field

Examination Findings 14-2
Brachial Plexus Trauma

Examination Segment	Clinical Findings
History of Current Condition	*Onset:* Acute *Pain characteristics:* Pain in the trapezius and deltoid, radiating into the arm *Other symptoms:* Paresthesia along distribution of the involved nerve(s) *Mechanism:* **Brachial plexus stretch:** Lateral bending of the cervical spine and depression of the opposite shoulder, resulting in tension on the brachial plexus; symptoms occur on the side **opposite** the lateral bend **Brachial plexus compression:** Extension and lateral bending of the cervical spine, resulting in the entrapment of the cervical nerve roots; symptoms occur on the side *toward* the lateral bend *Risk factors:* History of repeated brachial plexus trauma; stenosis of the intervertebral foramen; degenerative changes in the cervical spine
Functional Assessment	Grip strength may be diminished, and, initially, the patient will not voluntarily move the involved arm.
Inspection	The involved arm hangs limply at the patient's side but resolves with time.
Palpation	Palpation of the cervical spine is necessary to rule out the possibility of a vertebral fracture or dislocation. Possible tenderness over Erb's point
Joint and Muscle Function Assessment	*AROM:* Initially, AROM of the cervical spine and affected limb is diminished. Return of motor function usually begins minutes after the onset of injury. *MMT:* Muscles innervated by the involved nerve are weak (grade 3/5 or lower). Strength typically returns quickly. *PROM:* Pain is increased with lateral flexion (brachial plexus stretch test).
Joint Stability Tests	*Stress tests:* Not applicable *Joint play:* Not applicable
Selective Tissue Tests	Brachial plexus stretch tests, cervical compression and distraction tests, and Spurling test
Neurological Screening	A complete upper quarter screen is necessary to identify the involved cervical nerve roots or peripheral nerves.
Vascular Screening	Within normal limits
Imaging Techniques	Plain film radiographs, CT, or MR images may be obtained to rule out stenosis of the intervertebral foramen.
Differential Diagnosis	Cervical spine fracture, herniated disc, cervical spine instability, transient quadriplegia, rotator cuff tear, AC joint pathology, TOS, injury to another peripheral nerve (e.g., long thoracic), scapular fracture, proximal humerus fracture,[55] "burning hands syndrome" (indicative of central spinal cord syndrome)[2]
Comments	The presence of a cervical fracture or dislocation must be ruled out before initiating the tests for brachial plexus pathology. All sensory, motor, and reflex test results must be normal and equal before allowing athletes to return to competition.

AC = acromioclavicular; AROM = active range of motion; CT = computed tomography; MMT = manual muscle test; MR = magnetic resonance; PROM = passive range of motion; TOS = thoracic outlet syndrome

Table 14-11 Jackson/Lohr Method of Grading Brachial Plexus Neuropathy

Grade	Characteristics
I	Motor and sensory function return within a matter of minutes.
II	Muscle strength is degraded for at least 3 weeks but resolves by 6 months.
III	Motor and sensory deficits persist longer than 1 year.

management section in this chapter. Rehabilitation of patients with brachial plexus trauma includes strengthening of the cervical musculature, biofeedback exercises, functional exercise programs, cervical ROM exercises, and reeducation of the upper extremity muscles that may have been affected.[65] This set of exercises should also be used to prevent the onset of brachial plexus trauma and other cervical spine injuries.

Athletes must not be allowed to return to competition until all symptoms have cleared. They must have full ROM, a full return of sensation, and normal strength throughout the affected extremity.

Thoracic Outlet Syndrome

The thoracic outlet anatomically comprises the interscalene triangle, the costoclavicular space, and the subcoracoid space, which is covered by the pectoralis minor muscle (Fig. 14-26). TOS is caused by pressure on the trunks and medial cord of the brachial plexus, the subclavian artery, or the subclavian vein (collectively known as the neurovascular bundle). TOS is categorized as either vascular (arterial or venous) or neurological (true neurological or disputed).[54,67]

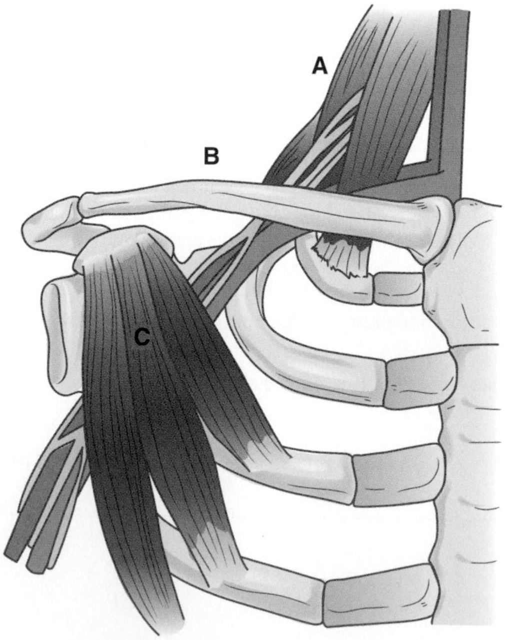

FIGURE 14-26 ■ Causes of thoracic outlet syndrome. Compression can occur (A) between the scalenes, (B) between the clavicle and the ribs (especially if a cervical rib is present), and (C) beneath the pectoralis minor.

Arterial TOS is the least common (less than 1%), followed by venous TOS (3% to 5%). Neurogenic TOS is by far the most prevalent.[54] TOS is most commonly diagnosed in patients between 20 and 50 years old, and women are more likely to develop neurogenic TOS; vascular TOS occurs equally in men and women.[67]

True neurological TOS is diagnosed based on objective diagnostic findings such as EMG activity. Disputed neurological TOS has similar symptoms but does not present with definitive diagnostic findings. Because TOS mimics several conditions and disputed neurogenic TOS is associated with no conclusive diagnostic tests, arriving at a diagnosis of TOS is often a process of exclusion. Cervical disc herniation, carpal tunnel syndrome, cubital tunnel syndrome, vascular occlusive disease, malignant tumors, multiple sclerosis, fibromyalgia, Raynaud disease, complex regional pain syndrome, and angina must be ruled out (Examination Findings 14-3).[54,55,68]

The etiology of TOS may be linked to the presence of a cervical rib (more common in women)[72] that places pressure on the neurovascular bundle as it is impinged between the clavicle and the first rib. The neurovascular structures can also be compressed between the pectoralis minor and rib cage or between the anterior and middle scalene muscles. Present in about 1% of the population, the cervical rib is a congenital outgrowth of the seventh cervical vertebra. This structure places pressure on the neurovascular bundle, especially when the shoulder complex is pulled inferiorly, such as when carrying a heavy bag in the hand. The presence of a cervical rib in isolation from other causative factors rarely leads to the clinical signs and symptoms of TOS.[67,73]

The neurovascular bundle passes between the clavicle and the first thoracic rib and is therefore susceptible to pressure on its anterior surface. Poor posture, drooping shoulders that depress the clavicles, forward shoulder posture, prolonged pressure on the upper surfaces of the first rib (such as wearing a backpack), or acute trauma may lead to the onset of TOS. The incidence of TOS is increased in athletes who perform repetitive overhead movements such as when throwing or swimming.

Complaints and clinical findings associated with TOS range from dramatic vascular engorgement to mild, intermittent symptoms associated with sustained postures (functional TOS).[74] The signs and symptoms of TOS may be neurological or vascular in nature. Neurological symptoms commonly occur along the distribution of the medial cord of the brachial plexus (C8 and T1). Generally, clinical symptoms are produced along the distribution of the ulnar nerve; decreased function along the median nerve may also be noted.

Vascular signs and symptoms reflect the specific structure being obstructed. Occlusion of the subclavian artery

Selective Tissue Tests 14-10
Brachial Plexus Traction Test

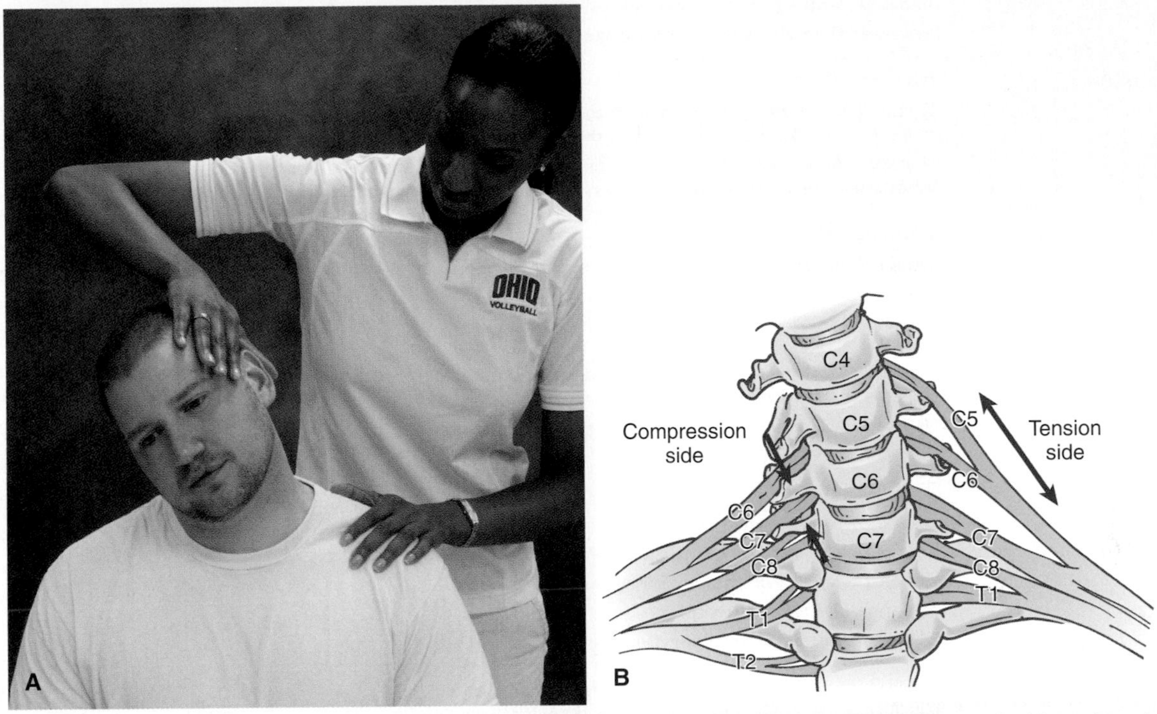

The examiner duplicates the MOI and replicates the patient's symptoms (A). Pain radiates down the patient's left shoulder when a traction injury exists and down the patient's right shoulder when a compression injury exists (B). This test should be performed in each direction.

Patient Position	Seated or standing
Position of Examiner	Standing behind the patient
Evaluative Procedure	One hand is placed on the side of the patient's head; the other hand is placed over the AC joint, stabilizing the trunk. The cervical spine is laterally bent and the opposite shoulder depressed.
Positive Test	Reproduction of pain and/or paresthesia symptoms throughout the involved upper extremity
Implications	Brachial plexus neurapraxia *Radiating pain on the side opposite the lateral bending:* Tension (stretching) of the brachial plexus *Radiating pain on the side toward the lateral bending:* Compression of the cervical nerve roots between two vertebrae
Comments	This test should not be performed until the possibility of a cervical fracture or significant instability has been ruled out.
Evidence	Absent or inconclusive in the literature

AC = acromioclavicular

Examination Findings 14-3
Thoracic Outlet Syndrome

Examination Segment	Clinical Findings
History of Current Condition	*Onset:* *Vascular:* Arterial – gradual or spontaneous; Venous – gradual or spontaneous; generally worse with activity *Neurogenic:* Gradual. May be exacerbated by sustained positioning or compression (such as when wearing a backpack) *Pain characteristics:* *Vascular:* With an arterial cause, pain tends to occur distally (e.g., in the hand) rather than in the cervical region; a venous cause results in pain in the chest and throughout the upper extremity. *Neurogenic:* Achy pain may be described in the lateral cervical spine, shoulder, axillary, periscapular region, and arm; some patients describe nocturnal pain, while others describe increased symptoms during the day. *Other symptoms:* *Vascular:* With an arterial onset, numbness in a nonradicular pattern; venous causes result in a feeling of heaviness, especially after activity *Neurogenic:* Numbness or paresthesia in a nonradicular pattern (generally in lower plexus); occipital headache; cold intolerance (sympathetic response) *Mechanism:* Vascular (arterial, venous): Arterial insufficiency and/or venous obstruction; possible history of vigorous and/or repetitive arm activity or an insidious onset *Neurogenic:* Acute neck injury (e.g., whiplash mechanism); insidious *Risk factors:* Cervical rib; use of a backpack; participation in activities that require repetitive overhead movements; tightness of pectoralis minor
Functional Assessment	Repeating movements may be necessary to induce symptoms. Increased complaints of symptoms during overhead motions *Neurogenic:* Decreased dexterity Observe for decreased clavicular mobility during shoulder elevation.
Inspection	Rounded shoulders and forward head posture may be noted. *Vascular (arterial):* Pallor and/or cyanosis in the involved arm *Vascular (venous):* Pooling edema; distended veins in the shoulder and chest *Neurogenic:* Atrophy of thenar eminence (Gilliatt-Sumner hand)
Palpation	Confirmation of the inspection findings of pooling edema and/or distended veins Spasm of the scalene muscle may be palpated or observed.[69] Decreased skin temperature may be noted in both vascular and neurogenic TOS. *Neurogenic:* Point tenderness at Erb's point
Joint and Muscle Function Assessment	*AROM:* Cervical rotation combined with lateral flexion may reveal tightness of the scalenes. *Neurogenic:* Cervical rotation to opposite side and overhead movements may provoke symptoms.[70] *MMT:* **Neurogenic:** Weakness of the intrinsic muscles of the hand *PROM:* **Neurognic:** Symptoms may be provoked during overhead motions.
Joint Stability Tests	*Stress tests:* Not applicable *Joint play:* SC and AC joint play may be hypomobile, contributing to restricted clavicular motion.
Selective Tissue Tests	Adson, Allen, Military Brace, Roos
Neurological Screening	*Neurogenic:* Sensory loss along the lower trunk (C8, T1); upper limb tension test
Vascular Screening	*Vascular (arterial):* Diminished or absent pulse in the involved arm; >20 mm Hg decrease in arterial blood pressure relative to the uninvolved side
Imaging Techniques	Radiographs will confirm or rule out the presence of a cervical rib. Ultrasonography to identify arterial or venous insufficiency Angiography for arterial TOS MRI more accurately identifies the presence of causative factors for TOS than clinical tests.[71]
Differential Diagnosis	Cervical disc herniation, carpal tunnel syndrome, cubital tunnel syndrome, vascular occlusive disease, malignant tumors, multiple sclerosis, fibromyalgia, Raynaud disease, complex regional pain syndrome, and angina
Comments	Nerve conduction studies and electromyography are used to diagnose true neurological TOS; these tests will be negative with disputed neurological TOS. Patients who present with vascular symptoms should be immediately referred to a physician. Selective tissue test findings yield a high rate of false-positive results.

AC = acromioclavicular; AROM = active range of motion; MMT = manual muscle test; MRI = magnetic resonance imaging; PROM = passive range of motion; SC = sternoclavicular; TOS = thoracic outlet syndrome presents signs and symptoms typical of decreased blood flow. Blockage of the subclavian vein is characterized by edema in the distal upper extremity and, if untreated, may result in thrombophlebitis.

A thorough postural examination and an examination of movement patterns are warranted to detect underlying causes. Rounded shoulders, increased thoracic kyphosis, decreased clavicular movement, and decreased mobility of the first rib may all contribute to the development of TOS.

The underlying principle for TOS selective tissue tests is related to provoking symptoms by placing pressure on the neurovascular bundle. **Adson's test** attempts to depress the shoulder complex and place the medial cord of the brachial plexus, the subclavian artery, and the subclavian vein on stretch while simultaneously placing pressure on the bundle from the anterior scalene muscle (Selective Tissue Test 14-11). TOS caused by the pectoralis minor muscle may be detected via the **Allen test** (Selective Tissue Test 14-12). Costoclavicular etiology is tested via the **costoclavicular syndrome test (military brace position)** (Selective Tissue Test 14-13). The **Roos test** has demonstrated accuracy in identifying the presence of TOS resulting from either neurological or vascular abnormalities (Selective Tissue Test 14-14). Each of these tests can be positive by virtue of a diminishing radial pulse or reproduction of neurological symptoms. Because arterial TOS is rare, reproduction of symptoms (as opposed to a diminishing pulse) is a more meaningful positive finding. When clusters of these tests are positive, the likelihood of TOS increases.[67] In addition, the upper limb tension test (see Selective Tissue Test 14-1) may also reproduce neurological symptoms.[67,70]

Neurological TOS mimics many symptoms of distal nerve entrapment, such as carpal tunnel syndrome, and, in fact, neurological TOS may contribute to the development of distal neuropathies. This so-called double-crush pathology occurs because a proximal nerve compression makes the distal nerve more susceptible to entrapment.[67] A detailed neurological examination is warranted.

Positive test results for TOS are not necessarily definitive of any underlying pathology. Patients who test positive for TOS need to be referred to a physician for further evaluation.

Thoracic Outlet Syndrome Intervention Strategies

The management of TOS depends on the involved structures and the location of the entrapment. Early recognition and prompt treatment of vascular TOS is necessary. With arterial TOS, surgical intervention often occurs to decompress the subclavian artery. With venous TOS, **thrombolytic therapy** is usually necessary to dissolve the clot, followed by rehabilitation to restore normal movement patterns.

Neurological TOS is generally managed conservatively, with initial interventions targeting atypical postures and reducing overhead movements and positions. Patients who complain of nocturnal symptoms should not sleep with their arms over their head. Postural awareness training and the use of ergonomically correct positioning, especially while driving, using a computer, or participating in any repetitive activity, is indicated. For patients with positive upper limb tension tests, the use of ***nerve gliding*** may help decrease adhesions restricting normal brachial plexus movement. Botulinum toxin (Botox®) injected into the scalene has been used to decrease constricting spasm.[75]

Surgical decompression may be warranted for true neurological TOS if conservative interventions fail.[72,75]

Thoracic Spine Pathologies

The thoracic spine is relatively well protected compared with the cervical and thoracic spinal regions. Pathology in the upper thoracic spine mimics cervical spine conditions, while lower thoracic spine pathologies behave more like lumbar spine conditions. Disc pathology is less common in the thoracic spine, probably due to the limited available motion. Thoracic spine pathology, especially with rib involvement, can affect breathing, making deep breaths painful and exercise difficult. Symptoms of many pathologies, such as cancer and gall bladder and gastroesophageal conditions, include referred pain to the thoracic or scapular region, making careful screening even more important.[76]

The articulations of the ribs with T1–T10 provide potential sites of pain. Hypomobility or hypermobility of the costovertebral articulations can result in sharp, well-localized pain that is exacerbated with rotation and radiates anteriorly to the chest. Coughing and sneezing can make symptoms worse. Painful posterior–anterior joint play as described for the lumbar vertebrae may be painful, but detecting differences in mobility is not reliable.

The intercostal and paraspinal muscles in the thoracic region are the common sites of tears and hypersensitive trigger points, generally brought on by repetitive overload mechanisms. These trigger points are palpable, defined areas or bands of point tenderness and increased tissue density.

Scheuermann's Kyphosis

Scheuermann's kyphosis results when the vertebral bodies wedge anteriorly, creating an abnormally rounded spine. With a strong genetic component, **Scheuermann's disease** affects boys and girls equally and generally becomes apparent during the teenage years (13 to 16 years old).[77] The problem is attributed to osteochondrosis of the vertebral bodies and is often found in conjunction with scoliosis. The diagnosis is made with radiographs, and **Schmorl's nodes** are a common associated finding.

Adolescents with Scheuermann's kyphosis appear to have an increased thoracic or thoracolumbar kyphosis with a compensatory increase in lumbar lordosis and cervical lordosis. These individuals describe local pain in the

Thrombolytic therapy The use of medicines that dissolve blood clots

Scheuermann's disease A disease process involving the vertebral bodies of the thoracic spine

Selective Tissue Tests 14-11
Adson's Test for Thoracic Outlet Syndrome

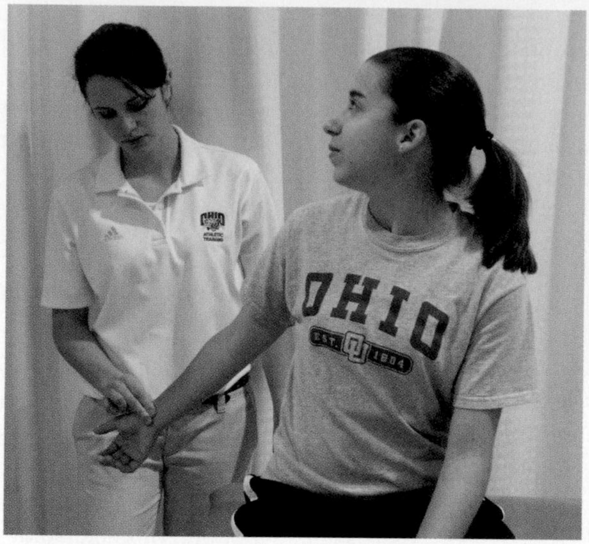

Identifies possible occlusion of the medial cord of the brachial plexus, subclavian artery, and subclavian vein secondary to entrapment between the anterior and middle scalenes.

Patient Position	Sitting The shoulder abducted to 30° The elbow extended with the thumb pointing upward The humerus externally rotated
Position of Examiner	Standing behind the patient One hand positioned so that the radial pulse is palpable
Evaluative Procedure	While still maintaining a feel for the radial pulse, the examiner externally rotates and extends the patient's shoulder while the face is rotated toward the involved side and the patient extends the neck. The patient is instructed to inhale deeply and hold the breath.
Positive Test	The radial pulse disappears or markedly diminishes as compared with the opposite side. Reproduction of symptoms
Implications	The subclavian artery and/or brachial plexus is being occluded between the anterior and middle scalene muscles and the pectoralis minor.
Evidence	

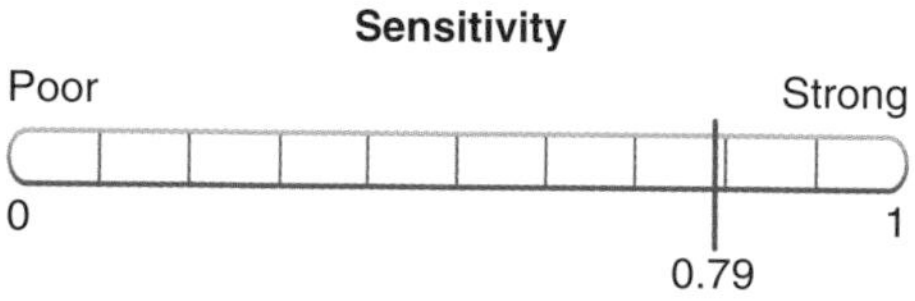

LR+: 3.29

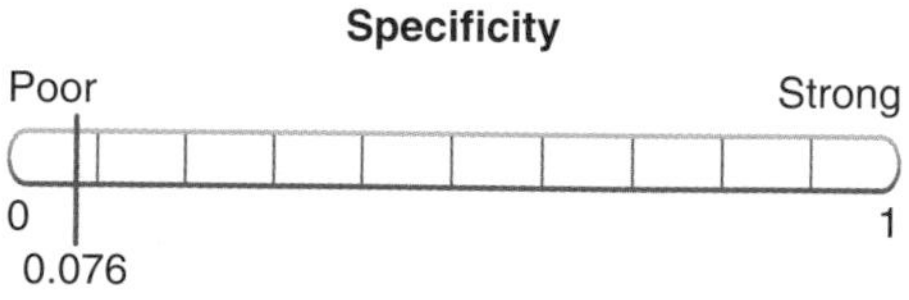

LR−: 0.28

Selective Tissue Tests 14-12
Allen Test for Thoracic Outlet Syndrome

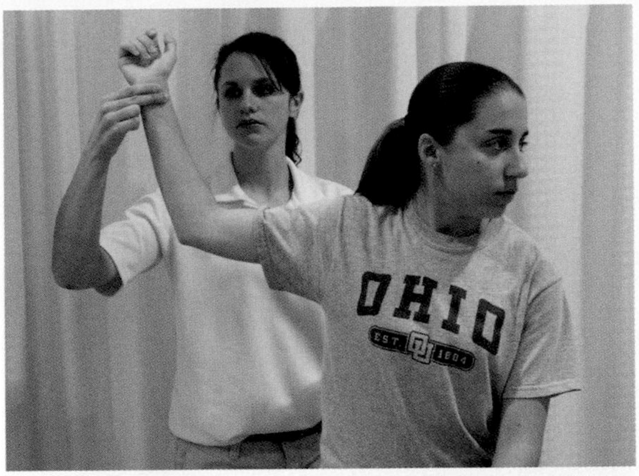

Identifies possible occlusion of the subclavian artery and vein caused by compression from the pectoralis minor.

Patient Position	Sitting The head facing forward
Position of Examiner	Standing behind the patient One hand positioned so that radial pulse is felt
Evaluative Procedure	The elbow is flexed to 90° while the clinician abducts the shoulder to 90°. The shoulder is then passively horizontally abducted and placed into external rotation. The patient then rotates the head toward the opposite shoulder.
Positive Test	The radial pulse disappears or neurological symptoms are reproduced.
Implications	The pectoralis minor muscle is compressing the neurovascular bundle.
Evidence	Absent or inconclusive in the literature

thoracic region, as well as hamstring, iliopsoas, and anterior shoulder girdle tightness.

Scheuermann's Kyphosis Intervention Strategies

Generally self-limiting, patients with flexible curves are managed with stretching exercises and strengthening of the trunk extensors and core stabilizers. Some patients may also be braced; however, this intervention requires high patient compliance and is associated with loss of correction once the brace is removed. Surgical correction may be needed for those with prolonged pain, progressive curves, loss of function, or debilitating self-perception.[77]

Thorax Pathologies

The MOI of the thorax may involve the superficial tissues, ribs, heart, or lungs. Likewise, the signs and symptoms of injury to the superficial tissues may mask trauma to the underlying structures.

Rib Fractures

The lateral and anterior portions of ribs 5–9 are most commonly fractured. The upper two ribs are protected by the clavicle and the mass of the pectoralis major muscle. The upper six or seven ribs are protected on their posterior aspect by the scapula, decreasing the incidence of rib trauma in these areas, although fractures of the upper ribs can occur.[78] The floating ribs have only a posterior attachment on the vertebrae, allowing them to bend and absorb the force of an impact. In sports such as football, the upper ribs are protected by shoulder pads and players in certain positions protect the lower ribs by wearing a "flak jacket" type of padding. Most rib fractures are the result of a single traumatic blow, but repetitive stresses and explosive muscle contractions may lead to a stress fracture of a rib.[79]

In cases of a rib fracture, the chief complaint is pain directly at the fracture site that worsens and radiates with deep inspirations, coughing, sneezing, and movement of the torso. The patient may assume a comfortable posture by leaning toward the side of the fracture and may actively splint the fracture site by holding the painful area to limit the amount of chest wall movement during inspiration. Respirations are usually shallow and rapid to minimize chest movement. Palpation of the area produces pain over

Selective Tissue Tests 14-13
Military Brace Position for Thoracic Outlet Syndrome

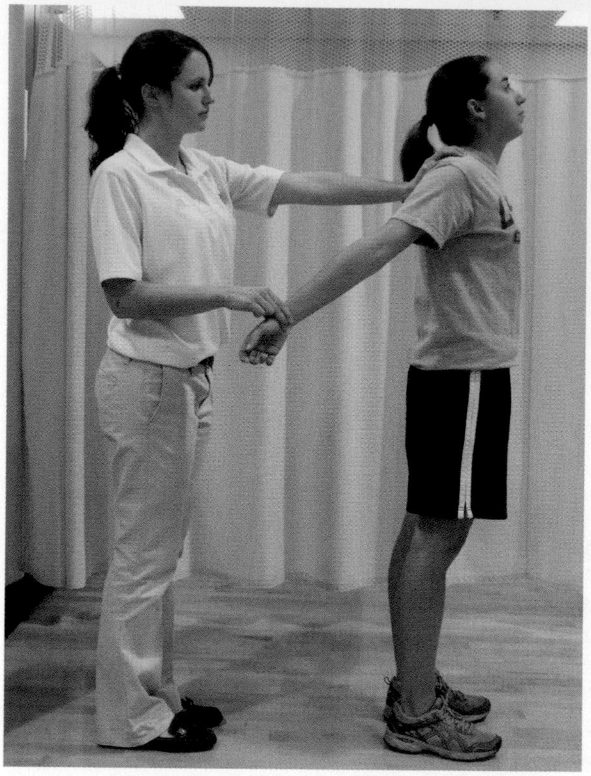

Identifies occlusion of the subclavian artery or brachial plexus by the shoulder's costoclavicular structures.

Patient Position	Standing The shoulders in a relaxed posture The head looking forward
Position of Examiner	Standing behind the patient One hand positioned to locate the radial pulse on the involved extremity
Evaluative Procedure	The patient retracts and depresses the shoulders as if coming to military attention. The humerus is extended and abducted to 30°. The neck and head are hyperextended.
Positive Test	The radial pulse disappears or neurological symptoms are reproduced.
Implications	The subclavian artery and/or lower trunks of the brachial plexus are being blocked by the costoclavicular structures of the shoulder.
Evidence	Absent or inconclusive in the literature

Selective Tissue Tests 14-14
Roos Test (or EAST–Elevated Arm Stress Test) for Thoracic Outlet Syndrome

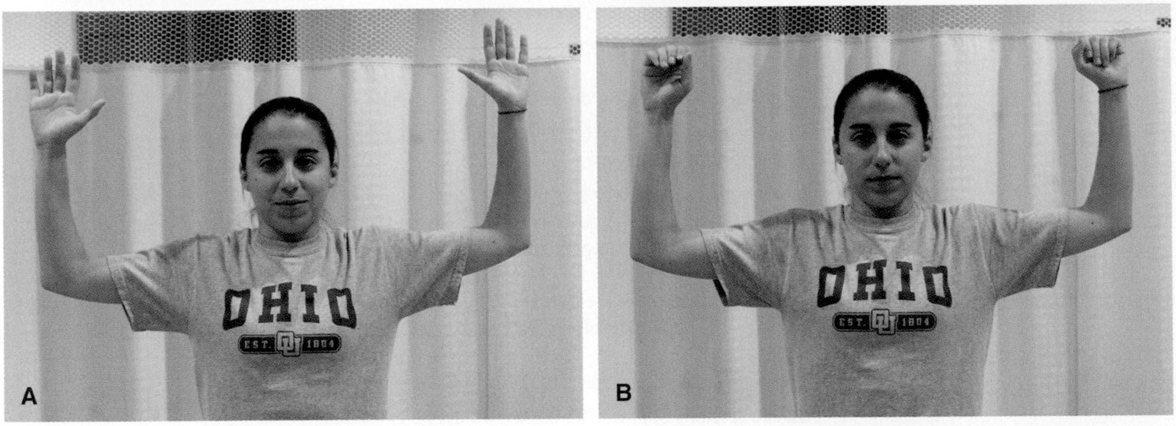

Identifies the presence of TOS of neurological or vascular etiology.

Patient Position	Sitting or standing The shoulders are abducted to 90°, and the humerus is externally rotated. The elbows are flexed to 90°.
Position of Examiner	Standing in front of the patient
Evaluative Procedure	The patient rapidly opens and closes both hands for 3 minutes. **(A) (B)**
Positive Test	Inability to maintain the testing position Replication of sensory and/or motor symptoms in the extremity
Implications	Vascular or neurological TOS
Evidence	

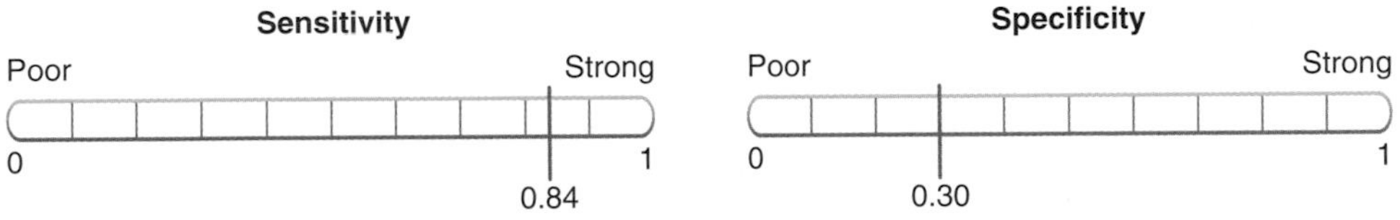

LR+: 1.20 **LR−: 0.53**

the site of the injury, and deformity of the bone or crepitus may also be noted (Examination Findings 14-4). The suspicion of a rib fracture can be confirmed through the **rib compression test** (Selective Tissue Test 14-15). This test should not be performed if a fracture is evident via simple palpation.

A blow in the anteroposterior direction usually results in an outward dispersion of forces along the ribs, forcing the fractured rib segments outward as well. Blows to the lateral rib cage have a higher incidence of inwardly projecting fractures, possibly leading to a pneumothorax or hemothorax (Box 14-1).[80] Fractures of the first and second ribs, often associated with cervical trauma, may occlude the underlying vasculature.[78,80] Unrecognized rib fractures can result in a nonunion, seriously impairing the patient's ability to move the trunk.[81]

The ribs are also subject to stress fractures, especially in sports such as rowing, swimming, and golf.[79,85] Most commonly occurring in the first rib (where the anterior scalene inserts) or in the posterolateral portion of ribs 4–9 at the origin of the serratus anterior, stress fractures are the result of sudden increases in training, improper biomechanics, or a change in equipment.[86] The signs and symptoms of rib stress fractures cause them to be misidentified as injury of the erector spinae or intercostal muscles or as osteochondritis or chostochondritis.[86] Stress fractures typically begin with vague discomfort in the thoracic region. They progress to sharp, localized pain that is often posterior and may worsen with deep breaths.

Rib Fracture Intervention Strategies

The possible complications warrant that all patients with suspected rib fractures be referred to a physician for further

Examination Findings 14-4
Acute Rib Fractures

Examination Segment	Clinical Findings
History of Current Condition	*Onset:* Acute *Pain characteristics:* Over a discrete area of the ribs *Other symptoms:* Difficulty breathing; if applicable, the signs of a pneumothorax or hemothorax may also be present. *Mechanism:* Direct blow; when the force occurs in the anteroposterior direction, the fracture has the tendency to displace outwardly. A blow from the lateral side results in the fractured ribs being displaced inwardly, threatening the lungs and other internal organs.
Functional Assessment	Movement of the torso—either through active motion or from deep respiration, coughing, or sneezing—produces pain along the fracture site; also possible limited torso movement.
Inspection	Initial inspection should rule out an open fracture. Possible splinting posture; the patient holds the injured area or leans toward the injured side. Discoloration and swelling may be visible over the injury site.
Palpation	Point tenderness over the area of impact Deeper palpation may reveal crepitus or identification of the fracture.
Joint and Muscle Function Assessment	*AROM:* Pain is elicited with trunk motion. *MMT:* Pain is elicited during testing of muscles attached to the ribs. *PROM:* Pain is elicited when stress is placed on the involved ribs.
Joint Stability Tests	*Stress tests:* Not applicable *Joint play:* Not applicable
Selective Tissue Tests	Rib compression test (contraindicated in the presence of an obvious fracture or lung trauma)
Neurological Screening	Within normal limits
Vascular Screening	Within normal limits
Imaging Techniques	Plain radiographs are usually sufficient to identify acute rib fractures. Stress fracture may be identified using a bone scan. MR or CT images may be used to rule out concurrent injury to the lungs or other organs.
Differential Diagnosis	Costochondral injury, erector spinae injury (for stress fractures), pneumothorax, hemothorax
Comments	Bony fragments that are displaced inward may jeopardize the integrity of the lungs and other internal organs.

AROM = active range of motion; CT = computed tomography; MMT = manual muscle test; MR = magnetic resonance; PROM = passive range of motion

evaluation and a definitive diagnosis. Rib fractures are managed by controlling the inflammatory response. Pain may be addressed with ice, medication, or both. A rib belt can be used to limit the amount of rib and chest motion that accompanies breathing and other activities of daily living. If deep breathing has been impaired, rehabilitation may involve the use of a spirometer to improve lung function (see Review of Systems, p. 28).[80]

The management of stress fractures includes avoiding aggravating activities and a gradual increase in activity intensity as symptoms abate.

Costochondral Injury

A costochondral injury is usually caused by overstretching the costochondral junction as the arm is forced into hyperflexion and horizontal abduction, potentially separating the costocartilage from the ribs. The signs of costochondral injury are similar to those of rib fractures, but the pain is anteriorly located at the costal–cartilage junction (see Examination Findings 14-4). The patient has immediate pain at the injury site and may report hearing a "snap" or "pop" at the time of injury. Pain is increased with deep breathing, coughing, sneezing, and movement. As with rib fractures,

Selective Tissue Tests 14-15
Compression Test for Rib Fractures

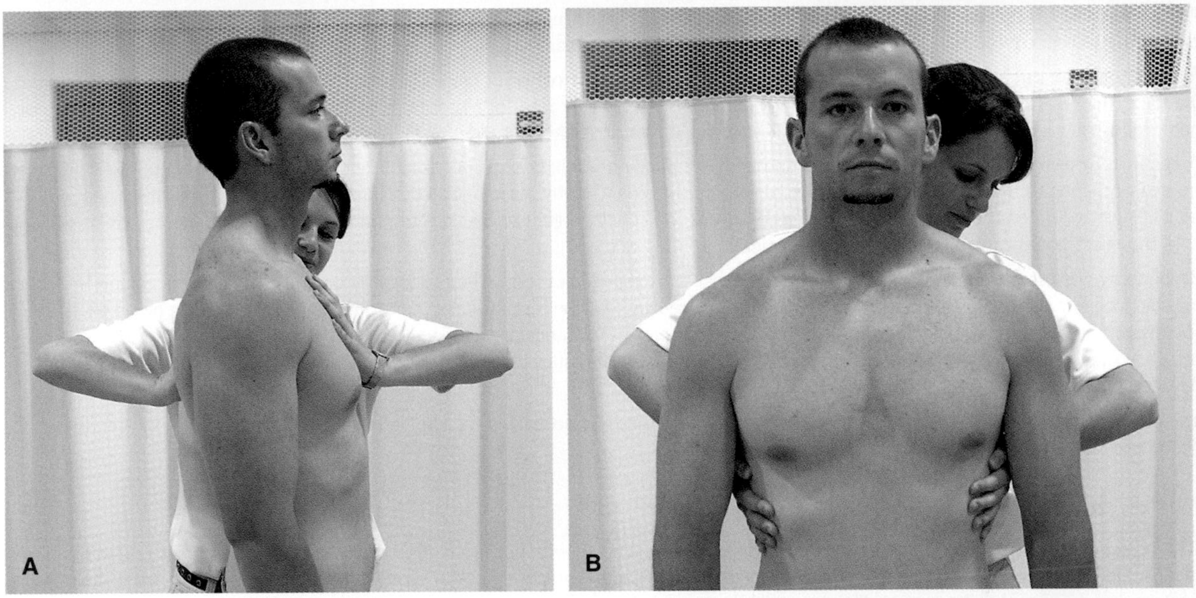

Manual compression causes deformation of the rib cage, causing pain in the presence of a rib fracture. (A) Anterior–posterior compression; (B) lateral compression. Costochondral injury may produce a false-positive result.

Patient Position	Seated or standing
Position of Examiner	Standing in front of the patient with the hands on opposite sides of the rib cage
Evaluative Procedure	The examiner compresses the rib cage in an anteroposterior direction and quickly releases the pressure. The rib cage is then compressed from the patient's side, and the pressure is quickly released.
Positive Test	Pain in the rib cage isolated to the fracture site
Implications	Damage to the rib cage, including the possibility of a fracture, contusion, or costochondral separation
Comments	Do not perform this test in the presence of palpable rib deformity or crepitus.
Evidence	Absent or inconclusive in the literature

the patient guards the area through body positioning and splinting with the hands. Swelling is often present, and palpation reveals point tenderness over the site of the trauma as well as deformity if the rib has separated from the cartilage.

Costochondral Injury Intervention Strategies

Patients with costochondral injuries are managed similarly to those with rib fractures, with the protocol focused on decreasing pain, controlling inflammation, and eliminating unnecessary movement of the rib cage.

Splenic Injury

Located on the left side of the body at the level of ribs 9–11, the **spleen** is a solid, fragile organ that is supported by ligaments attaching it to the kidney, colon, stomach, and diaphragm (Fig. 14-27). The largest of the lymphatic organs, its primary function is to produce and destroy blood cells during times of systemic infection. During certain disease states, such as **mononucleosis**, the spleen becomes engorged with blood, causing it to protrude below the ribs' protective bony cover, increasing the risk of injury. When the spleen is traumatized, surgical removal may be necessary. If the spleen is removed, its functions are assumed by the liver and bone marrow.

The spleen may be injured when the abdomen receives a blunt blow such as when a person falls on a ball or other object. The subsequent force delivered to the spleen can result in possible contusion or laceration. An inflamed spleen, which can occur in patients with mononucleosis, pneumonia, or other systemic infections, is predisposed to

Mononucleosis A disease state caused by an abnormally high number of mononuclear leukocytes in the bloodstream

Box 14-1 Lung Pathologies

Pneumothorax

A pneumothorax is the accumulation of air in the pleural cavity that disrupts the lung's ability to expand and draw in oxygen. The decreased oxygen intake reduces the amount of oxygen absorbed into the bloodstream, resulting in hypoxia and the development of respiratory distress.

A pneumothorax can be either open or closed. A **spontaneous pneumothorax** occurs when blebs rupture and allow air to leak into the pleural cavity or as the result of distal airway inflammation.[82] Mechanical causes of a spontaneous pneumothorax include blow to the rib cage, penetrating rib cage injury, improper breathing, or sneezing or can arise after surgery.[78,82-84]

A **tension pneumothorax** develops when a spontaneous pneumothorax fails to spontaneously close or as the result of blunt or penetrating trauma occurring to the chest. The result is that air enters the pleural cavity but cannot exit. The air within the pleural cavity continues to build up, placing pressure on the lung and causing it to collapse. If this condition goes unchecked, the subsequent pressure quickly affects the opposite lung, the heart, and the major arteries, leading to death.

Respiratory distress is a common finding in patients with a tension pneumothorax. The patient may complain of pain and shortness of breath or may be unable to speak, appearing agitated or anxious. Labored and shallow respirations accompany a rapidly decreasing blood pressure. Breath sounds, as assessed during auscultation, may be decreased or completely absent on the affected side. The skin may appear to be cyanotic, and the patient will become hypotensive and tachycardic. In extreme cases, the tissues between the ribs and clavicle are distended, and the trachea deviates away from the side of the trauma.

Immediate activation of the emergency system is needed for a tension pneumothorax. The patient should receive 100% oxygen, and decompression often occurs before transport to the hospital.

Hemothorax

A hemothorax is similar to—and often occurs concurrently with—a pneumothorax. In a hemothorax, respiratory distress is caused by a collection of blood in the pleural cavity. Bleeding occurs from an internal chest wound (e.g., a fractured rib lacerating a lung) or from the rupture of a blood vessel within the chest cavity. The signs and symptoms of a hemothorax are very similar, if not identical, to those of a pneumothorax. However, with a hemothorax, the person may cough up bloody sputum, hemoptysis. Refer to the "On-Field Management" section of this chapter for a description of the initial care of patients with this condition.

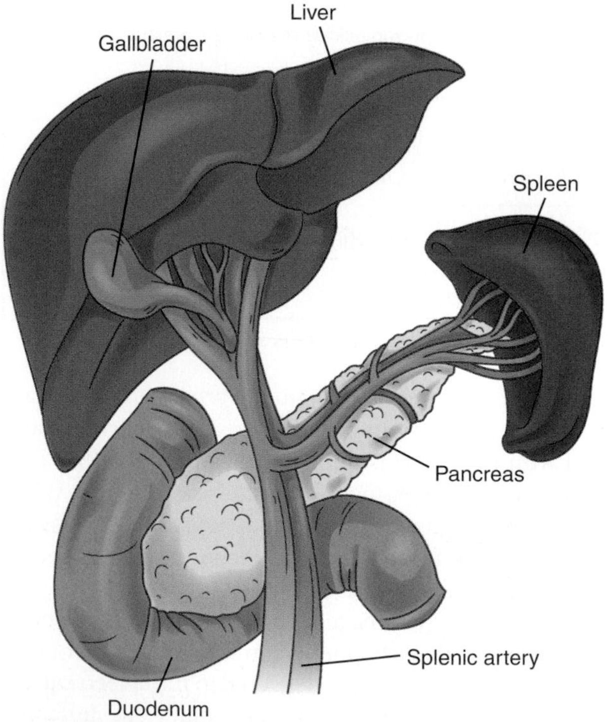

FIGURE 14-27 ■ Spleen. During illness, the spleen may become enlarged, causing it to become vulnerable to injury.

injury because of the organ's increased mass and decreased elasticity.[87] In patients with advanced disease states, such as mononucleosis, the spleen may spontaneously rupture without a history of blunt force.[88] Likewise, the time between physical trauma to the spleen and the onset of symptoms may be delayed for weeks, days, or years.[89]

The signs and symptoms of shock soon develop after acute spleen trauma. The telltale indicator of a ruptured spleen is the **Kehr's sign**, pain in the upper left quadrant and left shoulder. These symptoms are aggravated by movement, and the patient may vomit or describe being nauseated (Examination Findings 14-5). The vital signs are key indicators of **hemodynamic** changes.

If the patient vomits, attempt to observe the discharge to determine if it is undigested food, red from blood, or greenish from bile. Advise the patient with abdominal injury not to eat or drink because doing so may worsen the symptoms or complicate any surgical procedure that may need to be performed. Various imaging techniques, such as MRI and CT scans, are used to identify splenic trauma.[90]

* Practical Evidence

Determining return-to-play status for contact-sport athletes with mononucleosis should not rely on whether or not the spleen is palpable. Splenomegaly is palpable in only about 20% of persons who actually have the condition.[91]

Splenic Rupture Intervention Strategies

Patients suspected of a splenic injury require referral to a physician for immediate evaluation, observation, and treatment.

Bleb A large sac filled with air or fluid having the potential to rupture

Cyanotic Dark blue or purple tint to the skin and mucous membranes caused by a decreased oxygen supply

Sputum A substance formed by mucus, blood, or pus expelled by coughing or clearing the throat

Hemodynamic The process of blood circulating through the body

Examination Findings 14-5
Splenic Injury

Examination Segment	Clinical Findings
History of Current Condition	*Onset:* Acute, although the onset of symptoms may take hours *Pain characteristics:* Pressure experienced in the upper left quadrant, discrete area of referred pain in the anterior and posterior portions of the lower left quadrant and the upper left shoulder (**Kehr's sign**) *Other symptoms:* Feeling of "fullness" in the upper left quadrant and stomach *Mechanism:* Blow to the abdomen or thorax, compressing or jarring the spleen *Risk factors:* Mononucleosis, systemic infection
Functional Assessment	Pain in the upper left quadrant and shoulder aggravated by movement General unwillingness to move
Inspection	The impact site possibly showing signs of a contusion or rib fracture
Palpation	Cold and clammy skin with the onset of shock Tenderness in area over the impact site Distention of upper left quadrant
Review of Systems	*Cardiovascular:* Low blood pressure Increased heart rate *Respiratory:* Increased respiratory rate if in shock *Gastrointestinal:* Nausea and vomiting possible Abdominal rigidity *Genitourinary:* Within normal limits *Neurological:* Kehr's sign
Selective Tissue Tests	Not applicable
Imaging Techniques	MR or CT scan Diagnostic ultrasound
Differential Diagnosis	Liver trauma; kidney injury; rib fracture
Comments	Patients suffering from mononucleosis or other systemic infections are predisposed to spleen injury secondary to the enlargement and hardening of this organ. Concurrent injury to the left kidney must be ruled out. Symptoms of mononucleosis include fever, fatigue, swollen lymph nodes (adenopathy), tonsil/throat exudate, and sore throat.

CT = computed tomography; MR = magnetic resonance

Kidney Trauma

The kidneys sit well protected behind the lower ribs and spinal musculature. Forces of sufficient magnitude to traumatize the kidneys are often associated with concurrent injury to the lower ribs, lower thoracic vertebrae, upper lumbar vertebrae, or other internal organs. Any penetrating wounds most likely involve some of these structures as well.

Acute kidney injuries occur following blunt trauma to the upper lumbar and lower thoracic region. The only outward signs of a kidney contusion or laceration may be bruising or bleeding over the area of contact. The patient may complain of rib pain that increases in intensity during deep inspiration. Cases of severe internal bleeding also produce the signs and symptoms of shock. Palpation of the area generally reveals diffuse tenderness unless a rib is concurrently injured, at which time a more focused pain and crepitus are demonstrated (Fig. 14-28). With severe bleeding, guarding of the abdomen may reflexively occur because of pain (Examination Findings 14-6).

Hematuria is a diagnostic sign associated with an injured kidney; however, the absence of blood in the urine immediately after an injury does not rule out kidney trauma. Except in the case of severe bleeding within the kidney, the urine may not seem noticeably discolored to the unaided eye, and bleeding can be detected only via laboratory analysis of a urine sample collected after the trauma occurs.

Kidney Trauma Intervention Strategies

The use of CT scans or contrast imaging of the urinary tract may be required for a definitive diagnosis. The potential

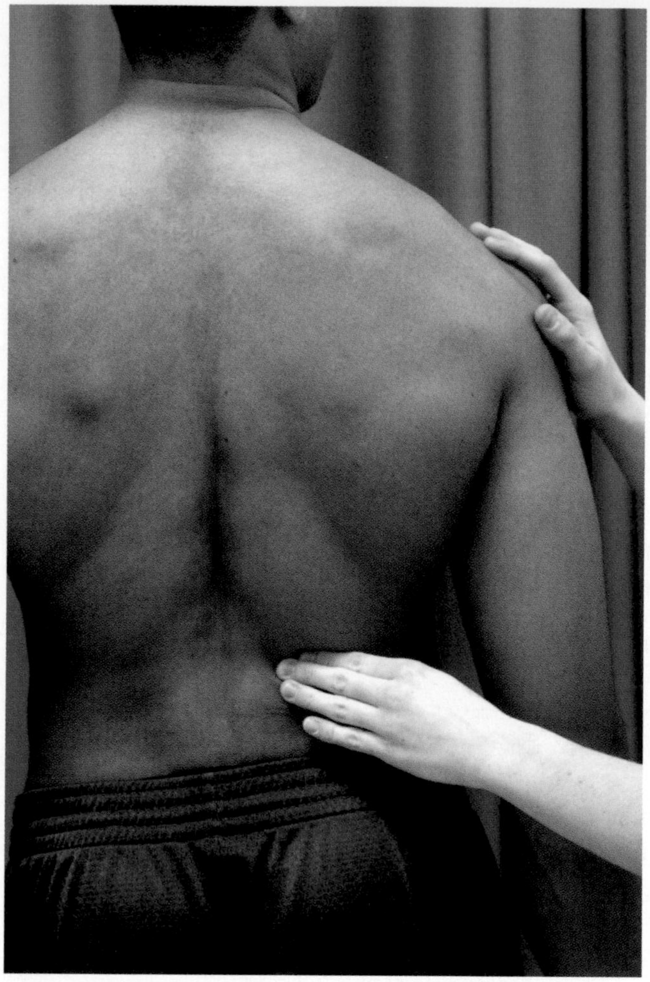

FIGURE 14-28 ■ Palpation of the right kidney. After an injury, the area overlying the kidneys may become tender to the touch or reveal crepitus secondary to a rib fracture.

loss of a kidney warrants that individuals demonstrating any of these signs and symptoms be immediately referred to a physician.

Commotio Cordis

Commotio cordis, a "cardiac concussion," is an instantaneous cardiac arrest caused by a nonpenetrating blow to the chest in a person with an otherwise healthy heart that does not result in injury of the overlying structures.[92-94] The most frequent cause of commotio cordis is being struck in the chest by a projectile such as a ball or a puck, followed by automobile accidents and domestic (child) abuse.[92,95] The pliability of the chest during childhood more easily transmits the force to the heart, but individuals of any age may be affected.

The onset of commotio cordis is influenced by the type, location, force, and timing of the impact.[92] Of these factors, the timing of the impact is most crucial to its onset. A precordial impact delivered within 30 and 15 milliseconds before the peak of the T wave can trigger ventricular fibrillation (Fig. 14-29).[92,96]

The vulnerable area of the chest wall is a silhouette of the cardiac profile directly anterior to the heart.[93,96] The force of the blow is believed to activate mechanosensitive ion channels by triggering mechanoelectrical coupling. While high-velocity forces such as being struck by a lacrosse ball or hockey puck can trigger the cardiac **arrhythmia**, commotio cordis can also be the result of relatively low-velocity forces such as a thrown baseball. The incidence of occurrence is greater when using solid-core objects than those that are air-filled (e.g., soccer ball, football).[93]

The signs and symptoms of commotio cordis—those of cardiac arrest—occur immediately after the blow or may be delayed by several seconds, followed by cardiac arrhythmia, most frequently ventricular fibrillation.[92,94,97] Although the survival rate for commotio cordis is only about 15%, successful resuscitation and subsequent survival using on-site CPR and an automated external defibrillator have been documented.[93,95,96,98] When CPR, including defibrillation, is initiated within 3 minutes after the trauma, the survival rate is 25%; when initiating CPR is delayed for more than 3 minutes, the survival rate drops to 3%.[93]

Commotio Cordis Intervention Strategy

The immediate intervention for commotio cordis is the use of an automated external defibrillator to restore the heart's normal rhythm. Without this intervention, death soon occurs. The poor survivability and limited management options have led to emphasis being placed on the prevention of commotio cordis, especially in young athletes. Many youth leagues have changed to using softer balls and require that batters and those at other at-risk positions wear chest protectors. However, cases of commotio cordis have still occurred with these preventive measures in place, primarily because the chest protector was not properly fitted.[98]

On-Field Evaluation and Management of Cervical and Thoracic Spine and Thorax Injuries

All injuries to the spinal column requiring an on-field evaluation must be treated as possibly life threatening until spinal cord involvement and serious injury have been ruled out. Bilateral symptoms in the upper extremities or symptoms in the lower extremities should alert the examiner to the potential of spinal cord involvement. Chapter 20 discusses the evaluation and management of patients with potentially catastrophic spinal cord injuries.

Because trauma to the thorax and abdomen is most often the result of acute, high-velocity impact, the need for on-field evaluation of these conditions is commonplace. At first, injuries to the internal organs may produce only the signs and symptoms of a contusion overlying the impact

Arrhythmia Loss of the normal heart rhythm; an irregular heart rate

Examination Findings 14-6
Contused or Lacerated Kidney

Examination Segment	Clinical Findings
History of Current Condition	*Onset:* Acute *Pain characteristics:* Posterolateral portion of the upper lumbar and lower thoracic region *Mechanism:* Blunt trauma or penetrating injury to the kidney (e.g., contusive forces, fractured rib impaling the kidney)
Functional Assessment	General unwillingness to move
Inspection	Contusion or laceration in the impacted area may be present.
Palpation	Tenderness over the impact site Abdominal rigidity may occur.
Review of Systems	*Cardiovascular:* Hypotension *Respiratory:* Breathing may become rapid. *Genitourinary:* Macroscopic or microscopic blood may be present in the urine. Possible pain with urination. *Neurological:* Within normal limits
Selective Tissue Tests	Not applicable
Imaging Techniques	Contrast CT scan
Differential Diagnosis	Rib fracture; muscle strain or contusion; urinary tract infection
Comments	The traumatic forces may also result in a rib fracture or costochondral injury. Trauma to the spleen must be ruled out with injury to the left kidney; liver trauma must be ruled out with injury to the right kidney. Patients suspected of suffering from a kidney injury should immediately be referred to a physician.

CT = computed tomography

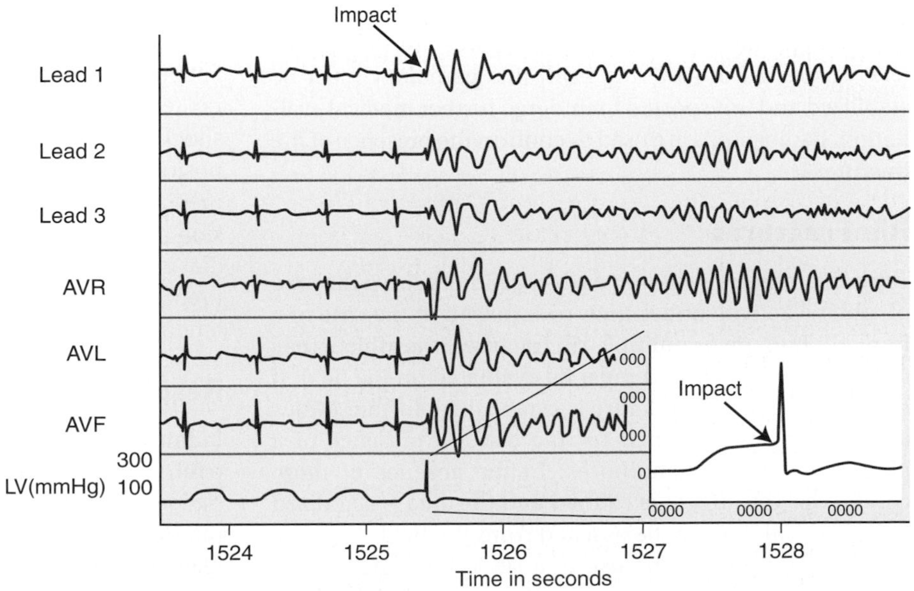

FIGURE 14-29 ■ Electrocardiogram demonstrating ventricular fibrillation caused by a blunt impact to the chest wall during vulnerable zone of repolarization (10–30 ms before the T-wave peak).

area. As blood collects within the viscera, outward symptoms of the underlying condition are produced.

Brachial Plexus Injury

Typically, athletes with a brachial plexus injury leave the field of play under their own power, with the involved arm dangling limp at the side. The head may be held in a position to relieve any stress placed on the brachial plexus as the result of spasm of the trapezius muscle. The athlete's signs and symptoms (see Examination Findings 14-2) are usually transient in nature. After a thorough evaluation to rule out the possibility of trauma to the cervical vertebrae, the cervical spine should be treated with ice packs to decrease pain and spasm.

The athlete should demonstrate a normal neurological examination without weakness and with full pain-free ROM before returning to activity. Any continuation of the signs and symptoms precludes further participation until the athlete is cleared by a physician to return to play.

Thoracic Spine

Forced flexion or lateral bending of the thoracic spine places compressive forces on the anterior aspect of the vertebral bodies in the lower thoracic spine. The thoracic spine can be compressed by an axial load, distraction (flexion force), or a rotational force being placed on the cervical spine.[99] In most instances, neurological function is normal, leaving the on-field determination of a possible fracture to be based on the MOI and point tenderness over the affected vertebra. If the fracture goes unrecognized, pain and stiffness in the thoracic region and pain during deep inspiration may be reported. Although it is a rare occurrence, fractured thoracic vertebra may puncture the esophagus[100] or the aorta.[101]

Although most thoracic spine fractures are stable, athletes suspected of suffering from this pathology must be stabilized and transported to undergo further medical evaluation. Radiographs are used to confirm the presence of the fracture.

Rib Fractures

Typically, athletes suffering a rib cage injury leave the area of athletic activity under their own power. In the case of a frank rib fracture or multiple rib fractures, the athlete may not be able to move and must be evaluated on the field. If the presence of a rib fracture is established, further evaluation must be performed to rule out the presence of a pneumothorax or hemothorax. In the absence of these conditions, the athlete is calmed and the area is stabilized before the athlete can be assisted from the field. The area may be stabilized by the use of a rib belt or, more commonly, by wrapping the ipsilateral arm to the side of the athlete with a swathe (Fig. 14-30). The athlete can then be assisted off the field and transported to a medical facility for further evaluation.

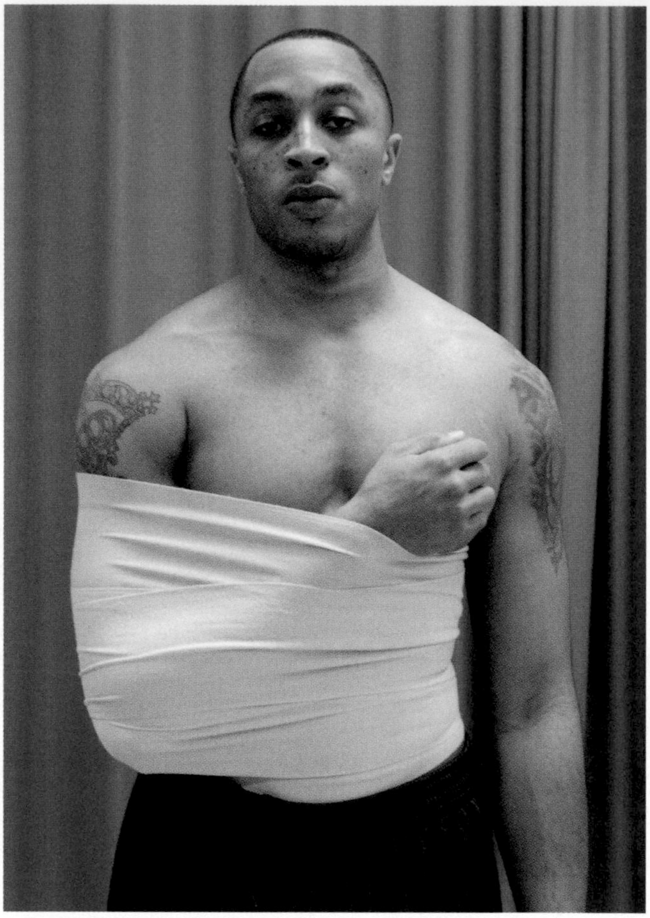

FIGURE 14-30 ■ Immobilization of the rib cage through the use of a swath. The arm of the involved side may be immobilized to reduce pain that is secondary to movement of the shoulder.

Pneumothorax and Hemothorax

Patients suspected of having a pneumothorax or hemothorax require continuous vital sign monitoring, treatment for shock, and placement on the affected side in a semireclined position, if possible. Provide supplemental oxygen. The immediate and potentially life-saving management of a tension pneumothorax includes insertion of a large-bore needle into the space between the second and third ribs. Prepare to assist with respiration if needed and activate the emergency medical system.

Respiratory Distress

Pulmonary problems include difficulty with respiration, or pain, or both. The difficulty in breathing may cause the patient to panic. Although pain may occur secondary to pulmonary obstruction, these problems are typically recognized by the shear labor required for breathing. Excruciating, deep thoracic pain that develops in the middle and upper back is the most distinctive early sign of developing an aortic aneurysm, the typical cause of death associated with **Marfan syndrome** (Box 14-2).[102]

Box 14-2
Marfan Syndrome

Diagnostic Findings

Musculoskeletal Examination

Arm span greater than the person's height

Elongated metacarpal and metatarsal bones, causing the hands and feet to appear disproportionately large

Thoracic kyphosis

Scoliosis

Systemic joint laxity

Pectus excavatum ("sunken chest" or depression of the sternum)

High arched palate

Ophthalmologic

Dislocation of the eye lens

Myopia

Cardiovascular

Dilated aortic root

Aortic regurgitation

Mitral valve prolapse

Aortic insufficiency murmur

An inherited condition, Marfan syndrome is characterized by cardiovascular, musculoskeletal, and ocular abnormalities. Although Marfan syndrome is a disease of the body's connective tissue, failure of the cardiac system usually leads to death. The connective tissue providing strength to the aorta is decreased, causing weakness that results in the formation of an aneurysm. Even when the syndrome is recognized and the individual is removed from strenuous activity, the person can suffer rupture of an aortic aneurysm, causing immediate death.[102,103]

Cardiac testing may produce various abnormalities, the most common being an abnormal aorta and multivalvular deformities, leading to prolapse of the valves and aortic valve regurgitation.

Suspicion of Marfan syndrome warrants a full medical examination. Although medical clearance is determined on a case-by-case basis, individuals who have Marfan syndrome are restricted from participating in vigorous physical activity. An absolute disqualifying condition is an enlarged aortic root, a predisposition to aortic rupture.[103,104]

REFERENCES

1. Olson, S, et al: Tender point sensitivity, range of motion and perceived disability in subjects with neck pain. *J Orthop Sports Phys Ther*, 30:13, 2000.
2. Chang, D, and Bosco, JA: Cervical spine injuries in the athlete. *Bull NYU Hosp Jt Dis*, 64:119, 2006.
3. Scifert, J, et al: Spinal cord mechanics during flexion and extension of the cervical spine: a finite element study. *Pain Physician*, 5:394, 2002.
4. Dalton, D: The vertebral column. In Levangie, PK, and Norkin, CS. *Joint Structure and Function: A Comprehensive Analysis*, ed 5. Philadelphia, PA: FA Davis, 2011.
5. da C_rte, FC, and Neves, N: Cervical spine instability in rheumatoid arthritis. *Eur J Orthop Surg Traumatol*, 24 (Suppl 1):S83, 2014.
6. Moore, KL, and Dalley, AF: Summary of cranial nerves. In *Clinically Oriented Anatomy*, ed 5. Philadelphia, PA: Lippincott Williams & Wilkins, 2006, pp 1124-1155.
7. Young, BA, et al: Thoracic costotransverse joint pain patterns: a study in normal volunteers. *BMC Musculoskelet Disord*, 9:140, 2008.
8. Pietrobon, R, et al: Standard scales for measurement of functional outcome for cervical pain or dysfunction: a systematic review. *Spine*, 27:515, 2002.
9. Heintz, MM, et al: Multimodal management of mechanical neck pain using a treatment based classification system. *J Man Manip Ther*, 16:217, 2008.
10. Fritz, JM and Brennan, GP: Preliminary examination of a proposed treatment-based classification system for patients receiving physical therapy interventions for neck pain. *Phys Ther*, 87:513, 2007.
11. Sizer, PS, Brismée, J, and Cook, C: Medical screening for red flags in the diagnosis and management of musculoskeletal spine pain. *Pain Pract*, 7:53, 2007.
12. Fjelhner, A, et al: Interexaminer reliability in physical examination of the cervical spine. *J Manipulative Physiol Ther*, 22:511, 1999.
13. Vlaeyen, JWS, and Linton, SJ: Fear-avoidance and its consequences in chronic musculoskeletal pain: a state of the art. *Pain*, 85:317, 2000.
14. Childs, JD, et al: Screening for vertebrobasilar insufficiency in patients with neck pain: manual therapy decision-making in the presence of uncertainty. *J Orthop Sports Phys Ther*, 35:300, 2005.
15. Bertilson, B, et al: Pain drawing in the assessment of neurogenic pain and dysfunction in the neck/shoulder region: inter-examiner reliability and concordance with clinical examination. *Pain Med*, 8:134, 2007.
16. Asavasopon, S, Jankoski, J, and Godges, JJ: Clinical diagnosis of vertebrobasilar insufficiency: resident's case problem. *J Orthop Sports Phys Ther*, 35:645, 2005.
17. Wainner, RS, et al: Reliability and diagnostic accuracy of the clinical examination and patient self-report measures for cervical radiculopathy. *Spine*, 28:52, 2003.
18. Wrisley, DM, et al: Cervicogenic dizziness: a review of diagnosis and treatment. *J Orthop Sports Phys Ther*, 30:755, 2000.
19. Richter, RR, and Reinking, MF: How does evidence on the diagnostic accuracy of the vertebral artery test influence teaching of the test in a professional physical therapist education program? *Phys Ther*, 85:589, 2005.
20. Norkin, CC, and White, DJ: *Measurement of Joint Motion: A Guide to Goniometry*. Philadelphia, PA: FA Davis, 2009, p 346.
21. Williams, MA, et al: A systematic review of reliability and validity studies of methods for measuring active and passive cervical range of motion. *J Manipulative Physiol Ther*, 33:138, 2010.
22. Pool, JJ, et al: The interexaminer reproducibility of physical examination of the cervical spine. *J Manipulative Physiol Ther*, 27:84, 2004.
23. Dall-Alba, PT, et al: Cervical range of motion discriminates between asymptomatic persons and those with whiplash. *Spine*, 26:2090, 2001.
24. Cook, CE: Manual therapy of the thoracic spine. In Cook, CE: *Orthopedic Manual Therapy: An Evidence-based Approach*, ed 2. Upper Saddle River, NJ: Pearson Education, 2012.
25. Edmondston, SJ, et al: Reliability of isometric muscle endurance tests in subjects with postural neck pain. *J Manipulative Physiol Ther*, 31:348, 2008.
26. Reese, NB: *Muscle and Sensory Testing*. St. Louis, MO: Elsevier Saunders, 2005, p 203.
27. Domenech, MA, et al: The deep flexor endurance test: normative data scores in healthy adults. *PM R*, 3:105, 2011.

28. Edmondston, S, et al: Endurance and fatigue characteristics of the neck flexor and extensor muscles during isometric tests in patients with postural neck pain. *Man Ther*, 16:332, 2011.
29. de Koning, CHP, et al: Clinimetric evaluation of methods to measure muscle functioning in patients with non-specific neck pain: a systematic review. *BMC Musculoskelet Disord*, 9:142, 2008.
30. Mitchell, J, et al: Is cervical spine rotation, as used in the standard vertebrobasilar insufficiency test, associated with a measurable change in intracranial vertebral artery blood flow? *Man Ther*, 9:220, 2004.
31. Davis, DS, et al: Upper limb neural tension and seated slump tests: the false positive rate among healthy young adults without cervical or lumbar symptoms. *J Man Manip Ther*, 16:136, 2008.
32. Kleinrensink, GL, et al: Upper limb tension tests as tools in the diagnosis of nerve and plexus lesions: anatomical and biomechanical aspects. *Clin Biomech*, 15:9, 2000.
33. Walsh, MT: Upper limb neural tension testing and mobilization: fact, fiction, and a practical approach. *J Hand Ther*, 18:241, 2005.
34. Miller, TM, and Johnston, SC: Should the Babinski sign be part of the routine neurologic examination? *Neurology*, 65:1165, 2005.
35. Emery, SE: Cervical spondylitic myelopathy: diagnosis and treatment. *J Am Acad Orthop Surg*, 9:376, 2001.
36. Buijper, B, et al: Degenerative cervical radiculopathy: diagnosis and conservative treatment. A review. *Eur J Neuro*, 16:15, 2009.
37. Carette, S, and Fehlings, MG: Cervical radiculopathy. *N Engl J Med*, 353:4, 2005.
38. Triantafillou, KM, et al: Degenerative disease of the cervical spine and its relationship to athletics. *Clin Sports Med*, 31:509, 2012.
39. Malanga, GA, Landes, P, and Nadler, S: Provocative tests in cervical spine examination: historical basis and scientific analyses. *Pain Physician*, 6:199, 2003.
40. Anekstein, Y, and Smorgick, Y: What is the best way to apply the Spurling test for cervical radiculopathy? *Clin Orthop Relat Res*, 470:2566, 2012.
41. Tong, HC, Haig, AJ, and Yamakawa, K: The Spurling test and cervical radiculopathy. *Spine*, 27:156, 2002.
42. Eubanks, JD: Cervical radiculopathy: nonoperative management of neck pain and radicular symptoms. *Am Fam Physician*. 81:33, 2010.
43. D'Haen, B, et al: Chordoma of the lower cervical spine. *Clin Neurol Neurosurg*, 97:245, 1995.
44. Wainer, RS, and Gill, H: Diagnosis and nonoperative management of cervical radiculopathy. *J Orthop Sports Phys Ther*, 30:728, 2000.
45. Cook, C, et al: Clustered clinical findings for diagnosis of cervical spine myelopathy. *J Man Manip Ther*, 18:175, 2010.
46. Davidson, RI, Dunn, EJ, and Metzmaker, JN: The shoulder abduction test in the diagnosis of radicular pain in cervical extradural compressive monoradiculopathies. *Spine*, 6:441, 1981.
47. Moore, RA, et al: Amitriptyline for neuropathic pain and fibromyalgia in adults. *Cochrane Database Syst Rev*. 12:CD008242, 2012. doi:10.1002/14651858.CD008242.pub2
48. Boselie, T, et al: Arthroplasty versus fusion in single-level cervical degenerative disc disease: a Cochrane review. *Spine*, 38,E1069, 2013.
49. Cook, C, et al: Identifiers suggestive of clinical cervical spine instability: a Delphi study of physical therapists. *Phys Ther*, 85:895, 2005.
50. Olson, KA, and Joder, D: Diagnosis and treatment of cervical spine clinical instability. *J Orthop Sports Phys Ther*, 31:194, 2001.
51. Bransford, RJ, et al: Posterior fixation of the upper cervical spine: contemporary techniques. *J Am Acad Orthop Surg*, 19:63, 2011.
52. Kirpalani, D, and Mitra, R: Cervical facet joint dysfunction: a review. *Arch Phys Med Rehabil*, 89:770, 2008.
53. Sehgal, N, et al: Systematic review of diagnostic utility of facet (zygapophysial) joint injections in chronic spinal pain: an update. *Pain Physician*, 10:213, 2007.
54. Klaassen, Z, et al: Thoracic outlet syndrome: a neurological and vascular disorder. *Clin Anat*, 27:724, 2014.
55. Safran, MR: Nerve injury about the shoulder in athletes, part 2: long thoracic nerve, spinal accessory nerve, burners/stingers, thoracic outlet syndrome. *Am J Sports Med*, 32:1063, 2004.
56. Markey, KL, Di Benedetto, M, and Curl, WW: Upper trunk brachial plexopathy: the stinger syndrome. *Am J Sports Med*, 21:650, 1993.
57. Chao, S, Pacella, MJ, and Torg, JS: The pathomechanics, pathophysiology and prevention of cervical spinal cord and brachial plexus injuries in athletics. *Sports Med*, 40:59, 2010.
58. Speer, KP, and Bassett, FH: The prolonged burner syndrome. *Am J Sports Med*, 18:591, 1990.
59. Standaert, CJ, and Herring, SA: Expert opinion and controversies in musculoskeletal and sports medicine: stingers. *Arch Phys Med Rehabil*, 90:402, 2009.
60. Kitamura, T, et al: Brachial plexus stretching injuries: microcirculation of the brachial plexus. *J Shoulder Elbow Surg*, 4:118, 1995.
61. Levitz, CL, Reilly, PJ, and Torg, JS: The pathomechanics of chronic, recurrent cervical nerve root neurapraxia: the chronic burner syndrome. *Am J Sports Med*, 25:73, 1997.
62. Manchikanti, L, et al: An update of comprehensive evidence-based guidelines for interventional techniques in chronic spinal pain. Part II: guidance and recommendations. *Pain Physician*, 16(suppl):S49, 2013.
63. Reilly, PJ, and Torg, JS: Athletic injury to the cervical nerve roots and brachial plexus. *Operat Tech Sports Med*, 1:231, 1993.
64. Walker, AT, et al: Detection of nerve rootlet avulsion on CT myelography in patients with birth palsy and brachial plexus injury after trauma. *Am J Roentgenol*, 167:1283, 1996.
65. Bajuk, S, Jelnikar, T, and Ortar, M: Rehabilitation of patient with brachial plexus lesion and break in axillary artery. Case study. *J Hand Ther*, 9:399, 1996.
66. Kepler, CK, and Vaccaro, AR: Injuries and abnormalities of the cervical spine and return to play criteria. *Clin Sports Med*, 31:499, 2012.
67. Hooper, TL, et al: Thoracic outlet syndrome: a controversial clinical condition, part 1: anatomy, and clinical examination/diagnosis. *J Man Manip Ther*, 18:74, 2010.
68. Huang, JH, and Zager, EL: Thoracic outlet syndrome. *Neurosurgery*, 55:897, 2004.
69. Laulan, J, et al: Thoracic outlet syndrome: definition, aetiological factors, diagnosis, management and occupational impact. *J Occup Rehabil*, 21:366, 2011.
70. Sanders, RJ, Hammond, SL, and Rao, NM: Diagnosis of thoracic outlet syndrome. *J Vasc Surg*, 46:601, 2007.
71. Demirbag, D, et al: The relationship between magnetic resonance imaging findings and postural maneuver and physical examination tests in patients with thoracic outlet syndrome: results of a double-blind, controlled study. *Arch Phys Med Rehabil*, 88:844, 2007.
72. Ferrante, MAL: The thoracic outlet syndrome. *Muscle Nerve*, 45:780, 2012.
73. Walden, MJ, et al: Cervical ribs: identification on MRI and clinical relevance. *Clin Imaging*, 37:938, 2013.
74. Gillard, J, et al: Diagnosing thoracic outlet syndrome: contribution of provocative tests, ultrasonography, electrophysiology, and helical computer tomography in 48 patients. *Joint Bone Spine*, 68:416, 2001.
75. Hooper, TL, et al: Thoracic outlet syndrome: a controversial clinical condition, part 2: non-surgical and surgical management. *J Man Manip Ther*, 18:132, 2010.
76. Fruth, SJ: Differential diagnosis and treatment in a patient with posterior upper thoracic pain. *Phys Ther*, 86:254, 2006.
77. Tsirikos, AI, and Jain, AK: Scheuermann's kyphosis; current controversies. *J Bone Joint Surg Br*, 93:857, 2011.
78. Colosimo, AJ, et al: Acute traumatic first-rib fracture in the contact athlete. *Am J Sports Med*, 32:1310, 2004.
79. Miller, TL, Harris, JD, and Kaeding CC: Stress fractures of the ribs and upper extremities: causation, evaluation, and management. *Sports Med*, 43:665, 2013.

80. Feden, JP: Closed lung trauma. *Clin Sports Med*, 32:255, 2013.
81. Delos Reyes, AP, et al: Conservative management of esophageal perforation after a fall. *Int J Surg Case Rep*, 4:550, 2013.
82. Dotson, K, and Johnson, LH: Pediatric spontaneous pneumothorax. *Pediatr Emerg Care*, 28:215, 2012.
83. Partridge, RA, et al: Sports-related pneumothorax. *Ann Emerg Med*, 30:539, 1997.
84. Marnejon, T, Sarac, S, and Cropp, AJ: Spontaneous pneumothorax in weightlifters. *J Sports Med Phys Fitness*, 35:124, 1995.
85. Hosea, TM, and Hannafin, JA: Rowing injuries. *Sports Health*, 4:236, 2012.
86. Noonan, TJ, et al: Posterior rib stress fracture in professional baseball pitchers. *Am J Sports Med*, 35:654, 2007.
87. Rinderknecht, AS, and Pomerantz, WJ: Spontaneous splenic rupture in infectious mononucleosis: case report and review of the literature. *Pediatr Emerg Care*, 28:1377, 2012.
88. Lippstone, MB, et al: Spontaneous splenic rupture and infectious mononucleosis in a forensic setting. *Del Med J*, 70:433, 1998.
89. Fernandes, CM: Splenic rupture manifesting two years after diagnosis of injury. *Acad Emerg Med*, 3:946, 1996.
90. Tonolini, M, and Bianco, R: Nontraumatic splenic emergencies: cross-sectional imaging and triage. *Emerg Radiol*, 20:323, 2013.
91. Waninger, KN, and Harcke, HT: Determination of safe return to play for athletes recovering from infectious mononucleosis. *Clin J Sport Med*, 15:410, 2005.
92. McCroy, P: Commotio cordis: instantaneous cardiac arrest caused by a blow to the chest depends on the timing of the blow relative to the cardiac cycle. *Br J Sports Med*, 36:236, 2002.
93. Madias, C, et al: Commotio cordis—sudden cardiac death with chest wall impact. *J Cardiovasc Electrophysiol*, 18:115, 2007.
94. Bode, F, et al: Ventricular fibrillation induced by stretch pulse: implications for sudden death due to commotio cordis. *J Cardiovasc Electrophysiol*, 17:1011, 2006.
95. Salib, EA, et al: Efficacy of bystander cardiopulmonary resuscitation and out-of-hospital automated external defibrillation as life-saving therapy in commotio cordis. *J Pediatr*, 147:863, 2005.
96. Maron, BJ, Estes, NAM, and Link, MS: Task Force 11: commotio cordis. *JACC*, 45:1371, 2005.
97. Valani, R, Mikrogianakis, A, and Goldman, RD: Cardiac concussion (commotio cordis). *Can J Emerg Med*, 6:428, 2004.
98. Maron, BJ, et al: Death in a young athlete due to commotio cordis despite prompt external defibrillation. *Heart Rhythm*, 2:991, 2005.
99. Gertzbein, SD, et al: Thoracic and lumbar fractures associated with skiing and snowboarding injuries according to the AO comprehensive classification. *Am J Sports Med*, 40:1750, 2012.
100. Brouwers, MA, Veldhuis, EF, and Zimmerman, KW: Fracture of the thoracic spine with paralysis and esophageal perforation. *Eur Spine J*, 6:211, 1997.
101. Bakker, FC, Patka, P, and Haarman, HJ: Combined repair of a traumatic rupture of the aorta and anterior stabilization of a thoracic spine fracture: a case report. *J Trauma*, 40:128, 1996.
102. Leski, M: Sudden cardiac death in athletes. *South Med J*, 97:861, 2004.
103. Lorvidhaya, P, and Huang, SKS: Sudden cardiac death in athletes. *Cardiology*, 100:186, 2003.
104. Giese, EA, et al: The athletic preparticipation evaluation: cardiovascular assessment. *Am Fam Physician*, 75:1008, 2007.

SECTION 4

Upper Extremity Examination

As with the lower extremity, there are multiple patient-rated instruments for the upper extremity. The DASH and *Quick*-DASH are the most commonly used clinically. Functional tasks assessed are unique to the patient's activities. For example, a baseball pitcher may rate pain associated with throwing.

Disabilities of the Arm, Shoulder, and Hand (DASH)

This 30-item questionnaire is completed by the patient and results in a measurement of perceived physical function and symptoms associated with upper extremity pathology. The optional Work (four items) and Sport/Performing Arts (four items) modules have also been validated. Patients are asked to respond regarding their ability to perform certain activities on a 1 (No Difficulty) to 5 (Unable) scale over the previous week. The scoring algorithm is applied [(mean of all responses – 1) × 25] to arrive at a percentage score from 0 to 100. Higher scores represent increased disability. The Work and Sport/Performing Arts modules are scored separately. In the U.S. population, the average score is 10.1 (±14.7).[1]
The *Quick*DASH includes 11 items and can be used when a shorter version is preferred.

Minimum Detectable Change: DASH 8–15; *Quick*DASH – 13 points[2]
Minimal Clinically Important Difference: DASH = 13 (reported range 8–17); *Quick*DASH = 18 (reported range 16–20)[3]

Penn Shoulder Score (PSS)

Specific to the shoulder, the PSS contains three subscales. The Pain subscale requires the patient to report pain on a 0 to 10 scale during various conditions. The Satisfaction subscale uses the same 0 to 10 scale for the patient to describe the level of satisfaction with the current function. The Function subscale asks the patient to rate the extent of difficulty associated with different activities on a 4-point scale. The subscale scores are considered individually and in the aggregate from 0 to 100, with higher scores representing less disability. As with the DASH, the patient may achieve maximum scores on the PSS before achieving full participation status.[4]

Minimum Detectable Change: 12 points (5 for pain section; 2 for satisfaction section; 9 for function section)[5]
Minimal Clinically Important Difference: 11 points

Shoulder Pain and Disability Index (SPADI)

The SPADI can be used for patients with any shoulder pathology. To complete the SPADI, the patient responds to 13 statements on an 11-point numeric rating scale. Pain (five items) and function (eight items) subscores can also be calculated. Higher scores correlate with higher perceived pain and disability.

Minimum Detectable Change: 13 points (reported values range from 13–22)[2]
Minimal Clinically Important Difference: 13–23[2]

American Shoulder and Elbow Surgeons (ASES) Elbow Outcome Score

This region-specific instrument is designed to measure elbow function. The patient self-evaluates on 19 questions relating to pain, function, and satisfaction as well as a clinician-rated assessment of shoulder motion, strength, and stability. Scores are converted to a 0 to 100 range, with 100 representing optimal function.[6]

Minimum Detectable Change: Not reported
Minimal Clinically Important Difference: Not reported

Michigan Hand Outcomes Questionnaire (MHQ)

This region-specific instrument is used by patients with hand pathologies. The 37-item questionnaire includes six subscales: overall hand functioning, physical function with activities of daily living, pain, work performance, aesthetics, and patient satisfaction with function. The patient reports symptoms for the right and left hands, except for the pain and work performance subscales. Each subscale is scored separately, and an overall score from 0 to 100 is calculated by adding the six subscale scores. Higher scores represent less perceived disability.[7]

Minimal Clinically Important Difference: 11–23 (values vary by diagnosis)[8]

REFERENCES

1. Kennedy, CA, et al: *The DASH outcome measure user's manual* (ed 3). Toronto, Canada: Institute for Work & Health, 2011.
2. Angst, F, et al: Measures of adult shoulder function. Disabilities of the Arm, Shoulder, and Hand Questionnaire (DASH) and its short version (QuickDASH), Shoulder Pain and Disability Index (SPADI), American Shoulder and Elbow Surgeons (ASES) Society standardized shoulder assessment form, Constant (Murley) Score (CS), Simple Shoulder Test (SST), Oxford Shoulder Score (OSS), Shoulder Disability Questionnaire (SDQ), and Western Ontario Shoulder Instability Index (WOSI). *Arthritis Care Res*, 63(Suppl 11):S174, 2011.
3. Sorensen, AA, et al: Minimal clinically important differences of three patient-rated outcomes instruments. *J Hand Surg Am*, 38A:641, 2013.
4. Thigpen, C, and Shanley, E: Clinical assessment of upper extremity injury outcomes. *J Sport Rehabil*, 20:61, 2011.
5. Leggin, BG, et al: The Penn Shoulder Score: reliability and validity. *J Orthop Sports Phys Ther*, 36:138, 2006.
6. Smith, MV, et al: Upper extremity-specific measures of disability and outcomes in orthopaedic surgery. *J Bone Joint Surg Am*, 94:277, 2012.
7. Hoang-Kim, A, et al: Measuring wrist and hand function: common scales and checklists. *Injury*, 24:253, 2011.
8. Shauver, MJ, and Chung, KC: The minimal clinically important difference of the Michigan hand outcomes questionnaire. *J Hand Surg Am*, 34:509, 2009.

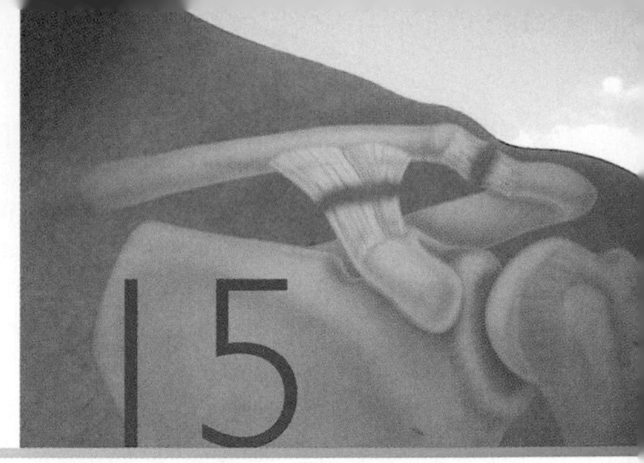

CHAPTER 15

Shoulder and Upper Arm Pathologies

The shoulder complex is perhaps the most complicated of the body's articulations because it must provide extensive yet precise range of motion (ROM) in all anatomical planes. The relationship between the glenohumeral (GH) joint and the scapula allows the humerus to be placed in 16,000 positions that can be differentiated in 1-degree increments.[1]

The shoulder complex lacks the intrinsic bony and ligamentous stabilizers that occur in other joints. Relying on its musculature to provide most of its stability, the shoulder complex in general, and specifically the GH joint, is inherently unstable. The GH joint, because of its poor bony stability and weak capsular structures, depends more on the proprioceptive and stabilizing function of its musculature than any other joint in the body.[2] Injury to the shoulder complex may occur from a direct force or secondary to forces transmitted proximally along the upper extremity. The shoulder complex also is predisposed to overuse conditions, especially in individuals participating in activities that require repeated overhead movements.

Clinical Anatomy

The upper extremity's only attachment to the axial skeleton is at the sternoclavicular (SC) joint. This configuration results in a mechanism whereby the arm is suspended from the torso by muscular attachments. The motions provided by the upper extremity arise from the intricate interactions of the four bones forming the shoulder girdle and the four articulations providing movement. Elevation describes the integrated movement of the glenohumeral, sternoclavicular, acromioclavicular, and scapulothoracic articulations as the arm is raised. Elevation can occur in the sagittal plane (flexion), frontal plane (abduction), and anywhere in between them.[3] The large ROM provided by the shoulder complex, especially the GH joint, is achieved at the expense of joint stability. Unlike the hip joint, which gains its stability through a deep ball-and-socket joint and strong ligamentous support (at the expense of mobility), the GH joint is characterized by shallow articular surfaces, inconsistent ligamentous support, and an increased reliance on dynamic support through muscle activity.

Bony Anatomy

The shoulder complex, formed by the sternum, clavicle, scapula, and humerus, may be likened to a series of hinges, pulleys, and levers working in unison to choreograph intricate motions in many anatomical planes (Fig. 15-1). A precise degree of ROM, strength, and coordination must be maintained to ensure efficient biomechanics.

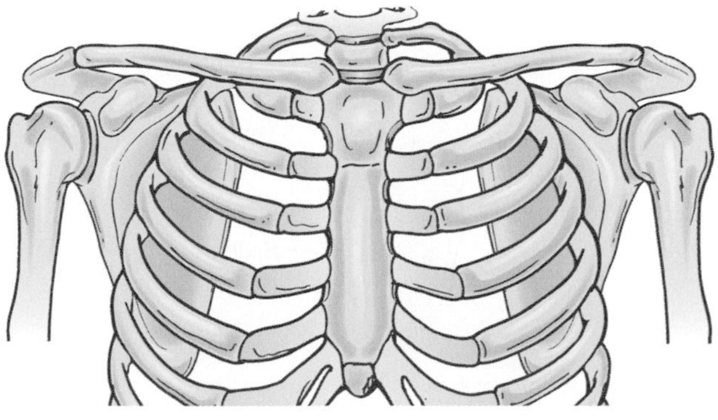

FIGURE 15-1 ■ Bones of the shoulder complex and glenohumeral joint.

The **manubrium** of the sternum serves as the site of attachment for each clavicle. Projecting above the body of the sternum, the superior surface of the manubrium is indented by the **jugular (suprasternal) notch**. Projecting off each side of the jugular notch is the **clavicular notch**, which accepts the medial head of the clavicle (Fig. 15-2).

Serving as a strut between the sternum and scapula, the **clavicle** elevates and rotates to maintain the alignment of the scapula, allowing for additional motion when the arm is raised and preventing excessive anterior displacement of the scapula. The proximal two-thirds of the clavicle is characterized by an anteriorly convex bend. The distal one-third begins to flatten while curving concavely to meet with the scapula (Fig. 15-3). The point at which the clavicle begins to transition from a convex to a concave bend, approximately two-thirds of the way along its shaft, is relatively weak and is a common site for fractures. The superior surface of the clavicle is not protected by muscle mass, making the bone susceptible to injury. The medial clavicular epiphysis is the last growth plate in the body to ossify and does not fully fuse until approximately the age of 18 to 20.[4]

Having no direct bony or ligamentous attachment to the axial skeleton, the **scapula** gains its attachment to the torso by way of the clavicle. Its anterior surface is held against the torso by atmospheric pressure and muscle attachments. The scapula's unique form gives rise to its unique function of serving as both a lever and a pulley.

Thin and triangular, the scapula's anterior costal surface is concave, forming the **subscapular fossa**. The **vertebral (medial) border** is marked by the **inferior** and **superior angles**. The posterior surface is distinguished by the horizontal **scapular spine**, which divides the scapula into the large **infraspinous fossa** below and the smaller **supraspinous fossa** above. On the lateral end of the scapular spine is the anteriorly projecting **acromion process**, which articulates with the clavicle. Projecting inferiorly and anteriorly to the acromion is the beak-shaped **coracoid process**. The infraspinous, supraspinous, and subscapular fossae merge on the axial border to form the glenoid fossa. Located below the acromion, this fossa articulates with the humeral head (Fig. 15-4).

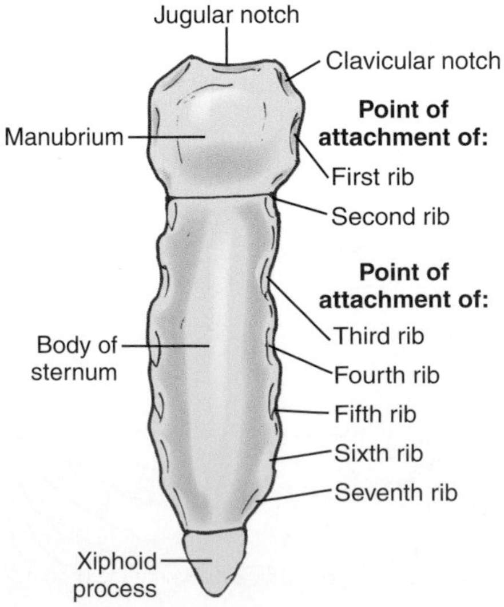

FIGURE 15-2 ■ The sternum, formed by the manubrium, body, and xiphoid process. In preadolescents, the junction between the manubrium and sternal body is pliable, but it fuses with age.

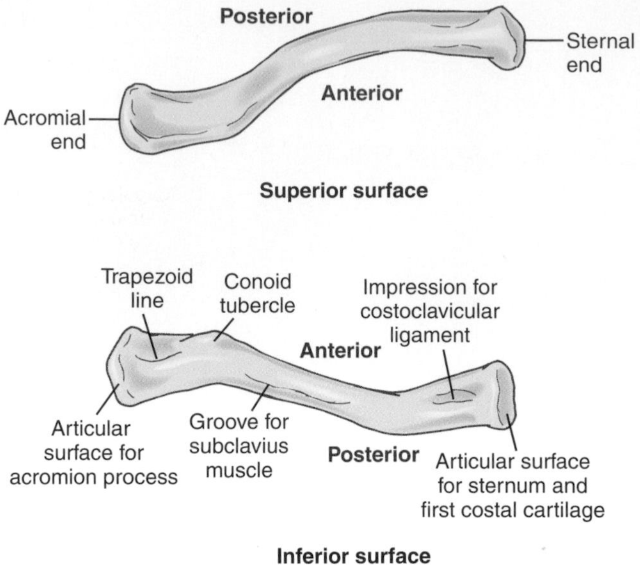

FIGURE 15-3 ■ Clavicle, superior and inferior views.

When the scapula is placed in its anatomical position, the glenoid fossa angles 30 degrees from the frontal plane, and its face assumes a downward direction (Fig. 15-5).[5] The angle assumed by the face of the glenoid fossa, the **plane of the scapula**, provides a more functional plane for motion than the cardinal sagittal or frontal planes. This angle, in conjunction with the position of the scapula, places the rotator cuff muscles in their optimal length–tension relationship. For example, when reaching for an item on an overhead shelf, it is more natural to lift the arm in the plane of the scapula rather than lifting the arm through the sagittal or frontal planes.

The proximal end of the **humerus** is characterized by the medially projecting **humeral head** from the **anatomical neck** (Fig. 15-6). Bisecting the upper quarter of the anterior surface of the humerus, the **bicipital groove** (intertubercular groove) forms a canal through which the long head of the biceps tendon (LHBT) passes. The lateral edge of the groove is formed by the **greater tuberosity**. The medial border is formed by the **lesser tuberosity**. The inferior borders of the greater and lesser tuberosities mark the **surgical neck**, a name derived because fractures at this location generally require surgical intervention. Laterally and slightly above the midshaft is the insertion site for the deltoid muscle group, the **deltoid tuberosity**. The distal structures of the humerus are covered in Chapter 16.

The **angle of inclination** is the relationship between the shaft of the humerus and the humeral head in the frontal plane, normally 130 to 150 degrees. In the transverse plane, the relationship between the shaft of the humerus and the

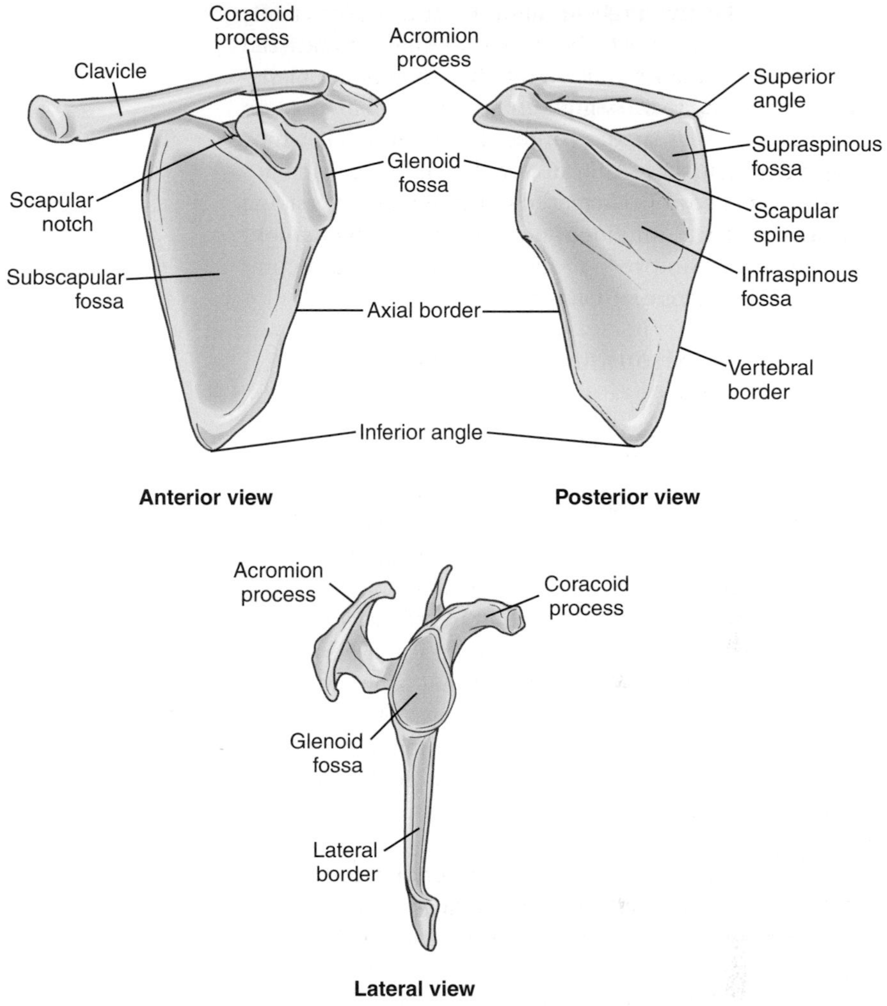

FIGURE 15-4 ■ Bony anatomy of the scapula, anterior (costal), posterior (dorsal), and lateral views, showing the relationship with the clavicle.

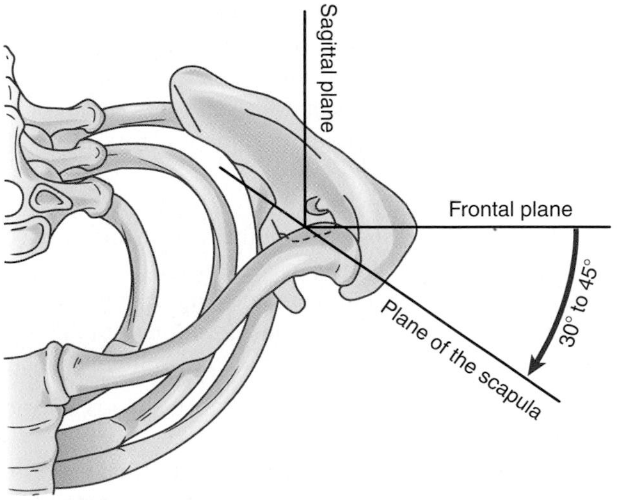

FIGURE 15-5 ■ Plane of the scapula. The face of the glenoid fossa sits at a 30° angle of horizontal adduction in the frontal plane. Movements within the plane of the scapula are more "natural" than movements in the cardinal plane.

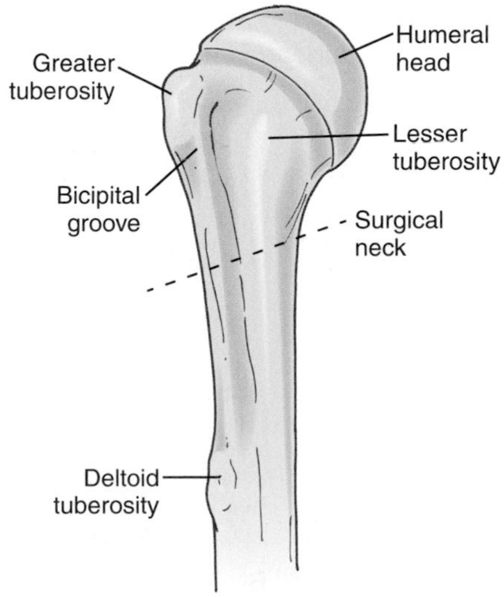

FIGURE 15-6 ■ The proximal humerus, showing the prominent bony landmarks.

humeral head is the **angle of torsion**, which varies greatly from individual to individual (Fig. 15-7).[6] The humeral head is retroverted (twisted posteriorly from the frontal plane) approximately 20 to 30 degrees to permit optimal function in the plane of the scapula.[6,7] Increased retroversion, which is thought to enhance performance and protect against injury, is associated with increased GH external rotation and decreased internal rotation. Throwers commonly demonstrate increased retroversion in their dominant arm compared with their nondominant arm.[6]

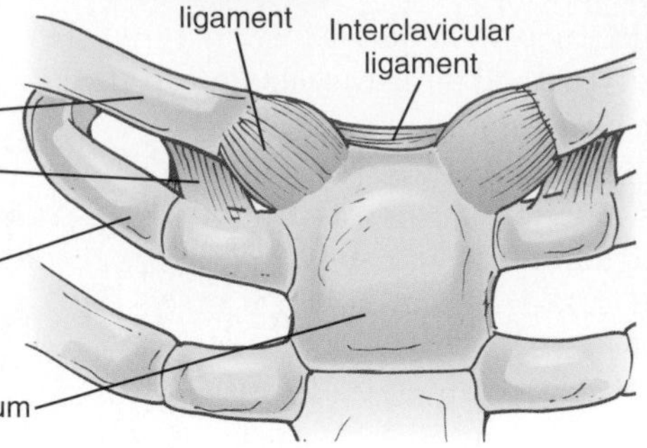

FIGURE 15-8 ■ Ligaments of the SC joint. Although the SC joint does not have inherent bony stability, the ligamentous arrangement provides great strength to the joint.

Joints of the Shoulder Complex

The motion of the GH joint is augmented by the SC and **acromioclavicular (AC)** joints and the movement between the scapula and the thorax. A change in the mobility or function at any of these associated joints decreases the function at the GH joint.

Sternoclavicular Joint

At the SC joint, the proximal portion of the clavicle meets the manubrium of the sternum and a portion of the first costal cartilage to form a gliding joint that allows three degrees of freedom of motion: (1) elevation and depression, (2) protraction and retraction, and (3) anterior and posterior rotation. The SC joint's functional axis lies lateral to the joint itself. Elevation and depression and protraction and retraction describe the movement at the lateral clavicle. Posterior rotation (where the inferior surface of the clavicle moves anteriorly) occurs on the long axis of the clavicle, with anterior rotation used to describe return to neutral from a posteriorly rotated position.[3]

The articulation between the manubrium and clavicle is inherently incongruent because the proximal end of the clavicle extends one-half of its width above the manubrium (Fig. 15-8). Although the overall stability of the joint is enhanced by the presence of a fibrocartilaginous disc, the SC joint has the poorest bony stability of any of the major joints. Its strong ligamentous structure and protected location, however, makes it one of the least frequently dislocated joints.[4] Surrounded by a synovial membrane, the SC joint is supported by the anterior and posterior SC ligaments, the costoclavicular ligament, and the interclavicular ligament.

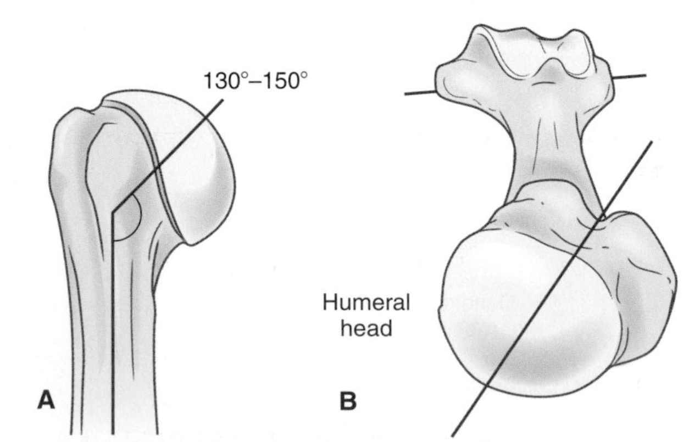

FIGURE 15-7 ■ Angular alignment of the humerus. (A) Angle of inclination representing the angle formed by the long axis of the humeral shaft and the axis of the humeral head. (B) Angle of torsion representing the relationship between the humeral condyles and the humeral head in the transverse plane.

The **sternoclavicular disc**, which has qualities similar to the menisci found in the knee, functions as a shock absorber. The upper portion of the disc is attached to the clavicle, and its lower portion is attached to the manubrium and first costal cartilage. This disc divides the joint into two articular cavities, one between the disc and the clavicle and a second between the disc and the manubrium.

The synovial membrane is reinforced by the **anterior** and **posterior sternoclavicular ligaments**. Whereas the anterior fibers resist posterior displacement of the clavicle on the manubrium, the posterior fibers resist anterior displacement. The costoclavicular ligament serves as an axis of clavicular elevation and depression and protraction and retraction.

The SC joints are joined to each other by the **interclavicular ligament**. Attaching to the superior proximal ends of the left and right clavicles, the ligament has a common connection on the superior border of the sternum. The interclavicular ligament resists downward movement of the clavicle and assists in dissipating force across the entire upper extremity.

The **costoclavicular ligament** (rhomboid ligament) arises from the superior aspect of the first rib and connects to the inferior aspect of the clavicle. Likewise, the posterior fibers limit elevation and medial movement of the clavicle. The anterior fibers resist clavicular elevation from the superior pull of the sternomastoid and sternohyoid muscles and limit medial translation of the clavicle.[3]

The Acromioclavicular Joint

The distal end of the clavicle meets the acromion process of the scapula to form the AC joint. A plane synovial joint, the AC joint allows a gliding articulation between the acromion and the clavicle, capable of 3 degrees of freedom of movement, each around an oblique axis: (1) internal and external rotation around a vertical axis, (2) upward and downward rotation around an axis perpendicular to the plane of th scapula, and (3) anterior and posterior **scapular tilting** around a horizontal axis. This articulation allows for the motion necessary to maintain the relationship between the scapula and the clavicle in the early and late stages of the GH joint's ROM.

Surrounded by a synovial membrane, the AC joint is supported by the AC ligament and the **coracoclavicular ligament**, which suspend the scapula from the clavicle (Fig. 15-9). A synovial disc is present between the clavicle and the acromion that disappears by the fourth decade of life.[8]

Divided into two separate bands, the superior and inferior portions of the AC ligament function to maintain continuity between the articulating surfaces of the acromion and clavicle. With much of its restraint in the horizontal plane, this ligament maintains stability by preventing the clavicle from riding up and over the acromion process.

Most of the AC joint's intrinsic stability arises from the coracoclavicular ligament, a structure extrinsic to the joint. Because of its direct connection to the scapula, the coracoclavicular ligament influences scapulohumeral motion.[8] This ligament is divided into two distinct portions: the lateral quadrilateral-shaped trapezoid ligament and the medial triangular-shaped conoid ligament. Separated by a bursa, the **trapezoid ligament** limits lateral movement of the clavicle over the acromion. The **conoid ligament** restricts superior movement of the clavicle. Acting jointly, these ligaments limit rotation of the scapula and provide some degree of horizontal stability. The conoid portion of the ligament is critical for the passive posterior rotation of the clavicle that occurs during shoulder elevation. A horizontal dislocation of the AC joint can occur with the coracoclavicular ligament remaining intact.

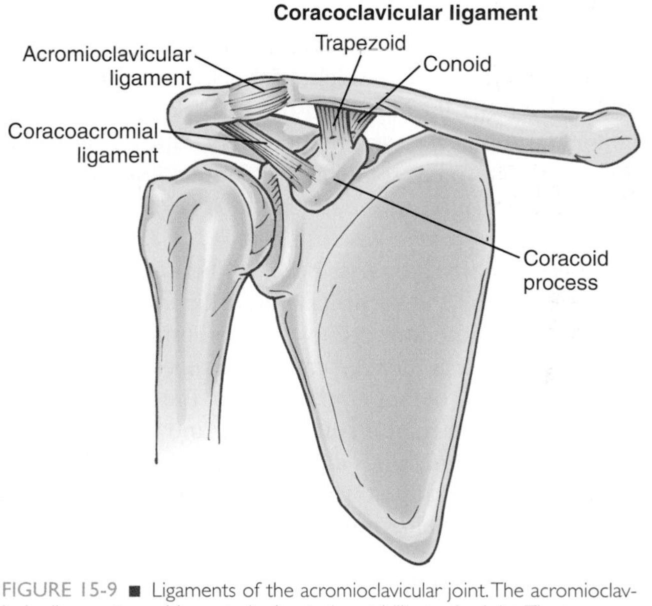

FIGURE 15-9 ■ Ligaments of the acromioclavicular joint. The acromioclavicular ligament provides anterior/posterior stability to the joint. The two portions of the coracoclavicular ligament prevent superior/inferior displacement of the clavicle on the scapula.

Scapular tilting Anterior tilting is marked by the inferior angle of the scapula moving away from the thorax while its superior border moves toward the thorax. The opposite occurs during posterior tilt.

The Scapulothoracic Articulation

The articulation between the scapula and the posterior rib cage is not a true anatomical joint because it lacks the typical synovial joint characteristics of connection by fibrous, cartilaginous, or synovial tissues. Fundamentally a soft tissue interface,[9] the scapulothoracic articulation moves only in response to AC and SC joint movement. For example, when the arm is abducted, the scapulothoracic articulation must upwardly rotate, externally rotate, and posteriorly tilt (Fig. 15-10).[3] Changes in mobility or stability at either the AC or SC joints influence the movement of the scapulothoracic articulation.

The Glenohumeral Joint

Formed by the head of the humerus and the scapula's glenoid fossa, the GH articulation is a ball-and-socket joint capable of three degrees of freedom of motion: flexion and extension, abduction and adduction, and internal and external rotation. Although not true anatomical motions,

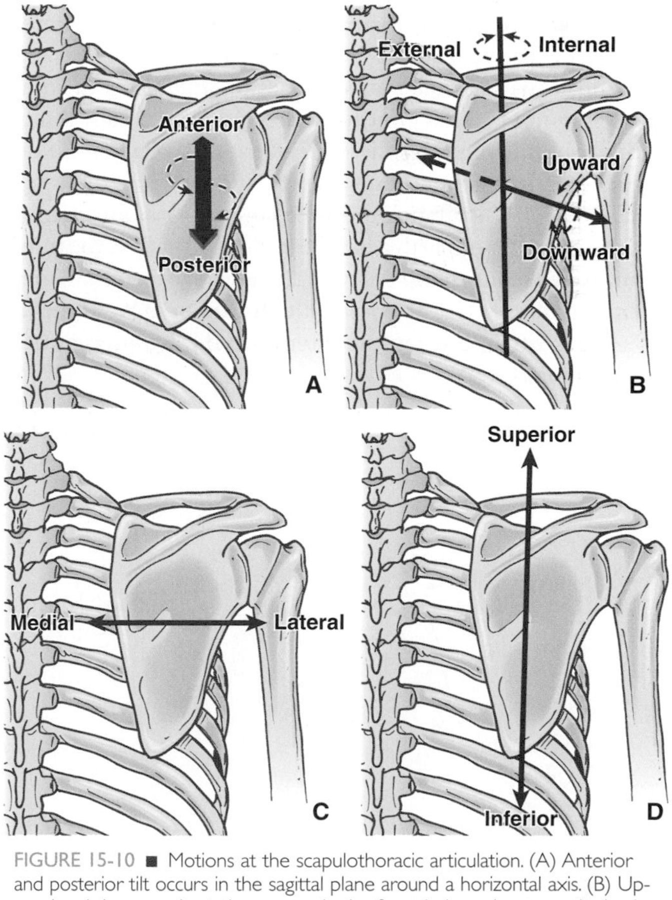

FIGURE 15-10 ■ Motions at the scapulothoracic articulation. (A) Anterior and posterior tilt occurs in the sagittal plane around a horizontal axis. (B) Upward and downward rotation occurs in the frontal plane about a sagittal axis. Internal and external rotation occurs in the transverse plane about a vertical axis. The scapula also translates (C) medially and laterally and (D) superiorly and inferiorly (elevation or "shrug"/depression). Scapular protraction describes the coupled motions of lateral translation and internal rotation. Scapular retraction is coupled medial translation and external rotation.

horizontal adduction and abduction (or horizontal flexion and extension) and circumduction also occur at the GH joint. Most upper extremity motions do not occur in a single isolated plane but, rather, are a combination of movements in two or more planes.

The GH joint is inherently unstable because of the relationship in the sizes of the articular surfaces of the glenoid fossa and the humeral head, a loose joint capsule, and relatively weak ligamentous support. The pear-shaped articulating surface of the glenoid fossa is significantly smaller than that of the humeral head and only vaguely resembles the ball-and-socket joint of the hip. The socket is somewhat deepened by the **glenoid labrum**, which also slightly increases the articular surface. Inserting on the scapula via a transitional fibrous cartilage, the remaining labrum is made up of collagen fibers with both a radial and circular orientation.[9,10] Disruption of the glenoid labrum is often associated with recurrent shoulder instability.

Possessing a volume twice the size of the humeral head, the joint capsule arises from the glenoid fossa and glenoid labrum to blend with the muscles of the rotator cuff. Studies on cadavers indicate that the laxity of the capsular arrangement allows the humeral head to be distracted 2 cm or more from the glenoid fossa.[11] The capsule is reinforced by the **glenohumeral ligaments** and the **coracohumeral ligament** (Fig. 15-11).

The three GH ligaments—superior, middle, and inferior—are not distinct joint structures but are actually thickenings in the joint capsule. The specific GH ligament that limits motion depends on the position of the humerus (Table 15-1). The inferior GH ligament possesses an anterior and posterior band with a hammock-like structure, the **inferior pouch**, connecting the two. The area between the superior and middle GH ligaments, the **foramen of Weitbrecht**, is a weak site in the capsule often torn during anterior GH dislocations.

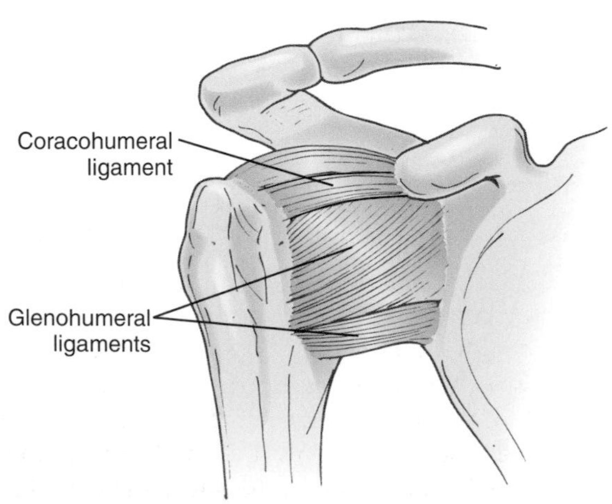

FIGURE 15-11 ■ Ligaments of the GH joint: the coracohumeral and GH ligaments. The GH ligament is divided into superior, middle, and inferior portions. To provide the necessary range of motion to the GH joint, these ligaments must be relatively lax. Much of the stability of this articulation is gained from its muscular arrangement.

Table 15-1 Ligaments Limiting Humeral Motion

Position of the Humerus	Ligamentous Structures Limiting Movement
External rotation in 0° abduction	Superior GH ligament Coracohumeral ligament
External rotation in 45° abduction	Middle GH ligament Anterior band of the inferior GH ligament
External rotation in 90° abduction	Inferior GH ligament
Internal rotation in 90° abduction	Posterior band of the inferior GH ligament
Inferior displacement in 0° abduction	Superior GH ligament Coracohumeral ligament
Inferior displacement in 90° abduction	Inferior GH ligament

GH = glenohumeral

Emanating from the coracoid process, the **coracohumeral ligament** merges with the superior capsule and the supraspinatus tendon on the greater tuberosity, limiting inferior translation of the humeral head when the arm is hanging at the side of the body.[3] The anterior fibers of this ligament limit extension, while the posterior fibers limit the amount of GH flexion. The coracohumeral ligament and the superior GH ligament limit external rotation of the humerus when the arm is at the side of the body.

When the humerus is hanging at rest in the anatomical position, the articular surfaces of the GH joint have very little contact. Much of the weight of the arm is supported by the superior GH ligament and the inferior portion of the glenoid labrum. When the humerus is abducted to 90 degrees and externally rotated, the entire joint capsule is wound tightly, placing the GH joint in its closed-packed position.

Superior to the humeral head is the **coracoacromial arch**, formed by the **coracoacromial ligament** that traverses from the inferior portion of the acromion process to the posterior portion of the coracoid process (Fig. 15-12). The arch protects the superior portion of the humeral head, the tendons of the rotator cuff muscles, and various bursae from trauma and provides a restraint against superior and anterior GH dislocations. The coracoacromial arch is also involved with shoulder impingement syndrome.

Muscles of the Shoulder Complex

The function of the shoulder complex and arm is controlled by two groups of muscles: those that act primarily on the scapula and those that function primarily on the humerus. Movements of the shoulder complex involve an intricate series of static and dynamic interactions between these two groups of muscles.

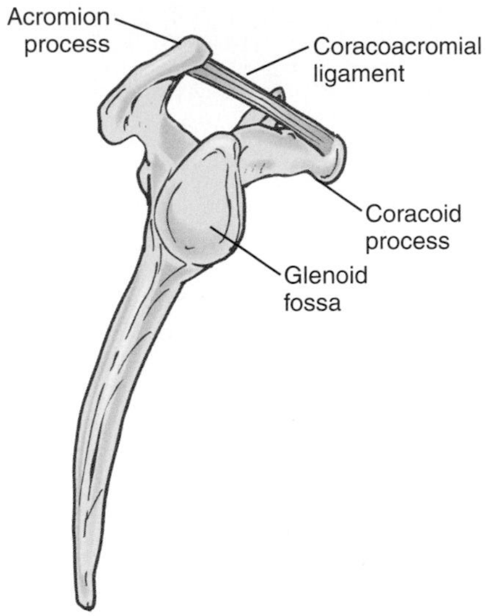

FIGURE 15-12 ■ Coracoacromial arch. The tendons of the rotator cuff, the long head of the biceps brachii tendon, and the subacromial bursa must fit between the space created between the coracoacromial ligament and the humeral head.

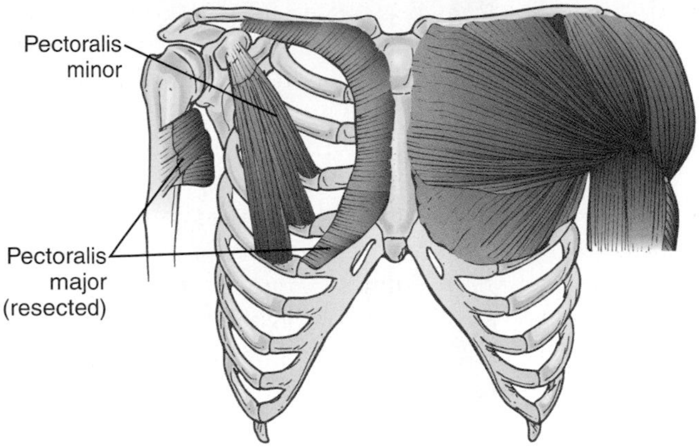

FIGURE 15-13 ■ Muscles of the chest

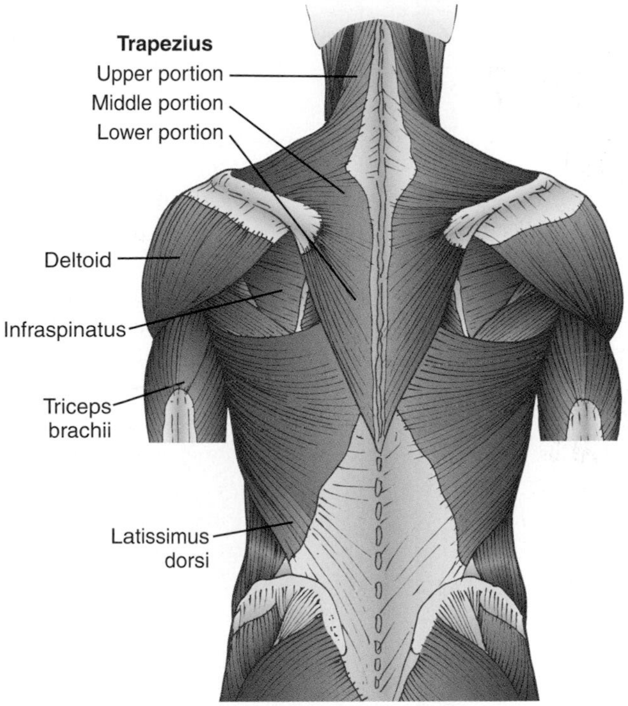

FIGURE 15-14 ■ Superficial posterior muscles acting on the scapula and GH joint.

Muscles Acting on the Scapula

The muscles acting on the scapula have two purposes: (1) to control positioning of the scapula's glenoid fossa to allow the shoulder complex increased ROM and (2) to stabilize the scapula on the thorax to provide the rotator cuff muscles with a stable base of support during contractions. The action, origin, insertion, and nerve supply for the muscles acting on the scapula are presented in Table 15-2.

Inserting on the scapula's vertebral border are the **rhomboid minor** and **rhomboid major**. These muscles retract the scapula toward the spine and elevate and downwardly rotate the scapula. The **levator scapulae** muscle acts to elevate and downwardly rotate the scapula. The **serratus anterior**, inserting on the costal surface of the vertebral border, upwardly rotates and protracts the scapula. Working segmentally, the serratus anterior's lower fibers depress the scapula, and the upper fibers elevate it. In addition, this muscle plays a primary function in stabilizing the scapula's vertebral border to the thorax. A weakness of the serratus anterior or injury to the long thoracic nerve innervating it can result in **scapular winging** where the vertebral border lifts away from the thorax. The pectoralis minor tilts the scapula anteriorly so that the inferior angle lifts away from the thorax (Fig. 15-13).

The **trapezius** muscle is divided into upper, middle, and lower segments (Fig. 15-14). Each of these three segments of the trapezius has a unique action on the scapula. The upper fibers elevate and upwardly rotate, the middle fibers retract, and the lower fibers depress and upwardly rotate the scapula. The lower trapezius may also assist to posteriorly tilt and externally rotate the scapula, both movements that open up the subacromial space.[12]

Two additional muscles have an indirect force on the scapula. The upper fibers from the **latissimus dorsi** depress the shoulder complex. The clavicular portion of the **pectoralis major** depresses the scapula by its attachment to the clavicle at the AC joint.

Muscles Acting on the Humerus

Motion at the shoulder complex can occur as GH motion. Generally, however, apparent motion at the shoulder joint is the result of the motion provided by the entire shoulder complex. The action, origin, insertion, and nerve supply for the muscles acting primarily on the humerus are presented in Table 15-3.

Four muscles arising off the scapula form the **rotator cuff** muscle group (Fig. 15-15). As a group, the rotator cuff internally and externally rotates the humerus and compresses and

Table 15-2 Muscles Acting Primarily on the Scapula

Muscle	Action	Origin	Insertion	Innervation	Root
Levator Scapulae	Scapular elevation and downward rotation. Extension of cervical spine Rotation of the c-spine	Transverse processes of cervical vertebrae C1–C4	Superior medial angle of the scapula	Dorsal scapular	C3, C4, C5
Rhomboid Major	Scapular retraction, elevation, and downward rotation	Spinous processes of T2, T3, T4, and T5	Vertebral border of scapula (lower two-thirds)	Dorsal scapular	C4, C5
Rhomboid Minor	Scapular retraction and elevation	Inferior portion of the ligamentum nuchae Spinous processes C7 and T1	Vertebral border of scapula (near the medial border of the scapular spine)	Dorsal scapular	C4, C5
Serratus Anterior	Scapular upward rotation and protraction Scapular depression (lower fibers) Scapular elevation (upper fibers) Fixation of the scapula to the thorax	Anterior portion of 1st–8th or 9th ribs Aponeuroses of the intercostal muscles	Costal surfaces of the: • Superior angle of scapula • Vertebral border of scapula Inferior angle of scapula	Long thoracic	C5, C6, C7
Trapezius (upper one-third)	Scapular elevation and upward rotation Rotation of c-spine to the opposite side Extension of c-spine	Occipital protuberance Superior nuchal line of the occipital bone Upper portion of the ligamentum nuchae Spinous process of C7	Distal/lateral one-third of clavicle Acromion process Scapular spine	Accessory	CN XI
Trapezius (middle one-third)	Scapular retraction Fixation of thoracic spine	Lower portion of the ligamentum nuchae Spinous processes of the 7th cervical vertebra and T1–T5	Acromion process Spine of the scapula (superior, lateral border)	Accessory	CN XI
Trapezius (lower one-third)	Scapular depression, upward rotation and retraction; external rotation and posterior tipping of the scapula	Spinous processes and supraspinal ligaments of T8–T12	Spine of the scapula (medial portion)	Accessory	CN XI
Pectoralis Minor	Scapular anterior tilt	Costal cartilages of ribs 6–7 Anterior portion of 3rd–5th ribs	Coracoid process of scapula	Lateral pectoral	C7, C8, T1

Table 15-3 Muscles Acting Primarily on the Humerus

Muscle	Action	Origin	Insertion	Innervation	Root
Biceps Brachii	Flexion Abduction	Long head: Supraglenoid tuberosity of scapula Short head: Coracoid process of scapula	Radial tuberosity and aponeurosis	Musculocutaneous	C5, C6
Coracobrachialis	Flexion Adduction	Coracoid process	Medial shaft of the humerus, adjacent to the deltoid tuberosity	Musculocutaneous	C6, C7
Deltoid (anterior one-third)	Flexion Abduction Horizontal adduction Internal rotation	Lateral one-third of the clavicle	Deltoid tuberosity	Axillary	C5, C6
Deltoid (middle one-third)	Abduction Flexion	Acromion process	Deltoid tuberosity	Axillary	C5, C6
Deltoid (posterior one-third)	Extension Horizontal abduction Abduction External rotation	Spine of the scapula	Deltoid tuberosity	Axillary	C5, C6
Infraspinatus	External rotation Horizontal abduction Humeral head stabilization	Infraspinous fossa of the scapula	Lateral portion of the greater tuberosity of the humerus GH joint capsule	Suprascapular	C5, C6
Latissimus Dorsi	Extension Internal rotation Adduction Depression of shoulder girdle	Spinous processes of T6–T12 and the lumbar vertebrae via the lumbodorsal fascia Posterior iliac crest	Floor of the bicipital groove of the humerus	Thoracodorsal	C6, C7, C8
Pectoralis Major	Adduction Horizontal adduction Humeral flexion (clavicular segment) Internal rotation Depression of the shoulder girdle (clavicular fibers)	Medial one-half of the clavicle Anterolateral portion of the sternum Costal cartilages of ribs 6–7	Greater tuberosity of the humerus	Lateral and medial pectoral	C6, C7, C8

Continued

Table 15-3 Muscles Acting Primarily on the Humerus—cont'd

Muscle	Action	Origin	Insertion	Innervation	Root
Subscapularis	Internal rotation Humeral head stabilization	Anterior surface (subscapular fossa) and axillary border of the scapula	Lesser tuberosity of the humerus Ventral portion of the GH capsule	Upper and lower subscapular	C5, C6, C7
Supraspinatus	Abduction External rotation Humeral head stabilization	Supraspinous fossa (medial two-thirds) of the scapula	Medial aspect of the greater tuberosity GH joint capsule	Suprascapular	C4, C5, C6
Teres Major	Extension Internal rotation Adduction	Inferior angle of scapula Lower one-third of the axillary border of the scapula	Medial lip of the bicipital groove	Lower subscapular	C5, C6, C7
Teres Minor	External rotation Horizontal abduction	Lateral upper two-thirds of axillary border of the scapula	Lateral aspect of the greater tuberosity	Axillary	C5, C6
Triceps Brachii	Extension (long head) Adduction	Long head: Infraglenoid tuberosity of scapula Lateral head: Lateral and posterior surface of the proximal one-half of the humerus Medial head: Distal two-thirds of medial and posterior humerus	Olecranon process of ulna	Radial	C6, C7, C8

GH = glenohumeral

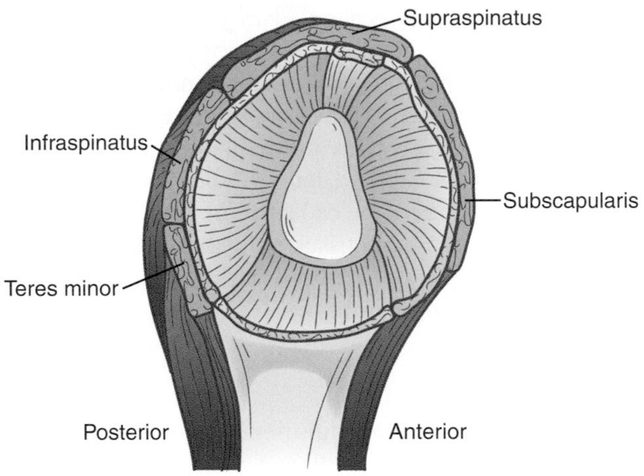

FIGURE 15-15 ■ Muscles of the rotator cuff relative to the glenoid fossa.

centralizes the humeral head in the glenoid fossa, limiting extraneous movement and maintaining optimal efficiency. During the later stages of abduction, the rotator cuff muscle group also provides a downward pull on the humeral head, allowing for its unimpeded passage under the acromion. The **subscapularis muscle** is the only member of the rotator cuff group that internally rotates the humerus. The **supraspinatus** assists in abducting and externally rotating the humerus in addition to compressing the humeral head in the fossa. The remaining two members of the rotator cuff, the **infraspinatus** and **teres minor**, externally rotate the humerus and provide some assistance during horizontal abduction. In addition, the teres minor assists during extension of the GH joint. The eccentric contractions of the infraspinatus and teres minor muscles decelerate the humerus at the end of overhead throwing motions. Closely associated with the muscles of the rotator cuff is the teres major, which assists with internal rotation, adduction, and extension of the humerus.

Although having a common insertion on the deltoid tuberosity of the humerus, each section of the **deltoid muscle group** should be considered independently. As a whole, the deltoid muscle group is the prime mover during abduction. Considered as individual units, the **anterior fibers** flex the GH joint and horizontally adduct and internally rotate the humerus. The **middle fibers** serve to abduct the humerus. The **posterior fibers** act to extend, horizontally abduct, and externally rotate the humerus. The deltoid group and the upper fibers of the trapezius merge at the AC joint and assume the role of secondary stabilizers of this articulation.

During abduction, a **force couple** is formed between the line of pull between the rotator cuff (specifically the supraspinatus) and the deltoid muscle group. The line of force created by the deltoid's contraction tends to pull the head of the humerus upward against the inferior portion of the acromion process and the coracoacromial ligament. In the early stages of abduction, the rotator cuff's angle of pull must be sufficient to hold the head of the humerus against the glenoid fossa. After the humerus moves past 90 degrees, the rotator cuff's angle of pull changes so that its force slides the humeral head inferiorly on the glenoid fossa, creating clearance to pass under the acromion process and the coracoacromial ligament (Fig. 15-16). A damaged or weak rotator cuff group or dysfunction of the scapulothoracic muscles changes the dynamics of the force couple, resulting in the impingement of the rotator cuff and long head of the biceps brachii tendon between the humeral head, subacromial bursa, and acromion process.

The **pectoralis major** is divided into two portions, the clavicular portion and the sternal portion, each having a common insertion on the greater tuberosity (see Fig. 15-13). As a whole, the pectoralis major adducts, horizontally adducts, and internally rotates the humerus. The clavicular portion flexes, internally rotates, and horizontally adducts the humerus. The sternal portion depresses the shoulder girdle and assists in horizontal adduction.

The **latissimus dorsi** has a broad origin on the lumbar spine, thoracodorsal fascia, and iliac crest. Inserting on the intertubercular groove of the humerus, the latissimus dorsi adducts, internally rotates, and extends the humerus. Attaching to the infraglenoid tuberosity of the scapula, the **long head of the triceps brachii** is an adductor and extensor of the humerus, especially when the elbow is flexed.

The **coracobrachialis** acts on the humerus as a flexor and adductor. Both heads of the **biceps brachii** have an attachment on the scapula (Fig. 15-17). Both heads assist in

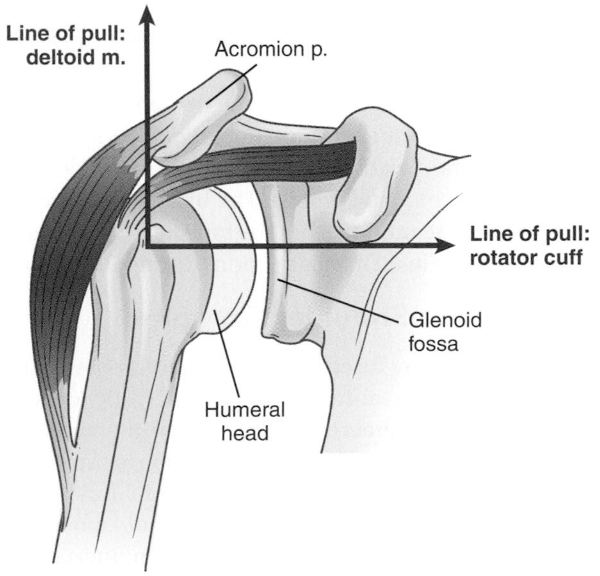

FIGURE 15-16 ■ Scapulohumeral force couple. Contraction of the deltoid muscle pulls the humeral head upward. To prevent contact between the humeral head and the acromion process during abduction, the supraspinatus, assisted by the remaining rotator cuff muscles, must hold the humeral head close to the glenoid fossa and, when the humerus approaches 90° of abduction, provides leverage to glide the humerus inferiorly.

Force couple Coordination between dynamic and isometric contractions of opposing muscle groups to perform a movement of a joint

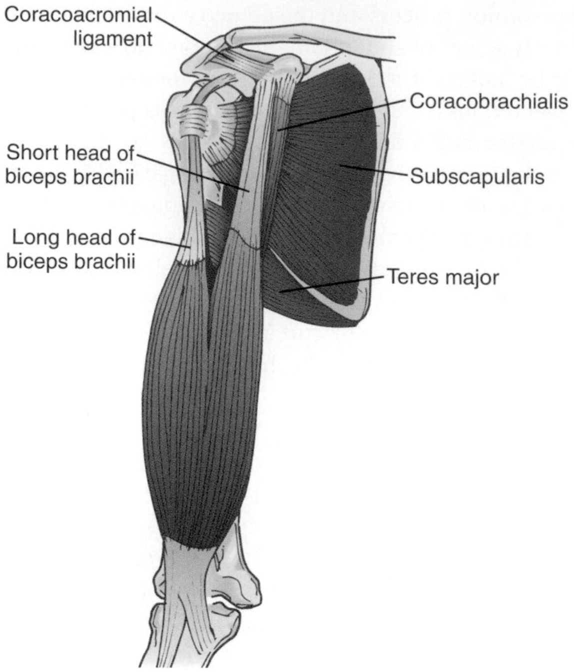

FIGURE 15-17 ■ Coracobrachialis and attachment of the long and short heads of the biceps brachii muscle.

GH flexion and, when the humerus is externally rotated, the long head assists in GH abduction. The short head attaches to the coracoid process, and the long head passes through the bicipital groove to attach on the supraglenoid tuberosity, its attachment blending in with the superior labrum. Stability within the bicipital groove is maintained by the **transverse humeral ligament**, lined by a capsular sheath emanating from the GH capsule. An inflammatory response or damage to the transverse humeral ligament results in pain and disrupts the normal mechanics of the GH joint.

The long head of the biceps enters the joint capsule between the supraspinatus and subscapularis muscles. Although the capsule is penetrated, the tendon does not enter the synovial membrane of the articulation. During the motions of humeral flexion and abduction, the tendon must slide within the bicipital groove. The biceps produces little force during these motions, but the long head tendon stabilizes the humeral head in all directions during GH motion.[13]

Bursae of the Shoulder Complex

Although commonly fused into a single unit referred to as the subacromial bursa, two bursae are actually located at the GH joint: the **subacromial bursa** and the **subdeltoid bursa**. The subacromial bursa is located above the superior surface of the supraspinatus tendon and lubricates the movement of the overlying fibers of the deltoid muscle, acting as a secondary joint cavity.[14] When the humerus is elevated, the bursa buffers the supraspinatus tendon against its contact with the acromion process and the coracoacromial ligament. When the bursa becomes inflamed, the structures within the subacromial space become compressed, potentially leading to rotator cuff impingement.

Clinical Examination of Shoulder Injuries

Because of the interrelationship of the shoulder complex to the cervical and thoracic spine, torso, abdomen, and elbow, clinicians must consider this interdependence in the examination process. Likewise, distal pathology, such as elbow pain, may arise from or be causative of dysfunction at the shoulder. Chapter 14 discusses pain that originates from the cervical spine and describes visceral pain referred into the shoulder and upper arm.

History

Determine the onset and duration of the condition and identify the location of pain. Because the shoulder and upper arm are common sites for referred or radiating pain from orthopedic or visceral origins, a complete examination of the cervical spine, thorax, and abdomen may be indicated, particularly when a patient presents with a vague history of injury to the shoulder complex (see Fig. 15-14). The arm of the dominant hand is subject to more repetitive forces throughout the day and is therefore more susceptible to injury.

The use of standardized outcome measures, described in the introductory section, helps establish a baseline from which to measure progress during rehabilitation and identifies the impact of the condition on the patient's life.

The following information should be obtained during the history-taking process so that the mechanism of injury, influence of prior or current other injuries, structures involved in the injury, and nature of the pain can be determined.

Past Medical History

A history of previous injury to the SC, AC, or GH joints can alter the biomechanics of the shoulder complex. Injury to related body parts such as the cervical and thoracic spine, ribs, and thorax can also influence mechanics and should be investigated. Because cervical spine pathology can result in referred or radiating pain to the shoulder, the previous injury history of the cervical spine must be ascertained, especially if the patient describes an uncertain cause of shoulder pain.

History of the Present Condition

- **Location of the pain:** The examination begins by localizing the area and type of pain. Shoulder pathology typically produces pain within the GH joint that may project laterally into the upper arm or medially into the trapezius. Pain that begins in the neck and radiates into the upper arm, forearm, or hand implicates cervical nerve root involvement.

✻ Practical Evidence

Patients with rotator cuff pathology or subacromial bursitis typically describe pain in the anterior and lateral shoulder whereas chronic acromioclavicular pathology is commonly associated with pain into the upper trapezius region, especially at night.[15-17]

Examination Map

HISTORY

Past Medical History

History of Present Condition

Mechanism of injury

Onset of symptoms

Location of pain

FUNCTIONAL ASSESSMENT

Athletic or other daily tasks that provoke symptoms

Throwing (as indicated)

INSPECTION

Inspection of the Anterior Structures

Level of the shoulders

Position of the head

Position of the arm

Contour of the clavicles

Acromion process

Deltoid muscle groups

Humerus

Inspection of the Posterior Structures

Vertebral column

Position of the scapula

Muscle development

Position of the humerus

PALPATION

Palpation of the Anterior Structures

Jugular notch

Sternoclavicular joint

Clavicular shaft

Acromion process

Acromioclavicular joint

Coracoid process

Humeral head

Greater tuberosity

Lesser tuberosity

Bicipital groove

Humeral shaft

Pectoralis major

Pectoralis minor

Coracobrachialis

Deltoid muscle group

Biceps brachii

- Long head
- Short head

Palpation of the Posterior Structures

Spine of the scapula

Superior angle

Inferior angle

Rotator cuff

- Infraspinatus
- Teres minor
- Supraspinatus

Teres major

Rhomboids

Levator scapulae

Trapezius

Latissimus dorsi

Posterior deltoid

Triceps brachii

JOINT AND MUSCLE FUNCTION ASSESSMENT

Goniometry

- Flexion
- Extension
- Abduction
- Internal rotation
- External rotation
- Horizontal abduction
- Horizontal adduction

Active Range of Motion

Apley scratch test

Flexion/extension

Abduction/adduction

- Drop arm test

Internal and external rotation

Horizontal adduction/abduction

Manual Muscle Tests

Gerber lift-off test

Flexion/extension

Abduction/adduction

Internal/external rotation

Horizontal abduction/adduction

Scapular muscles

- Retraction and downward rotation
- Retraction
- Protraction and upward rotation
- Depression and retraction
- Elevation

Passive Range of Motion

Flexion

Extension

Abduction

Adduction

Internal rotation

External rotation

Horizontal abduction

Horizontal adduction

JOINT STABILITY TESTS

Joint Play Assessment

Sternoclavicular joint

Acromioclavicular joint

Glenohumeral joint

NEUROLOGICAL EXAMINATION

Upper Quarter Screen

VASCULAR EXAMINATION

Distal Pulses

Capillary Refill

REGION-SPECIFIC PATHOLOGIES AND SELECTIVE TISSUE TESTS

Sternoclavicular Joint

Acromioclavicular Joint

Acromioclavicular traction test

Acromioclavicular compression test

Glenohumeral Joint

Anterior instability

- Apprehension test
- Relocation test
- Anterior release test

Posterior instability

- Posterior apprehension test
- Jerk test

Inferior instability

- Sulcus sign

Multidirectional instability

Rotator Cuff Pathology

Impingement syndrome

- Neer impingement test
- Hawkins impingement test
- Drop arm test

Rotator cuff tendinopathy

- Empty can test

Subacromial Bursitis

Biceps Tendon Pathology

Bicipital tendinopathy

- Yergason's test
- Speed's test

SLAP lesions

- Active compression test
- Anterior slide test
- Compression–rotation test

SLAP = superior labrum anterior to posterior

- **Onset:** The onset of pain often indicates the underlying pathology. Pain with an acute onset may indicate a fracture, GH joint dislocation or subluxation, tendon rupture, or an AC sprain. Inflammatory conditions of the shoulder complex, such as tendinopathies, bursitis, or osteoarthritis, usually have an insidious onset. In these cases, pain may first be noticed after activity and then progresses to pain during activity and, eventually, constant pain.
- **Activity and injury mechanism:** An external force applied to the shoulder complex, such as a direct blow or joint force beyond normal limits, results in acute soft tissue or bony injury. A history of repetitive overhead motion activities such as throwing, swimming, or hitting a tennis ball may indicate an overuse condition such as rotator cuff tendon degeneration.
- **Symptoms:** The symptoms to be noted include resting pain, pain with movement, and dysfunction of the shoulder complex. The patient may describe the shoulder as "going out of place," indicating GH instability; decreased velocity or poor accuracy when throwing; or discomfort when performing overhand motions, indicating inflammatory conditions. Question the patient about pain or muscle spasm in the cervical region or radiating pain and altered sensation or numbness possibly indicating nerve pathology. Pain when sleeping on the involved side is often associated with rotator cuff injury.

The preceding list is not all inclusive for the questions to be asked during the history-taking process. The scope of the questions expands for cases involving an insidious onset. When an acute traumatic injury is being assessed, the history-taking process should become more focused based on the mechanism of injury.

Functional Assessment

Observe the patient's willingness to move the involved limb throughout the examination. Does the patient raise the involved arm when removing the shirt or jacket or does the arm remain at the side with the clothing dropped down over it? Unwillingness to move the arm may indicate apprehension or a more severe condition.

Observe the patient performing relevant functional activities, such as reaching for an object or throwing, and note any pain-provoking motions or adaptations to reduce symptoms. For example, during abduction patients suffering from supraspinatus tendinopathy may laterally flex the trunk to the same side to limit activity of the supraspinatus. Examine the scapular position and motion during elevation (see Assessment of Dynamic Scapular Function).

Box 15-1 presents the phases of the pitching motion and relates the structures involved with each. About half the energy for throwing is generated from arm and shoulder action; the remaining energy comes from lower extremity and trunk rotation, further illustrating how weakness in one region can impact another. With overhead-throwing athletes, the arm position that produces pain and throwing deficits yields information regarding the possible underlying pathology[17,18]:

- **Pain on follow-through:** Possible rotator cuff pathology
- **Pain in cocked position:** Instability or impingement
- **Pain in deceleration:** SLAP (superior labrum anterior to posterior) lesion, biceps tendon pathology
- **Loss of control and/or velocity:** Often proportional to the severity of the condition. Loss of control associated with early ball release is suggestive of internal impingement. Complaints of loss of velocity are associated with a limitation in internal rotation.

Inspection

The patient should wear clothing that allows full inspection of both shoulders and the cervical, thoracic, and lumbar spine.

Inspection of the Anterior Structures

- **Level of the shoulders:** Observe the height of the AC joints, the clavicle, and the SC joints. These should align bilaterally, but the dominant shoulder may appear slightly lower than the nondominant one (Fig. 15-18).

  A painful shoulder [hcb1]is often held in its resting position of slight abduction in the plane of the scapula. Asymmetry may occur secondary to unilateral hypertrophy or atrophy of the larger muscles or in the presence of scoliosis (see the "Inspection of the Posterior Structures" section). Bilaterally raised shoulders may result from well-developed upper trapezius muscles or unwanted spasm in these muscle groups. Shoulders that are abnormally depressed bilaterally may occur as a result of decreased upper trapezius muscle tone. Bilaterally or unilaterally depressed shoulder complexes can place pressure on the arterial, venous, and nervous supply of the arm, predisposing the patient to **thoracic outlet syndrome** (see Chapter 14). Rounded shoulders can indicate tightness of the pectoralis major and minor muscles and result in changes in scapular position.
- **Position of the head:** Observe the position of the head, which is normally upright. A head that is side bent or rotated may indicate muscle spasm, pressure on a cervical nerve root, or stretching of the cervical nerves. Conditions relating to the cervical spine and its nerve network are discussed in Chapter 14.
- **Position of the arm:** Note whether the arm is splinted alongside the body or if it simply hangs limp at the side. Traumatic shoulder injuries are often voluntarily splinted with the humerus along the lateral portion of the rib cage and the forearm supported across the chest. Brachial plexus injuries are characterized by the arm's hanging limply at the side (see Chapter 14). With GH dislocations, the humerus is locked into a fixed position.

Box 15-1
Phases of Pitching

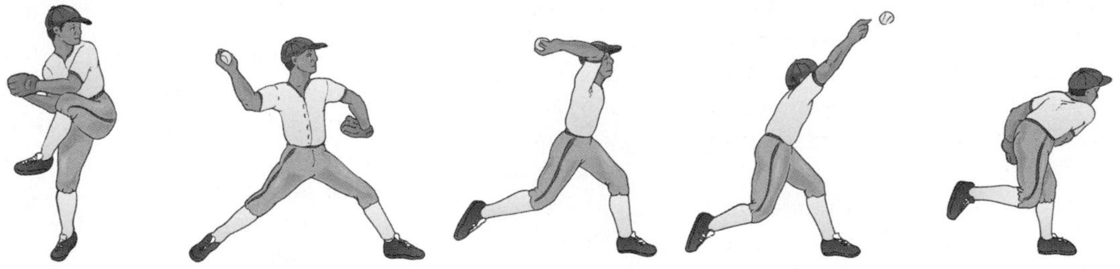

	Wind-up	Cocking	Acceleration	Deceleration	Follow through
Glenohumeral Joint Position	Neutral	90° abduction Maximum external rotation	90° abduction Internally rotating	90° abduction Internally rotating	Horizontal adduction Internally rotating
Glenohumeral Joint Stresses	Low joint stresses	Anterior joint capsule Inferior joint capsule	Anterior joint capsule	Posterior joint capsule Distraction of GH joint	Posterior joint capsule Distraction of GH joint
Elbow Position	Some degrees of flexion	Approximately 90° flexion Increased valgus forces on the elbow	90° flexion moving into extension	20°–30° flexion moving into extension	Extension
Center of Gravity	Over pivot foot	Over pivot foot	Between pivot foot and plant foot	Over plant foot	Forward of plant foot
Accelerating Muscle Activity	Deltoid Supraspinatus Infraspinatus/Teres minor Serratus anterior (rotates scapula) Trapezius (rotates scapula)		Anterior deltoid Subscapularis Pectoralis major Latissimus dorsi Triceps brachii Serratus anterior (stabilizes scapula) Trapezius (stabilizes scapula)		
Decelerating Muscle Activity	Anterior deltoid Subscapularis Pectoralis major Latissimus dorsi			Posterior deltoid Supraspinatus Biceps Brachialis Serratus anterior (scapula) Trapezius (scapula) Rhomboids	

GH = glenohumeral

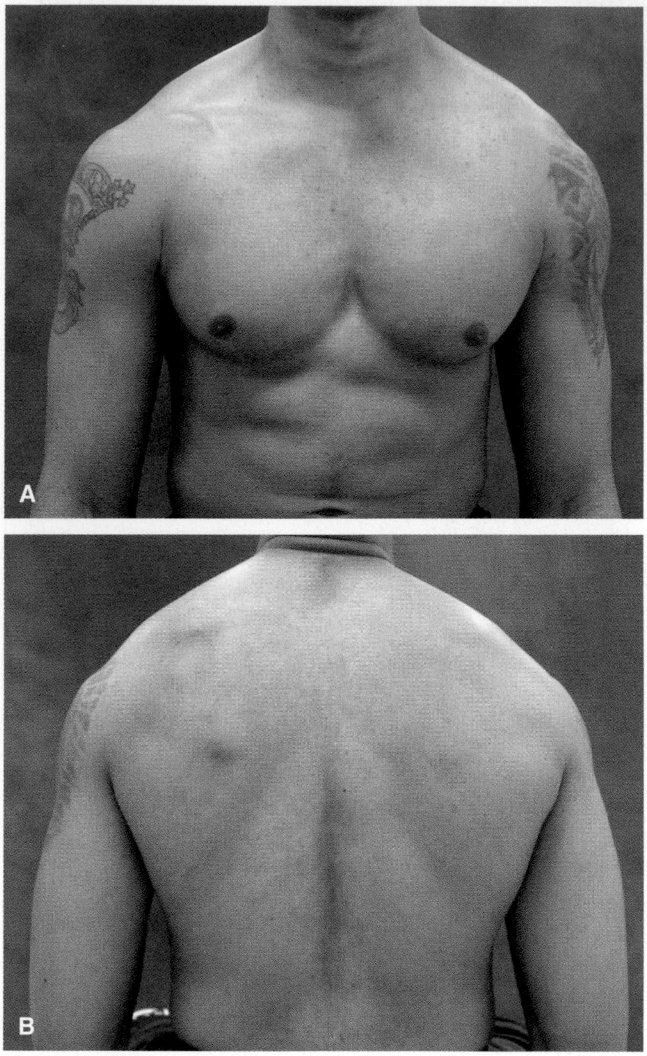

FIGURE 15-18 ■ (A) Anterior and (B) posterior view of the shoulders. Note that the shoulder of the dominant right arm hangs lower than the shoulder of the nondominant arm.

- **Contour of the clavicle:** Inspect the clavicle, easily visible in thin patients or those with well-defined upper body musculature. Observe the SC joint, the shaft of the clavicle, and the clavicle's termination at the AC joint for symmetry and compare them bilaterally.

  In adults, acute traumatic conditions involving the clavicle are typically identifiable during the inspection process. SC or AC joint sprains may be marked by a gross deformity at the articulation, with one side having a more predominant protrusion than the other side. Any previous history involving these joints must be established because deformity may be residual from past trauma.

  Complete clavicular fractures are indicated by a clear deformity of the shaft (Fig. 15-19). Although these fractures usually occur at the juncture between the concave and convex bends (the distal third of the shaft), they can occur anywhere along the clavicle. Patients suffering from a fractured clavicle tend to support the involved arm next to the body and rotate the head to the opposite side.

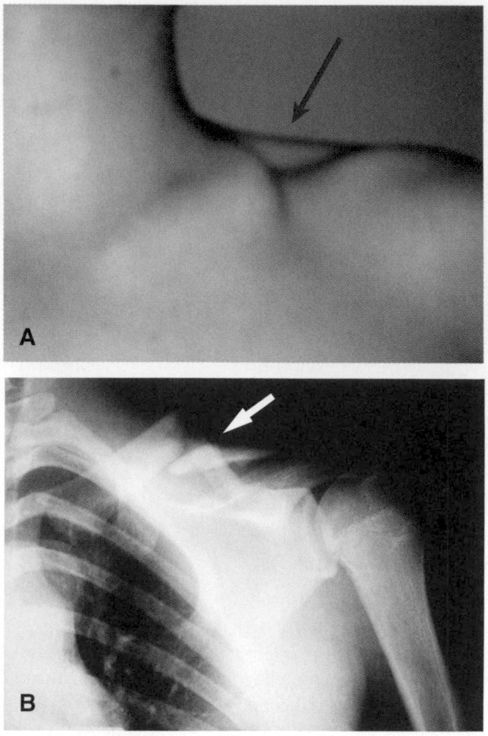

FIGURE 15-19 ■ Fracture of the left clavicle. (A) Inspection showing gross deformity. (B) Anterior–posterior.

- **Acromion process:** The junction between the clavicle and the acromion process usually appears smooth and even. Look for the presence of a **step deformity,** the clavicle riding above the acromion process indicating an AC sprain (**see Acromioclavicular Joint Sprains**). This finding is confirmed via palpation (**piano key sign**) and during stress testing (**AC traction test**).
- **Symmetry of the deltoid muscle groups:** Note the bilateral symmetry of the deltoid muscle group. Normally, this muscle group has a rounded contour. The deltoid of the dominant arm may be hypertrophied compared with the deltoid of the nondominant side. Atrophy of this muscle group may indicate a lack of use of the involved arm or may reflect pathology to the C5 and C6 nerve roots (axillary nerve involvement).

  A dislocated GH joint disrupts the contour of the deltoid group by flattening the area passing over the head of the humerus (Fig. 15-20). With anterior dislocations, the humeral head rests just below the coracoid process. Distal pulses should always be checked when a GH dislocation is suspected. The absence of a distal pulse indicates potentially catastrophic impingement of the vascular bundle supplying the arm, wrist, and hand and requires immediate referral for further medical attention.
- **Anterior humerus and biceps brachii muscle group:** Note the shape and contour of the biceps brachii and any unilateral bulges within the muscle. A **long head**

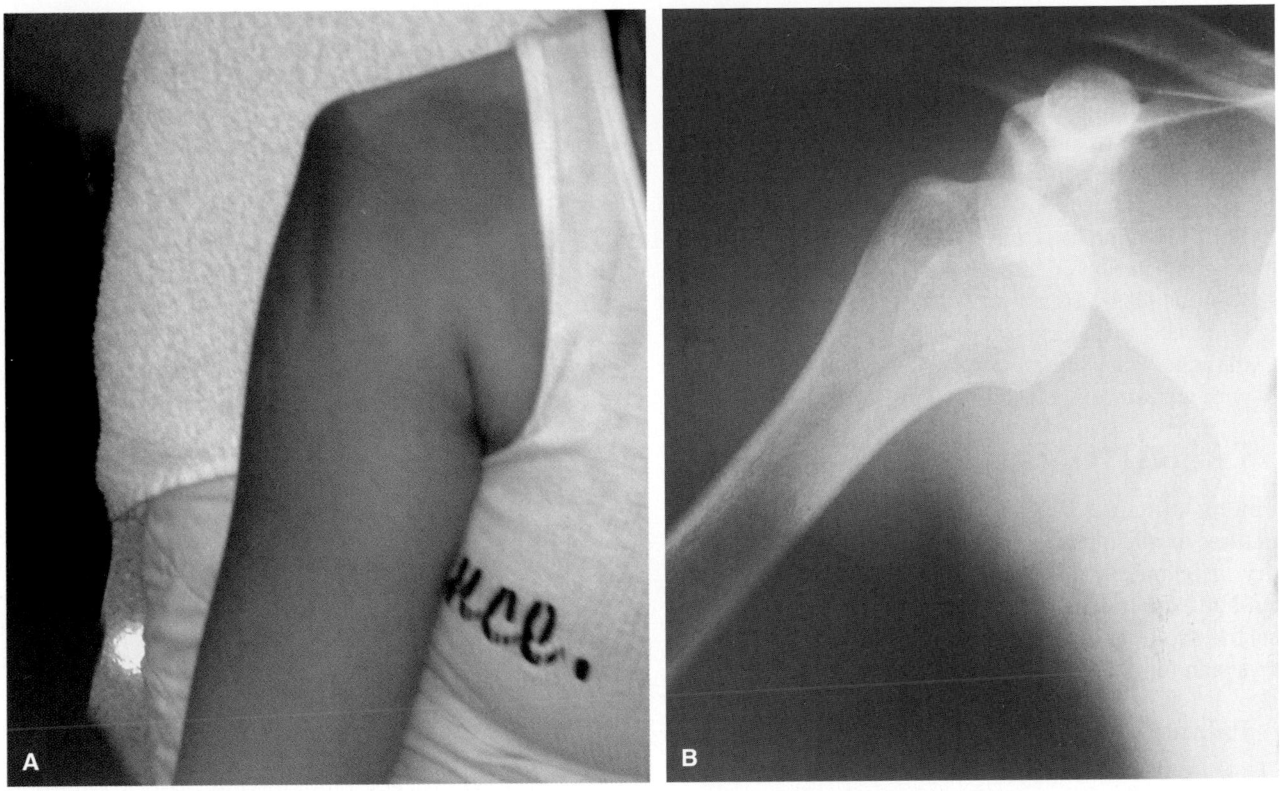

FIGURE 15-20 ■ (A) Photograph of an anterior GH dislocation. (B) Radiograph of an anterior GH dislocation (right shoulder, anterior oblique view).

of the biceps tendon rupture is characterized by the muscle's shortening away from the involved structure (Fig. 15-21). A careful inspection of the entire muscle is necessary because the distal tendon can rupture from its insertion at the elbow, causing deformity.

Inspection of the Posterior Structures

- **Alignment of the vertebral column:** Inspect the alignment of the cervical, thoracic, and lumbar spine to evaluate for scoliosis. This malady can cause altered biomechanics of the shoulder complex.
- **Position of the scapulae:** Observe the vertebral borders of both scapulae, which usually rest an equal distance from the spinous processes of the thoracic vertebrae. The superior angle normally sits at the level of the T3 or T4 spinous process and the inferior angle at the T7 or T8 spinous process. The most medial aspect of the scapular spine is located at the level of the third thoracic vertebra. In the anatomical position, the scapula is in full contact with the thorax. The dominant-side scapula often rests lower and further laterally away from the spine compared with the nondominant side.

  Sprengel's deformity, a congenitally undescended scapula, may occur on one scapula or both. A high-riding scapula may indicate poorly developed or malformed scapular elevators. The clinical ramifications of this condition vary from little or no dysfunction to extreme disability.

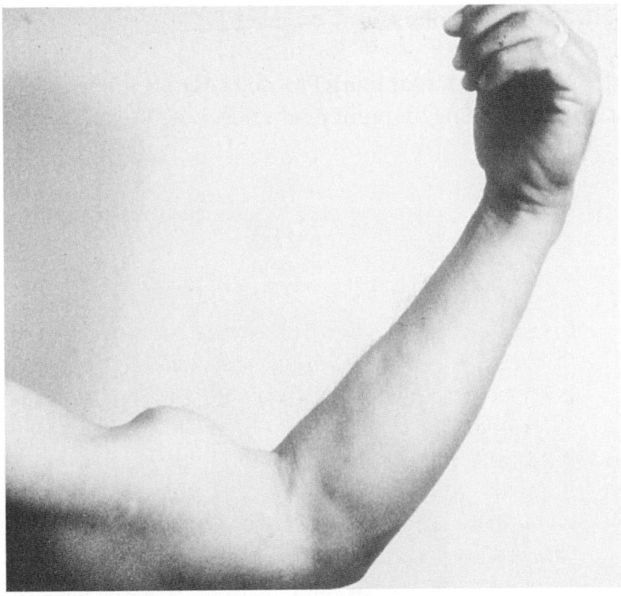

FIGURE 15-21 ■ Rupture of the long head of the biceps brachii tendon.

- **Muscle development:** Inspect the posterior musculature for symmetry on each side. The superficial muscles of well-developed individuals are usually easily identifiable, as are the prominent bony landmarks. Any spasm, deformity, or discoloration of the musculature or skin should be noted as well.

  Observe the prominence of the scapular spine. Atrophy of the supraspinatus or infraspinatus muscles makes the spine of the scapula more visible and palpable. Chronic rotator cuff tears are classically marked by the wasting of the infraspinatus muscle.[19] The scapular stabilizers should also be observed for symmetry (refer to Fig. 15-33).

- **Position of the humerus:** Check patients with acute shoulder injuries for possible posterior GH dislocation, although it is rare. The head of the humerus, when posteriorly dislocated, usually rests on the infraspinous fossa. This injury is associated with possible bony and articular surface injury and neurovascular damage. This condition may be masked by in patients with well-developed shoulder muscles.

PALPATION

The bony structures are palpated prior to the soft tissue structures to rule out fractures, dislocations, and gross joint injury. If palpation reveals any gross deformity, the limb should be examined for neurological and vascular compromise, the shoulder immobilized, and the patient referred to a physician for a definitive diagnosis.

Palpation of Anterior Shoulder

1 **Jugular notch:** Begin the palpation process by locating the **jugular notch** on the manubrium. Palpate the common junction provided by the interclavicular ligament between the SC joints.

2 **Sternoclavicular joint:** Proceed laterally to identify the **SC joint**, checking for point tenderness over the articulation or a prominence or depression of the clavicle, indicating an anteriorly or posteriorly dislocated joint. A **posterior SC dislocations is a medical emergency** because posterior displacement of the clavicle may jeopardize the integrity of the neurovascular structures directly posterior to the joint or may place pressure on the trachea, lung, or both.

3 **Clavicular shaft:** From the SC joint, continue to palpate laterally along the **clavicular shaft**, noting any deformity, crepitus, or pain. The superior surface is easily palpable because of the absence of muscle attachments. Healed clavicular fractures may be marked by palpable bony callus formation over the healed fracture site.

4 **Acromion process and AC joint:** As the clavicle extends laterally, expect that it may become less palpable in patients who have well-developed deltoid muscles. The **acromion process** may be more easily located by palpating to the lateral end of the scapular spine.

If a step deformity is observed during the observation phase of the examination, note for bobbing of the clavicle when downward pressure is applied, the **piano key sign**, to determine the integrity of the coracoclavicular ligaments.

5 **Coracoid process:** From the most concave portion of the clavicle, move approximately 1 inch (2.54 cm) inferior to it to locate the **coracoid process**. Feel for the coracoid process just above and behind the tendon of the pectoralis major. To confirm that the coracoid process has been located, passively move the GH joint through 15 to 30 degrees of flexion and extension and abduction and adduction. No movement of the coracoid process should be felt within this

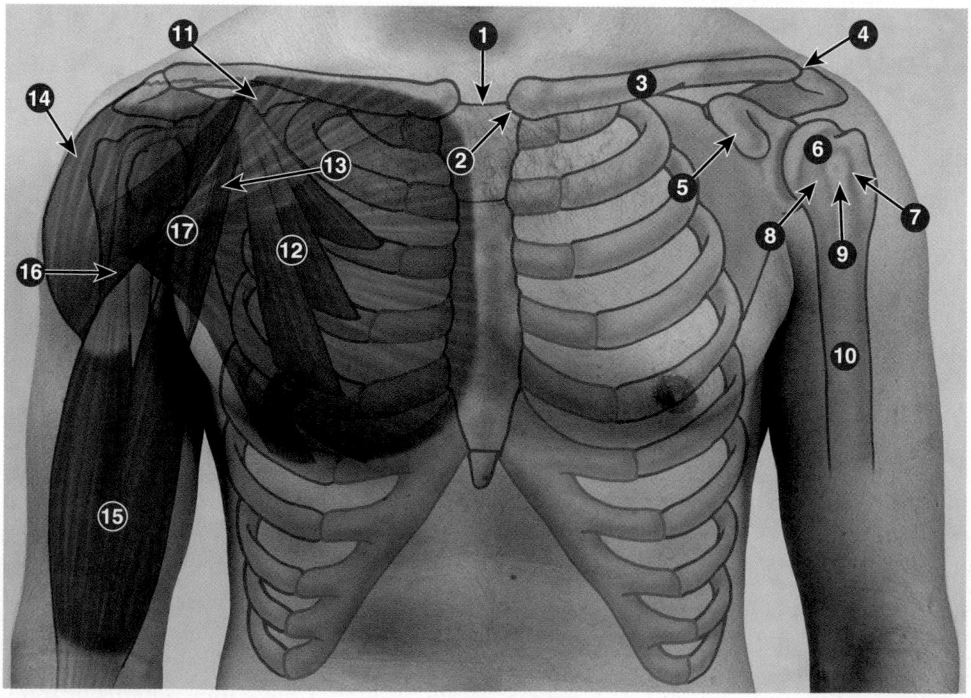

ROM. If movement is felt beneath the fingers, the humeral head is most probably being palpated. In this case, move the fingers medially and attempt this procedure again.

The coracoid process serves as the point of insertion for the pectoralis minor and is the origin of the short head of the biceps brachii tendon and the coracobrachialis muscle. In addition, it provides a source of attachment for several ligaments. Apply pressure carefully when palpating this area because it is easily irritated.

6 **Humeral head:** Moving laterally from the acromion process, palpate the anteromedial portion of the **humeral head** in the axilla posterior to the tendon of pectoralis major. The relationship of the humeral head to the glenoid fossa must be determined. Direct palpation of the humeral head may not be possible in patients with well-developed shoulder musculature. However, an anteriorly or inferiorly displaced humeral head is easily palpable.

7 **Greater tuberosity:** Locate the **greater tuberosity** in the anatomical position approximately one finger breadth inferior to the lateral edge of the anterior portion of the acromion process. This structure is more easily palpated by passively extending the humerus, causing the greater tuberosity to move from beneath the acromion process.

8 **Lesser tuberosity:** With the humerus externally rotated to ease palpation, locate the medial border of the bicipital groove formed by the **lesser tuberosity**.

9 **Bicipital groove:** Externally rotate the humerus to make the **bicipital groove** more palpable. The groove is felt as an indentation in the bone just medial to the greater tuberosity. Gently palpate this area along its length to elicit any tenderness caused by pathology of the LHBT or damage to the transverse humeral ligament. Note that this area is typically tender and should be compared with the opposite side to determine a relative difference in pain.

10 **Humeral shaft:** The **humeral shaft** is more easily palpated along its medial and lateral borders under the belly of the biceps brachii and brachioradialis muscles.

11 **Pectoralis major:** Locate the **pectoralis major** on the anterior thoracic cavity. Palpate this muscle as it flares into its tendon, noting the integrity and any point tenderness as it crosses the GH capsule and attaches on the greater tuberosity of the humerus.

12 **Pectoralis minor:** Attempt to palpate the tendon insertion on the coracoid process of the **pectoralis minor**. Located beneath the pectoralis major, the bulk of the pectoralis minor is not palpable.

13 **Coracobrachialis:** Locate the **coracobrachialis** muscle as it originates off the coracoid process. It may be palpable at this point. Its body and insertion lie deep to the superficial musculature of the humerus and are therefore difficult to palpate. Gentle resistance to forward flexion with the elbow flexed makes this structure more prominent.

14 **Deltoid group:** Palpate each of the three portions of the **deltoid** from its unique origin to the common insertion on the humerus.

15–17 **Biceps brachii:** From the belly of the **(15) biceps brachii**, palpate each of the two heads. Feel for the long head of the biceps **(16)** as it travels through its passage in the bicipital groove under the transverse humeral ligament until it passes beneath the anterior deltoid. Palpate the biceps' short head **(17)** along its length as it passes beneath the pectoralis major tendon and attaches on the coracoid process.

Palpation of Posterior Shoulder

1 **Spine of the scapula:** Locate the **spine of the scapula** by finding the acromion process. Palpate posteriorly along the bony surface of the acromion to meet with the scapular spine. This most posterior aspect of the acromion as it meets the scapular spine comprises the posterior scapular angle. Continue palpation medially along the length of the spine to its termination along the scapula's vertebral border.

2 **Superior angle:** From the vertebral border, palpate upward to find the **superior angle** of the scapula. This landmark may be obstructed by muscle mass of the upper portion of the trapezius and levator scapulae.

3 **Inferior angle:** Moving inferiorly along the vertebral border, feel for the apex of the **inferior angle** of the scapula. Ask the patient to touch the inferior angle of the opposite scapula from below, causing the scapula undergoing examination to wing and making the inferior angle and the lower portions of the vertebral and axial borders more easily palpable.

4–6 **Rotator cuff:** Palpate the mass of three of the four **rotator cuff** muscles on the scapula. Palpate the **(4)** infraspinatus, **(5)** teres minor, and **(6)** supraspinatus (partially covered by the trapezius) along their lengths until they disappear beneath the mass of the deltoid. By passively extending the GH joint from the anatomical position, the greater tuberosity becomes prominent, allowing for the palpation of supraspinatus and subscapularis insertions on the humerus. Although the individual tendons are not distinguishable from each other, any pain or tenderness elicited during palpation should be noted because it may indicate rotator cuff pathology. Only the tendinous insertion of the subscapularis muscle is directly palpable.

7 **Teres major:** Locate the origin and body of the **teres major** muscle immediately inferior to the teres minor. The

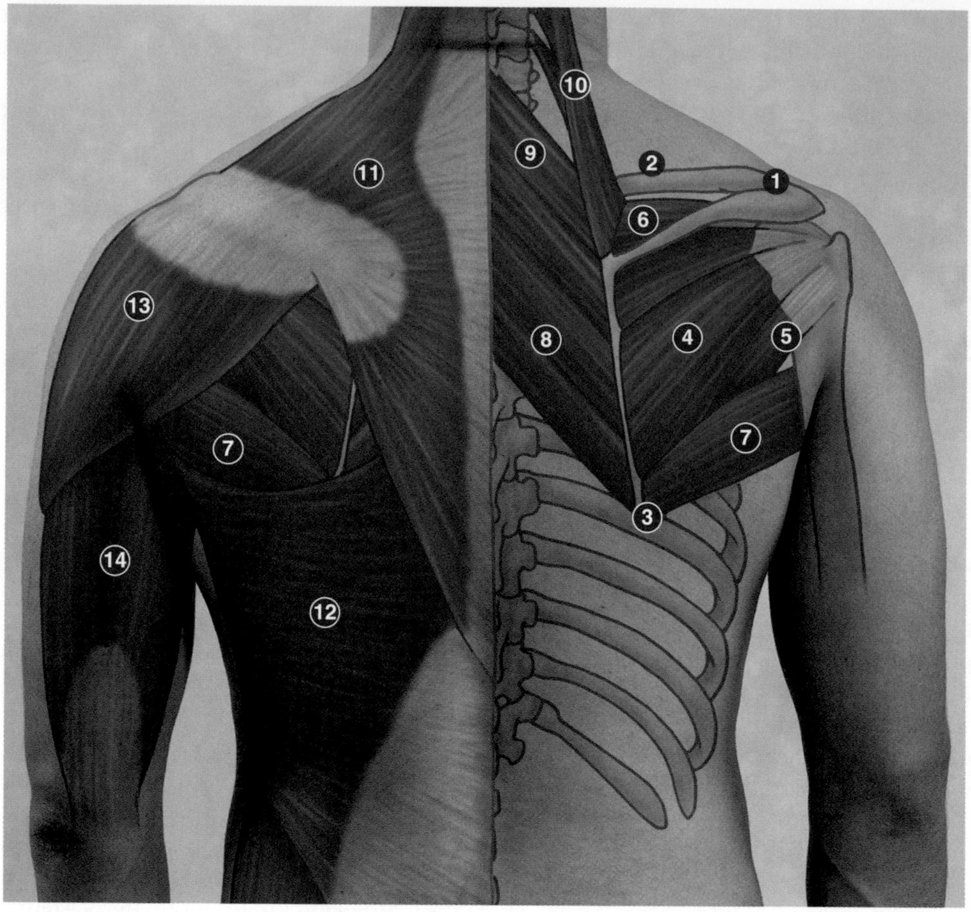

insertion of this muscle cannot be directly palpated. This muscle is a common site for trigger points in swimmers and in athletes who participate in sports with overhead movements. Note any hypersensitive areas.

8–9 Rhomboid: The (8) **rhomboid major** and (9) **rhomboid minor** cannot be directly palpated and are indistinguishable from each other except for their relative locations.

10 Levator scapulae: Although it is largely covered by the upper portion of the trapezius muscle, palpate the origin of the **levator scapulae** on the transverse processes of the first through the fourth cervical vertebrae to its insertion on the medial border of the scapula, just inferior to the superior angle.

11 Trapezius: Palpate the **trapezius** muscle relative to its upper, middle, and lower portions. This muscle is the most superficial of the muscles acting on the scapula and therefore overlies the levator scapulae and the rhomboid muscle group.

12 Latissimus dorsi: Locate the **latissimus dorsi** tendon inferior to the teres major. Follow this tendon through the axilla to its attachment on the floor of the bicipital groove.

13 Posterior deltoid: Palpate the **posterior** portion of the **deltoid** muscle group, noting for atrophy, spasm, or localized areas of pain.

14 Triceps brachii: Palpate the long head of the **triceps brachii** tendon superiorly until the insertion disappears under the posterior deltoid.

Joint and Muscle Function Assessment

The motion occurring at the GH, AC, and SC joints, as well as the motion of the scapula, is evaluated during functional assessment, keeping in mind the interrelationship among these articulations. A deficit at one joint affects the motion of the others. These functional tests must not be performed when severe traumatic injuries such as fractures, joint dislocation, or complete muscle tears are suspected.

The amount of motion that the GH joint is capable of producing depends on the position of the greater and the lesser tuberosities relative to the scapula's bony structures. To achieve complete abduction, the humerus must externally rotate to allow the greater tuberosity to clear under the acromion process. The motion of flexion does not depend on relative internal or external rotation of the humerus because the greater tuberosity depresses inferiorly and passes beneath the acromion process.[20]

Goniometric evaluation of shoulder ROM is presented in Goniometry 15-1 through 15-3. Although horizontal abduction and adduction can be measured goniometrically,

Goniometry 15-1
Shoulder Goniometry: Flexion and Extension

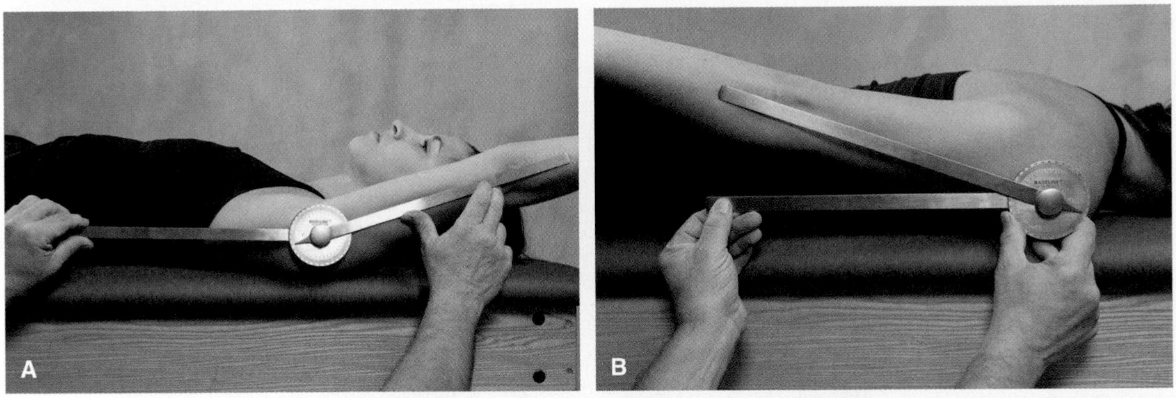

GH Flexion (0–120°)
Elevation Through Flexion (0–180°)

GH Extension (0 to 60°)

Total Excursion (GH extension-flexion): 60°–0°–120°

Patient Position	**Supine** The head is rotated to the opposite side.	**Prone** The head is rotated to the opposite side. Place the elbow in slight flexion.

Goniometer Alignment

Fulcrum	Aligned lateral to the acromion process	Aligned lateral to the acromion process
Proximal Arm	The stationary arm is aligned parallel to the thorax.	The stationary arm is aligned parallel to the thorax.
Distal Arm	The movement arm is centered over the midline of the lateral humerus.	The movement arm is centered over the midline of the lateral humerus.
Comments	To isolate GH flexion, stabilize the scapula at its lateral border. Perform the measurement at the point where the scapula begins to move.	Stabilize the scapula on its posterior surface to isolate GH extension. Allow the elbow to flex when measuring extension.

GH = glenohumeral

Goniometry 15-2
Shoulder Goniometry: Abduction

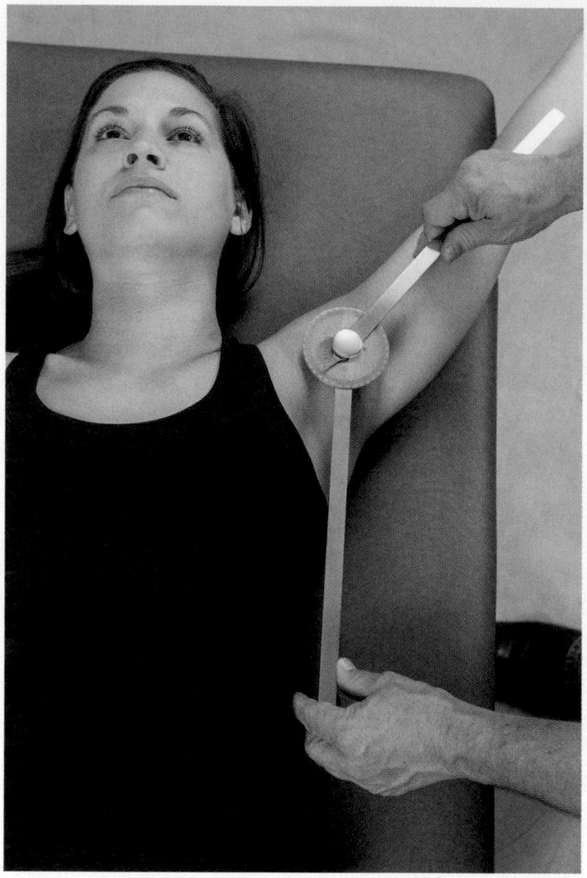

GH Abduction (0–120°)
Elevation Through Abduction (0–180°)

Patient Position	Supine

Goniometer Alignment

Fulcrum	Anterior to the acromion process
Proximal Arm	The stationary arm is aligned parallel to the long axis of the torso.
Distal Arm	The movement arm is centered over the midline of the anterior humerus.
Comments	To isolate GH abduction, stabilize the scapula at its lateral border. Perform the measurement at the point where the scapula begins to move. Adduction is not normally measured.

GH = glenohumeral

Goniometry 15-3
Shoulder Goniometry: Internal and External Rotation

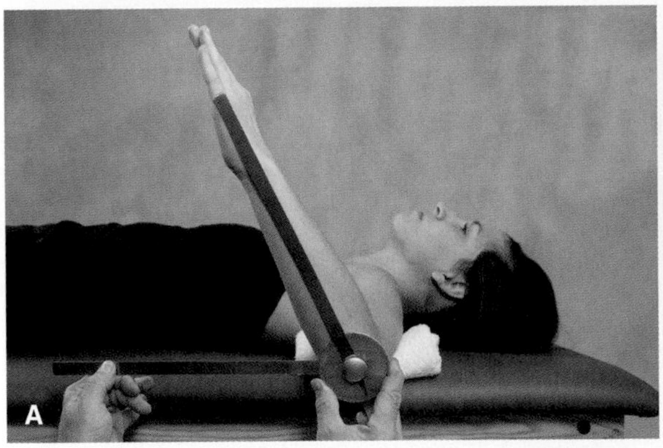

Internal Rotation (0–90°)

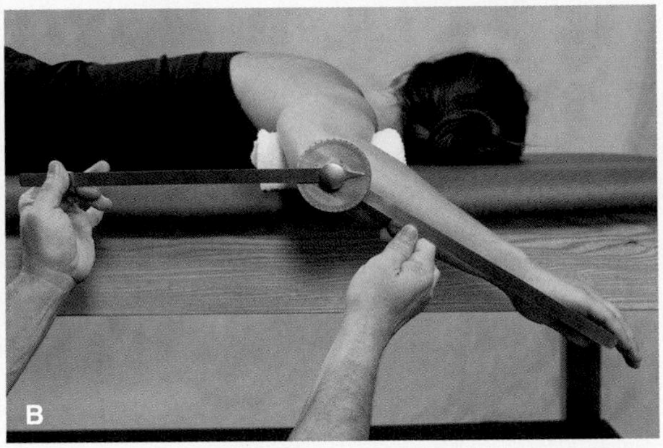

External Rotation (0–100°)

	Internal Rotation	External Rotation
Patient Position	Supine with the shoulder abducted to 90° and the elbow flexed to 90° A towel may be needed under the distal humerus to maintain this position.	Prone with the shoulder abducted to 90° and the elbow flexed to 90° A towel may be needed under the distal humerus to maintain this position.

Goniometer Alignment

Fulcrum	Centered lateral to the olecranon process
Proximal Arm	The stationary arm is aligned perpendicular to the floor or parallel to the tabletop.
Distal Arm	The movement arm is centered over the long axis of the ulna.
Comments	Anterior instability may result in pain and/or apprehension at the end range of external rotation (the apprehension test). To isolate GH motion, stabilize the scapula during external rotation. Scapular stabilization is provided by the body weight during internal rotation.

GH = glenohumeral

gross assessments of these motions are commonly obtained using bilateral comparison.

Active Range of Motion

The muscles acting on the scapulothoracic articulation are presented in Table 15-4 and those acting on the glenohumeral joint in Table 15-5. An evaluation of the aggregate motion available to the shoulder complex can be quickly determined through the **Apley scratch test** (Box 15-2). Each of the three components of this test should be compared bilaterally to determine a decrease in the ROM, pain, and the willingness to move.

- **Flexion and extension:** The shoulder complex is capable of producing 220 to 240 degrees of movement in the sagittal plane (Fig. 15-22). The majority of this ROM, accounting for 170 to 180 degrees of motion from the anatomical position, is provided by flexion. The remaining 50 to 60 degrees occur from the limb's moving from the anatomical position to extension.

Table 15-4 Muscles Contributing to Scapular Movements

Elevation	Protraction	Upward Rotation
Levator scapulae Rhomboid major Rhomboid minor Serratus anterior (upper portion) Trapezius (upper portion)	Serratus anterior	Serratus anterior Trapezius (upper and lower portion)
Depression	**Retraction**	**Downward Rotation**
Serratus anterior (lower portion) Trapezius (lower portion) Pectoralis major (clavicular portion)	Rhomboid major Rhomboid minor Trapezius (middle fibers) Trapezius (lower fibers)	Rhomboid major Rhomboid minor Levator scapulae

Table 15-5 Muscles Contributing to Humeral Movements

Flexion	Adduction	Horizontal Adduction	Internal Rotation
Biceps brachii	Coracobrachialis	Deltoid (anterior one-third)	Deltoid (anterior one-third)
Coracobrachialis	Latissimus dorsi	Coracobrachialis	Latissimus dorsi
Deltoid (anterior one-third)	Pectoralis major	Pectoralis major	Pectoralis major
Deltoid (middle one-third)	Teres major		Subscapularis
Pectoralis major (clavicular fibers)	Triceps brachii		Teres major
Extension	Abduction	Horizontal Abduction	External Rotation
Deltoid (posterior one-third)	Biceps brachii	Deltoid (posterior one-third)	Deltoid (posterior one-third)
Latissimus dorsi	Deltoid (anterior one-third)	Infraspinatus	Infraspinatus
Teres major	Deltoid (middle one-third)	Teres minor	Teres minor
Triceps brachii (long head)	Deltoid (posterior one-third)		Supraspinatus
	Supraspinatus		

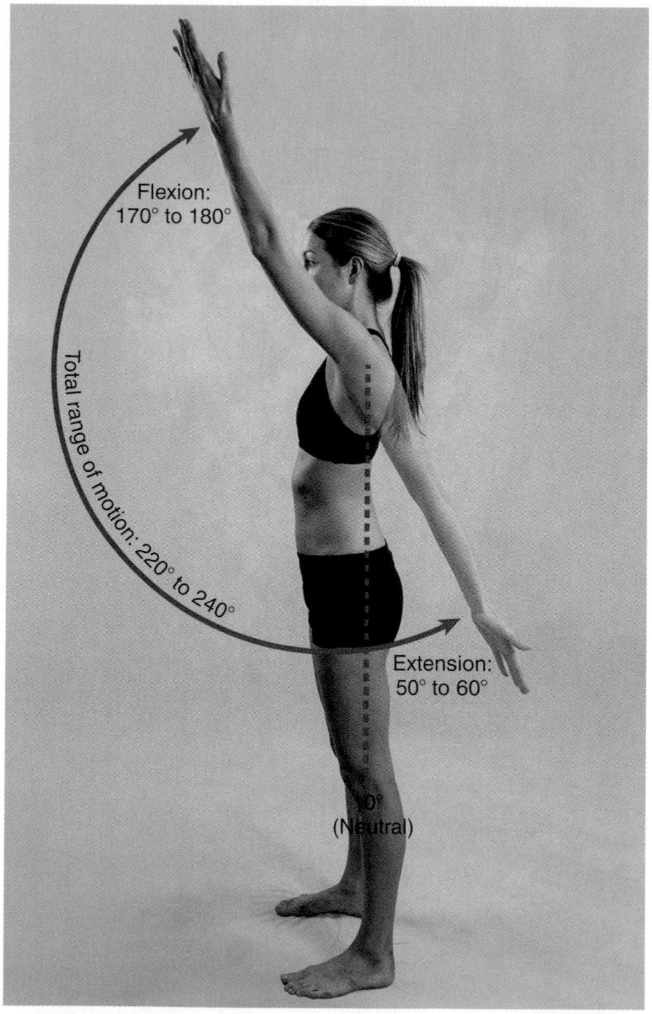

FIGURE 15-22 ■ Range of motion for shoulder flexion and extension.

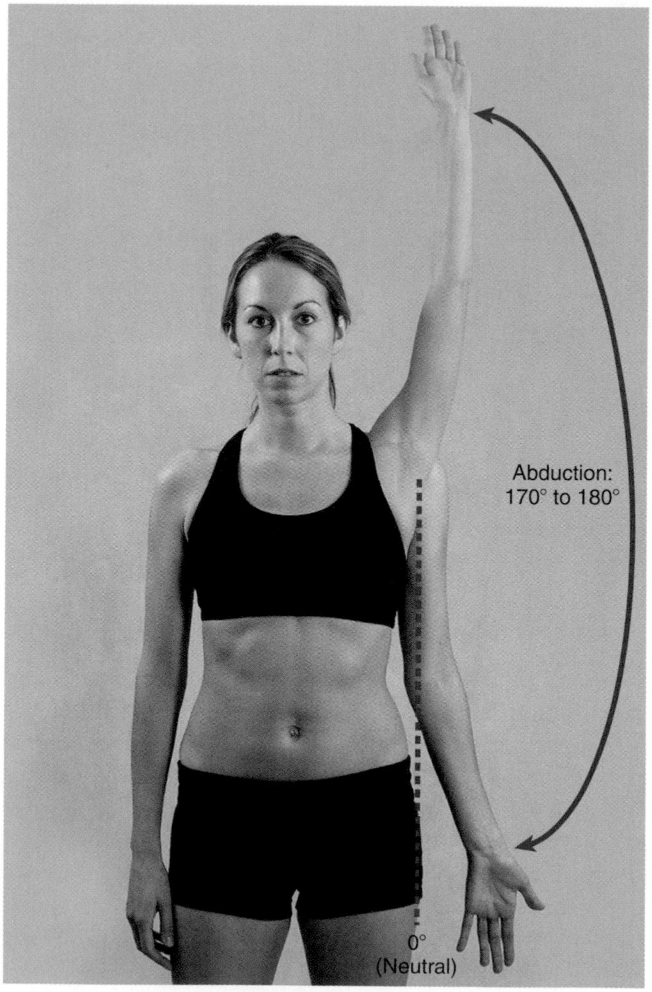

FIGURE 15-23 ■ Range of motion for shoulder abduction and adduction.

- **Abduction and adduction:** Occurring in the frontal plane, the normal ROM for abduction is 170 to 180 degrees (Fig. 15-23). The motion of adduction is blocked in the anatomical position, and any further movement requires that the GH joint be flexed or extended so that the humerus can pass in front of or behind the torso. The patient's ability to control adduction should be noticed. An arm that falls uncontrollably from 90 degrees of abduction indicates a positive **drop arm test** for rotator cuff pathology (Selective Tissue Test 15-1).[21]

Box 15-2
Apley Scratch Tests

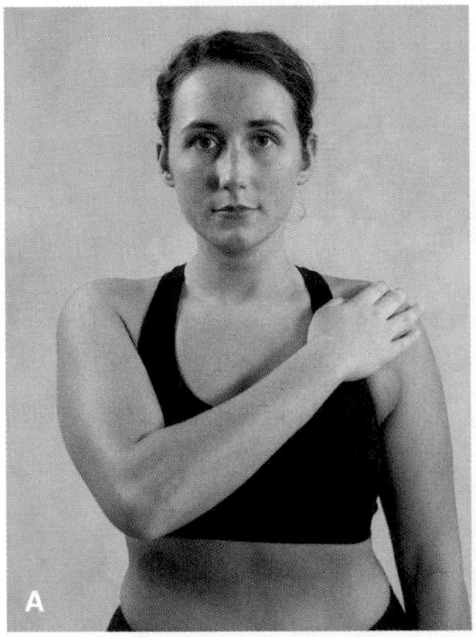

The patient touches the opposite shoulder by crossing the chest.

Motions produced: GH horizontal adduction, and internal rotation; scapular protraction

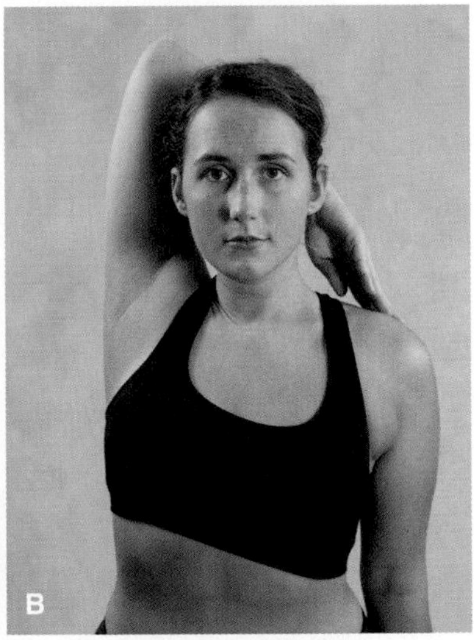

The patient reaches behind the head and touches the shoulder from behind.

Motions produced: GH abduction and external rotation; scapular elevation and upward rotation

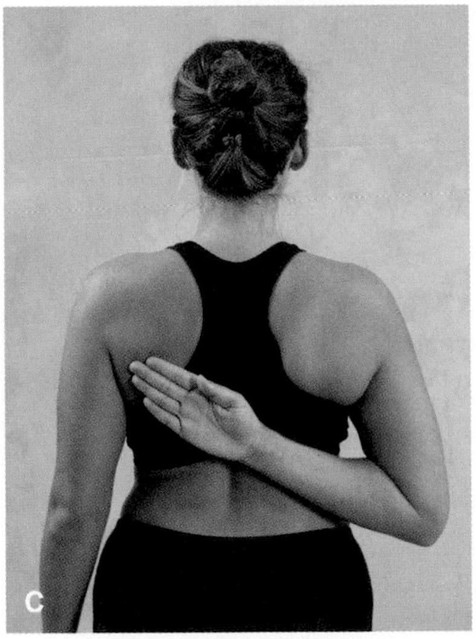

The patient reaches behind the back and touches the opposite scapula.

Motions produced: GH adduction and internal rotation; scapular retraction and downward rotation

The amount of internal GH rotation is determined by measuring the distance up the spinal column the patient can reach and comparing this result with that of the opposite shoulder.

GH = glenohumeral

Selective Tissue Tests 15-1
Drop Arm Test for Rotator Cuff Tendinopathy

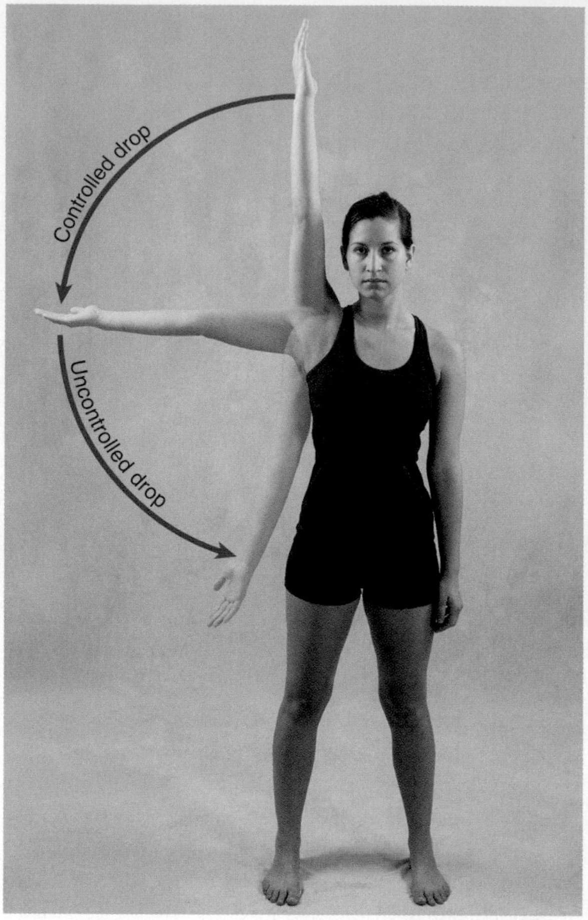

The drop arm test determines the patient's ability to control humeral motion via an eccentric contraction as the arm is slowly lowered from full abduction to adduction.

Patient Position	Standing or sitting The humerus fully abducted. The supraspinatus is emphasized when the humerus is internally rotated.
Position of Examiner	Standing lateral to, or behind, the involved extremity
Evaluative Procedure	The patient slowly lowers the arm to the side.
Positive Test	The arm falls uncontrollably from a position of approximately 90° abduction to the side. Severe pain may also be described.
Implications	The inability to lower the arm in a controlled manner is indicative of lesions to the rotator cuff, especially the supraspinatus.
Modification	If the patient is able to lower the arm in a controlled manner through the ROM, a derivative of the drop arm test may be implemented: The patient holds the humerus in 90° abduction. The examiner applies gentle pressure on the distal forearm. A positive test result causes the arm to fall against the side of the body, indicating lesions to the rotator cuff.
Evidence	

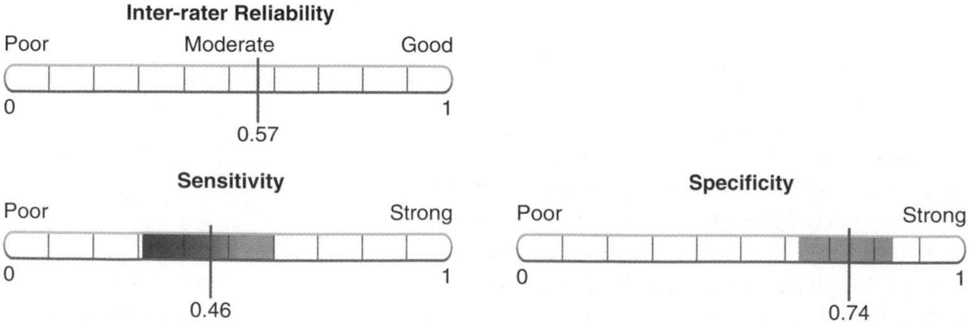

LR+: 1.67–2.27–2.86

LR−: 0.58–0.71–0.85

ROM = range of motion

The patient may describe an area within the ROM that elicits pain. This painful arc, usually occurring between 60 and 120 degrees of abduction, may be indicative of impingement of the rotator cuff musculature although its diagnostic value is limited when used in isolation.[22]

Practical Evidence

The clinical usefulness of the drop arm test is improved when the results are combined with the findings of other tests. A positive drop arm test with an associated painful arc and a weak infraspinatus manual muscle test (MMT) increase the probability of a full-thickness rotator cuff tear to 91%.[22]

- **Internal and external rotation:** Internal and external rotation is assessed in both the neutral position and in 90 degrees of abduction. In the neutral position, the humeral head and the greater tuberosity are allowed to rotate beneath the acromion without interference. During internal rotation, the torso blocks the motion. External rotation in this position, usually 40 to 50 degrees, is less than when the humerus is abducted 90 degrees. This motion is limited by the superior GH and coracohumeral ligaments.

  When abducted to 90 degrees so that the greater and lesser tuberosities can clear the structures of the scapula, the GH joint can obtain an increased amount of internal and external rotation (Fig. 15-24). With the humerus in 90 degrees of abduction with the elbow flexed to 90 degrees, the normal ROM in this position is 80 to 90 degrees of external rotation and 70 to 80 degrees of internal rotation. These motions are restricted by the inferior GH ligament.

  The amount of available motion is assessed bilaterally, with deficits assessed by having the patient reach behind and up the back, with right to left results compared (Fig. 15-25). These assessments are more representative of functional motion than standard goniometry and may help identify asymmetry and contributing underlying impairments.

Practical Evidence

High school baseball players with an internal rotation ROM deficit of 25 degrees or more are four times more likely to sustain an upper extremity injury.[23]

- **Horizontal adduction and abduction:** The neutral position for horizontal adduction and abduction is 90 degrees of abduction with the arm flexed at a 30-degree angle from the torso in the plane of the scapula (see Fig. 15-5). Occurring in the horizontal plane, the expected ROM is 120 degrees of horizontal adduction and 45 degrees of horizontal abduction relative to the plane of the scapula. Tightness of the posterior capsule can limit the amount of horizontal adduction.

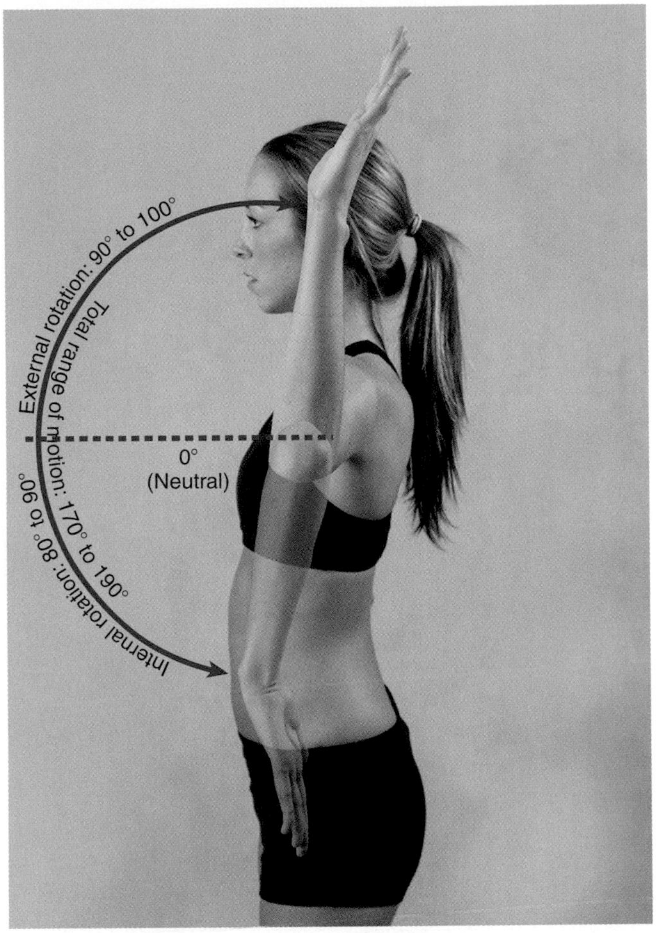
External rotation: 90° to 100°
Total range of motion: 170° to 190°
0°
(Neutral)
Internal rotation: 80° to 90°

FIGURE 15-24 ■ Range of motion for shoulder internal rotation and external rotation.

Manual Muscle Testing

Manual muscle testing begins with screening active range of motion (AROM) followed by the addition of resistance to detect pain or weakness associated with more specific muscle involvement. While resistance can be applied throughout the range, the results are equivocal because several structures are stressed. The use of an isometric (or break) test in the midrange of motion may minimize other causes of pain and weakness (Manual Muscle Tests 15-1 through 15-4). The **Gerber lift-off test** is a sensitive method of isolating the subscapularis (Selective Tissue Test 15-2).[24-27]

Scapular Movements

Observation of scapular movement combined with strength assessment of the scapular stabilizers is an integral component to detecting scapulothoracic dyskinesis. This process is described in the Assessment of Dynamic Scapular Function section. Manual muscle testing of the scapular muscles is presented in Manual Muscle Tests 15-5 through 15-9.

Passive Range of Motion

Passive range of motion (PROM) assessment helps detect the nature of any joint restriction by detecting the quality

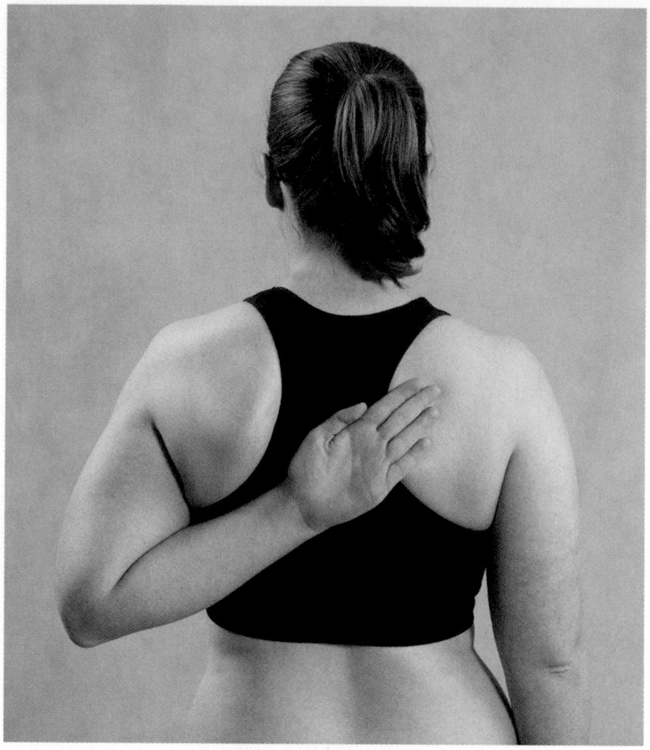

FIGURE 15-25 ■ Method of checking for shoulder internal rotation as recommended by the American Academy of Orthopaedic Surgeons.

and quantity of motion coupled with an assessment of end-feel (Table 15-6). Scapular stabilization is important to differentiate GH motion from shoulder girdle motion. Glenohumeral capsule involvement results in a characteristic pattern of restriction, with external rotation and abduction being limited initially. Patients who present with equal limitations in active and passive motion may have **adhesive capsulitis**, or a frozen shoulder. Usually affecting those older than age 50, adhesive capsulitis commonly has an idiopathic onset characterized initially by sporadic pain and progressing to constant pain and capsular restriction.

- **Flexion and extension:** PROM may be isolated to the GH joint or may encompass the entire motion allowed by the shoulder complex. To isolate the GH joint, the scapula must be stabilized to prevent its contribution to shoulder motion. When the entire motion provided by the shoulder complex is evaluated, the thorax must be stabilized. Each of these two methods of stabilization is more easily accomplished with the patient lying supine during flexion and prone during extension.

  Flexion should have a firm end-feel for both GH and shoulder complex motions. During GH flexion, the terminal motion is checked by the tightening of the GH capsule (especially the coracohumeral ligament and the posterior capsular fibers) and the teres minor, teres major, and infraspinatus muscles. The muscles attaching to the anterior portion of the humerus, especially the pectoralis major and the latissimus dorsi, normally limit flexion of the entire shoulder complex.

  The two types of passive extension result in a firm end-feel. During isolated GH extension, the coracohumeral ligament and the anterior joint capsule become taut. During extension of the shoulder complex, the pectoralis major (clavicular fibers) and serratus anterior muscles contribute to the end-feel.

  Pain occurring at the end-range of passive flexion may indicate impingement of the supraspinatus tendon, long head of the biceps brachii, or the subacromial bursa between the inferior portion of the acromion process and the humeral head. Pain during passive extension may result from damage to the anterior portion of the GH capsule or the coracohumeral ligament.
- **Abduction and adduction:** As in the case of flexion and extension, abduction is the result of motion arising from the shoulder complex or isolated to its pure GH movement. When attempting to isolate GH abduction, the scapula is stabilized to prevent its upward rotation and elevation. To restrict motion to the shoulder complex, the thorax is stabilized to eliminate lateral bending of the spine. Passive abduction may be examined with the patient sitting or supine.

  The normal ROM resulting from purely GH movement has a firm end-feel because of the stress placed on the inferior GH ligament, the inferior capsule, and the pectoralis major and latissimus dorsi muscles. During abduction arising from the entire shoulder complex, the rhomboids and the middle and lower fibers of the trapezius muscle contribute to the end-feel.

  PROM measurements and end-feels are not normally taken for adduction because of the humerus striking the body. However, hyperadduction may be measured by moving the arm in front of the torso. Note for the presence of a painful arc, indicating rotator cuff impingement, during passive motion from abduction

Table 15-6 Glenohumeral Joint Capsular Patterns and End-Feels

Capsular Pattern: External Rotation, Abduction, Internal Rotation

End-Feels:	
Elevation	Firm or hard
Extension	Firm
Flexion	Firm
Abduction	Firm or hard
Horizontal Abduction	Firm
Horizontal Adduction	Firm or soft
Internal Rotation	Firm
External Rotation	Firm

Manual Muscle Test 15-1
Shoulder Flexion and Extension

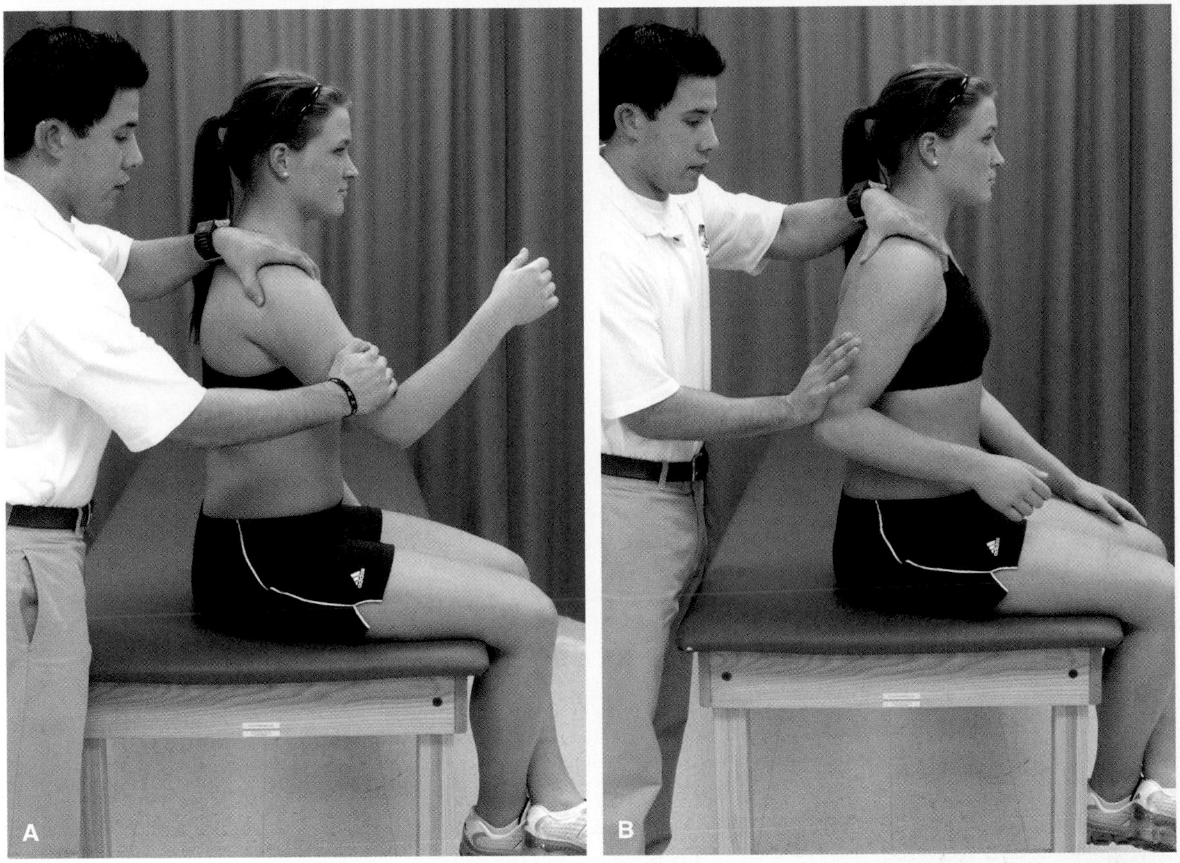

	Flexion	Extension
Patient Position	Seated	
Test Position	Glenohumeral joint flexed about 45°	Glenohumeral joint in slight extension
Stabilization	Superior aspect of the shoulder	
Resistance	Distal anterior humerus, just proximal to the cubital fossa	Distal posterior humerus, just proximal to the olecranon
Primary Movers (Innervation)	Anterior deltoid (C5, C6)	Latissimus dorsi (C6, C7, C8) Teres major (C5, C6, C7)
Secondary Movers (Innervation)	Pectoralis major (clavicular portion) (C6, C7, C8, T1) Coracobrachialis (C6, C7) Middle deltoid (C5, C6) Biceps brachii (C5, C6)	Posterior deltoid (C5, C6) Triceps brachii (long head) (C6, C7, C8, T1)
Substitution	Trunk extension, scapular elevation	Scapular protraction (from pectoralis minor), trunk rotation
Comments		Maintain elbow extension to minimize contributions from the triceps.

Manual Muscle Test 15-2
Shoulder Abduction and Adduction

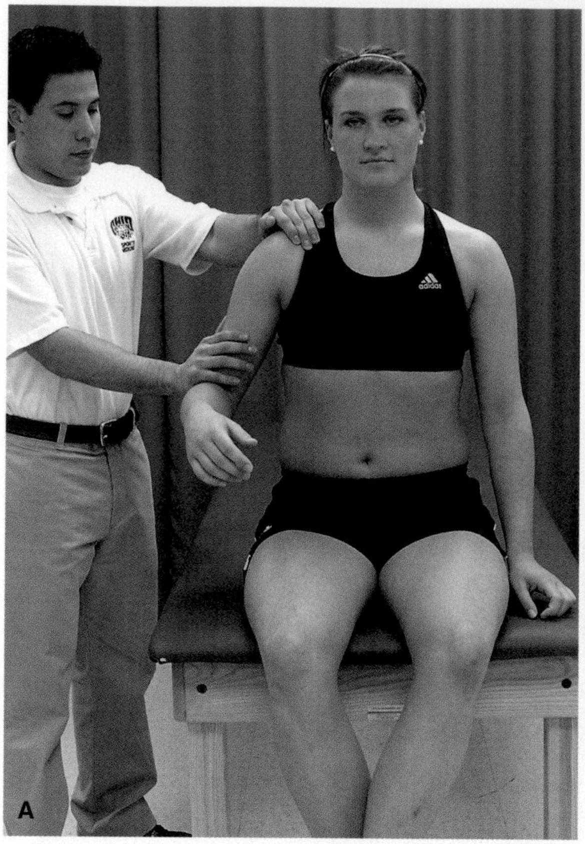

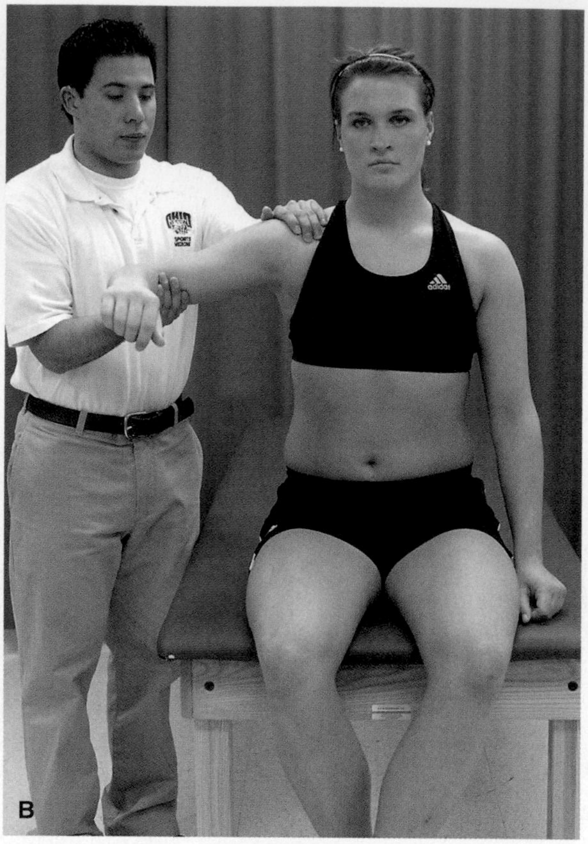

	Abduction	Adduction
Patient Position	Seated	Seated or supine
Test Position	The glenohumeral joint abducted to approximately 30°	The glenohumeral joint abducted to approximately 80°
Stabilization	Superior shoulder	Superior shoulder
Resistance	Distal humerus, just proximal to the lateral epicondyle	Distal humerus, just proximal to the medial epicondyle
Primary Movers (Innervation)	Deltoid muscle group (C5, C6) Supraspinatus (C4, C5, C6)	Pectoralis major (C6, C7, C8, T1) Latissimus dorsi (C6, C7, C8) Teres major (C5, C6, C7)
Secondary Movers (Innervation)		Coracobrachialis (C6, C7) Triceps brachii (C6, C7, C8, T1)
Substitution	Scapular elevation, external rotation, trunk lateral flexion to same or opposite side	Trunk lateral flexion to same side
Comments		Better isolation of the primary movers is achieved by testing shoulder extension and horizontal adduction.

Manual Muscle Test 15-3
Shoulder Internal and External Rotation

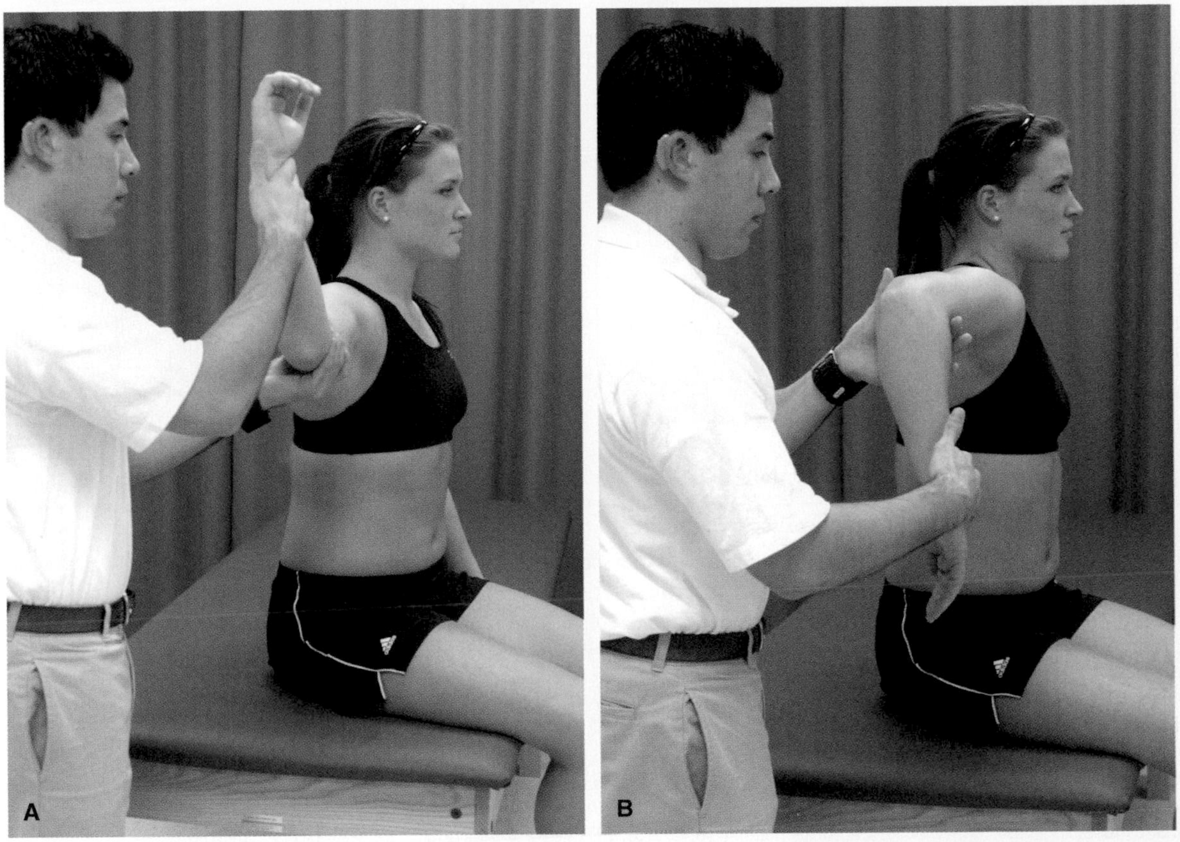

	Internal Rotation (A)	External Rotation (B)
Patient Position	Prone to improve stabilization; seated (shown) is also an option	Prone to improve stabilization. Seated (shown) is also an option.
Test Position	The GH joint is in neutral position or abducted to 90° and slightly internally rotated. The elbow is flexed to 90°.	The GH joint is in neutral position or abducted to 90° and slightly externally rotated. The elbow is flexed to 90°.
Stabilization	The distal humerus is stabilized just proximal to the elbow.	The distal humerus is stabilized just proximal to the elbow.
Resistance	Anterior distal forearm	Posterior distal forearm
Primary Movers (Innervation)	Subscapularis (C5, C6, C7)	Infraspinatus (C5, C6) Teres minor (C5, C6)
Secondary Movers (Innervation)	Teres major (C5, C6, C7) Pectoralis major (C6, C7, C8, T1) Latissimus dorsi (C6, C7, C8) Anterior deltoid (C5, C6)	Posterior deltoid (C5, C6)
Substitution	Elbow extension, scapular protraction	Elbow extension, scapular depression
Comments	The Gerber lift-off test is also used to assess subscapularis pathology.	

GH = glenohumeral

Manual Muscle Test 15-4
Shoulder Horizontal Adduction and Abduction

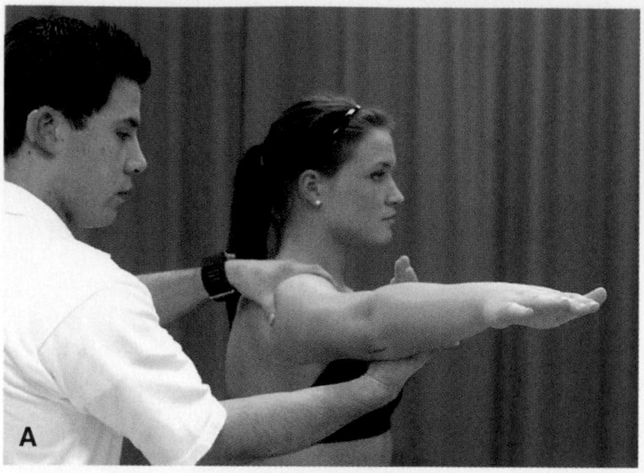

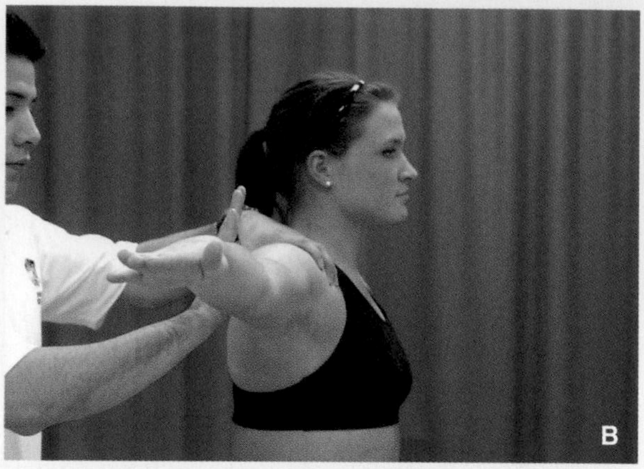

	Horizontal Adduction (A)	Horizontal Abduction (B)
Patient Position	Seated or supine Stabilization is improved with the patient supine. The GH joint is abducted to 90°.	Seated or prone Stabilization is improved with the patient prone. The GH joint is abducted to 90°.
Test Position	Slight horizontal adduction	Slight horizontal abduction
Stabilization	Scapula	Scapula
Resistance	Anterior portion of the distal humerus	Posterior portion of the distal humerus
Primary Mover (Innervation)	Pectorals major (C6, C7, C8, T1)	Posterior deltoid (C5, C6)
Secondary Movers (Innervation)	Anterior deltoid (C5, C6) Coracobrachialis (C6, C7)	Infraspinatus (C5, C6) Teres minor (C5, C6)
Substitution	Trunk rotation	Scapular retraction Trunk rotation

GH = glenohumeral

Selective Tissue Tests 15-2

Gerber Lift-off Test (Internal Rotation Lag Sign) for Subscapularis Pathology

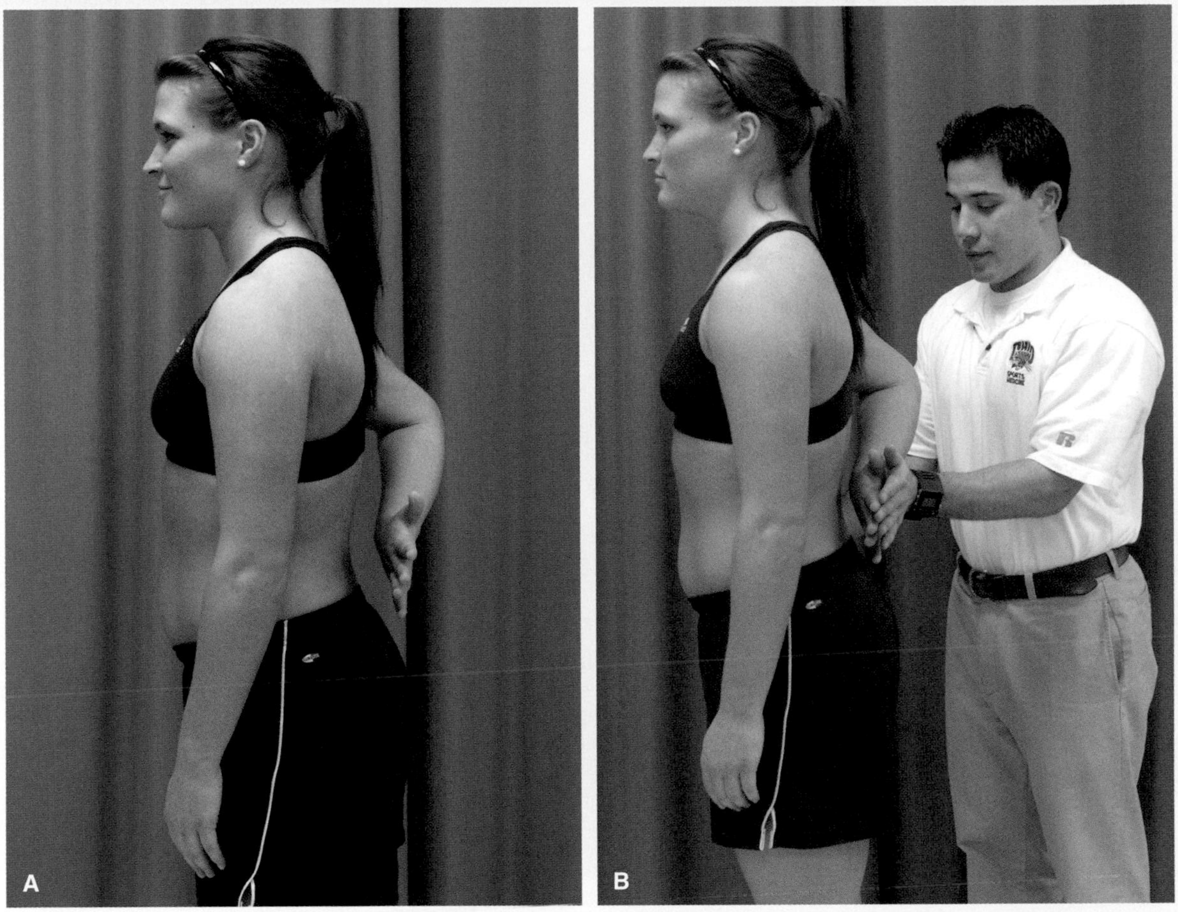

The Gerber lift-off test is a modification of a subscapularis manual muscle test..

Patient Position	(A) Standing with the GH joint internally rotated and extended, and the elbow flexed The dorsal surface of the hand is placed against the midlumbar spine.
Position of Examiner	Standing behind the patient
Evaluative Procedure	The patient attempts to actively lift the hand off the spine while the humerus stays in extension.
Positive Test	Inability to lift the hand off the back
Implications	Positive test findings are associated with tears or weakness of the subscapularis muscle. Possible C5, C6, C7 nerve root pathology
Modification	(B) Resistance can be applied to the patient's palm.
Comments	Test should be performed only if the patient has sufficient internal rotation to reach the sacral region or above. Do not allow compensatory motions such as GH extension. The high sensitivity of this test in detecting full-thickness tears of the subscapularis indicates that the patient is unlikely to have the condition if the test is negative.
Evidence	

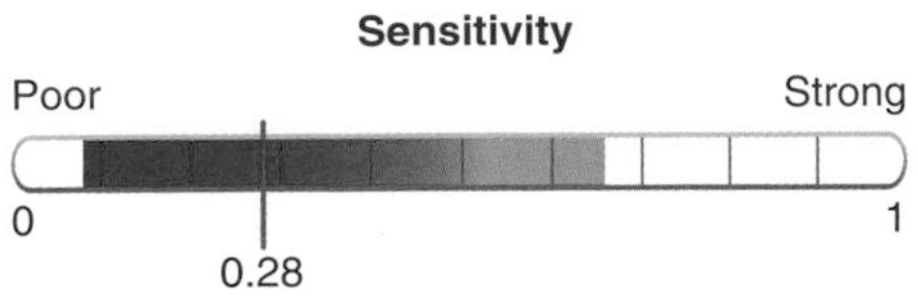

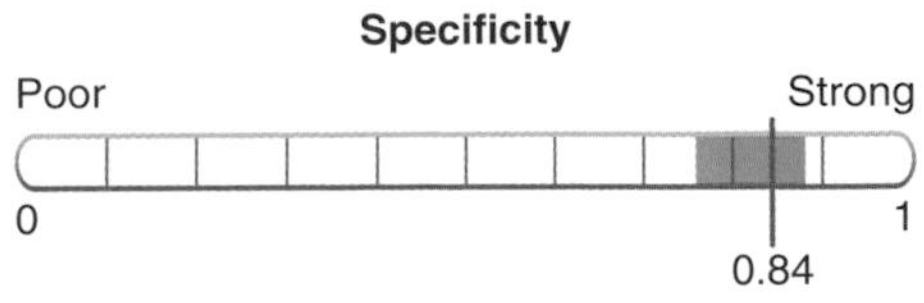

LR+: 0.34–1.48–2.26

LR−: 0.38–0.83–1.15

GH = glenohumeral

Manual Muscle Test 15-5
Scapular Retraction and Downward Rotation

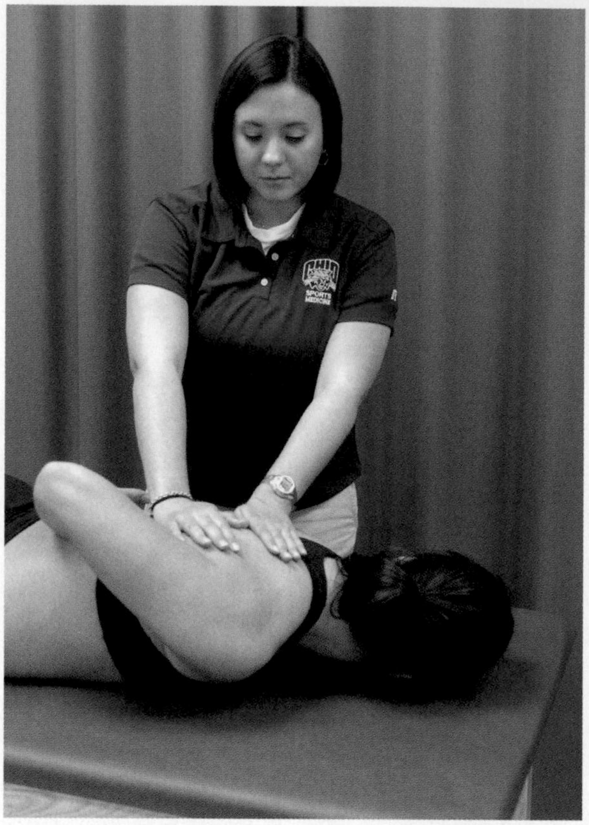

Patient Position	Prone. Rotating the head towards the side being tested decreases tension from the levator scapulae.
Test Position	The arm being tested is behind the patient's back, with the glenohumeral joint internally rotated and the elbow flexed.
Stabilization	Trunk
Resistance	Vertebral scapular border as the patient attempts to lift the hand off the back
Primary Movers (Innervation)	Rhomboid major (C4, C5) Rhomboid minor (C4, C5)
Secondary Mover (Innervation)	Middle trapezius (CN XI)
Substitution	Trunk rotation, glenohumeral extension, anterior tilting of the scapula
Comments	Note the application of resistance on the scapula, which differentiates this from the Gerber lift-off test (see Selective Tissue Test 15-2).

Manual Muscle Test 15-6
Scapular Retraction

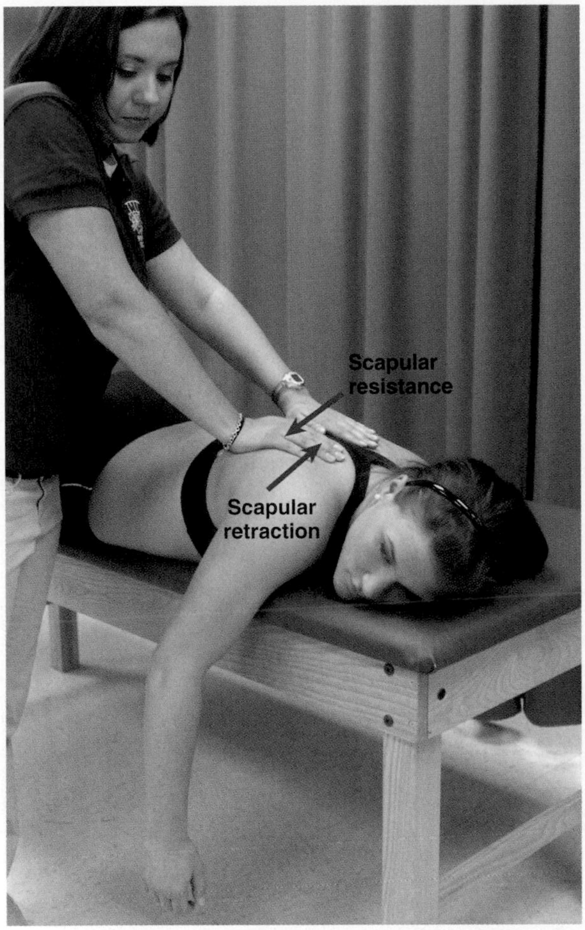

Patient Position	Prone
Test Position	The elbow is extended, and the glenohumeral joint is flexed to 90°. The scapula is in a slightly retracted position.
Stabilization	Trunk
Resistance	Vertebral border of the scapula
Primary Movers (Innervation)	Middle trapezius (CN XI) Rhomboids (C4, C5)
Secondary Mover (Innervation)	Upper and lower trapezius
Substitution	Trunk rotation, glenohumeral horizontal abduction

Manual Muscle Test 15-7
Scapular Protraction and Upward Rotation

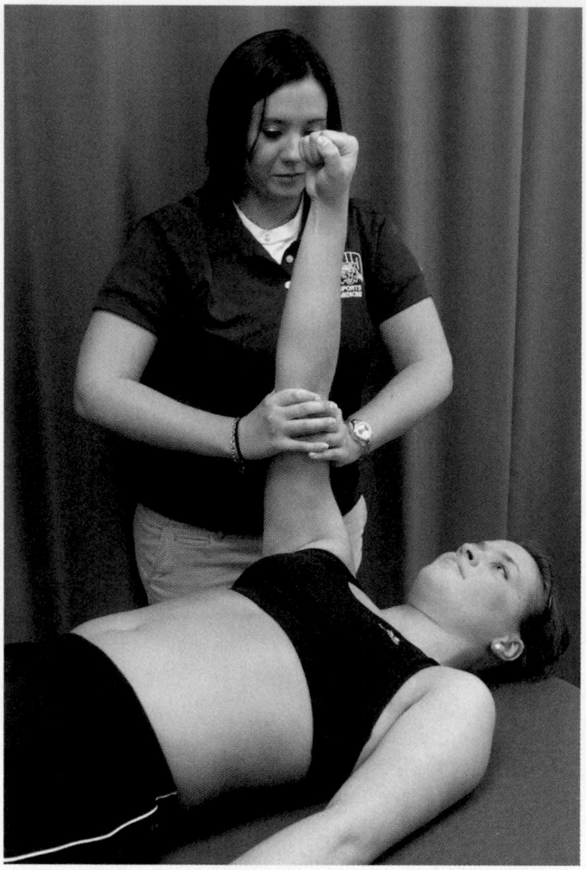

Patient Position	Supine
Test Position	The glenohumeral joint is flexed to 90°. The patient is instructed to "punch the ceiling," causing the scapula to protract and upwardly rotate.
Stabilization	Trunk
Resistance	Distal humerus, proximal to elbow
Primary Mover (Innervation)	Serratus anterior (C5, C6, C7)
Secondary Movers (Innervation)	Pectoralis minor (C7, C8, T1) Trapezius (CN XI)
Substitution	Horizontal adduction and trunk rotation
Comments	Observe the patient performing a wall push-up to functionally assess the serratus anterior.

Manual Muscle Test 15-8
Scapular Depression and Retraction

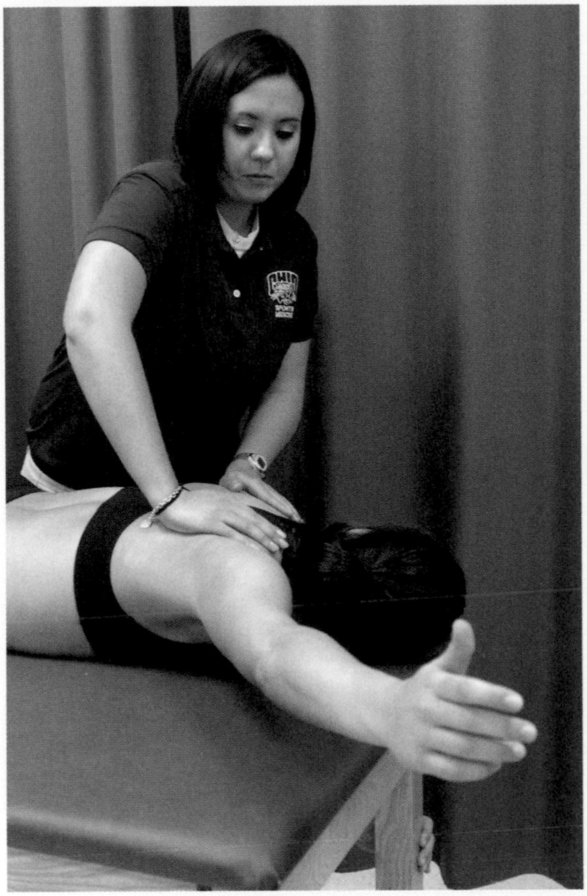

Patient Position	Prone
Test Position	The glenohumeral joint being tested is abducted to 135° with the forearm supinated and the patient's head rotated to the side opposite that being tested. Tell the patient: "Raise your arm."
Stabilization	Trunk
Resistance	Scapula in upward and outward direction
Primary Mover(s) (Innervation)	Lower trapezius (CN XI)
Secondary Mover (Innervation)	Middle trapezius (CN XI)
Substitution	Trunk rotation; glenohumeral extension
Comments	Patients suffering from impingement may be unable to achieve this test position. In this case, position the arm at the side and instruct the patient to bring the scapula "down and in."

Manual Muscle Test 15-9
Scapular Elevation

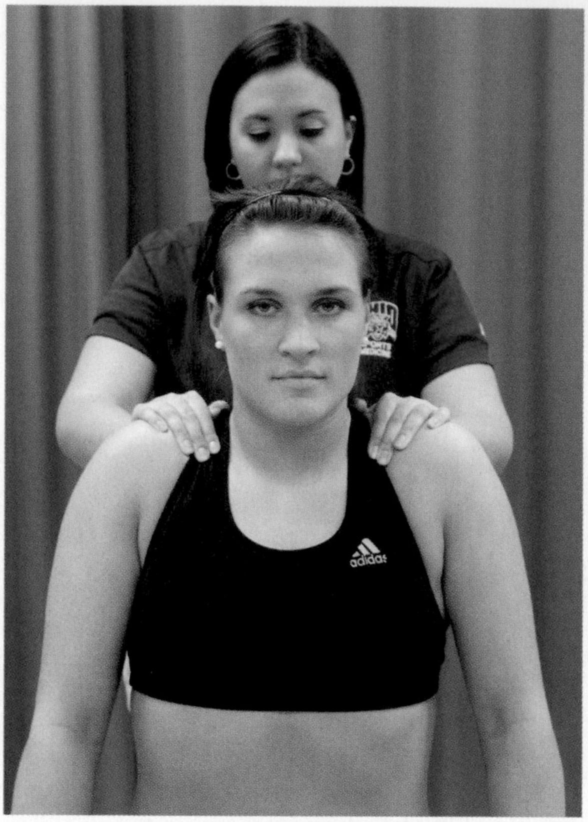

Patient Position	Seated
Test Position	Seated. The patient assumes a shoulder shrug position.
Stabilization	Trunk
Resistance	Pushing down on the superior aspect of the shoulder
Primary Movers (Innervation)	Upper trapezius (CN XI) Levator scapulae (C3, C4, C5)
Secondary Mover (Innervation)	Not applicable
Substitution	Trunk rotation or side-bending

to adduction. Pain experienced during both passive abduction and passive adduction may indicate inflammation of the subacromial structures.

- **Internal and external rotation:** PROM for rotation of the humerus is measured with the GH joint abducted to 90 degrees and the elbow flexed to 90 degrees. These motions can be tested with the patient in the seated or supine positions although scapular stabilization is more easily accomplished with the patient supine. To isolate rotation at the GH joint, the scapula is stabilized to prevent contributions from the scapulothoracic articulation. When measuring motion produced by the shoulder complex, stabilize the thorax to prevent flexion or extension of the spine (Fig. 15-26).

  The firm end-feel associated with normal internal rotation is caused by tightening of the posterior fibers of the GH capsule and the infraspinatus and teres minor muscles. During internal rotation with the scapula unstabilized, the rhomboid muscle group and the middle and lower fibers of the trapezius contribute to the end-feel.

  During external rotation, the GH ligaments, the coracohumeral ligament, and the joint capsule wind tight, resulting in a firm end-feel for both isolated GH movements and the shoulder complex as a whole. Muscular contributions lending to the end-feel for GH external rotation include the subscapularis, pectoralis major, latissimus dorsi, and teres major muscles.

  Athletes who perform overhand motions, such as baseball players, javelin throwers, tennis players, and quarterbacks, often have an increased range of external rotation and decreased internal rotation. Both of these changes alter the mechanics of the shoulder complex, but the total amount of ROM remains the same (e.g., decreased internal rotation is compensated for by increased external rotation).[28]

  Examination of passive external rotation and extension must be delayed until the end of the assessment procedure when a GH dislocation, subluxation, or chronic instability is suspected. In such instances, the examination proceeds with great care. Passive external rotation of the GH joint is the same procedure as the **apprehension test** (see Anterior Glenohumeral Instability).

  The GH joint is palpated during passive internal and external rotation to determine the presence of crepitus, which may indicate rotator cuff or bicipital tendinitis and subacromial bursitis, or "clicks," which may indicate a labral tear.

- **Horizontal adduction and abduction:** To isolate GH motion, the scapula must be stabilized to prevent medial and lateral translation. During evaluation of the entire shoulder complex, the torso is stabilized so that spinal motion does not contribute to motion of the shoulder.

  Horizontal adduction, also called cross-body adduction, may have a soft end-feel because of soft tissue approximation when the pectoralis major, biceps, and anterior deltoid muscles are well developed. A soft end-feel also may be found in obese individuals. A firm end-feel with the scapula stabilized is associated with stretching of the posterior GH capsule and tension developed by the posterior deltoid muscle. Pain at the end-range of horizontal adduction is also associated with AC joint pathology. A restriction may be indicative of GH impingement.

  A firm end-feel is expected during horizontal abduction because of the tightening of the anterior GH capsule and the middle and inferior GH ligaments. Some tension may also be developed by the anterior deltoid and pectoralis major.

Joint Stability Tests

The integrity of the ligaments and capsules of the shoulder complex is determined via joint play and stress testing. Because of the relative difficulty in manipulating the clavicle and their inherent joint stability, the findings for tests for SC and AC joint instability are more subtle than the findings for the other joints in the body. Generally, the findings are positive only in the more severe cases. These tests are contraindicated when a fracture or joint dislocation is suspected.

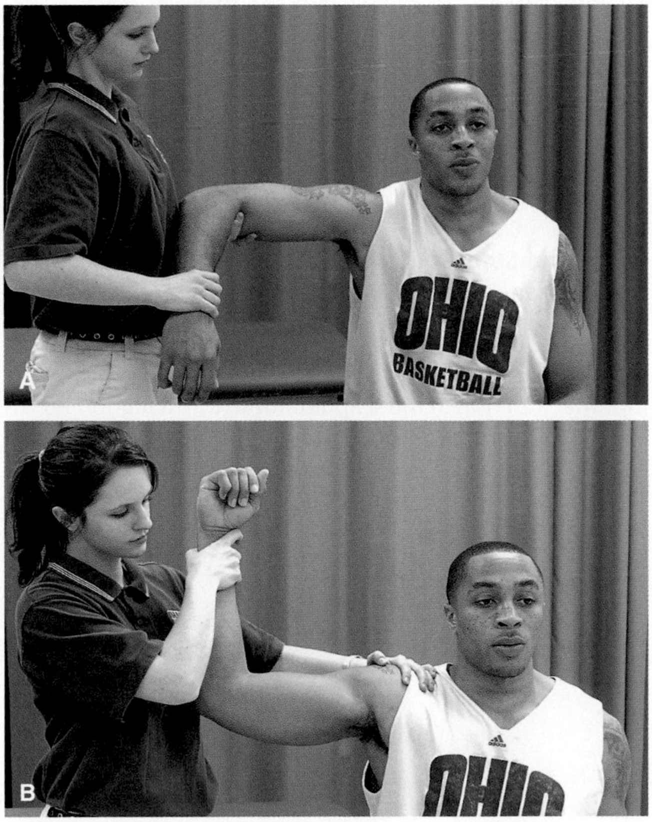

FIGURE 15-26 ■ Passive range of motion assessment of (A) internal rotation and (B) external rotation. See the text for information on how to isolate glenohumeral motion.

Sternoclavicular Joint Play

To determine the stability of the SC joint, position the patient supine, and, while sitting at the head of the patient, grasp the clavicle just distal to the medial clavicular head (Joint Play 15-1).

Pain and/or hypermobility that are evoked during all movements may result from either damage to the SC joint disc or a complete disruption of the joint capsule.

Acromioclavicular Joint Play

With the patient supine, the AC joint is stressed by grasping the clavicle along its distal one-third and gliding the joint anteriorly, posteriorly, inferiorly, and superiorly, noting any pain, hypermobility, or hypomobility (Joint Play 15-2).

Glenohumeral Joint Play

Assessment of true GH glide involves the sliding of the humeral head relative to the glenoid fossa. The ligaments tested during this procedure are also stressed during many of the selective tissue tests used to determine GH laxity. Laxity and instability are not synonymous. A lax shoulder can still be functionally stable. Also, an unstable shoulder may not demonstrate laxity during joint play, especially when the patient is awake (not anesthetized) because of reflexive muscle guarding.

The joint play assessment is performed in three directions—i.e., anterior, posterior, and inferior—with the humerus in the neutral (open pack) position and the scapula stabilized (Joint Play 15-3). Superior glide is not tested because of the bony block formed between the humeral head and the coracoacromial arch.

Joint play is assessed in a plane perpendicular to the plane of the scapula. Therefore, anterior glide is not tested by drawing the humerus forward relative to the sagittal plane but, rather, forward relative to the face of the glenoid fossa.[30] The degree of laxity is based on the amount of translation relative to the opposite limb. Any situation in which the humeral head can be displaced past the labral rim warrants further examination by a physician. The Region-Specific Pathology section of this chapter discusses multidirectional instabilities.

GH joint play can be modified using the **load and shift technique**. During standard GH joint play assessment, the humerus is distracted from the glenoid fossa. During load and shift testing, an axial load is placed on the humerus, compressing the humeral head into the glenoid fossa, centering the joint in its anatomical position. The following scale is used during load and shift testing[31]:

Grade	Amount of Humeral Head Translation
Trace (0)	No translation of the humeral head
Grade I	Translation of the humeral head to the glenoid rim but not over it
Grade II	Translation of the humeral head over the glenoid rim, but the head spontaneously reduces
Grade III	Dislocation of the humeral head without spontaneous reduction

When a three-point grading scale is used, there is poor intra- and intertester reliability.[32] If the grading scale is modified to a two-point scale (the humerus does not subluxate or the humerus does subluxate), the reliability of the test greatly improves.[33]

Neurological Testing

Cervical nerve root trauma, brachial plexus injury, thoracic outlet syndrome, and other nerve pathologies can produce neurological symptoms in the shoulder and upper extremity (Fig. 15-27). An upper quarter neurological screen can be used to identify the involved nerve root (or roots) (see Neurological Screening 1-2). Chapter 14 describes the brachial plexus and the actual mechanisms and tests for cervical nerve root impingement and discusses visceral origins of referred pain into this area.

Vascular Testing

Compare distal pulses bilaterally when there is a possibility of compromised blood flow to the arm. Vascular thoracic outlet syndrome can result in sporadic decreased blood flow and associated symptoms of cold and numb hands (see p. 580). The axillary artery can be impinged by the displaced humeral head following a glenohumeral dislocation, necessitating quick reduction (see Initial Management of On-Field Shoulder Injuries).

Region-Specific Pathologies and Selective Tissue Tests

Because of the number of bones, muscles, articulations, ligaments, and other supporting structures associated with the shoulder complex, this region is susceptible to a wide range of injuries. This section presents major orthopedic and athletic injuries to each segment and describes the signs, symptoms, and special evaluative procedures used to reach the appropriate conclusions.

Scapulothoracic Articulation Pathology

Optimal function of the scapulothoracic articulation is critical to performance of the shoulder and upper extremity

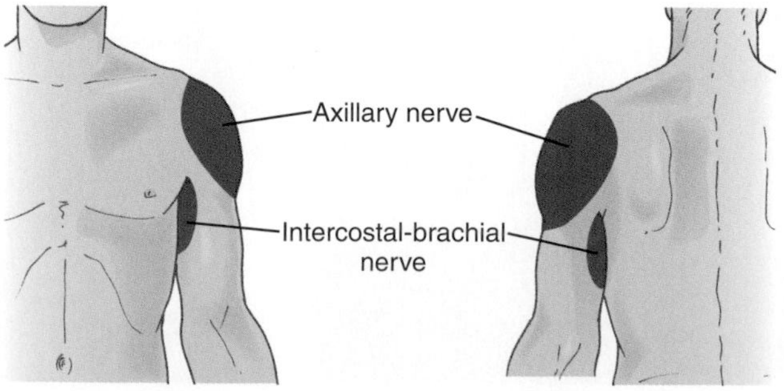

FIGURE 15-27 ■ Neuropathies of the shoulder and upper arm. Pain may also be referred to this area from the thorax (see Fig. 15-14) and the brachial plexus (see Chapter 14 and Neurological Screening 1-2).

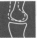

Joint Play 15-1
Sternoclavicular Joint Play

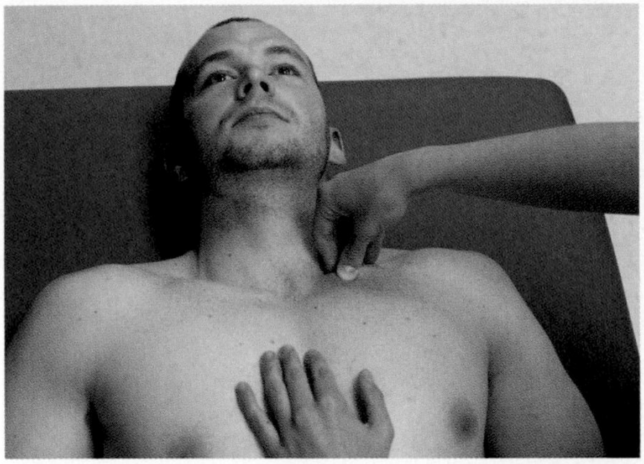

The proximal portion of the clavicle is manipulated to determine the amount of superior, anterior, and posterior motion available at the joint.

Patient Position	Supine or seated
Position of Examiner	Standing next to the patient, grasping the proximal clavicle
Evaluative Procedure	Apply a gliding pressure that forces the medial clavicle upward, anteriorly, and posteriorly relative to the sternum, noting pain, hypermobility, or hypomobility. Clavicular Motion — Structures Stressed Superior — Costoclavicular ligament (anterior and posterior fibers) Anterior — SC ligament (posterior fibers) Posterior — SC ligament (anterior fibers)
Positive Test	Pain, hypermobility, or hypomobility
Implications	Hypermobility: Laxity and/or sprain Hypomobility: Joint adhesions

SC = sternoclavicular

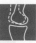

Joint Play 15-2
Acromioclavicular Joint Play

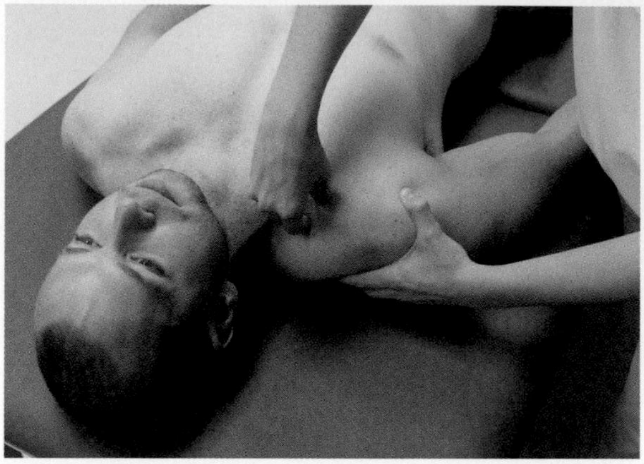

The distal portion of the clavicle is manipulated to determine the amount of inferior, superior, anterior, and posterior motion available at the acromioclavicular joint.

Patient Position	Seated or supine
Position of Examiner	Standing lateral to the patient, grasping the distal portion of the clavicle, just proximal to the AC joint. The opposite hand is stabilizing the acromion process via the scapula and scapular spine.
Evaluative Procedure	Apply a gliding pressure that forces the distal clavicle inferiorly, superiorly, anteriorly, and posteriorly relative to the scapula, noting pain or laxity elicited. The force should be directed perpendicular to the joint surfaces.

Clavicular Motion	Structures Stressed
Inferior	AC ligament (superior fibers)
Superior	Conoid ligament*
	Trapezoid ligament*
	AC ligament (inferior fibers)
Anterior	AC ligament
	Coracoclavicular ligament (in the absence of the AC ligament)
Posterior	Clavicle contacting acromion (posterior block)
	AC ligament
	*Portions of the coracoclavicular ligament

Positive Test	Pain, hypermobility, or hypomobility
Implications	Hypermobility: Laxity, sprain Hypomobility: Joint adhesions, osteophytes

AC = acromioclavicular

Joint Play 15-3
Glenohumeral Joint Play

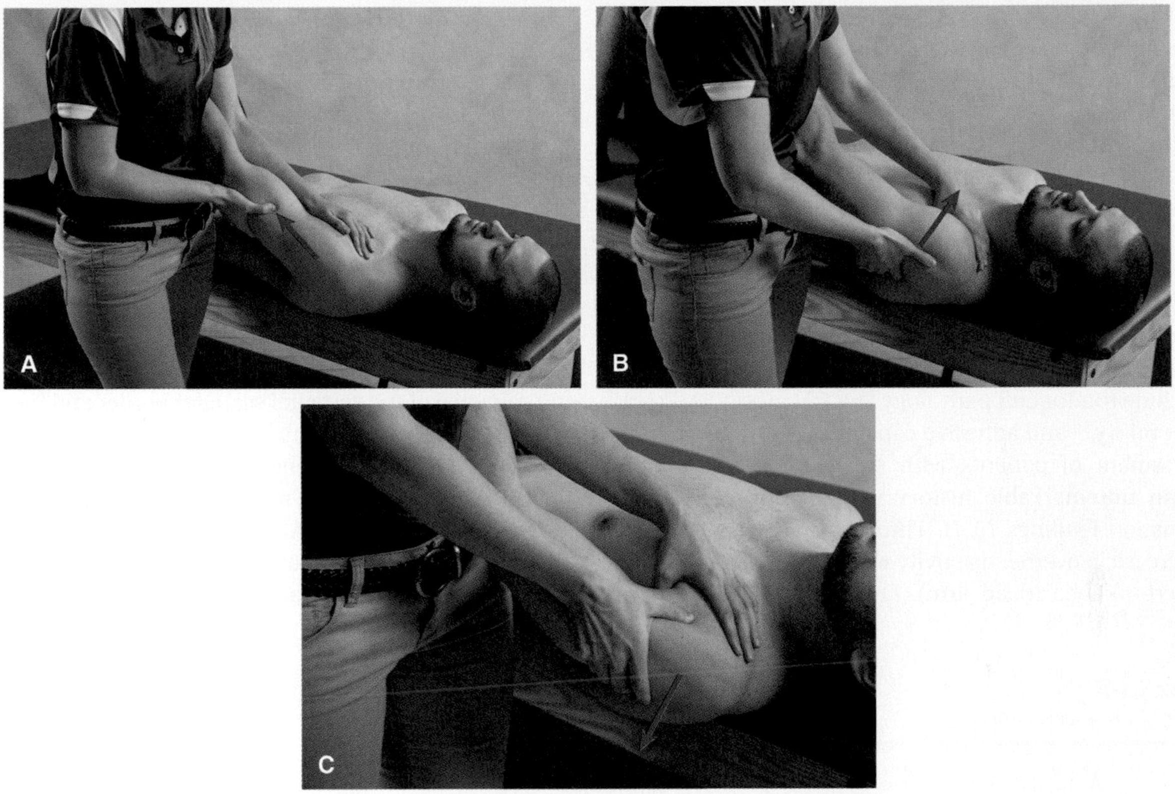

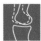

Glenohumeral joint play assesses the amount of mobility allowed by the joint capsule and ligaments.

Patient Position	Seated Place the patient's arm in the resting position (GH joint abducted to approximately 55° and flexed to approximately 30°). The examiner maintains the patient's arm in this position to assure relaxation.
Position of Examiner	*(A) Inferior glide:* One hand supports the arm to maintain the resting position. The opposite hand cups the superior aspect of the humerus. *(B) Anterior glide:* One hand stabilizes the scapula anteriorly by applying pressure to the coracoid process, reaching over the shoulder to the scapular body. The opposite hand applies force at the posterior aspect of the humerus. *(C) Posterior glide:* One hand stabilizes the scapula at the coracoid process and scapular body. The opposite hand applies force at the anterior aspect of the humeral head.
Evaluative Procedure	A gentle yet firm force is applied that distracts the joint (to take up the slack) and then moves the humeral head inferiorly, anteriorly, or posteriorly.
Positive Test	Pain, hypermobility, or hypomobility compared with the same direction on the opposite shoulder
Implications	Involvement of the static stabilizers of the GH joint: *(A)* Inferior: Inferior joint capsule, superior GH ligament, coracohumeral ligament *(B)* Anterior: Coracohumeral ligament, superior and middle GH ligaments, anterior joint capsule, labral tear *(C)* Posterior: Posterior joint capsule, labral tear
Modification	Stabilizing straps may be needed to achieve adequate scapular stabilization. Load and shift test: Center the humeral head in the fossa by applying an axial load while the patient's humerus is in 20° of abduction and 20° of forward flexion and the scapula is stabilized. Joint play is then assessed.
Comment	These results should be interpreted with caution and considered in light of the remaining exam because of the low interrater and intrarater reliability.[29] It is difficult to detect subtle changes (e.g., grade 0 and grade 1). The difference between the inferior glide joint play and the sulcus sign (see Selective Tissue Test 15-11) is that the sulcus sign is not performed in the resting position.

GH = glenohumeral

(Box 15-3). The scapula serves three basic roles: to provide a mobile and stable base for the humerus for GH mobility and stability, to position the glenoid fossa and acromial arch during humeral motion to avoid impingement, and to transfer kinetic energy between the upper extremity and the trunk. These roles are achieved by maintaining the humeral head centered within the glenoid fossa. Maintaining this relationship during humeral motion requires the scapulothoracic articulation to have adequate mobility, stability, and neuromuscular control.

Scapular dyskinesis describes poor scapular function, which may include abnormal motion, position, or stability. Dyskinesis is observed in patients with shoulder conditions that include rotator cuff pathology,[35-42] GH instability,[39,42-44] AC joint injury,[45] and adhesive capsulitis (Table 15-7).[46-49]

Assessment of patients with scapular dyskinesis may reveal an unremarkable history with an insidious onset (Examination Findings 15-1). Throwers may describe a recent increase in overhead activity with a loss of strength and poor performance (dead arm). Dyskinesis often becomes apparent during an assessment of associated GH or elbow pain. Pain may be localized over the coracoid process, pectoralis minor, superior and medial borders of the scapula, AC joint, posterior-lateral GH joint line, or subacromial space. Muscle spasm is often palpated or reported in the upper trapezius, posterior cervical, and levator scapulae musculature.

The assessment of scapular function begins with postural observation. Resting position of the scapula should be approximately 5 degrees of upward rotation, 40 degrees of internal rotation, and 15 degrees of anterior tilt. Abnormal position of the scapula often includes an excessively lower, protracted, and anteriorly tilted scapula (Fig. 15-28). The prominence of the vertebral scapular border and inferior angle may be secondary to thoracic kyphosis, cervical lordosis, scoliosis, a tight or shortened pectoralis minor or short head of the biceps, or posterior rotator cuff and capsular tightness.

Assessment of GH AROM and PROM may produce symptoms related to concurrent pathology. Measures of GH rotation and horizontal adduction may reveal a GIRD and

Box 15-3
Scapulothoracic Rhythm

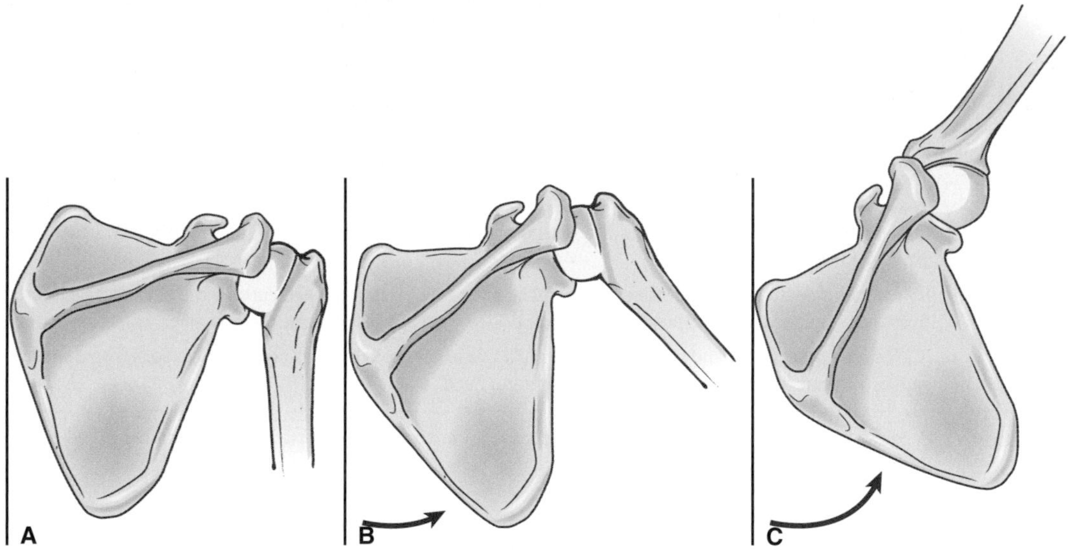

For the hand to obtain its maximal arc of motion, the GH and scapulothoracic articulations must combine their available ROMs. If the humeral head were rigidly fixated in the glenoid fossa in a manner eliminating GH movement, the humerus could still be elevated to 60 degrees through movement of the scapula via the AC and SC joints. For the humerus to be elevated to its maximum ROM of 180 degrees (relative to the thorax), the GH and scapulothoracic articulation must function together. Although a wide range of individual variability exists, an approximate 2:1 ratio is found between GH elevation and upward scapular rotation. For 180 degrees of humeral elevation to occur, 120 degrees is from GH movement, and 60 degrees is through upward rotation of the scapula.

The ratio of GH elevation to upward scapular rotation varies throughout humeral motion. Approximately the first 30 degrees of elevation is achieved primarily through GH motion, with the scapula setting (fixating) to provide stability for the contracting muscles. As humeral elevation reaches 90 degrees, the ratio between the GH joint and the scapula is approximately 1:1.[34] Towards full elevation, motion is again achieved primarily through the GH joint. Maintenance of this rhythm is based on the coordination of the prime movers of the humerus and the synergistic contractions of the scapular stabilizers.

Scapular dyskinesis An improperly moving scapula

Table 15-7 Association of Scapular Dyskinesis with Shoulder Pathologies

Pathology	Abnormal scapular function
Rotator cuff impingement/tear	The patient lacks scapular upward rotation, external rotation, and posterior tilt during arm elevation.[3,38,50]
	The scapular assistance test may decrease impingement symptoms.
	Manual scapular retraction may increase strength with the empty can test.[51]
	The relocation test may relieve symptoms of internal (posterior) impingement.
	Those with definite rotator cuff tears display increased upward rotation and lack posterior tilt.[50]
Superior labral lesion	The patient lacks scapular external rotation and posterior tilt during arm elevation.
	Manual scapular retraction may decrease symptoms during positive tests for superior labral lesions.[52]
AC sprain	Those with Type III-V AC sprains lack retraction at rest and during humeral elevation.[45]
GH MDI	The patient lacks scapular external rotation and posterior tilt during arm elevation.[53]
	Manual scapular retraction may increase strength with the empty can test.[51]

AC = acromioclavicular; GH = glenohumeral; MDI = multidirectional instability

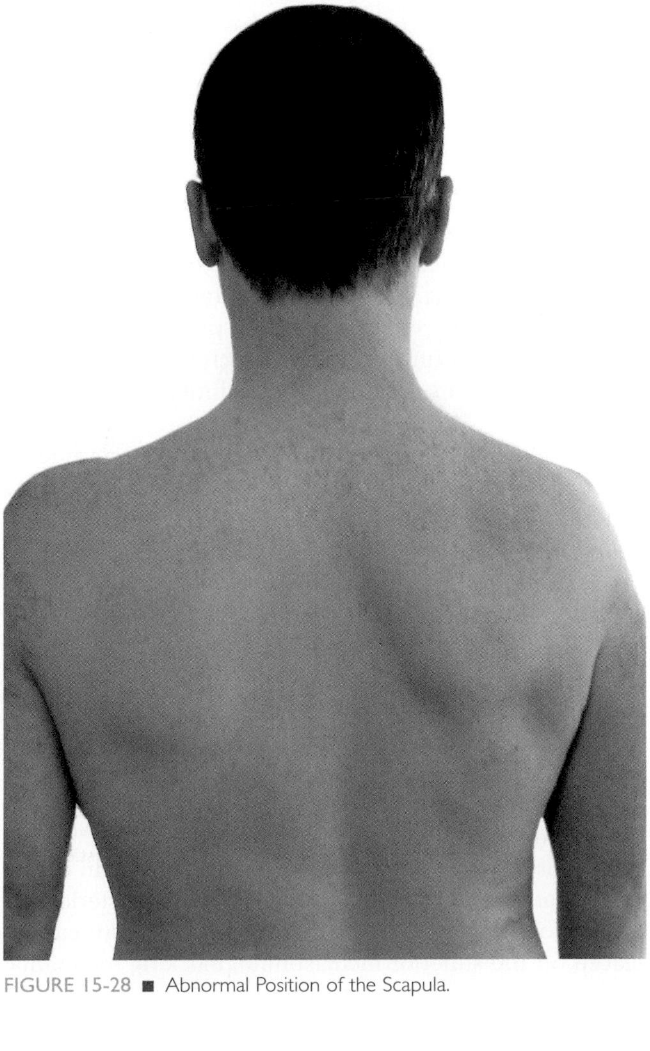

FIGURE 15-28 ■ Abnormal Position of the Scapula.

posterior shoulder tightness in overhead throwers. Manual muscle testing may suggest poor strength in the lower and middle trapezius, serratus anterior, or rotator cuff.

Assessment of Dynamic Scapular Function

Dynamic scapular function is assessed by standing behind the patient and observing multiple repetitions of bilateral forward humeral elevation and lowering in the sagittal plane and scapular plane (scaption) while holding 3- to 5-pound weights. Scapular motion is classified as abnormal (or dyskinetic) if there is obvious prominence of any aspect of the vertebral border or excessive upward translation (shrugging) in a majority of the repetitions. During forward humeral elevation, ideal scapular motion should include upward rotation and posterior tilting. The scapula should translate laterally and internally rotate slightly (protract) along the thorax as the humerus elevates to 90 degrees and then externally rotate and medially translate (retract) as the humerus continues to maximal elevation. These scapular motions should occur in reverse as the arm is lowered. To maintain the humeral head safely within the glenoid fossa during smooth and controlled repetitions of humeral elevation and lowering, the scapula should rotate with similar control and consistency. A lack of control or movement in any of these scapular motions may result in limited humeral motion, pain due to impingement, or a poor transfer of force through the kinetic chain.

Abnormal scapular internal rotation and posterior tilt may be observed during arm elevation as the vertebral scapular border and inferior angle lifting away from the thorax (scapular winging). The scapula fails to externally rotate and tilt posteriorly to retract the scapula during elevation above 90 degrees (Fig. 15-29). Abnormal scapular upward rotation is most often observed as a shrug during humeral elevation in an effort to elevate the acromion. Because asymmetry of scapular motion is observed in a large

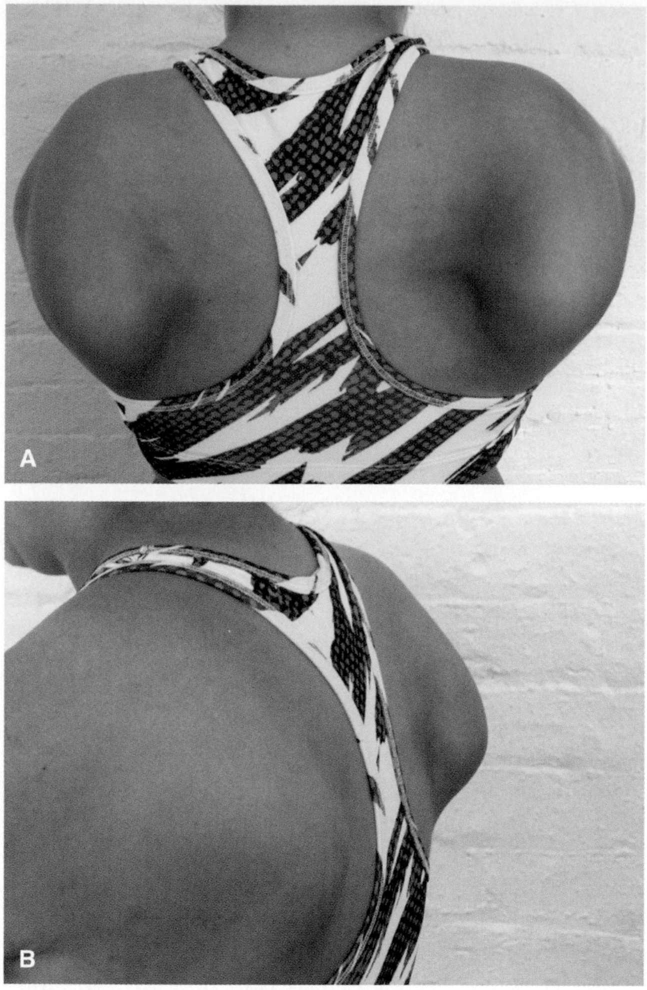

FIGURE 15-29 ■ Scapular winging. (A) Posterior view. (B) Oblique view. In the presence of a weakened serratus anterior muscle, or long thoracic nerve injury, performing a "push-up" against a wall causes the vertebral border of the scapula to lift off the thorax.

portion of asymptomatic individuals, the challenge is to recognize abnormal scapular function and correlate the observations with the symptoms presented.

Findings of abnormal scapular function should be followed by corrective maneuvers. These maneuvers may alter pathology-related symptoms and identify the role scapular dysfunction plays in the associated pathology or symptoms. A positive scapular assistance test (Selective Tissue Test 15-3) relieves symptoms produced during humeral elevation or improves upon the range of elevation.[54] This result suggests that poor scapular motion may have played a role in the associated pathology or symptoms and must be addressed in the management program. A positive scapular retraction test (Selective Tissue Test 15-4) is one in which applying manual stability and retraction improves strength or decreases symptoms.[54] This finding suggests that poor scapular stability failed to provide a stable base for the humerus. For these patients, management programs must aim to enhance scapular stability in retraction before addressing rotator cuff strength.

Scapulothoracic Articulation Intervention Strategies

Management of scapular dyskinesis varies depending on the levels of activity, dysfunction, and associated pathology. Patients with severe scapulothoracic dysfunction may need to discontinue aggravating activities until more normal control is restored. For other patients, the activity level may be maintained during management. Improving scapular function is a component of any comprehensive shoulder rehabilitation or conditioning program. Because the majority of force produced during overhead throwing is produced by the lower extremity, strength and stability of the legs, hips, and trunk must be assessed and established before addressing shoulder dysfunction.

Conservative treatment that focuses on correcting scapular dysfunction is very often able to return competitive overhead athletes to their preinjury level of performance within 4 months.[56] Patients must avoid aggravating motions or activity during early rehabilitation. Early treatment may include local modalities and manual therapy for pain, inflammation, and any spasms in the upper trapezius, posterior cervical, or levator scapulae musculature. Rehabilitation is founded on improving scapular position by increasing flexibility and establishing conscious appreciation and control of scapular position. Positive scapular assistance and/or retraction tests also help identify specific control deficits that must be addressed.

Sternoclavicular Joint Sprains

Injuries to the SC joint usually occur from indirect mechanisms such as falling on an outstretched arm or from an anterior or posterior force being placed on the lateral portion of the shoulder. Less frequently, traction forces, such as those experienced by gymnasts performing on the rings, high bar, or uneven bars in which the athlete is suspended by the arms, may disrupt the integrity of the joint capsule.

SC sprains are marked by pain during joint play movements. Protraction and retraction of the scapula can reproduce pain associated with ligamentous or disc damage. Functionally, patients suffering from SC sprains complain of pain with any shoulder movement that causes motion at the SC joint, particularly when the shoulders are compressed towards each other.

While dislocations can occur anteriorly, posteriorly, or superiorly, anterior dislocations are by far the most common and occur as a result of a posterior force to the clavicle, which results in the shoulder rolling backward.[8] Because of the rapid and extensive swelling associated with an SC joint dislocation, the direction of the dislocation may not be discernible via palpation.

Because of the potential threat to the subclavian artery, subclavian vein, trachea, and esophagus, posterior SC dislocations are a medical emergency.[4,8] Pressure can be placed on the superior mediastinum, blocking the cranial

Examination Findings 15-1
Scapular Dyskinesis

Examination Segment	Clinical Findings
History of Current Condition	*Onset:* Gradual; identified during examination for other pathology *Pain characteristics:* Localized over the coracoid process, pectoralis minor, superior and medial borders of the scapula, AC joint, posterior-lateral joint line or subacromial space; also possibly including the upper trapezius and posterior cervical musculature (secondary to trapezius spasm) *Risk factors:* The patient may describe a recent increase in overhead activity; dyskinesis may also be associated with other pathology.
Functional Assessment	Poor shoulder function during overhead activities with an associated loss of strength, power, or endurance
Inspection	Thoracic kyphosis, cervical lordosis, and/or scoliosis may be present. Dominant-side scapula may be positioned lower and more protracted than the nondominant arm at rest.
Palpation	May present with pain over the coracoid process, pectoralis minor, superior and medial borders of the scapula, posterior-lateral GH joint line or subacromial space, upper trapezius, and posterior cervical region
Joint and Muscle Function Assessment	*AROM:* Dysfunctional motion, position, or stability of the scapula observed during arm elevation or lowering. *MMT:* Decreased strength in lower and middle trapezius, serratus anterior; decrease in strength in rotator cuff secondary to the scapula failing to provide a stable base. Scapular retraction test may be positive. *PROM:* GH internal rotation deficit (GIRD) may be present in overhead throwers.
Joint Stability Tests	*Stress tests:* Not applicable *Joint play:* Joint play movements may reveal hypermobility of the AC, SC, or GH joint.
Selective Tissue Tests	Tests for rotator cuff impingement (subacromial or internal) or AC or labral pathology may be positive. Scapular assistance test may be positive.
Neurological Screening	Within normal limits
Vascular Screening	Symptoms resembling thoracic outlet syndrome may be reported.
Imaging Techniques	Within normal limits Typically, only suspicion of concurrent pathology warrants referral of these patients to a physician for imaging or assessment.
Differential Diagnosis	Cervical radiculopathy, suprascapular nerve syndrome, thoracic outlet syndrome, brachial plexus neuropathy/long thoracic nerve palsy

AC = acromioclavicular; AROM = active range of motion; GH = glenohumeral; MMT = manual muscle test; PROM = passive range of motion; SC = sternoclavicular

Selective Tissue Tests 15-3
Scapular Assistance Test

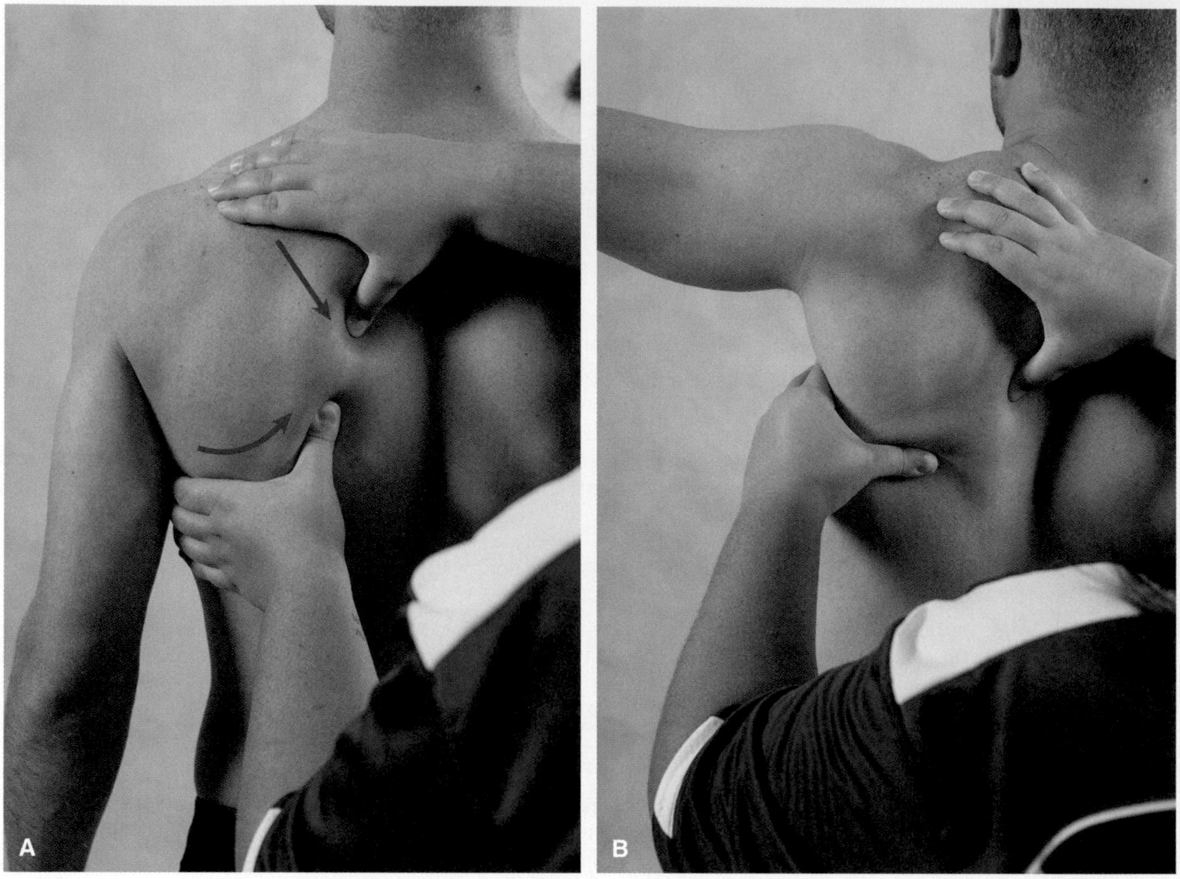

The scapular assistance test is a corrective maneuver designed to alter symptoms and identify the role of scapular dysfunction in the associated pathology.

Patient Position	Standing
Position of Examiner	Standing behind the involved side (A) One hand on the superior scapular border in position to assist the scapula with upward rotation, the other at the inferior angle in position to assist retraction (posterior tilt and external rotation)
Evaluative Procedure	(B) The patient elevates the humerus and any pain or limitation in motion is noted. Next, as the patient elevates the humerus, the examiner manually assists the scapula with retraction (posterior tilt and external rotation) and upward rotation.
Positive Test	The patient displays additional ROM or decreased symptoms.
Implications	Assisted scapular motion that improves ROM or symptoms suggests that poor scapular function may have played a role in the associated pathology or dysfunction and must be addressed in the management program.
Evidence	This test has good inter-rater reliability.[55]

Selective Tissue Tests 15-4
Scapular Retraction Test

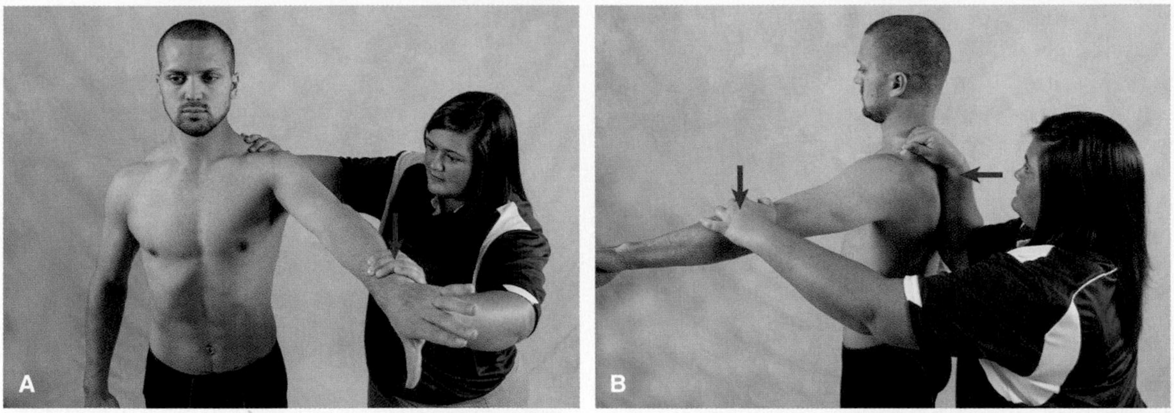

The scapular retraction test is a corrective maneuver designed to alter pathology-related symptoms and identify the role of scapular dysfunction in the associated pathology.

Patient Position	Standing
Position of Examiner	Standing behind the involved side
Evaluative Procedure	(A) The examiner performs a standard empty can manual muscle test for the supraspinatus, noting strength and symptoms. (B) The examiner places the scapula in a retracted position and provides manual stabilization with a forearm on the vertebral border and a hand on the superior border. The empty can test is repeated while maintaining the manual stabilization.
Positive Test	Supraspinatus strength is increased or symptoms diminished with manual stabilization.
Implications	Manual scapular stabilization and retraction that improves strength or symptoms suggests that poor scapular stability may have played a role in the associated pathology or dysfunction and must be addressed in the management program.
Comments	Manual scapular retraction may decrease symptoms during positive tests for superior labral lesions.[52] Manual scapular retraction may increase strength with the empty can test in patients with rotator cuff pathology or multi-directional glenohumeral instability.[51]
Evidence	Absent or inconclusive in the literature

vessels, trachea, and esophagus, producing dizziness, nausea, neurovascular symptoms in the upper extremity, dyspnea, and **dysphagia**. (Examination Findings 15-2).[57,58]

The clavicle's medial epiphysis does not completely fuse until approximately age 25. The signs and symptoms of a SC joint sprain or dislocation and those associated with an epiphyseal injury, a **pseudodislocation**, are similar; injuries to the growth plate must be ruled out in patients younger than 25 years old.[4,6] A definitive evaluation of the integrity of the SC joint can be made using CT. Plain radiographs often result in false-negative readings unless an oblique (serendipity) view is obtained.

SC Joint Sprain Therapeutic Interventions

The initial management of SC joint dislocations is closed reduction with the patient sedated.[59] An open reduction with concomitant joint stabilization is performed if the closed reduction fails. Early reduction is associated with improved outcomes.[59] Following a successful closed reduction, patients are managed with a period of immobilization in a figure-8 brace.

Treatment of mild and moderate SC joint sprains typically involves palliative measures to decrease the signs and symptoms of inflammation and allow the injury to heal. Ice and sling immobilization are used as necessary to decrease the traction on the joint. ROM for the cervical spine and upper extremity are incorporated initially. As the pain and swelling at the joint decrease, strengthening of the surrounding musculature is initiated with a progressive return to functional activities.

Acromioclavicular Joint Pathology

The AC joint can be injured acutely or become symptomatic as a result of repetitive stress or simple degeneration associated with aging. Acute injury to the AC joint occurs either directly or indirectly, with injury five times more common in men.[8] Commonly referred to as a "separated shoulder," a sprain of the AC ligament and/or the conoid and trapezoid segments of the coracoclavicular ligaments results in instability or dislocation of the joint. The more common direct force injury occurs when the person falls onto the acromion with the arm at the side. Indirect injury can occur when the person falls onto an outstretched arm, driving the humeral head into the acromion.[8] Classification of AC sprains is based on the structures involved, the degree of instability, and the direction in which the clavicle has been displaced relative to the acromion and coracoid process (Box 15-4).

Examination of patients with acute AC injuries reveals a history describing a direct or indirect mechanism (Examination Findings 15-3). Pain is primarily located over the superior anterior shoulder, anterolateral neck, and anterolateral deltoid.[60] On inspection, advanced sprains (Type II and above) normally result in noticeable displacement of the clavicle from the acromion process, creating a **step deformity** (Fig. 15-30). During palpation, the distal clavicle may depress and elevate, the **piano key sign,** indicating damage to the coracoclavicular ligament.

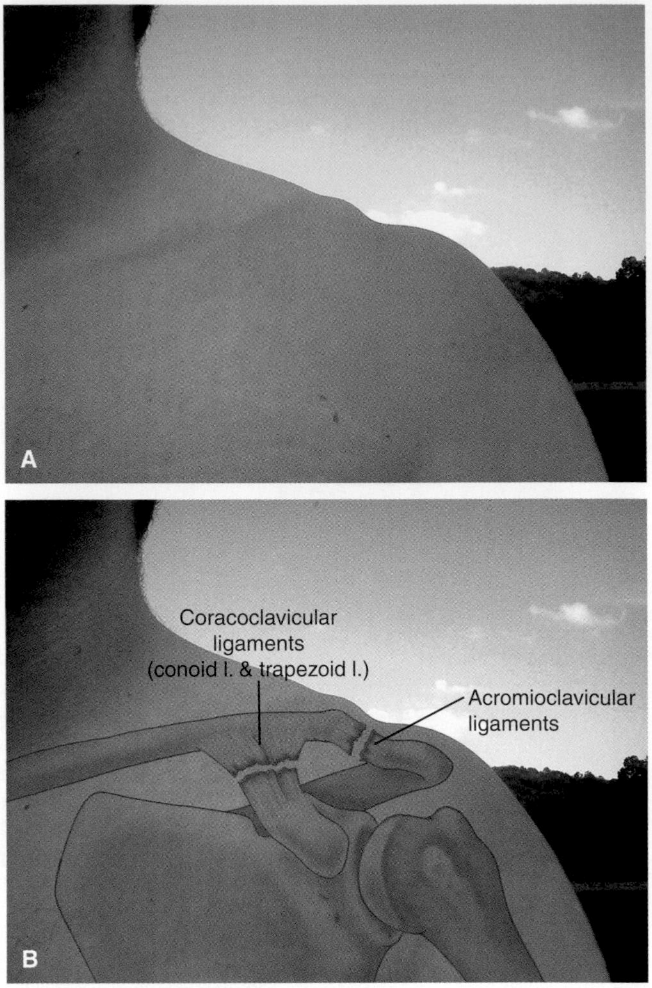

FIGURE 15-30 ■ Step deformity associated with an acromioclavicular joint sprain. (A) Gross inspection showing the rise in the distal clavicle. (B) Overlay showing the associated ligamentous trauma and associated structures. Depressing the distal clavicle and then releasing it results in the piano key sign.

Assessment of AROM and PROM produces pain on most movements, especially those occurring above 90 degrees and during the **Apley scratch test** (see Box 15-2). Passive and active horizontal adduction also elicit pain from the AC joint, especially at end-range, secondary to joint compression. The **acromioclavicular traction test** (Selective Tissue Test 15-5) reveals trauma to the coracoclavicular ligament, and the **AC compression test** (Selective Tissue Test 15-6) reproduces horizontal AC instability.

Patients displaying a hypermobile AC articulation should be referred to a physician for evaluation because, in some instances, fractures of the distal clavicle may clinically mimic a dislocation of the AC joint. The AC joint is best visualized radiographically with an oblique, or Zanca, view.[8,60] Stress radiographs can be used to differentiate between injuries that are isolated to the AC ligament and those that include the coracoclavicular ligament. Magnetic resonance imaging (MRI)

Dysphagia Difficulty with swallowing or the inability to swallow

Examination Findings 15-2
Sternoclavicular Joint Injury

Examination Segment	Clinical Findings
History of Current Condition	*Onset:* Acute *Pain characteristics:* Limited to the SC joint area *Other symptoms:* Pressure on the underlying neurovascular network can cause paresthesia in the upper extremity. Pressure on the esophagus and trachea may impede swallowing and breathing. *Mechanism:* Indirect force applied to the joint through the clavicle, such as falling on an outstretched arm, or anteriorly or posteriorly directed forces exerted on the anterolateral or posterolateral shoulder
Functional Assessment	Pain is increased with any shoulder motion that causes movement at the SC joint.
Inspection	Dislocations are marked by displacement of the clavicular head anteriorly, superiorly, or posteriorly. First- and second-degree sprains may present with localized swelling over the joint; discoloration may or may not be present. The patient's neck may be tilted toward the involved joint. Venous congestion of the involved arm, neck, and head may occur with posterior dislocation.
Palpation	Obvious joint displacement may be felt, although this finding is often obscured by swelling. Pain at the SC joint
Joint and Muscle Function Assessment	For first- and second-degree sprains, pain is elicited at any point after 90° of elevation, after which the ligamentous structures are maximally taut. Pain may be elicited during scapular protraction and retraction. *AROM:* Increased pain with flexion and abduction *MMT:* Isometric testing should not be painful. *PROM:* Increased pain with flexion, abduction, and horizontal adduction
Joint Stability Tests	*Stress tests:* Ligamentous tests should not be performed on obvious dislocations. *Joint play:* Joint play movements elicit pain for first-degree sprains; second- and third-degree sprains are marked by hypermobility.
Selective Tissue Tests	None
Neurological Screening	Within normal limits
Vascular Screening	Increased pain during early phases of elevation
Imaging Techniques	Anterior/posterior radiographs may be inconclusive; an oblique (serendipity) view will help visualize the displacement. CT is the imaging of choice.
Differential Diagnosis	Proximal clavicle fracture, sternal fracture, first rib fracture, medial clavicle epiphyseal injury, pneumothorax
Comments	Posterior SC dislocations are considered medical emergencies because of the potential threat to the underlying neurovascular structures, the esophagus, and trachea. Fractures of the medial one-third of the clavicle can produce a pseudodislocation. The medial end of the clavicle is the last long bone epiphysis to close.

AROM = active range of motion; CT = computed tomography; MMT = manual muscle test; PROM = passive range of motion; ROM = range of motion; SC = sternoclavicular

Box 15-4
Classification System for Acromioclavicular Joint Sprains

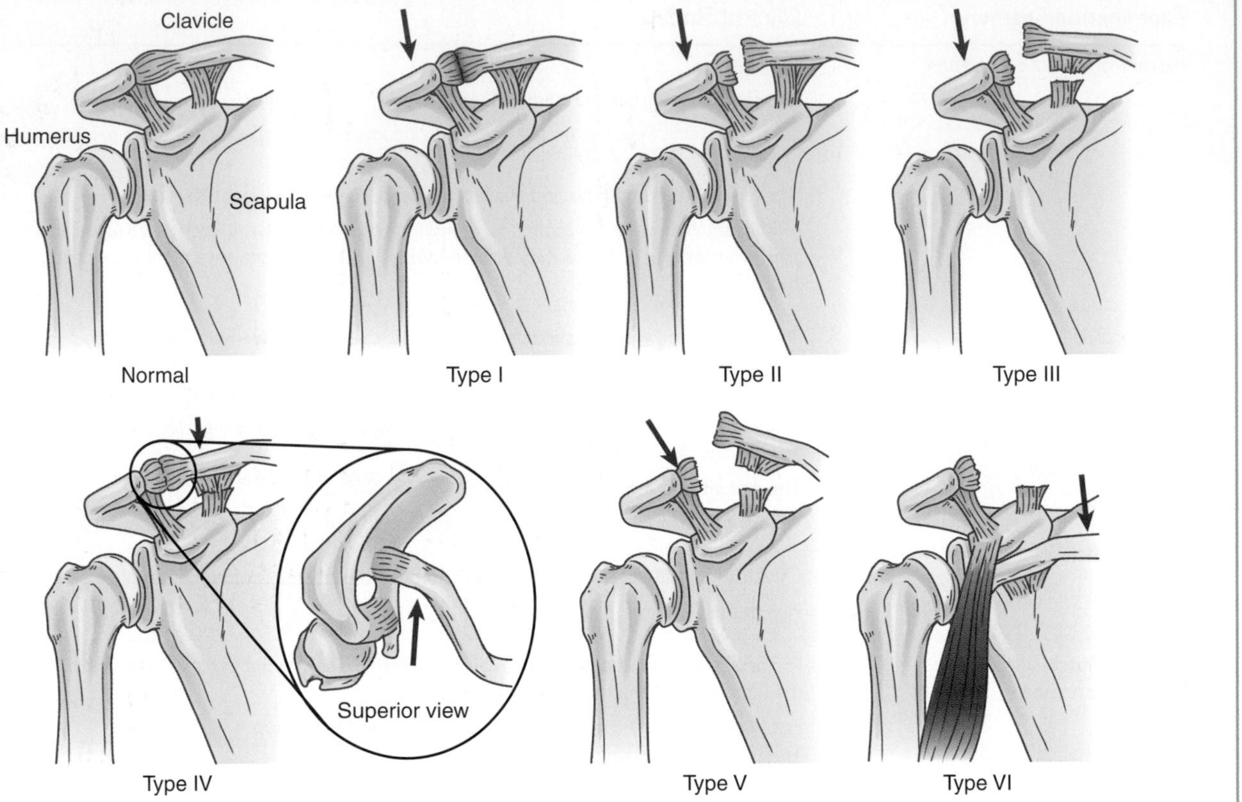

Grade	Structures Involved	Signs and Symptoms
Type I	Slight to partial damage of the AC ligament and capsule	Point tenderness over the AC joint; no laxity or deformity noted
Type II	Rupture of the AC ligament and partial damage to the coracoclavicular ligament	Slight laxity and deformity of the AC joint Slight step deformity
Type III	Complete tearing of the AC and coracoclavicular ligaments; possible involvement of the deltoid and trapezius fascia	Obvious dislocation of the distal end of the clavicle from the acromion process
Type IV	Complete tearing of the AC and coracoclavicular ligaments and tearing of the deltoid and trapezius fascia	Posterior clavicular displacement into the insertion of the upper fibers of the trapezius
Type V	Same as Type IV	Displacement of the involved clavicle from the acromion one to three times the height of the clavicle as compared with the opposite limb; clavicle posteriorly displaced with stripping away of the deltoid-trapezius aponeurosis
Type VI	Same as Type IV	Displacement of the clavicle inferiorly under the coracoid (possible involvement of the brachial plexus)

AC = acromioclavicular

Examination Findings 15-3
Acromioclavicular Joint Sprains

Examination Segment	Clinical Findings
History of Current Condition	*Onset:* Acute *Pain characteristics:* Superior anterior shoulder at the AC joint, anterolateral neck, and anterolateral deltoid *Mechanism:* Falling on the point of the shoulder, landing on the AC joint Force applied longitudinally to the clavicle, such as falling on an outstretched arm
Functional Assessment	Increased pain with overhead motions
Inspection	Displacement of the clavicle may be obvious. Step deformities indicate damage to the coracoclavicular ligament.
Palpation	Superior displacement of the clavicle that is reduced with manual pressure (piano key sign)
Joint and Muscle Function Assessment	*AROM:* Pain with elevation of the humerus and during protraction and retraction of the scapula *MMT:* Decreased strength secondary to pain for all muscles having attachment on the acromion or clavicle *PROM:* Pain produced during elevation of the humerus owing to movement at the AC joint; increased pain with horizontal adduction
Joint Stability Tests	*Stress tests:* Not applicable *Joint play:* Joint play movements reveal hypermobility of the AC joint.
Selective Tissue Tests	AC traction test, AC compression test
Neurological Screening	Within normal limits
Vascular Screening	Within normal limits
Imaging Techniques	AP radiograph to rule out associated clavicular or scapular fracture (primarily the coracoid process) and/or displacement between the acromion and clavicular Stress radiographs are rarely required to identify AC joint dislocations.
Differential Diagnosis	Distal clavicle fracture, scapular fracture (coracoid), rotator cuff pathology, SLAP lesions
Comments	Fractures of the distal clavicle may present with the clinical signs and symptoms of an acromioclavicular joint sprain.

AC = acromioclavicular; AP = anteroposterior; AROM = active range of motion; MMT = manual muscle test; PROM = passive range of motion; SLAP = superior labrum anterior to posterior

may be helpful to capture associated GH joint injury, which occurs in up to 30% of acute AC joint injuries.[62]

Chronic AC joint pain is more prevalent in those over the age of 50 and may be the result of a degenerative process within the articulation, previous injury, or aging. Its symptoms may be easily confused with rotator cuff symptoms and may result in, or be caused by, rotator cuff injuries.[63] Pain is produced when the arm is internally rotated or abducted, the AC joint is stressed, or when the GH joint is placed in the classic impingement position of forward flexion and abduction.[64] Pain arising from the AC joint can be differentiated from that arising from the subacromial structures by its location. AC joint pain is localized to the AC joint, while subacromial space pathology tends to cause pain in the deltoid region.[65] During chronic AC joint degeneration, many of the signs and symptoms of an acute AC joint injury are present, but there is no history of trauma to the AC joint. Although the joint may be painful on palpation, instability is not generally demonstrated. Radiographic examination may show degenerative changes within the joint's articulating space, although bone scans are more sensitive in detecting change.[61]

AC Joint Pathology Therapeutic Interventions

For patients suffering from grade I and II AC sprains and those with chronic joint degeneration, conservative management

Selective Tissue Tests 15-5
Acromioclavicular Traction Test

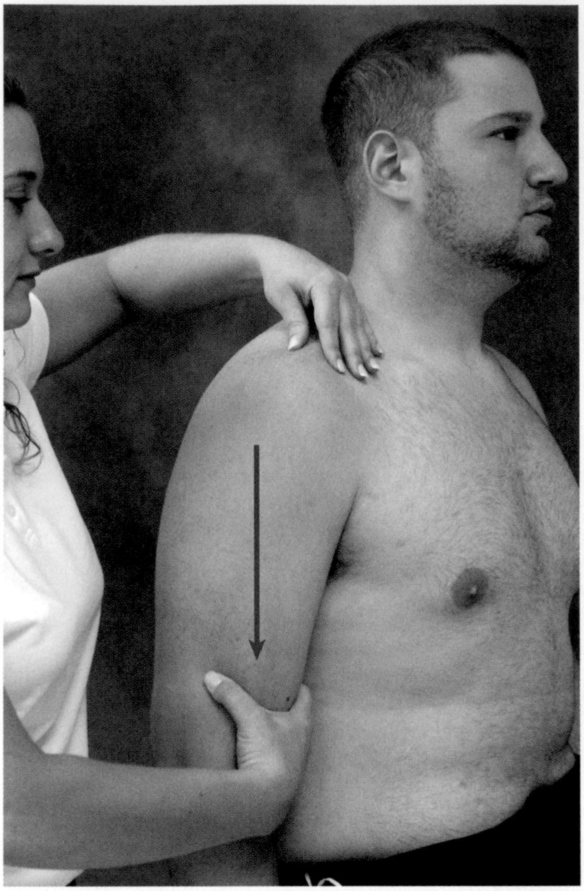

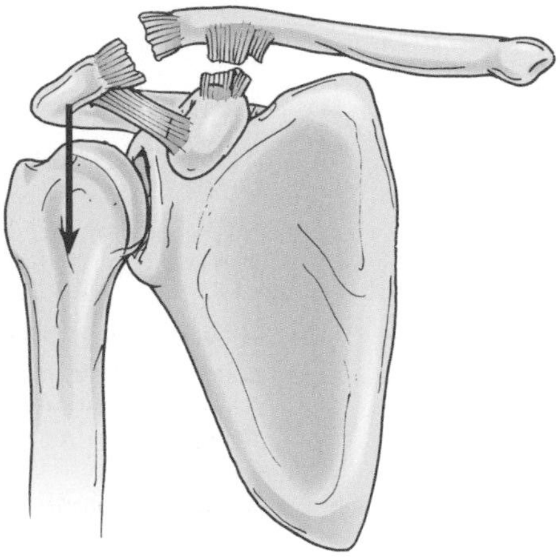

The principle behind the AC traction test is similar to a stress radiograph used to diagnose AC laxity.

Patient Position	Sitting or standing The arm hanging naturally from the side
Position of Examiner	Standing lateral to the involved side The clinician grasps the patient's humerus proximal to the elbow. The opposite hand gently palpates the AC joint.
Evaluative Procedure	The examiner applies a downward traction on the humerus.
Positive Test	The humerus and scapula move inferior to the clavicle, causing a step deformity, pain, or both.
Implications	Sprain of the AC or coracoclavicular ligaments (see Box 15-4 for grades).
Comments	Patients displaying positive AC traction test results should be referred to a physician for follow-up radiographic stress testing and to rule out a clavicular fracture.
Evidence	Absent or inconclusive in the literature

AC = acromioclavicular

Selective Tissue Tests 15-6
Acromioclavicular Compression Test

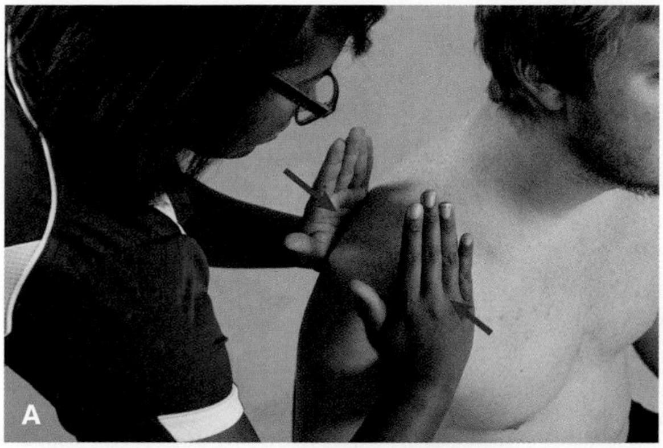

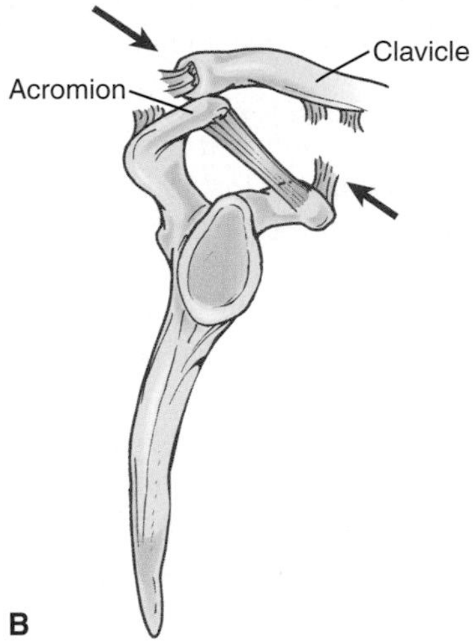

The AC compression test attempts to displace the clavicle from the acromion process, stressing the coracoclavicular and acromioclavicular ligaments. (A) Clinical technique. (B) Illustration demonstrating displacement of the clavicle relative to the acromion process.

Patient Position	Sitting or standing with the arm hanging naturally at the side
Position of Examiner	Standing on the involved side with the palm of one hand on the posterior acromion and the palm of the other hand on the anterior clavicle
Evaluative Procedure	The examiner squeezes the hands together, compressing the AC joint.
Positive Test	Pain at the AC joint or excursion of the clavicle over the acromion process
Implications	Damage to the AC ligament and possibly the coracoclavicular ligament
Modification	Place a thumb on the posterolateral aspect of the acromion process and the index and middle fingers of the same or opposite hand on the midpoint of the clavicle.[61] An anterosuperior force is applied with the thumb and an inferior force on the clavicle. A positive test is marked by pain.
Evidence	

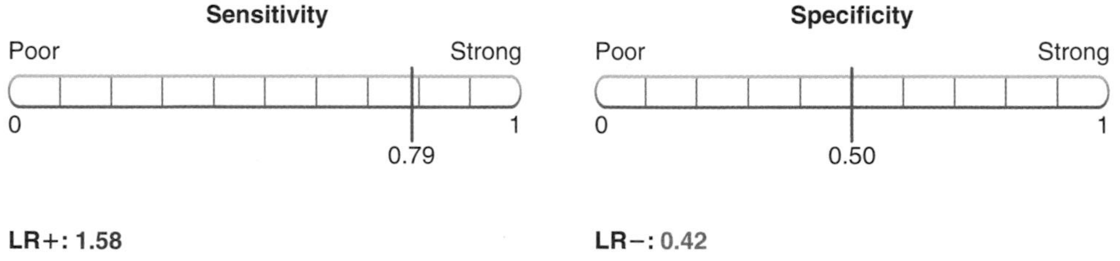

AC = acromioclavicular

is usually recommended. Conservative management for acute injuries consists of immobilization only as necessary for pain control and progressive increase in ROM and strengthening activities. Individuals with chronic joint pain are treated with symptomatic interventions such as nonsteroidal antiinflammatory medications and strengthening exercises focusing on scapular stability. Ultrasound-guided local corticosteroid injections can provide short-term relief of symptoms, but they do not alter the long-term progression of the condition.[66,67]

For patients with Type III and higher AC joint injuries, surgical or conservative management is used, with the decision made on a case-by-case basis depending on the patient's desired type and level of activity. Conservative management consists of a short period of immobilization for pain control followed by early ROM and strengthening exercises. Surgical intervention for Type III injuries may follow if symptoms persist; however, long-term outcomes are similar between those treated operatively and those treated nonoperatively.[8]

Glenohumeral Instability

The GH joint may present with instability anteriorly, posteriorly, inferiorly, or in multiple planes. It is the result of ligamentous or labral pathology, capsular instability, or muscular weakness. The severity of the laxity is graded based on **joint play movements**, the relative displacement of the humeral head on the glenoid fossa.

The primary passive supports of the GH joint have been described as being the GH ligaments, the joint capsule, and the coracohumeral ligament, which provide stability, limit the extremes of motion, and align the humeral head during movement.[68] These passive restraints are augmented by the rotator cuff and other GH musculature to provide coordinated motion of the shoulder complex. Because of the close relationship between the passive and dynamic stabilizers, dynamic compensation can mask GH instability (Table 15-8).[69]

Anterior Instability

Anterior instability is the result of laxity of the anterior stabilizing structures such as the middle GH ligament and, more specifically, the anterior band of the inferior GH ligament.[68] Instability can be acquired through repetitive overload or following an acute episode of subluxation or dislocation. Laxity of the superior and middle GH ligaments, large tears or weakness of the rotator cuff musculature, and dysfunction of the LHBT may also contribute to anterior GH instability.[70] The rotator interval, located in the anterior capsule at the anterior border of the supraspinatus and the superior border of the subscapularis, is a potential area of capsular weakness leading to instability.[71]

Nontraumatic Anterior Instability

Repetitive throwing creates an anterior shear force across the GH joint that may lead to stretching of the static structures and a resulting increased demand on dynamic stabilization via the GH and scapular stabilizing musculature. As throwing continues, dynamic stabilization is insufficient, and symptoms of weakness and instability result. Impingement is a common consequence of this excessive mobility (see Rotator Cuff Pathology, p. 664).

Examination techniques are designed to provoke or alleviate pain and/or the sensation of instability. Passive external rotation of the humerus must be performed with caution, especially when the shoulder is in 90 degrees of flexion as this replicates the **apprehension test for anterior instability** (Selective Tissue Test 15-7). Positive apprehension test results are followed up with the **relocation test for anterior instability** (Selective Tissue Test 15-8), in which posteriorly directed manual pressure is applied on the anterior humeral head to add external stability. The **anterior release (surprise) test** can be performed following the relocation test and is performed by suddenly releasing the posterior pressure applied during the relocation test. The anterior release test should not be performed if gross instability (i.e., subluxation or dislocation) is evident during the apprehension and relocation tests.

> *** Practical Evidence**
>
> Positive findings on any two of the apprehension, relocation, and anterior release ("surprise") tests are highly predictive of anterior instability.[72-74]

Traumatic Anterior Instability

The GH joint typically dislocates in an anterior direction following excessive external rotation and abduction of the humerus. The patient may describe the episode as the shoulder going out and relocating, or the joint may stay displaced. Management of acute GH dislocation is described in the On-Field Management section. Dislocation can damage static, dynamic, neurological, and vascular structures and often leads to residual instability or risk of repeat injury. The inferior GH ligament may be avulsed from the labrum or may be avulsed along with a portion of the labrum, forming a **Bankart lesion**. Bankart lesions are difficult to identify clinically, with the primary complaints being pain or a sensation of instability as the humeral head moves against the anterior labrum during GH joint play assessment, load and shift testing, or external rotation of the humerus. The axillary nerve can be stretched as it crosses the anterior joint, and patients may report paresthesia at the lateral upper arm following dislocation. A Hill-Sachs lesion, a bony defect of the posterior humeral head, can occur as the humeral head shears over the glenoid rim (Fig. 15-31). In patients who report that the shoulder dislocated but spontaneously relocated, the lesion may be present on radiographic examination. The lesion itself is rarely symptomatic but may lead to early degeneration of the GH joint.

Following an acute injury, selective tissue tests for anterior GH instability may be helpful in determining whether or not the joint dislocated and spontaneously reduced. These tests are not necessary following a known episode of dislocation.

Anterior Instability Intervention Strategies

Nontraumatic anterior instability is usually managed nonoperatively unless a mechanical explanation such as a torn labrum is discovered. Whether or not to surgically restore stability following anterior dislocation depends on multiple factors including the patient's desired level of activity and age. Conservative management consists of a brief period of immobilization for pain control followed by a gradual strengthening program focusing on maintaining solid scapular position by strengthening the anterior dynamic stabilizers.

Table 15-8 Differential Findings of Chronic Glenohumeral Instability

	Anterior Instability	Posterior Instability	Multidirectional Instability
Onset	Insidious	Chronic	Insidious or chronic
Functional Limitations	Diffuse ache during ADLs along with the unstable sensation when brought into abduction with external rotation	Diffuse ache during ADLs; the patient reports that the shoulder feels unstable when it is brought across the body or when loaded posteriorly, such as during a push-up or bench press.	Pain in the shoulder that increases with ADLs; the patient reports decreased athletic performance and nonspecific pain with activity.
Mechanism	A specific mechanism of injury may be described, but chronic anterior instability is often caused by repetitive microtrauma involving external rotation when the GH joint is abducted to 90°.	Patient may describe a specific mechanism of injury, but chronic posterior instability is generally caused by repetitive microtrauma involving longitudinal force on the length of the humerus while internally rotated and the GH joint flexed to 90° and horizontally adducted.	Congenital or acquired from repetitive overhead activity.[69] A sensation of instability may be described during the midrange of motion.
Inspection	A flattened deltoid is possible as chronic cases can cause atrophy of the deltoid muscle group and the scapular muscles. Possible atrophy of the rotator cuff muscles	Chronic cases can cause atrophy of the deltoid muscle group, rotator cuff muscles, and scapular muscles.	Chronic cases can cause atrophy of the deltoid muscle group and the scapular muscles.
Palpation	Tenderness of the anterior GH joint	Tenderness of the posterior GH joint	Tenderness in the anterior GH joint
Joint and Muscle Function Assessment			
AROM	Decreased external rotation secondary to sensation of instability and/or pain	Decreased internal rotation	Possible limitation at the end-ranges of motion secondary to a sensation of instability
MMT	Pain and weakness when assessing external rotation	Pain and weakness when assessing internal rotation	Pain and weakness when assessing internal and external rotation
PROM	Decreased external rotation secondary to sensation of instability and/or pain	Decreased internal rotation	Limited end-range due to pain and instability
Stress Tests/Joint Play	Increased anterior glide, although it may not appear increased to the contralateral side due to the bilateral nature of instability in chronic cases	Increased posterior glide, although it may not appear increased to the contralateral side due to the bilateral nature of instability in chronic cases	Increased glide in all directions
Selective Tissue Tests	Apprehension, relocation, and surprise tests	Posterior apprehension test; test for posterior instability in the plane of the scapula Jerk test	Apprehension test; Relocation test; Posterior apprehension test; Test for posterior instability in the plane of the scapula; positive sulcus sign
Comments	Chronic cases may have a predisposition to bilateral involvement. Chronic atraumatic instability usually occurs in patients younger than 30 years old.	Chronic cases may have a predisposition to bilateral involvement. Chronic atraumatic instability usually occurs in patients younger than 30 years old.	Chronic cases may have a predisposition to bilateral involvement. Multidirectional instability usually manifests itself in patients younger than 30 years old.

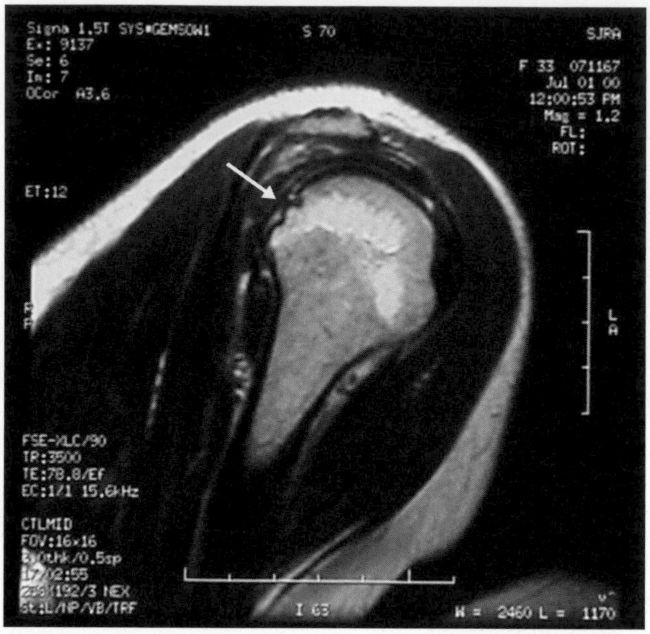

FIGURE 15-31 ■ An MRI of a Hill–Sachs lesion.

Because repeated dislocations can increase soft tissue and bony injury and the high frequency of repeat dislocations for some groups, surgery following initial dislocation is commonly recommended. In young males, the recurrence rate of anterior dislocations is between 80% and 90%, especially when a Bankart lesion is present.[77,78] Surgery to repair the Bankart lesion and augment the GH ligaments is associated with a return to the patient's desired level of function.[78]

*** Practical Evidence**

The rate of reoccurrence for anterior dislocations varies by age: 15 to 25 years old = 80% to 90%; 25 to 40 years old = 20% to 30%; >40 years old = 10% to 15%.[78]

Posterior Instability

Like anterior GH instability, posterior GH instability can result from repetitive injury or as a result of an acute, dislocating episode. Acutely, this type of instability most often occurs when the humerus is flexed and internally rotated while a longitudinal posterior force is placed through the arm. Repetitive forces that force the humeral head posteriorly such as blocking during football and forces that distract the posterior GH joint surfaces, such as the follow-through during throwing, can create instability. Weakness or fatigue of the subscapularis and infraspinatus can magnify symptoms when their ability to stabilize is reduced.

Patients with posterior instability complain of pain with maneuvers that require horizontal adduction, such as the follow-through phase of throwing and positions that load the posterior joint, such as during the bench press.[79,80] The **posterior apprehension test** (Selective Tissue Test 15-9) and **jerk test** (Selective Tissue Test 15-10) are used to evaluate posterior GH instability. The jerk test (posterior stress test) is used to detect posteroinferior instability of the GH joint by applying an axial load to the humerus as it is horizontally adducted. A clunk that is either painful or pain free will occur as the head of the humerus slides off the fossa. A painless clunk is associated with instability, while a painful clunk is associated with a labral tear.[79,81]

Acute Posterior Dislocation

Although they account for only about 3% of all GH dislocations, posterior GH dislocations are difficult to diagnose, likely because of the relatively high frequency of associated proximal humeral fracture.[82] Following a suspicious mechanism of a posteriorly directed force with the humerus flexed and adducted, inspection will reveal a prominent coracoid process on the involved side, and the patient will be unable to externally rotate the joint.[82] Following a subluxation, provocative tests such as the posterior apprehension test and jerk test may provide further evidence of the underlying condition.

Posterior Instability Intervention Strategies

Conservative treatment is generally the first line of intervention for those with posterior instability. Rehabilitation emphasizes restoration strength and endurance of the infraspinatus muscle. Surgical intervention is considered when a specific structural pathology such as a posterior labral tear is detected.[80,82]

Inferior/Multidirectional Instability

The primary restraint against inferior translation of the GH joint depends on the position of the humerus. In the neutral position, the primary restraint against inferior translation is the superior GH ligament, with little or no assistance provided by the coracohumeral ligament. When the humerus is abducted to 45 degrees in neutral rotation, the anterior portion of the inferior GH ligament is the primary restraint; this position also permits the greatest amount of translation. After further abducting the humerus to 90 degrees, the entire inferior GH ligament is responsible for restricting inferior displacement, but the posterior band is perhaps the most important restraint.[83] The presence of rotator cuff tears or weakness also increases inferior GH laxity.[84] Superior translation of the humeral head is limited by the presence of the coracoacromial arch and the acromion process.

Multidirectional instabilities (MDIs) are a combination of two or more unidirectional instabilities. The etiology of the MDI is important to determine for the correct intervention. The patient with a congenital MDI will present with generalized hyperlaxity of the shoulders and other joints and have no history of trauma. Those with acquired MDI typically participate in overhead activities that impose repetitive microtrauma. These individuals are symptomatic with their activities and present with less laxity than those

Selective Tissue Tests 15-7
Apprehension Test for Anterior Glenohumeral Laxity

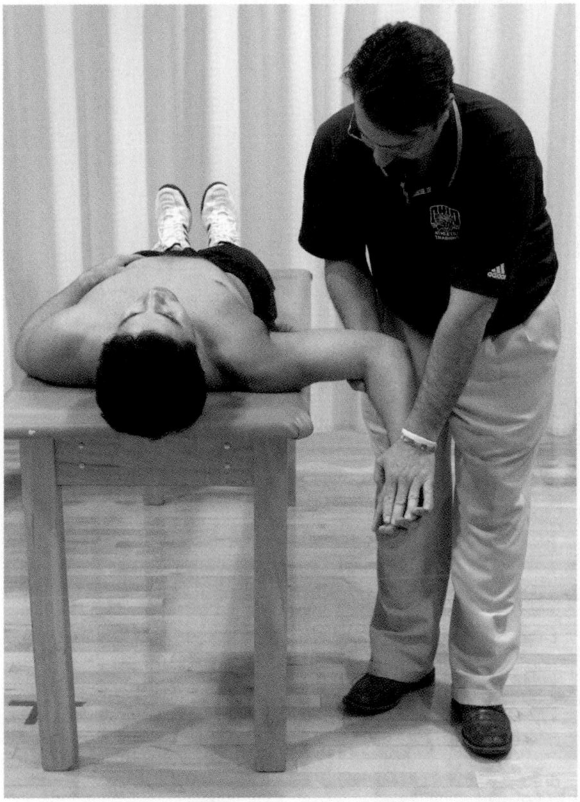

The apprehension test, passive external rotation of the GH joint, places the joint in the closed-pack position and replicates the mechanism of injury for anterior GH dislocations.

Patient Position	Supine, standing, or sitting The GH joint is abducted to 90°, and the elbow is flexed to 90°.
Position of Examiner	Positioned in front of or beside the patient on the involved side The examiner supports the humerus at midshaft while grasping the forearm proximal to the wrist.
Evaluative Procedure	While supporting the humerus at 90° abduction, the examiner passively externally rotates the GH joint by slowly applying pressure to the anterior forearm.
Positive Test	The patient displays apprehension that the shoulder may dislocate and resists further movement. Pain is centered in the anterior capsule of the GH joint.
Implications	The anterior capsule, inferior GH ligament, or glenoid labrum have been compromised, allowing the humeral head to dislocate or subluxate anteriorly on the glenoid fossa. Apprehension coupled with pain is often associated with instability secondary to rotator cuff pathology.[18] Pain in the deep posterior shoulder may be associated with internal impingement.[18]
Comments	Pressure should be applied gradually and the test terminated at the first sign of apprehension. Do not perform this test when there is obvious dislocation or subluxation of the GH joint. The relocation test is usually performed following a positive apprehension test (see Selective Tissue Test 15-8).
Evidence	

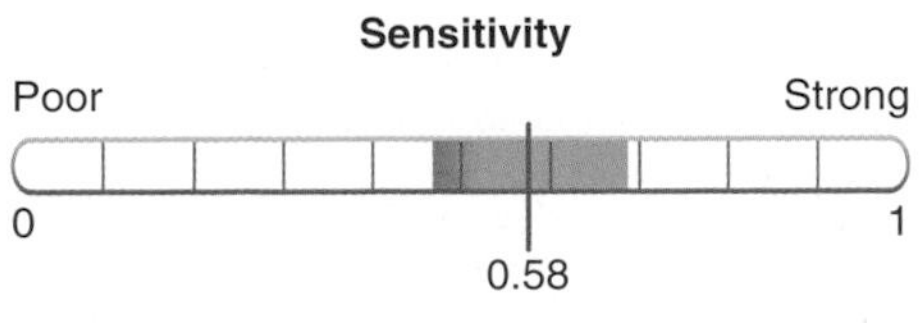

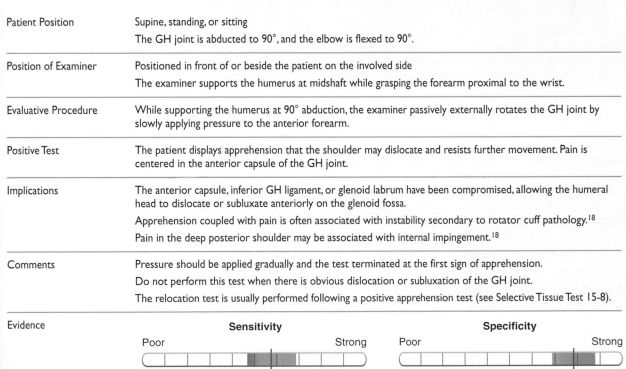

LR+: 1.60–8.85–16.10

LR−: 0.40–0.57–0.75

GH = glenohumeral

Selective Tissue Tests 15-8

Relocation and Anterior Release Tests for Anterior Glenohumeral Laxity

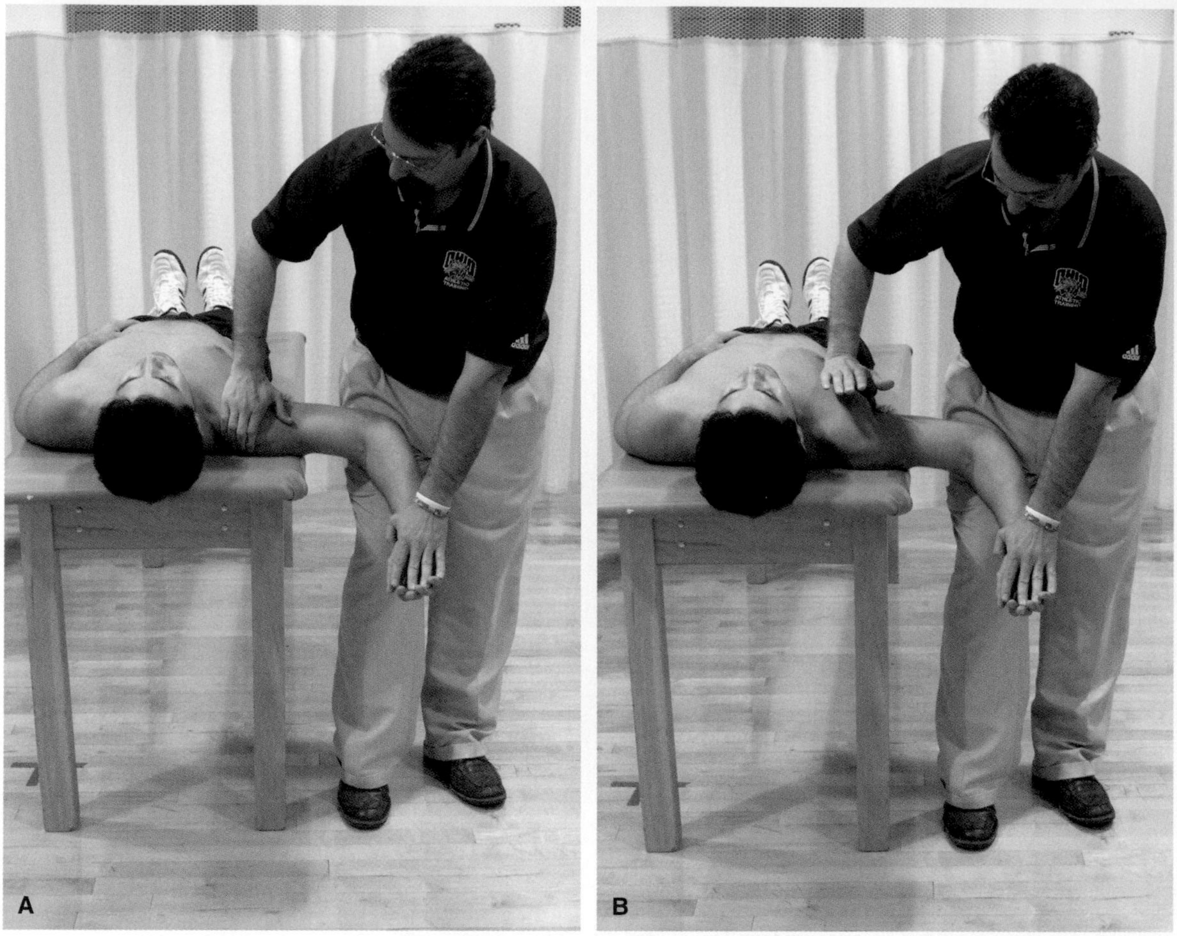

Performed after a positive apprehension test (see Selective Tissue Test 15-7), the relocation test uses manual pressure to maintain alignment and stability of the GH joint as it moves into external rotation (A). The anterior release test determines apprehension when the pressure applied during the apprehension test is suddenly released (B). The anterior release test, also known as the surprise test, should be performed with caution.

Patient Position	Supine The GH joint is abducted to 90°. The elbow is flexed to 90°.
Position of Examiner	Standing beside the patient, inferior to the humerus on the involved side The forearm is grasped proximal to the wrist to provide leverage during external rotation of the humerus. The opposite hand is held over the humeral head.
Evaluative Procedure	*(A) Relocation test:* With the patient's arm in the original position, the examiner applies a posterior force to the head of the humerus and maintains that force while externally rotating the humerus. *(B) Anterior release test ("Surprise!" test):* With the GH in external rotation during the relocation test, the examiner removes the hand applying the posterior pressure.
Positive Test	*Relocation test:* Decreased pain or increased ROM (or both) compared with the anterior apprehension test *Anterior release test:* Apprehension and/or pain when the anterior stabilizing pressure from the relocation test is removed
Implications	*Relocation test:* A positive test result supports the conclusion of increased laxity in the anterior capsule owing to capsular damage or labrum tears. The manual pressure applied by the examiner increases the stability of the anterior portion of the GH capsule, allowing more external rotation to occur. *Anterior release test:* By its nature, the anterior release test reproduces the apprehension test. Its clinical use is not recommended.

Selective Tissue Tests 15-8
Relocation and Anterior Release Tests for Anterior Glenohumeral Laxity—cont'd

Comments

The relocation test is usually performed after a positive anterior apprehension test. The anterior release test is usually performed after a positive relocation test.

The apprehension test and the relocation test may also be positive in the presence of internal impingement.

Positive findings with the relocation test (e.g., pain reduction) may also be associated with a SLAP lesion, as tension on the disrupted LHBT is reduced.[75,76]

The relocation test adds little predictive value in detecting anterior shoulder instability. It has more predictive value when the posterior force reduces the feeling of apprehension rather than pain.

Evidence

Relocation Test (Anterior Instability)

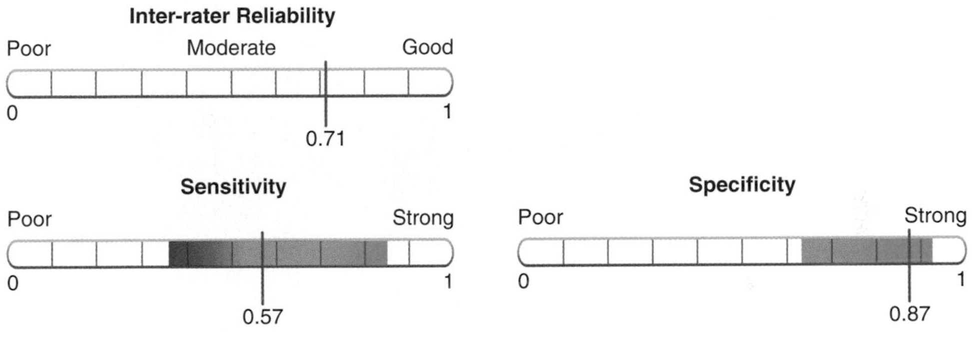

LR+: 1.00–4.50–7.44 **LR−: 0.17–0.43–1.00**

Relocation Test (SLAP Lesion)

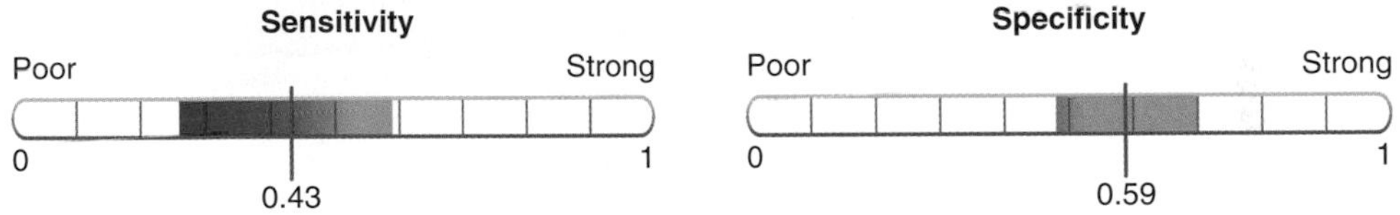

LR+: 0.68–1.13–1.58 **LR−: 0.53–1.11–1.68**

Anterior Release (Anterior Instability)

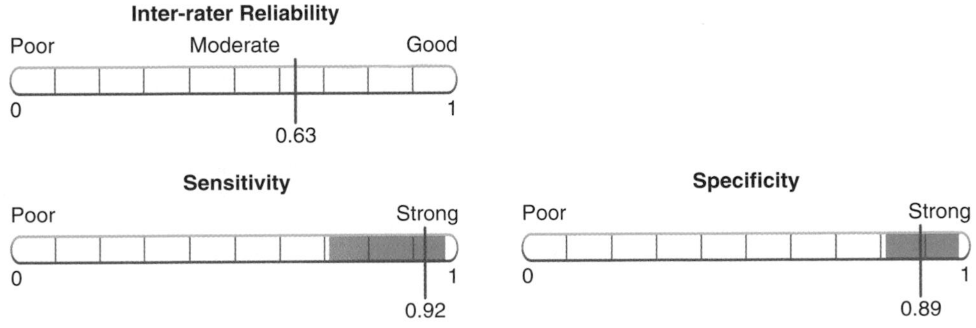

LR+: 5.43–8.36–11.29 **LR−: 0.05–0.09–0.29**

GH = glenohumeral; ROM = range of motion; LHBT = long head of the biceps tendon; SLAP = superior labrum anterior to posterior

Selective Tissue Tests 15-9
Posterior Apprehension Test for Glenohumeral Laxity

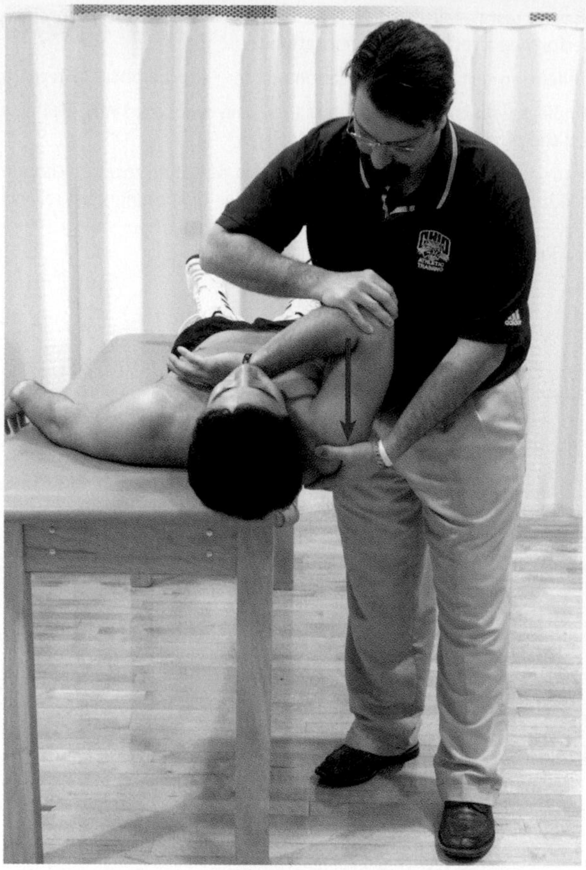

The humeral head is moved posteriorly on the glenoid fossa. In the presence of posterior GH laxity or instability, the patient will be apprehensive and guard against the test.

Patient Position	Sitting or supine The shoulder is flexed to 90°, and the elbow is flexed to 90°. The GH joint being tested is off to the side of the table.
Position of Examiner	Standing on the involved side One hand grasps the forearm. The opposite hand stabilizes the posterior scapula.
Evaluative Procedure	The examiner applies a longitudinal force to the humeral shaft, forcing the humeral head to move posteriorly on the glenoid fossa. The examiner may choose to alter the amount of flexion and rotation of the humerus.
Positive Test	The patient displays apprehension and produces muscle guarding to prevent the shoulder from subluxating posteriorly.
Implications	Laxity in the posterior GH capsule, torn posterior labrum
Modification	The Jerk test is a modification of the Posterior Apprehension Test (see Selective Tissue Test 10-15).
Evidence	

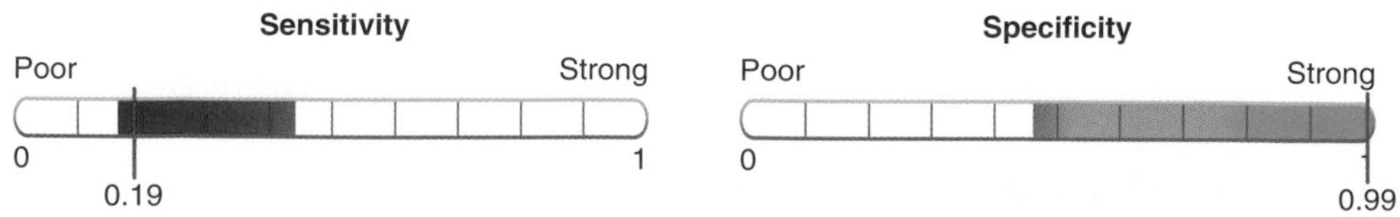

LR+: 0.37–7.36–21.50

LR−: 0.62–0.95–1.84

GH = glenohumeral

Selective Tissue Tests 15-10
Jerk (Posterior Stress) Test for Labral Tears

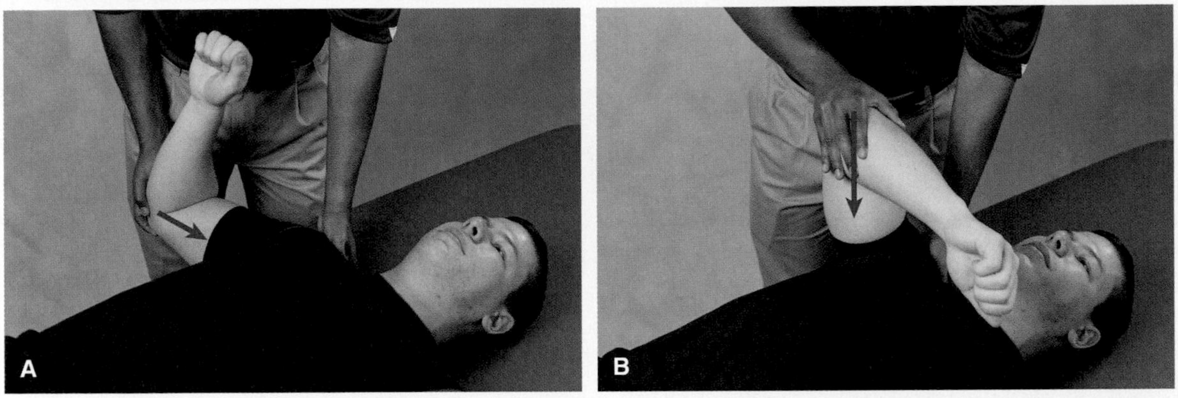

A posterior force is applied to the GH joint. Pain is associated with posteroinferior instability; a clunk is associated with a tear of the glenoid labrum.

Patient Position	Supine or seated. The supine position provides better scapular stabilization.
Position of Examiner	Behind the patient One hand stabilizes the scapula. The opposite hand holds the affected arm at 90° of flexion and internal rotation and applies an axial load to the humerus **(A)**.
Evaluative Procedure	The affected arm is passively horizontally adducted while the examiner maintains the axial load to the humerus **(B)**.
Positive Test	Clunk that may or may not be painful
Implications	Posteroinferior instability with or without posteroinferior labral tear
Comments	A painful clunk is frequently associated with a posteroinferior labral tear that must be surgically repaired. Patients with a painless clunk respond well to nonsurgical treatment.[79]
Evidence	

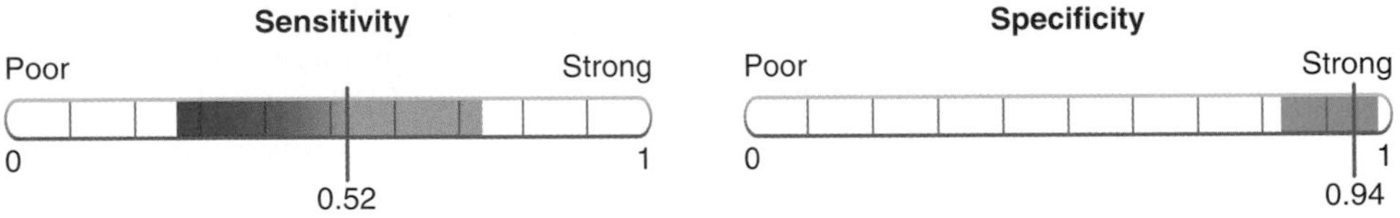

LR+: 1.71–19.80–36.50

LR−: 0.28–0.53–0.90

with congenital MDI. Evaluation of shoulder instability must be performed carefully to differentiate between unidirectional and multidirectional instabilities.

The **sulcus sign** is used to identify the presence of multidirectional instability (Selective Tissue Test 15-11). If the shoulder demonstrates laxity in the neutral position, it can be assumed to be lax in all positions. A positive sulcus sign with the humerus flexed to 90 degrees may indicate inferior instability.

Multidirectional Instability Intervention Strategies

Treatment of only one of the unidirectional instabilities in the presence of a multidirectional instability can worsen the condition because only one aspect of the joint is reinforced, potentially increasing the chance of instability in the other involved planes. MDI is generally managed conservatively with an emphasis on retraining and strengthening the scapular stabilizers and rotator cuff. Those with acquired MDI who can compensate by avoiding positions that recreate their instability are most likely to benefit from surgical stabilization.[69]

Rotator Cuff Pathology

The space between the superior GH joint and the coracoacromial ligament is occupied by the supraspinatus and infraspinatus tendons, the subacromial bursa, the superior capsule, the labrum, and the long head of the biceps. A cause-and-effect relationship exists between pathology of any or all of these structures and encroachment, or impingement, in this space. Impingement is characterized as being external (or in the subacromial space) or internal (between the humeral head and the glenoid) (Table 15-9).

Subacromial Impingement

Subacromial, or external, impingement of the rotator cuff muscles occurs when there is decreased space through which the rotator cuff tendons pass under the coracoacromial arch. In its initial stages, the impingement often results in the inflammation of the rotator cuff tendons. Likewise, inflammation of the rotator cuff tendons results in the enlargement of the tendons, decreasing the subacromial space and increasing the likelihood of impinging the tendons (see Table 15-9). This sequence of events creates a closed cycle in which one condition exacerbates the other. When allowed to proceed unchecked, the ultimate outcome is a shoulder with greatly diminished function. To athletes participating in overhead sports or workers who perform repetitive overhead movements, impingement syndrome or rotator cuff pathology can be career threatening.

The rotator cuff tendons (primarily the supraspinatus and infraspinatus tendons), the long head of the biceps brachii tendon, the subacromial bursa, the GH joint capsule, and the head of the humerus are compressed in the space between the acromion process and the humeral head (Fig. 15-32). Primary subacromial impingement occurs when a structural cause such as a hooked acromion encroaches on the subacromial space (Box 15-5). Secondary subacromial impingement results when weakness, laxity, fatigue, motion restriction, or a combination of these factors results in a limited space. Decreased strength or fatigue leads to decreased humeral head depression as the humerus is brought into overhead positions, causing impingement of the structures. Impingement can occur anywhere along the coracoacromial arch and under the AC joint.

A relationship between poor scapular biomechanics and subacromial impingement syndromes has been suggested (see Scapular Dyskinesis). In this case, the scapula does not upwardly and externally rotate or posteriorly tilt appropriately to allow the tendons of the rotator cuff muscles and the LHBT to pass beneath the coracoacromial arch.[86] In addition, during elevation, activation of the middle and lower trapezius muscles is delayed in those with impingement symptoms. This pattern is consistent with excessive scapular elevation and anterior tilting that further decreases the

Table 15-9 Types of Impingement

Force	Source
Primary Subacromial Impingement	Irregularly shaped acromion Spur formation on acromion Os acromiale
Secondary Subacromial Impingement	Loss of humeral head depression/stabilization Poor posture Repetitive overhead movement Scapular dyskinesis GH instability Supraspinatus hypertrophy[85]
Internal impingement	Glenohumeral internal rotation deficit (GIRD) GH instability High volume of throwing or other repetitive overhead activity Occupation requiring repetitive overhead activity

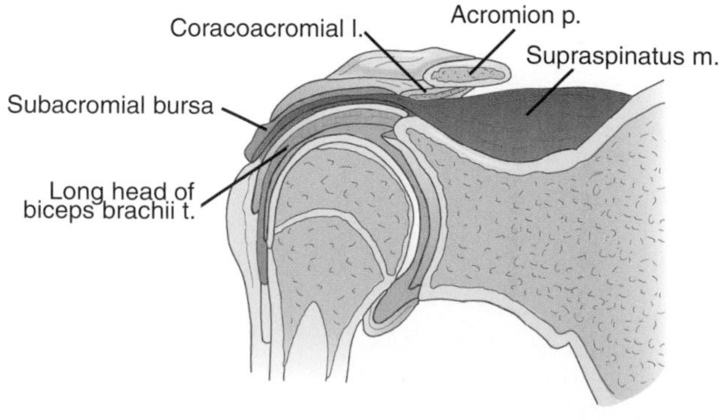

FIGURE 15-32 ■ Structures involved in subacromial impingement syndrome. If the humeral head does not depress during abduction, the long head of the biceps brachii, the subacromial bursa, and the supraspinatus tendon are impinged between the coracoacromial arch and the head of the humerus.

Selective Tissue Tests 15-11
Sulcus Sign for Inferior Glenohumeral Laxity

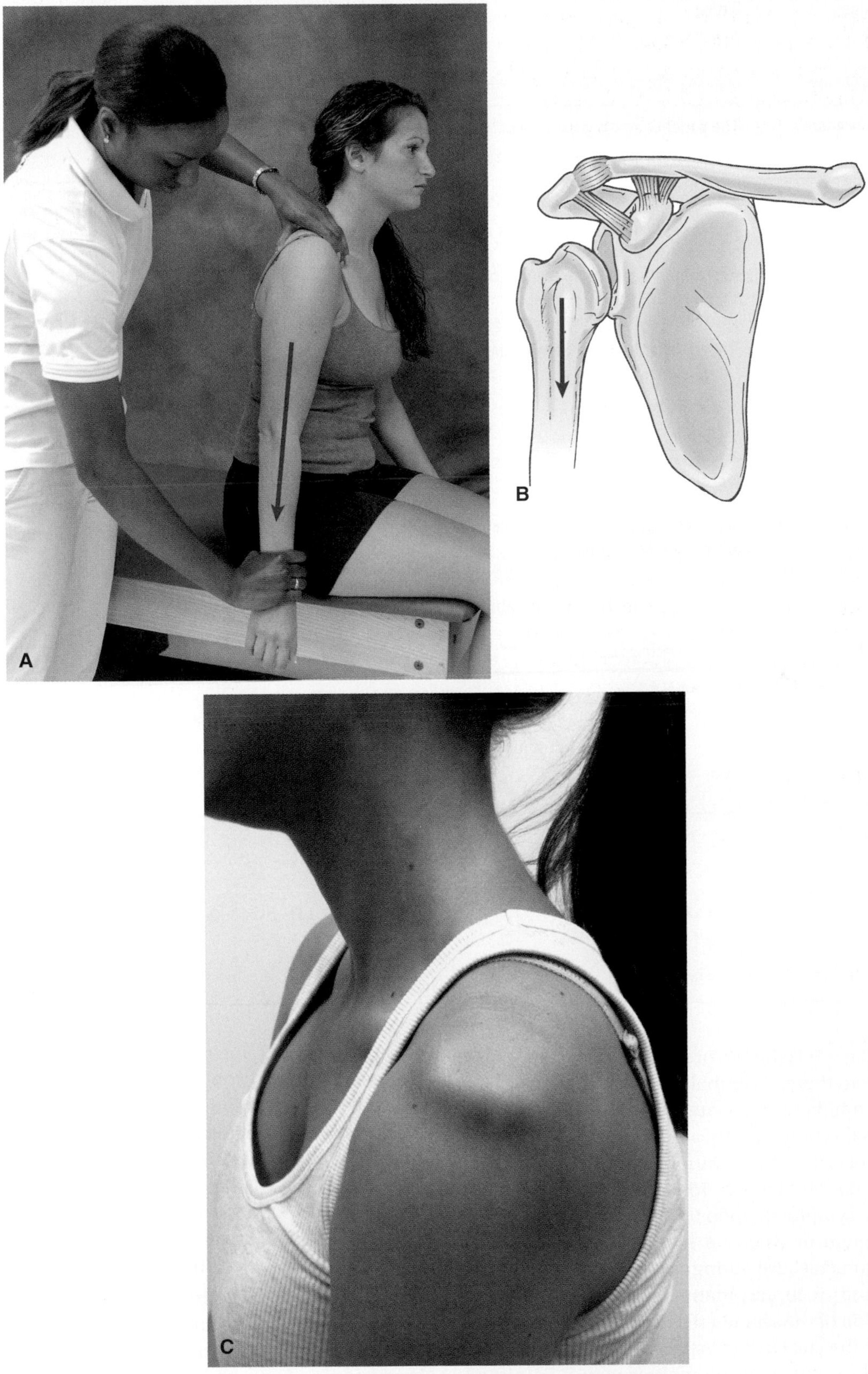

The sulcus sign determines the amount of inferior glide of the humeral head when traction is applied to the humerus. (C)

Continued

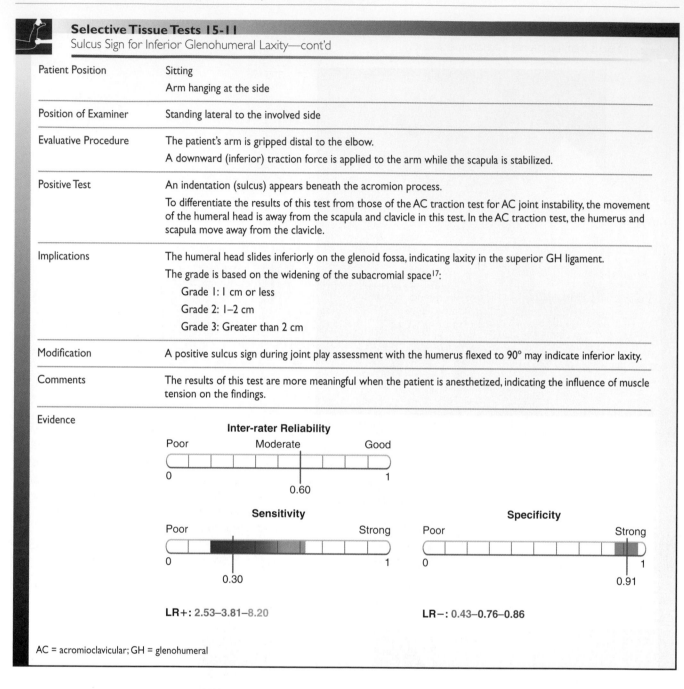

Selective Tissue Tests 15-11
Sulcus Sign for Inferior Glenohumeral Laxity—cont'd

Patient Position	Sitting Arm hanging at the side
Position of Examiner	Standing lateral to the involved side
Evaluative Procedure	The patient's arm is gripped distal to the elbow. A downward (inferior) traction force is applied to the arm while the scapula is stabilized.
Positive Test	An indentation (sulcus) appears beneath the acromion process. To differentiate the results of this test from those of the AC traction test for AC joint instability, the movement of the humeral head is away from the scapula and clavicle in this test. In the AC traction test, the humerus and scapula move away from the clavicle.
Implications	The humeral head slides inferiorly on the glenoid fossa, indicating laxity in the superior GH ligament. The grade is based on the widening of the subacromial space[17]: Grade 1: 1 cm or less Grade 2: 1–2 cm Grade 3: Greater than 2 cm
Modification	A positive sulcus sign during joint play assessment with the humerus flexed to 90° may indicate inferior laxity.
Comments	The results of this test are more meaningful when the patient is anesthetized, indicating the influence of muscle tension on the findings.
Evidence	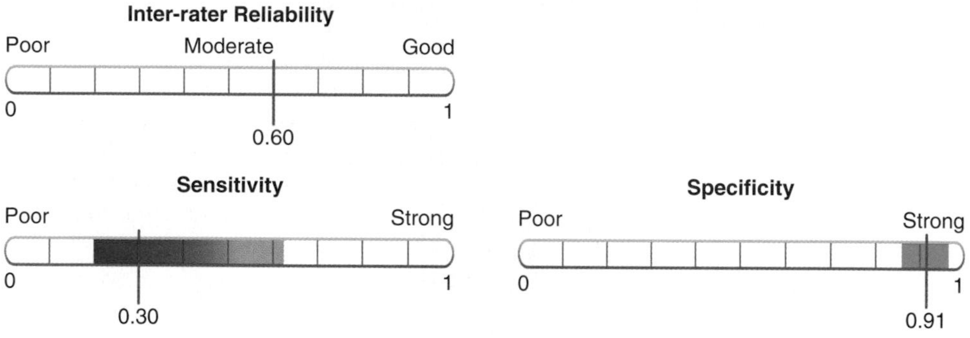

LR+: 2.53–3.81–8.20

LR−: 0.43–0.76–0.86

AC = acromioclavicular; GH = glenohumeral

subacromial space.[86] Tightness of the pectoralis minor may also contribute to these abnormal mechanics.[87]

The chief complaint associated with subacromial impingement is pain during overhead movements and an associated painful arc with elevation in the plane of the scapula (Examination Findings 15-4). The patient may describe a relief of symptoms when the GH joint is maintained in slight abduction or when an inferiorly gliding force is applied to the humeral head during elevation.[88] Atrophy of the infraspinatus and/or supraspinatus muscles may be noted during inspection of the scapula (Fig. 15-33). An injection of anesthetic into the subacromial space with subsequent relief of symptoms is indicative of impingement.[22] In relaxed stance, the patient may present with a forward shoulder posture indicative of decreased thoracic mobility in extension.[89] Greater thoracic spine extension is associated with greater shoulder ROM.[89] Common evaluative tests used to evaluate for subacromial impingement or its underlying causes include the **Neer impingement test** (Selective Tissue Test 15-12), the **Hawkins (Kennedy-Hawkins) impingement test** (Selective Tissue Test 15-13), the **drop arm test** (see Selective Tissue Test 15-1), passive horizontal adduction (which decreases the subacromial space), and manual muscle tests for the infraspinatus and supraspinatus.

Subacromial Impingement Intervention Strategies

Patients with subacromial impingement often respond well to conservative treatment focused on addressing identified impairments. Strengthening the rotator cuff to maximize dynamic stabilization, restoration of scapular kinematics, improved thoracic extension mobility through joint

Box 15-5
Classification of Acromion Shapes

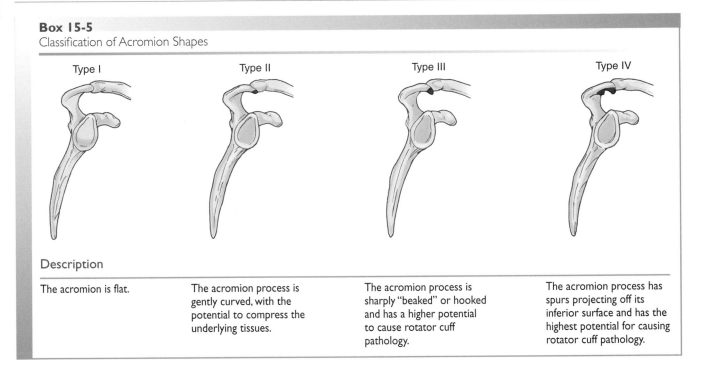

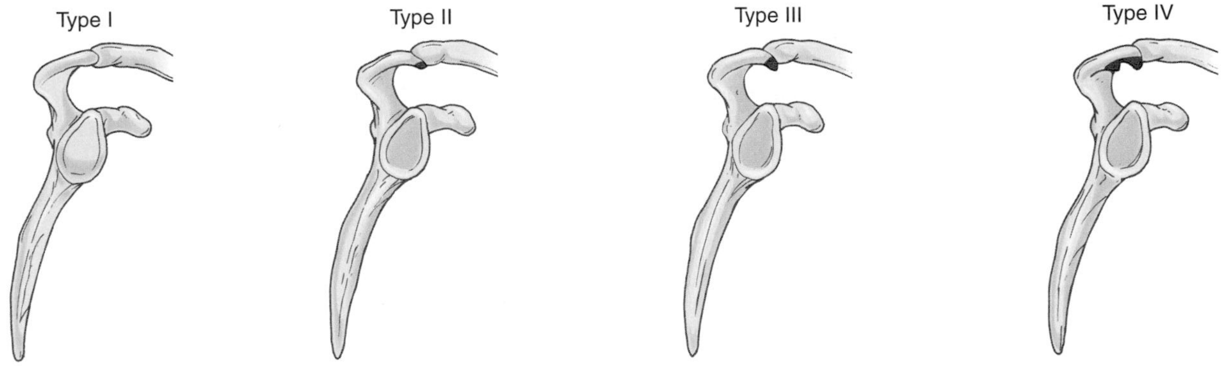

Description

The acromion is flat.	The acromion process is gently curved, with the potential to compress the underlying tissues.	The acromion process is sharply "beaked" or hooked and has a higher potential to cause rotator cuff pathology.	The acromion process has spurs projecting off its inferior surface and has the highest potential for causing rotator cuff pathology.

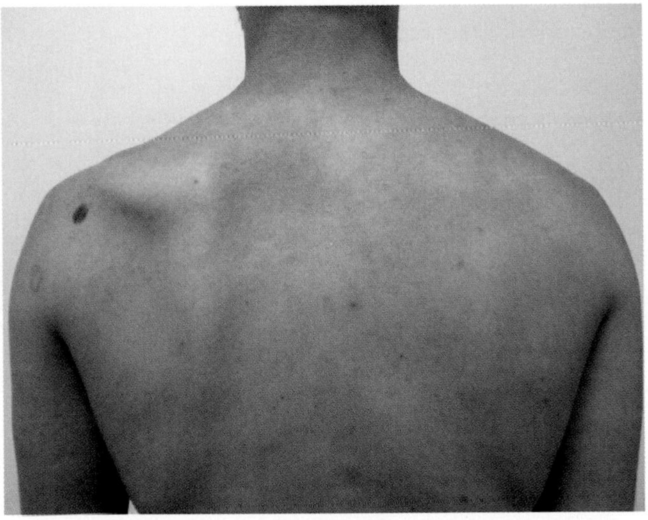

FIGURE 15-33 ■ Atrophy of the left infraspinatus. Note the prominent left scapular spine, suggesting atrophy of the infraspinatus and, possibly, the supraspinatus muscles. This finding can be a long-term consequence of rotator cuff pathology.

mobilization, targeted stretching, and activity modification are all potential components of the treatment plan.[89] Surgical intervention to increase the subacromial space may be warranted when a primary cause such as a hooked acromion is identified.

*** Practical Evidence**

When examined collectively, positive findings from the Kennedy-Hawkins test coupled with a painful arc and pain and weakness with a manual muscle test of the infraspinatus strongly predict the presence of subacromial impingement (positive likelihood ratio = 10.56).[22]

Internal Impingement

The most common type of internal impingement, posterosuperior impingement involves pathology of the undersurface, or articular side, of the infraspinatus and the supraspinatus; it occurs when these tendons twist and are compressed against the glenoid during abduction and external rotation of the GH joint.[90] Internal impingement is strongly associated with a **glenohumeral internal rotation deficit** (GIRD) and anterior instability.[91,92] GIRD, with associated tightness of the posterior inferior GH ligament, results in a superior translation of the humeral head during elevation, further decreasing available space. Patients with internal impingement complain of posterior shoulder pain that worsens with activity. Complaints of loss of control and velocity when throwing are common. Tightness of the posterior capsule, as evidenced by restricted posterior joint play, restricted horizontal adduction, and restricted internal rotation, causes increased and earlier superior and anterior migration of the humeral head and are common examination findings.[92,93] The relocation test may reduce symptoms by recentering the humeral head in the glenoid fossa.

Internal Impingement Intervention Strategies

Conservative treatment of internal impingement consists of improving scapular control, improving thoracic extension, stretching the posterior structures to reduce GIRD, and improving dynamic control of the GH joint. Surgical options include anterior stabilization to reduce humeral head migration. Simple debridement of the rotator cuff is not associated with a good outcome.[92]

Rotator Cuff Tendinopathy

Rotator cuff tendinopathy typically presents with a slow onset of the symptoms. Pathology ranges from acute tendinitis

Examination Findings 15-4
Subacromial Impingement Syndrome

Examination Segment	Clinical Findings
History of Current Condition	*Onset:* Insidious *Pain characteristics:* Beneath the acromion process and radiating to the lateral arm *Other symptoms:* The patient may complain of popping and clicking, depending on involvement of bursa and rotator cuff musculature. *Mechanism:* Repetitive overhead motion impinging the rotator cuff muscles (especially the supraspinatus) and LHBT between the humeral head and coracoacromial arch *Risk factors:* Increased anterior laxity, irregularly shaped acromion (curved or hooked), subacromial spurs, scapular dyskinesis, rotator cuff weakness
Functional Assessment	Increased pain with overhead motions; may be coupled with compensatory scapulothoracic movement, with early and excessive scapular elevation and/or decreased posterior tilting during arm-raising maneuvers
Inspection	The shoulder may be postured for comfort by holding the arm in slight abduction. A forward shoulder posture where the scapula rests in a protracted position and the humerus is internally rotated is frequently associated with impingement.
Palpation	Tenderness exists beneath the acromion process, over the supraspinatus insertion at the greater tuberosity, and over the bicipital groove.
Joint and Muscle Function Assessment	*AROM:* Active abduction in an arc of motion from about 70°–120° results in pain. *MMT:* Pain and/or weakness with elevation in plane of scapula (empty can or full can test) and external rotation *PROM:* Increased pain at the end-range of elevation Pectoralis minor tightness is often associated with impingement.
Joint Stability Tests	*Stress tests:* A complete ligamentous and capsular screen is necessary to rule out GH and AC laxity. *Joint play:* GH hypermobility and/or hypomobility may be present; decreased thoracic spine mobility
Selective Tissue Tests	The Neer and Hawkins impingement tests are usually painful.
Neurological Screening	Within normal limits
Vascular Screening	Within normal limits
Imaging Techniques	Radiographs to rule out a primary cause of impingement, including a hooked acromion or osteophyte
Differential Diagnosis	Labral tears, SLAP lesions, rotator cuff tendinopathy, subacromial bursitis, long head of the biceps tendinopathy
Comments	Impingement may occur secondary to GH instability in younger patients. The degenerative response caused by rotator cuff impingement, if untreated, can lead to rotator cuff tears. Temporary relief of symptoms associated with an injection of anesthetic into the subacromial space is indicative of impingement.[22]

AC = acromioclavicular; ADLs = activities of daily living; AROM = active range of motion; GH = glenohumeral; LHBT = long head of the biceps tendon; MMT = manual muscle test; PROM = passive range of motion; SLAP = superior labrum anterior to posterior

after an abrupt change in level of activity to the more common chronic degenerative change in the tissue. Actual tears in the cuff can be partial or complete, with partial tears occurring on the bursal side or articular side of the cuff.

In the early stages of rotator cuff tendinopathy, the chief complaint is pain deep within the shoulder in the subacromial area after activity. The symptoms then progress to pain during activity and, finally, to constant pain with most activities of daily living. Factors contributing to the onset of rotator cuff pathology include a muscle imbalance between the internal and external rotators, capsular laxity, poor scapular control, and subacromial or internal impingement.

The shoulder is predisposed to rotator cuff tendinopathy by the relatively poor vascularization of the tendons, a fact that hastens the degenerative process and hinders the healing process.[90] The supraspinatus tendon is the most susceptible

Selective Tissue Tests 15-12
Neer Impingement Test

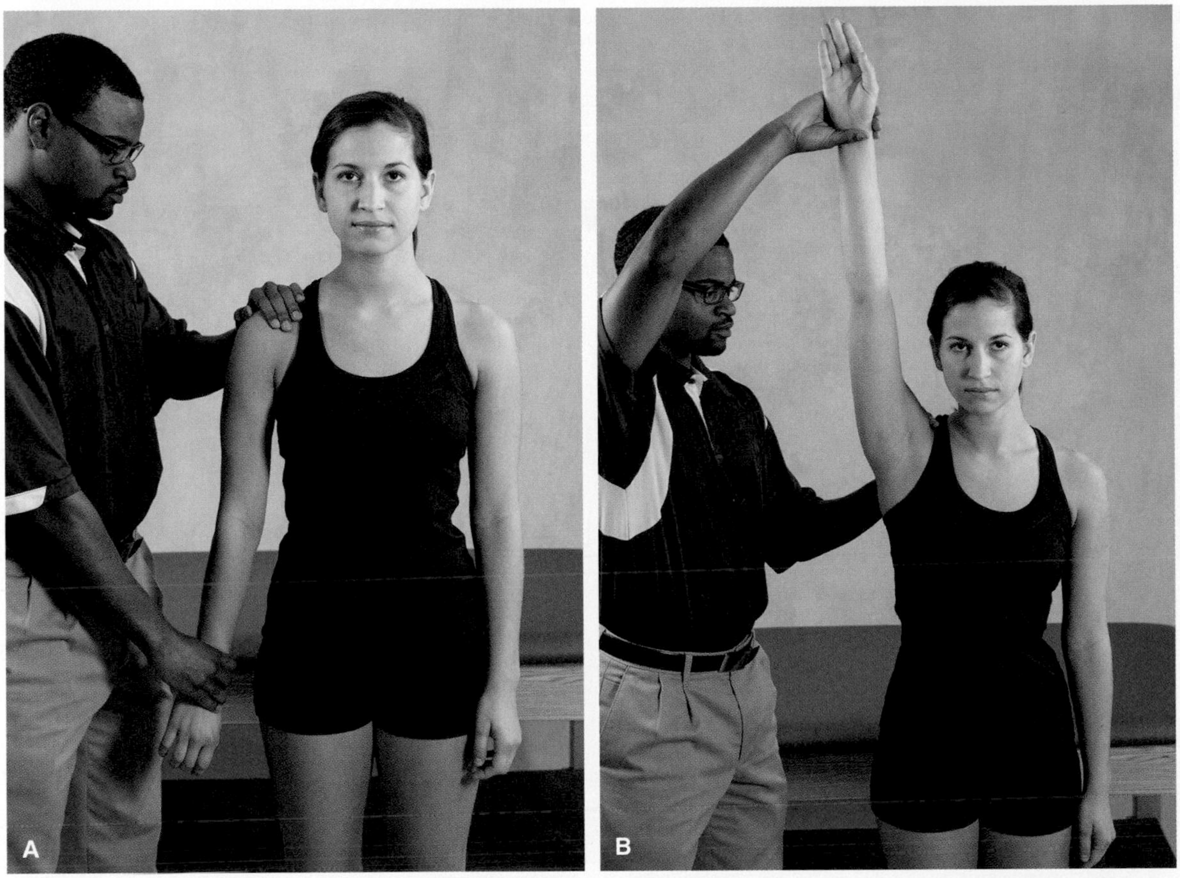

The patient's arm is passively moved through flexion to reproduce the symptoms of rotator cuff impingement, usually between 90° and 180° of flexion.

Patient Position	Standing or sitting The shoulder, elbow, and wrist begin in the anatomical position.
Position of Examiner	(A) Standing lateral or forward to the involved side One hand stabilizes the scapula. The opposite hand grasps the patient's arm distal to the elbow joint.
Evaluative Procedure	(B) With the elbow extended, the humerus is placed in internal rotation, and the forearm is pronated. The GH joint is moved through forward flexion as the scapula is stabilized.
Positive Test	Pain in the anterior or lateral shoulder, in the range of 90° to full elevation
Implications	Pathology is present in the rotator cuff group (especially the supraspinatus) or the long head of the biceps brachii tendon. The test motion impinges these structures between the greater tuberosity and the inferior side of the acromion process and coracoacromial ligament.

Continued

Selective Tissue Tests 15-12
Neer Impingement Test—cont'd

Comments	In cases of bursal involvement only (i.e., the rotator cuff is not damaged), the sensitivity improves to 0.86, but the specificity decreases to 0.49 (LR+ = 1.69).[22]
Evidence	Impingement

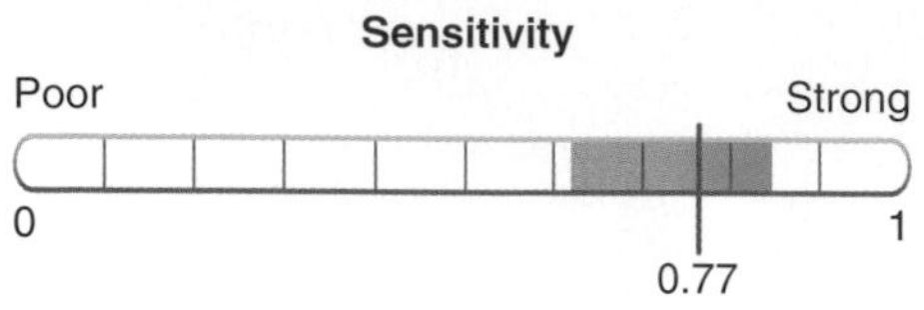

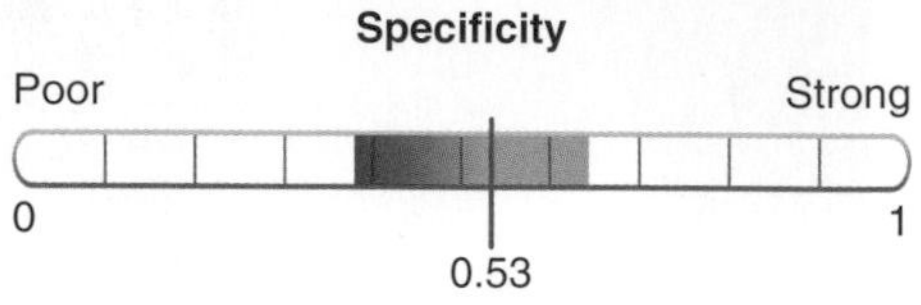

LR+: 1.06–1.68–1.91

LR−: 0.36–0.40–0.75

SLAP Lesion

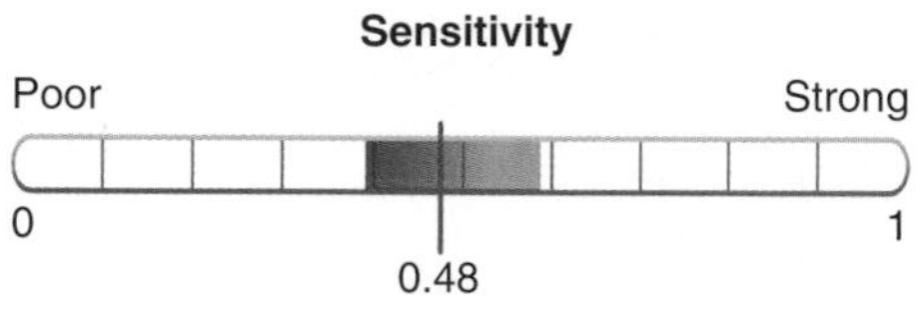

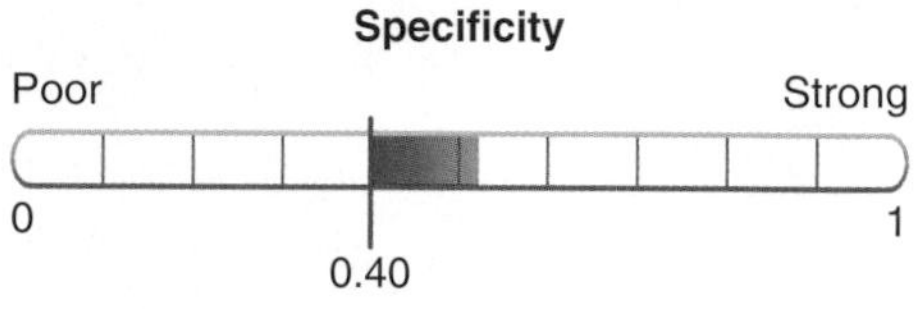

LR+: 0.72–0.98–1.05

LR−: 0.96–1.03–1.43

GH = glenohumeral

of the rotator cuff group to inflammatory conditions, especially at the convergence zone of the anterior and posterior circumflex arteries, just proximal to the greater tuberosity.[90] In addition to its poor blood supply, pressure is placed on this tendon by the humeral head "wringing" it dry of blood and other vital nutrients.

The shape and location of the acromion process may also precipitate the onset of rotator cuff pathology. The rate of rotator cuff pathology is markedly increased when the lateral acromion angle is less than 70 degrees, forming an acromial spur.[90] Shoulders that are affected by chronic rotator cuff pathology are also characterized by an increased number of acromial osteophytes (see Box 15-5).[94]

The posterior rotator cuff muscles, the infraspinatus and teres minor, play an important role in the throwing motion. In addition to externally rotating the humerus during the cocking phase of the throw, these muscles eccentrically contract to decelerate the arm during the follow-through phase. The eccentric contraction can lead to microtearing or inflammation of these muscles, eventually giving way to larger tears.

The relative severity of rotator cuff pathology is based on the presence of tearing within the tendons (Examination Findings 15-5). Tears to the tendons may result from a single traumatic force or, more commonly and especially in the older population, from the accumulation of microtrauma (overuse injuries). **Partial-thickness tears** are short longitudinal lesions in the tendon, initially involving the superficial or midsubstance fibers. Tears most commonly occur in the supraspinatus tendon.[95] Partial-thickness tears can occur on the articular side or subacromial side of the rotator cuff. Subacromial tears are more associated with subacromial impingement, while articular-side tears are associated with internal impingement.[95] When partial-thickness tears go untreated, a **full-thickness tear** may develop (full-thickness tears may also develop secondary to a single traumatic force). Severe dysfunction of the supraspinatus or infraspinatus muscles may lead to atrophy that is visible during inspection of the scapula.

During the lowering motion from full abduction to adduction, individuals suffering from tears in the rotator cuff tendons are unable to control the rate of fall after the humerus reaches 90 degrees of abduction as demonstrated by the **drop arm test** (see Selective Tissue Test 15-1). The **empty can test**, the manual muscle test for the supraspinatus, isolates the supraspinatus tendon for weakness or pain (Selective Tissue Test 15-14). Because the supraspinatus contributes so little to general abduction strength, the empty can test may not be able to detect subtle changes in strength resulting from tears in the tendon. The test is most useful in determining the presence of large rotator cuff tears.[15,97] Subscapularis tears can be detected using the Gerber lift-off test to isolate internal rotation. In this test, the hand is positioned in the small of the back, and the

Selective Tissue Tests 15-13

Hawkins (Kennedy-Hawkins) impingement test

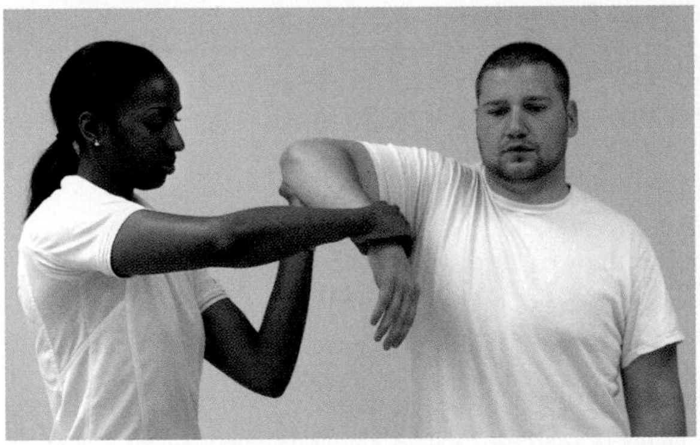

With the GH joint abducted to 90° in the scapular plane, the humerus is internally rotated to reproduce the symptoms of rotator cuff impingement.

Patient Position	Sitting or standing The shoulder, elbow, and wrist are in the anatomical position.
Position of Examiner	Standing lateral or in front of the involved side Grasp the patient's arm at the elbow joint.
Evaluative Procedure	With the elbow flexed, the GH joint is elevated to 90° in the scapular plane. The humerus is then internally rotated until pain is experienced or scapular rotation is felt or observed.
Positive Test	Pain with motion, especially near the end ROM
Implications	Pathology is present in the rotator cuff group (especially the supraspinatus) or the long head of the biceps brachii tendon. The motion of the test impinges these structures between the greater tuberosity and the inferior side of the acromion process.
Comments	If the humerus is moved towards the sagittal plane, the probability of eliciting a false-positive result secondary to AC joint pathology increases.
Evidence	Impingement

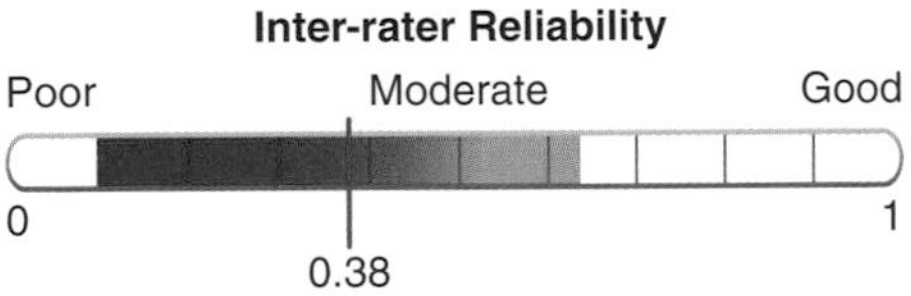

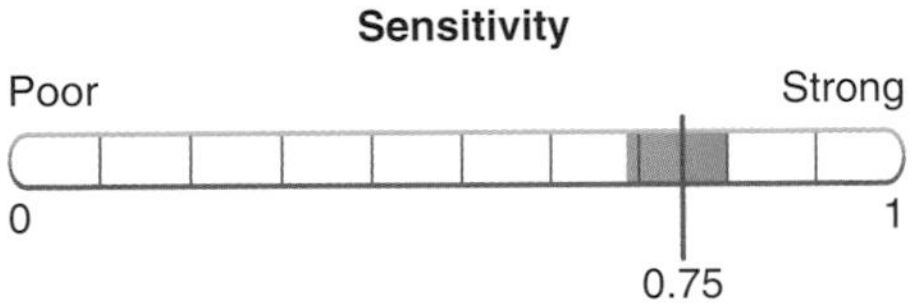

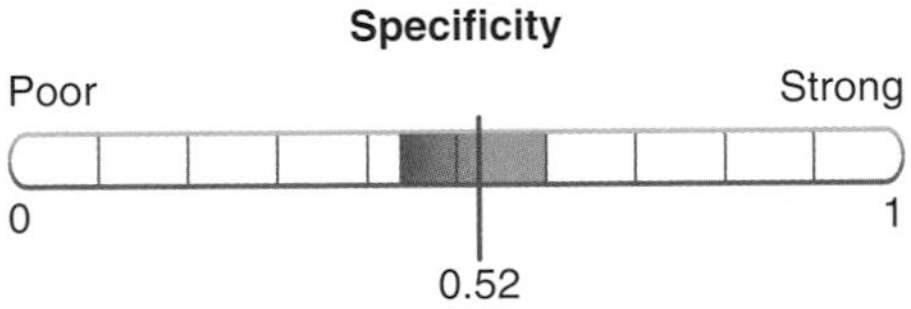

LR+: 1.27–1.88–2.49

LR−: 0.39–0.52–0.64

SLAP Lesion

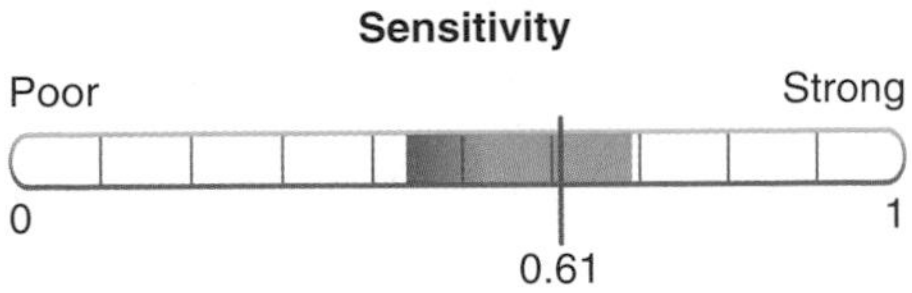

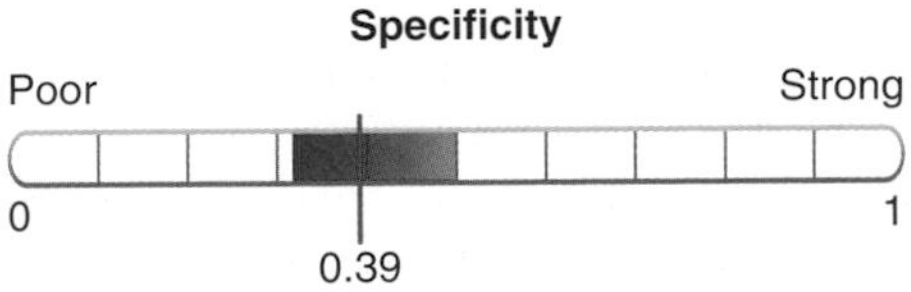

LR+: 0.72–0.95–1.17

LR−: 0.76–1.08–1.28

AC = acromioclavicular; GH = glenohumeral; ROM = range of motion

Examination Findings 15-5
Rotator Cuff Tendinopathy

Examination Segment	Clinical Findings
History of Current Condition	*Onset:* Insidious or acute *Pain characteristics:* Deep within the shoulder beneath the acromion process. Pain usually radiates into the lateral arm. *Other symptoms:* Clicking during certain GH motions *Mechanism:* **Insidious:** Chronic impingement or degeneration of the rotator cuff tendons over time due to aging; a single traumatic episode may cause the final rupture of a weakened tendon. **Acute:** Dynamic overloading of the tendon *Risk factors:* Subacromial impingement, internal impingement, acromion changes, repetitive overhead motion, repetitive eccentric loading, scapular dyskinesis
Functional Assessment	Pain during overhead motions. During elevation, scapula may excessively protract, elevate, or anteriorly tip.
Inspection	In chronic cases, atrophy of the infraspinatus and/or supraspinatus
Palpation	Tenderness in the subacromial space and at the insertion of the supraspinatus tendon into the greater tuberosity
Joint and Muscle Function Assessment	*AROM:* Painful between 70° and 120° of elevation, especially in abduction *MMT:* Pain and/or weakness with abduction, internal rotation, external rotation, and elevation in the plane of the scapula *PROM:* Decreased pain compared with AROM, except in positions of impingement
Joint Stability Tests	*Stress tests:* Tests to rule out GH and AC laxity and impingement *Joint play:* Joint play to assess for hyper- or hypomobility
Selective Tissue Tests	Drop arm test Impingement tests may be positive.
Neurological Screening	Within normal limits
Vascular Screening	Within normal limits
Imaging Techniques	The standard radiographic series consists of scapular plane AP, internal rotation, external rotation, and transscapular and axillary views to rule out rotator cuff tears and bony abnormalities. A subacromial space of less than 7 mm is indicative of a full-thickness cuff tear. MRI has a sensitivity of 0.95 and specificity of 0.95 in identifying rotator cuff tears, degeneration, and partial thickness tears.[96] MR arthrography, ultrasonography
Differential Diagnosis	AC joint degeneration, subacromial impingement, internal impingement, labral tear, long head of the biceps tendinopathy, capsulitis
Comments	A history of rotator cuff tendinopathy often precedes a rotator cuff tear.

AC = acromioclavicular; AP = anteroposterior; AROM = active range of motion; GH = glenohumeral; MMT = manual muscle test; MR = magnetic resonance; MRI = magnetic resonance imaging; PROM = passive range of motion

Selective Tissue Tests 15-14
Empty Can Test for Supraspinatus Pathology

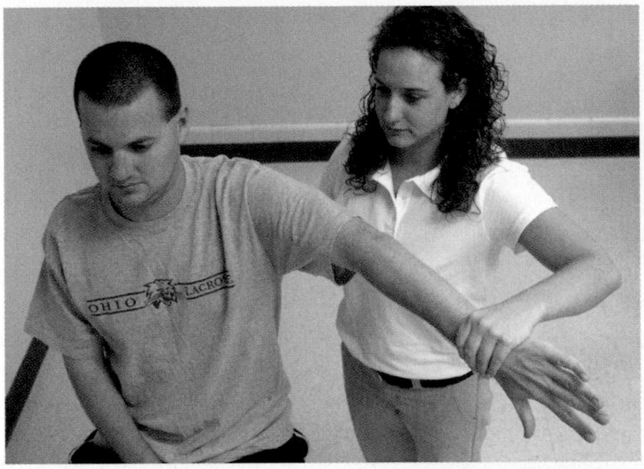

The empty can test is actually a manual muscle test for the supraspinatus muscle. A positive test often indicates subacromial impingement or a lesion to the musculotendinous unit.

Patient Position	Sitting or standing The glenohumeral joint is abducted to 90° in the scapular plane, the elbow extended, and the humerus internally rotated and the forearm pronated so that the thumb points downward.
Position of Examiner	Standing facing the patient One hand is placed on the superior portion of the midforearm to resist the motion of abduction in the scapular plane.
Evaluative Procedure	The evaluator resists abduction (applies a downward pressure).
Positive Test	Weakness and/or pain accompanying the movement
Implications	The supraspinatus tendon is weak, impinged, or partially or fully torn.
Modification	This test can be performed with the humerus externally rotated and the forearm supinated so that the thumb is facing upward, the full can test.
Comments	The empty can and full can tests are about equally accurate in detecting supraspinatus tears. Because the full can test is less pain provoking of impingement symptoms, its use is recommended.[98] Pain in the absence of weakness does not help detect partial-thickness tears or tendinopathy.[99]

Evidence

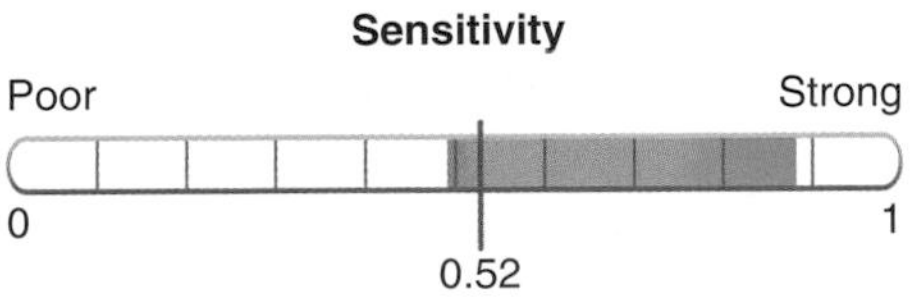

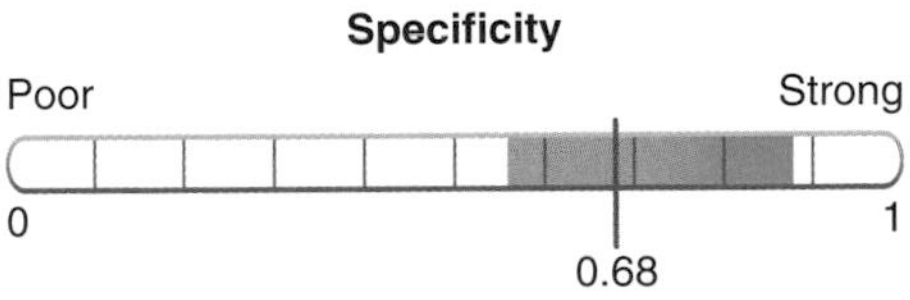

LR+: 1.37–2.36–3.94

LR−: 0.21–0.60–0.90

patient is asked to lift the hand straight off the back. With a reported 100% specificity, a positive finding is conclusive for a subscapularis tear.

✻ Practical Evidence

The diagnostic accuracy of the shoulder examination improves when the results are grouped by positive findings. Weakness during the empty can test, weakness in external rotation, and a positive impingement sign are associated with a rotator cuff tear 98% of the time.[21] A positive drop arm test, an associated painful arc, and weakness in external rotation are also highly predictive of a rotator cuff tear.[22]

Subacromial Bursitis

Chronic rotator cuff impingement or rotator cuff tears, if untreated, ultimately lead to inflammation of the subacromial bursa and still further encroachment of the subacromial space. Since they often occur concurrently, it is difficult to differentiate between rotator cuff pathology and subacromial bursitis. Subacromial bursitis causes positive results from impingement tests and tests for supraspinatus tendinopathy as the three conditions are often related.

Rotator Cuff Pathology Intervention Strategies

As with the management of the different types of impingement, nonsurgical approaches to managing patients with rotator cuff tendinopathies emphasize an approach that addresses impairments that alter function and modification of activity as necessary. Strengthening must focus on the scapular musculature, the rotator cuff, and other shoulder muscles. The strength and use of the legs and trunk also must be analyzed.

Surgery may be required for rotator cuff tears that limit participation. Based on the pathology, especially the size of any rotator cuff tear, the physician determines if surgery is done arthroscopically, with a mini-open technique (small scar over the superior aspect of the shoulder), or full-open repair. Most small to medium-sized tears can be repaired with arthroscopy or the mini-open technique.

Post-operatively, rehabilitation is dictated by the type of surgery required. Although débridement of the subacromial space and rotator cuff can progress based on the patient's tolerance, rotator cuff repairs require careful use of active and resisted motions in the repaired tissues for a period of 6 to 8 weeks to allow healing to occur.

Biceps Tendon Pathology

The LHBT provides very little force in moving the GH joint. Because of its insertion into the glenoid labrum and intraarticular nature, pathology of this structure can impact the joint's function. During normal overhead movements, the tendon slides within its sheath, which is located in the bicipital groove.

Bicipital Tendinopathy

Bicipital tendon pathology may result from rotator cuff dysfunction, from overuse of the biceps brachii muscle, or from subacromial impingement. The transverse humeral ligament, which holds the tendon in the bicipital groove, may become stretched or torn as the result of sudden forceful extension or external rotation of the shoulder accompanied by elbow flexion. Disruption of the transverse humeral ligament can cause the LHBT to sublux from the bicipital groove, especially when the elbow is flexed and the humerus is externally rotated.

Yergason's test can reproduce subluxation of the LHBT or cause pain in the presence of bicipital tendinopathy or a labral tear (Selective Tissue Test 15-15). Pain caused by a subluxating tendon can be differentiated by **Speed's test**, which only has positive test results in the presence of bicipital tendinopathy (Selective Tissue Test 15-16). MRI can also be used to differentiate between the two conditions.[100]

Bicipital Tendinopathy Intervention Strategies

Bicipital and rotator cuff tendinopathies often occur simultaneously. Conservative rehabilitation includes decreasing inflammation with the use of oral medications and activity modification. Stretching and strengthening of the shoulder complex muscles should progress in a manner similar to that used for rotator cuff tendinopathies. Recalcitrant bicipital tendinopathy can be managed operatively with a tenotomy (cutting the tendon) or tenodesis (repositioning the tendon). Both procedures are associated with favorable outcomes, although the tenotomy is associated with a worse cosmetic result.

Superior Labrum Anterior to Posterior Lesions

SLAP lesions are tears of the superior aspect of the glenoid labrum that extend anteriorly and posteriorly to the biceps insertion.[105] Table 15-10 presents one classification system for SLAP lesions. Type I lesions are most frequently associated with rotator cuff degeneration; GH instability is often the precursor to Type III and IV lesions. Type II lesions, the

Table 15-10 Classification of SLAP Lesions

Type	Pathology
I	Degenerative fraying of the labrum near the insertion of the LHBT
II	Avulsion of the glenoid labrum with an associated tear of the LHBT Type II SLAP lesions have been further classified relative to the detachment of the labrum[106]: • Isolated to the anterior aspect • Isolated to the posterior aspect • Appearing in both aspects
III	A bucket-handle tear of the labrum with displacement of the fragment; no involvement of the LHBT
IV	Bucket-handle tear of the labrum with associated tearing of the LHBT

LHBT = long head of the biceps tendon; SLAP = superior labrum anterior to posterior

Selective Tissue Tests 15-15
Yergason's Test

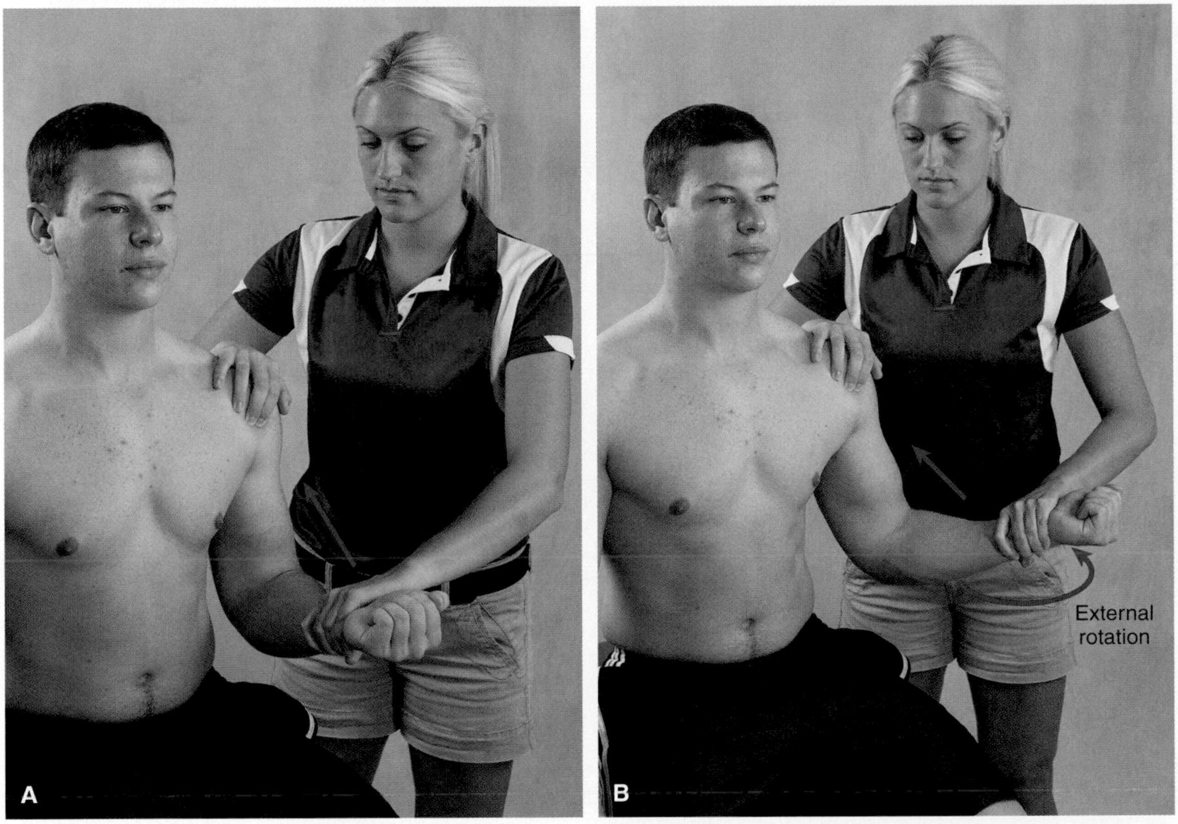

Yergason's test identifies the presence of pathology to the LHBT within the bicipital groove or the presence of a SLAP lesion. Palpate the tendon as it passes through the bicipital groove to identify lesions involving this area.

Patient Position	Sitting or standing GH joint in the anatomical position The elbow is flexed to 90°. The forearm is positioned so that the lateral border of the radius faces upward (neutral position).
Position of Examiner	Lateral to the patient on the involved side, lightly palpating the bicipital groove The elbow is stabilized inferiorly and maintained close to the thorax. The forearm is stabilized proximal to the wrist.
Evaluative Procedure	The patient provides resistance while the examiner concurrently moves the GH joint into external rotation while resisting forearm supination and elbow flexion.
Positive Test	Pain or snapping (or both) in the bicipital groove Pain at the superior glenohumeral joint (SLAP lesion)
Implications	*Primary:* Snapping or popping in the bicipital groove indicates a tear or laxity of the transverse humeral ligament. This pathology prevents the ligament from maintaining the long head of the tendon in its groove. *Secondary:* Pain with no associated popping in the bicipital groove may indicate bicipital tendinopathy.
Modification	Resist elbow flexion as the humerus moves into external rotation.

Continued

Selective Tissue Tests 15-15
Yergason's Test—cont'd

Comments	False-positive findings may be the result of rotator cuff impingement.[101] Pain in the superior glenohumeral region is weakly predictive of SLAP lesions.[102]
Evidence	*LHBT Pathology*

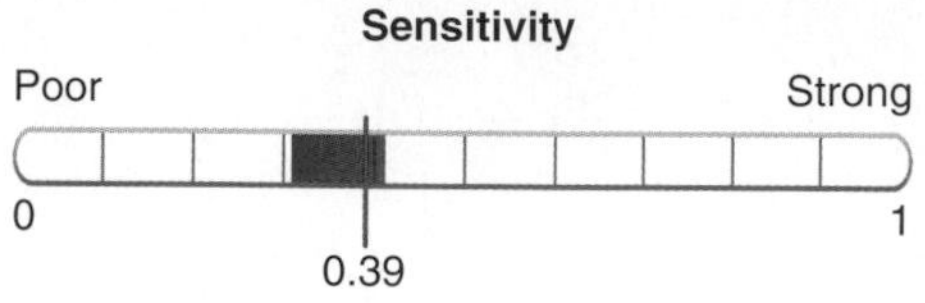

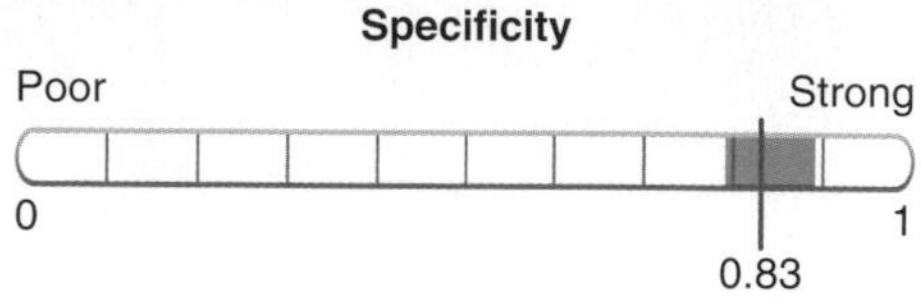

LR+: 1.95–2.32–2.75

LR−: 0.73–0.74–0.79

SLAP Lesion

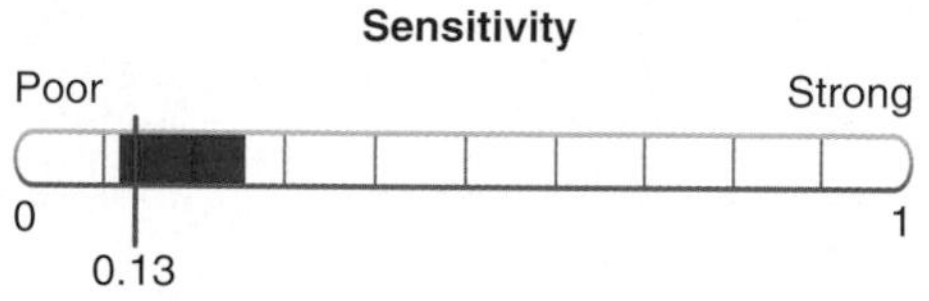

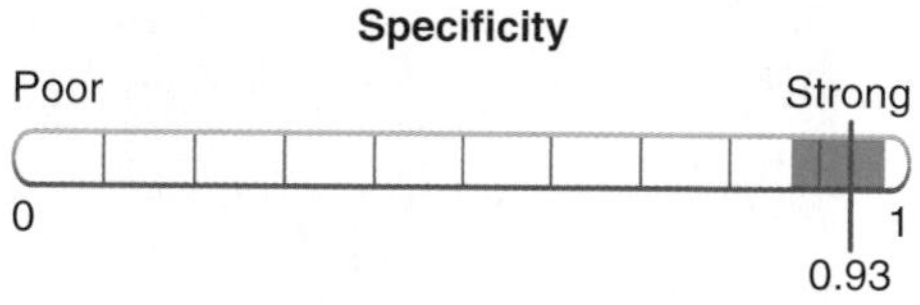

LR+: 1.04–1.89–2.38

LR−: 0.87–0.94–0.97

GH = glenohumeral; LHBT = long head of the biceps tendon; SLAP = superior labrum anterior to posterior

most common type, are age dependent. In younger patients, Type II lesions tend to clinically resemble those of Type III and IV lesions in adults; in older patients, Type II lesions more closely resemble Type I.[106] SLAP lesions are most confidently confirmed during arthroscopy, but magnetic resonance arthrograms can also be used.[105]

Tension of the LHBT, such as that experienced during the follow-through phase of pitching when the biceps works to decelerate the elbow, pulls the labrum away from the glenoid fossa. Other compression and inferior traction mechanisms can also produce SLAP lesions.[105,107] The LHBT contacting the rotator cuff when the arm is in the cocked position has been associated with posterior-superior tears.[106] Type II lesions can occur by the LHBT being peeled back caused by tendon torsion created as the arm is brought into abduction and external rotation.[105]

With an acute or gradual onset, SLAP lesions present with clinically inconsistent symptoms and are frequently associated with concurrent pathology (Examination Findings 15-6).[105,107] The chief complaint is of pain between the AC joint and coracoid process during overhead arm movement that is relieved by rest.[105] Throwing athletes report "dead arm" symptoms and a loss of throwing control and velocity.

Selective tissue tests to evaluate for the presence of SLAP lesions: (1) attempt to reproduce symptoms by recreating tensile forces on the LHBT or (2) apply compressive forces on the labrum. The **active compression test (O'Brien test)** (Selective Tissue Test 15-17),[108] **anterior slide test** (Selective Tissue Test 15-18), and **compression-rotation test (grind test)** (Selective Tissue Test 15-19) are among the many used clinically. The stated clinical usefulness of these techniques varies widely by investigator[74-76,109-112] with more recent analyses questioning the diagnostic utility of any of them—either alone or grouped together.[107] Reproduction of symptoms with the Yergason's test, Neer impingement sign, Speed's test, and the relocation test may or may not add predictive value to the diagnosis of SLAP lesions.[76,102,109]

Tests for SLAP tend to yield false-positive results because of the presence of concurrent GH or AC pathologies. In other cases, procedures may produce pain caused by a SLAP lesion but be negative for the pathology being tested. For example, the Neer impingement test may be negative for rotator cuff involvement but evoke pain caused by a SLAP lesion.[113]

SLAP Lesion Intervention Strategies

Symptomatic SLAP lesions require surgical repair.[105] Postoperative management of a patient with a SLAP lesion depends on whether the tear was debrided or repaired. Although cases of debridement can usually progress as tolerated, repairs of SLAP lesions progress more slowly. Most importantly after a surgical SLAP repair, contraction of the biceps tendon and other traction forces from the tendon placed on the repair must be controlled for 6 to 8 weeks.

Selective Tissue Tests 15-16

Speed's Test for Long Head of the Biceps Brachii Tendinopathy

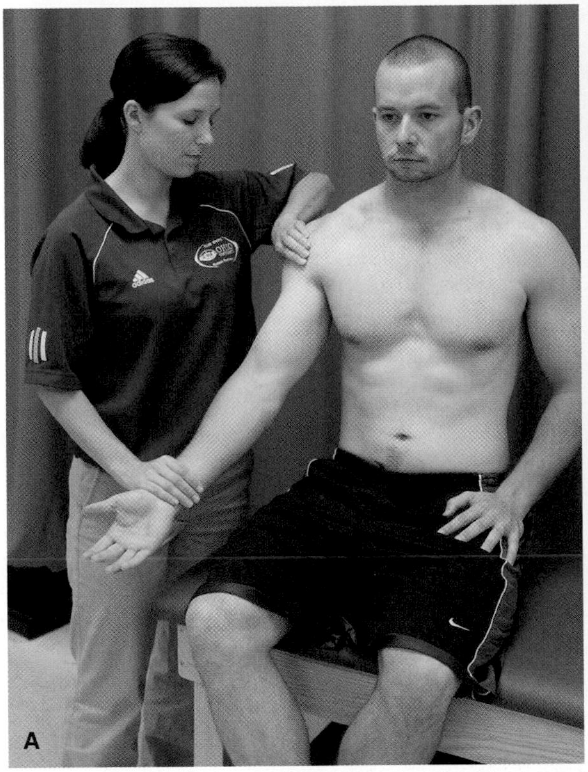

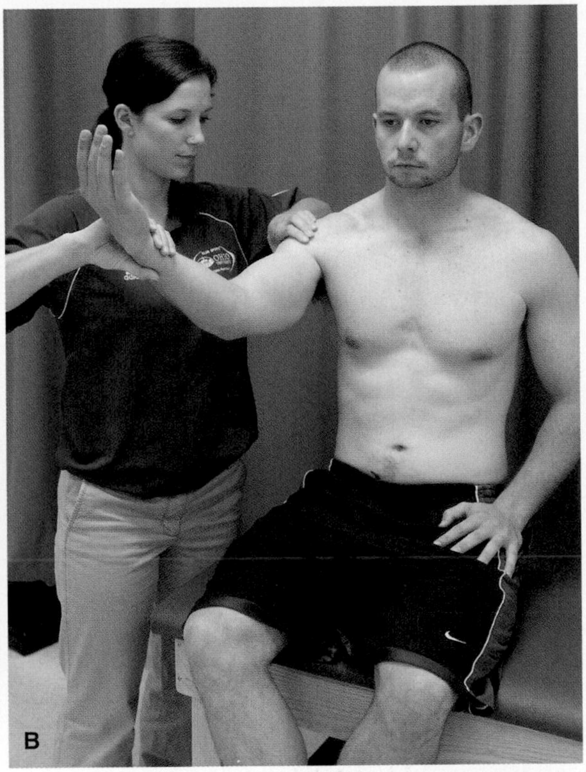

Resisted shoulder flexion with the elbow extended (A) or shoulder flexion and elbow flexion (B) elicit pain in the bicipital groove in the presence of long head of the biceps tendinopathy, a disruption of the transverse humeral ligament, or a SLAP lesion.

Patient Position	Sitting or standing The elbow is extended. The GH joint is in neutral position or slightly extended to stretch the biceps brachii.
Position of Examiner	Standing lateral to and in front of the involved limb The fingers of one hand are positioned over the bicipital groove while stabilizing the shoulder. The forearm is stabilized proximal to the wrist.
Evaluative Procedure	The clinician resists flexion of the GH joint while palpating for tenderness over the bicipital groove. Allow the patient to move through flexion ROM.
Positive Test	Pain along the long head of the biceps brachii tendon, especially in the bicipital groove or at the superior shoulder
Implications	Inflammation of the LHBT as it passes through the bicipital groove Possible tear of the transverse humeral ligament with concurrent instability of the LHBT as it passes through the bicipital groove SLAP lesion (with pain at the superior shoulder)
Modification	The active Speed's test where the examiner resists elbow flexion and forward flexion simultaneously may also be helpful in the detection of SLAP lesions.[103]

Continued

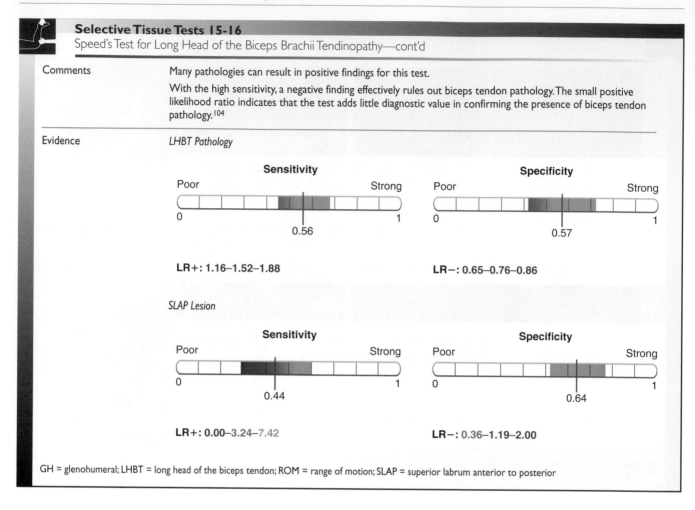

Selective Tissue Tests 15-16
Speed's Test for Long Head of the Biceps Brachii Tendinopathy—cont'd

Comments	Many pathologies can result in positive findings for this test. With the high sensitivity, a negative finding effectively rules out biceps tendon pathology. The small positive likelihood ratio indicates that the test adds little diagnostic value in confirming the presence of biceps tendon pathology.[104]
Evidence	*LHBT Pathology*

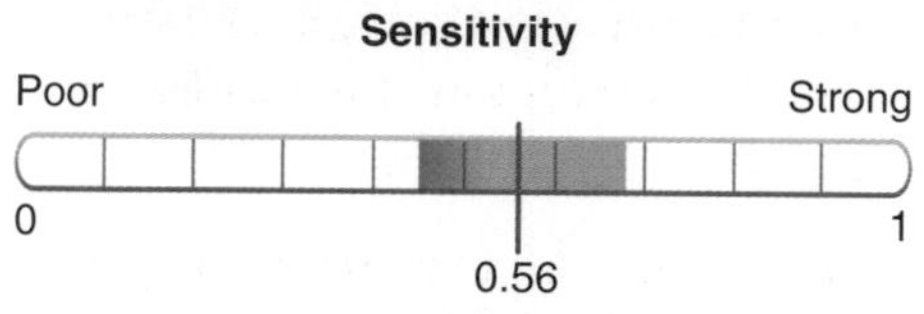

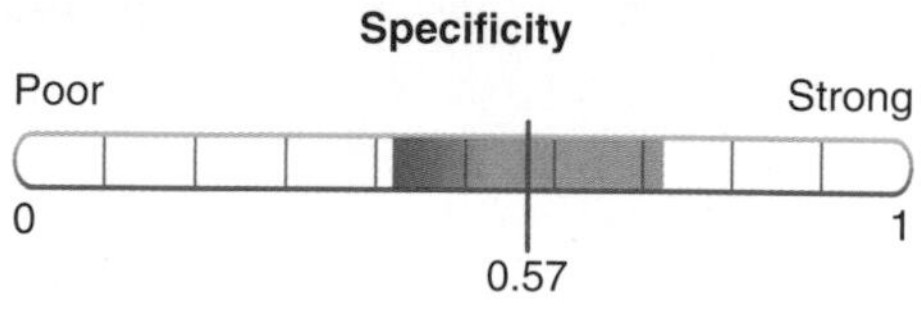

LR+: 1.16–1.52–1.88

LR−: 0.65–0.76–0.86

SLAP Lesion

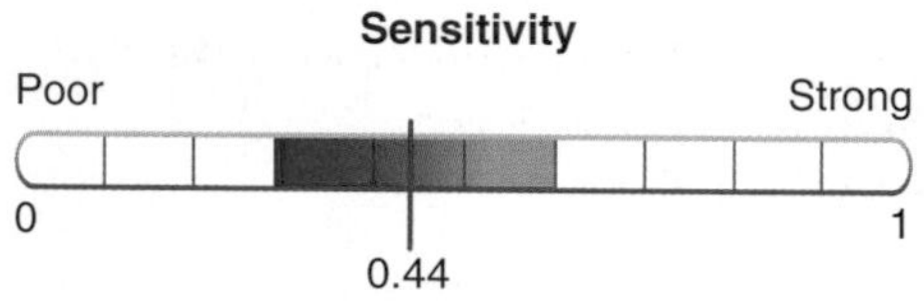

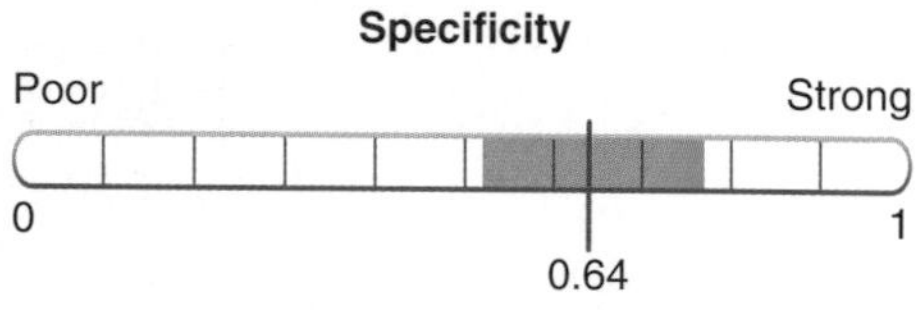

LR+: 0.00–3.24–7.42

LR−: 0.36–1.19–2.00

GH = glenohumeral; LHBT = long head of the biceps tendon; ROM = range of motion; SLAP = superior labrum anterior to posterior

Adhesive Capsulitis

Affecting primarily individuals 40 to 70 years old and primarily in women, adhesive capsulitis is a painful shoulder condition associated with loss of ROM in all planes.[107,114] While its etiology is poorly understood, adhesive capsulitis (also known as frozen shoulder) has no identifiable cause, although individuals with diabetes are predisposed to the condition. A four-stage progression of the condition has been described: (1) pain at night; pain referred to deltoid insertion; (2) severe night pain and stiffness; (3) profound stiffness; pain at the end-range of motion; (4) profound stiffness with minimal pain.[114] The diagnosis is generally made via exam; imaging may be helpful in ruling out other conditions such as tumors, arthritis, fractures, and cervical nerve compression.

Adhesive Capsulitis Intervention Strategies

Adhesive capsulitis is described as self-limiting in that the condition usually resolves on its own over a period of several months to years.[107,114] Oral steroids, steroid injections, manipulation under anesthesia, nerve blocks, and ROM exercises and joint mobilization have all been used to help resolve the condition.

On-Field Examination of Shoulder Injuries

The most important conditions to be ruled out during the on-field evaluation of injuries to the shoulder complex are fractures and dislocations, which may often be confirmed through visual inspection or palpation of the area. When a humeral fracture or GH joint dislocation is suspected, the presence of a distal pulse must be determined. The absence of this pulse warrants the athlete's immediate transportation to a hospital.

Pain radiating through the shoulder and into the arm may indicate damage to one or more cervical nerve roots. A complete evaluation of the cervical or thoracic spine must be performed first when the mechanism of injury or description of the symptoms implicates possible cervical spine trauma (see Chapter 20). The athlete is not moved until the possibility of spinal injury has been eliminated. Trauma to the spleen or myocardial dysfunction may also refer pain into the shoulder.

The on-field evaluation of patients with shoulder injuries is complicated by the presence of shoulder pads in sports such as football, ice hockey, and lacrosse. The examiner must become familiar with how to work around these pads

Examination Findings 15-6
SLAP Lesions

Examination Segment	Clinical Findings
History of Current Condition	*Onset:* Acute or resulting from repetitive microtrauma *Pain characteristics:* Pain in the superior portion of the shoulder Increased pain in position of 90° of abduction and 90° of external rotation Pain is typically not described at rest. *Other symptoms:* Patient may complain of clicking or catching. *Mechanism:* Landing on an outstretched arm, GH instability, overhead motions *Risk factors:* GH instability; posterior GH hypomobility
Functional Assessment	Complaints of inability to perform (e.g., decreased throwing velocity, decreased accuracy); increased pain with late cocking phase of throwing
Inspection	Forward shoulder posture The scapula is protracted at rest.
Palpation	Point tender at posterior GH joint, just inferior to acromion process
Joint and Muscle Function Assessment	*AROM:* Limited internal rotation and horizontal adduction *MMT:* Pain with shoulder and elbow flexion *PROM:* Limited horizontal adduction Limited internal rotation
Joint Stability Tests	*Stress tests:* Not applicable *Joint play:* Hypomobile posterior GH glide consistent with internal impingement
Selective Tissue Tests	Active compression test Anterior slide test Compression–rotation (grind) test
Neurological Screening	Within normal limits
Vascular Screening	Within normal limits
Imaging Techniques	MR arthrography, arthroscopy (anatomical variants make MR less accurate)[105]
Differential Diagnosis	Rotator cuff pathology; LHBT tendinopathy; internal impingement, acromioclavicular pathology, subacromial impingement, Bankart lesion

AROM = active range of motion; GH = glenohumeral; LHBT = long head of the biceps tendon; MMT = manual muscle test; MR = magnetic resonance; PROM = passive range of motion; SLAP = superior labrum anterior to posterior

Selective Tissue Tests 15-17
Active Compression Test (O'Brien Test)

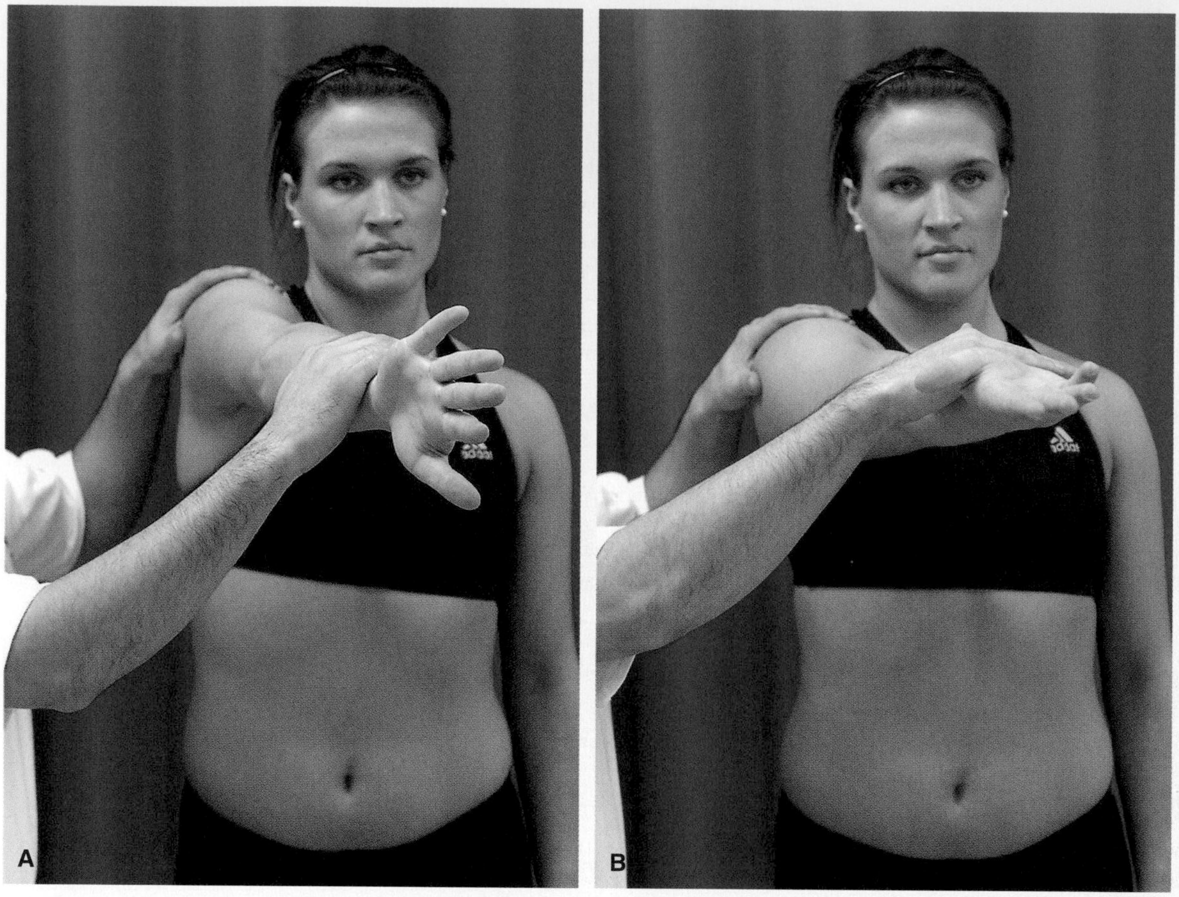

An isometric contraction with the humerus flexed to 90° and horizontally adducted once with the humerus internally rotated (A) and then again with the humerus externally rotated (B). Depending on the positions in which pain is produced, a positive test may indicate a labral tear, AC joint pathology, or a SLAP lesion.

Patient Position	Standing The GH joint is flexed to 90° and horizontally adducted 15° from the sagittal plane. The humerus is in full internal rotation, elbow extended, and the forearm pronated **(A)**.
Position of Examiner	In front of the patient One hand is placed over the superior aspect of the patient's distal forearm.
Evaluative Procedure	The patient isometrically resists the examiner's downward force. The test is repeated with the humerus externally rotated and the forearm supinated **(B)**.
Positive Test	Pain that is experienced with the arm internally rotated is decreased during external rotation: 1. Pain or clicking within the GH joint may indicate a labral tear. 2. Pain at the AC joint may indicate AC joint pathology. Positive SLAP lesion tests are confirmed with pain relief when the hand is supinated; pain with cross-armed horizontal adduction is used to confirm AC pathology.[17]
Implications	SLAP lesion AC joint pathology

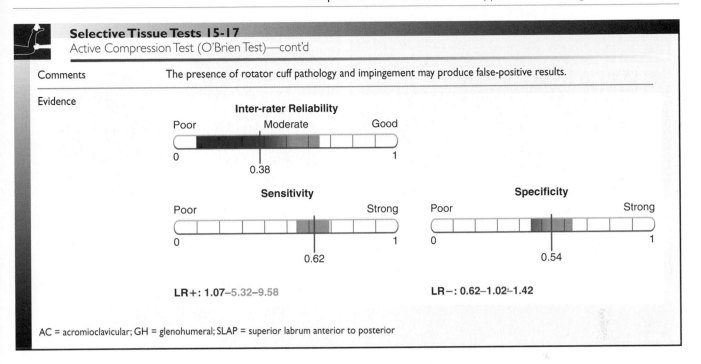

Selective Tissue Tests 15-17
Active Compression Test (O'Brien Test)—cont'd

Comments	The presence of rotator cuff pathology and impingement may produce false-positive results.
Evidence	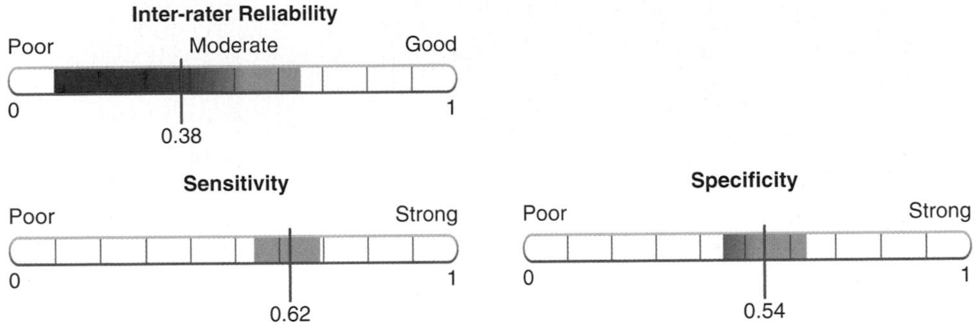 LR+: 1.07–5.32–9.58 LR−: 0.62–1.02–1.42

AC = acromioclavicular; GH = glenohumeral; SLAP = superior labrum anterior to posterior

and, if necessary, how to remove them without further aggravating the injury.

Equipment Considerations

Palpation Under the Shoulder Pads

Shoulder pads have at least one cantilever that arches over the acromion process and the deltoid muscle group. The space provided by the cantilever provides enough room to reach under the jersey and palpate the humeral head, AC joint, and distal clavicle. By unfastening the strap that passes beneath the axilla and loosening the sternal fasteners, more room may be created. It is also possible to palpate the proximal structures of the shoulder complex by entering the shoulder pads from the neck opening.

Because the clinician is palpating these structures without actually being able to see them, care must be used when applying pressure. The initial palpation must be performed gently, following the contours of the shoulder complex while checking for gross deformity.

Removal of the Shoulder Pads

Certain injuries such as AC or SC joint sprains, GH dislocations, or clavicular fractures require the removal of the shoulder pads to further evaluate the condition, begin treatment of the area, or transport the athlete. This must be done with as little movement of the injured extremity as possible to prevent further insult to the injured structures.

If the athlete's jersey is loose fitting, first remove the uninjured arm from the sleeve. After this is completed, slide the shirt up and over the head and then drop it down over the injured arm. In many cases, it is easier to remove the shirt and shoulder pads as a single unit (Fig. 15-34). If the shirt is extraordinarily tight fitting or is a practice jersey or if it is a medical emergency, cut the shirt off the athlete.

On-Field History

- **Location of pain:** Trauma to the AC joint is described as pain localized to the upper shoulder, possibly projecting into the deltoid. Pain that involves the upper trapezius and radiates into the shoulder and arm and is also accompanied by weakness may indicate brachial plexus involvement.
- **Mechanism of injury:** A force that internally or externally rotates the GH joint can result in a GH subluxation or dislocation, especially if the humerus was abducted at the time of the injury. Falling on the tip of the shoulder or landing on an outstretched arm can result in a clavicular fracture, AC sprain, or SC sprain.

On-Field Inspection

- **Arm posture:** The position of the shoulder, humerus, and arm can provide useful clues to the possible pathology.
  - **Arm splinted against the torso:** The humerus' being splinted against the ribs with the forearm supported across the body and the athlete's head looking away from the involved side can indicate a clavicular fracture or AC joint pathology.
  - **Arm hanging limply at the side:** The arm's dangling limply to the side often indicates brachial plexus pathology (see Chapter 14).
  - **Arm "locked":** The humerus' being locked in various positions can indιχate a GH dislocation, with the position of the arm providing evidence of the direction of

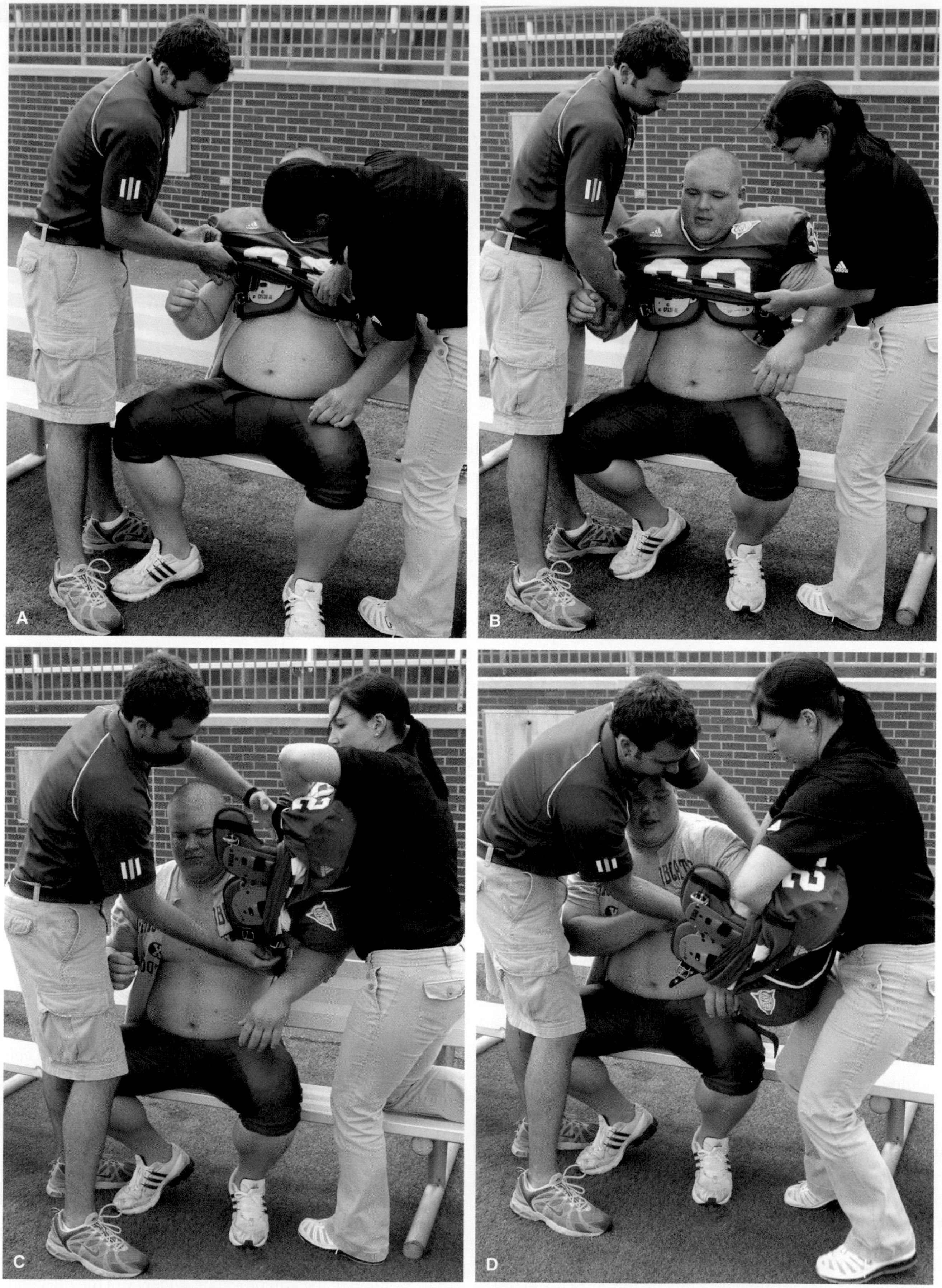

FIGURE 15-34 ■ Removing shoulder pads (the athlete's left arm is injured). (A) Unsnap the chest straps. (B) Pull the shirt off the uninjured arm. (C) Lift the shoulder pads and shirt over the athlete's head. (D) Slide the shoulder pads from around the injured arm.

Selective Tissue Tests 15-18
Anterior Slide Test

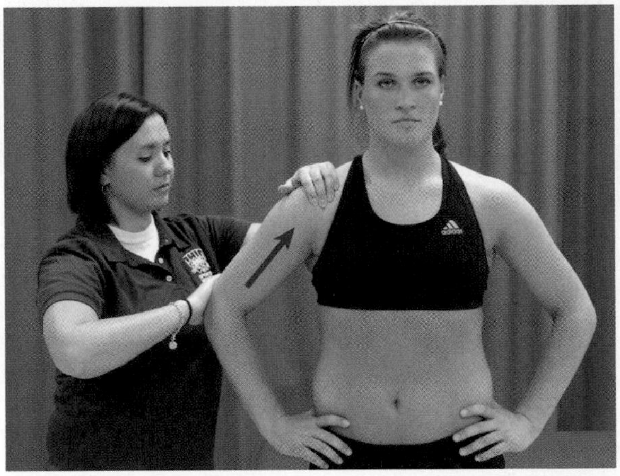

The anterior slide test creates an anteriorly and superiorly directed force that would result in humeral head translation or impingement if a labral tear is present.

Patient Position	Seated or standing Hands on hips with thumbs pointing posteriorly
Position of Examiner	Behind the patient One hand is placed over the shoulder with the index finger lateral to the acromion and over the GH joint. The opposite hand is behind the elbow on the test side.
Evaluative Procedure	An anterior and slightly superior force is applied longitudinally through the humerus. The patient resists, or pushes back, against this force.
Positive Test	Shoulder pain or pop or click under the examiner's index finger Patient report of reproduction of symptoms
Implications	SLAP lesion
Comments	A positive anterior slide test partnered with patient complaints of "popping" or "clicking" are strongly associated with a labral tear.[112]
Evidence	

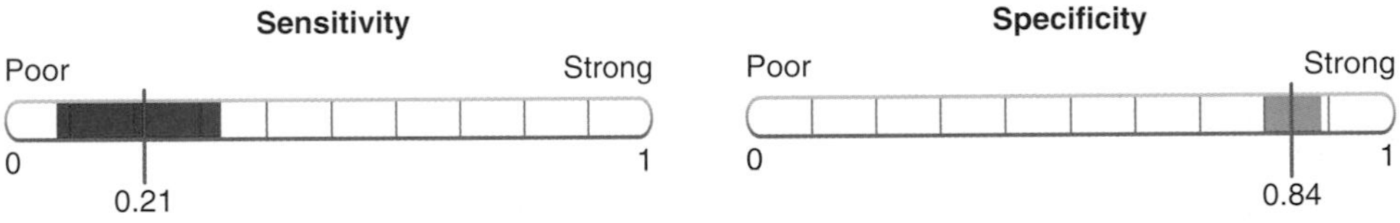

LR+: 0.19–2.26–4.34

LR−: 0.79–0.95–1.10

GH = glenohumeral; SLAP = superior labrum anterior to posterior

Selective Tissue Tests 15-19
Compression-Rotation (Grind) Test

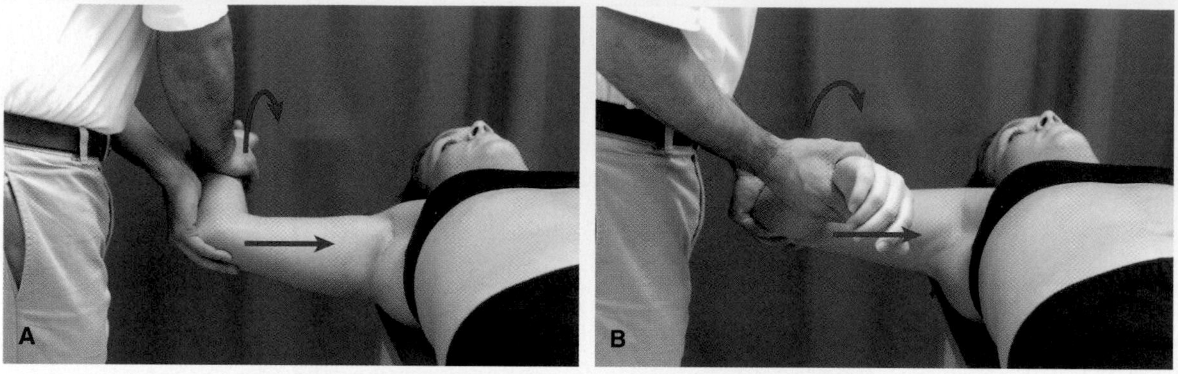

This test is designed to compress the labrum, resulting in reproduction of painful symptoms.

Patient Position	Supine The shoulder is abducted to 90°. The elbow is flexed to 90°.
Position of Examiner	At the test side of the patient
Evaluative Procedure	The examiner maintains an axial load on the humerus while internally and externally rotating the GH joint.
Positive Test	Reproduction of symptoms
Implications	SLAP lesion
Modification	The crank test incorporates a similar mechanism with the arm positioned in maximum forward flexion.
Evidence	

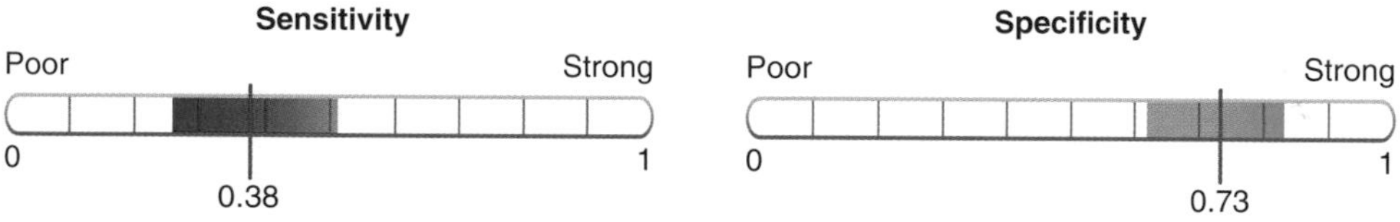

LR+: 0.80–3.32–5.85

LR−: 0.68–0.88–1.08

GH = glenohumeral; SLAP = superior labrum anterior to posterior the dislocation. If it is abducted and externally rotated, suspect an anterior GH dislocation; inferior dislocations are marked by a limited amount of abduction. If it is adducted and internally rotated, suspect posterior GH dislocation.

- **Gross deformity:** Initial inspection of the shoulder complex may be hindered by shoulder pads and jerseys. Gross deformity may be identified during palpation or visually after the equipment has been removed.

On-Field Palpation

- **Position of the humeral head:** If the GH joint is dislocated, the humeral head can be palpated sitting anterior, posterior, or inferior relative to the glenoid fossa.
- **AC joint alignment:** The AC joint is palpated for any abnormal motion, including the piano key sign.
- **Clavicle:** Fractures of the clavicle are often readily apparent. If no visible sign of a fracture is present, palpate the length of the clavicle to identify subcutaneous discontinuity or areas of point tenderness.
- **Sternoclavicular joint:** The SC joint is palpated for bilateral symmetry and continuity.
- **Humerus:** The length of the humerus is palpated for signs of a fracture, especially in the area of the surgical neck.

On-Field Neurological Tests

Brachial plexus injuries cause pain, numbness, and paresthesia in the upper extremity, but the trauma actually involves the cervical spinal nerve roots (see Chapter 14).

Initial Management of On-Field Shoulder Injuries

The following is suggested protocol for the initial management of major injuries to the shoulder complex and upper arm. In emergencies or when proper splinting materials are not available, the athlete's jersey may be used as a sling or the hand can be tucked into the belt of the pants (Fig. 15-35).

Scapular Fractures

Although rare, scapular fractures in football players have been reported.[115] Incidence of scapular fractures is highest among players who wear relatively small shoulder pads. Fractures may occur to the body of the scapula, but most often in the glenoid fossa, glenoid neck, or coracoid process secondary to a GH dislocation. Any athlete suffering from a GH dislocation also needs a radiographic evaluation to rule out a secondary fracture to the glenoid or coracoid process.

To prevent motion, suspected scapular fractures are managed by immobilizing the arm on the affected side in a comfortable position. The athlete then is transported for further medical evaluation.

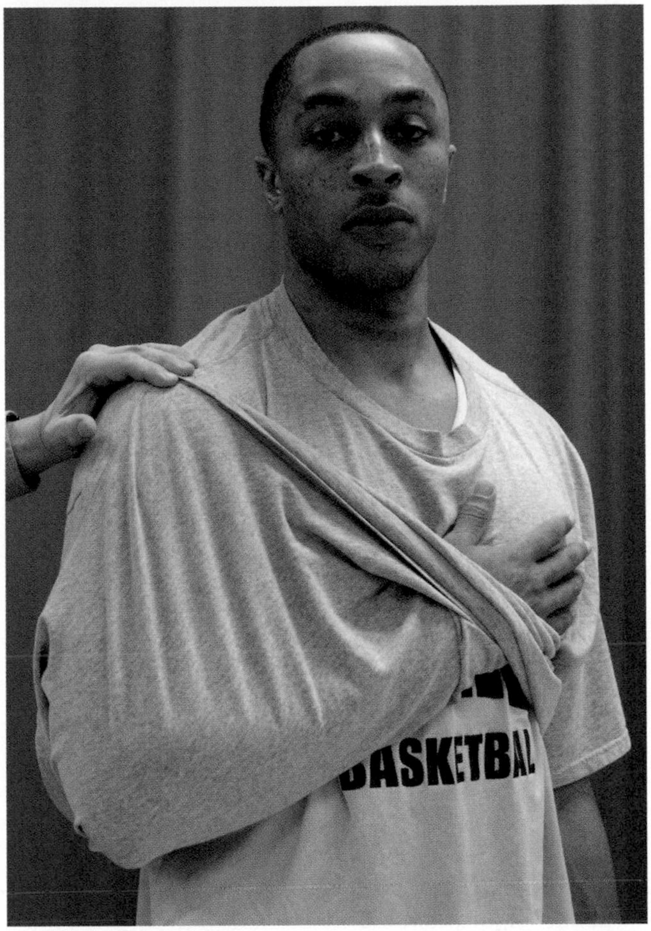

FIGURE 15-35 ■ A temporary sling can be made by pulling the shirt up and over the involved arm.

Clavicular Injuries

Clavicular Fractures

When fractures of the clavicle are suspected, the arm must be immobilized to prevent movement of the fractured segments. The athlete also is transported to a physician for a definitive diagnosis. Displaced fractures of the medial one-third of the clavicle may require emergency surgery due to neurovascular compromise.[116]

The shoulder may be immobilized using a sling or triangular bandage. A sling and swath approach may be more comfortable for the athlete by taking the weight of the arm off the involved clavicle. The use of figure-8 bandages for stabilization is discouraged as their use is associated with greater pain with no difference in functional outcome or appearance.[117] In adults, most distal fractures are managed nonoperatively. Surgical intervention may be indicated with extensive displacement.[117,118]

Sternoclavicular Joint Injuries

The immediate concern with SC dislocations is the potential compromise to the underlying structures from a posterior dislocation.[8] Neurological and vascular examinations of the extremity and carotid artery on the involved side must be performed immediately. Any absent or diminished findings are considered a medical emergency. The involved arm is immobilized using the procedure described for clavicular fractures, and the athlete is immediately transported to an emergency medical facility. To avoid placing pressure on the structures posterior to the SC joint, the athlete must not be transported in the supine position.

Acromioclavicular Joint Injuries

Athletes displaying the signs and symptoms of an AC joint sprain require immobilization in a position that lessens the displacement between the clavicle and the acromial process. Initially, this may be achieved by using a foam pad with a hard shell held in place over the acromial process by a spica wrap and a sling supporting the weight of the arm.

Athletes suffering from AC joint contusions, in addition to the standard modality protocol, need to have the joint protected with additional padding during activity. Such protection may be obtained by using a foam doughnut pad with a hard shell held in place by an elastic spica wrap or elastic tape.

Glenohumeral Dislocations

Because of the possibility of a dislocated humeral head causing additional trauma to the blood and nerve supply to the arm, it is important to monitor the distal pulses, check for circulation in the fingertips, and perform a sensory screen of the involved arm. Absence of a pulse indicates a medical emergency.

Reduction of anterior glenohumeral dislocations should occur as quickly as possible by qualified personnel to minimize damage and reduce the patient's pain and suffering. Reduction of acute anterior glenohumeral dislocations is obtained by slightly abducting and internally rotating the arm while applying gentle longitudinal traction. Other reduction techniques include applying longitudinal traction while moving the arm into abduction[119] and also rotating the scapula to align the glenoid while the patient is prone.

If reduction is not possible, the athlete's shoulder should be fixed in its assumed position using a sling and towel or any other available materials. It is important to keep the wrist and hand easily accessible so that the pulses may be rechecked.

Forced reduction of the humeral head may damage the glenoid fossa, the coracoid process, or the neurovascular structures in the area. After reduction, assess distal pulse and AROM, avoiding external rotation and abduction. Stabilize the shoulder using a sling and refer the athlete for further examination.

Humeral Fractures

Fractures of the humeral shaft and neck are often marked by extreme pain, dysfunction, and obvious deformity. Most humeral fractures occur as the result of a high-impact force. Spontaneous fractures occurring during pitching also have been reported.[120] Fractures in the region of the surgical neck can threaten the radial nerve. Fractures of the humeral head may occur secondary to GH dislocations and therefore initially go unnoticed because of the attention placed on the joint.

Fractures of the humeral shaft are splinted in the position they are found, using a moldable aluminum splint or a vacuum splint. The wrist and fingers remain exposed so that the radial pulse, circulation to the fingers, and sensation of the fingers can be monitored. The athlete is transported supine or on a stretcher. An immediate physician referral is indicated.

REFERENCES

1. Perry, J: Normal upper extremity kinesiology. *Phys Ther*, 58:265, 1978.
2. Nyland, JA, Caborn, DN, and Johnson, DL: The human glenohumeral joint: a proprioceptive and stability alliance. *Knee Surg Sports Traumatol Arthrosc*, 6:50, 1998.
3. Ludewig, PM, and Borstead, JD: The shoulder complex. In: Levangie, PK, and Norkin, CC. *Joint Structure and Function*. Philadelphia, PA: FA Davis, 2011.
4. Groh, GI, and Wirth, MA: Management of traumatic sternoclavicular joint injuries. *J Am Acad Orthop Surg*, 19:1, 2011.
5. Culham, E, and Peat, M: Functional anatomy of the shoulder complex. *J Orthop Sports Phys Ther*, 18:342, 1993.
6. Whiteley, RA, et al: Sports participation and humeral torsion. *J Orthop Sports Phys Ther*, 39:256, 2009.
7. Neumann, DA: *Kinesiology of the Musculoskeletal System: Foundations for Physical Rehabilitation*. St. Louis, MO: Mosby, 2002.
8. Bontempo, NA, and Mazzocca, AD: Biomechanics and treatment of acromioclavicular and sternoclavicular joint injuries. *Br J Sports Med*, 44:361, 2010.
9. Hurov, J: Anatomy and mechanics of the shoulder: review of current concepts. *J Hand Ther*, 22:328, 2009.
10. Tischer, T, et al: Arthroscopic anatomy, variants, and pathologic findings in shoulder instability. *Arthroscopy*, 27:1434, 2011.
11. Hsu, AT, Chiu, JF, and Chang, JH: Biomechanical analysis of distraction mobilization of the glenohumeral joint: a cadaver study. *Man Ther*, 14:381, 2009.
12. Reinold, MM, Escamilla, R, and Wilk, KE: Current concepts in the scientific and clinical rationale behind exercises for glenohumeral and scapulothoracic musculature. *J Orthop Sports Phys Ther*, 39:105, 2009.
13. Elser, F, et al: Anatomy, function, injuries, and treatment of the long head of the biceps brachii tendon. *Arthroscopy*, 27:581, 2011.
14. Precerutti, M, et al: US anatomy of the shoulder: pictorial essay. *J Ultrasound*, 13:179, 2010.
15. Itoi, E, et al: Are pain location and physical examinations useful in locating a tear site of the rotator cuff? *Am J Sports Med*, 34:256, 2006.
16. Chronopoulos, E, et al: Diagnostic value of physical tests for isolated chronic acromioclavicular lesions. *Am J Sports Med*, 32:655, 2004.
17. Baker, CL, and Merkley, MS: Clinical evaluation of the athlete's shoulder. *J Athl Train*, 35:256, 2000.
18. Meister, K: Injuries to the shoulder in the throwing athlete. Part One: biomechanics/Pathophysiology/Classification of injury. *Am J Sports Med*, 28:265, 2000.
19. Harris, JD, et al: Predictor of pain and function in patients with symptomatic, atraumatic full-thickness rotator cuff tears: a time-zero analysis of a prospective patient cohort enrolled in a structured physical therapy program. *Am J Sports Med*, 40:359, 2012.
20. Ludewig, PM, and Borstead, JD: The shoulder complex. In: Levangie, PK, and Norkin, CC (eds): *Joint Structure and Function: A Comprehensive Analysis* (ed 4). Philadelphia, PA: FA Davis, 2005, p 233.
21. Murrell, GA, and Walton, JR: Diagnosis of rotator cuff tears. *Lancet*, 357:769, 2001.

22. Park, HB, et al: Diagnostic accuracy of clinical tests for the different degrees of subacromial impingement syndrome. *J Bone Joint Surg*, 87-A:1446, 2005.
23. Shanley, E: Shoulder range of motion measures as risk factors for shoulder and elbow injuries in high school softball and baseball players. *Am J Sports Med*, 39:1997, 2011.
24. Gerber, C, and Krushell, RJ: Isolated rupture of the tendon of the subscapularis muscle: clinical features in 16 cases. *J Bone Joint Surg*, 73(B):389, 1991.
25. Kelly, BT, Kadrmas, WR, and Speer, KP: The manual muscle examination for rotator cuff strength: an electromyographic investigation. *Am J Sports Med*, 24:581, 1996.
26. Greis, PE, et al: Validation of the lift-off test and analysis of subscapularis activity during maximal internal rotation. *Am J Sports Med*, 24:589, 1996.
27. Hertel, R, et al: Lag signs in the diagnosis of rotator cuff rupture. *J Shoulder Elbow Surg*, 5:307, 1996.
28. Angloague, PA, et al: Glenohumeral range of motion and lower extremity flexibility in collegiate-level baseball players. *Sports Health*, 4:25, 2012.
29. Levy, AS, et al: Intra- and interobserver reproducibility of the shoulder laxity examination. *Am J Sports Med*, 58:272, 1999.
30. Speer, KP: Anatomy and pathomechanics of shoulder instability. *Oper Tech Sports Med*, 1:252, 1993.
31. Hawkins, RJ, and Bokor, DJ: Glenohumeral instability. In: Rockwood, CA, and Masten, FA (eds): *The Shoulder* (vol 1) (ed 4). Philadelphia, PA: WB Saunders, 2009, pp 687-688.
32. Levy, AS, et al: Intra- and interobserver reliability of the shoulder laxity examination. *Am J Sports Med*, 27:460, 1999.
33. McFarland, EG, et al: Posterior shoulder laxity in asymptomatic athletes. *Am J Sports Med*, 24:468, 1996.
34. Doody, SG, and Waterland, JC: Shoulder movements during abduction in the scapular plane. *Arch Phys Med Rehabil*, 51:595, 1970.
35. Hebert, LJ, et al: Scapular behavior in shoulder impingement syndrome. *Arch Phys Med Rehabil*, 83:60, 2002.
36. Laudner, KG, Stanek, JM, and Meister, K: Differences in scapular upward rotation between baseball pitchers and position players. *Am J Sports Med*, 35:2091, 2007.
37. Lukasiewicz, AC, et al: Comparison of 3-dimensional scapular position and orientation between subjects with and without shoulder impingement. *J Orthop Sports Phys Ther*, 29:574, 1999.
38. McClure, PW, et al: Shoulder function and 3-dimensional scapular kinematics in people with and without shoulder impingement syndrome. *Phys Ther*, 86:1075, 2006.
39. Warner, JJP, et al: Scapulothoracic motion in normal shoulders and shoulders with glenohumeral instability and impingement syndrome: a study using Moiré topographic analysis. *Clin Orthop Relat Res*, 285:191, 1992.
40. Myers, JB, et al: Scapular position and orientation in throwing athletes. *Am J Sports Med*, 33:263, 2005.
41. Mell, AG, et al: Effect of rotator cuff pathology on shoulder rhythm. *J Shoulder Elbow Surg*, 14:S58, 2001.
42. Paletta, GA, et al: Shoulder kinematics with two-plane x-ray evaluation in patients with anterior instability or rotator cuff tearing. *J Shoulder Elbow Surg*, 6:516, 1997.
43. Ogston, JB, and Ludewig, PM: Differences in 3-dimensional shoulder kinematics between persons with multidirectional instability and asymptomatic controls. *Am J Sports Med*, 35:1361, 2007.
44. von Eisenhart-Rothe, R, et al: Pathomechanics in atraumatic shoulder instability: scapular positioning correlates with humeral head centering. *Clin Orthop Relat Res*, 433:82, 2005.
45. Gumina, S, et al: Scapular dyskinesis and sick scapula syndrome in patients with chronic type III acromioclavicular dislocation. *Arthroscopy*, 25:40, 2009.
46. Fayad, F, et al: Three-dimensional scapular kinematics and scapulohumeral rhythm in patients with glenohumeral osteoarthritis or frozen shoulder. *J Biomech*, 41:326, 2008.
47. Lin, J, et al: Effect of shoulder tightness on glenohumeral translation, scapular kinematics, and scapulohumeral rhythm in subjects with stiff shoulders. *J Orthop Res*, 24:1044, 2006.
48. Rundquist, PJ, et al: Correlation of 3-dimensional shoulder kinematics to function in subjects with idiopathic loss of shoulder range of motion. *Phys Ther*, 85:636, 2005.
49. Vermeulen, HM, et al: Measurement of three dimensional shoulder movement patterns with an electromagnetic tracking device in patients with a frozen shoulder. *BMJ*, 61:115, 2002.
50. Graichen, H, et al: Three-dimensional analysis of shoulder girdle and supraspinatus motion patterns in patients with impingement syndrome. *J Orthop Res*, 19:1192, 2001.
51. Kibler, WB, et al: Evaluation of apparent and absolute supraspinatus strength in patients with shoulder injury using the scapular retraction test. *Am J Sports Med*, 34:1643, 2006.
52. Kibler, WB, et al: Clinical utility of traditional and new tests in the diagnosis of biceps tendon injuries and superior labrum anterior and posterior lesions in the shoulder. *Am J Sports Med*, 37:1840, 2009.
53. Ludewig, PM, and Reynolds, JF: The association of scapular kinematics and glenohumeral joint pathologies. *J Orthop Sports Phys Ther*, 39:90, 2009.
54. Kibler, WB, and McMullen, J: Scapular dyskinesis and its relation to shoulder pain. *J Am Acad Orthop Surg*, 11:142, 2003.
55. Rabin, A, et al: The intertester reliability of the scapular assistance test. *J Orthop Sports Phys Ther*, 36:653, 2006.
56. Burkhart, SS, et al: The disabled throwing shoulder: spectrum of pathology part III: the SICK scapula, scapular dyskinesis, the kinetic chain, and rehabilitation. *Arthroscopy*, 19:641, 2003.
57. Wirth, MA, and Rockwood, CA: Acute and chronic traumatic injuries of the sternoclavicular joint. *J Am Acad Orthop Surg*, 4:268, 1996.
58. Jougon, JB, et al: Posterior dislocation of the sternoclavicular joint leading to mediastinal compression. *Ann Thorac Surg*, 61:711, 1996.
59. Glass, ER, et al: Treatment of sternoclavicular joint dislocations: a systematic review of 251 dislocations in 24 case series. *Trauma*, 70:1294, 2011.
60. Mazzocca, AD, et al: Evaluation and treatment of acromioclavicular joint injuries. *Am J Sports Med*, 35:316, 2007.
61. Walton, J, et al: Diagnostic values of tests for acromioclavicular joint pain. *J Bone Joint Surg Am*, 86-A:807, 2004.
62. Pauly, S, et al: Prevalence and patterns of glenohumeral injuries among acute high-grade acromioclavicular joint injuries. *J Shoulder Elbow Surg*, 22:760, 2013.
63. Gartsman, GM: Arthroscopic resection of the acromioclavicular joint. *Am J Sports Med*, 21:71, 1993.
64. Gartsman, GM, et al: Arthroscopic acromioclavicular joint resection: an anatomical study. *Am J Sports Med*, 19:2, 1991.
65. Carter, T, et al: Intertester reliability of a classification system for shoulder pain. *Physiotherapy*, 98:40, 2012.
66. Borbas, P, et al: The influence of ultrasound guidance on the rate of success of AC joint injection: an exploratory study on human cadavers. *J Shoulder Elbow Surg*, 21:1694, 2012.
67. Soh, E, et al: Image-guided versus blind corticosteroid injections in adults with shoulder pain: a systematic review. *BMC Musculoskelet Disord*, 12:137, 2011.
68. Omoumi, P, et al: Glenohumeral joint instability. *J Magn Reson Imaging*, 33:2, 2011.
69. Gaskill, TR, et al: Management of multidirectional instability of the shoulder. *J Am Acad Orthop Surg*, 19:758, 2011.
70. Eckenrode, BJ, et al: Anatomic and biomechanical fundamentals of the thrower shoulder. *Sports Med Arthrosc Rev*, 20:2, 2012.

71. Levine, WM, and Flatow, EL: The pathophysiology of shoulder instability. *Am J Sports Med,* 28:910, 2000.
72. Lo, IK, et al: An evaluation of the apprehension, relocation and surprise tests for anterior shoulder instability. *Am J Sports Med,* 32:301, 2004.
73. Farber, AJ, et al: Clinical assessment of three common tests for traumatic anterior shoulder instability. *J Bone Joint Surg,* 88(A):1467, 2006.
74. Guanche, CA, and Jones, DC: Clinical testing for tears of the glenoid labrum. *Arthroscopy,* 19:517, 2003.
75. Tripp, BL, et al: Functional multijoint position reproduction acuity in overhead throwing athletes. *J Athl Train,* 41:146, 2006.
76. Parentis, MA, et al: An evaluation of the provocative tests for superior labral anterior posterior lesions. *Am J Sports Med,* 34:265, 2006.
77. Brophy, RH, and Marx, RG: The treatment of traumatic anterior instability of the shoulder: nonoperative and surgical treatment. *Arthroscopy,* 25:298, 2009.
78. Boone, JL, and Arciero, RA: First-time anterior shoulder dislocation: has the standard changed? *Br J Sports Med,* 44:355, 2010.
79. Kim, SH, et al: Painful jerk test: a predictor of success in nonoperative treatment of posteroinferior instability of the shoulder. *Am J Sports Med,* 32:1849, 2004.
80. Van Tongel, A, et al: Posterior shoulder instability: current concepts review. *Knee Surg Sports Traumatol Arthrosc,* 19:1547, 2011.
81. Kim, S-H, et al: The Kim test: a novel test for posteroinferior labral lesion of the shoulder—a comparison to the jerk test. *Am J Sports Med,* 33:1188, 2005.
82. Kowalsky, MS, and Levine, WN: Traumatic posterior glenohumeral dislocation: classification, pathoanatomy, diagnosis, and treatment. *Orthop Clin N Am,* 39:519, 2008.
83. Warner, JJP, et al: Static capsuloligamentous restraints to superior-inferior translation of the glenohumeral joint. *Am J Sports Med,* 20:675, 1992.
84. Hsu, HC, et al: Influence of rotator cuff tearing on glenohumeral stability. *J Shoulder Elbow Surg,* 6:413, 1997.
85. Sein, ML, et al: Shoulder pain in elite swimmers: primarily due to swim-volume-induced supraspinatus tendinopathy. *Br J Sports Med,* 44:105, 2010.
86. Struyf, F, et al: Scapular positioning and movement in unimpaired shoulders, shoulder impingement syndrome, and glenohumeral instability. *Scand J Med Sci Sports,* 21:352, 2011.
87. Borstad, JD, and Ludewig, PM: The effect of long versus short pectoralis minor resting length on scapular kinematics in healthy individuals. *J Orthop Sports Phys Ther,* 35:227, 2005.
88. Corso, G: Impingement relief test: an adjunctive procedure to traditional assessment of shoulder impingement syndrome. *J Orthop Sports Phys Ther,* 22:183, 1995.
89. Tate, AR, et al: Comprehensive impairment-based exercise and manual therapy intervention for patients with subacromial impingement syndrome: a case series. *J Orthop Sports Phys Ther,* 40:474, 2010.
90. Seitz, AL, et al: Mechanisms of rotator cuff tendinopathy: intrinsic, extrinsic, or both? *Clin Biomech,* 26:1, 2011.
91. Kibler, WB, et al: Glenohumeral internal rotation deficit: pathogenesis and response to acute throwing. *Sports Med Arthrosc Rev,* 20:34, 2012.
92. Castagna, A, et al: Posterior superior internal impingement: an evidence-based review. *Br J Sports Med,* 44:382, 2010.
93. Cowderoy, GA, et al: Overuse and impingement syndromes of the shoulder in the athlete. *Magn Reson Imaging Clin N Am,* 17:577, 2009.
94. Cuomo, F, et al: The influence of acromioclavicular joint morphology on rotator cuff tears. *J Shoulder Elbow Surg,* 7:555, 1998.
95. Matava, MJ, et al: Partial-thickness rotator cuff tears. *Am J Sports Med,* 33:1405, 2005.
96. Wilson, JJ, and Best, TM: Common overuse tendon problems: a review and recommendations for treatment. *Am Fam Physician,* 72:811, 2005.
97. Jobe, FW, et al: Anterior capsulolabral reconstruction of the shoulder in athletes in overhand sports. *Am J Sports Med,* 19:428, 1991.
98. Itoi, E, et al: Which is more useful, the "full can test" or the "empty can test" in detecting the torn supraspinatus tendon? *Am J Sports Med,* 27:65, 1999.
99. Holtby, R, and Razmjou, H: Validity of the supraspinatus test as a single clinical test in diagnosing patients with rotator cuff pathology. *J Orthop Sports Phys Ther,* 34:194, 2004.
100. Zanetti, M, et al: Tendinopathy and rupture of the tendon of the long head of the biceps brachii muscle: evaluation with MR arthrography. *Am J Rotentgenol,* 170:1557, 1998.
101. Caliş, M, et al: Diagnostic values of clinical diagnostic tests in subacromial impingement syndrome. *Ann Rheum Dis,* 59:44, 2000.
102. Holtby, R, and Razmjou, H: Accuracy of the Speed's and Yergason's tests in detecting biceps pathology and SLAP lesions: comparison with arthroscopic findings. *Arthroscopy,* 20:231, 2004.
103. Wilk, KE, et al: Current concepts in the recognition and treatment of superior labral (SLAP) lesions. *J Orthop Sports Phys Ther,* 35:273, 2005.
104. Bennett, WF: Specificity of the Speed's test: arthroscopic technique for evaluating the biceps tendon at the level of the bicipital groove. *Arthroscopy,* 14:789, 1998.
105. Powers, R: SLAP lesions: how to recognize and treat this debilitating shoulder injury. *JAAPA,* 24:32, 2011.
106. Kim, TK, et al: Clinical features of the different types of SLAP lesions: an analysis of one hundred and thirty-nine cases. *J Bone Joint Surg,* 85(A):66, 2003.
107. Cook, C, et al: Diagnostic accuracy of five orthopedic clinical tests for diagnosis of superior labrum anterior posterior (SLAP) lesions. *J Shoulder Elbow Surg,* 21:13, 2012.
108. O'Brien, SJ, et al: The active compression test: a new and effective test for diagnosing labral tears and acromioclavicular joint abnormalities. *Am J Sports Med,* 26:610, 1998.
109. Stetson, WB, and Templin, K: The crank test, the O'Brien test, and routine magnetic imaging scans in the diagnosis of labral tears. *Am J Sports Med,* 30:806, 2002.
110. McFarland, EG, et al: Clinical assessment of three common tests for superior labral anterior-posterior lesions. *Am J Sports Med,* 30:810. 2002.
111. Kibler, WB: Specificity and sensitivity of the anterior slide test in throwing athletes with superior glenoid labral tears. *Arthroscopy,* 11:296, 1995.
112. Walsworth, MK, et al: Reliability and diagnostic accuracy of history and physical examination for diagnosing glenoid labral tears. *Am J Sports Med,* 36:162, 2007.
113. Alessandro, DF, et al: Superior labral lesions: diagnosis and management. *J Athl Train,* 35:286, 2000.
114. Ewald, A: Adhesive capsulitis: a review. *Am Fam Physician,* 83:417, 2011.
115. Cain, TE, and Hamilton, WP: Scapular fractures in professional football players. *Am J Sports Med,* 20:363, 1992.
116. Quillen, DM, et al: Acute shoulder injuries. *Am Fam Physician,* 70: 1947, 2004.
117. Pandya, NK, et al: Displaced clavicle fractures in adolescents: facts, controversies, and current trends. *J Am Acad Orthop Surg,* 20:498, 2012.
118. Banerjee, R, et al: Management of distal clavicle fractures. *J Am Acad Orthop Surg,* 19:392, 2011.
119. Sayegh, FE, et al: Reduction of acute anterior dislocations: a prospective randomized study comparing a new technique with the Hippocratic and Kocher methods. *J Bone Joint Surg Am,* 91:2775, 2009.
120. Branch, T, et al: Spontaneous fractures of the humerus during pitching: a series of 12 cases. *Am J Sports Med,* 20:468, 1992.

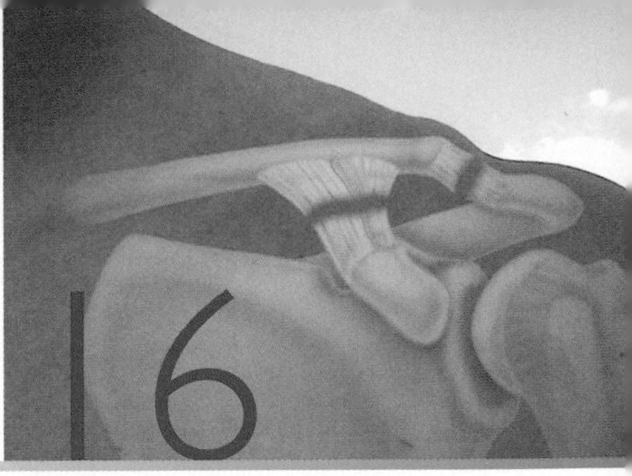

CHAPTER 16

Elbow and Forearm Pathologies

Serving as the link between the powerful movements of the shoulder and the **fine motor control** of the hand, the elbow is often overlooked as an area of potentially disabling injury. Even minor injuries to the elbow can severely hamper the ability to perform the most rudimentary movements. Fractures or other trauma involving the elbow or forearm can result in impairment of the neurovascular structures supplying the wrist, hand, and fingers. Additionally, pathology at the shoulder can influence movement patterns and stresses at the elbow. Therefore, examination of the elbow and forearm is often expanded to include the hand and shoulder.

Clinical Anatomy

The humerus, radius, and ulna form the elbow joint. The radius and ulna continue on to form the proximal and distal radioulnar joints of the forearm. The distal end of the humerus flares to form the medial and lateral epicondyles, with the medial epicondyle larger than the lateral. Between the epicondyles lie the capitulum and the trochlea, the articulating surfaces for the radius and ulna. Separated from the trochlea by the trochlear groove, the **capitulum** forms the lateral humeral articulating surface on the distal border of the **lateral epicondyle**. Unlike the trochlea, the dome-shaped capitulum does not extend to the posterior aspect of the humerus. Located immediately above the capitulum, the **radial fossa** is an indentation in the lateral epicondyle that accepts the radial head during elbow flexion (Fig. 16-1). The distal end of the humerus is anteriorly rotated 30 degrees relative to the humeral shaft.

The **ulna** forms the medial border of the forearm. Proximally, the ulna articulates with the humerus and radius. The proximal border of the ulna is formed by the **olecranon process**, a projection that fits into the humeral **olecranon fossa** during complete extension of the elbow.

Fine motor control Specific control of the muscles allowing for completion of small, delicate tasks

The **semilunar notch**, an indentation lined with articular cartilage, fits snugly around the humeral trochlea. The distal border of the semilunar notch is formed by the **coronoid process**. The ulnar coronoid process is received by the **coronoid fossa** of the humerus during elbow flexion. Lateral and slightly distal to the coronoid process, the **radial notch** is an indentation that accepts the radial head to form the **proximal radioulnar joint** (Fig. 16-2).

Located on the thumb-side of the forearm, the **radius** is lateral to the ulna when the body is in its anatomical position. The proximal articulating surface, the **radial head**, is disk shaped and concave to allow gliding and rotation on the capitulum, significantly enhancing the elbow's stability.[1] The border of the proximal radius is also covered with articular cartilage to allow it to rotate on the ulna. Distal to the radial head is the **bicipital tuberosity** (radial tuberosity), the insertion site for the biceps brachii. The **radial shaft** is triangular in shape and broadens medially and laterally at its distal end. The **radial styloid process** projects off the lateral border

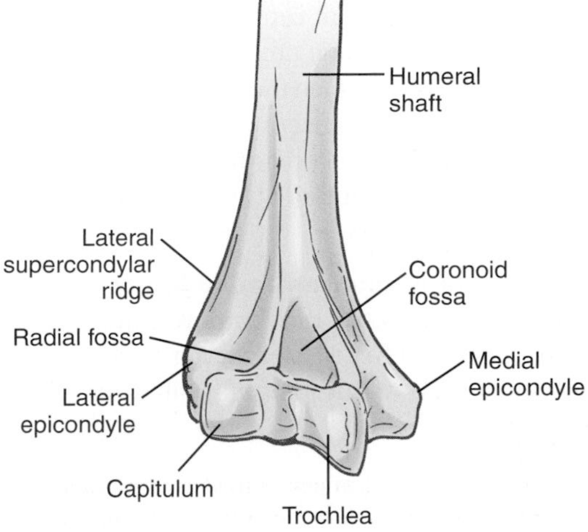

FIGURE 16-1 ■ Bony anatomy of the distal humerus. The trochlea articulates with the ulna; the capitulum, with the radial head.

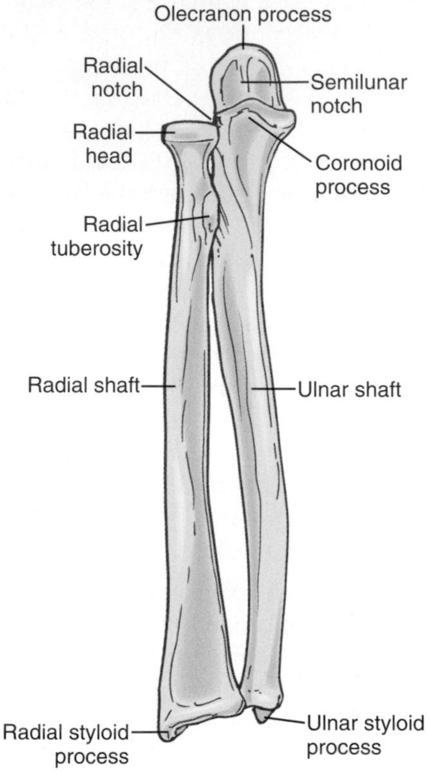

FIGURE 16-2 ■ Bony anatomy of the radius and ulna.

of the distal radius. **Lister's tubercle** projects off the dorsal surface of the distal radius.

Articulations and Ligamentous Support

To function properly, the elbow relies on the integrity of four individual articulations: the humeroulnar joint, humeroradial joint, proximal radioulnar joint, and distal radioulnar joint. The elbow relies on its bony configuration and ligamentous structure for support. Bony stability formed by the relationship between the olecranon and the olecranon fossa is greatest between 0 degrees and 20 degrees and beyond 120 degrees of flexion. Within this range, the ligaments are the primary restraints against valgus and varus stresses.[2] The three proximal joints share a common joint capsule, such that injury at one joint impacts function at the others. This interrelationship is particularly problematic when the elbow is immobilized.

Elbow flexion and extension occur at the humeroulnar and humeroradial joints. Forearm **supination** and **pronation** occur at the humeroradial, superior radioulnar, and inferior radioulnar joints.

Humeroulnar and Humeroradial Joints

A modified hinge joint, the **humeroulnar articulation** allows for 1 degree of freedom of movement: flexion and extension. The design of this joint may allow up to 5 degrees of internal rotation of the ulna on the humerus, but this motion is an accessory one.

Also a modified hinge joint, the **humeroradial joint** permits 2 degrees of freedom of movement: (1) flexion and extension as the radial head glides over the capitulum and (2) rotation of the radius on the capitulum during the movements of pronation and supination.

Proximal and Distal Radioulnar Joints

The **proximal radioulnar joint** is formed by the convex radial head and the concave radial notch of the ulna. The **distal radioulnar joint** is formed by an articular disk between the radius and ulna where the concave ulnar notch of the radius articulates with the convex region of the ulna. The radioulnar joints have 1 degree of freedom of movement, pronation, and supination. Their alignment is maintained by an interosseous membrane between the bones, classifying them as syndesmotic joints. During pronation, proximal joint motion occurs as the radius rotates within the radial notch of the ulna, causing the radius to cross over the ulna (Fig. 16-3). The reverse occurs during supination.

Ligamentous Support

Valgus support of the medial elbow is obtained from the **ulnar collateral ligament** (UCL), also referred to as the medial collateral ligament. The UCL is divided into three unique sections: the anterior, transverse, and posterior bundles

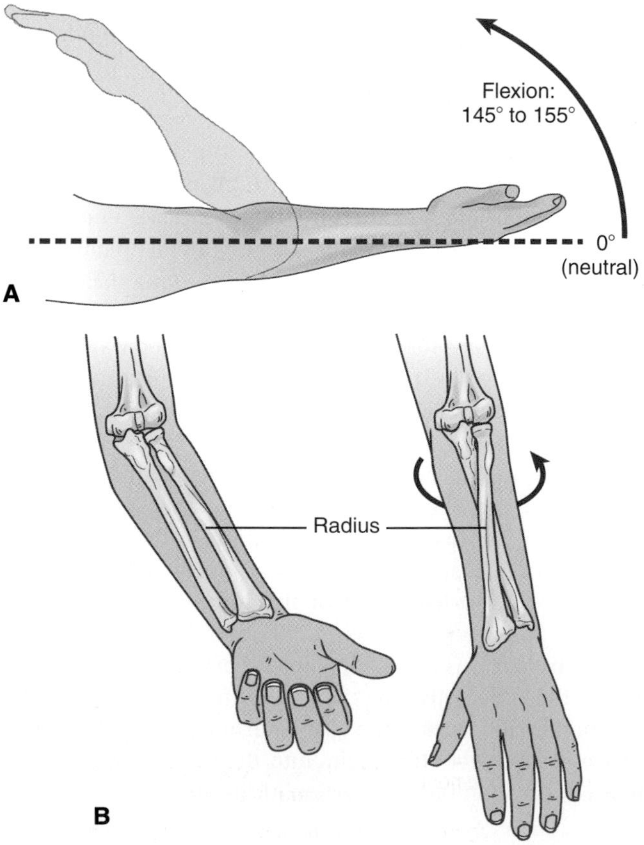

FIGURE 16-3 ■ Motion at the elbow. (A) Elbow flexion and extension. (B) Forearm pronation and supination. Pronation involves a palm down position; supination is the palm up position.

Supination (forearm) Movement at the radioulnar joints allowing for the palm to turn upward, as if holding a bowl of soup

Pronation (forearm) Movement at the radioulnar joints allowing for the palm to be turned downward

(Fig. 16-4). The **anterior bundle** originates from the inferior surface of the medial epicondyle and passes anterior to the axis of rotation to insert on the medial aspect of the coronoid process. Unlike the other elbow ligaments, the anterior bundle is easily distinguishable from the joint capsule. Taut throughout the elbow's range of motion (ROM), this band is the primary restraint against valgus force. The anterior bundle is further divided into anterior and posterior bands. The anterior band resists valgus stress until about 90 degrees of flexion; the posterior band is the primary restraint when the elbow is flexed beyond 60 degrees and is primarily stressed in overhead-throwing athletes.[3] The **transverse bundle**, originating from the medial epicondyle and inserting on the coronoid process, does not cross the axis of the elbow and therefore provides little, if any, medial support.[2] Inserting on the olecranon process, the **posterior bundle** is taut in flexion beyond 90 degrees and is subject to stress only if the anterior bundle is completely disrupted.[3]

Lateral support of the elbow is derived from the radial collateral, annular, lateral ulnar collateral, and the accessory lateral collateral ligaments (Fig. 16-5). The **lateral ulnar collateral ligament** (LUCL) is the most important lateral stabilizing structure. Arising from the middle of the lateral epicondyle and inserting on the tubercle of the ulna, the LUCL provides lateral support of the ulna that is independent of the other lateral ligaments. Disruption of this ligament results in rotatory instability of the elbow joint.

The radial collateral ligament (RCL) is a thickened area in the lateral joint capsule between the lateral epicondyle and the annular ligament. In addition to resisting varus stresses, the RCL assists in maintaining the close relationship between the humeral and radial articulating surfaces.

Encircling the radial head, the annular ligament is a fibro-osseous structure that permits internal and external rotation of the radial head on the capitulum of the humerus. Both ends of the annular ligament attach to the coronoid process and form four-fifths of a circle. The remaining one-fifth of the circle is formed by the radial notch. This articulation receives additional support from the attachment of the RCL and the fibrous attachment of the supinator muscle. The distal end of the annular ligament narrows to conform to the shape of the radial head, preventing the radius from sliding distally.

At the end-range of supination, the anterior fibers of the annular ligament become taut; at the end of pronation, the posterior fibers are taut. When a varus stress is applied to the elbow, the accessory collateral ligament assists the annular ligament and the RCL to prevent the radius from separating from the ulna.

Interosseous Membrane

A dense band of fibrous connective tissue, the fibers of the interosseous membrane run obliquely from the radius to the ulna and span the distance between the proximal and distal radioulnar joints (Fig. 16-6). This fibrous arrangement

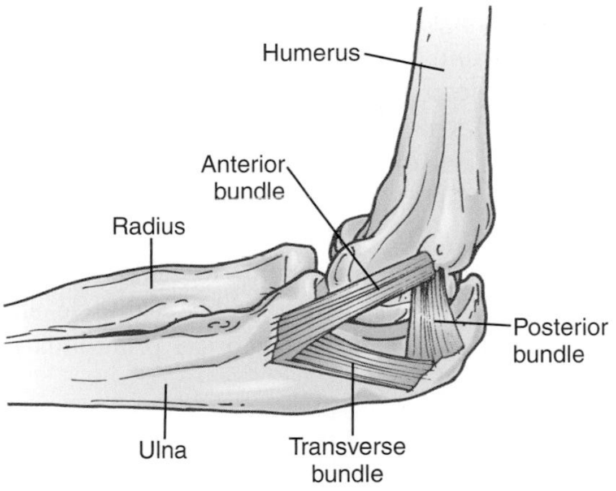

FIGURE 16-4 ■ Ulnar collateral ligament complex. This ligament is formed by the anterior bundle, the posterior bundle, and the transverse bundle.

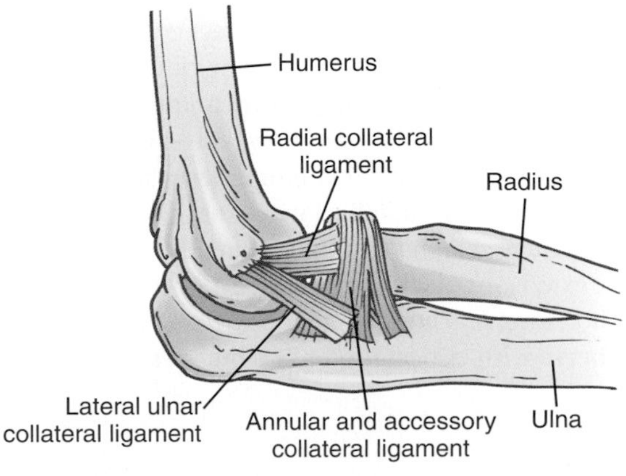

FIGURE 16-5 ■ Lateral ligaments of the elbow. This group is formed by the radial collateral ligament, the lateral ulnar collateral ligament, and the annular ligament. The annular ligament maintains the articulation between the proximal radius and ulna.

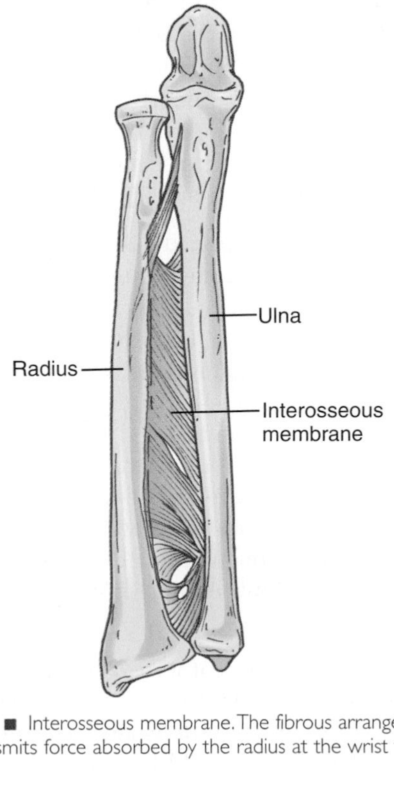

FIGURE 16-6 ■ Interosseous membrane. The fibrous arrangement of this structure transmits force absorbed by the radius at the wrist to the ulna.

serves as a stabilizer against axial forces applied to the wrist, transmitting force from the radius to the ulna. This force is then transmitted to the humerus. The interosseous membrane also serves as an attachment site for many of the muscles acting on the wrist and hand. Dislocation of the proximal or distal radioulnar joint may also injure the interosseous membrane.[1]

Muscular Anatomy

The muscles inserting on the proximal radius and ulna act to flex or extend the elbow and pronate or supinate the forearm. Many of the prime movers of the wrist and hand originate from the humeral epicondyles and the proximal radius and ulna. The actions, origins, insertions, and innervation of the muscles producing elbow and forearm motion are presented in Table 16-1. Chapter 17 discusses the muscles acting on the wrist and hand.

Elbow Flexor and Supinator Group

The **biceps brachii**, **brachialis**, and **brachioradialis** are the primary elbow flexors. The relative position (pronated, supinated, or neutral) of the forearm determines which of the muscles provides the primary contribution to the movement. The biceps brachii is the prime elbow flexor when the forearm is supinated; when the forearm is pronated, the brachialis is the prime flexor.[4] The contribution of the biceps brachii to forearm supination increases with the amount of elbow flexion until approximately 90 degrees where the maximum length–tension relationship is reached.[4] When the forearm is in its neutral position (radial side upward), the brachioradialis is the primary elbow flexor. The **supinator** is assisted by the biceps brachii during forceful supination. The brachioradialis contributes to both pronation and supination when the forearm is at the end of the opposite motion (i.e., the brachioradialis contributes to pronation when the forearm is fully supinated). The lateral bulk of the forearm muscles is formed by the extensor carpi radialis longus, extensor carpi radialis brevis, extensor carpi ulnaris, and extensor digitorum communis muscles (Fig. 16-7).

Elbow Extensor and Pronator Group

The **triceps brachii** and **anconeus** extend the elbow, with the anconeus stabilizing the ulna during pronation and supination of the forearm (Fig. 16-8). The primary pronator muscles of the forearm are the **pronator teres**, arising from just above the medial epicondyle of the humerus and inserting on the anterolateral aspect of the radius, and the **pronator quadratus**, located on the distal forearm running obliquely from the medial aspect of the ulna to the radius. The remaining medial bulk of the proximal forearm is formed by the flexor carpi radialis, palmaris longus, flexor digitorum superficialis, and flexor carpi ulnaris muscles, which are discussed in Chapter 17.

Nerves

Three primary nerves cross the elbow: the median nerve, ulnar nerve, and radial nerve. Their relatively superficial course across the elbow and in the distal portion of the forearm predisposes them to acute traumatic injury; their anatomical locations predispose them to entrapment-type conditions (Fig. 16-9).

Median Nerve

Crossing the anterior elbow in the same path as the brachial artery, the median nerve travels deep within the forearm muscles to follow the flexor digitorum superficialis down the middle of the anterior forearm. As it approaches the wrist, the median nerve becomes superficial once again as it passes between the flexor digitorum superficialis and flexor carpi radialis tendons (beneath the palmaris longus) to pass through the carpal tunnel and enter the hand. With the exception of the flexor carpi ulnaris and the medial portion of the flexor digitorum profundus, the median nerve supplies all of the wrist flexor muscles and the pronator teres and pronator quadratus. Shortly after crossing the elbow joint, the **anterior interosseous nerve** projects off the median nerve to pass under the two heads of the pronator teres.

Ulnar Nerve

The ulnar nerve enters the elbow via the **arcade of Struthers**, located approximately 8 cm proximal to the medial epicondyle, and then passes between the olecranon process and the medial epicondyle.[2] After superficially crossing the joint line, it courses deep to follow the ulnar artery to the middle of the forearm. At this point, it moves medial to the flexor carpi ulnaris tendon and crosses the wrist joint superficial to the flexor retinaculum, traveling between the pisiform bone and the hook of the hamate bone (**tunnel of Guyon**) to provide sensory and motor innervation to the hand. The ulnar nerve innervates the flexor carpi ulnaris muscle and the medial portion of the flexor digitorum profundus in the forearm.

Radial Nerve

The radial nerve courses distally on the posterior aspect of the humerus and then crosses the lateral aspect of the elbow's joint line between the brachioradialis and brachialis muscles. Then it diverges into the superficial and deep branches approximately 1.3 cm proximal to the radiohumeral joint. The **superficial branch**, the direct continuation of the radial nerve, provides sensation to the dorsum of the wrist, hand, and thumb. The **deep branch** (deep radial nerve) passes through the radial tunnel and the extensor carpi radialis brevis muscle to provide motor innervation exclusively to the extensor carpi radialis longus and brevis, supinator, brachioradialis, extensor pollicis longus, abductor pollicis longus, extensor pollicis brevis, and extensor digitorum muscles. Therefore, it is possible to injure the deep branch of the radial nerve with critical motor loss but no sensory loss.

Bursae

Several bursae are found in the elbow region, but few have clinical significance. The **subcutaneous olecranon bursa**, located between the olecranon process and the skin, is susceptible to trauma and infection. This bursa is usually

Table 16-1 Muscles Acting on the Elbow and Forearm

Muscle	Action	Origin	Insertion	Innervation	Root
Anconeus	Elbow extension Stabilization of ulna during pronation and supination	Posterior surface of the lateral epicondyle	Lateral border of the olecranon process	Radial	C7, C8
Biceps Brachii	Elbow flexion Forearm supination Shoulder flexion	Long head: Supraglenoid tuberosity of scapula Short head: Coracoid process of scapula	Radial tuberosity	Musculocutaneous	C5, C6
Brachialis	Elbow flexion	Distal one-half of anterior humerus	Coronoid process of ulna Ulnar tuberosity	Musculocutaneous	C5, C6
Brachioradialis	Elbow flexion Forearm pronation May assist with forearm supination	Lateral supracondylar ridge of humerus	Styloid process of radius	Radial	C5, C6
Extensor Carpi Radialis Brevis	Wrist extension Radial deviation	Lateral epicondyle via the common extensor tendon Radial collateral ligament	Base of the 3rd metacarpal	Radial	C6, C7
Extensor Carpi Radialis Longus	Wrist extension Radial deviation	Supracondylar ridge of humerus	Radial side of the 2nd metacarpal	Radial	C6, C7
Extensor Carpi Ulnaris	Wrist extension Ulnar deviation	Lateral epicondyle via the common extensor tendon	Ulnar side of the base of the 5th metacarpal	Deep radial	C6, C7, C8
Extensor Digitorum Communis	Wrist extension MCP extension PIP extension	Lateral epicondyle via the common extensor tendon	Into the dorsal surface of the base of the middle and distal phalanges of each of the four fingers	Deep radial	C6, C7, C8
Flexor Carpi Radialis	Forearm pronation Wrist flexion Radial deviation Elbow flexion	Medial epicondyle via the common flexor tendon	Palmar aspect of the bases of the 2nd and 3rd metacarpal bones	Median	C6, C7
Flexor Carpi Ulnaris	Wrist flexion Ulnar deviation Elbow flexion	Humeral head: Medial epicondyle via the common flexor tendon Ulnar head: Medial border of the olecranon; proximal two-thirds of the posterior ulna	Pisiform Hamate Palmar aspect of the base of the 5th metacarpal	Ulnar	C8, T1
Flexor Digitorum Profundus	DIP flexion PIP flexion Wrist flexion	Anteromedial proximal three-fourths of the ulna and associated interosseous membrane	Bases of the distal phalanges of the 2nd through 5th digits	Lateral: Median nerve Medial: Ulnar nerve	C8, T1

Continued

Table 16-1 Muscles Acting on the Elbow and Forearm—cont'd

Muscle	Action	Origin	Insertion	Innervation	Root
Flexor Digitorum Superficialis	PIP flexion MCP flexion Wrist flexion	Humeral head: Medial epicondyle via the common flexor tendon; ulnar collateral ligament Ulnar head: Coronoid process Radial head: Oblique line of radius	Middle phalanges of the 2nd through 5th digits	Median	C7, C8, T1
Palmaris Longus	Wrist flexion	Medial epicondyle via the common flexor tendon	Flexor retinaculum Palmar aponeurosis	Median	C6, C7
Pronator Quadratus	Forearm pronation	Anterior surface of the distal one-fourth of the ulna	Lateral portion of the distal one-fourth of the radius	Anterior interosseous nerve	C8, T1
Pronator Teres	Forearm pronation Elbow flexion	Humeral head: Proximal to the medial epicondyle of the humerus Ulnar head: Coronoid process	Middle one-third of the lateral radius	Median	C6, C7
Supinator	Forearm supination	Lateral epicondyle Radial collateral ligament Annular ligament Supinator crest of the ulna	Proximal one-third of the radius	Deep radial	C6, C7, C8
Triceps Brachii	Elbow extension Shoulder extension	Long head: Infraglenoid tuberosity of the scapula Lateral head: Posterolateral surface of the proximal one-half of the humeral shaft Medial head: Posteromedial surface of the humerus	Olecranon process of the ulna	Radial	C7, C8

DIP = distal interphalangeal; MCP = metacarpophalangeal; PIP = proximal interphalangeal

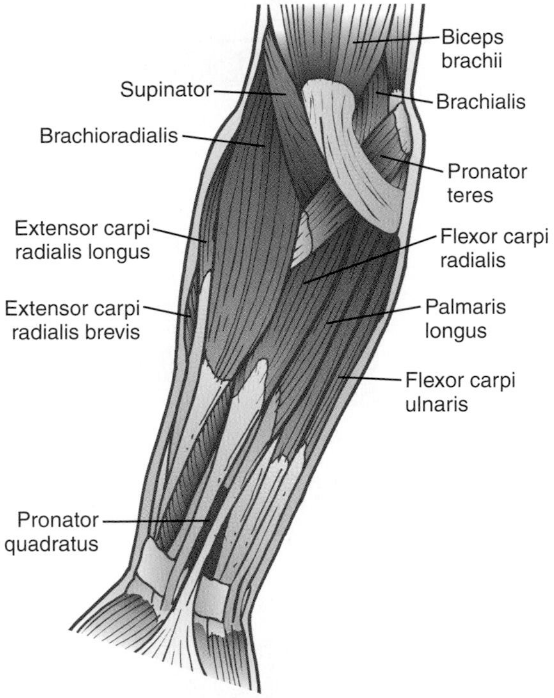

FIGURE 16-7 ■ Anterior muscles of the forearm. These muscles serve primarily to flex the elbow, wrist, and fingers and rotate the forearm.

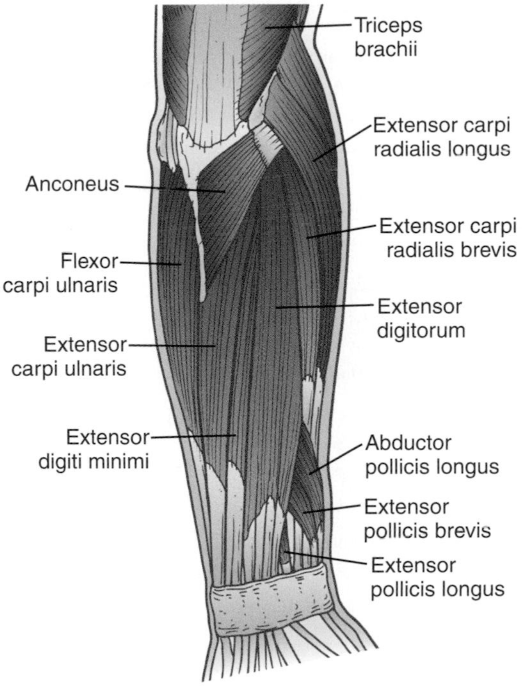

FIGURE 16-8 ■ Posterior muscles of the forearm. These muscles serve to extend the wrist and fingers.

injured after a direct blow to the olecranon process. The other significant bursa is the **subtendinous olecranon bursa**. This structure is located between the tendon of triceps brachii and the olecranon process and may become inflamed secondary to repetitive stresses applied to the joint.

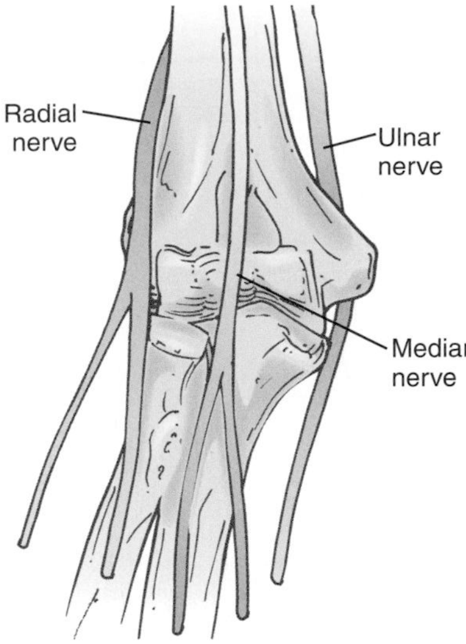

FIGURE 16-9 ■ Anterior view of the primary nerves crossing the elbow.

Clinical Examination of the Elbow and Forearm

The elbow has interdependence with the cervical and thoracic spine and shoulder as well as the wrist, hand, and fingers. The elbow may be traumatized by valgus or varus forces, forced hyperextension, direct blows to the olecranon process or the epicondyles, or, most commonly, secondary to overuse from the inherently unnatural motion of throwing or other activities requiring repetitive motion. The stresses placed on the elbow are increased when improper technique is used or when an individual compensates for shoulder pain or decreased ROM by altering elbow motion. Neuropathies of the ulnar, median, and/or radial nerves (and their branches) may originate from the cervical spine.

History

A thorough history includes questioning regarding any pain or functional limitations in the cervical, shoulder, and wrist and hand regions, as impairments in these regions can impact function at the elbow. For example, weakness of the scapular stabilizers of the shoulder may result in increased forces at the elbow. Question the patient regarding any changes in sensation or temperature, which may signal vascular or nerve compromise. To begin to identify a treatment strategy, identify the impact of the condition on the patient's life and resulting activity limitations.

Past Medical History

- **Previous history:** Pain that is associated with seasonal athletic activity may be related to poor conditioning. Patients with nontraumatic origin of pain or suspected of having radicular symptoms emanating from the cervical region require investigation about a history of previous trauma, paresthesia, strength loss, or other dysfunction in this area.

Examination Map

HISTORY

Past Medical History

- General medical health

History of the Present Condition

- Location and onset of symptoms
- Mechanism of injury

FUNCTIONAL ASSESSMENT

Athletic or other daily tasks that provoke symptoms

- Throwing

INSPECTION

Inspection of the Anterior Structures

- Carrying angle
- Cubital fossa

Inspection of the Medial Structures

- Medial epicondyle
- Flexor muscle mass

Inspection of the Lateral Structures

- Alignment of the wrist and forearm
- Cubital recurvatum
- Extensor muscle mass

Inspection of the Posterior Structures

- Bony alignment
- Olecranon process and bursa

PALPATION

Palpation of the Anterior Structures

- Biceps brachii
- Cubital fossa
- Brachioradialis
- Wrist flexor group
  - Pronator teres
  - Flexor carpi radialis
  - Palmaris longus
  - Flexor carpi ulnaris

Palpation of the Medial Structures

- Medial epicondyle
- Ulna
- Ulnar collateral ligament

Palpation of the Lateral Structures

- Lateral epicondyle
- Radial head
- Radial collateral ligament
- Capitulum
- Annular ligament
- Lateral ulnar collateral ligament

Palpation of the Posterior Structures

- Olecranon process
- Olecranon fossa
- Triceps brachii
- Anconeus
- Ulnar nerve
- Wrist extensors
  - Extensor carpi ulnaris
  - Extensor carpi radialis brevis
  - Extensor carpi radialis longus
- Finger extensors
  - Extensor digitorum
  - Extensor digiti minimi
- Thumb musculature
  - Extensor pollicis brevis
  - Abductor pollicis longus
- Radial tunnel

JOINT AND MUSCLE FUNCTION ASSESSMENT

Goniometry

- Flexion
- Extension
- Pronation
- Supination

Active Range of Motion

- Flexion
- Extension
- Pronation
- Supination

Manual Muscle Tests

- Flexion
- Extension
- Pronation
- Supination

Passive Range of Motion

- Flexion
- Extension
- Pronation
- Supination

JOINT STABILITY TESTS

Stress Testing

- Valgus stress test
- Varus stress test

Joint Play Assessment

- Humeroulnar
- Radioulnar
- Humeroulnar radiohumeral

NEUROLOGICAL EXAMINATION

Upper Quarter Screen

VASCULAR EXAMINATION

Distal Pulses

Capillary Refill

REGION-SPECIFIC PATHOLOGIES AND SELECTIVE TISSUE TESTS

Elbow Dislocations

Fractures About the Elbow

Elbow Sprains

- Ulnar collateral ligament
  - Moving valgus stress test
- Valgus extension overload
- Posterolateral rotatory instability
  - Posterolateral rotatory instability test
- Radial collateral ligament

Osteochondritis Dissecans of the Capitulum

Epicondylalgia

- Lateral epicondylalgia
  - Tennis elbow test
- Medial epicondylalgia

Distal Biceps Tendon Rupture

- Hook test
- Biceps squeeze test

Nerve Pathology

- Ulnar nerve pathology
- Radial nerve pathology
- Median nerve pathology

Forearm compartment syndrome

- **General medical health:** A history of other medical conditions needs to be ascertained. Certain vascular problems, neurological involvement, or systemic diseases may predispose the elbow to inflammatory or degenerative injuries or illnesses. Osteoporosis is associated with an increased risk of forearm and wrist fractures.[5]

History of the Present Condition

The onset and location of the symptoms are among the most important history findings surrounding elbow pathology. Determining the cause-and-effect relationship between the mechanism and the onset of the symptoms is helpful in developing a successful treatment plan. In addition, because the elbow may be the site of radicular symptoms from the cervical nerve roots, all other possible sources of pain must be ruled out.

- **Location of the symptoms:** Begin the examination by localizing the area of pain, the type of pain, and any dysfunction that is reported, remembering the possibility of these symptoms being referred by pathology that is proximal or distal to the elbow (Table 16-2). Localized pain suggests the presence of specific soft tissue pathology; nondescript pain suggests a neurological or vascular cause.[2] Radicular pain usually presents with symptoms localized within the distribution of a peripheral nerve or nerve root. Nerve entrapment around the elbow may result in symptoms in the hand and forearm.
- **Onset of the symptoms:** Elbow pain may have an acute or chronic onset. Traumatic injury is traced to a specific onset of pain and symptoms. Chronic conditions of the elbow may initially produce minor symptoms related to activity but can rapidly progress to constant pain during all activities of daily living (ADLs).
- **Mechanism of injury:** The elbow is well protected at the side of the body and is not subjected to an overburden of harmful stress during everyday life. The elbow can be acutely injured by the high amount of stress generated while throwing or during weight lifting. Acute injury can occur if the hand is planted on the ground and forces are transmitted across the joint.

Most elbow injuries tend to be caused by repetitive low-load stresses. Throwing a ball or using a racquet can cause stresses capable of resulting in tendinopathy or neuritis in the elbow. Adolescents are vulnerable to repetitive stress injuries at open growth plates as stresses are transmitted across these areas. Question athletes who are involved in throwing activities about the level of activity, including the number of throws, time span in which the throws occurred, and any changes in the throwing technique. The use of computers, musical instruments, or machinery that requires repetitive wrist and finger motions may also produce symptoms or exacerbate the current symptoms.

✻ Practical Evidence

Adolescent pitchers who throw high-velocity pitches and participate in showcase events are more likely to sustain serious injuries.[6,7]

- **Technique:** Overuse injuries commonly lead to suspicion of improper technique or poor elbow biomechanics or weak muscles. Ask the patient about changes in technique or equipment or increases in the intensity or duration of play. Although frequently cited as a causative factor in elbow problems for tennis players, inappropriate grip size in tennis does not alter muscle activation strength.[8] However, a further biomechanical analysis of elbow function during the pain-causing activity may be needed.
- **Associated sound and sensations:** An elbow that chronically locks, clicks, or pops during movement may indicate osteochondritis dissecans or an unstable joint.

Functional Assessment

Patients with an acutely injured elbow will frequently cradle the elbow to their side, keeping the joint in the resting position of approximately 70 degrees of flexion to minimize stresses.

Observe the patient performing common daily tasks and those tasks that provoke symptoms. Limitations in elbow motion result in characteristic adaptations at the shoulder and at the wrist and hand. For example, a limitation in elbow extension may result in increased scapular protraction during elevation. Patients with limited pronation or supination

Table 16-2 Possible Pathology Based on the Location of Pain

	Location of Pain			
	Lateral	Anterior	Medial	Posterior
Soft Tissue Injury	Annular ligament sprain Radial collateral ligament sprain Radiocapitellar chondromalacia Lateral epicondylalgia (tennis elbow) Radial head dislocation Radial nerve pathology	Biceps brachii tendinopathy Rupture of the biceps brachii tendon Median nerve trauma Anterior capsule sprain	Ulnar collateral ligament sprain Medial epicondylalgia Ulnar nerve pathology	Olecranon bursitis Triceps brachii tendinopathy Triceps tendon rupture
Bony Injury	Avulsion of the common extensor tendon Lateral epicondyle fracture Radius fracture Radial head fracture Radial head dislocation	Osteochondral fracture Avulsion of the biceps brachii tendon	Avulsion of the common flexor tendon Medial epicondyle fracture Ulna fracture Osteophyte formation	Fracture of the olecranon process Osteophyte formation

may compensate with increased internal and external glenohumeral motion, respectively.

Throwing athletes with medial elbow instability frequently complain of pain during the late cocking and acceleration phases of throwing, as these periods invoke the most stresses on the ulnar collateral ligament (see Box 15-1).[9]

Inspection

The upper arm, elbow, and forearm are inspected for evidence of contusions, ecchymosis, scars, and swelling. These conditions can place pressure on the radial, median, and ulnar nerves, causing symptoms to radiate to the forearm and hand.

Inspection of the Anterior Structures

- **Carrying angle:** The angle formed by the long axis of the humerus and ulna, the carrying angle, ranges from 13 to 16 degrees of valgus in women and 11 to 14 degrees in adult men (note that there is a wide range of normative data reported for the "normal" angle).[2,10,11] Usually, this angle is reduced or entirely eliminated during flexion. With the elbow fully extended and the forearm supinated, note the presence of an increased carrying angle, **cubitus valgus**, or a decreased angle, **cubitus varus** (Fig. 16-10).
- Baseball pitchers may exhibit cubitus valgus in the throwing arm, with an angle of 15 or more degrees, an adaptation to repeated valgus loading during the throwing motion.[2] Other deviations of this angle may reflect a fracture of one or more bones or their epiphyseal plates. Cubitus varus may be associated with ulnar neuropathy, avascular necrosis, osteoarthritis, posterolateral rotatory instability, and other conditions.[12]
- **Cubital fossa:** Swelling within the cubital fossa can place pressure on the local neurovascular structures, raising the suspicion of injury to the nearby soft tissues, including the distal biceps tendon (Fig. 16-11).

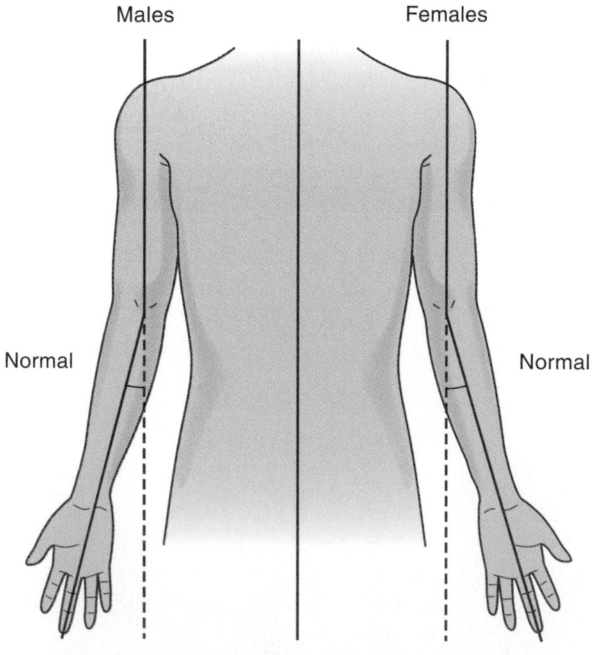

FIGURE 16-10 ■ Angular relationships at the elbow. On average, women have an increased angle between the midline of the forearm and the humerus (the "carrying angle") relative to men. Long-term participation in overhand throwing sports increases this angle in the dominant arm.

Inspection of the Medial Structures

- **Medial epicondyle:** The medial epicondyle is the most prominent structure on the medial aspect of the elbow, but it may become masked by excessive swelling.
- **Flexor muscle mass:** The wrist flexor muscle mass is observable along the medial aspect of the elbow and forearm. The mass widens approximately 2 to 3 inches below the elbow. Loss of girth along the medial forearm may occur secondary to prolonged immobilization or disuse associated with long-term tendinopathy.

Inspection of the Lateral Structures

- **Alignment of the wrist and forearm:** The wrist should be centered on the forearm. Compression of the radial nerve as it crosses the elbow joint can inhibit the wrist extensors, resulting in drop-wrist syndrome (see Chapter 17).[2]
- **Cubital recurvatum:** The alignment of the forearm and humerus when the elbow is fully extended is noted. Although normally a straight line, extension beyond 0 degrees (cubital recurvatum) is common, especially in women (Fig. 16-12).
- **Extensor muscle mass:** The wrist extensor muscle mass is observable along the lateral aspect of the elbow and forearm. The mass widens approximately 1 to 2 inches below the elbow. Loss of girth along the lateral forearm can occur secondary to prolonged immobilization or disuse after long-term tendinopathy or radial nerve involvement.

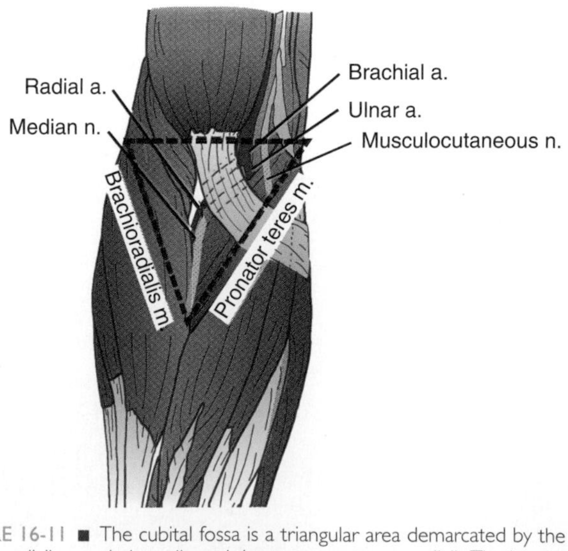

FIGURE 16-11 ■ The cubital fossa is a triangular area demarcated by the brachioradialis muscle laterally and the pronator teres medially. The brachial artery and its two subdivisions (the radial and ulnar arteries), the median nerve, and the musculocutaneous nerve pass through this fossa.

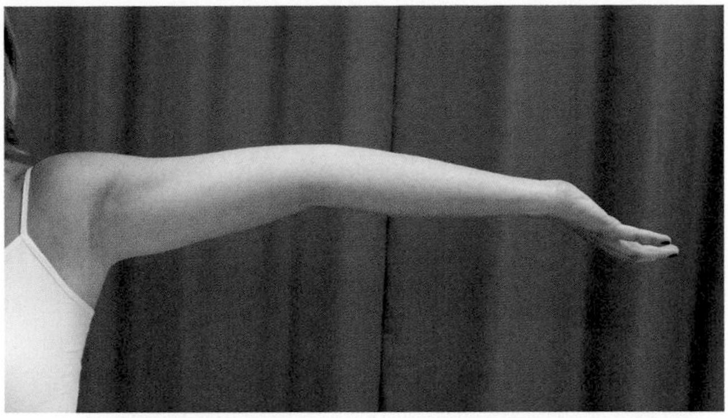

FIGURE 16-12 ■ Cubital recurvatum. A normal hyperextension of the elbow.

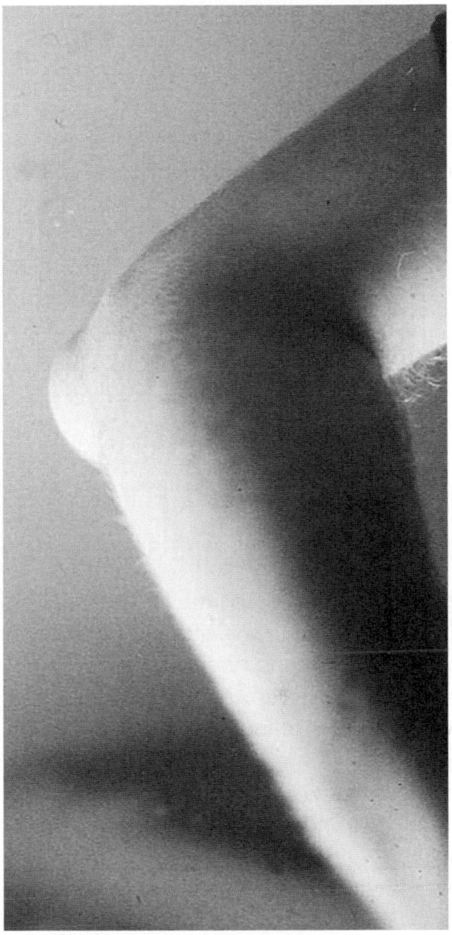

FIGURE 16-13 ■ Inflammation of the subcutaneous olecranon bursa. This structure is often traumatized by a direct blow to the olecranon process.

Inspection of the Posterior Structures

- **Bony alignment:** When the elbow is flexed to 90 degrees, the medial epicondyle, lateral epicondyle, and olecranon process form an isosceles triangle. When the elbow is extended, these structures typically lie within a straight line. Deviation from this alignment may reflect bony pathology.
- **Olecranon process and bursa:** Flexion of the elbow makes the bony contour of the olecranon process visible. Acute injury or infection may cause the olecranon bursa to rupture or swell, masking the outline of the olecranon (Fig. 16-13).

PALPATION

Many of the structures of the upper extremity insert or originate at the elbow, making careful, precise palpation a must for the examiner. Tenderness elicited with palpation must be correlated with other subjective and physical objective findings. Some areas, such as the radial head, may be tender in the uninjured elbow.

Palpation of the Anterior Structures

1 **Biceps brachii:** Palpate the muscle belly of the **biceps brachii** along the anterior aspect of the humerus until its tendon inserts onto the radius. The tendon is more easily recognized if the elbow is held in 90 degrees of flexion. The distal biceps brachii tendon can be ruptured with a forceful eccentric contraction, resulting in deformity of the muscle.

2 **Cubital fossa:** Passing within the **cubital fossa**, palpate the brachial artery medial to the biceps brachii tendon. In some individuals, the median nerve can be palpated within the fossa. The musculocutaneous nerve also passes through this area but cannot be palpated because it runs underneath the pronator teres muscle (see Fig. 16-11).

3 **Brachioradialis:** The **brachioradialis** is the most lateral of the elbow flexor muscles. To palpate the brachioradialis, place the forearm in the neutral position and resist elbow flexion. Palpate the length of the brachioradialis muscle from its attachment on the lateral supracondylar ridge to the

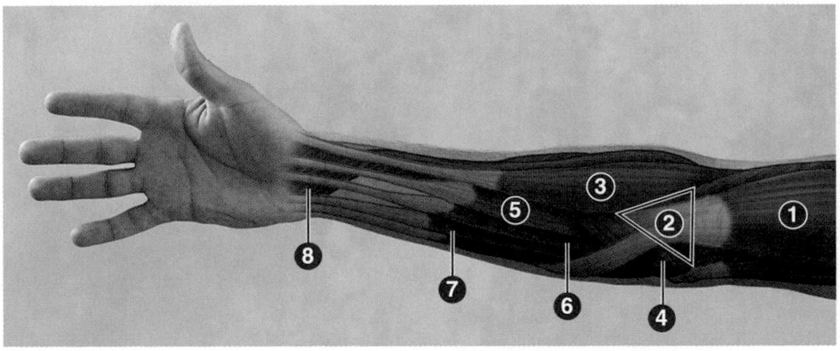

distal attachment on the radial styloid process. The distal tendon of the brachioradialis is also the site to assess the deep tendon reflex of the C6 nerve root.

4-7 Medial muscles: Near their origin, the muscles originating from the medial epicondyle cannot be distinguished from one another. The **(4) pronator teres** is the most proximal of this group. As the other muscles progress distally, the individual tendons of the **(5) flexor carpi radialis**, **(6) palmaris longus** (absent in some individuals), **(7)** and the **flexor carpi ulnaris** become identifiable as they near the wrist. Figure 16-14 presents a method to identify these muscles.

8 Pronator quadratus: Laying deep to the wrist and finger flexors, palpate the area over the **pronator quadratus** muscle on the distal aspect of the anterior forearm.

Palpation of the Medial Structures

1 Medial epicondyle: Locate the **medial epicondyle**, prominent along the distal aspect of the humerus as it flares away from the shaft of the bone. The common wrist flexor tendon attaches at the epicondyle; palpation of the epicondyle elicits exquisite tenderness in the presence of the medial epicondylalgia.

2 Ulna: Identify the base of the **ulna**, located distal to the elbow's medial joint space. The shaft is prominent throughout its length, especially along its medial and posterior (dorsal) surfaces. The anterior aspect of the shaft can be palpated along the distal two-thirds of its length as it arises from beneath the mass of the wrist flexors to its point of articulation with the wrist.

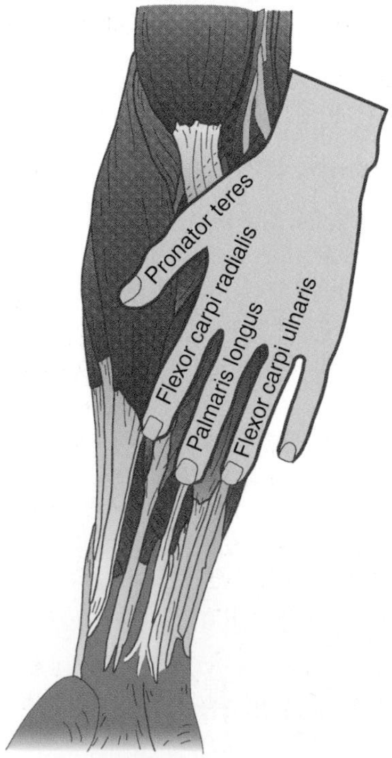

FIGURE 16-14 ■ Method of approximating the superficial muscles of the forearm flexors.

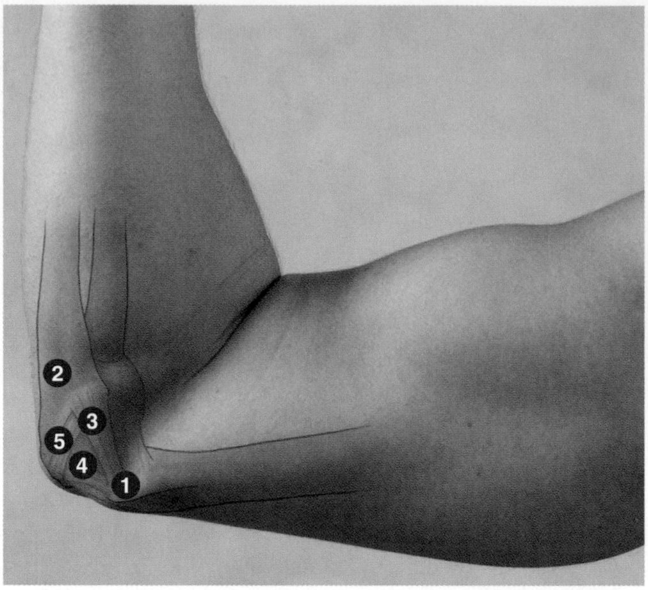

3-5 Ulnar collateral ligament (UCL): To uncover the **UCL** from the more superficial flexor-pronator muscles, have the patient flex the elbow to between 50 and 70 degrees.[9] The anterior band **(3)** of this ligament can be directly palpated as it crosses the angle formed by the humerus and ulna. Continue around the medial aspect of the elbow to palpate the area over the posterior **(4)** and transverse bundles **(5)** of the UCL, although these are usually not distinguishable.

Palpation of the Lateral Structures

1 Lateral epicondyle: Smaller than the medial epicondyle, identify the **lateral epicondyle**, prominent as it projects from the distal end of the humerus. Palpate this structure for tenderness caused by pathology of the common origin of the wrist extensors.

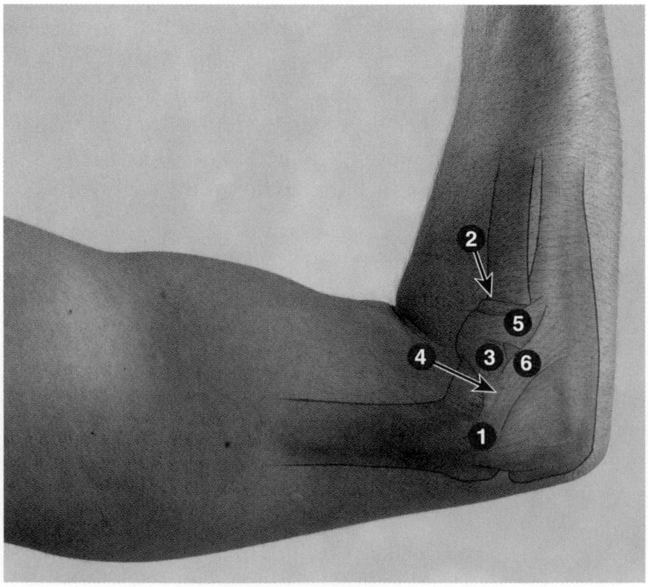

Palpation of the Lateral Structures

2 Radial head: Moving slightly distal from the lateral joint line, locate and palpate the head of the radius underneath the posterior aspect of the wrist extensor muscles. It becomes more identifiable as it rolls beneath the examiner's finger as the forearm is pronated and supinated. During flexion and extension of the elbow, the **radial head** moves with the forearm.

3 Radial collateral ligament (RCL): Locate the **RCL** between the radial head and the lateral epicondyle. Although the RCL is not normally identifiable, its length is palpated for tenderness.

4 Capitulum: Moving proximally from the radial head across the joint line, find the rounded **capitulum**. While passively pronating and supinating the forearm with the elbow flexed to various degrees, palpate the capitulum and radial head for the presence of crepitus, which indicates radiocapitular chondromalacia.[13]

5 Annular ligament: Although the **annular ligament** cannot be identified directly during palpation, palpate the area overlying the radial head for evidence of tenderness or swelling.

6 Lateral ulnar collateral ligament (LUCL): Move superiorly and anteriorly from the radial head to locate the **LUCL** as it crosses the lateral joint line. Passively extending the forearm may make this structure more palpable.

Palpation of the Posterior Structures

1 Olecranon process: Locate the ulna's **olecranon process**, the prominent rounded bone on the posterior aspect of the elbow. Palpate this structure for tenderness and mobility. A forced hyperextension of the elbow or a direct backward fall on the elbow may cause a fracture. The olecranon bursa is not palpable unless it is inflamed, in which case it can potentially result in a large amount of swelling and tenderness and mask the underlying bone.

2 Olecranon fossa: With the elbow partially flexed and the triceps muscle relaxed, palpate the **olecranon fossa** on the posterior humerus, located just superior to the olecranon process. Posteromedial tenderness resulting from impingement is associated with valgus extension overload.

3 Triceps brachii: Slightly flex the elbow to make the fibers of the **triceps brachii** tendon stand out from its attachment on the olecranon. The posterolateral portion of this muscle is formed by the lateral head of the triceps and the posteromedial portion by the long head. The medial head runs deep to the long head but becomes palpable over the medial aspect of the distal humerus. The length of the triceps brachii is palpated for tenderness or deformity.

4 Anconeus: Palpate the **anconeus** between the lateral epicondyle and the olecranon process. This area will feel "full" in the presence of a joint effusion, synovitis, infection, or intra-articular fracture.[2]

5 Ulnar nerve: With the elbow in full extension, palpate the sulcus formed by the medial epicondyle and the medial border of the olecranon process for the **ulnar nerve**, identifiable as a thin, cordlike structure. Determine if the ulnar nerve can be displaced from the sulcus by gently moving it medially and laterally. Inflammation of the nerve may result in a positive Tinel's sign, burning, pain, or paresthesia along the medial border of the forearm and little finger during palpation. Also palpate the ulnar nerve as the elbow is flexed and extended to determine if the nerve subluxates out of its groove.

6-8 Wrist extensors: Resist wrist extension with the fingers relaxed to make the **(6) extensor carpi ulnaris**, **(7) extensor carpi radialis brevis**, and **(8) extensor carpi radialis longus** muscles become prominent. With the forearm pronated, the wrist extensors can be palpated distal to the lateral epicondyle. The superficial muscle is the extensor carpi radialis longus; the inferior is the extensor carpi radialis brevis.

9-10 Finger extensors: Resist finger extension to make the **(9) extensor digitorum** and **(10) extensor digiti minimi** muscles prominent.

11-12 Thumb musculature: Ask the patient to extend and abduct the thumb to more easily identify the **(11) extensor pollicis brevis** and **(12) abductor pollicis longus muscles**.

13 Radial tunnel: Place the patient's forearm in neutral. Approximately as long as four fingertips, the **radial tunnel** can be located on the posterior aspect of the forearm on a line anterior to the radiohumeral joint to the forearm's midpoint. Patients who demonstrate the clinical signs of lateral epicondylalgia but are more sensitive to palpation over the radial tunnel should also be examined to rule out radial tunnel syndrome.[14]

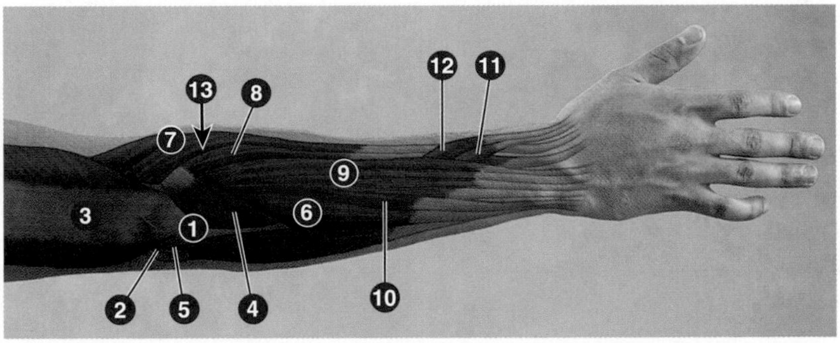

Joint and Muscle Function Assessment

The motions at the elbow joints are limited to flexion and extension and pronation and supination. Testing of strength and length of the wrist and long finger flexors and extensors is routinely included in an examination of the elbow, as these structures are closely associated with elbow, wrist, and hand function. Entrapment of the median, radial, or ulnar nerve around the elbow may manifest with distal symptoms. Chapter 17 describes muscle function at the wrist and hand.

Goniometry 16-1 and 16-2 describe the measurement of elbow flexion and extension and forearm pronation and supination. Baseball pitchers typically demonstrate reduced flexion and extension on the dominant side, although this change is not associated with a change in function.[15]

Active Range of Motion

- **Flexion and extension:** Occurring in the sagittal plane around a coronal axis, most of the elbow's ROM is composed of flexion, ranging between 145 and 155 degrees from the neutral position. Extension is usually limited at 0 degrees by the olecranon process, but hyperextension is common (see Fig. 16-12).

  In the population as a whole, extension beyond 0 degrees may be congenital and is considered normal when it occurs bilaterally. Throwing athletes may acquire unilateral cubital recurvatum as the result of prolonged, repetitive forces that result in ligamentous laxity.

  Loss of full extension is often one of the first signs of elbow pathology. Examine the patient for associated crepitus or other mechanical blockage that prevents full elbow extension.[2]
- **Pronation and supination:** The neutral position for forearm pronation and supination is the thumb and radius pointing upward. The total ROM is 170 to 180 degrees, with approximately 90 degrees of motion in each direction. This movement occurs in the transverse plane around the longitudinal axis relative to the anatomical position.

Goniometry 16-1
Elbow Goniometry: Flexion and Extension

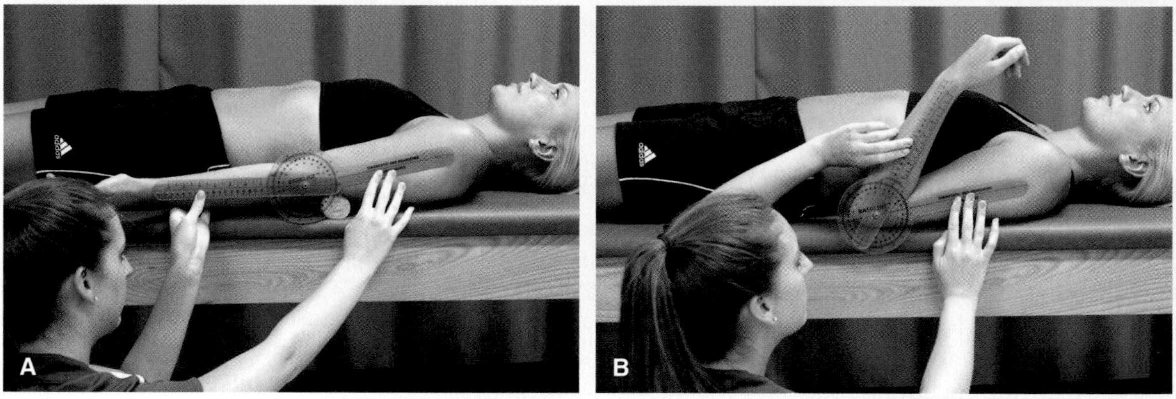

Extension to Flexion (0°–145° to 155°)

Patient Position	Supine with the humerus close to the body, the shoulder in the neutral position, and the forearm supinated A bolster is placed under the distal humerus to measure extension.

Goniometer Alignment

Fulcrum	Centered over the lateral epicondyle
Proximal Arm	The stationary arm is aligned with the long axis of the humerus, using the acromion process as the proximal landmark.[16]
Distal Arm	The movement arm is aligned with the long axis of the radius, using the styloid process as the distal landmark.

Evidence

Inter-rater Reliability

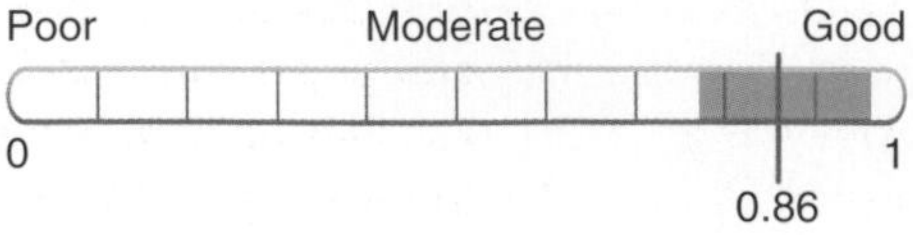

Intra-rater Reliability

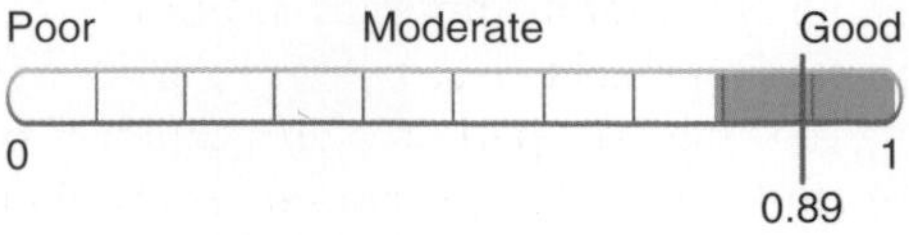

Goniometry 16-2

Elbow Goniometry: Pronation and Supination

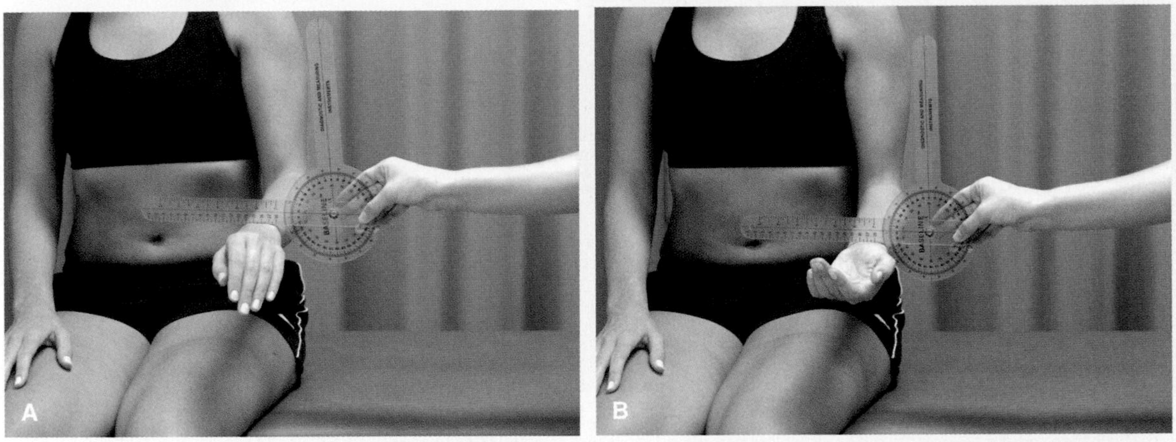

Pronation to Supination (90°–0°–90°)

	Pronation	Supination
Patient Position	Sitting with the humerus held against the torso The elbow is flexed to 90°.	
Goniometer Alignment		
Fulcrum	Centered lateral to the ulnar styloid process	
Proximal Arm	Align the stationary arm parallel to the midline of the humerus.	
Distal Arm	The movement arm is positioned across the dorsal portion of the forearm, proximal to the radiocarpal joint.	The movement arm is positioned across the ventral portion of the forearm, proximal to the radiocarpal joint.
Modifications	The movement arm is aligned parallel to a pencil held in the hand, using the 3rd metacarpal as the axis.[17] This method captures a more functional range by incorporating movement at the wrist. Both measurement strategies demonstrate high inter- and intrarater reliability.[18]	
Evidence		

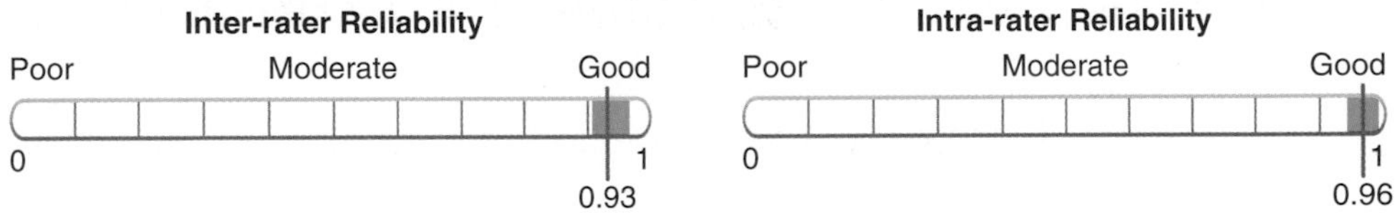

Manual Muscle Testing

Manual muscle testing (MMT) procedures are presented in Manual Muscle Tests 16-1 and 16-2. Because of the interrelated functioning of the elbow and wrist and hand musculature, assuring relaxation of the wrist and hand during testing of the elbow muscles is important to the validity of the manual muscle test.

Even injured patients are capable of overpowering the clinician during pronation and supination testing. An alternative method of resisting pronation and supination is to use a 1-inch-diameter dowel (Fig. 16-15).

Passive Range of Motion

- **Flexion and extension:** Position the elbow in extension with the forearm supinated and the shoulder joint stabilized to prevent compensatory motion (Fig. 16-16). Flex the elbow until soft tissue approximation between the bulk of the biceps brachii muscle and the muscles of the anterior forearm limits the motion, creating a soft end-feel. A hard end-feel during passive flexion is indicative of osteophyte formation or a loose body in the joint.[9] Extension produces a hard end-feel by the bony contact between the olecranon process and the olecranon fossa (Table 16-3).

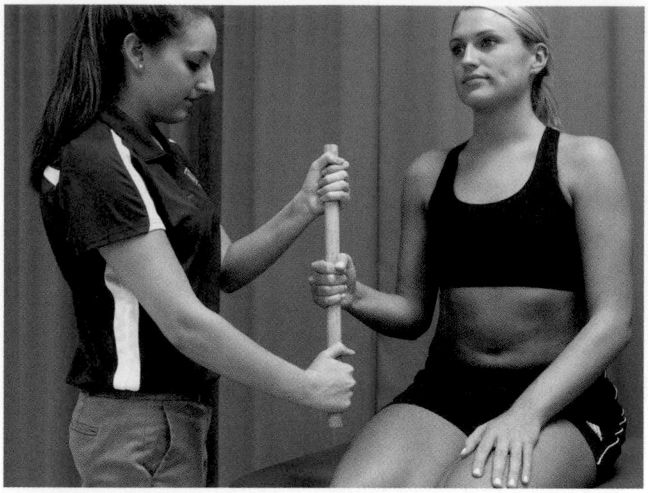

FIGURE 16-15 ■ Alternate method for assessing pronation and supination strength. The patient grasps the middle of the dowel as if holding a hammer. The examiner then applies resistance to both ends of the dowel as the patient pronates and supinates the forearm. This test for pronation and supination is more functionally oriented than the clinical test, but the patient is more likely to compensate using humeral movements.

Table 16-3 **Passive Range of Motion**

Elbow: Ulnohumeral and Radiohumeral Joint Capsular Patterns and End-Feels	
Capsular Pattern: Flexion, Extension	
Extension	Hard
Flexion	Soft
Elbow: Superior Radioulnar Joints	
Capsular Pattern: Supination and Pronation Equally	
Radioulnar supination	Firm
Radioulnar pronation	Hard or firm
Forearm: Distal Radioulnar Joint	
Capsular Pattern: Supination and Pronation Equally	
Radioulnar supination	Firm
Radioulnar pronation	Firm

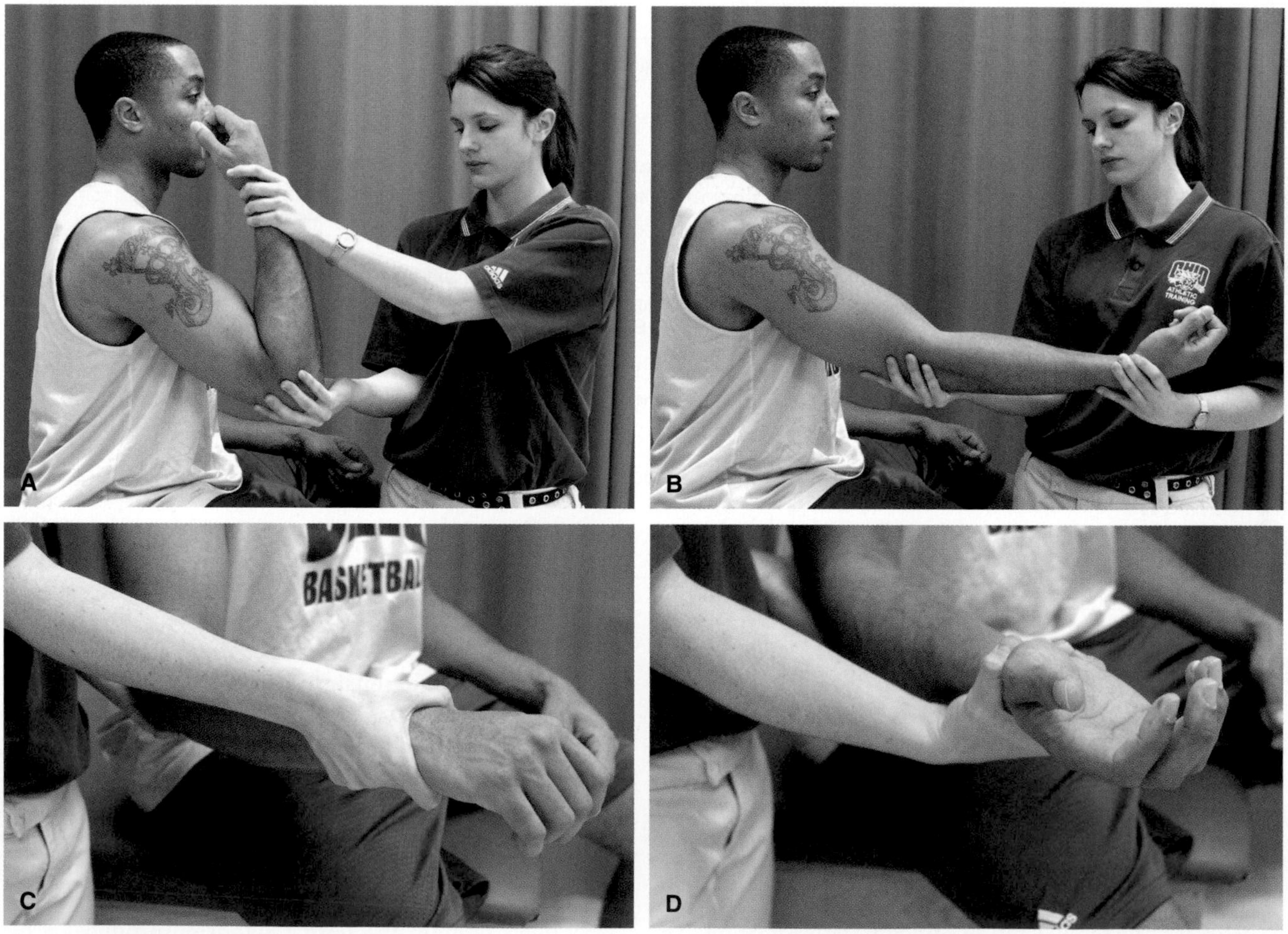

FIGURE 16-16 ■ Passive range of motion for (A) flexion and (B) extension and (C) pronation and (D) supination.

Manual Muscle Test 16-1
Elbow Flexion and Extension

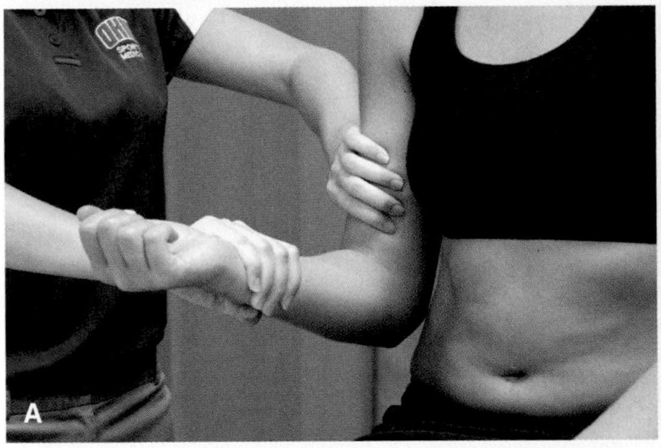

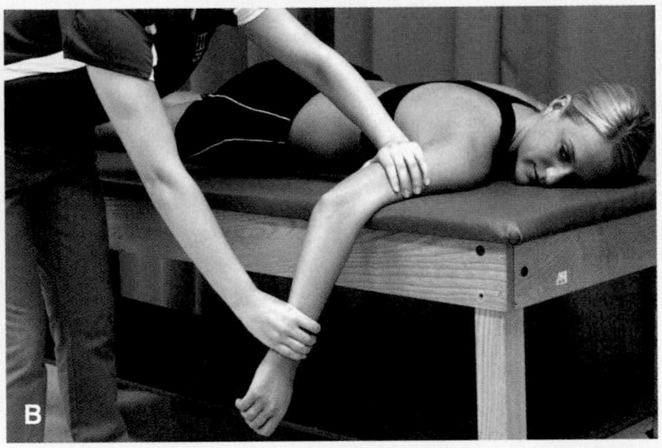

	Flexion	Extension
Patient Position	Sitting, standing, or supine	Prone
Test Position	The shoulder in the neutral position; the elbow in midrange To emphasize a specific muscle during the test: Forearm supinated Forearm pronated Forearm in midposition	The shoulder is abducted to 90°. The elbow is in mid-range and the forearm pronated.
Stabilization	Anterior humerus, being careful not to compress the involved muscles	Posterior humerus, being careful not to compress the involved muscles
Resistance	Over the distal forearm	Over the posterior aspect of the distal forearm
Primary Movers (Innervation)	Forearm supinated: Biceps brachii (C5,C6) Forearm pronated: Brachialis (C5,C6) Forearm neutral: Brachioradialis (C5,C6)	Triceps brachii (C7,C8)
Secondary Mover (Innervation)	Flexor carpi ulnaris (C8,T1)	Anconeus (C7,C8)
Substitution	Wrist and finger flexion, shoulder elevation	Wrist and finger extension, glenohumeral horizontal abduction, scapular retraction
Comments	The patient should keep the fingers relaxed.	An alternative test position is supine, with the shoulder flexed to 90° and the elbow flexed.

- **Pronation and supination:** Position the shoulder in the neutral position and flex the elbow to 90 degrees. Support the forearm so that the radius and thumb are pointing upward and the elbow is stabilized against the torso to prevent shoulder motion (Fig. 16-16). During pronation, the end-feel may be hard as the radius and ulna contact each other or firm secondary to stretching of the proximal and distal radioulnar ligaments and the interosseous membrane. Supination normally meets with a firm end-feel caused by the stretching of the proximal and distal radioulnar ligaments and the interosseous membrane.

Joint Stability Tests

Stress Testing

Single-plane instability of the elbow joint can be tested only in the frontal plane when the joint is not fully extended. Valgus and varus stress ligamentous testing of the fully extended elbow is meaningless in detecting ligamentous instability because the olecranon process is locked securely within its humeral fossa. However, laxity demonstrated in this position may indicate an epiphyseal or olecranon fracture.

- **Stress tests for medial ligament laxity:** The anterior bundle of the UCL is the primary restraint of the

Manual Muscle Test 16-2
Pronation and Supination

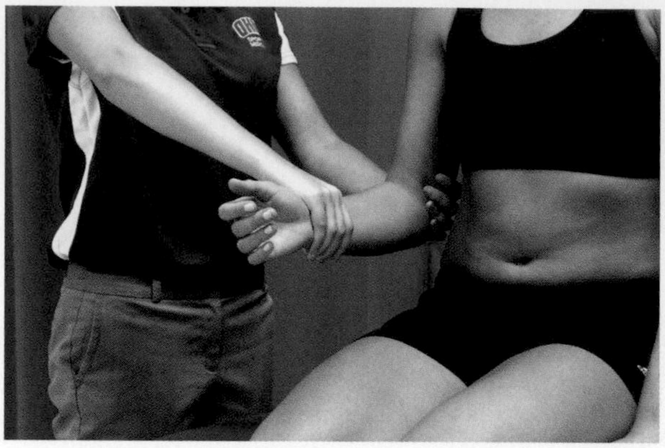

	Pronation	Supination
Patient Position	Seated	
Test Position	The shoulder is in the neutral position and the elbow flexed to 90°. The thumb is facing upward.	
Stabilization	Proximal to the elbow to prevent abduction or adduction of the glenohumeral joint	
Resistance	Resistance is applied to the ventral surface of the forearm.	Resistance is applied to the dorsal surface of the forearm.
Primary Movers (Innervation)	Pronator quadratus (C8,T1) Pronator teres (C6,C7)	Biceps brachii (C5,C6)
Secondary Movers (Innervation)	Brachioradialis (C5,C6) Flexor carpi radialis (C6,C7)	Brachioradialis (C5,C6) Supinator (C6,C7,C8)
Substitution	Finger flexion, wrist flexion, glenohumeral internal rotation	Wrist extension, glenohumeral external rotation
Comments	A more functional assessment of pronation and supination strength is performed by having the patient grip the examiner's hand and rotating. The brachioradialis assists in returning the forearm to neutral from a pronated or supinated position. Weakness with pronation is commonly associated with C6 radiculopathy.[19]	

medial elbow against valgus stress. Trauma to this structure is assessed using the **valgus stress test** (Stress Test 16-1). Detecting laxity is clinically difficult because the joint only opens a few millimeters, even when the ligament is ruptured.[20] Injury to the other medial ligaments is unlikely without first damaging the anterior bundle of the UCL.

- **Stress tests for lateral ligament laxity:** Less common than medial ligament laxity, straight-plane varus laxity of the elbow occurs when the RCL is damaged. Involvement of the annular ligament, ALCL, or LUCL increases the laxity by allowing the radial head to separate from the ulna. The integrity of these structures is determined through varus stress tests (Stress Test 16-2).

Joint Play

If passive flexion and extension at the elbow or pronation and supination at the forearm is restricted, examination of the accessory motions is warranted. The common joint capsule of all three elbow articulations means that restriction at all three joints is possible in the event of elbow injury (Joint Play 16-1).

Neurological Testing

The muscles innervated by the brachial plexus range from the shoulder into the elbow, forearm, and hand, and neurological testing often incorporates a complete upper-quarter screen (see Neurological Screening 1-2). Nerve impingement occurring in the cervical or shoulder region can result

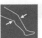

Stress Test 16-1
Valgus Stress Test

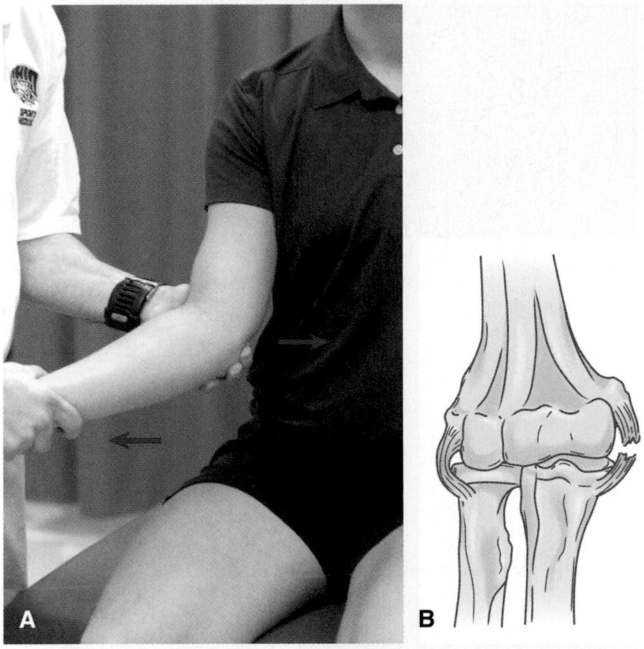

The valgus stress test determines the integrity of the UCL. (Also see the Moving Valgus Stress Test [Selective Tissue Test 16-1].)

Patient Position	Standing, sitting, or supine The glenohumeral joint is in neutral. The elbow is flexed 10°–25°.
Position of Examiner	Standing lateral to the joint being tested One hand supports the lateral elbow with the fingers reaching behind the joint to palpate the medial joint. The opposite hand grasps the distal forearm.
Evaluative Procedure	A valgus force is applied to the joint. The procedure is repeated with the elbow in various degrees of flexion.
Positive Test	Increased laxity compared with the opposite side, or pain, or both
Implications	Sprain of the ulnar collateral ligament, especially the anterior bundle Laxity beyond 60° of flexion also implicates involvement of the posterior bundle. Laxity in full extension is indicative of an olecranon or humeral fracture.
Modification	The patient can be positioned with the glenohumeral joint in external rotation for better stabilization. This position should be avoided in patients with anterior glenohumeral instability.
Comments	Laxity may also indicate epiphyseal injury.
Evidence	

Sensitivity

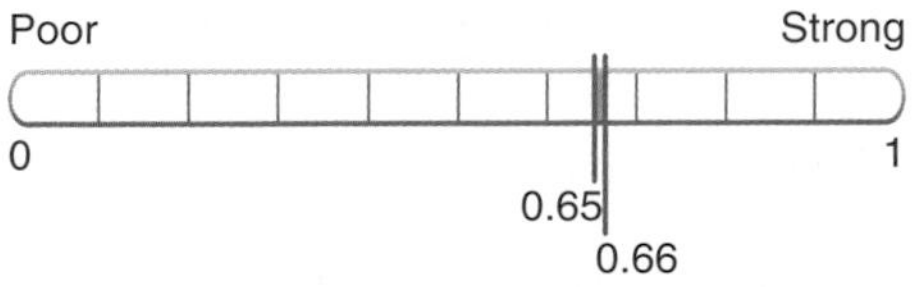

Specificity

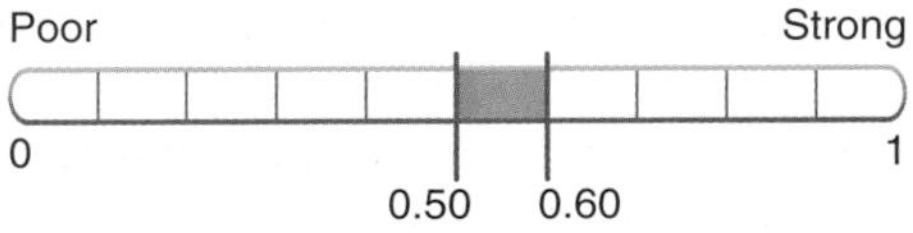

LR+: 1.70–19.00

LR−: 0.57–0.70–0.82

Stress Test 16-2
Varus Stress Test

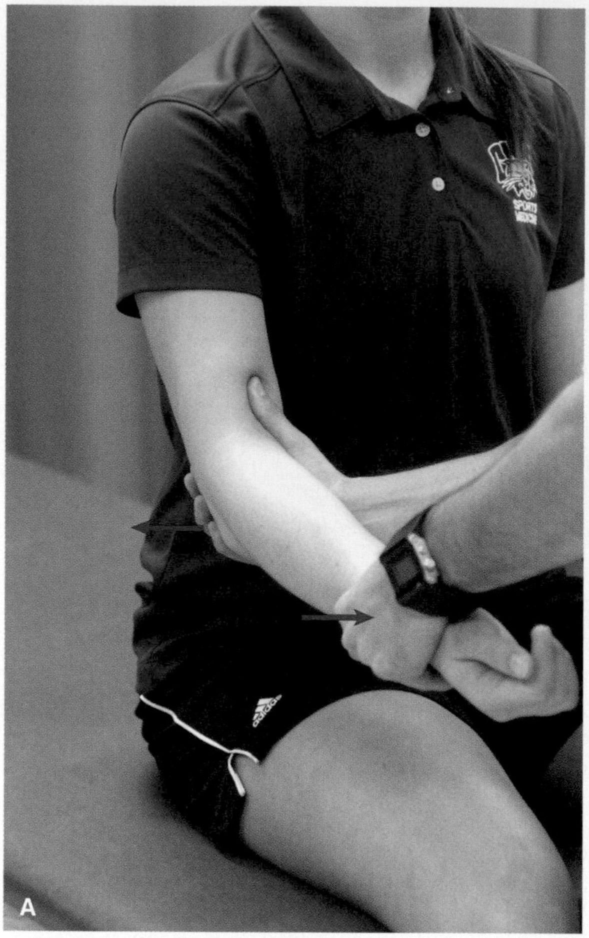

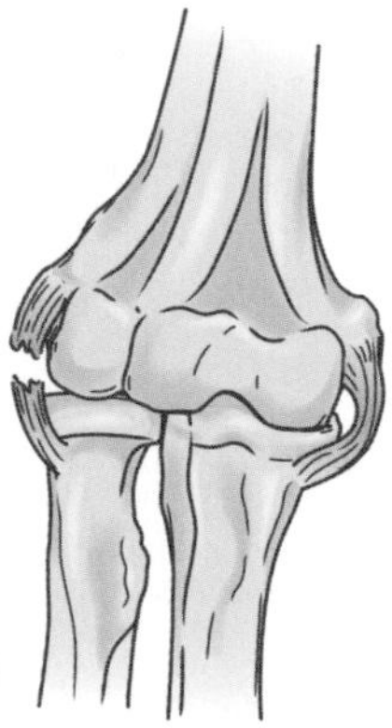

The varus stress test determines the integrity of the RCL.

Patient Position	Standing or sitting The elbow is flexed to 25°. The glenohumeral joint is in neutral.
Position of Examiner	Standing medial to the joint being tested One hand supports the medial elbow with the fingers reaching behind the joint to palpate the lateral joint line. The opposite hand grasps the distal forearm.
Evaluative Procedure	A varus force is applied to the elbow. This process is repeated with the joint in various degrees of flexion.
Positive Test	Increased laxity compared with the opposite side and/or pain is produced
Implications	Moderate laxity reflects trauma to the RCL. Gross laxity may also indicate damage to the annular or LUCL, causing the radius to displace from the ulna.
Comments	Laxity may also indicate bony or epiphyseal injury.
Evidence	Absent or inconclusive in the literature

LUCL = lateral ulnar collateral ligament; RCL = radial collateral ligament

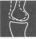

Joint Play 16-1
Elbow Joint Play

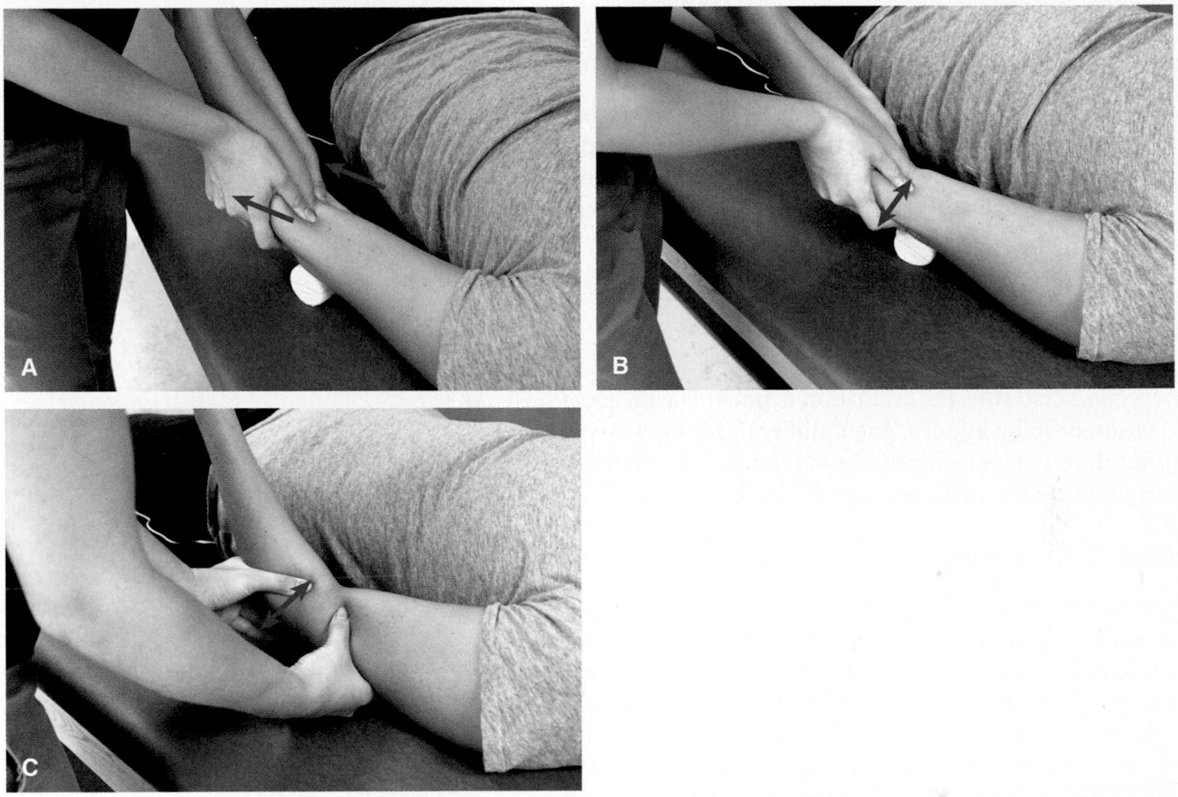

Joint play at the elbow assesses the amount of mobility allowed by the joint capsule and ligaments.

Patient Position	**(A) Humeroulnar:** Supine; elbow in about 70° of flexion and the forearm supinated about 10° **(B) Radioulnar:** Sitting or supine; elbow in 70° of flexion and 35° of supination **(C) Radiohumeral:** Sitting or supine; elbow extended and forearm supinated
Position of Examiner	At the side of the patient
Evaluative Procedure	**Humeroulnar:** The examiner places thumbs on the proximal ulna while stabilizing the distal forearm between his/her forearm and body and then applies a distracting force to the elbow. **Radioulnar:** The examiner stabilizes the proximal ulna and applies an anterior and then posterior force at the radial head. **Radiohumeral:** The examiner stabilizes the proximal humerus and applies an anterior and then posterior force at the radial head.
Positive Test	Hypomobility, hypermobility, or pain
Implications	Restrictions in all articulations may accompany loss of physiological elbow motion. Hypomobility at the radioulnar joint is associated with restricted supination and pronation.
Comments	Note that only the patient's position differs when assessing the radioulnar and radiohumeral articulations. The pressure needed to grasp the patient's radial head may be painful in noninjured patients. Joint movement is easier to detect in the posterior direction.

in disruption of the sensory or motor function (or both) in the elbow, forearm, and hand. Likewise, nerve trauma in the elbow refers its symptoms into the wrist, hand, and fingers (Fig. 16-17).

Vascular Testing

In cases of suspected or apparent fractures about the elbow, elbow dislocation, or compartment syndrome, the integrity of distal blood supply must be identified. Confirm the presence of the ulnar and radial pulses and capillary refill (see Selective Tissue Test 1-2).

Region-Specific Pathologies and Selective Tissue Tests

This section discusses the evaluation of patients with acute and chronic elbow injuries. The number of selective tissue tests for the elbow is relatively limited compared with those associated with the other joints described in this text.

Elbow Dislocations

Elbow dislocations result in obvious deformity, loss of function, extreme pain, and occasionally hysteria from the patient. Large forces are required to cause an elbow dislocation, typically requiring an axial force through the forearm while the elbow is slightly flexed and the forearm is supinated. This load creates a rotational and compressive force that often damages the posterolateral corner and the anterior bundle of the ulnar collateral ligament.[21] The forearm is displaced posteriorly or posterolaterally relative to the humerus in approximately 90% of the cases (Fig. 16-18).[22] Rarely, the elbow will dislocate in an anterior or lateral direction.[21]

The majority of elbow dislocations involve only soft tissue damage. However, complex dislocations involve soft tissue injury and a fracture of the distal humerus, radial head and neck, olecranon, or coronoid process.[21] Because of the possibility of fracture, radiographs must be obtained following reduction. The terrible triad of the elbow includes a posterior dislocation, fracture of the radial head, and fracture of the coronoid and is associated with a worse outcome when compared with a dislocation that involves only soft tissue trauma.[21,23,24] Swelling forms rapidly, possibly masking the underlying deformity if there is a delay in evaluating the condition (Examination Findings 16-1). Because of the potential compromise of the blood vessels and nerves crossing the joint, the patient's distal neurovascular function must be assessed. Up to 20% of patients report symptoms from the ulnar nerve or anterior interosseous branch of the median nerve. These neuropathies usually resolve with conservative management. Compartment syndromes may also result.[25]

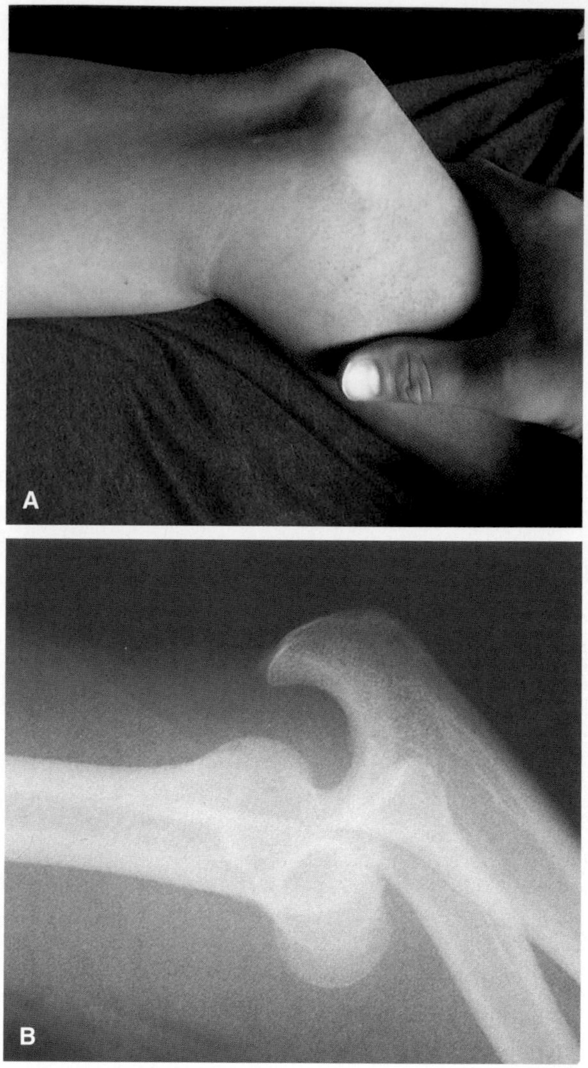

FIGURE 16-18 ■ Posterior dislocation of the elbow. This condition results in obvious deformity of the joint. Note that the humeroulnar and humeroradial joints are involved. (A) Inspection findings. (B) Radiographic view.

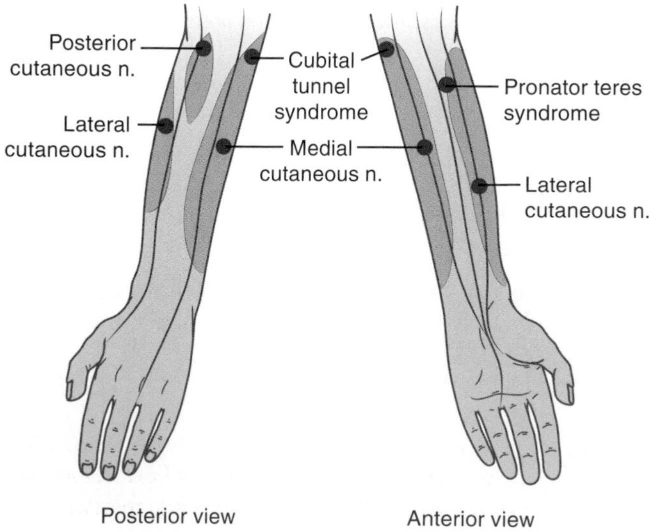

FIGURE 16-17 ■ Local neuropathies of the elbow, forearm, and hand. Correlate these findings with those of an upper quarter neurological screen (see Neurological Screening 1-2).

*** Practical Evidence**

Most cases of posterolateral rotatory instability occur following a dislocation of the elbow.[24]

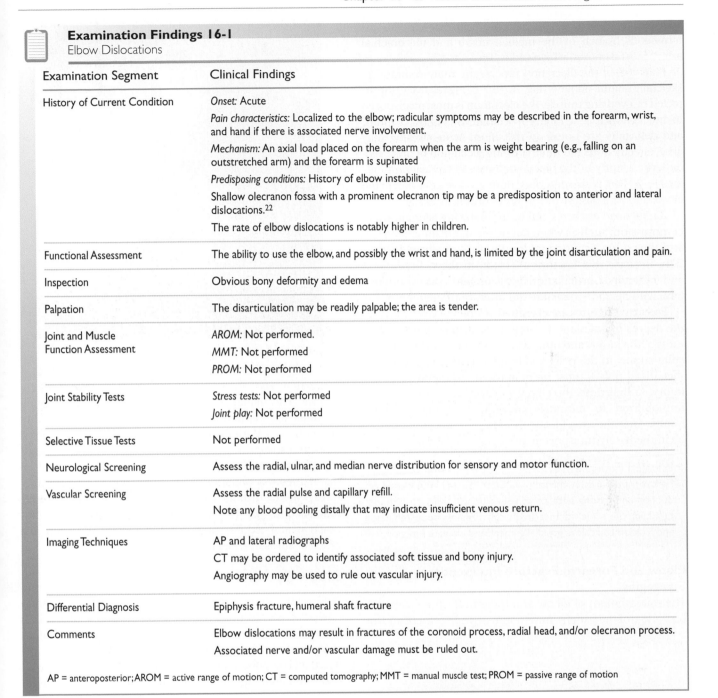

Examination Findings 16-1
Elbow Dislocations

Examination Segment	Clinical Findings
History of Current Condition	*Onset:* Acute *Pain characteristics:* Localized to the elbow; radicular symptoms may be described in the forearm, wrist, and hand if there is associated nerve involvement. *Mechanism:* An axial load placed on the forearm when the arm is weight bearing (e.g., falling on an outstretched arm) and the forearm is supinated *Predisposing conditions:* History of elbow instability Shallow olecranon fossa with a prominent olecranon tip may be a predisposition to anterior and lateral dislocations.[22] The rate of elbow dislocations is notably higher in children.
Functional Assessment	The ability to use the elbow, and possibly the wrist and hand, is limited by the joint disarticulation and pain.
Inspection	Obvious bony deformity and edema
Palpation	The disarticulation may be readily palpable; the area is tender.
Joint and Muscle Function Assessment	*AROM:* Not performed. *MMT:* Not performed *PROM:* Not performed
Joint Stability Tests	*Stress tests:* Not performed *Joint play:* Not performed
Selective Tissue Tests	Not performed
Neurological Screening	Assess the radial, ulnar, and median nerve distribution for sensory and motor function.
Vascular Screening	Assess the radial pulse and capillary refill. Note any blood pooling distally that may indicate insufficient venous return.
Imaging Techniques	AP and lateral radiographs CT may be ordered to identify associated soft tissue and bony injury. Angiography may be used to rule out vascular injury.
Differential Diagnosis	Epiphysis fracture, humeral shaft fracture
Comments	Elbow dislocations may result in fractures of the coronoid process, radial head, and/or olecranon process. Associated nerve and/or vascular damage must be ruled out.

AP = anteroposterior; AROM = active range of motion; CT = computed tomography; MMT = manual muscle test; PROM = passive range of motion

Elbow Dislocation Intervention Strategies

Reduction of elbow dislocations can be performed either on the field or in the emergency room by trained personnel. Gross instability of the posterolateral corner may be present near or at full extension and often necessitates surgical repair. Following reduction, ROM should be assessed to determine stability. Neurovascular function should also be assessed postreduction, and individuals displaying any findings associated with vascular compromise (e.g., diminished distal pulse, compartment syndrome symptoms) should receive immediate treatment.

Following reduction of simple dislocations, patients are generally placed in a hinged brace to allow early active ROM but avoid valgus and varus forces. Periods of complete immobilization are brief (1 to 5 days), with longer periods associated with worse outcomes.[21]

Fractures About the Elbow

Supracondylar fractures are almost exclusively found in adolescents and result from a fall directly onto a flexed elbow or a hyperextension mechanism. When displaced, angular deformity occurs, with the distal fragment almost always displaced dorsally in an extension-type fracture pattern.[26] Individuals with displaced supracondylar fractures should be carefully assessed for neurovascular integrity, with the anterior interosseous branch of the median nerve and the brachial artery most commonly involved.[26]

Fractures of the olecranon process are more common in skeletally mature patients (Fig. 16-19).[6] Being relatively unprotected by overlying muscle, the olecranon is most predisposed to direct blows such as falling on a flexed elbow. Pain, crepitus, and deformity are noted on palpation. Acute swelling may arise directly from the trauma to the olecranon or arise secondary to injury of the olecranon bursa (Examination Findings 16-2). Pain is also described during active extension of the elbow and with passive overpressure during extension.

Radial head fractures can occur following a longitudinal compression, such as when falling on an outstretched arm, and they often occur concurrently with an elbow dislocation. Because this fracture affects both the radiohumeral and radioulnar articulations, the patient will experience pain with flexion/extension and pronation/supination.

Forearm fractures are classified as open or closed and by the degree of angulation, rotation, or displacement. Fractures of the radius and ulna may compromise the neurovascular supply to the wrist and hand (Fig. 16-20). Because of this, distal pulses must be monitored constantly after the injury. At that time, the elbow, forearm, and wrist must be immobilized to minimize movement of the fractured bones. After the area has been stabilized, the athlete must be immediately transported and treated for shock.

*** Practical Evidence**

Forearm fractures in children are often treated with closed reduction and casting because of young bone's ability to remodel. In adults, the same fracture frequently requires open reduction and fixation to achieve good alignment and ultimate function.[27,28]

Elbow and Forearm Fracture Intervention Strategies

The management of elbow and forearm fractures depends on the age of the patient, the amount of displacement and/or angulation, and whether or not the fracture crosses a joint surface. The management decision is based on restoring anatomical congruency so that long-term function is not compromised. With displaced or angulated fractures, closed reduction and casting is often the first-line treatment. Surgical fixation may be necessary if the reduction cannot be maintained.[28] A benefit of surgical fixation of forearm fractures, whether through a plate or intramedullary nail, is early mobilization.[29] By their nature, olecranon fractures are intra-articular and require anatomical alignment to restore the articular surfaces (see Figure 16-19).[6]

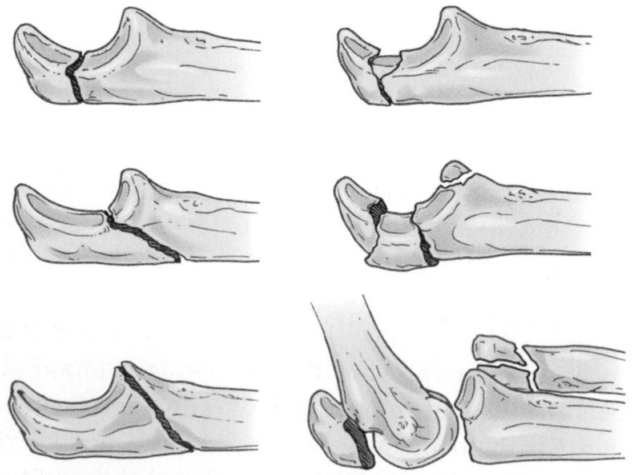

FIGURE 16-19 ■ Fractures of the olecranon process. All fractures involving the olecranon process are intra-articular. Management involves the restoration of joint congruency.

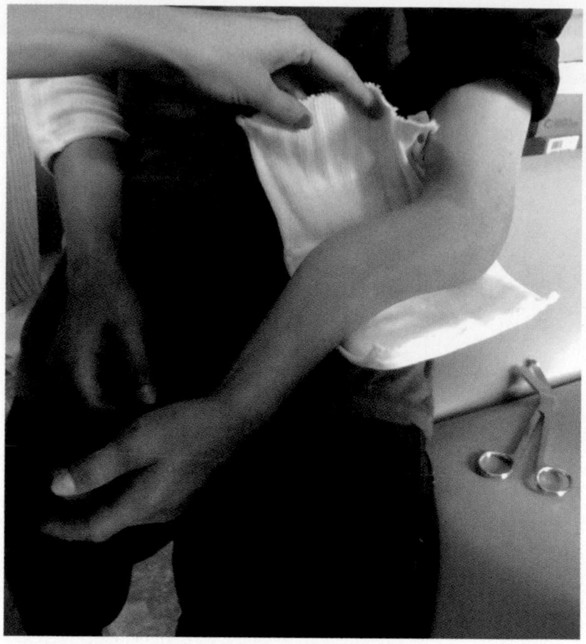

FIGURE 16-20 ■ Fracture of the radial and ulnar shafts.

Elbow Sprains

Because the elbow is stabilized by the locking of the olecranon process in its fossa when the joint is extended, strain is placed on the ligaments when the elbow is flexed. A valgus or varus stress from a blow or forceful motion delivered to a flexed elbow is dissipated by the collateral ligaments. The elbow's collateral ligament structure and bony arrangement create a mechanism whereby tensile forces on one side of the joint result in compressive forces on the opposite side.[30]

Trauma becomes more complex when a rotational component is added to the elbow. When a valgus or varus force is placed on an extended elbow, the olecranon process, in addition to the collateral ligament, must be evaluated for injury. A hyperextension mechanism can stress the elbow's anterior capsule or compress the posterior structures.

Ulnar Collateral Ligament

The UCL is stressed secondary to a valgus loading of the humeroulnar joint. Acutely, this stress results from a force delivered to the lateral elbow or from repetitive throwing that ultimately leads to attenuation and then failure. Valgus

Examination Findings 16-2
Fractures About the Elbow

Examination Segment	Clinical Findings
History of Current Condition	*Onset:* Acute *Pain characteristics:* Localized to the elbow *Mechanism:* Fall onto the elbow, falling on an outstretched arm, hyperextension *Predisposing conditions:* Skeletal immaturity, osteoporosis
Functional Assessment	The ability to use the elbow, and possibly the wrist and hand, is limited by the fracture and pain.
Inspection	Although fractures around the elbow may result in obvious deformity, distal humeral fractures, coronoid process fractures, olecranon process fractures, and radial head fractures may not have evident bony displacement. Swelling and ecchymosis may be noted.
Palpation	Point tender over the fracture site (excluding intra-articular fractures)
Joint and Muscle Function Assessment	Do not perform in the presence of obvious fracture. *AROM:* Limited by pain and possible instability *MMT:* Painful and weak with muscle attachment on involved bone *PROM:* Pain with movement; olecranon process fractures elicit pain with passive overpressure. Radial head fractures elicit pain with pronation and supination.
Joint Stability Tests	Do not perform if a fracture is suspected. *Stress tests:* Apparent ligamentous laxity may be caused by bony instability. *Joint play:* Apparent increased joint mobility may be caused by bony instability.
Selective Tissue Tests	Not applicable
Neurological Screening	Assess the radial, ulnar, and median nerve distribution for sensory and motor function.
Vascular Screening	Assess the radial pulse and capillary refill. Note any blood pooling distally that may indicate insufficient venous return.
Imaging Techniques	AP and lateral radiographs are used to identify the magnitude and direction of the fracture. The fat pad sign, representing bleeding into the joint, may be noted on radiographs.
Differential Diagnosis	Elbow dislocation, biceps tendon rupture, collateral ligament sprain
Comments	Distal humeral fractures are often intra-articular. The fracture may be open. Concurrent dislocation of the elbow may occur.

AP = anteroposterior; AROM = active range of motion; MMT = manual muscle test; MRI = magnetic resonance imaging; PROM = passive range of motion

loading of the UCL occurs during normal athletic movements and is significantly increased during the overhand-throwing motion. The force generated during this motion is so great that the UCL cannot tolerate the tension on its own. As a result, the UCL must rely on the triceps brachii, the wrist flexor–pronator muscles, and the anconeus to provide dynamic stabilization to counteract the valgus force placed on this joint.[10] The LUCL can also be injured if the force is sufficient. When the forces generated during the cocking and acceleration phases of throwing are greater than the tensile strength of the UCL, insidious tearing of the ligament begins.[20] Tensile forces on the medial elbow also produce compressive forces on the lateral structures, warranting examination of the lateral bony structures (see Valgus Extension Overload).[2]

The chief complaint is pain on the medial aspect of the elbow that intensifies with motion. Compression of the radial nerve may produce radicular pain in the forearm and dorsal surface of the hand. Tensile forces placed on the ulnar nerve can cause paresthesia in the distal ulnar nerve distribution. Swelling may be present on the anterior, medial, and posterior borders of the joint. In most medial sprains, the anterior bundle of the UCL is traumatized. Tenderness, which has high sensitivity but poor specificity in detecting UCL damage, is noted along its length from the medial epicondyle to the coronoid process.[31] If the elbow is flexed past 60 degrees, the posterior bundle may also be painful. ROM testing may reveal pain secondary to stretching of the ligaments or from joint instability. A limitation in passive glenohumeral internal rotation is often present.[20] Valgus stress testing demonstrates pain and laxity at various degrees of flexion (Examination Findings 16-3). The **moving valgus stress test** identifies UCL instability within the range of maximal dynamic pressure, normally between 120 and 70 to 80 degrees, closely approximating the late cocking and early acceleration phases of throwing (Selective Tissue Test 16-1).[2,32,33] Because of the relationship of the ulnar nerve to the medial elbow, a neurological examination of the forearm, wrist, hand, and fingers may also be required. Additionally, examination of the entire kinetic chain is warranted; scapular dyskinesis and hip weakness and/or inflexibility are also associated with the development of UCL pathology.[20]

- **Valgus extension overload:** Attenuation of the anterior bundle of the UCL leads to **valgus extension overload (VEO)**, a collection of tensile, shear, and compressive forces that result from mild UCL laxity.[35] In addition to tensile stresses on the ulnar nerve and UCL, compressive and shear forces are created at the radial head and posterior medial olecranon process. Consequences of this compression and shear include osteophyte formation and loose bodies on the posterior medial olecranon process and fossa and loose bodies at the radiohumeral articulation. This collection of forces begins with medial laxity as a result of repetitive throwing. Potential symptoms of VEO include posteromedial and lateral elbow pain, along with ulnar nerve paresthesia as the nerve is stretched. Extending the elbow while applying a valgus stress will replicate the mechanism and may recreate symptoms associated with VEO.[35]
- **Elbow posterolateral rotatory instability:** Tears of the LUCL permit a transient rotational subluxation of the radius and ulna relative to the humerus, **posterolateral rotatory instability**, causing external rotation of the radius and ulna, and valgus opening of the elbow (Fig. 16-21).[10,12,36] This results in the radius and ulna acting as a single unit as they rock away from the articulating surfaces of the humerus. A classic complaint of patients with an insufficiency of the LUCL is an ability or reluctance to push out of a chair and fully extend the elbow with the forearms supinated and the arms abducted greater than shoulder width (**chair sign**).[2] In addition, patients will be unable to fully extend or be apprehensive in performing a push-up from the floor with the forearms supinated and the arms abducted greater than shoulder width (**push-up sign**).[24,37] Clinically, patients with this condition may be evaluated through the **posterolateral rotatory instability test** (Selective Tissue Test 16-2).

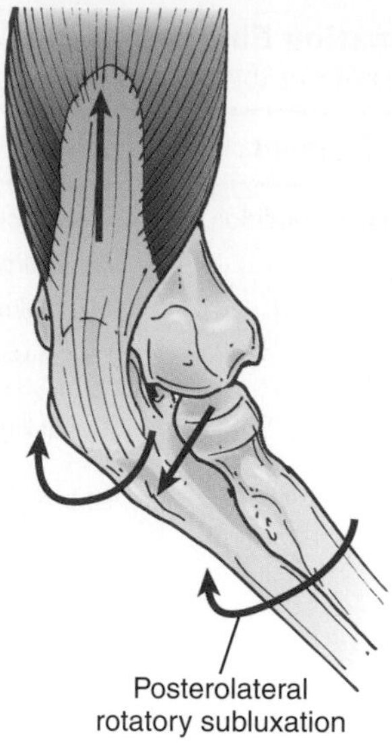

FIGURE 16-21 ■ Posterolateral rotational subluxation of the radius. Contraction of the triceps brachii against resistance results in a varus stress and external rotation of the ulna. This causes the radius to externally rotate. The subluxation occurs when the radial head rotates off the capitulum.

✱ Practical Evidence

A patient's inability to perform a push-up or to push out of a chair (with the forearms supinated and greater than shoulder-width apart) is a better indicator of posterolateral rotatory instability than the posterolateral rotatory instability (pivot shift) test in an unanesthetized patient.[37]

Ulnar Collateral Ligament Sprain Intervention Strategies

In cases of chronic overload to the medial side of the elbow, the initial treatment is to alleviate any repetitive forces on the elbow. Local modalities are helpful to decrease pain and inflammation. ROM is progressed in a pain-free manner. Strengthening of the muscles surrounding the joint is performed to assist in stabilizing the elbow against valgus forces. ROM deficits at the shoulder or hip should be addressed, with particular attention to restoration of normal internal rotation at the glenohumeral joint. Strengthening of the trunk, shoulder, and hip musculature is often indicated in addition to specific instruction in throwing mechanisms to minimize valgus forces.

✱ Practical Evidence

To reduce valgus forces on the elbow, throwing instructions should include strategies for trunk rotation occurring later in the throwing sequence, reduced shoulder external rotation, and increased elbow flexion. Sidearm throwing should be discouraged.

Surgery to reconstruct the medial elbow with a palmaris longus autograft may be necessary to fully restore function in the throwing athlete with valgus instability. The surgery has a generally successful outcome in returning throwing athletes to full activity in about a year.[20,31]

Examination Findings 16-3
Ulnar Collateral Ligament Sprain

Examination Segment	Clinical Findings
History of Current Condition	*Onset:* Acute or insidious *Pain characteristics:* Medial aspect of elbow *Mechanism:* Acute: Valgus stress placed on the ulnar collateral ligament Insidious: Repeated activities that exert tensile stresses on the medial aspect of the elbow, creating valgus loading (e.g., throwing) *Predisposing conditions:* Internal rotation deficits in the throwing athlete; cubital valgus;[20] taller and heavier baseball player[20]
Functional Assessment	Overhand-throwing athletes will describe a significant decrease in velocity, accuracy, and/or endurance. Pain during late cocking or early acceleration phase
Inspection	Effusion may be present in the anterior, medial, and posterior aspects of the elbow. Edema may extravasate distally if the capsule is torn. Ecchymosis may be present over the medial aspect of the elbow. Scapular dyskinesis may be observed during active motion.
Palpation	Palpation of the medial elbow from the medial epicondyle to the coronoid process may elicit tenderness and crepitus.
Joint and Muscle Function Assessment	*AROM:* Elbow motion is limited secondary to pain because of stretching of the ligaments or joint instability, especially moving into extension. Wrist flexion is painful. *MMT:* Decreased strength and pain in wrist flexors *PROM:* Pain elicited at end-range of supination and extension Extension may be limited by a flexion contracture in chronic cases. Wrist extension is painful at the end-range. Decreased glenohumeral internal rotation
Joint Stability Tests	*Stress tests:* Valgus testing at 10°–25° of flexion demonstrates increased laxity and pain at the medial elbow and may elicit paresthesia in the ulnar nerve distribution. Testing at other degrees of flexion (e.g., 45°, 60°, and 90°) may elicit symptoms. *Joint play:* Humeroulnar, radiohumeral, radioulnar
Selective Tissue Tests	Posterolateral rotatory instability test of the elbow Moving valgus stress test
Neurological Screening	Sensory and motor testing of the ulnar and radial nerve distributions Tinel's sign at the ulnar nerve may be positive if the nerve has been traumatized.
Vascular Screening	Within normal limits
Imaging Techniques	Valgus stress radiographs may be obtained. An opening of the medial joint line greater than 2 to 3 mm is consistent with instability.[3,34] Ligament disruption and surrounding soft tissue involvement is visualized via MRI. Asymptomatic overhead-throwing athletes may demonstrate increased medial opening on stress radiographs.[32]
Differential Diagnosis	Pronator muscle tear, supinator muscle sprain, arthritis, ulnar neuropathy, flexor carpi radialis tear, flexor carpi ulnaris tear, cubital tunnel syndrome

AROM = active range of motion; MMT = manual muscle test; MRI = magnetic resonance imaging; PROM = passive range of motion

Selective Tissue Test 16-1
Moving Valgus Stress Test

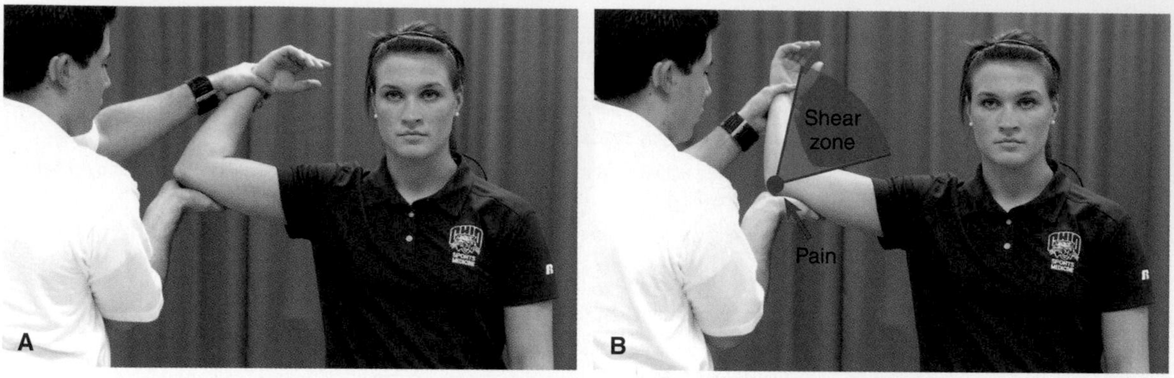

The moving valgus stress test places tensile forces on the UCL through elbow flexion and extension to identify dynamic elbow instability.

Patient Position	Sitting
Position of Examiner	The shoulder is abducted to 90°. The elbow is flexed to the end of the ROM.
Position of Examiner	Standing next to the patient One hand stabilizes the distal humerus. The opposite hand grasps the ulnar side of the distal forearm.
Evaluative Procedure	(A) The examiner externally rotates the glenohumeral joint and applies a valgus force on the elbow. (B) The examiner extends the elbow to approximately 30° while maintaining a valgus force on the joint, noting the position(s) in which pain is evoked. The examiner then moves the elbow from extension into flexion while maintaining a valgus stress on the joint.
Positive Test	Pain at the medial elbow that reproduces functional pain, often producing an apprehension response AND Pain that occurs between 120° and 70° (representing the position of the late cocking and early acceleration throwing phases) A positive test is marked by the reproduction of pain at the same point in the ROM during both the flexion and extension segments of the examination.
Implications	Partial tear or attenuation of the UCL
Comments	Shoulder pathology may elicit pain during this procedure. Do not perform in the presence of known GH instability.
Evidence	

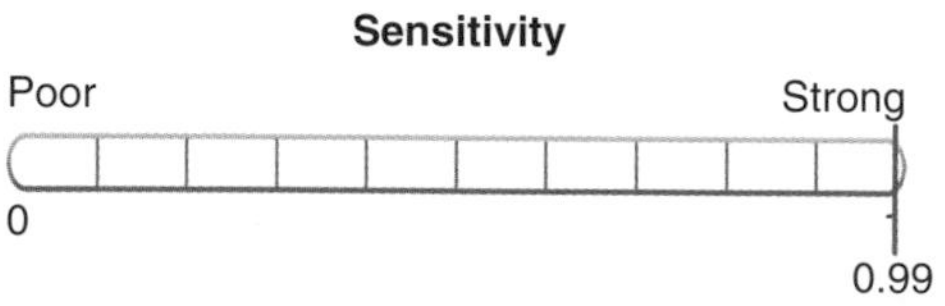

LR+: 3.96

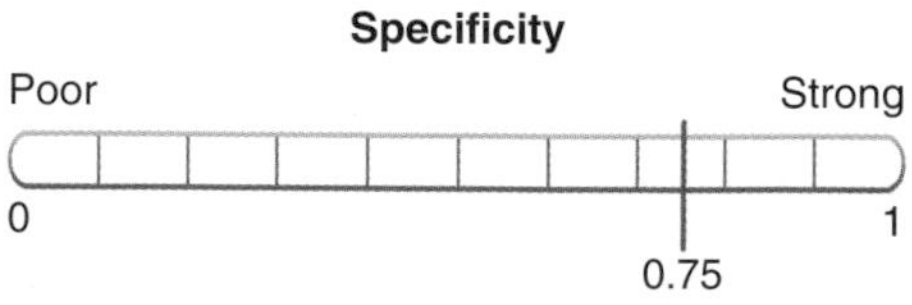

LR−: 0.01

GH = glenohumeral; ROM = range of motion; UCL = ulnar collateral ligament

Selective Tissue Test 16-2
Posterolateral Rotatory Instability Test (Pivot Shift)

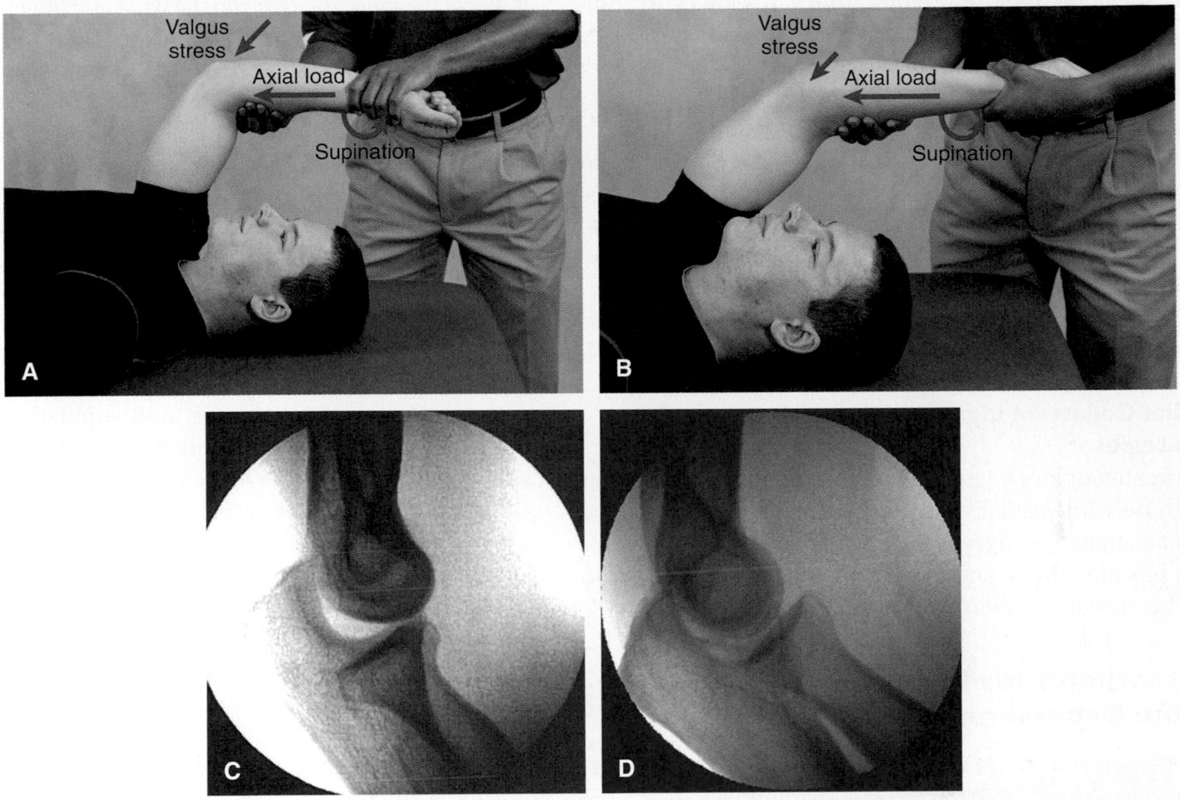

Test for posterolateral instability of the elbow. (A) Starting position of elbow flexion, forearm pronation, and a valgus and axial load at the elbow. (B) The elbow is then extended and the forearm supinated while maintaining a valgus force an axial load. The patient is then returned to the starting position. (C) Fluoroscopic view of the subluxated radiocapitellar joint. (D) Reduction of the joint.

Patient Position	Supine The shoulder and elbow are flexed to 90°, and the forearm is fully supinated.
Position of Examiner	Standing at the head of the patient One hand grasps the proximal forearm, and the other hand grasps the distal forearm at the wrist **(A).**
Evaluative Procedure	While applying a valgus stress and axial compression, the elbow is extended, and the forearm is maintained in full supination **(B)**. The elbow is then returned to the flexed position **(A)**.
Positive Test	The elbow subluxates as it is extended **(C)** and can be felt to reduce as it is flexed **(D)**.
Implications	Chronic instability of the elbow
Comments	When performed with the patient under anesthesia, the posterolateral rotatory instability test was positive only when the entire lateral collateral ligament was sectioned.[36]
Evidence	

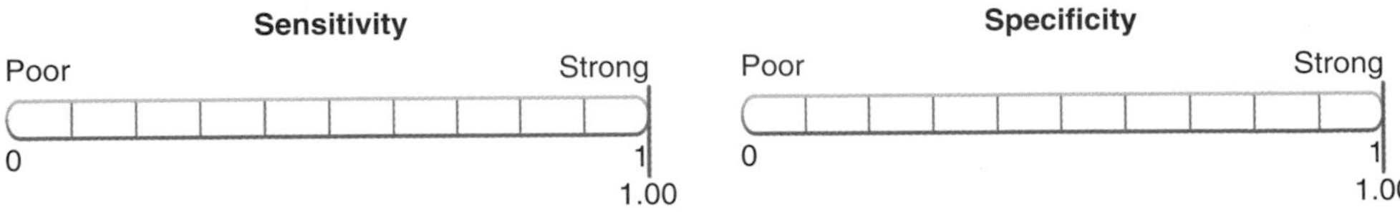

LR−: 0.00

Radial Collateral Ligament

Injury to the RCL complex is rare because, in most positions, the body shields the elbow from varus forces. In addition, the stresses placed on the elbow joint during throwing and racquet sports are absorbed by the UCL and the wrist extensor muscles.

Varus forces placed on the lateral elbow ligaments can result in trauma to the RCL and, possibly, the annular ligament. Trauma to the RCL or its component parts (see Fig. 16-5) results not only in varus laxity but it may also disrupt the articulation between the radial head and the capitulum. The signs and symptoms of RCL sprains are similar to those of UCL trauma but may be compounded by pain, laxity, or weakness during pronation and supination.

Radial Collateral Ligament Sprain Intervention Strategies

The treatment for patients with RCL sprains is similar to that for those with medial elbow sprains. With radial collateral sprains, strengthening focuses on the wrist extensors, supinators, brachioradialis, and the surrounding elbow muscles to provide dynamic stabilization against varus stresses.

Osteochondritis Dissecans of the Capitulum

Osteochondritis dissecans of the capitulum develops gradually because of increased valgus loading with overhead throwing. The resulting valgus load on the elbow places compressive and shear forces on the capitulum and radial head.[38] Osteochondritis dissecans develops secondary to disrupted blood flow to the area, creating an osteochondral defect over time. Osteochondritis dissecans is frequently associated with other orthopedic conditions such as osteochondral fracture, avascular necrosis, and detached bony fragments.[38]

The patient complains of "dull" lateral elbow pain that increases with activity. In throwing athletes, pain is increased during the late cocking and acceleration phase. The patient holds the elbow in a flexed position, and passive extension may be restricted.[2] Symptoms may increase while an axial load is placed on the forearm during passive pronation and supination. Palpation yields tenderness over the capitulum, lateral epicondyle, and lateral joint line. Radiographic examination and/or ultrasonic imagining reveal either a nondisplaced fragmented defect or a loose body within the joint.

Osteochondritis Dissecans of the Capitulum Intervention Strategies

If the fragment has not separated, rest along with a progressive program of ROM and strengthening is used. A loose body warrants surgical intervention to remove the fragment and curettage the defect. In either case, the return to previous athletic endeavors is guarded, especially in the throwing athlete.

Epicondylalgia

Both the lateral and medial epicondyles serve as the origin for many of the muscles acting on the wrist and fingers. Although commonly used, the term epicondylitis does not accurately capture most conditions at these origins; chronic pathology is more likely a degenerative tendinosis than an actual inflammatory tendinitis condition. The term epicondylalgia is a broader description to capture pain in the medial and lateral epicondyles.

Lateral Epicondylalgia

Inflammation or repetitive stresses at the lateral epicondyle irritates the common attachment of the wrist extensor group (extensor carpi ulnaris, extensor carpi radialis brevis, extensor digitorum communis, and supinator). Although any or all of these muscles may be involved, the extensor carpi radialis brevis is the muscle most commonly affected. Underlying the extensor carpi radialis longus, the brevis has a broad origin from the common extensor tendon on the lateral epicondyle, lateral collateral ligament, annular ligament, and associated muscular fascia.[10] Repeated, forceful eccentric contractions of the wrist extensor muscles result in the accumulation of degenerative forces at their attachment site, creating microtears.[10,39] The relatively small area of attachment for these muscles causes a great force load to be applied to the bone as these muscles contract.

Lateral epicondylalgia is prevalent in racquet sports, affecting more than half of all regular tennis players, leading to its colloquial name, "tennis elbow." Most common in individuals older than 40 years of age, the chief complaint and most significant clinical finding is pain over the lateral epicondyle, decreased grip strength, and pain with gripping (Examination Findings 16-4).[40,41] In patients who play racquet sports, the symptoms are increased during backhand strokes. Other risk factors for lateral epicondylalgia include rotator cuff pathology, de Quervain's disease, carpal tunnel syndrome, oral corticosteroid therapy, and smoking.[42]

Inspection of the painful area may reveal swelling, and palpation of the area may produce pain. Active wrist extension, especially with the elbow extended, results in pain that worsens with resisted motion.[43] Pain elicited during passive stretching of the extensor muscles and resisted finger extension have also been demonstrated to be reliable indicators of this condition.[41] Active and passive wrist flexion, elbow extension, and forearm pronation, all of which stretch the common extensor tendon, are routinely limited for the patient with lateral epicondylalgia.[37] Manual muscle testing reveals weakness of the grip musculature (including wrist extensors and flexors) as well as elbow flexors and extensors. Because the dominant arm is usually involved, strengths deficits may be underestimated. The **tennis elbow test** is sensitive to even mild cases of lateral epicondylalgia (Selective Tissue Test 16-3). Entrapment of the radial nerve may produce symptoms that are similar to lateral epicondylalgia, and proximal nerve root compression of C6 should also be considered in the differential diagnosis.

Examination Findings 16-4
Lateral Epicondylalgia

Examination Segment	Clinical Findings
History of Current Condition	*Onset:* Insidious *Pain characteristics:* Lateral epicondyle and proximal portion of the common tendons of the wrist extensors; radicular pain into the wrist extensor muscles is possible with advanced cases. *Mechanism:* Overuse syndrome involving repeated, forceful wrist extension; radial deviation, supination, or grasping in an overhand position; repeated eccentric loading of the wrist extensor muscles *Predisposing conditions:* Rotator cuff pathology, de Quervain's disease, carpal tunnel syndrome, smoking, oral corticosteroid therapy[42] Inexperience or newness in playing racquet sports[30] Occupation requiring prolonged computer use or greater than 1 hour per day of repetitive flexing and straightening the elbow[44,45]
Functional Assessment	Pain and weakness or compensatory movement with activities that require gripping or repetitive elbow flexion and extension Decreased grip strength as measured on a dynamometer[46] Pain and weakness with activities requiring combined elbow flexion and wrist extension motions In racquet sports, pain is worsened with the backhand stroke and may be related to improper size of the racquet handle grip or a racquet that is too tightly strung.
Inspection	Swelling possibly present over the lateral epicondyle
Palpation	Pain and possible crepitus over the lateral epicondyle and proximal portion of the common wrist extensor tendon
Joint and Muscle Function Assessment	*AROM:* Pain with combined wrist extension and elbow flexion; radial deviation also possibly painful Pronation and supination may be limited in patients with chronic lateral epicondylalgia.[30] *MMT:* Pain with wrist extension and MCP joint extension when elbow is extended; weakness may also be noted at the shoulder and with elbow flexion and extension.[47] *PROM:* Pain at the end-range of passive wrist flexion, especially with elbow extended Limitation in wrist flexion with the elbow extended
Joint Stability Tests	*Stress tests:* Unremarkable *Joint play:* Restricted radioulnar and radiohumeral glide
Selective Tissue Tests	Test for lateral epicondylalgia ("tennis elbow" test)
Neurological Screening	Rule out radial nerve or proximal cervical nerve root entrapment.
Vascular Screening	Within normal limits
Imaging Techniques	Plain radiography is used to image (or rule out) osteophyte formation, arthritis, osteochondritis dissecans, or fracture.[43,48] Diagnostic ultrasound may demonstrate thickening in the tendon.[43,48] MRI can image tendon degeneration.[43,48]
Differential Diagnosis	Radial tunnel syndrome, arthritis, acute epicondylar fracture, stress fracture; cervical radiculopathy
Comments	Lateral epicondylalgia, LCL, and/or radial nerve pathology may occur in any combination.[30]

AROM = active range of motion; LCL = lateral collateral ligament; MCP = metacarpophalangeal; MMT = manual muscle test; MRI = magnetic resonance imaging; PROM = passive range of motion

Selective Tissue Test 16-3
Test for Lateral Epicondylalgia ("Tennis Elbow" Test)

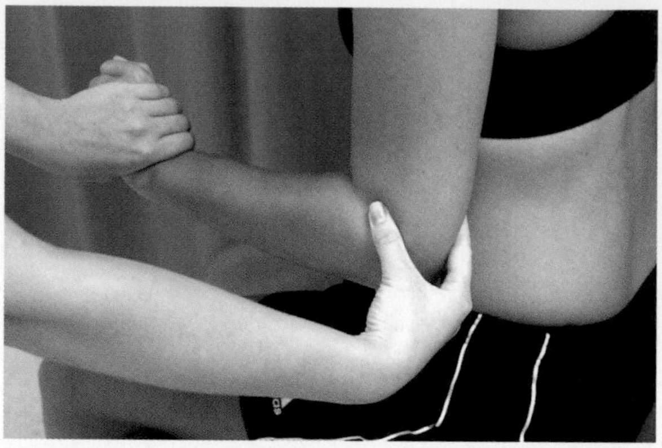

The test for lateral epicondylalgia involves resisted wrist extension while palpating the lateral epicondyle.

Patient Position	Seated with the tested elbow flexed to 90°, the forearm pronated, and the fingers flexed
Position of Examiner	Standing lateral to the patient with one hand positioned over the dorsal aspect of the wrist and hand
Evaluative Procedure	The examiner resists wrist extension while palpating the lateral epicondyle and common attachment of the wrist extensors.
Positive Test	Pain at the lateral epicondyle
Implications	Lateral epicondylalgia ("tennis elbow")
Modification	This test may also be performed with the elbow in extension.
Comments	This is the MMT for wrist extension performed through a full ROM instead of midrange.
Evidence	Absent or inconclusive in the literature

MMT = manual muscle test; ROM = range of motion

Lateral Epicondylalgia Intervention Strategies

Treatment of lateral epicondylalgia involves avoiding the activities that aggravate the condition. Oral anti-inflammatory medications and local anti-inflammatory modalities may reduce pain but do not otherwise affect the condition. Local corticosteroid injections may be beneficial for short-term gains in pain reduction, although structured rehabilitation or simply waiting produces better long-term outcomes.[33,37,43] Patients who have occupations that require extensive computer use have worse outcomes than those in other occupations.[44] Therapeutic exercises involve stretching and strengthening around the elbow with the main focus on the wrist extensor group. Shoulder strengthening should be performed if indicated.[47] The use of "tennis elbow" straps can eliminate pain and other symptoms associated with lateral epicondylagia.[49,50,51]

As the patient recovers, a return to the initial activities creating the condition may require an assessment of the equipment being used (e.g., racquet size and stiffness, ergonomic assessment of computer workstation) and the technique being used. Many patients who develop this condition from athletic participation may benefit from a lesson with an expert to improve their techniques. Activity modifications that reduce or eliminate repetitive contraction of the wrist extensors may be beneficial.

Medial Epicondylalgia

Activities involving the swift, powerful snapping of the wrist and pronation of the forearm load the medial epicondyle. As with its lateral counterpart, medial epicondylalgia involves point tenderness at the origin of the pronator teres, flexor carpi radialis, palmaris longus, and flexor carpi ulnaris tendon on the medial epicondyle. The length of the pronator teres muscle also may be tender, and the patient's grip strength may be markedly decreased (Examination Findings 16-5).[52] In young baseball pitchers, the tension buildup in the medial epicondyle

Examination Findings 16-5
Medial Epicondylalgia

Examination Segment	Clinical Findings
History of Current Condition	*Onset:* Insidious *Pain characteristics:* Medial epicondyle and the proximal portion of the adjacent wrist flexor and pronator muscles *Mechanism:* Repeated, forceful flexion or pronation of the wrist (or both) *Predisposing conditions:* Repeated activities that eccentrically load the medial elbow muscles (e.g., throwing, golfing)
Functional Assessment	Patient may demonstrate decreased grip strength. Pain or compensatory movement with activities requiring gripping or repetitive elbow flexion and extension
Inspection	Swelling in the area over the medial epicondyle
Palpation	Point tenderness and crepitus over the medial epicondyle; tenderness in the proximal portion of the wrist flexor group, especially the pronator teres
Joint and Muscle Function Assessment	*AROM:* Pain during wrist flexion; wrist extension possibly resulting in pain secondary to stretching the involved muscles *MMT:* Decreased strength and pain during testing of the wrist flexors and forearm pronators *PROM:* Pain at the end-range of wrist extension, especially with the elbow extended
Joint Stability Tests	*Stress tests:* Unremarkable *Joint play:* Unremarkable
Selective Tissue Tests	Not applicable
Neurological Screening	Sensory and motor tests to identify potential ulnar nerve neuropathy Upper quarter screen to identify cervical radiculopathy
Vascular Screening	Within normal limits
Imaging Techniques	Plain radiography is used to image (or rule out) osteophyte formation, arthritis, osteochondritis dissecans, or fracture.[48] Diagnostic ultrasound may demonstrate thickening in the tendon.[48] MRI can image tendon degeneration.[48]
Differential Diagnosis	Ulnar neuropathy, medial epicondylalgia, arthritis, acute epicondylar fracture, stress fracture, cervical radiculopathy
Comments	Medial epicondylalgia, UCL, and/or ulnar nerve trauma may occur in any combination.[30]

AROM = active range of motion; MMT = manual muscle test; MRI = magnetic resonance imaging; PROM = passive range of motion; UCL = ulnar collateral ligament

may result in avulsion of the common tendon from its attachment site, sometimes called "Little Leaguer's elbow" (Fig. 16-22).[7] Radiographic changes involving separation or fragmentation of the medial epicondyle are commonly detected in Little League pitchers and catchers, although the individuals may or may not complain of pain.[53] Medial epicondylalgia may cause neuropathy of the ulnar nerve, causing symptoms to radiate into the medial forearm and fingers.[54]

Medial Epicondylalgia Intervention Strategies

The treatment of patients with medial epicondylalgia follows the interventions described for those with lateral epicondylalgia.

Distal Biceps Tendon Rupture

Biceps tendon ruptures are most common in males older than age 40.[4,24,55] The incidence of rupture is 7.5 times greater in patients who smoke than in those with no history of smoking.[55] The tendon and its aponeurosis degrades with time, ultimately resulting in a spontaneous rupture of the tendon, often occurring in the hypovascular zone between the proximal and distal blood supply.[4] Most biceps tendon ruptures involve the avulsion of the bicipital (radial) tuberosity, a diagnosis made using radiographs, magnetic resonance imaging (MRI), or computed tomography (CT) scans.

The mechanism of injury involves the eccentric loading of the biceps brachii when the elbow is flexed to

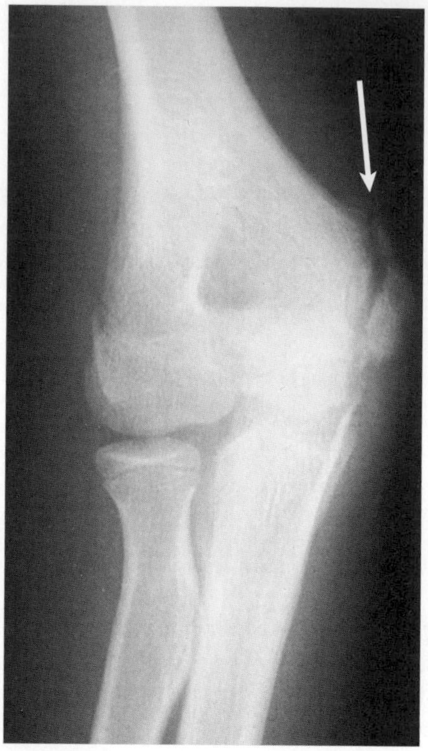

FIGURE 16-22 ■ Avulsion of the origin of the wrist flexor muscles, "Little Leaguer's elbow." This condition can mimic medial epicondylalgia.

90 degrees.[4,56,57] Ruptures are classified as being complete or partial. Clinically, the distal tendon is still palpable along its length when it is partially ruptured.

*** Practical Evidence**

The biceps squeeze test, similar to the Thompson test for the Achilles tendon, may be used to assess for a distal biceps tendon rupture and has a high sensitivity. With the patient's elbow flexed to 60 to 80 degrees, squeeze the biceps and observe for forearm supination.[58]

Rupture of the distal biceps tendon is debilitating because of the loss of strength during elbow flexion and supination. The patient reports immediate pain and the sensation of a "pop" within the elbow. A loss of arm strength during elbow flexion and forearm supination is also apparent. Inspection of the cubital fossa reveals swelling and ecchymosis. A palpable defect in the distal biceps tendon may also be noted. Active and passive ROM may remain within normal limits, but a definitive decrease in strength during Manual Muscle Test for elbow flexion and supination is present (Examination Findings 16-6). Clinically, in addition to observing the rupture, distal biceps tendon ruptures can be identified using the **hook test** (Selective Tissue Test 16-4).[59]

Distal Biceps Tendon Rupture Intervention Strategies

Although biceps tendon ruptures may be managed conservatively, surgical repair is the preferred method of treatment for both complete and partial ruptures.[4,50,60,61] Postsurgical rehabilitation consists of a progressive return of elbow extension combined with passive elbow flexion with minimal immobilization. Full ROM is expected after 8 weeks, after which strengthening exercises are integrated.[58]

Nerve Pathology

The peripheral nerves emanating from the brachial plexus can be compromised by chronic entrapment, repetitive tension, or trauma. Anatomical structures including the **arcade of Struthers**, intramuscular fascia, tunnels beneath ligaments, and bony tracts through which the nerve passes are common sites for entrapment.[62] Postinjury fibrosis or postsurgical scarring can also compress the nerve. Abnormal tension resulting from instability, such as when the ulnar nerve is stretched secondary to medial elbow laxity, can result in nerve symptoms. Acute trauma can directly damage the nerves. With humeral fractures, the radial nerve is damaged around 12% of the time.[63]

The anatomic tunnels through which the ulnar, radial, and median nerves pass can result in entrapment symptoms. Inhibition of these nerves in the area of the elbow causes the symptoms to radiate distally, resulting in dysfunction in the wrist, hand, and fingers. This dysfunction is characterized by paresthesia, decreased grip strength, and the inability to actively extend the wrist, depending on the nerve involved (Examination Findings 16-7). Figure 16-23 presents the sensory distribution of these nerves in the hand.

Examination of a patient with unexplained neurological symptoms in the elbow, forearm, wrist, and/or hand should include a thorough examination of the cervical region.

Ulnar Nerve Pathology

Cubital tunnel syndrome describes a collection of ulnar-nerve symptoms that may result from ulnar-nerve instability, direct blow, prolonged leaning on the elbow, or repetitive elbow flexion.[64] The superficial nature of the ulnar nerve makes it susceptible to contusing forces and also to

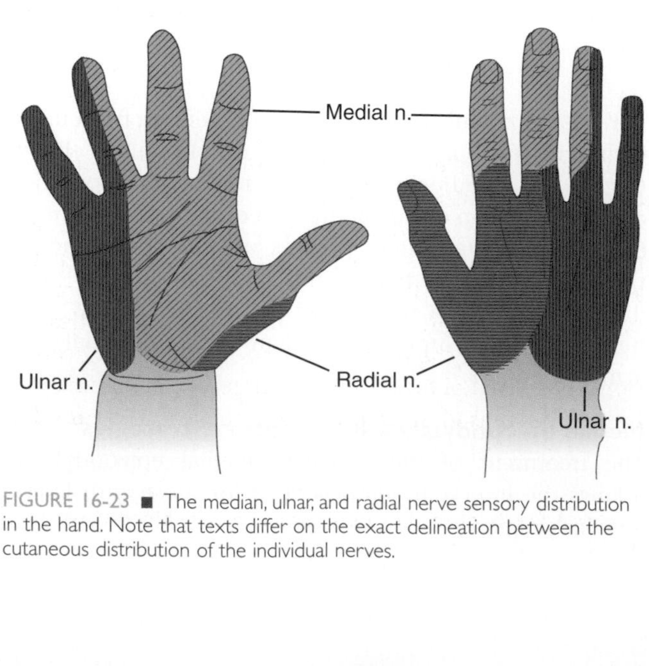

FIGURE 16-23 ■ The median, ulnar, and radial nerve sensory distribution in the hand. Note that texts differ on the exact delineation between the cutaneous distribution of the individual nerves.

Examination Findings 16-6
Distal Biceps Tendon Rupture

Examination Segment	Clinical Findings
History of Current Condition	*Onset:* Acute *Pain characteristics:* Pain in the cubital fossa that decreases over time *Mechanism:* Eccentric loading of the biceps brachii while the elbow is flexed *Predisposing conditions:* More commonly seen after the third decade of life as the tensile strength of the tendon decreases A history of cigarette smoking Anabolic steroid use **Statin** use[56]
Functional Assessment	Patient will describe or demonstrate weakness in activities that require lifting.
Inspection	Swelling and ecchymosis in the cubital fossa
Palpation	Palpable defect in the distal biceps tendon that may be obscured by swelling; the lesion may be more easily recognized if the patient attempts to hold the elbow in 90° of flexion. The defect is more difficult to detect when the aponeurosis is intact than when it is ruptured along with the tendon.
Joint and Muscle Function Assessment	*AROM:* Possibly within normal limits or slightly decreased during elbow flexion and extension and forearm pronation and supination secondary to pain *MMT:* Decreased strength for elbow flexors and forearm supinators *PROM:* Within normal limits; a partial tearing of the tendon may produce pain at the end-range of elbow extension and pronation as the remaining fibers are stretched.
Joint Stability Tests	*Stress tests:* Unremarkable *Joint play:* Unremarkable
Selective Tissue Tests	Hook test
Neurological Screening	Radial neuropathy may arise secondary to the trauma or the surgical technique.
Vascular Screening	Within normal limits
Imaging Techniques	Radiographs, MRI, or CT scans are obtained to determine if an avulsion of the radial tuberosity has occurred and to rule out concomitant fractures.
Differential Diagnosis	Biceps tendon tear, avulsion fraction of the radial tuberosity
Comments	The long head of the biceps tendon may rupture in the shoulder.

AROM = active range of motion; CT = computed tomography; MMT = manual muscle test; MRI = magnetic resonance imaging; PROM = passive range of motion

subluxation, while the traction forces associated with throwing also make it vulnerable to pathology.

Pathology of the ulnar nerve manifests its symptoms through decreased sensory and motor function in the hand and fingers. Patients will complain of increased symptoms at night and with prolonged elbow flexion. Acute trauma of the ulnar nerve causes a burning sensation in the medial forearm, little finger, and ring finger as well as decreased strength of the finger flexor muscles, lumbricals, interossei, thumb abductors, and flexor carpi ulnaris. Numbness on the dorsal aspect of the hand is indicative of ulnar neuropathy in the area of the elbow. Numbness on only the palmar side of the ulnar nerve distribution is indicative of ulnar nerve compression distal to the tunnel of Guyon where the nerve diverges into palmar and dorsal branches.[62]

Chronic neurological deficit to these muscles causes the hand to deviate radially during flexion and results in the inability to maintain adduction of the little finger, leaving it resting in an abducted position (**Wartenberg's sign**).[55] This deficit also inhibits the individual's ability to make a fist because of a lack of flexion in the fourth and fifth distal

Statin: A family of medications used to reduce blood cholesterol levels.

Selective Tissue Test 16-4
Hook Test for Distal Biceps Tendon Rupture

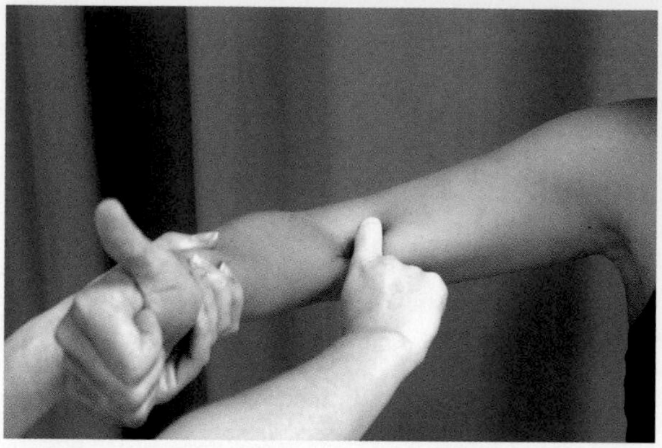

The hook test attempts to snag the distal biceps tendon. If the tendon cannot be "hooked," it is indicative of a distal rupture.

Patient Position	Sitting or standing The shoulder is abducted to 90°, and the elbow is flexed to 90°.
Position of Examiner	Standing beside the patient
Evaluative Procedure	The examiner resists forearm supination while attempting to hook the distal biceps tendon with a finger.
Positive Test	The inability to catch the distal biceps tendon with the finger
Implications	Rupture of the distal biceps tendon
Comments	In uninjured individuals, the distal biceps tendon can be identified as a cordlike structure crossing the center of the cubital fossa.

Evidence

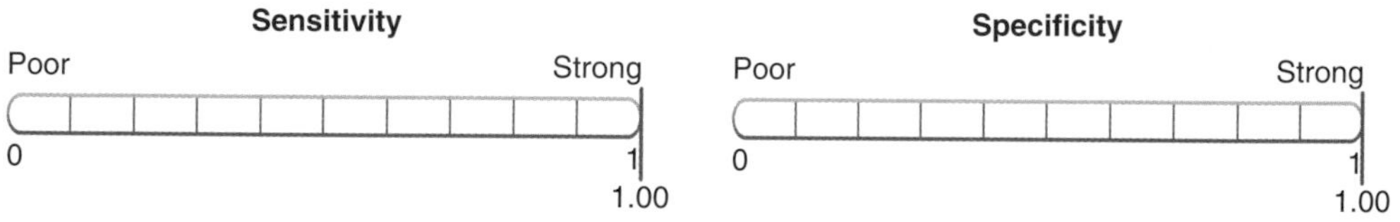

LR−: 0.00

Examination Findings 16-7
Nerve Pathology at the Elbow

Examination Segment	Clinical Findings
History of Current Condition	*Onset:* Insidious *Pain characteristics:* **Ulnar nerve:** Medial aspect of the elbow and forearm **Radial nerve:** Proximal dorsal forearm, wrist extensor region **Median nerve:** Anterior (ventral) forearm *Other symptoms:* Numbness or paresthesia radiating into the nerve patterns (see Fig. 16-23): **Ulnar nerve:** Medial forearm, little finger, and medial one-half of ring finger **Radial nerve:** Lateral first metacarpal, dorsal lateral hand, distal forearm **Median nerve:** Ventral lateral hand (thumb to lateral one-half of ring finger), ventral lateral forearm Symptoms may radiate from the elbow into the shoulder and cervical spine. *Mechanism:* Compression, traction, or inflammation of the nerve *Predisposing conditions:* Arthritis of the epicondylar groove or osteophytes can result in insidious nerve irritation. Diabetes Circulatory impairments Fractures
Functional Assessment	The function of the elbow, wrist, and hand may deteriorate with time.
Inspection	Swelling may be associated with concomitant injury.
Palpation	Pain or paresthesia may be elicited when palpating around the course of the nerve.
Joint and Muscle Function Assessment	*AROM:* May be limited following prolonged symptoms *MMT:* Weakness in the muscles serviced by the involved nerve *PROM:* Increased symptoms when nerve is maximally tensioned
Joint Stability Tests	*Stress tests:* As needed to rule out underlying instability placing additional tension on nerve *Joint play:* As needed to rule out underlying instability placing additional tension on nerve
Selective Tissue Tests	Tinel's sign
Neurological Screening	Complete upper quarter screen is warranted to assess for cervical involvement. Electrodiagnostic studies may be required to definitively diagnose the condition.
Vascular Screening	Within normal limits
Imaging Techniques	AP, oblique, and lateral views are used to identify neuropathy caused by bony defects.
Differential Diagnosis	Cervical radiculopathy, lateral epicondylalgia, carpal tunnel syndrome, complex regional pain syndrome
Comments	A nerve can be compressed at multiple points along its path.

AP = anteroposterior; AROM = active range of motion; MMT = manual muscle test; PROM = passive range of motion interphalangeal (DIP) joints, characterized by a **clawhand** position (see Chapter 17).

Radial Nerve Pathology

The radial nerve is often injured by deep lacerations of the elbow or secondary to fractures of the humerus or radius. The posterior interosseous nerve, the deep branch of the radial nerve, is dedicated to motor function of the thumb's extensors, wrist extensors, finger extensors, and supinators. Thus, there is no sensory loss associated with trauma to this nerve segment. If the superficial branch is lacerated or entrapped, sensory loss or paresthesia results on the posterior forearm and hand. Inflammation or irritation of the ulnar and radial nerves as they cross the elbow joint can be detected through Tinel's sign (Fig. 16-24).

Entrapment of the radial nerve, **radial tunnel syndrome** (RTS), also known as supinator syndrome, clinically resembles lateral epicondylalgia.[65] RTS differs from epicondylalgia in that its symptoms are located more distally on the forearm. RTS can persist for more than 6 months with tenderness over the radial tunnel. Compression of the radial nerve distal to the elbow usually results in weak finger extension but normal wrist extension strength. Activities requiring repetitive supination and elbow extension are often associated with the onset of RTS.

Median Nerve Pathology

The median nerve is typically injured or compressed on the distal portion of the forearm. However, pressure in the cubital fossa may compress the nerve as it crosses the joint line. The most common clinical manifestation of median nerve involvement, **carpal tunnel syndrome**, is discussed in Chapter 17. A branch of the median nerve, the anterior interosseous nerve, can become compressed by the pronator teres, causing **pronator teres syndrome**.[2] This syndrome is characterized by the patient's inability to pinch the tips of the thumb and index fingers together.

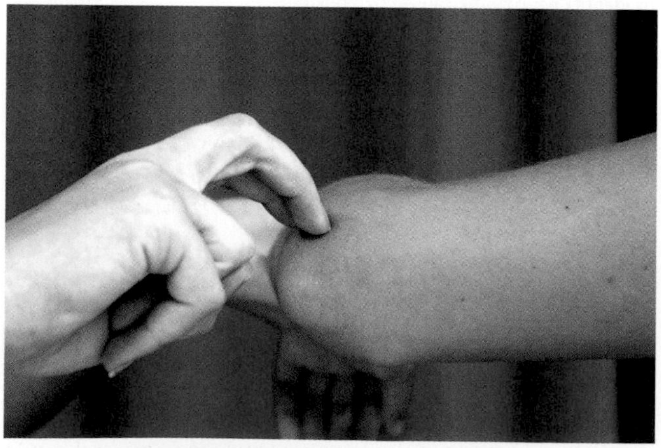

FIGURE 16-24 ■ Tinel's sign for neuropathy. In the presence of neuropathy, tapping on the ulnar (shown) or radial nerve results in a burning sensation in the hand. This test is associated with a high rate of false positives.

*** Practical Evidence**

The median nerve may be compressed by the interosseous membrane, producing only motor deficits of the flexor digitorum profundus, flexor pollicis longus, and pronator quadratus.[2]

Nerve Pathology Intervention Strategies

Nerve entrapment syndromes are managed by identifying and alleviating the underlying cause of the compression or tension. Although surgical intervention is often needed, in many cases the entrapment can be reduced via stretching and soft tissue mobilization.

Forearm Compartment Syndrome

The forearm contains three identifiable compartments: the volar, dorsal, and carpal tunnel.[66] Increased pressure within these compartments, possibly the result of hypertrophic muscles, hemorrhage, or fractures of the midforearm, distal radius, or supracondylar area, increases the risk for compromising circulation and neurological function of the hand.[67] As in the lower leg, forearm compartment syndromes can be acute or exertional; exertional syndromes subside with cessation of the offending activity.

In its early stages, forearm compartment syndrome is marked most often by swelling. Pain and neurological symptoms may or may not be present. Motor involvement, while rare, is associated with a worse outcome following surgery.[66] Untreated compartment syndromes may result in the development of **Volkmann's ischemic contracture** (see Chapter 17). Because signs and symptoms are unreliable, referral for pressure readings are warranted if a compartment syndrome is suspected.[66]

Forearm Compartment Syndrome Intervention Strategies

Fasciotomy surgery is often required to relieve the increased intracompartmental pressure. Associated with a high rate of complications, fasciotomies should be performed within 6 to 12 hours to optimize the outcome.[66]

On-Field Examination of Elbow and Forearm Injuries

In most instances, acute injuries of the elbow do not require an on-field evaluation and subsequent management of the condition. The exceptions to this are elbow dislocations and fractures of the forearm or humerus. In many of these cases, the athlete remains down on the playing surface.

Clawhand Positioning characterized by hyperextension of the metacarpophalangeal joints and flexion of the middle and distal phalanges resulting from trauma to the median and ulnar nerves

On-Field History

After the possibility of a fracture or dislocation has been ruled out, the circumstances surrounding the injury must be established:

- **Position of the arm:** When the hand is supporting the body weight, the arm is in a closed kinetic chain. Blows to the forearm, elbow, or humerus must be absorbed by the elbow's supportive structures, increasing the suspicion of acute ligamentous injuries.
- **Type of force involved:** The nature of the force delivered to the elbow must be determined. Landing on the palm of the hand delivers a longitudinal force up the radius that is transferred to the ulna by the interosseous membrane. A force to the lateral side of the elbow places stress on the UCL, and a medial force stresses the RCL. A force from the posterior aspect of the elbow results in hyperextension of the joint and places shear forces on the olecranon process. A blunt force places compressive forces on the tissues beneath the location of the impact.

On-Field Inspection

The primary tool in the evaluation of these conditions is inspection of the injured area. Elbow dislocation and forearm or humeral fractures tend to result in gross deformity, but displaced radial and ulnar fractures are also apparent.

- **Alignment of forearm and wrist:** Observe the length of the radius and ulna for gross deformity and note the relationship between the forearm and wrist. A complete fracture of either of the long bones may alter the wrist's position relative to the forearm.
- **Posterior triangle of the elbow:** Note the alignment of the medial epicondyle, lateral epicondyle, and the olecranon process. These structures should form an isosceles triangle when the elbow is flexed to 90 degrees. Any deviation of this relationship may indicate a dislocation. In the event of a posterior dislocation, the olecranon process becomes overly prominent. If either condition exists, the evaluation must be terminated immediately, and the athlete must be referred to a physician after appropriate immobilization.

On-Field Palpation

Palpation is performed to confirm the suspicion of injury established during the history-taking process while also ruling out any other gross trauma.

- **Alignment of the elbow:** Palpate the medial epicondyle, lateral epicondyle, and olecranon for tenderness, crepitus, and improper alignment.
- **Collateral ligaments:** Palpate the RCL and UCL along their lengths to identify any pain or crepitus along these structures. Crepitus at the ligament's origin or insertion may indicate an avulsion.
- **Radius and ulna:** Palpate the length of the radius and ulna for tenderness, deformity, or false joints indicative of a fracture.

On-Field Joint and Muscle Function Tests

Before deciding whether to splint the arm, the athletic trainer must establish the athlete's willingness and ability to move the elbow:

- **Active range of motion:** Ask the athlete to wiggle the fingers, move the wrist through flexion and extension and radial and ulnar deviation, and then through forearm pronation and supination and elbow flexion and extension. The inability to perform any one of these steps or significant pain with these motions warrants the immobilization of the elbow, forearm, and wrist before the athlete is removed from the field. If the patient can fully extend the elbow, it is unlikely that an elbow fracture is present.[68]
- **Manual muscle tests:** Although this portion of the examination can be delayed until the athlete is removed to the sideline, establish a baseline of strength for future comparison. Nerve root compression may result in a short-term loss of strength that rapidly returns to normal.
- **Passive range of motion:** After the athlete has displayed the ability to actively and willingly move the elbow, passively move the joint through its ROMs. Osteochondral fractures cause a premature endpoint in the ROM. Fractures of the olecranon process cause pain at the terminal range of extension.

On-Field Neurological Tests

The immediate evaluation of elbow injuries may necessitate the neurological assessment of the forearm and hand. Refer to the section of this chapter on neurological testing and see Figure 16-22.

On-Field Management of Elbow and Forearm Injuries

The most significant elbow injuries facing athletic trainers during the on-field evaluation are dislocations of the elbow joint and fractures of the forearm. These conditions require careful management to prevent further trauma to the involved structures and protect the neurovascular network supplying the hand.

Elbow Dislocations

Reduction of elbow dislocations can be performed either on the field or in the emergency room by trained personnel. If reduction is going to occur in the emergency room, the elbow is immobilized in the position in which it is found, while still allowing the distal pulse to be monitored. Concomitant injury to the glenohumeral joint, proximal humerus, and wrist must be ruled out. The athlete must be immediately transported for further medical treatment by a physician.

Fractures About the Elbow

Fractures of the radius and ulna may compromise the neurovascular supply to the wrist and hand. Because of this, distal pulses must be monitored constantly after the injury. The elbow, forearm, and wrist must be immobilized to minimize movement of the fractured bones. After the area has been stabilized, the athlete must be immediately transported and monitored for shock.

REFERENCES

1. Smith, AM, et al: Radius pull test: predictor of longitudinal forearm instability. *J Bone Joint Surg*, 84(A):1970, 2002.
2. Hsu, SH, et al: Physical examination of the athlete's elbow. *Am J Sports Med*, 40:699, 2012.
3. Chen, FS, Rokito, AS, and Jobe, FW: Medial elbow problems in the overhead-throwing athlete. *J Am Acad Orthop Surg*, 9:99, 2001.
4. Ramsey, ML: Distal biceps tendon injuries: diagnosis and management. *J Am Acad Orthop Surg*, 7:199, 1999.
5. McClung, MR: Do current management strategies and guidelines adequately address fracture risk? *Bone*, 38:S13, 2006.
6. Hak, DJ, and Golladay, GJ: Olecranon fractures: treatment options. *J Am Acad Orthop Surg*, 8:266, 2000.
7. Fleisig, GS, et al: Risk of serious injury for young baseball pitchers: a 10-year prospective study. *Am J Sports Med*, 39:253, 2011.
8. Hatch, GF, et al: The effect of tennis racket grip size on forearm muscle firing patterns. *Am J Sports Med*, 34:1997, 2006.
9. Cain, EL, et al: Elbow injuries in throwing athletes: a current concepts review. *Am J Sports Med*, 31:621, 2003.
10. Brabston, EW, Genuario, JW, and Bell, J: Anatomy and physical examination of the elbow. *Oper Tech Orthop*, 19:190, 2009.
11. Goldfarb, CA, et al: Elbow radiographic anatomy: measurement techniques and normative data. *J Shoulder Elbow Surg*, 21:1236, 2012.
12. O'Driscoll, SW, et al: Tardy posterolateral rotatory instability of the elbow due to cubitus varus. *J Bone Joint Surg*, 83:1358, 2001.
13. Andrews, JR, et al: Physical examination of the thrower's elbow. *J Orthop Sports Phys Ther*, 17:269, 1993.
14. Ekstrom, RA, Holden, R: Examination of and intervention for a patient with chronic lateral elbow pain with signs of nerve entrapment. *Phys Ther*, 82:1077, 2002.
15. Wright, RW, et al: Elbow range of motion in professional baseball pitchers. *Am J Sports Med*, 34:190, 2006.
16. Chapleau, J, et al: Validity of goniometric elbow measurements: comparative study with a radiographic method. *Clin Orthop Relat Res*, 469:3134, 2011.
17. Gajdosik, RL: Comparison and reliability of three goniometric methods for measuring forearm supination and pronation. *Percept Mot Skills*, 93:353, 2001.
18. Karagiannopoulos, C, Sitler, M, and Michlovitz, S: Reliability of two functional goniometric methods for measuring forearm pronation and supination active range of motion. *J Orthop Sports Phys Ther*, 33:523, 2003.
19. Rainville, J, et al: Assessment of forearm pronation strength in C6 and C7 radiculopathies. *Spine*, 32:72, 2007.
20. Hariri, S, and Safran, MR: Ulnar collateral ligament injury in the overhead athlete. *Clin Sports Med*, 29:619, 2010.
21. McCabe, MP, and Savoie, FH: Simple elbow dislocations: evaluation, management, and outcomes. *Phys Sportsmed*, 40:62, 2012.
22. Cohen, MS, and Hastings, H: Acute elbow dislocation: evaluation and management. *J Am Acad Orthop Surg*, 6:15, 1998.
23. Ring, D, Jupiter, JB, and Zilberfarb, J: Posterior dislocation of the elbow with fractures of the radial head and coronoid. *J Bone Joint Surg*, 84(A):547, 2002.
24. Lin, K-Y, et al: Functional outcomes of surgical reconstruction for posterolateral rotatory instability of the elbow. *Injury*, 43:1657, 2012.
25. Carter, SJ, et al: Orthopedic pitfalls in the ED: neurovascular injury associated with posterior elbow dislocations. *Am J Emerg Med*, 28:960, 2010.
26. Allen, SR, Hang, JR, and Hau, RC: Review article: paediatric supracondylar humeral fractures: emergency assessment and management. *Emerg Med Australas*, 22:418, 2010.
27. Arnander, MWT, and Newman, KJH: Forearm fractures. *Surgery*, 24:426, 2006.
28. Zlotolow, DA: Pediatric forearm fractures: spotting and managing the bad actors. *JHS*, 37A:363, 2012.
29. Jones, DB, and Kakar, S: Adult diaphyseal forearm fractures: intramedullary nail versus plate fixation. *J Hand Surg Am*, 36:1216, 2011.
30. Hume, PA, Reid, D, and Edwards, T: Epicondylar injury in sport: epidemiology, type, mechanisms, assessment, management, and prevention. *Sports Med*, 36:151, 2006.
31. Timmerman, LA, Schwartz, ML, and Andrews, JR: Preoperative evaluation of the ulnar collateral ligament by magnetic resonance imaging and computed tomography arthrography: evaluation in 25 baseball players with surgical confirmation. *Am J Sports Med*, 22:26, 1994.
32. O'Driscoll, SWM, Lawton, RL, and Smith, AM: The "moving valgus stress test" for medial collateral ligament tears of the elbow. *Am J Sports Med*, 33:231, 2005.
33. Smidt, N, et al: Corticosteroid injections, physiotherapy, or a wait-and-see policy for lateral epicondylitis: a randomised controlled trial. *Lancet*, 359:657, 2002.
34. Chen, AL, et al: Imaging of the elbow in the overhead throwing athlete. *Am J Sports Med*, 31:466, 2003.
35. Dugas, J: Valgus extension overload: diagnosis and treatment. *Clin Sports Med*, 29:645, 2010.
36. Dunning, CE, et al: Ligamentous stabilizers against posterolateral rotatory instability of the elbow. *J Bone Joint Surg*, 83(A):1823, 2001.
37. Bisset, L, et al: Mobilisation with movement and exercise, corticosteroid injection, or wait and see for tennis elbow: randomized trial. *BMJ*, 333:939, 2006.
38. Takahara, M, et al: Early detection of osteochondritis dissecans of the capitellum in young baseball players: report of three cases. *J Bone Joint Surg*, 80(A):892, 1998.
39. Lieber, RL, Ljung, BO, and Friden, J: Sarcomere length in wrist extensor muscles: changes may provide insights into the etiology of chronic lateral epicondylitis. *Acta Orthop Scand*, 68:249, 1997.
40. Smidt, N, et al: Interobserver reproducibility of the assessment of severity of complaints, grip strength, and pressure pain thresholds in patients with lateral epicondylitis. *Arch Phys Med Rehabil*, 83:1145, 2002.
41. Bhargava, AS, Eapen, C, and Kumar, SP: Grip strength measurements at two different wrist extension positions in chronic lateral epicondylitis: comparison of involved vs. uninvolved side in athletes and nonathletes: a case-control study. *Sports Med Arthrosc Rehabil Ther Technol*, 2:22, 2010.
42. Titchener, AG, et al: Risk factors in lateral epicondylitis (tennis elbow): a case-control study. *J Hand Surg Eur Vol*, 38:159, 2013..
43. Behrens, SB, et al: A review of modern management of lateral epicondylitis. *Phys Sportsmed*, 40:34, 2012.
44. Waugh, EJ, Jaglal, SB, and Davis, AM: Computer use associated with poor long-term prognosis of conservatively managed lateral epicondylalgia. *J Orthop Sports Phys Ther*, 34:770, 2004.

45. Walker-Bone, K, et al: Occupation and epicondylitis: a population-based study. *Rheumatology*, 51:305, 2012.
46. Pienimä, TT, Siira, PT, and Vanharanta, H: Chronic medial and lateral epicondylitis: a comparison of pain, disability, and function. *Arch Phys Med Rehabil*, 83:317, 2002.
47. Coombes, BK, Bisset, L, Vicenzio, B: Elbow flexor and extensor muscle weakness in lateral epicondylalgia. *Br J Sports Med*, 46:449, 2012.
48. Wilson, JJ, and Best, TM: Common overuse tendon problems: a review and recommendations for treatment. *Am Fam Physician*, 72:811, 2005.
49. Garg, R, et al: A prospective randomized study comparing a forearm strap brace versus a wrist splint for the treatment of lateral epicondylitis. *J Shoulder Elbow Surg*, 19:508, 2010.
50. Jafarian, FS, Demneh, ES, and Tyson, SF: The immediate effect of orthotic management on grip strength of patients with lateral epicondylosis. *J Orthop Sports Phys Ther*, 39:484, 2009.
51. Ng, GY, and Chan, HL: The immediate effects of tension counterforce forearm brace on neuromuscular performance of wrist extensor muscles in subjects with lateral humeral epicondylosis. *J Orthop Sports Phys Ther*, 34:72, 2004.
52. Rosenberg, N, Soudry, M, and Stahl, S: Comparison of two methods for the evaluation of treatment in medial epicondylitis: pain estimation vs grip strength measurements. *Arch Orthop Trauma Surg*, 124:363, 2004.
53. Hang, DW, Chao, CM, and Hang, Y-S: A clinical and roentgenographic study of Little League elbow. *Am J Sports Med*, 32:79, 2004.
54. Gong, HS, et al: Musculofascial lengthening for the treatment of patients with medial epicondylitis and coexistent ulnar neuropathy. *J Bone Joint Surg*, 92(B):823, 2010.
55. Safran, MR, Graham, SM: Distal biceps tendon ruptures: incidence, demographics, and the effect of smoking. *Clin Orthop Relat Res*, 404:275, 2002.
56. Sawidou, C, and Moreno, R: Spontaneous distal biceps tendon ruptures: are they related to statin administration? *Hand Surg*, 17:167, 2012.
57. D'Arco, P, et al: Clinical, functional, and radiographic assessments of the conventional and modified Boyd-Anderson surgical procedures for repair of distal biceps tendon ruptures. *Am J Sports Med*, 26:254, 1998.
58. Rineer, CA, Ruch, DS: Elbow tendinopathy and tendon ruptures: epicondylitis, biceps and triceps ruptures. *J Hand Surg*, 34A:566, 2009.
59. O'Driscoll, SW, Goncalves, LBJ, and Dietz, P: The hook test for distal biceps tendon avulsion. *Am J Sports Med*, 35:1865, 2007.
60. Grewal, R, et al: Single versus double-incision technique for the repair of acute distal biceps tendon ruptures: a randomized clinical trial. *J Bone Joint Surg*, 94(A):1166, 2012.
61. Bosman, HA, Fincher, M, and Saw, N: Anatomic direct repair of chronic distal biceps brachii tendon rupture without interposition graft. *J Shoulder Elbow Surg*, 21:1342, 2012.
62. Posner, MA: Compressive ulnar neuropathies at the elbow: I. etiology and diagnosis. *J Am Acad Orthop Surg*, 6:282, 1998.
63. Shao, YC, et al: Radial nerve palsy associated with fractures of the shaft of the humerus. *J Bone Jt Surg (Br.)*, 87-B:1647, 2005.
64. Hutchison, RL, and Rayan, G: Diagnosis of cubital tunnel syndrome. *J Hand Surg Am*, 36: 1519, 2011.
65. Stanley, J: Radial tunnel syndrome: a surgeon's perspective. *J Hand Ther*, 19:180, 2006.
66. Duckworth, AD, et al.: Acute compartment syndrome of the forearm. *J Bone Joint Surg Am*, 94:e63(1), 2012.
67. Kalyani, BS, et al: Compartment syndrome in the forearm: a systematic review. *J Hand Surg*, 36A:535, 2011.
68. Docherty, MA, Schwab, RA, and Ma, OJ: Can elbow extension be used as a test of clinically significant injury? *South Med J*, 95:539, 2002.

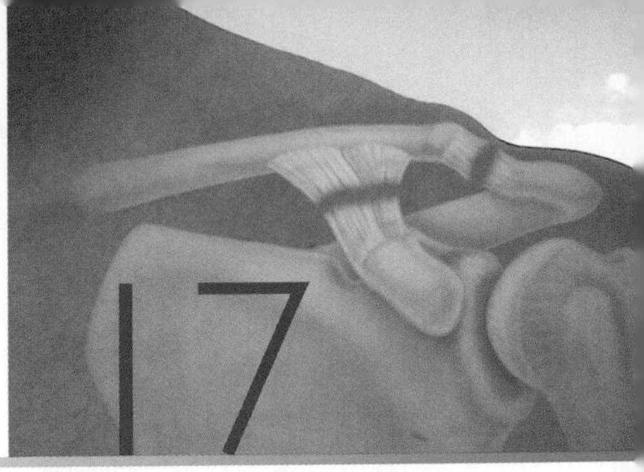

CHAPTER 17

Wrist, Hand, and Finger Pathologies

The shoulder is equipped for mobility and gross placement of the arm in space. The elbow is equipped for stability. The wrist, hand, and fingers, the final links in the chain, are perfectly equipped for strength and precision. Injury to this area includes impairment of gross and fine motor movements. The extent of an individual's participation restrictions after injury to these areas depends on the nature of necessary tasks and whether or not the dominant extremity is involved. In football, a hand injury that has little consequence to a lineman could be disabling to a quarterback or wide receiver.

Clinical Anatomy

The distal portions of the radius and ulna, eight carpal bones, five metacarpals, and 14 phalanges, form the skeleton of the wrist, hand, and fingers (Fig. 17-1). The **distal radius** broadens to form a small **ulnar notch** on its medial surface to accept the ulnar head, and the **radial styloid process** projects off its anterolateral border. The **ulnar head** is more circular, with the **ulnar styloid process** arising from its medial surface.

Having unusual shapes and irregular surfaces, the **carpal bones** are aligned in two rows (Fig. 17-2). From the radial to ulnar sides, the proximal row consists of the scaphoid, lunate, triquetrum, and pisiform bones. The distal row is formed by the trapezium, trapezoid, capitate, and hamate bones. In the distal carpal row, the trapezium articulates with the first **metacarpal**, the trapezoid with the second metacarpal, the capitate with the third metacarpal, and the fourth and fifth metacarpals with the hamate. The pisiform "floats" on the triquetrum, acting as a sesamoid bone to improve the mechanical efficiency of the flexor carpi ulnaris muscle. The scaphoid is the most commonly fractured of the carpals, and the lunate is the most commonly dislocated.

Much of the length of the hand is formed by the metacarpals, numbered from I (thumb) to V (little finger). Shaped similarly to long bones, the proximal articulating surfaces are concave to accept the convex surface of the carpals. The distal surfaces are convex to accept the concave surface of the proximal phalanx of each of the fingers. Each finger (except the thumb, which has only a proximal and distal phalanx) has a **proximal**, **middle**, and **distal** phalanx. The proximal aspect of these bones is referred to as the base, and the distal aspect is referred to as the head.

Two small sesamoid bones are located over the palmar aspect of the distal end of the first metacarpal (see Fig. 17-2). These mobile bones change the mechanical line of pull of the flexor pollicis brevis, abductor pollicis brevis, and adductor pollicis muscles to improve thumb function.

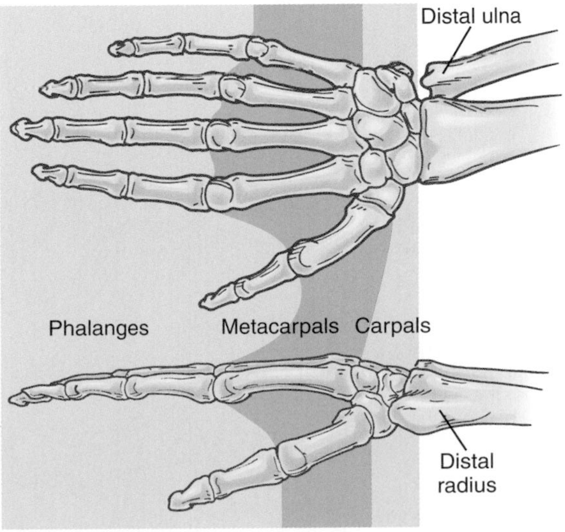

FIGURE 17-1 ■ Bones of the wrist and hand, formed by the radius and ulna, 8 carpals, 5 metacarpals, and 14 phalanges.

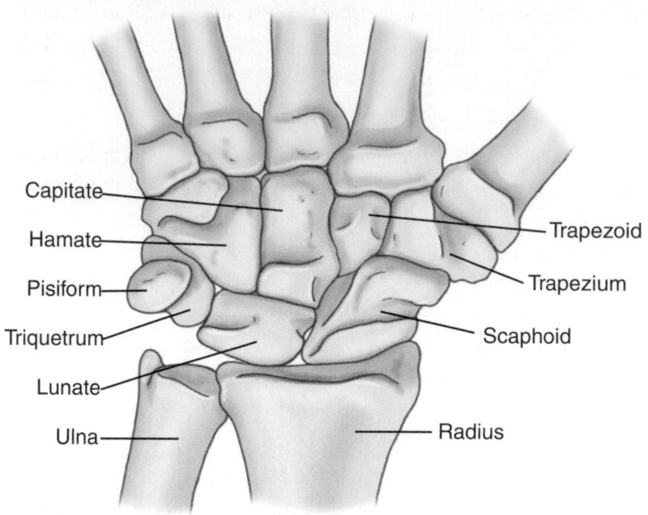

FIGURE 17-2 ■ Carpal bones of the hand (palmar view).

Articulations and Ligamentous Support

The motion produced by the wrist, hand, and fingers occurs through the interaction of multiple joints. Several force couples among each joint's associated muscles facilitate the precise coordination needed at the wrist and hand. An overview of the interactions involving specific joints is described in this section.

Distal Radioulnar Joint

The distal radioulnar articulation, formed by the ulnar head and the ulnar notch of the radius, allows 1 degree of freedom of movement: pronation and supination. The distal and proximal radioulnar joints work together to produce those motions. Restriction of motion at either of these joints limits pronation and supination of the entire forearm. At the distal radioulnar joint, pronation and supination are produced by the radius' gliding around the ulna.

Radiocarpal Joint

The radiocarpal articulation is an ellipsoid joint that provides 2 degrees of freedom of movement: flexion and extension and radial and **ulnar deviation**. The joint is formed by the distal end of the radius' articulation with the scaphoid and lunate. Through its connection to the distal radius, the triangular fibrocartilage functionally extends this joint to incorporate the triquetrum.

The joint is covered by a fibrous capsule reinforced by ligamentous thickenings (Fig. 17-3). The **radial collateral ligament** (RCL), originating off the styloid process and inserting on the scaphoid and trapezium, limits ulnar deviation and becomes taut when the wrist is at the extreme ranges of flexion and extension.

The **palmar radiocarpal ligament** originates from the anterior surface of the distal radius and courses obliquely and medially to split into three individual segments, each named for the bone to which it attaches: the **radiocapitate ligament**, **radiotriquetral ligament**, and **radioscaphoid ligament**.[1] As a unit, these ligaments maintain the alignment of the associated joint structures and limit hyperextension of the wrist.

The **dorsal radiocarpal ligament** is the only major ligament on the dorsal surface of the wrist (Fig. 17-4). Arising from the posterior surface of the distal radius and styloid process, this ligament attaches to the lunate and triquetrum to limit wrist flexion.

The ulna is buffered from the proximal row of carpals by the **triangular fibrocartilaginous complex (TFCC)**. The TFCC is composed of the articular disc (or central fibrocartilage), the dorsal and palmar distal radioulnar ligaments, the ulnolunate and ulnotriquetral ligaments, the subsheath surrounding the extensor carpi ulnaris tendon, and the meniscus homolog (meaning like a meniscus), which attaches the fibrocartilage to the triquetrum (Fig. 17-5).[2,3] The TFCC dissipates stresses imposed on the forearm during loading by extending the radiocarpal articulation, stabilizes

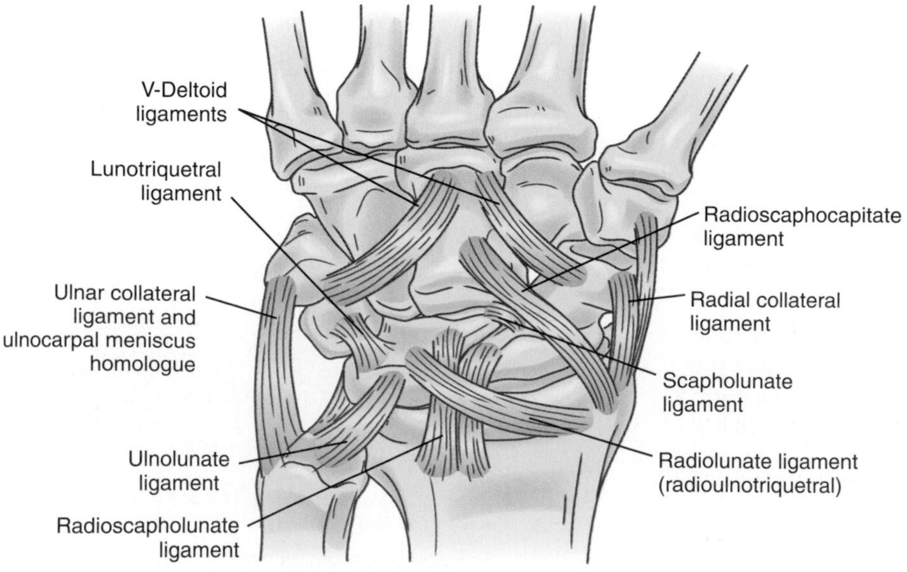

FIGURE 17-3 ■ Palmar (volar) ligaments of the left wrist and hand. Note the three bands of the palmar radiocarpal ligament: radioscaphocapitate, radiolunate, and radioscapholunate ligaments.

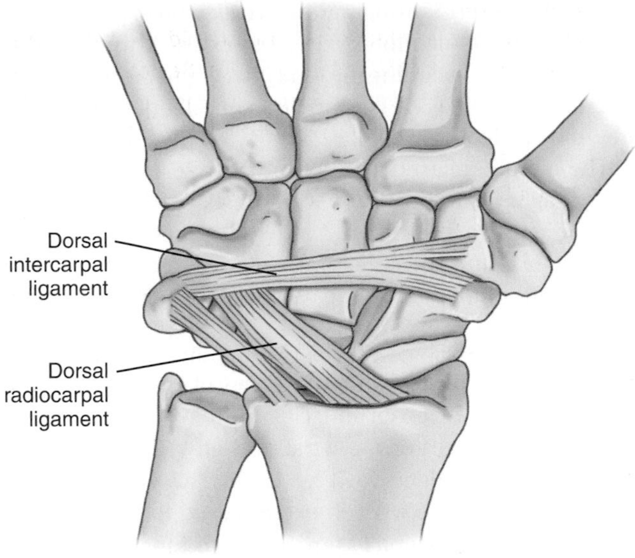

FIGURE 17-4 ■ Dorsal ligaments of the right wrist and hand. Note the horizontal "V" configuration of these ligaments that adds to radiocarpal stability.

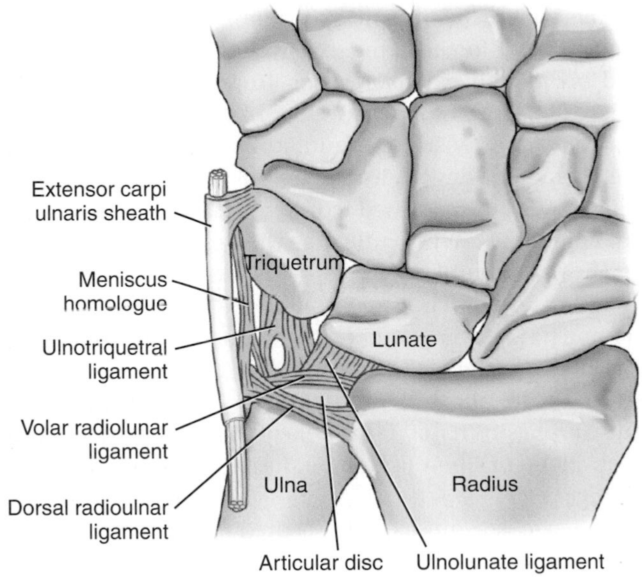

FIGURE 17-5 ■ The triangular fibrocartilage complex (TFCC). Several ligaments and other fibrous structures attach to the fibrocartilage. As a unit the TFCC provides support to the distal radioulnar joint. L = lunate; TQ = triquetrum. Courtesy of Norkin, CC, and Levangie, PK: *Joint Structure and Function: A Comprehensive Analysis*, ed 4. Philadelphia: FA Davis, 2005.

the distal radioulnar joint, and provides stability during pronation and supination.[2]

The **ulnar collateral ligament (UCL)** arises from the ulna's styloid process and attaches on the medial aspect of the triquetrum dorsally and on the pisiform palmarly. This ligament checks **radial deviation** and becomes taut at the end-ranges of flexion and extension. The small palmar ulnocarpal ligament originates from the distal ulna, blends in with the UCL, and attaches to the lunate and triquetrum.

Intercarpal Joints

Capsular and interosseous ligaments bind the carpal bones tightly together. Each carpal bone is fixated to its contiguous carpal in the same row by small palmar, dorsal, and **interosseous ligaments**. The capsular ligaments arise from the radius and insert on the individual carpals.[4] This ligamentous arrangement allows for very little gliding movement between the bones adjacent to one another within a row.

The interosseous C-shaped **scapholunate** and **lunotriquetral** ligaments span the dorsal and palmar aspects of the palmar edges of the scaphoid, lunate, and triquetrum (Fig. 17-6). The palmar segments of these ligaments are stronger than the dorsal. The relationship of the lunate between the scaphoid and the triquetrum results in the lunate exerting a flexion force through the scapholunate ligament and an extension force through the lunotriquetral ligament.[5] Disruption of one of these carpals and/or its associated ligament can result in profound dysfunction of the carpal group's biomechanics.

Midcarpal Joints

The proximal and distal carpal rows are separated by a single joint cavity with small fibrous ligamentous-type projections connecting the carpal rows. This structure allows limited gliding movements of flexion and extension and radial and ulnar deviation that are needed to obtain normal wrist flexion and extension.

Carpometacarpal Joints

Each of the first three metacarpals articulates primarily with a single carpal: metacarpal I with the trapezium and metacarpal III with the capitate. The broad base of the second metacarpal articulates primarily with the trapezoid but also has an articulation with the trapezium and capitate. The fourth and fifth metacarpals articulate with the hamate to form one of the **carpometacarpal (CMC) joints** (see Fig. 17-2).

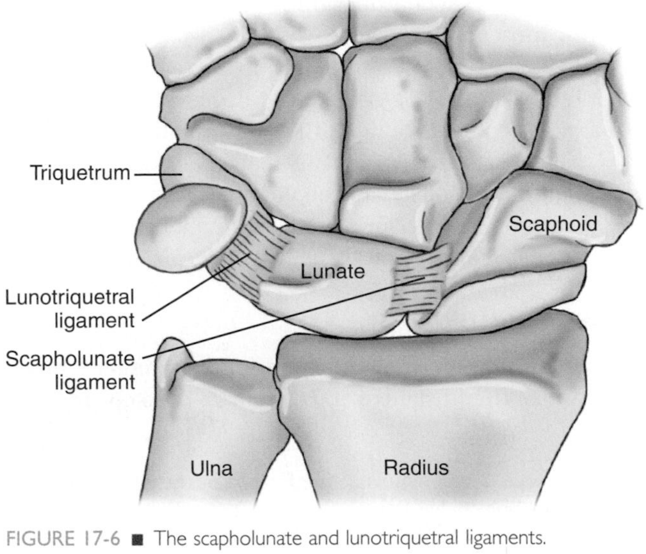

FIGURE 17-6 ■ The scapholunate and lunotriquetral ligaments.

Ulnar deviation Movement of the hand toward the ulnar side of the forearm

Dorsal The posterior aspect of the hand and forearm relative to the anatomical position

Radial deviation Movement of the hand toward the radial (thumb) side

The first CMC joint, that of the thumb, has a synovial cavity separate from the lateral four joints. Classified as a saddle joint, the first CMC joint is capable of 2 degrees of freedom of movement: flexion and extension and abduction and adduction. An accessory rotational component occurs concurrently with these motions, allowing for **opposition**, a combined movement that allows the thumb to touch each of the four fingers (the return motion from opposition is **reposition**).

The CMC joints II, III, and IV are **plane synovial joints** that have 1 degree of freedom of movement: flexion and extension. The fifth CMC joint has 2 degrees of movement: flexion and extension and abduction and adduction. Several small ligaments support these joints and allow progressively more motion with each medial joint. The second and third CMC joints are practically immobile, but the fourth and fifth have greater mobility, allowing the hand to strongly grip.

Metacarpophalangeal and Interphalangeal Joints

The condyloid metacarpophalangeal joints are capable of 2 degrees of freedom of movement: flexion and extension and abduction and adduction. The five metacarpophalangeal (MCP) articulations represent the union between the concave articular surface of the proximal phalanx of each finger and the convex articular surface of the associated metacarpal. The lateral four fingers have maximum abduction and adduction excursion when the MCP joint is in full extension.

Support against valgus and varus forces is provided by pairs of collateral ligaments running obliquely from the dorsal aspect of the side of the metacarpal to the palmar aspect of the phalanx. As the fingers are flexed, these ligaments tighten, limiting the amount of abduction and adduction available to the joint in this position. This feature makes gripping less dependent on dynamic stability.

The palmar aspect of the MCP joints is reinforced by a thick fibrocartilaginous **palmar ligament**. The dorsal aspects of the lateral four MCP joints are reinforced by the expansion of the extensor hood. Reinforcement is also provided by the deep transverse metacarpal ligament. These strong bands limit abduction and adduction and reinforce the palmar ligaments. MCP hyperextension is primarily limited by the intrinsic musculature.[6]

With one on the thumb and two on the remaining fingers, the interphalangeal (IP) joints have 1 degree of freedom: flexion and extension. Like the MCP joints, the IP joints have a thick palmar ligament (volar plate) that restricts extension and radial and ulnar collateral ligaments that restrict abduction and adduction. The shallow bony configuration of the IP joints results in a reliance on soft tissue structures for stability.

Muscular Anatomy

The muscles of the wrist and hand function under a broad spectrum of circumstances and demands. The same muscles that are used to grip strongly are also called on to perform the most delicate of fine motor skills. The extrinsic muscles acting on the wrist, including the long muscles of the fingers, are described in Table 17-1. The intrinsic muscles of the hand are presented in Table 17-2.

The natural, relaxed position of the hand and fingers is one of slight flexion with the wrist in slight extension. This positioning is caused by the relative shortness of the finger flexors. This concept is demonstrated by noting how the fingers continue to flex as the wrist is passively extended.

Extensor Muscles

Located on the posterolateral portion of the forearm, the wrist and finger extensor muscles form six compartments in the dorsal aspect of the wrist and are primarily innervated by the radial nerve (Fig. 17-7). The wrist extensor muscles stabilize the wrist in extension so that the refined finger flexors are optimally positioned to function. Figures 16-6 and 16-7 show the locations of these muscles relative to the forearm, and Figures 17-8 and 17-9 show the locations of their insertions on the wrist and hand.

The superficial muscles originating on the posterior humerus and forearm, the **extensor carpi radialis longus and brevis** and **extensor carpi ulnaris**, are the primary wrist extensors. The **extensor digitorum communis (EDC)**, the primary extensor of the interphalangeal (IP) joints of the lateral four fingers, assists in wrist extension. The brachioradialis is also located in the superficial compartment, but it does not directly influence wrist movement.

The deep compartment contains the thumb's extensors, the **extensor pollicis longus** and the **extensor pollicis brevis**, and its primary abductor, the **abductor pollicis longus**. The long extensor of the second finger, the **extensor indicis**, is also located in this compartment. The remaining deep muscle, the **supinator**, is capable of supinating the forearm at all angles of elbow flexion but has no action on the hand or fingers.

The extensor muscles are secured to the posterior portion of the distal radius and ulna by the **extensor retinaculum**. This strong, transverse band increases the efficiency of the muscles' pull and prevents "bow stringing" when the wrist is extended.

Flexor Muscles

The anteromedial forearm is also divided into two compartments, superficial and deep. The superficial compartment houses the wrist's flexor muscles, the **flexor carpi radialis**, **palmaris longus** (absent in approximately 12% to 15% of the population), and **flexor carpi ulnaris**. The **flexor digitorum superficialis (FDS)**, responsible for flexion of the four proximal interphalangeal (PIP) joints, and the **pronator teres** are also located in this compartment. The location of these muscles is presented in Figure 16-6, and their insertions on the wrist and hand are presented in Figure 17-9. The deep compartment is formed by the **flexor digitorum profundus (FDP)**, flexing both the PIP and distal interphalangeal (DIP) joints; the **flexor pollicis longus**; and the **pronator quadratus**.

Plane synovial joint A synovial joint formed by the gliding between two or more bones

Table 17-1 Extrinsic Muscles Acting on the Wrist and Hand

Muscle	Action	Origin	Insertion	Innervation	Root
Abductor Pollicis Longus	1st CMC joint abduction 1st CMC joint extension Assists in radial deviation of the wrist	Posterior surface of the distal ulna Posterior surface of the distal radius Adjoining interosseous membrane	Radial side of the base of the 1st metacarpal	Median	C6, C7
Extensor Carpi Radialis Brevis	Wrist extension Radial deviation	Lateral epicondyle via the common extensor tendon Radial collateral ligament	Base of the 3rd metacarpal	Radial	C6, C7
Extensor Carpi Radialis Longus	Wrist extension Radial deviation	Supracondylar ridge of humerus	Radial side of the base of the 2nd metacarpal	Radial	C6, C7
Extensor Carpi Ulnaris	Wrist extension Ulnar deviation	Lateral epicondyle via the common extensor tendon	Ulnar side of the base of the 5th metacarpal	Deep radial	C6, C7, C8
Extensor Digiti Minimi	5th MCP joint extension 5th DIP and PIP extension, working with the lumbricals and interossei	Lateral epicondyle via the common extensor tendon Deep antebrachial fascia	To the middle and distal phalanx of the 5th finger via the extensor digitorum tendon	Radial	C6, C7, C8
Extensor Digitorum Communis	Wrist extension MCP extension IP extension Radial deviation of the wrist	Lateral epicondyle via the common extensor tendon	Dorsal surface of the proximal base of the middle and distal phalanges of each of the four fingers	Deep radial	C6, C7, C8
Extensor Indicis	2nd MCP extension (index finger) 2nd DIP and PIP extension, working with the lumbricals and interossei	Posterior surface of the ulna, distal to the extensor pollicis longus Interosseous membrane	To the middle and distal phalanx of the index finger via the extensor digitorum tendon	Radial	C6, C7, C8
Extensor Pollicis Brevis	1st MCP joint extension 1st CMC joint extension 1st CMC joint abduction Assists in wrist radial deviation	Posterior surface of the distal radius Adjoining interosseous membrane	Dorsal surface of the base of the proximal phalanx of the thumb	Deep radial	C6, C7
Extensor Pollicis Longus	1st IP joint extension 1st MCP joint extension 1st CMC joint extension Assists in wrist extension Assists in wrist radial deviation	Posterior surface of the middle one third of the ulna Adjoining interosseous membrane	Dorsal surface of the base of the distal phalanx of the thumb	Deep radial	C6, C7, C8
Flexor Carpi Radialis	Wrist flexion Forearm pronation Radial deviation	Medial epicondyle via the common flexor tendon	Bases of the 2nd and 3rd metacarpals	Median	C6, C7

Continued

Table 17-1 Extrinsic Muscles Acting on the Wrist and Hand—cont'd

Muscle	Action	Origin	Insertion	Innervation	Root
Flexor Carpi Ulnaris	Wrist flexion Ulnar deviation	Humeral head • Medial epicondyle via the common flexor tendon Ulnar head • Medial border of the olecranon • Proximal two-thirds of the posterior ulna	Pisiform Hamate 5th metacarpal	Ulnar	C8, T1
Flexor Digitorum Profundus	DIP flexion PIP flexion Wrist flexion	Anteromedial proximal three-fourths of ulna and associated interosseous membrane	Bases of the medial phalanges of digits II–V	Palmar interosseous	C8, T1
Flexor Digitorum Superficialis	PIP flexion MCP flexion Wrist flexion	Humeral head • Medial epicondyle via the common flexor tendon • Ulnar collateral ligament Ulnar head • Coronoid process Radial head • Oblique line of radius	Sides of the middle phalanges of digits II–V	Median	C7, C8, T1
Flexor Pollicis Longus	1st IP joint flexion 1st MCP joint flexion Assists in wrist flexion	Anterior surface of the radius Adjoining interosseous membrane Coronoid process of ulna	Palmar surface of the base of the distal phalanx of the thumb	Palmar interosseous	C8, T1
Palmaris Longus	Wrist flexion	Medial epicondyle via the common flexor tendon	Flexor retinaculum Palmar aponeurosis	Median	C6, C7

CMC = carpometacarpal; DIP = distal interphalangeal; IP = interphalangeal; MCP = metacarpophalangeal; PIP = proximal interphalangeal

Table 17-2 Intrinsic Muscles Acting on the Hand

Muscle	Action	Origin	Insertion	Innervation	Root
Abductor Digiti Minimi	Abduction of the 5th finger Assists in opposition	Tendon of flexor carpi ulnaris Pisiform	By two slips into the 5th finger • Ulnar side of the base of the proximal phalanx • Ulnar border of the extensor expansion	Ulnar	C8, T1
Abductor Pollicis Brevis	1st CMC joint abduction 1st MCP joint abduction Assists in opposition	Flexor retinaculum Trapezium Scaphoid	Radial surface of the base of the proximal phalanx of the thumb Via a slip into the extensor expansion	Median	C6, C7
Adductor Pollicis	1st CMC joint adduction 1st MCP joint adduction 1st MCP joint flexion Assists in opposition	Capitate bone Bases of 2nd and 3rd metacarpals Palmar surface of 3rd metacarpal	Ulnar surface of the base of the proximal phalanx of the thumb Via a slip into the extensor expansion	Deep palmar branch	C8, T1
Dorsal Interossei	Abduction of the 3rd, 4th, and 5th fingers Assists in MCP flexion Assists in extension of the IP joints	Thumb • Ulnar border of 1st metacarpal • Radial border of 2nd metacarpal 2nd, 3rd, and 4th fingers • Adjacent sides of metacarpals	Thumb • Radial border of the 2nd finger • Radial side of the 3rd finger 3rd • Ulnar side of 3rd finger 4th • Ulnar side of 4th finger	Deep palmar branch	C8, T1
Flexor Digiti Minimi	5th MCP joint flexion Assists in opposition	Hook of the hamate bone Flexor retinaculum	Ulnar border of the proximal phalanx of the 5th finger	Ulnar	C8, T1
Flexor Pollicis Brevis.	1st MCP joint flexion 1st CMC joint flexion Assists in opposition	Flexor retinaculum Trapezoid Capitate	Radial surface of the base of the proximal phalanx Via a slip into the extensor expansion	Median Deep palmar branch	C6, C7 C8, T1
Lumbricals	Flexion of the 2nd through 5th MCP joints Extension of the PIP and DIP joints	1st and 2nd: • Radial surface of flexor profundus tendons 3rd: • Adjacent sides of flexor profundus tendons of 3rd and 4th fingers 4th: • Adjacent sides of flexor profundus tendons of the 4th and 5th fingers	Radial border of the extensor tendons of the respective digits	1st and 2nd: Median 3rd and 4th: Deep palmar branch	C6, C7 C8, T1

Continued

Table 17-2 Intrinsic Muscles Acting on the Hand—cont'd

Muscle	Action	Origin	Insertion	Innervation	Root
Opponens Digiti Minimi	Opposition of the 5th finger	Hook of the hamate bone Flexor retinaculum	Ulnar border of the length of the 5th metacarpal	Ulnar	C8,T1
Opponens Pollicis	Thumb opposition	Flexor retinaculum Trapezium	Length of the 1st metacarpal	Median	C6, C7
Palmar Interossei	Adducts 1st, 2nd, 4th, and 5th fingers Assists in flexion of the MCP joints	Thumb • Ulnar border of the 1st metacarpal 2nd: • Ulnar border of the 2nd metacarpal 3rd: • Radial border of the 4th metacarpal 4th: • Radial border of the 5th metacarpal	Thumb • Ulnar border of thumb 2nd: • Ulnar side of 2nd finger 3rd: • Radial side of ring finger • Radial side of little finger	Deep palmar branch	C8,T1

CMC = carpometacarpal; DIP = distal interphalangeal; IP = interphalangeal; MCP = metacarpophalangeal; PIP = proximal interphalangeal

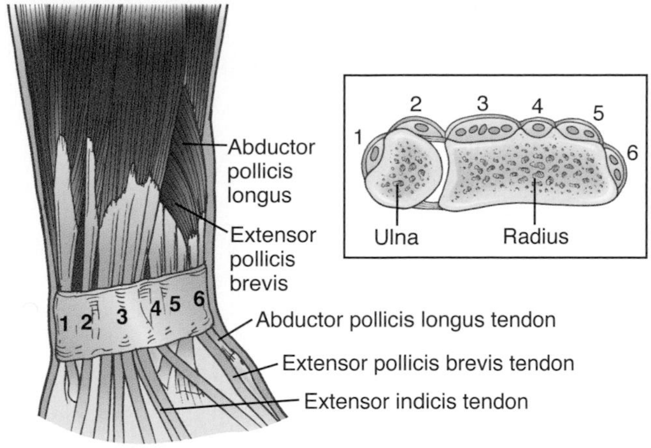

FIGURE 17-7 ■ Extensor compartment. Each group passes beneath the extensor retinaculum and contained within a compartment. From ulnar to radial: 1, extensor digiti minimi; 2, extensor carpi ulnaris; 3, extensor digitorum communis and extensor indicus; 4, extensor pollicis longus; 5, extensor carpi radialis longus and extensor carpi radialis brevis; 6, abductor pollicis longus and extensor pollicis brevis.

The flexor muscles are innervated by the **median nerve**. The exceptions are the flexor carpi ulnaris and the fourth and fifth portions of the FDP. These are supplied by the **ulnar nerve**.

Palmar Muscles

The hand's intrinsic muscles are grouped into the thenar, central, hypothenar, and adductor interosseous compartments. The **thenar eminence**, the mass found over the thumb's palmar surface, is formed by the **abductor pollicis brevis**, **flexor pollicis brevis**, and **opponens pollicis** muscles and the tendon of the **flexor pollicis longus muscle** (Fig. 17-10). On the ulnar aspect, the fleshy mound at the base of the little finger, the **hypothenar eminence**, contains the **abductor digiti minimi**, **flexor digiti minimi brevis**, and the **opponens digiti minimi muscles**.

The tendons of FDS and FDP pass through the central compartment. Proximally, the FDP lies directly underneath the FDS tendon. Near the distal phalanx, the FDS splits into two sections, allowing the profundus tendon to become superficial while the FDS tendons pass posteriorly and laterally to insert on the distal phalanx. This divergence results in the FDP's ability to flex the MCP, PIP, and DIP joints. The FDS only acts on the MCP and PIP joints.

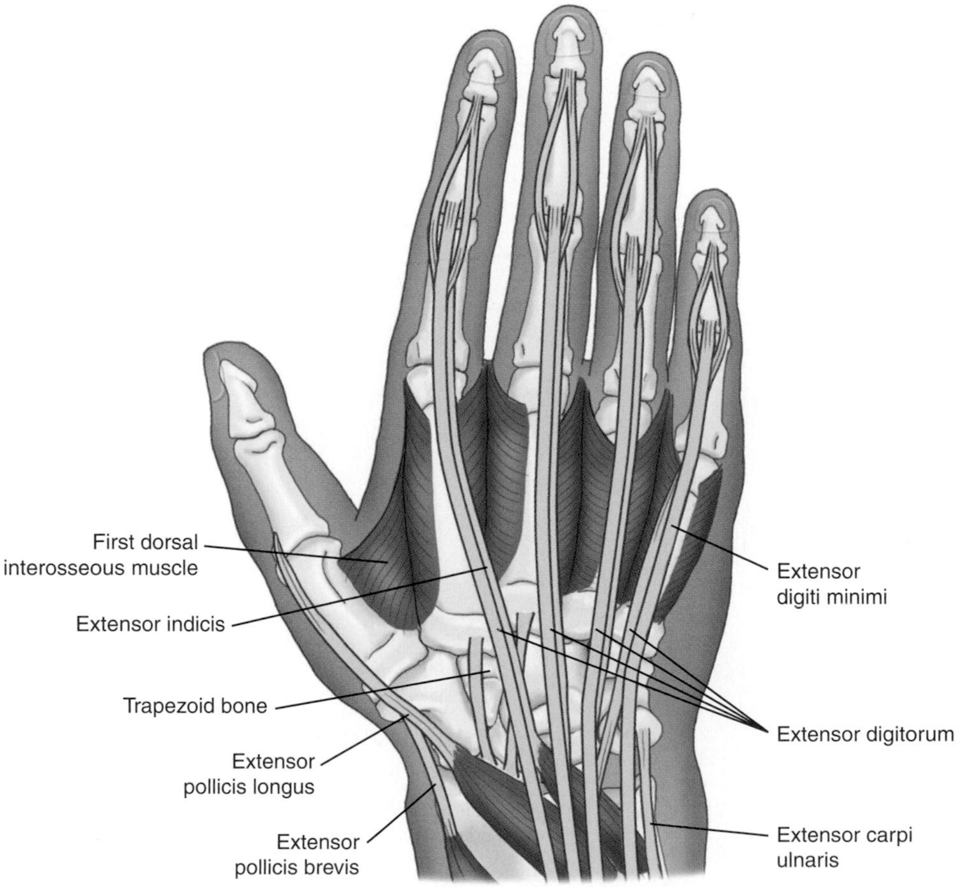

FIGURE 17-8 ■ Intrinsic muscles of the dorsal hand and attachments of the long finger extensors.

To prevent bowstringing, a series of pulleys restrain and guide the tendons as they travel across the length of the fingers (Fig. 17-11). During flexion and extension of the fingers, the flexor tendons require almost four times as much excursion as the extensor tendons.[7] The **annular pulleys**

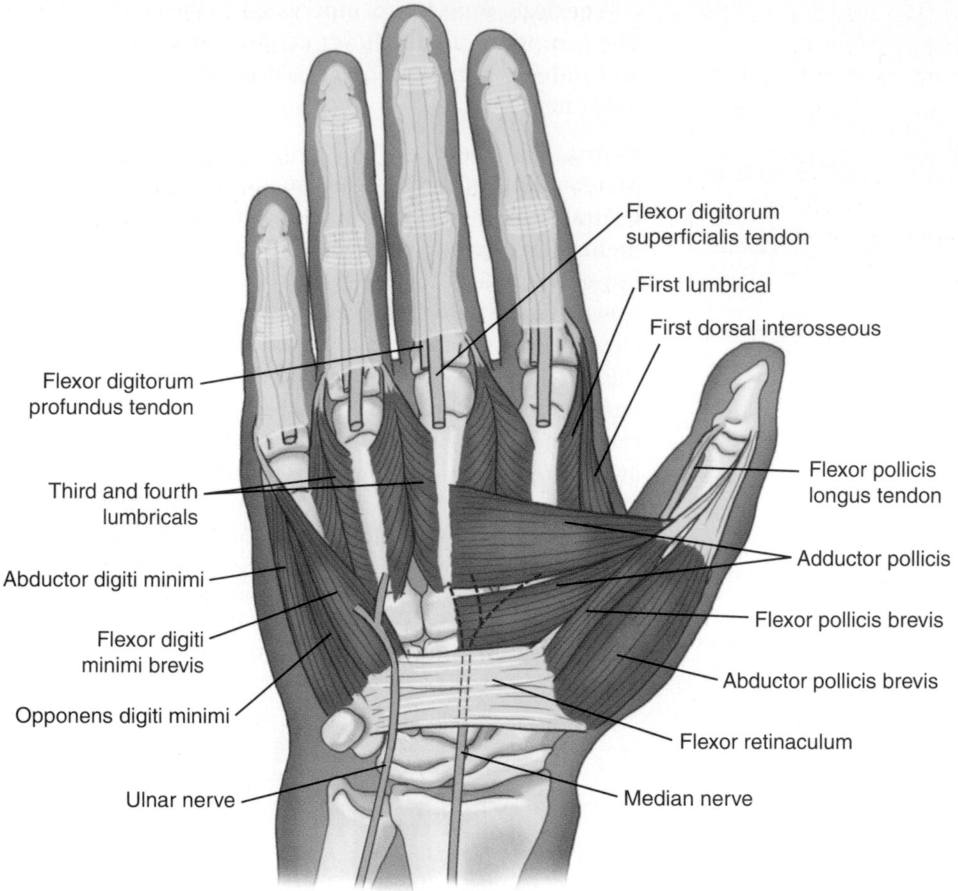

FIGURE 17-9 ■ Intrinsic palmar muscles and long finger flexors. Note the location of the ulnar and median nerves.

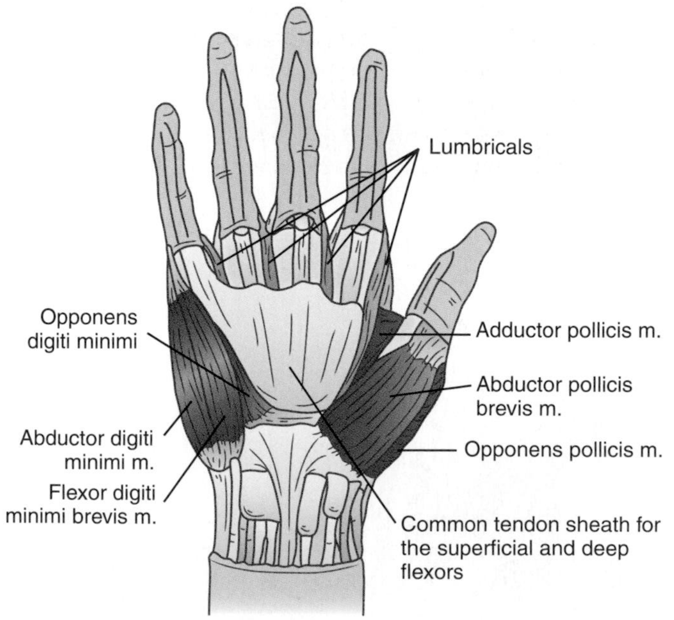

FIGURE 17-10 ■ Intrinsic muscles of the thumb and little finger.

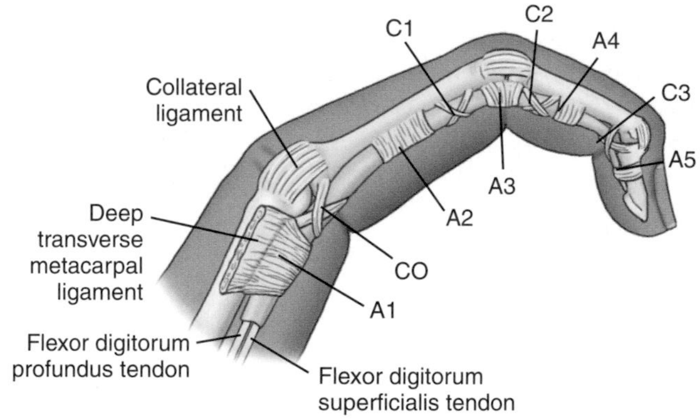

FIGURE 17-11 ■ The flexor pulley system. The annular pulleys (A's) hold the tendons close to the bone. The cruciate pulleys (C's) are flexible to allow full flexion of the finger.

arise from the palmar aspects of the MCP, PIP, and DIP joints. Numbered from proximal to distal, the annular pulleys act as tunnels through which the tendons pass to maintain their alignment with the finger. The **cruciate pulleys**, also numbered from proximal to distal, are more pliable and collapse to allow the annular pulleys to move towards each other during finger flexion. The **palmar aponeurosis pulley**, located on the distal aspect of the metacarpal, is the most proximal member of the pulley system.[7]

Four **lumbrical** muscles originate off the FDP tendons, cross the MCP joint on the palmar side, and cross dorsally to insert on the extensor hood. Lumbricals 1 and 2 are **unipennate** and originate on the radial side of the FDP. Lumbricals 3 and 4 are **bipennate**, with heads originating on the radial

Unipennate A muscle whose fibers attach to one side of a tendon
Bipennate A muscle whose fibers attach to both sides of a tendon

side of one FDP and the ulnar side of the adjacent FDP. Because of their attachment on the extensor hood, the lumbrical muscles serve to flex the MCP joints and extend the PIP and DIP joints. The entire central compartment is covered by the **palmar aponeurosis** (volar plate).

The palmar adductor interosseous compartment fills the void between metacarpals. The webspace between the thumb and index finger is filled by the **adductor pollicis muscle**. Three spaces between the remaining metacarpals are filled by three palmar and four dorsal interosseous muscles. Using the third metacarpal as the midline reference, the palmar interossei adduct the fingers, and the dorsal interossei abduct them. The palmar interossei have no attachment on the third finger.

Nerves

Three peripheral nerves provide motor and sensory input to the wrist and hand. Proximal entrapment of these nerves can manifest itself with symptoms in the wrist and hand.

Ulnar Nerve

The ulnar nerve travels superficially through the palmar aspect of the wrist just medial to the carpal tunnel and then passes through Guyon's canal formed by the hamate and pisiform. At its end, the ulnar nerve divides into superficial and deep branches. The superficial branch provides sensory input to the palmar surface of the little finger and medial one-half of the ring finger. The deep branch innervates the muscles of the hypothenar eminence, the medial two lumbricals, the interossei, and the adductor pollicis.[8]

Median Nerve

Following its course with the FDS through the forearm, the median nerve travels through the carpal tunnel lateral and divides into the motor and palmar digital branches.[9] The motor branches supply the muscles of the thenar eminence. The palmar digital branch provides sensation to the palmar surface of the thumb, index finger, middle finger and to the lateral one-half of the index finger in addition to innervating the lateral two lumbricals.[9]

Radial Nerve

The radial nerve divides into motor (posterior interosseous nerve) and sensory branches (superficial radial nerve) in the proximal forearm. The posterior interosseous nerve innervates the wrist and finger extensors. The superficial radial nerve travels down the dorsal forearm and supplies sensation to the dorsal hand.[10]

The Carpal Tunnel

Many of the anterior muscles acting on the wrist and fingers cross the radiocarpal joint through the carpal tunnel (Fig. 17-12). A fibro-osseous structure, the tunnel's floor is formed by the proximal carpal bones. Its roof is formed by the transverse carpal ligament. Ten structures pass through the tunnel: the median nerve, the flexor pollicis longus tendon, the four tendons of the FDS, and the four FDP tendons. Inflammation of these structures compresses the median nerve, resulting in paresthesia in the median nerve distribution in the palmar aspect of the second, third, and fourth fingers. Grip strength is decreased because of pain and inhibition of the motor nerves supplying the thumb's flexors and opposition muscles.

Clinical Examination of Injuries to the Wrist, Hand, and Fingers

An evaluation of the elbow, shoulder, and cervical spine may be warranted when a patient's described activity restrictions, history, or symptoms suggest involvement of these structures. For example, proximal nerve entrapment may result in decreased sensation and strength in the hand. The impact of the condition on the patient's life must be ascertained.

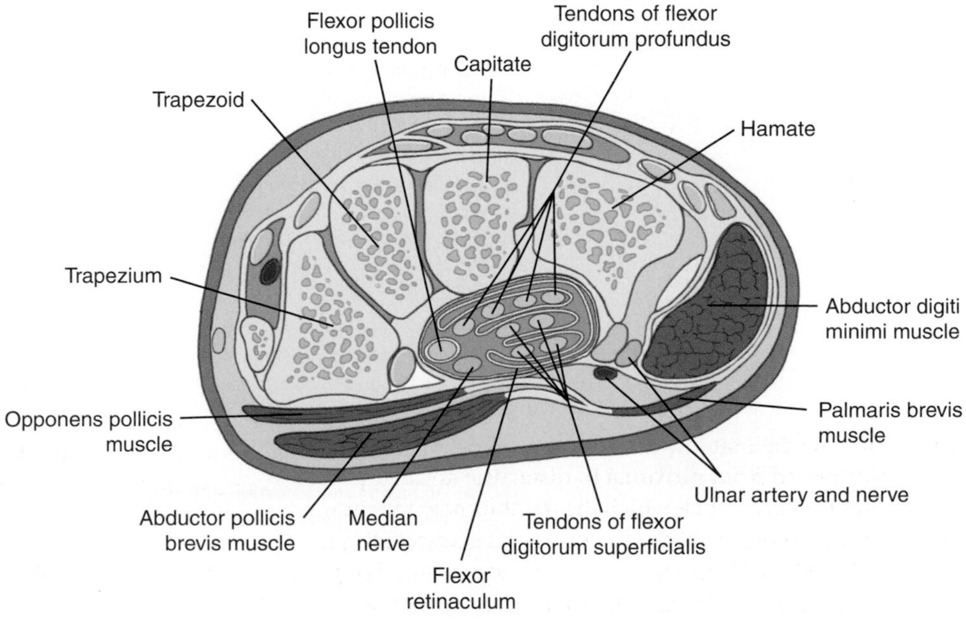

FIGURE 17-12 ■ The carpal tunnel. Inflammation of the tendons passing through the carpal tunnel increases the volume within this fixed space. If the volume continues to increase, the median nerve is compressed, resulting in neurological symptoms in the hand.

Examination Map

HISTORY

Past Medical History

Previous injury history

General medical health

History of the Present Condition

Location of pain

Mechanism of injury

Onset and severity of symptoms

Changes in activity

FUNCTIONAL ASSESSMENT

Daily or athletic tasks that are associated with reproduction or exacerbation of symptoms.

Throwing (if indicated)

INSPECTION

General Inspection

Wrist and hand posture

Gross deformity

Palmar creases

Lacerations or scars

- Russell's sign

Inspection of the Wrist and Hand

Continuity of the radius and ulna

Continuity of the carpals and metacarpals

Alignment of the MCP IP joints

Ganglion cyst

Inspection of the Thumb and Fingers

Skin and fingernails

Subungual hematoma

Felon

Paronychia

Alignment of fingernails

Muscle contour

Finger posture

PALPATION

Palpation of the Palmar Wrist

Radius

Flexor carpi radialis

Palmaris longus

Carpal tunnel

Ulna

Flexor carpi ulnaris

Triangular fibrocartilage complex

Pisiform

Hamate

Palpation of the Dorsal Wrist

Ulna

Ulnar styloid process

Ulnar collateral ligament

Extensor carpi ulnaris

Lister's tubercle

Distal radius/styloid process

Radial collateral ligament

Scaphoid

Lunate

Triquetrum

Trapezium

Capitate

Trapezoid

Extensor carpi radialis brevis

Extensor carpi radialis longus

Palpation of the Hand

Thenar eminence

Central compartment

Hypothenar compartment

Metacarpals

MCP Collateral ligaments

Phalanges

IP joint collateral ligaments

Thenar webspace

Extensor digitorum

Extensor pollicis longus

Abductor pollicis longus

Abductor pollicis brevis

JOINT AND MUSCLE FUNCTION ASSESSMENT

Wrist

Goniometry

Active range of motion

- Flexion and extension
- Radial and ulnar deviation

Manual Muscle Tests

- Flexion and extension
- Radial and ulnar deviation

Passive Range of Motion

- Flexion and extension
- Radial and ulnar deviation

Thumb

Goniometry

Active Range of Motion

- Flexion and extension
- Abduction and adduction

Manual Muscle Tests

- Flexion and extension
- Abduction and adduction
- Opposition

Passive Range of Motion

- Flexion and extension
- Abduction and adduction
- Opposition and reposition

Fingers

Goniometry

Active Range of Motion

- Flexion and extension - MCP joints
- Abduction and adduction - MCP joints
- Flexion and extension - IP joints

Manual Muscle Tests

- PIP flexion
- Abduction and adduction - MCP joints
- Flexion and extension
- Grip dynamometry

Passive Range of Motion

- Flexion and extension - MCP joints
- Abduction and adduction - MCP joints
- Flexion and extension of the IP joints

JOINT STABILITY TESTS

Stress Testing

Wrist

- Radial collateral ligament
- Ulnar collateral ligament

Finger (PIP and DIP)

- Radial collateral ligament
- Ulnar collateral ligament

Joint Play Assessment

Wrist

- Radial glide
- Ulnar glide
- Dorsal glide
- Palmar glide

Hand

- Intercarpal glide

NEUROLOGICAL EXAMINATION

Upper Quarter Screen

Tinel's Sign

REGION-SPECIFIC PATHOLOGIES AND SELECTIVE TISSUE TESTS

Wrist Pathologies

Distal forearm fracture

- Colles' fracture
- Smith's fracture

Scaphoid fracture

- Scaphoid compression test

Preiser's disease

Hamate fracture

Perilunate/lunate dislocation

- Dissociative carpal instability
- Kienböck's disease

Wrist sprains

- Watson test

Triangular fibrocartilage complex injury

Carpal tunnel syndrome

- Phalen's test

Hand Pathologies

Metacarpal fractures

Finger Pathologies

Collateral ligament injuries

Boutonnière deformity

- Pseudoboutonnière deformity

Finger fractures

Tendon ruptures and avulsion fractures

Thumb Pathologies

De Quervain's disease

- Finkelstein's test

Thumb sprains

MCP joint dislocations

Thumb fractures

History

Past Medical History

- **Previous history:** Determine the previous history of injury and any resulting loss of function. Wrist instabilities may result from a seemingly resolved prior trauma.
- **General medical health:** Question the patient about a history of other disorders. Systemic diseases such as gout or rheumatoid arthritis often affect the wrist and fingers before the other joints in the body.[11] This area is often the first to be affected by **peripheral vascular disease (PVD)** or **Raynaud's phenomenon**. Vascular insufficiencies may result in a sensation of coolness and thickness in the hand. Chronic wrist pain is a common complaint among people with diabetes and associated neuropathies.[12] Pregnancy increases the risk of acquiring carpal tunnel syndrome.[13]

History of the Present Condition

- **Location of pain:** Because the structures of the wrist and hand are so close to one another, enough details should be gained during the history-taking process to localize the symptoms as specifically as possible. Trauma to the cervical spine, shoulder, elbow, and forearm can radiate symptoms into the wrist and hand. Injury to the median, ulnar, and radial nerves can radiate symptoms into their specific sensory or motor distributions in the hand (Fig. 17-13).
- **Mechanism of injury:** In the case of acute trauma, identify the mechanism of injury to localize the injured structure or structures. Ask patients describing an injury of insidious onset about activities that increase or decrease the symptoms. When evaluating patients with hand injuries that have an insidious onset, pay particular attention to specific postures that may be assumed for long periods of time, such as when working at a computer.
- **Relevant sounds or sensations:** Question the patient about any sounds or sensations experienced. Fractures, dislocations, and tendon pathology such as a **trigger finger** may have an associated popping sound accompanied by a sensation of snapping (Box 17-1). "Clicking" on the ulnar side of the wrist is often associated with TFCC tears.
- **Duration of symptoms:** Correlate the injury mechanism with the duration of symptoms. Nagging wrist pain that does not decrease in severity may indicate a **scaphoid fracture**, a tear of the TFCC, or carpal instability.
- **Description of symptoms:** "Aching" symptoms are often associated with tendinopathies. "Burning" or "tingling" sensations suggest neurological or vascular involvement.
- **Changes in activity:** Question the patient regarding any changes in positioning associated with activities of daily living (ADLs) or sport activities. Sustained postures, such as those associated with working at a computer, may predispose an individual to tendinopathies of the wrist flexors or extensors. Tendon pathology is often associated with atypical manual activities.[15] Technique changes or adopting new activities such as rowing may overstress tissues, leading to acute or chronic pathologies.

Functional Assessment

When observing the patient's replication of activities that produce pain or during specific functional testing, compensation for a lack of mobility in the distal arm is demonstrated by using extra motion at the elbow and shoulder. Several pathologies such as a fracture, scapholunate instability, carpal dislocation, or carpal tunnel syndrome limit grip strength and cause the patient to describe an increase in symptoms with ADLs such as opening a door, brushing teeth, or shaking hands. The patient may be able to voluntarily reproduce subluxation at the distal radioulnar joint or at the scapholunate joint.[11]

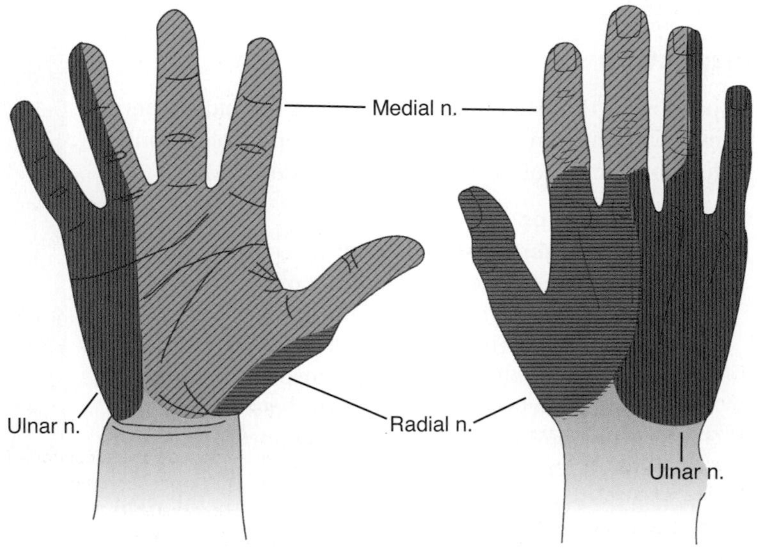

FIGURE 17-13 ■ Nerve distribution in the hand.

Box 17-1
Trigger Finger

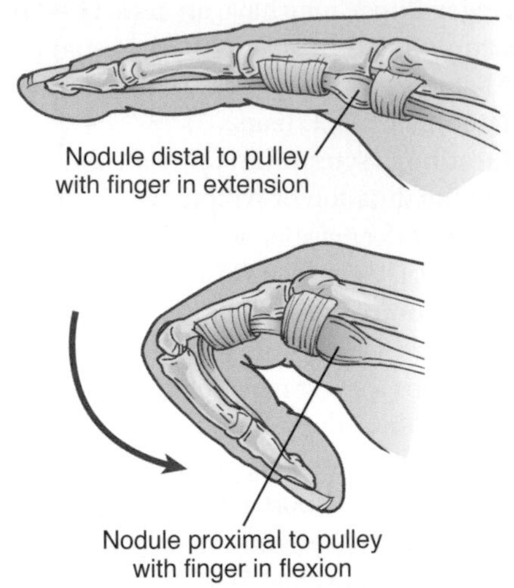

Trigger finger, a degenerative process, is the result of stenosing tenosynovitis that leads to the formation of a nodule in a flexor tendon, most frequently affecting the flexor digitorum profundus or flexor pollicis longus.[14] Normal flexion and extension of the MCP joint are affected as the nodule passes proximal to the A1 pulley (see Fig. 17-10) during flexion and distal to this pulley during extension. The finger will hesitate and then "snap" as the nodule is wedged beneath the pulley, often resulting in an audible pop as it passes through the opening.

More prevalent in females than males and in those with diabetes, trigger finger may affect multiple digits and occur bilaterally. The patient may be hesitant or unable to make a fist.[15] Initially, the nodule and joint motion are painless, but discomfort increases with time. Although the restriction to motion is occurring at the MCP joint, the patient may describe the PIP joint being involved. As the nodule enlarges, the nodule will become palpable and painful to the touch.

If the diagnosis is made early, trigger finger is sometimes successfully treated using injected anti-inflammatory medication. Significantly enlarged nodules, thickening of the A1 pulley, and/or the formation of adhesions within the sheath may require surgical correction, which has a high rate of success.[15]

Inspection

Inspection of the wrist, hand, and fingers should be performed with the arm exposed and, when applicable, should include inspection of the elbow and shoulder.

General Inspection

- **Posturing of the wrist and hand:** The natural, relaxed posture of the wrist and hand is that of mild extension of the wrist and slight flexion of the hand, with a subtle arch in the palm. The absence of this arch may indicate an avulsion of one or more finger flexors or atrophy of the hand's intrinsic muscles in the case of chronic injuries or prolonged nerve compression (Inspection Findings 17-1). Trauma to the structures that lie between the cervical spine and wrist may cause the wrist and hand to assume an abnormal posture such as **Volkmann's ischemic contracture**. Inhibition of the radial nerve may cause paralysis of the wrist and finger extensors and cause **drop-wrist deformity**, resulting in an inability to extend the wrist.
- **Gross deformity:** Dislocation of the MCP or IP joints results in obvious deformity of the joint's articulating surfaces (Fig. 17-14). A fracture of the metacarpal shows as a discontinuity along the usually flat dorsal surface of

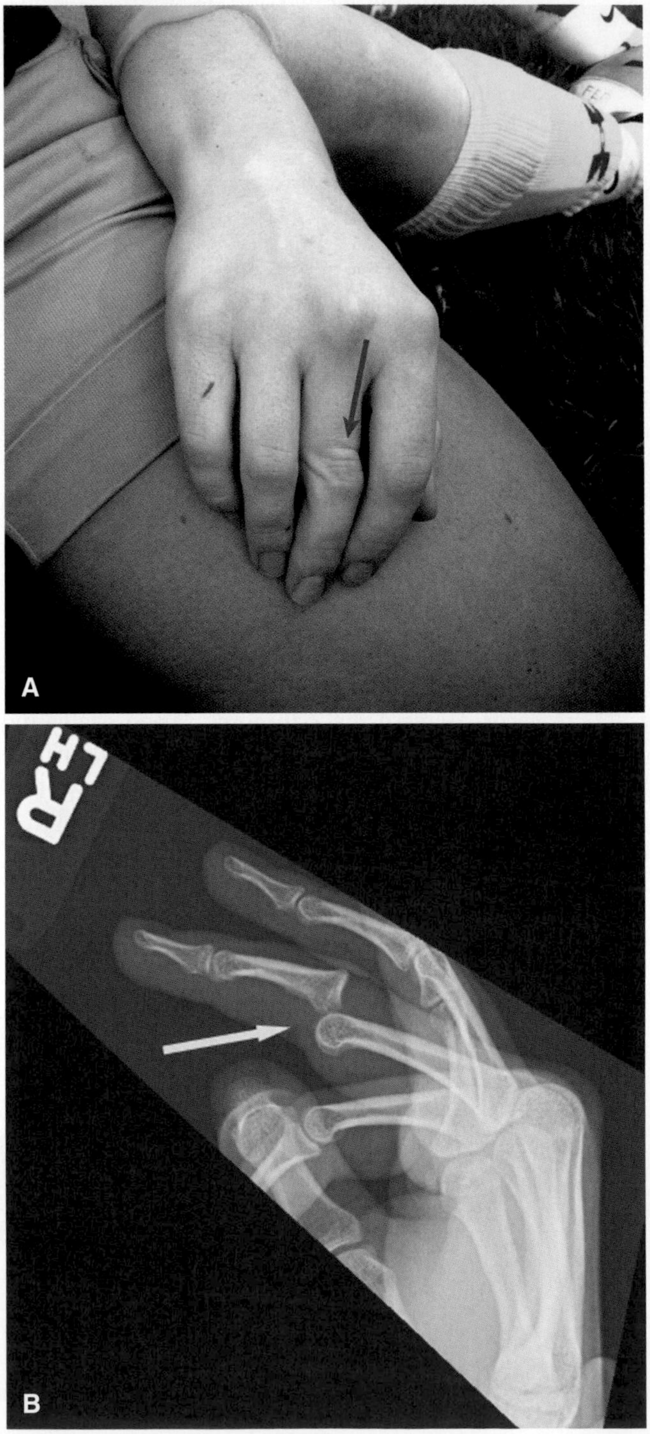

FIGURE 17-14 ■ Dislocation of the proximal interphalangeal joint of the middle finger. (A) As seen during inspection. (B) Radiograph (medial view, right hand) of the same injury demonstrating dorsal displacement of the middle phalanx.

	Ape Hand	Bishop's Deformity	Claw Hand
	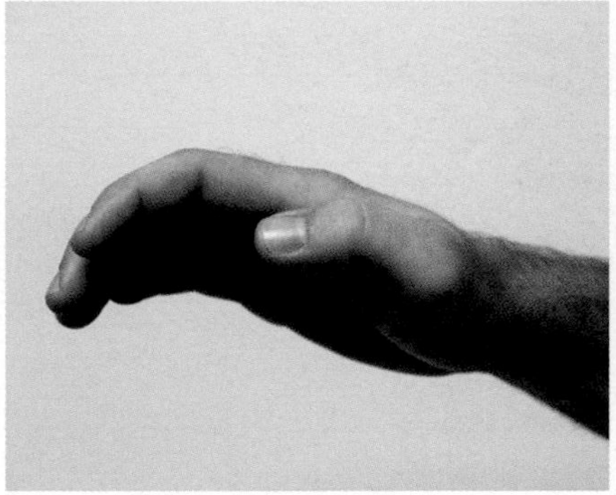	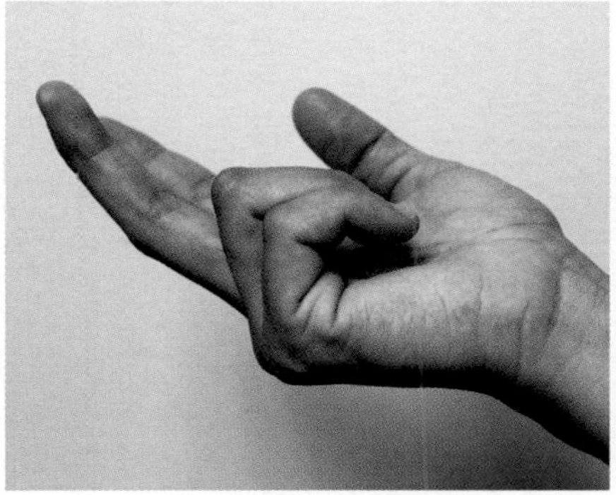	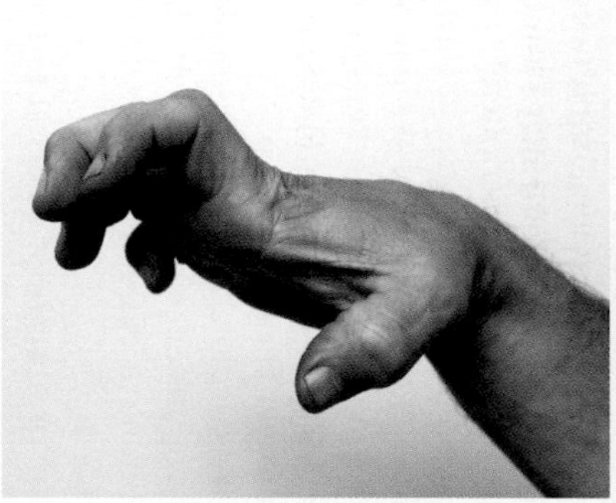
Impairments	Weakness and atrophy of the muscles of the thenar eminence result in overemphasis of the extensor muscles, which pull the thumb parallel with the fingers. Opposition and flexion of the MCP and IP are weakened.	Weakness and atrophy of the hypothenar, interossei, and medial two lumbricals cause the medial fingers to assume a resting posture of flexion in the PIP and DIP joints. Extension of these joints is limited.	Weakness and atrophy of the hand intrinsic muscles result in extension of the MCP joint and flexion of the PIP and DIP joints.
Pathology	Median nerve neuropathy	Inhibition of the ulnar nerve; also known as "Benediction deformity"	Ulnar and median nerve neuropathy
	Dupuytren's Contracture	**Swan-Neck Deformity**	**Volkmann's Ischemic Contracture**
	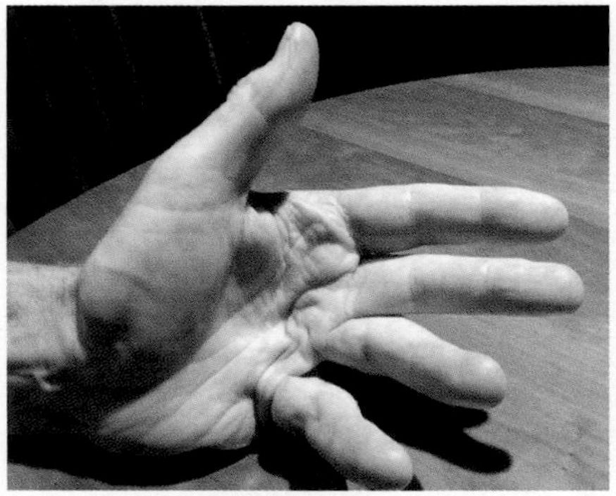	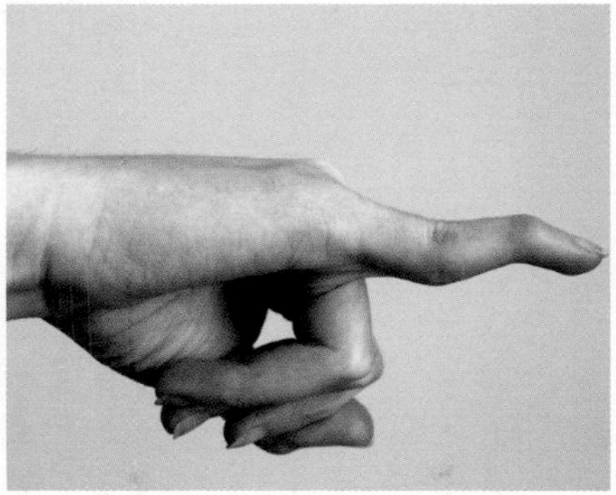	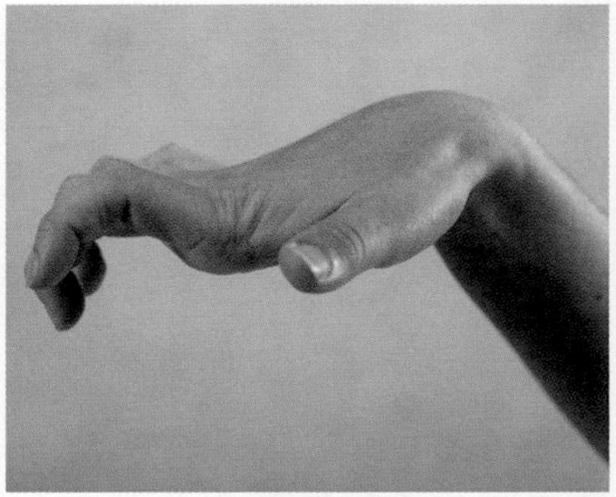
Impairments	Involved finger(s) assume(s) excessively flexed resting position. Inability to passively or actively extend the MCP and PIP joints of the involved finger	Characterized by flexion of the MCP and DIP joints and hyperextension of the PIP joint	Flexion contraction of the wrist and fingers (claw fingers) resulting in limited extension at these joints
Pathology	Flexion contracture of the MCP and PIP joints is caused by a shortening or adhesion (or both) of the palmar fascia. This hereditary condition most commonly affects the 4th and 5th fingers.	Can be caused by a wide range of pathologies, including volar plate injuries, malunion fractures of the middle phalanx, trauma to the finger flexor or extensor muscles, or rheumatoid arthritis.	A decrease in the blood supply to the forearm muscles; Volkmann's contracture can occur after a forearm fracture, fracture or dislocation of the elbow, or forearm compartment syndrome.

AROM = active range of motion; DIP = distal interphalangeal; IP = interphalangeal; MCP = metacarpophalangeal; PIP = proximal interphalangeal the hand. Fractures of the distal radius and/or ulna may result in a visible deformity. Also observe the dorsal area overlying the lunate for an abnormal contour that may indicate a dislocation (palmar-side dislocations are less easily observed).

- **Palmar creases:** Swelling in one or more of the hand compartments can obliterate the normal palmar creases.
- **Wounds or scars:** The superficial nature of the wrist and hand tendons and nerves makes them vulnerable to even minor cuts. Prior lacerations or surgery may have permanently injured the underlying structures, resulting in paresthesia or the loss of function in one or more fingers. Skin laceration over a joint, especially those caused by a bite, should be referred to a physician for prophylactic antibiotic treatment. Closely monitor puncture wounds to the palmar surface of the fingers. The flexor tendon sheath is vulnerable to infection and must be managed aggressively to avoid a poor outcome.[16]

  Abrasions, small cuts, or callosities over the dorsal surface of the MCP or IP joints, **Russell's sign**, can be one of the few outward signs of bulimia. These lesions are caused by repeated contact with the teeth during self-induced vomiting.[17]

Inspection of the Wrist and Hand

- **Alignment of the MCP joints:** Look for the MCP joints to be normally aligned relative to the noninvolved side. A depressed or shortened metatarsal head may indicate a metacarpal fracture.
- **Ganglion cyst:** Note any collection of fluid or the formation of a mass. A benign collection of thick fluid within a tendinous sheath or joint capsule, ganglion cysts are commonly found in the wrist and hand complex (Fig. 17-15). When the cyst becomes symptomatic, pain is caused by motion, and the ganglion is tender to the touch and hardens with time. Patients with symptomatic cysts should be referred to a physician for further evaluation and treatment.

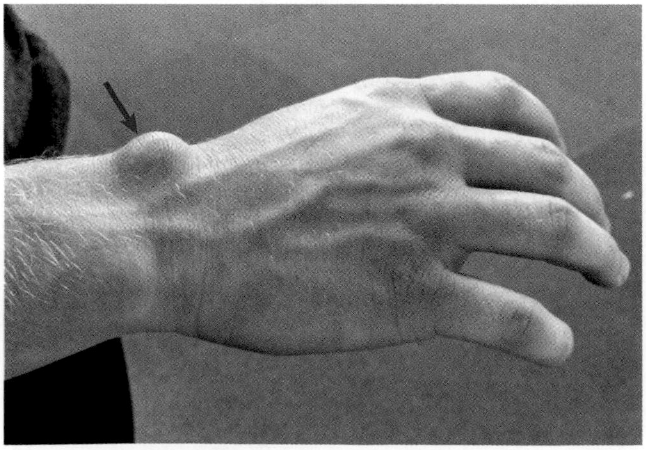

FIGURE 17-15 ■ Ganglion cyst of the wrist extensor tendon. These deformities, caused by a build-up of fluid within the tendon's sheath or joint capsule, are often asymptomatic.

Inspection of the Thumb and Fingers

- **Inspection of the skin and fingernails:** Trophic changes such as discoloration and changes in hair patterns or skin and nail texture may indicate peripheral vascular disease, complex regional pain syndrome, or Raynaud's phenomenon. Clubbing or cyanosis of the nail sometimes indicates pulmonary disease, Marfan syndrome, cardiovascular disorder, or other disease states.
- **Subungual hematoma:** The formation of a hematoma is characterized by discoloration beneath the fingernail. Observe for the presence of the crescent-shaped lumina. If the **lumina** is absent, the fingernail will eventually fall off.
- **Felon:** An infection or abscess at or distal to the DIP joints, a felon arises secondary to contusions or lacerations. The distal end of the finger is red, enlarged, tender to the touch, and warm. Felons must be treated with antibiotics to prevent them from spreading proximally in the finger and hand.
- **Paronychia:** An infection around the periphery of the fingernail, a paronychia results in redness, swelling, and possible drainage around the nailbed (Fig. 17-16). A paronychia should be treated with warm soaks. A physician may prescribe oral antibiotics or drain the affected area.
- **Individual finger deformities:** Irregular posture of one finger may indicate an acute injury or previous trauma (Inspection Findings 17-2). Deformities along the shaft of the bone may indicate a fracture; deformities at the joint indicate a dislocation.

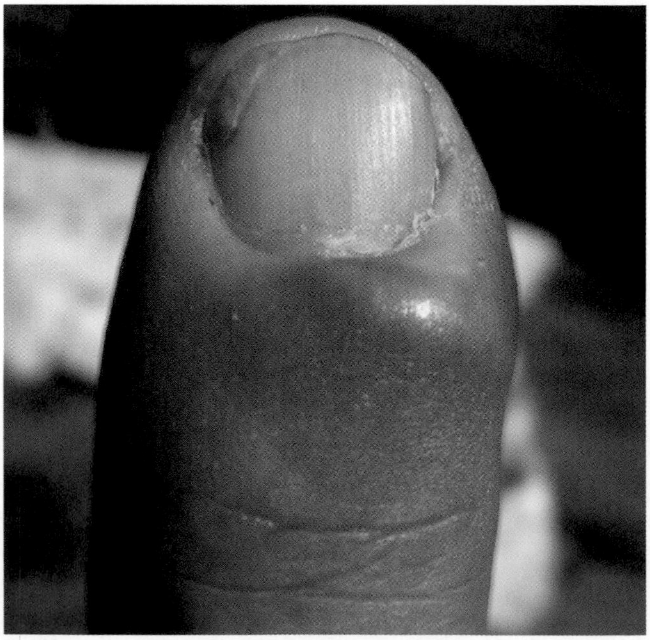

FIGURE 17-16 ■ A paronychia, infection of the fingernail bed.

Lumina The growth plate of a fingernail or toenail

Finger Deformities

	Jersey Finger	Mallet Finger*	Boutonnière Deformity*
Observation	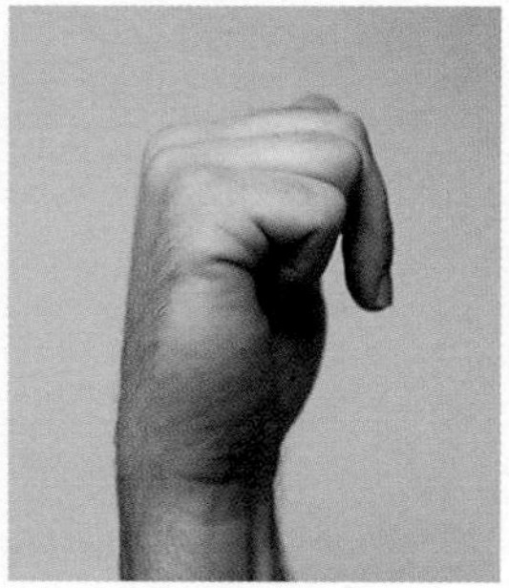	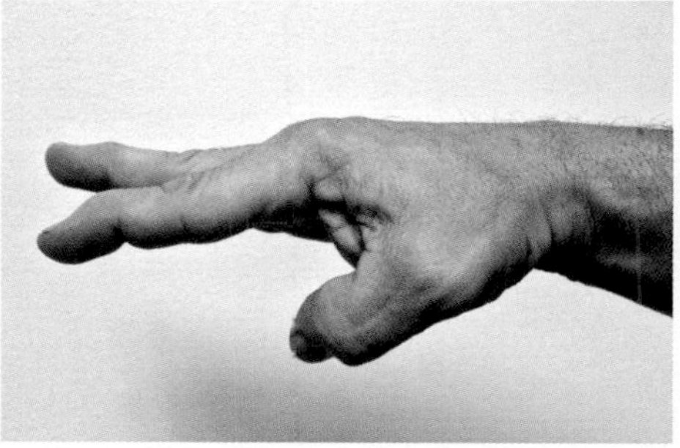	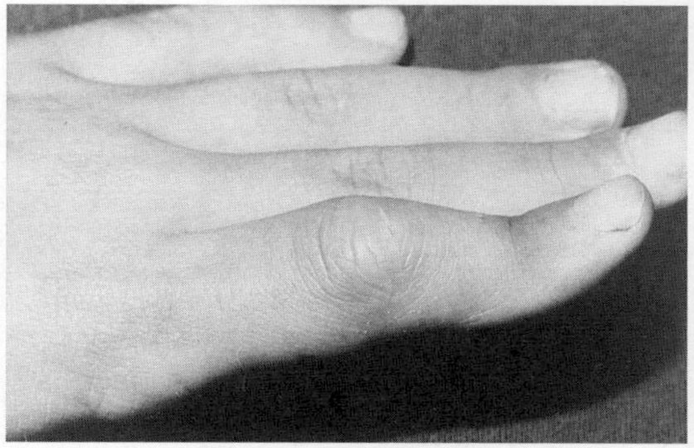
Illustration	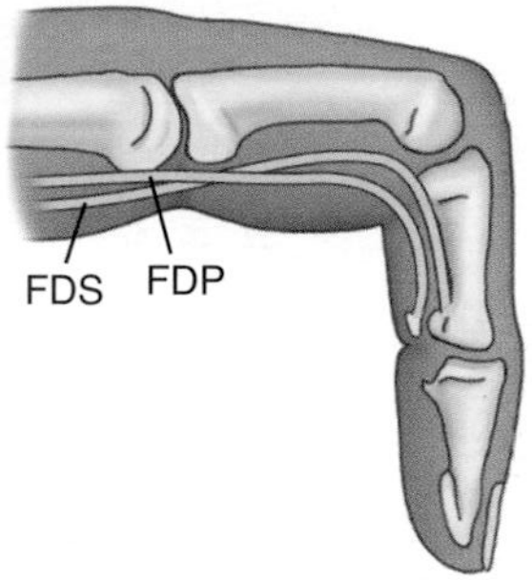	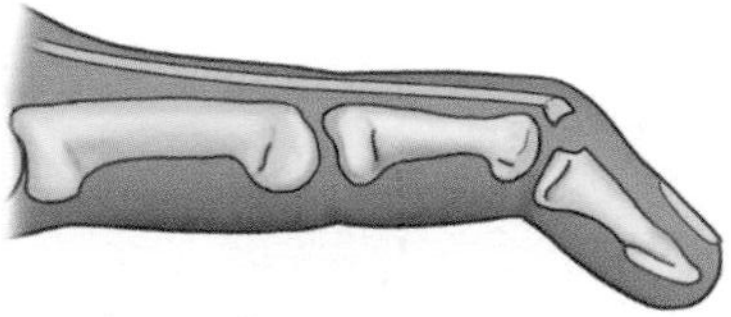	Boutonnière Deformity 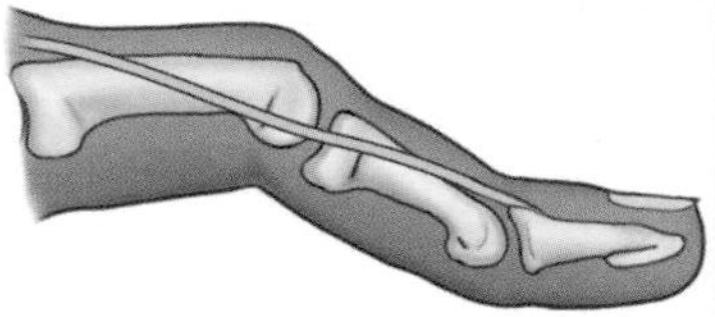 Pseudoboutonnière Deformity 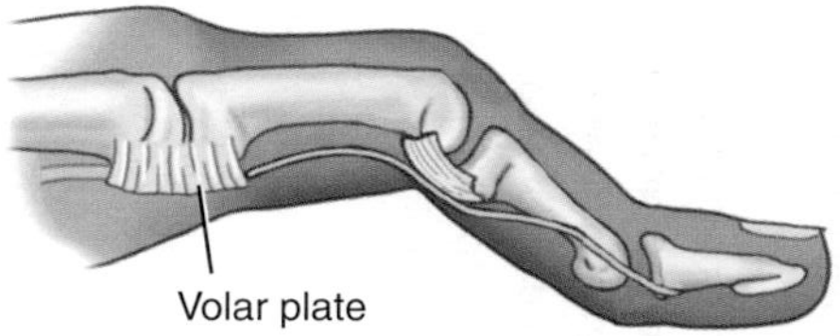
Pathology	Avulsion or rupture of the FDP tendon	Avulsion or rupture of the extensor digitorum tendon	Avulsion or rupture of the extensor digitorum tendon Pseudoboutonnière deformity: A rupture of the volar plate
Impairment	Inability to actively flex the DIP joint	Inability to actively extend the DIP, which assumes the posture of 25°–35° of flexion	Extension of the MCP and DIP joints and flexion of the PIP joint; acutely, the PIP joint can be passively extended in those with boutonnière deformities, but active PIP extension is absent. In pseudoboutonnière deformities, passive and active PIP extension is limited.

DIP = distal interphalangeal; FDP = flexor digitorum profundus; MCP = metacarpophalangeal; PIP = proximal interphalangeal
*Photo courtesy of Stanley, BG, and Tribuzi, SM: *Concepts in Hand Rehabilitation*. Philadelphia, PA: FA Davis, 1992.

- **Muscle contour:** Atrophy of the muscles of the thenar eminence is associated with prolonged compression of the median nerve, frequently associated with carpal tunnel syndrome. Entrapment of the ulnar nerve proximal or at the level of the pisiform (before Guyon's canal) may result in atrophy of the hypothenar eminence.
- **Finger alignment:** During finger flexion, the lateral four fingers usually assume approximately the same alignment, pointing to the scaphoid. A finger that deviates from the rest may indicate a spiral fracture of a phalanx or metacarpal.

PALPATION

Detailed palpation of the muscles that originate on the elbow and act on the wrist and hand is described in Chapter 16. Many of the structures of the wrist, hand, and fingers can be palpated from both the palmar and dorsal aspects.

Palpation of the Palmar (Anterior) Wrist

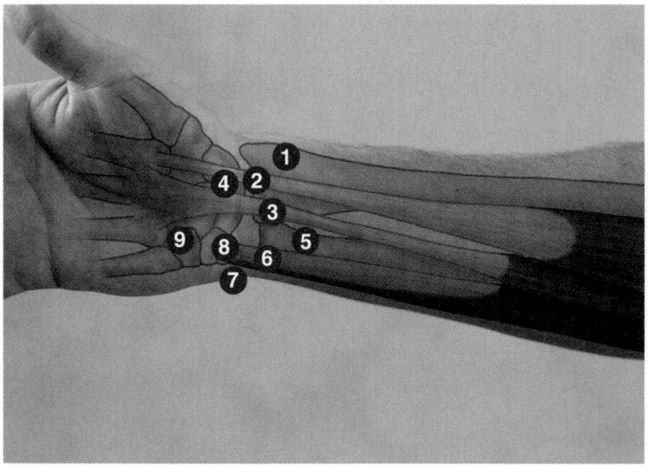

1 Radius: Palpate the distal **radius** as it forms the primary articulation with the proximal row of carpals.

2 Flexor carpi radialis (FCR): The tendon of the **FCR** is palpable just lateral to the tendon of the palmaris longus and is made more prominent by having the patient flex and radially deviate the wrist.

3 Palmaris longus: Absent in 12% to 15% of the population, the **palmaris longus** is more easily identified when the thumb and fifth finger are opposed and the wrist is flexed (Schaeffer test) (Fig. 17-17).[18]

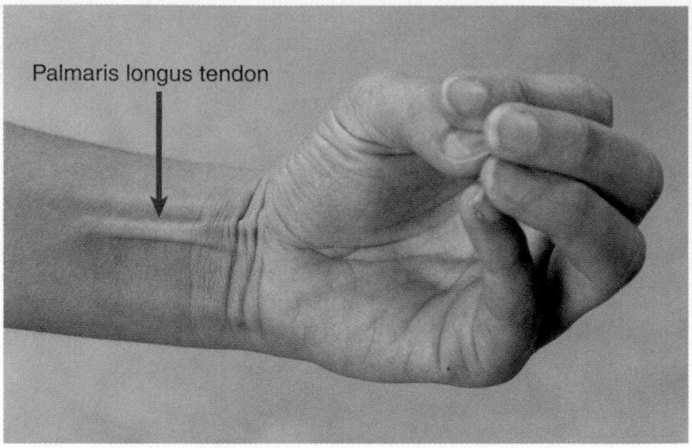

FIGURE 17-17 ■ The Schaeffer test. The palmaris longus tendon becomes prominent during wrist flexion and opposition of the thumb and little finger.

4 Carpal tunnel: Palpate the area of the **carpal tunnel** for edema, tissue thickening, or tenderness of the long finger flexor tendons or transverse ligament (see Fig. 17-12).

5 Ulna: Palmarly, the distal **ulna** is palpable at its most medial aspect. The lateral aspect is obscured by the wrist and finger flexor tendons. In the event of a fracture, bony displacement may be noted.

6 Flexor carpi ulnaris (FCU): The **FCU** fans out to insert on the pisiform, hook of the hamate, and base of the fifth metacarpal. Its tendon is easily palpated on the medial wrist when the wrist is flexed.

7 TFCC: Just distal to the ulna, the **TFCC** is most accessible at the medial-most wrist.

8 Pisiform: The **pisiform**, a sesamoid bone that lies directly anterior to the triquetrum, is prominent as a small, rounded protuberance at the proximal hypothenar eminence. This bone is mobile when the wrist is passively flexed as it lies in the tendon of the flexor carpi ulnaris.

9 Hamate: Identify the **hamate** by its palmarly projecting hook. Locate the center of the ulna and palpate immediately across the joint line, distal and lateral to the pisiform. The hook of the hamate feels like a hard palmar projection that moves with the hand as the wrist is flexed.

Palpation of the Dorsal (Posterior) Wrist

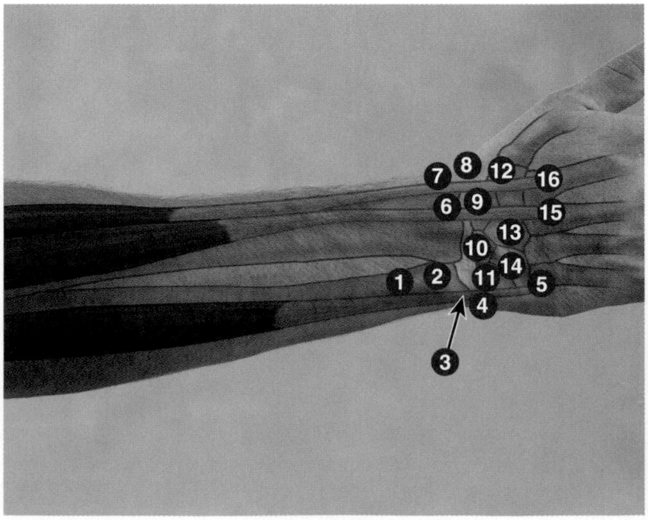

1 Ulna: The dorsal aspect of the distal two-thirds of the **ulna** is superficial from the point where it emerges from the bulk of the wrist flexors. As the ulna approaches the wrist articulation, the **(2) ulnar head** becomes prominent and palpable on its anterior, medial, and posterior borders.

3 Ulnar styloid process: The **ulnar styloid process** is palpated on the distal posteromedial border for tenderness or crepitus.

4 Ulnar collateral ligament (UCL): The wrist's **UCL** is palpated as it arises from the styloid process and crosses the joint space to attach to the triquetrum dorsally and the pisiform palmarly.

5 Extensor carpi ulnaris (ECU): The **ECU** is more prominent when the wrist is extended.

6 Lister's tubercle: Serving as a fulcrum for the extensor pollicus longus, **Lister's tubercle** is a small protuberance on the dorsal aspect of the radius that serves as a pulley for the extensor pollicus longus. Flexing the wrist makes the tubercle more prominent.

7 Distal radius/styloid process: The **styloid process** is located on the most **distal** aspect of the **radius.**

8 Radial collateral ligament (RCL): Locate the **RCL** from its attachment on the radial styloid process; this structure is palpated as it crosses the joint line to its attachment on the scaphoid.

9 Scaphoid: Locate the **scaphoid** bone, which serves as the floor of the anatomic snuffbox, making it easily identifiable and a good starting point for palpating the carpals. Actively extending the thumb and first metacarpal makes the abductor pollicis longus, extensor pollicis brevis, and extensor pollicis longus more distinct. The scaphoid is located within these two boundaries (Fig. 17-18). To differentiate between the scaphoid and trapezium bones, palpate the wrist just distal from the radius while the wrist is ulnarly deviated. The scaphoid bone will be felt to "pop" into position under the finger. The distal tuberosity of the scaphoid can be palpated on the palmar side of the hand.

10 Lunate: Return to the scaphoid bone and then move medially toward the ulna. The **lunate** is prominent across the joint line from the medial radial head, approximately in line with the third metacarpal. Locate the lunate by first finding Lister's tubercle on the dorsal aspect of the distal radius. From there palpate distally and slightly medially to locate a depression in the joint line. The lunate will fill this void as the patient's wrist is passively flexed. The space between the scaphoid and lunate, the scapholunate interval is a frequent site of sprains and is palpable 1.5 cm distal to Lister's tubercle.[13]

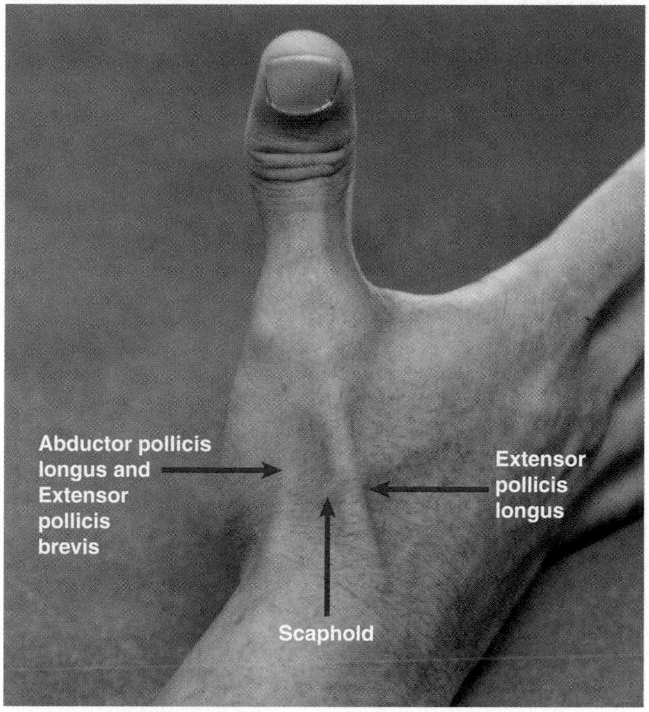

FIGURE 17-18 ■ Borders of the anatomical snuffbox.

11 Triquetrum: Palpate the **triquetrum** along the most proximal aspect of the hand approximately one finger's breadth distal to the ulnar styloid process. The triquetrum is the second most commonly fractured carpal bone.[19] The hamate and pisiform are palpated on the palmar aspect of the wrist.

12 Trapezium: Locate and palpate the **trapezium** between the scaphoid bone and the thumb's metacarpal.

13 Capitate: Move toward the thumb side of the hand to locate the **capitate**, just proximal to the base of the third metacarpal on the palmar aspect of the hand.

14 Trapezoid: Locate the **trapezoid** lying at the base of the second metacarpal. This structure is more easily palpated from the dorsal aspect of the hand.

15 Extensor carpi radialis brevis (ECRB): Palpate the **ECRB** at its insertion on the base of the third metacarpal.

16 Extensor carpi radialis longus (ECRL): Acting in concert with the ECRB to extend the wrist, the **ECRL** insertion is palpable at the base of the second metacarpal. Resisted wrist extension makes both the ECRL and ECRB more palpable.

Palpation of the Hand

The intrinsic muscles of the hand cannot be individually identified during palpation. The palpation of these structures is broken down into compartmental zones: thenar eminence, central compartment, and hypothenar eminence.

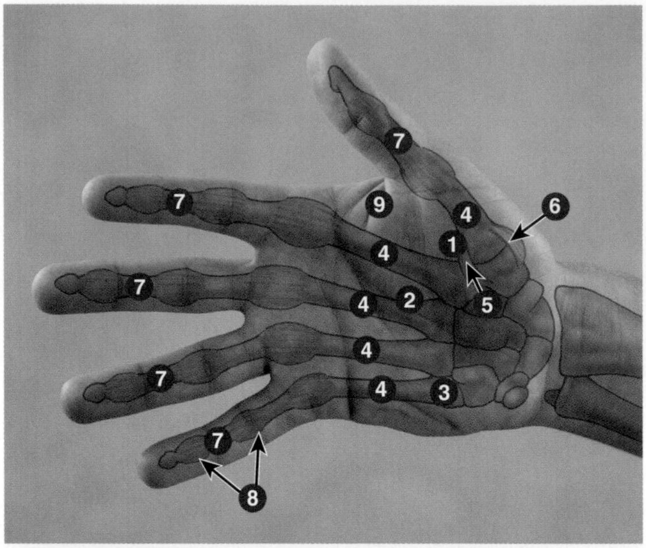

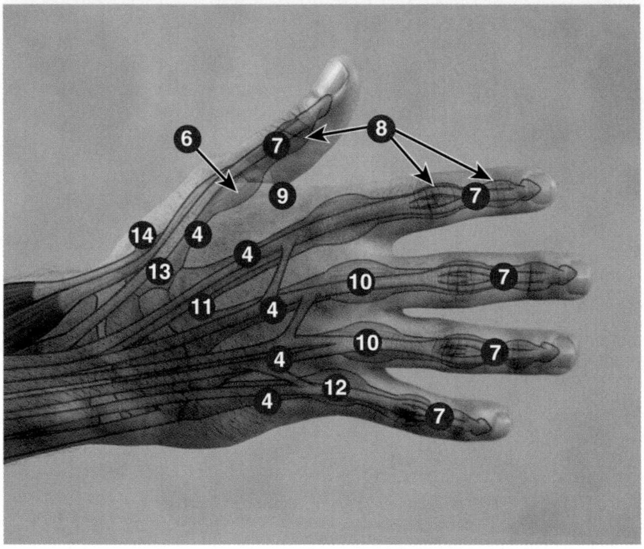

1 **Thenar eminence:** The small but prominent muscles of the **thenar eminence** are palpated near the base of the thumb. The opponens pollicis sits deep within the compartment, covered by the abductor pollicis brevis and the flexor pollicis brevis muscles and the tendon of the flexor pollicis longus tendon. Note any atrophy, which may result from prolonged compression of the median nerve.

2 **Central compartment:** Lying between the thenar and hypothenar compartments, the palmar aponeurosis is the most superficial structure within the **central compartment**. Palpation along the metacarpals may reveal the fingers' flexor tendons.

3 **Hypothenar compartment:** The **hypothenar** mass is palpated along the ulnar border of the palm. The muscles within this area the components of the hypothenar compartment (i.e., abductor digiti minimi, flexor digiti minimi brevis, and opponens digiti minimi) cannot be individually identified via palpation.

4 **Metacarpals:** All five **metacarpals** are palpable along their entire length. Begin the palpation of each metacarpal at the MCP joint and proceed proximally to the CMC joint, noting for areas of pain, deformity, or crepitation.

5-6 **Collateral ligaments of the metacarpophalangeal joints:** The **(5) UCL** and **(6) RCL** of the thumb are relatively subcutaneous as they cross the first MCP joint. The RCL of the second MCP joint and the UCL of the fifth MCP joint are the only other collateral ligaments directly palpable.

7 **Phalanges:** Each **phalanx** of the fingers is palpated for the presence of pain, crepitus, or deformity. The flares adjoining the bases and heads with the shafts are frequent sites of avulsion fractures. A direct blow to the fingertip or forceful abduction or adduction to the IP joints are common fracture mechanisms.

8 **Collateral ligaments of the IP joints:** The **collateral ligaments** of each of the nine **IP joints** are easily palpated as they cross the joint line. Palpate these ligaments from their origin on the proximal bone to their insertion on the distal bone.

9 **Thenar webspace:** The adductor pollicis is palpated within the **thenar webspace** between the thumb and index finger and is more prominent if the thumb is actively extended.

10-12. **Extensor digitorum:** The tendons of the **extensor digitorum** are palpated along its distal length, where it becomes tendinous and splits into four tendons leading to the fingers. The little and index fingers have independent tendons, the **(11) extensor indicis** and the **(12) extensor digiti minimi**.

13 **Extensor pollicis longus (EPL):** Serving as the ulnar border of the anatomic snuffbox, the **EPL** is most prominent when the thumb is extended.

14 **Abductor pollicis longus and extensor pollicis brevis:** These muscles serve as the radial border of the anatomic snuffbox. The scaphoid is found between these tendons and the EPL tendon.

Joint and Muscle Function Assessment

A summary of the end-feels obtained from passive ROM (PROM) assessment of the wrist, hand, fingers, and thumb is presented in Table 17-3.

Wrist Joint and Muscle Function Assessment

The motions of pronation and supination of the forearm are described in Chapter 16. Measurement of wrist flexion/extension and radial/ulnar deviation is presented in Goniometry 17-1.

Table 17-3 Normal End-Feels Obtained During Passive Range of Motion Testing

Area	Motion	End-Feel	Tissues
Wrist	Flexion	Firm	Dorsal radiocarpal ligament and joint capsule
	Extension	Firm	Palmar radiocarpal ligament and joint capsule
	Radial deviation	Hard	Scaphoid striking styloid process of radius
	Ulnar deviation	Firm	Radiocarpal ligaments and tendons
Thumb (CMC)	Flexion	Soft	Approximation of thenar eminence and the palm
	Extension	Firm	Palmar joint capsule, flexor pollicis brevis, opponens pollicis, first dorsal interossei
	Abduction	Firm	Stretching of the webspace
	Adduction	Soft	Approximation of thenar eminence and palm
Fingers and Thumb (MCP)	Flexion	Hard	Proximal phalanx contacts the metacarpal
	Extension	Firm	Tension in the volar plate
	Abduction	Firm	Stretching of the collateral ligaments and webspace
	Adduction	Firm	Stretching of the collateral ligaments and webspace
Fingers (PIP)	Flexion	Hard	Proximal and middle phalanges contact
	Extension	Firm	Stretching of the volar plate
Fingers (DIP) and Thumb (IP)	Flexion	Firm	Tension in dorsal joint capsule and collateral ligaments
	Extension	Firm	Stretching of palmar joint capsule and volar plate

CMC = carpometacarpal; DIP = distal interphalangeal; IP = interphalangeal; MCP = metacarpophalangeal; PIP = proximal interphalangeal

Active Range of Motion

- **Flexion and extension:** A total of 155 to 175 degrees of motion occurs in the sagittal plane around a coronal (medial–lateral) axis. Flexion accounts for 80 to 90 degrees, and extension ranges from 75 to 85 degrees. The fingers should be relaxed to assess the maximum amount of motion. Holding the fingers extended while extending the wrist and flexed while flexing the wrist helps determine the length of the FDP/FDS and EDC, respectively.
- **Radial and ulnar deviation:** Approximately 55 degrees of motion are permitted through the range of radial and ulnar deviation. This motion occurs in the frontal plane around an anteroposterior axis. From the neutral position, 35 degrees of ulnar deviation and 20 degrees of radial deviation are permitted by the joint structure. Normally, the proximal carpal row smoothly moves from a flexed position to an extended position as the wrist moves from radial to ulnar deviation. In individuals with a midcarpal instability, this transition may be abrupt, resulting in a clunk as the wrist moves from radial to ulnar deviation.[20] "Clicking" during ulnar deviation can indicate a tear of the triangular fibrocartilage complex (see p. 784).

Manual Muscle Tests

It is difficult to differentiate between specific muscles during single-plane motions such as wrist extension and wrist flexion; therefore, the components of ulnar and radial deviation should be incorporated (Manual Muscle Test 17-1). The muscles that flex and radially deviate the wrist are primarily supplied by the median nerve. The ulnar nerve innervates the muscles that flex and ulnarly deviate the wrist. The muscles that extend and radially deviate the wrist are supplied by the deep radial nerve. Because resisting range of motion (ROM) throughout the range can provoke symptoms from tissues other than the muscle, an isometric test in the midrange of a movement is recommended to detect muscle weakness or pain.

Passive Range of Motion

- **Flexion and extension:** Position the wrist over the edge of the table with the elbow flexed to 90 degrees, the forearm pronated, and the hand facing downward. Stabilize the forearm to prevent pronation and supination. The fingers should be relaxed (Figs. 17-19A and B).
- **Radial and ulnar deviation:** With the wrist, hand, and forearm resting on the table to prevent extension and flexion, note the relative difference in motion between radial and ulnar deviation (Figs. 17-19C and D).

Thumb Joint and Muscle Function Assessment: Carpometacarpal Joint

The degrees of freedom of motion and the ROM allowed by the first CMC joint are markedly different from the other CMC joints (Goniometry 17-2). Although abduction and adduction of the fingers occur in the frontal plane, abduction and adduction of the CMC joint (palmar abduction and adduction) occur in the sagittal plane. Likewise, flexion and extension of the fingers occur in the sagittal plane. At

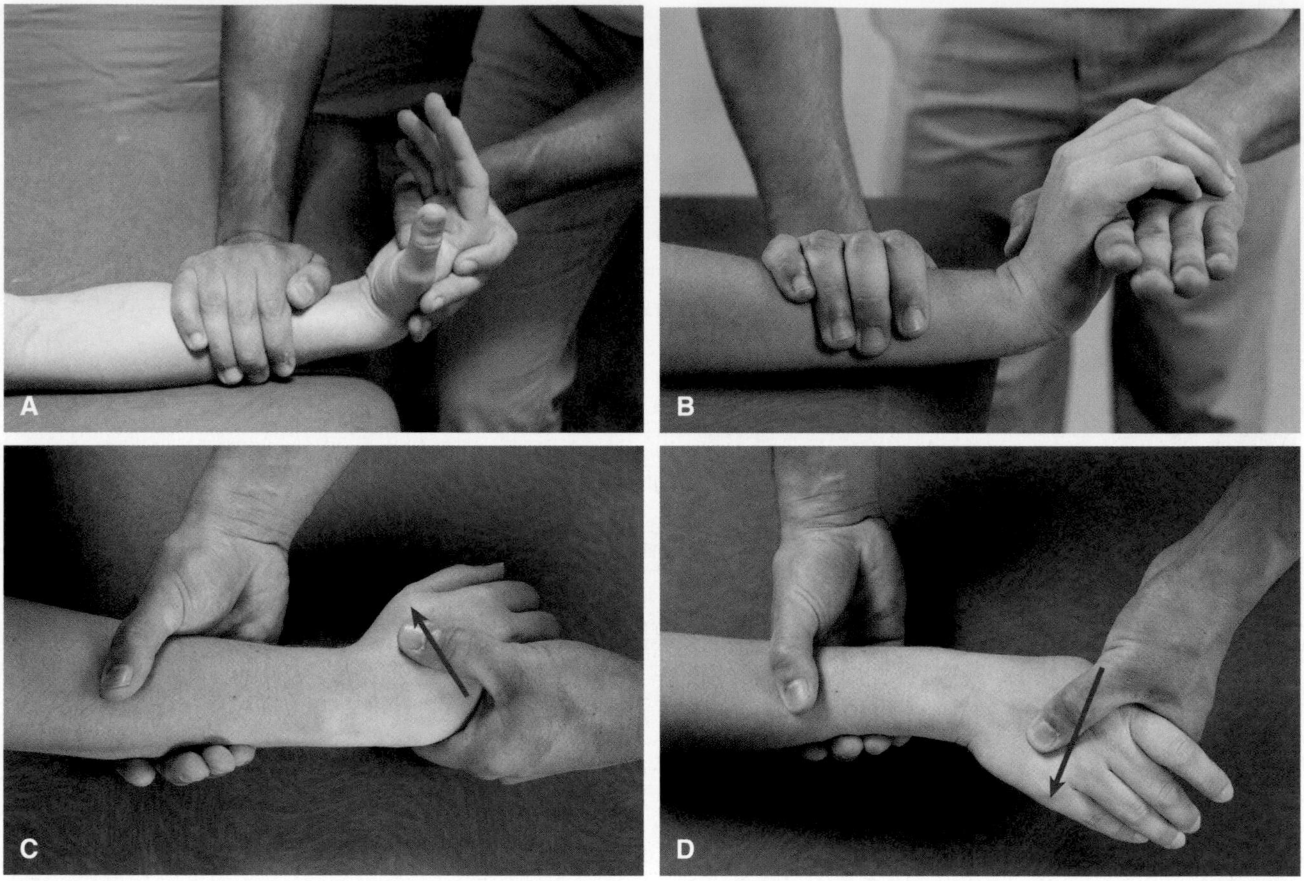

FIGURE 17-19 ■ Passive range of motion of the wrist: (A) flexion; (B) extension; (C) radial deviation; (D) ulnar deviation.

the CMC joint, these motions occur in the frontal plane. In functional terms, extension occurs when the thumb is put in a "hitchhiker position"; the CMC joint is placed in abduction when gripping a can.

Active Range of Motion

- **Flexion and extension:** Thumb CMC flexion and extension occur in the frontal plane around an anteroposterior axis. The majority of this motion, 60 to 70 degrees, is flexion (Fig. 17-20).
- **Abduction and adduction:** In the anatomical position, this motion occurs in the sagittal plane around a coronal axis at the CMC. Abduction accounts for the total motion of 70 to 80 degrees. True adduction is limited by the phalanx striking the second metacarpal.
- **Opposition:** Opposition is the combined motion of flexion, abduction, and rotation of the thumb and is demonstrated by touching the thumb to the little finger (see Fig. 17-17).

Manual Muscle Tests

Manual muscle tests (MMTs) for the muscles controlling the thumb are presented in Manual Muscle Tests 17-2, 17-3, and 17-4.

Passive Range of Motion

- **Flexion and extension:** Flexion and extension are measured with the forearm supinated and resting on a table with the wrist and IP joint in the neutral position. The carpal bones are stabilized to prevent wrist motion.
- **Abduction and adduction:** The medial forearm is rested on the table in the neutral position. The wrist, CMC, MCP, and IP joints are placed in 0 degrees of extension. Stabilization is provided to the carpal bones and second metacarpal.
- **Opposition:** The forearm is fully supinated, and the wrist is placed in its neutral position. The examiner brings the thumb and fifth finger toward each other. Normally, the two fingers should touch each other.

Finger Joint and Muscle Function Assessment

Each finger's range of motion, strength, and end-feel should be assessed independently (Goniometry 17-3).

Active Range of Motion

- **Flexion and extension of the MCP joints:** Flexion and extension of the MCP joints occur in the sagittal plane around a coronal axis. A maximum of 105 to 135 degrees of motion is allowed at the MCP joint, with 20 to 30 degrees occurring during extension and the remaining 85 to 105 degrees accounted for during flexion.
- Locking that occurs during finger flexion can indicate "**trigger finger**," adhesions in the flexor tendon sheath

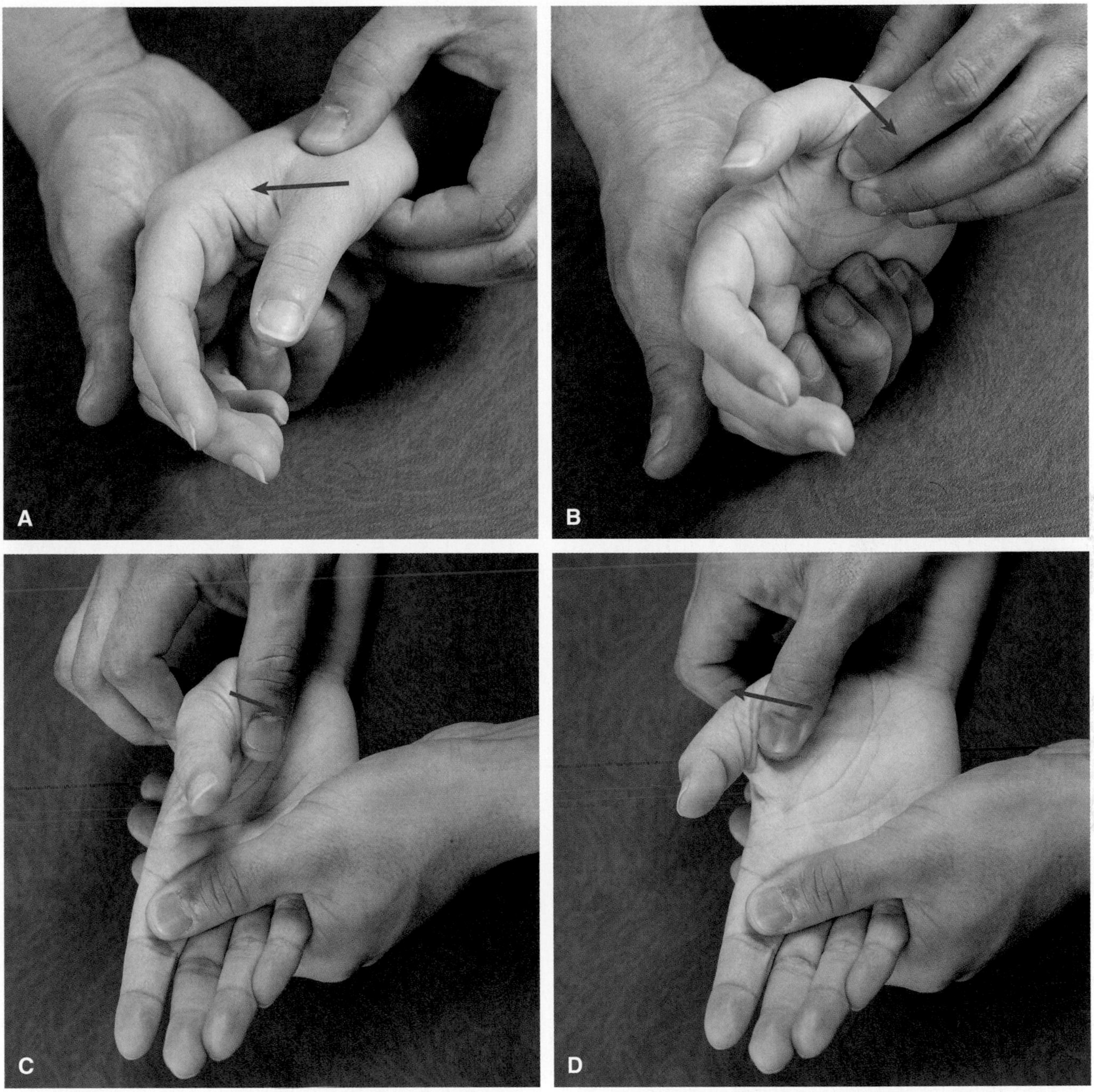

FIGURE 17-20 ■ Active range of motion of the first carpometacarpal joint: (A) CMC adduction, (B) CMC abduction, (C) CMC flexion, (D) CMC extension. Do not confuse CMC motion with motion produced by the MP joint.

(see Box 17-1). During active flexion, the sheath adheres to the surrounding tissues and requires additional effort to gain flexion. As the tendon releases, an audible snap is heard, and the finger snaps into flexion. During the latter stages of this condition, full flexion may be restricted.

- **Abduction and adduction of the MCP joints:** Twenty to 25 degrees of motion are allowed during abduction and the return motion of adduction. The movement occurs in the frontal plane around an anteroposterior axis with the third metacarpal serving as the reference point.
- **Flexion and extension of the IP joints:** Flexion and extension of the IP joints range from 80 to 90 degrees at the thumb, 100 to 110 degrees at the PIP, and 70 to 90 degrees at the DIP joints of the fingers.

Manual Muscle Tests

Manual Muscle Tests for the fingers are presented in Manual Muscle Tests 17-5, 17-6, and 17-7. A handheld dynamometer provides reliable information regarding grip strength (Selective Tissue Test 17-1), which increases until age 35 and then declines as aging continues.[21]

Goniometry 17-1
Wrist

	Flexion to Extension	Radial and Ulnar Deviation
	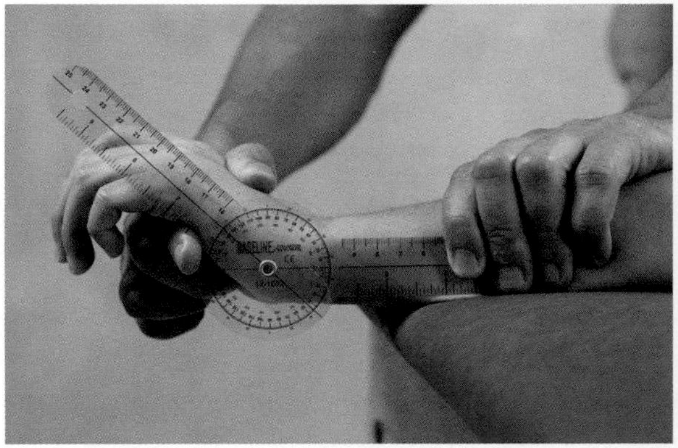 Flexion to Extension (90°–0°–85°)	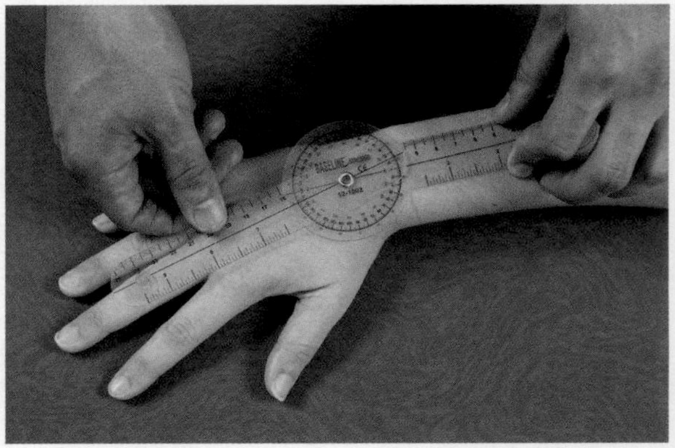 Radial and Ulnar Deviation (20°–0°–85°)
Patient Position	Forearm is pronated with the hand off the edge of the table. Elbow is flexed to 90°. During wrist flexion, the fingers are allowed to extend. During wrist extension, the fingers are allowed to flex.	Forearm is pronated with the hand resting on the table. Elbow is flexed to 90°.
Goniometer Alignment		
Fulcrum	Center the axis over the ulnar styloid process.	Center the axis over the dorsal surface of the capitate.
Proximal Arm	Align the stationary arm along the midline of the ulnar shaft.	Align the stationary arm along the midline of the forearm.
Distal Arm	Align the movement arm parallel to the longitudinal axis of the 5th metacarpal.	Align the movement arm over the 3rd metacarpal.
Comments	During measurement of PROM, apply the overpressure evenly at the dorsum of the metacarpals to avoid rotation at the wrist.	Avoid wrist extension during the measurement. Popping during ulnar deviation may be indicative of a tear of the TFCC.
Evidence	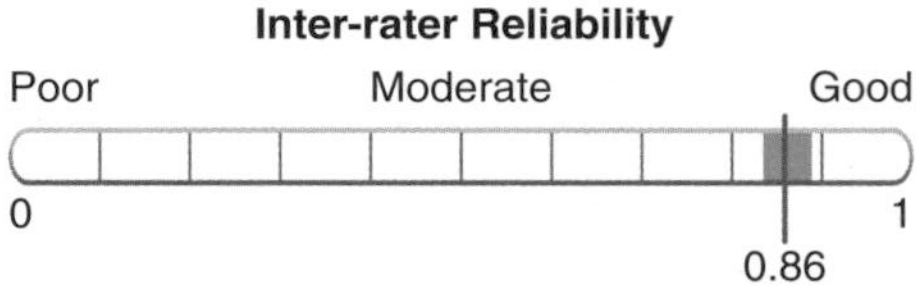 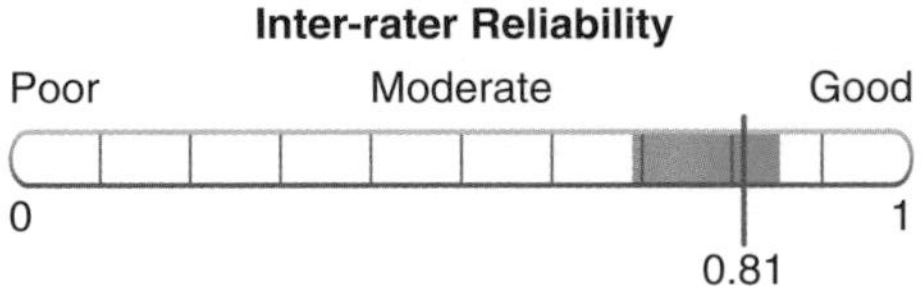	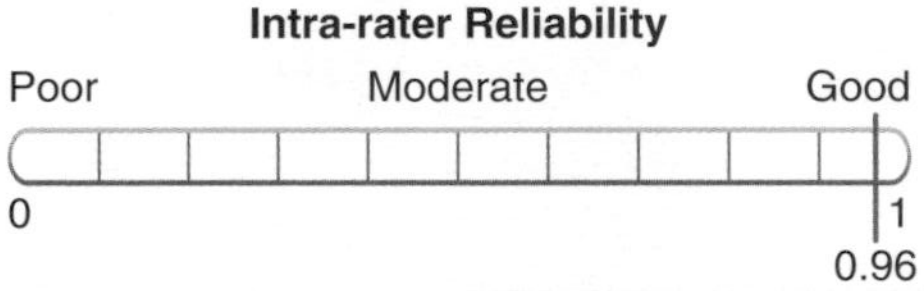 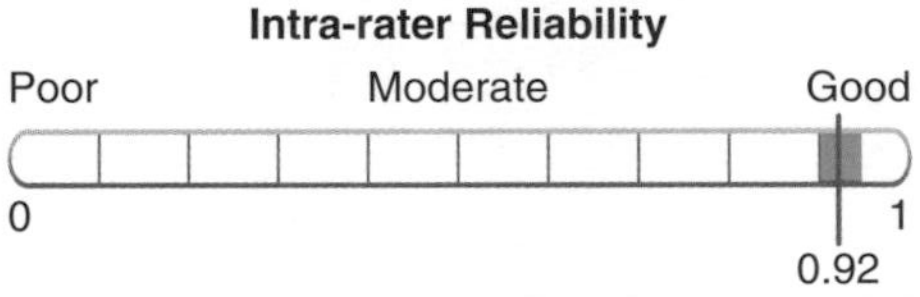

Manual Muscle Test 17-1
Wrist

	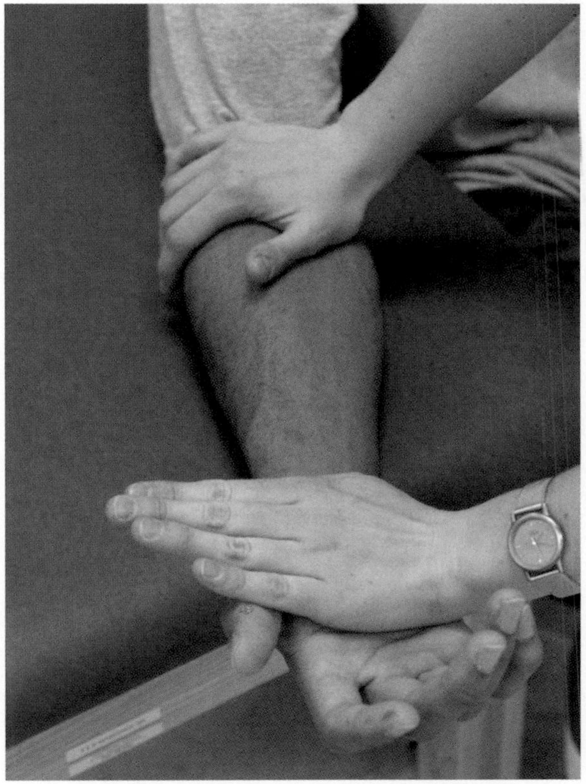 Flexion and Radial Deviation/Flexion and Ulnar Deviation	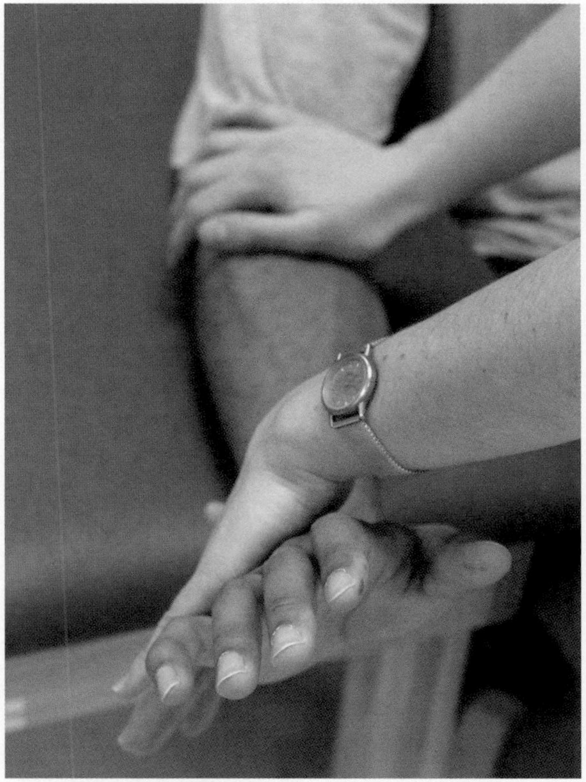 Extension and Radial Deviation/Extension and Ulnar Deviation
Patient Position	Seated	Seated
Test Position	The elbow is flexed to 90°, the forearm is supinated, and the wrist is slightly flexed off the end of the table and ulnarly deviated (FCU) or radially deviated (FCR).	The elbow is flexed to 90°. The forearm is pronated, and the wrist is slightly extended and radially deviated (ECRB/ECRL) or ulnarly deviated (ECU), with the fingers in a relaxed position.
Stabilization	Anterior portion of the mid-forearm	Posterior portion of the mid-forearm
Resistance	FCR: Thenar eminence FCU: Hypothenar eminence	Dorsal surface of the hand

Continued

Manual Muscle Test 17-1
Wrist—cont'd

Primary Movers (Innervation)	*Flexion and radial deviation:* Flexor carpi radialis (median: C6, C7) *Flexion and ulnar deviation:* Flexor carpi ulnaris (ulnar: C8, T1)	*Extension and radial deviation:* Extensor carpi radialis longus (radial: C6, C7) Extensor carpi radialis brevis (radial: C6, C7) *Extension and ulnar deviation:* Extensor carpi ulnaris (DR: C6, C7, C8)
Secondary Movers (Innervation)	*Flexion and radial deviation:* Flexor carpi ulnaris (ulnar: C8, T1) Palmaris longus (median: C6, C7) Flexor digitorum profundus (PI: C8, T1) Flexor digitorum superficialis (median: C7, C8, T1) Flexor pollicis longus (PI: C8, T1) *Flexion and ulnar deviation:* Flexor carpi radialis (median: C6, C7) Palmaris longus (median: C6, C7) Flexor digitorum profundus (ulnar: C8, T1) Flexor digitorum superficialis (Median: C7, C8, T1) Flexor pollicis longus (PI: C8, T1)	*Extension and radial deviation:* Extensor carpi ulnaris (DR: C6, C7, C8) Extensor digitorum communis (DR: C6, C7, C8) Extensor pollicis longus (DR: C6, C7, C8) *Extension and ulnar deviation:* Extensor carpi radialis longus (radial: C6, C7) Extensor carpi radialis brevis (radial: C6, C7) Extensor digitorum communis (DR: C6, C7, C8) Extensor pollicis longus (DR: C6, C7, C8)
Substitution	*Flexion and radial deviation:* Ulnar deviation, finger flexion *Flexion and ulnar deviation:* Radial deviation, finger flexion	*Extension and radial deviation:* Ulnar deviation, finger extension *Extension and ulnar deviation:* Radial deviation, finger extension
Comments	To minimize contributions from the FDS and FDP, the fingers should not flex during the test.	To minimize contributions from the extensor pollicis longus and extensor digitorum communis, instruct the patient to keep the fingers relaxed during the test.

DR = deep radial nerve; ECRB = extensor carpi radialis brevis; ECRL = extensor carpi radialis longus; ECU = extensor carpi ulnaris; FCR = flexor carpi radialis; FCU = flexor carpi ulnaris; FDP = flexor digitorum profundus; FDS = flexor digitorum superficialis; PI = palmar interosseous nerve

Goniometry 17-2
Thumb

	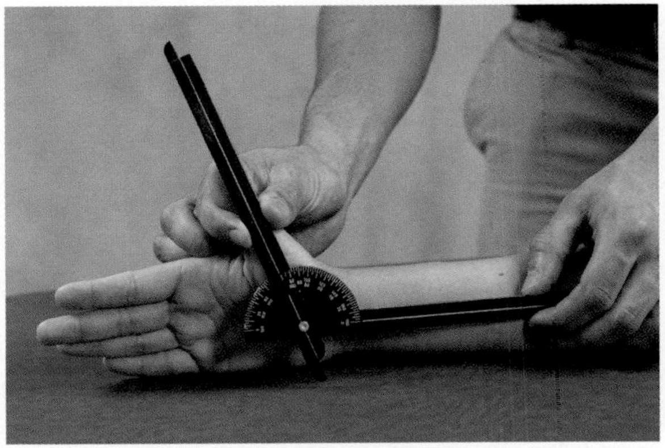 CMC Flexion/Extension (15°– 0°–20°)	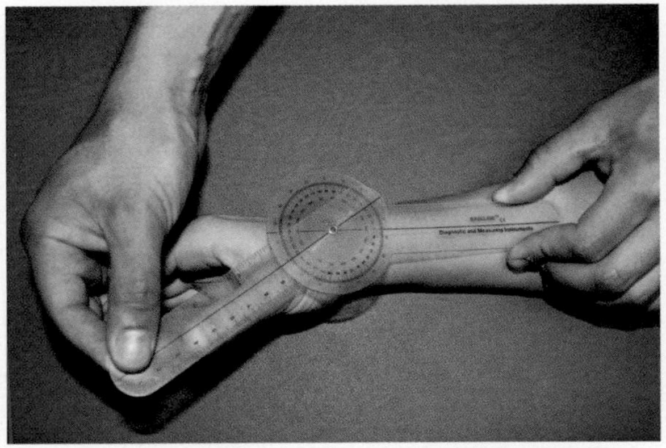 CMC Abduction (0°–70°)
Patient Position	The patient is sitting with the elbow flexed to 90°, and the forearm is in full supination. The forearm and hand are supported on the table. The wrist is in its neutral position.	The patient is seated with the elbow flexed to 90° and the forearm midway between supination and pronation. The forearm and hand are supported on the table. The wrist is in its neutral position.
Goniometer Alignment		
Fulcrum	Center the axis on the palmar aspect of the 1st CMC.	Center the axis on the lateral aspect of the radial styloid.
Proximal Arm	Align the stationary arm parallel to the shaft of the radius.	Align the stationary arm parallel to the shaft of the second metacarpal.
Distal Arm	Align the movement arm parallel to the shaft of the first metacarpal.	Align the movement arm parallel to the shaft of the first metacarpal.
Comments	Flexion and extension occur in the frontal plane. When measuring PROM, apply overpressure at the distal metacarpal instead of the proximal phalanx. The initial position of the goniometer is considered the start or position.	Abduction occurs at a right angle to the palm of the hand. When measuring PROM, apply overpressure at the distal metacarpal instead of the proximal phalanx. Stabilize the 2nd metacarpal. The initial position of the goniometer is considered the start or zero

CMC = carpometacarpal; PROM = passive range of motion

Manual Muscle Test 17-2

Thumb: MCP and IP Flexion and Extension

	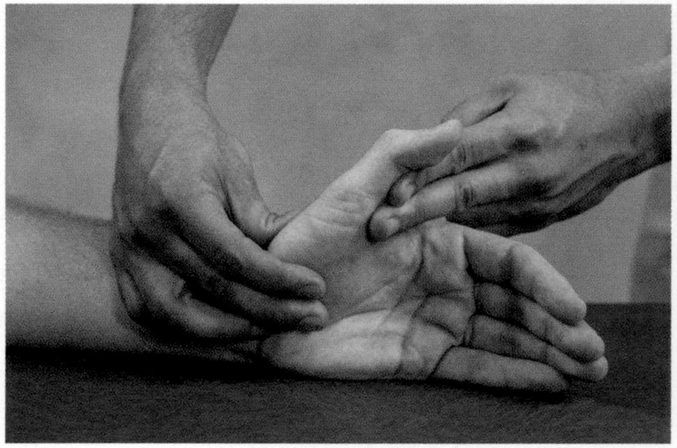 Flexion	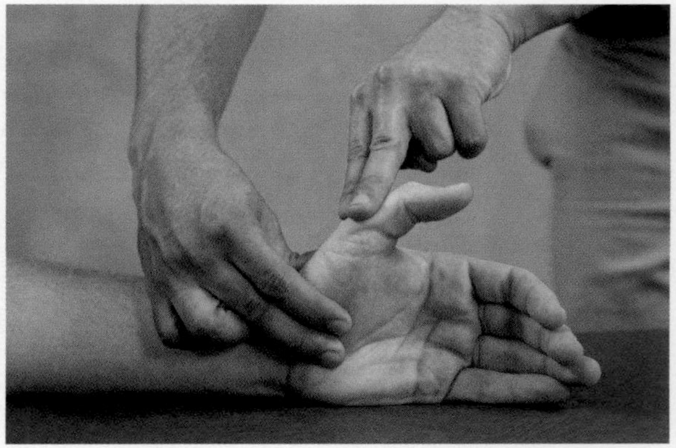 Extension
Patient Position	Seated, elbow flexed 90°, forearm supinated, and test hand resting on the tabletop	Seated, elbow flexed 90°, forearm in midposition resting on the tabletop
Test Position	MCP flexion: Wrist in neutral with MCP joint slightly flexed IP flexion: Wrist and MCP in neutral with IP joint slightly flexed	MCP extension: Wrist in neutral with MCP and IP joints flexed IP extension: Wrist in neutral with IP joint flexed
Stabilization	MCP flexion: First metacarpal IP flexion: Proximal phalanx	MCP extension: First metacarpal IP extension: Proximal phalanx
Resistance	MCP flexion: Palmar aspect, proximal phalanx IP flexion: Palmar aspect, distal phalanx	MCP extension: Dorsal aspect, proximal phalanx IP extension: Dorsal aspect: distal phalanx
Primary Movers (Innervation)	***MCP flexion:*** Flexor pollicis brevis (DPB: C6, C7, C8, T1) ***IP flexion:*** Flexor pollicis longus (PI: C8, T1)	***MCP extension:*** Extensor pollicis brevis (DR: C6, C7) ***IP extension:*** Extensor pollicis longus (DR: C6, C7, C8)
Secondary Movers (Innervation)	***MCP flexion:*** Flexor pollicis longus (PI: C8, T1) IP flexion: None	***MCP extension:*** Extensor pollicis longus (DR: C6, C7, C8) IP extension: None
Substitution	MCP flexion: Do not allow IP joint flexion.	MCP extension: Do not allow IP joint extension.

DR = deep radial nerve; DPB = deep palmar branch (median nerve); IP = interphalangeal; MCP = metacarpophalangeal; PI = palmar interosseous nerve

Manual Muscle Test 17-3
First Carpometacarpal Joint Abduction and Adduction

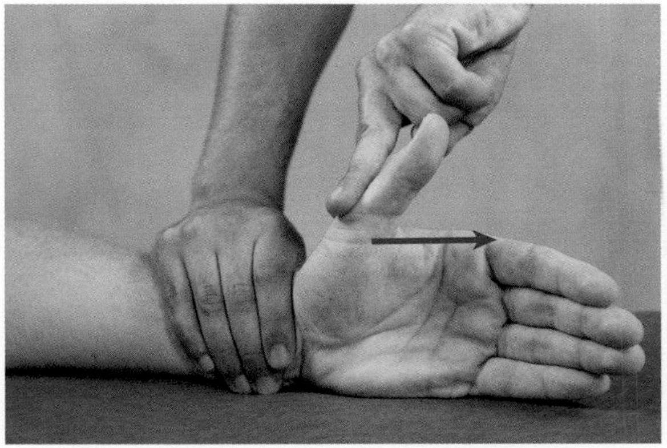

Abduction

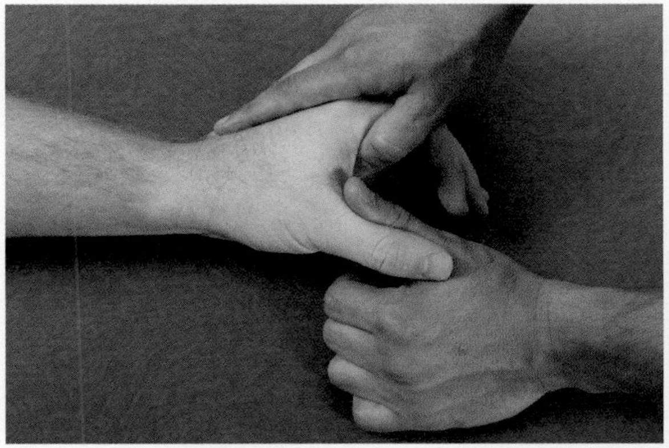

Adduction

	Abduction	Adduction
Patient Position	Seated; elbow flexed to 90°; forearm supinated with hand resting on tabletop	Seated; the elbow flexed to 90°; forearm supinated with hand resting on tabletop
Test Position	CMC in midrange of abduction	Thumb in palmar abduction with MCP and IP joints relaxed and slightly flexed
Stabilization	Wrist and lateral four metacarpals	Wrist and lateral four metacarpals
Resistance	Distal lateral aspect of 1st metacarpal	Medial border of the proximal phalanx
Primary Movers (Innervation)	Abductor pollicis brevis (median: C6, C7)	Adductor pollicis (DPB: C8, T1)
Secondary Movers (Innervation)	Abductor pollicis longus (median: C6, C7) Extensor pollicis brevis (DR: C6, C7)	Flexor pollicis brevis (DPB: C6, C7, C8, T1)
Substitution	Radial abduction	Not applicable
Comments	Provide resistance to abduction with the thumb at a 45° angle from the sagittal plane to better isolate the abductor pollicis longus. This is sometimes called radial abduction.	Maintain IP and MCP flexion during the test.

CMC = carpometacarpal; DR = deep radial nerve, DPB = deep palmar branch (median nerve); IP = interphalangeal; MCP = metacarpophalangeal

Manual Muscle Test 17-4
Opposition (First and Fifth Carpometacarpal Joint Flexion)

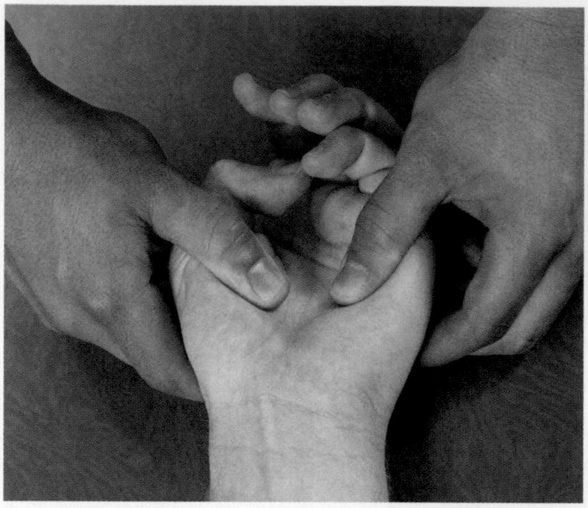

Patient Position	Seated; elbow flexed to 90°; forearm supinated with hand resting on tabletop
Test Position	The thumb and 5th fingers opposed
Stabilization	Not applicable
Resistance	The examiner attempts to separate the fingers, applying resistance at the distal 1st and 5th metacarpals.
Primary Movers (Innervation)	Opponens pollicis (median: C6, C7) Opponens digiti minimi (ulnar: C8, T1)
Secondary Movers (Innervation)	Abductor pollicis brevis (median: C6, C7) Flexor pollicis brevis (DPB: C6, C7, C8, T1)
Substitution	IP joint and wrist flexion

DPB = deep palmar branch (median nerve); IP = interphalangeal

Goniometry 17-3
Finger

	Flexion/Extension	Abduction/Adduction
	 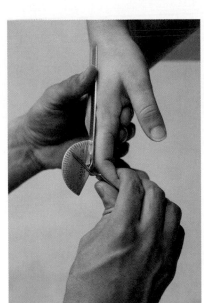 Flexion/Extension (MCP, PIP, and DIP) MCP = 90°–0°–45° PIP = 0°–100° (flexion) DIP = 0°–90° (flexion)	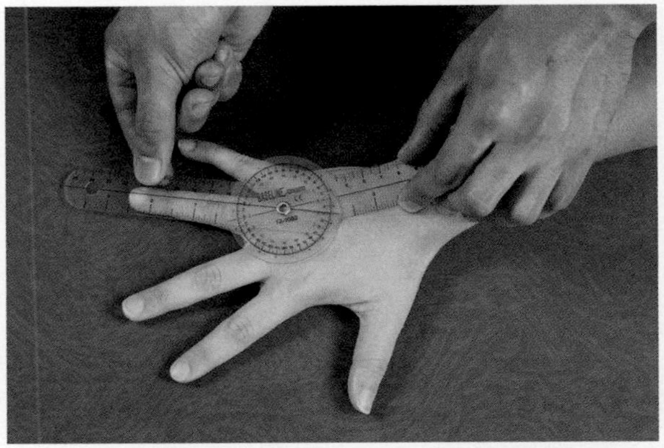 Abduction and Adduction (MCP)
Patient Position	The patient is sitting with the elbow flexed to 90° and the forearm in midposition. The forearm and hand are supported on the table. The wrist is in its neutral position.	The patient is sitting with the elbow flexed to 90° and the forearm pronated with the hand flat on the table. The wrist is in its neutral position.
Goniometer Alignment		
Fulcrum	Flexion: Positioned over the dorsal aspect of the joint being tested Extension: Positioned over the palmar aspect of the joint being tested	Positioned over the dorsal aspect of the MCP joint
Proximal Arm	The stationary arm is centered on the midline of the bone proximal to the joint being tested.	The stationary arm is aligned over the metacarpal of the joint being tested.
Distal Arm	The movement arm is centered on the midline of the bone distal to the joint being tested.	The movement arm is centered over the proximal phalanx of the joint being tested.
Comments	Stabilize the joints proximal to the joint being measured. Flexion and extension of the MCP of the index finger may be measured on the radial aspect. The same positioning is used to measure MCP and IP flexion and extension of the thumb.	Other fingers may need to be moved to permit full adduction.

DIP = distal interphalangeal; IP = interphalangeal; MCP = metacarpophalangeal; PIP = proximal interphalangeal

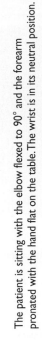

Manual Muscle Test 17-5
PIP and DIP Flexion

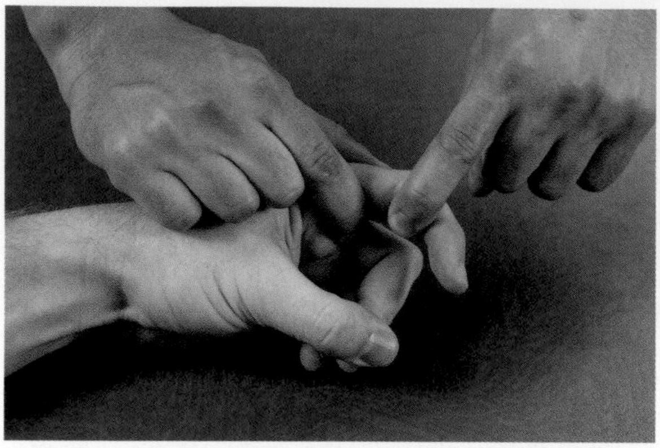
PIP Flexion

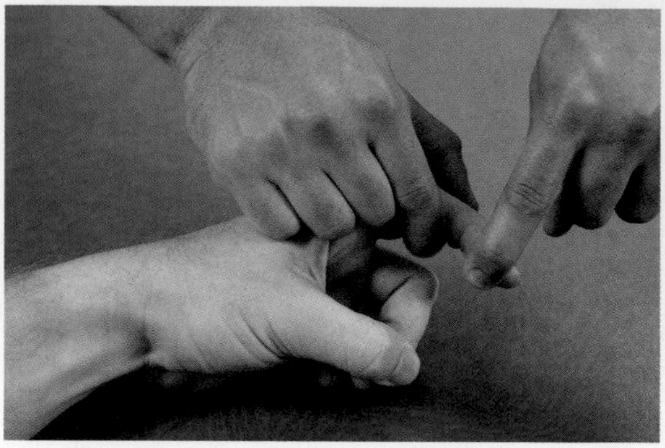
DIP Flexion

	PIP Flexion	DIP Flexion
Patient Position	Seated; forearm in supination and resting on table	Seated; forearm in supination and resting on table
Test Position	Test joint in midflexion	Test joint in flexion
Stabilization	Proximal phalanx	Middle phalanx
Resistance	Palmar surface, middle phalanx	Palmar surface, distal phalanx
Primary Movers (Innervation)	Flexor digitorum superficialis (C7, C8, T1)	Flexor digitorum profundus (C8, T1)
Secondary Movers (Innervation)	Flexor digitorum profundus (C8, T1)	None
Substitution	DIP flexion (FDP)	None
Comments	Maintain nontest fingers in extension to limit contribution from the FDP.[22]	

DIP = distal interphalangeal; FDP = flexor digitorum profundus; PIP = proximal interphalangeal

Manual Muscle Test 17-6
MCP Abduction and Adduction

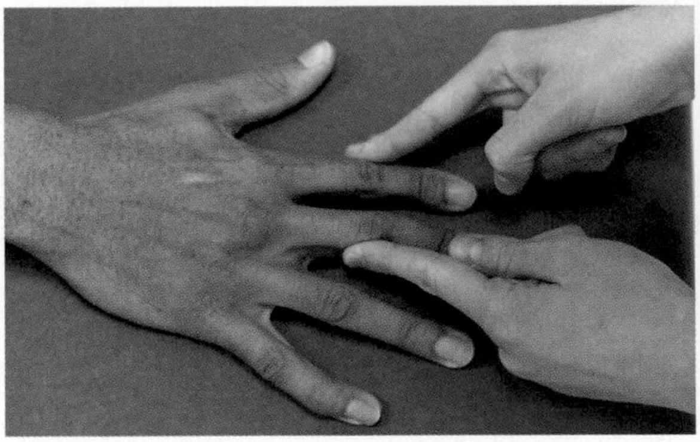

Abduction

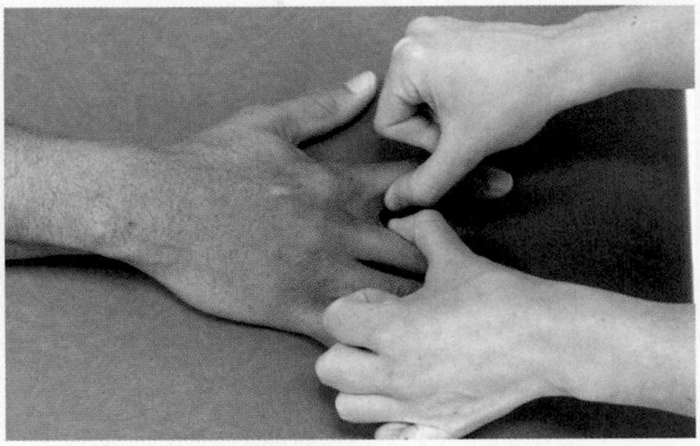

Adduction

	Abduction	Adduction
Patient Position	Seated; elbow flexed to 90°; forearm pronated and hand resting on table	Seated; elbow flexed to 90°; forearm supinated and hand resting on table
Test Position	Test joint in neutral position.	The MCP joints are abducted.
Stabilization	Dorsum of hand	Dorsum of hand
Resistance	Proximal phalanx of test finger	Proximal phalanx of test finger
Primary Movers (Innervation)	Dorsal interossei (C8, T1) Abductor digiti minimi (5th finger) (C8, T1)	Palmar interossei (C8, T1)
Secondary Movers (Innervation)	None	None
Substitution	MCP flexion	MCP flexion
Comments	To test all four dorsal interossei, apply resistance to abduction at the ulnar aspect of the ring finger, at the radial and ulnar aspect of the middle finger, and at the radial aspect of the index finger.	To test the three palmar interossei, apply resistance to adduction at the radial aspect of the little finger, the radial aspect of the ring finger, and the radial aspect of the index finger.

MCP = metacarpophalangeal

Manual Muscle Test 17-7
Finger MCP Extension and Flexion with IP Extension

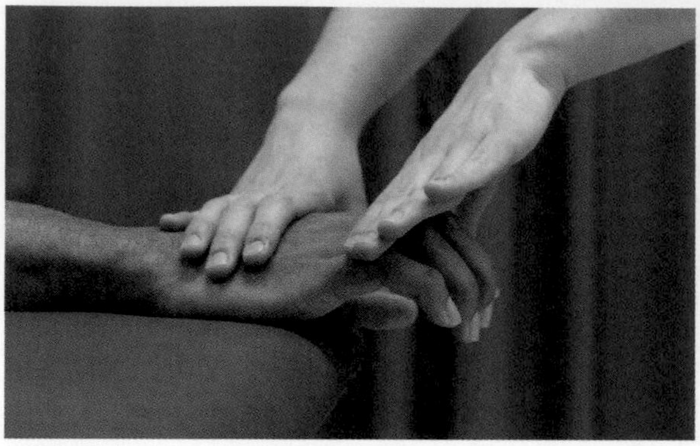

MCP Extension

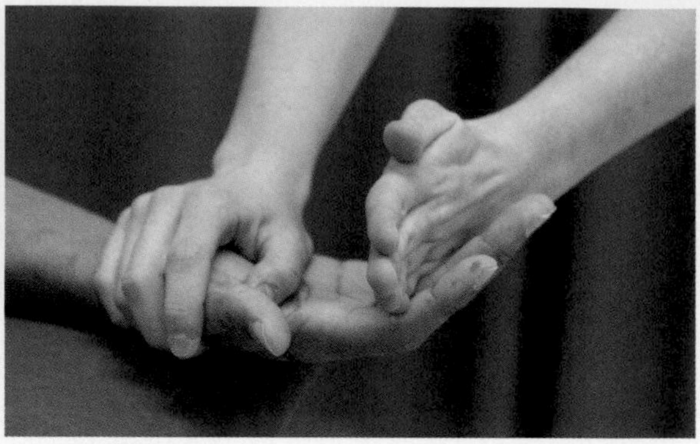

Flexion With IP Extension

	MCP Extension	Flexion With IP Extension
Patient Position	Seated; elbow in 90° of flexion; forearm pronated; wrist in neutral	Seated; elbow in 90° of flexion; forearm supinated and hand resting on the table
Test Position	MCP in extension and IP joints flexed	MCP and PIP joints are slightly flexed
Stabilization	Metacarpals	Metacarpals
Resistance	Dorsal aspect, proximal phalanx of the test finger	Palmar aspect, proximal phalanx (to resist MCP flexion); dorsal aspect, middle phalanx (to resist PIP extension)
Primary Movers (Innervation)	Extensor digitorum communis (C6, C7, C8) Extensor indicis (radial: C6, C7, C8) Extensor digiti minimi (radial: C6, C7, C8)	Lumbricals (C6, C7, C8, T1)
Secondary Movers (Innervation)	None	Flexor digiti minimi (Ulnar: C8, T1) Dorsal interossei (C8, T1) Palmar interossei (C8, T1)
Substitution	Wrist extension	Wrist flexion
Comments	Test MCP extension of all fingers at the same time. IP joint flexion should be maintained during the test. To assess for extensor digitorum communis tendon rupture, have the patient attempt to actively extend the involved joint while stabilizing the proximal segment.	Resist PIP extension and MCP flexion simultaneously. MCP flexion also occurs via the interossei. The flexor digiti minimi can be tested by resisting MCP flexion of the little finger.

IP = interphalangeal; MCP = metacarpophalangeal; PIP = proximal interphalangeal

Selective Tissue Test 17-1
Grip Dynamometry

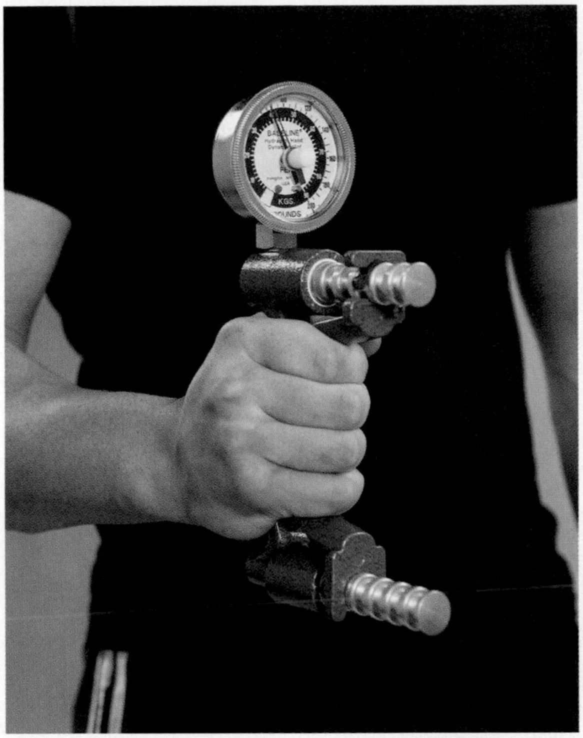

Use of a grip dynamometer provides a quantitative assessment of grip strength.

Patient Position	Holding the grip dynamometer with the elbow flexed to 90° and the radioulnar joint in its neutral position
Position of Examiner	Standing in front of the patient, viewing the dynamometer's gauge
Evaluative Procedure	The dynamometer is set at one of five specified settings (1, 1.5, 2, 2.5, and 3 inches). The patient squeezes the dynamometer's handle with maximum force at every setting, with adequate recovery time allowed between bouts. The values are recorded, and the test is repeated on the opposite hand.
Positive Test	More than 10% bilateral strength deficit compared with the opposite hand[21]
Implications	Pathology that inhibits grip strength; the underlying cause of the weakness must be determined.
Comments	Because of the wide range of variation in grip strength, the outcome of each of these tests is most meaningful when compared with a baseline measure. This test can be repeated three times at any one setting and the results averaged.
Evidence	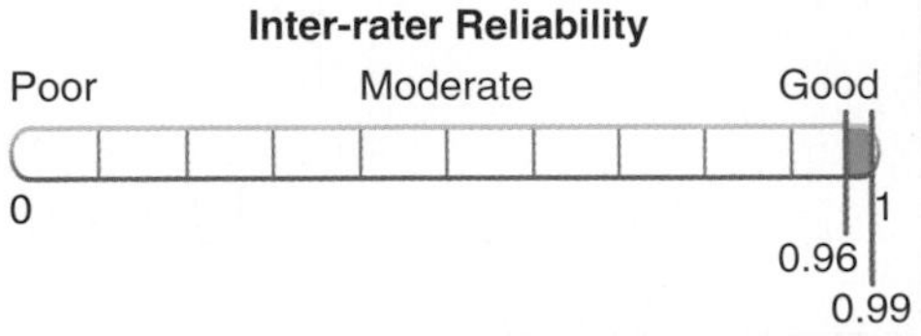

Passive Range of Motion

- **Flexion and extension of the MCP joints:** While stabilizing the metacarpal, grasp the proximal phalanx of the finger being tested (Figs. 17-21A and B).
- **Abduction and adduction of the MCP joints:** Grasp the finger over the PIP joint. The patient's arm is positioned so that the palm is resting flat against the table with the metacarpals stabilized to prevent wrist motion.
- **Flexion and extension of the interphalangeal joints:** With the MCP joint in neutral, stabilize the phalanx proximal to the joint being tested while applying force to the phalanx of the distal bone. The normal end-feel for the PIP joint is hard during flexion as the two phalanges contact each other, but a soft end-feel can occur by soft tissue approximation (Figs. 17-21C and D).

Joint Stability Tests

The ligaments of the wrist are stressed with overpressure during the evaluation of PROM (Table 17-4). Avulsion fractures of a ligament's attachment may produce positive results during stress testing. Because the fracture can involve the joint's articular surface, radiographs should be obtained to rule out bony pathology.

*** Practical Evidence**

Ligamentous testing of the carpal bones has limited usefulness. Positive findings of the intercarpal ligaments yield small to moderate positive likelihood ratios, thereby providing little diagnostic value.[23]

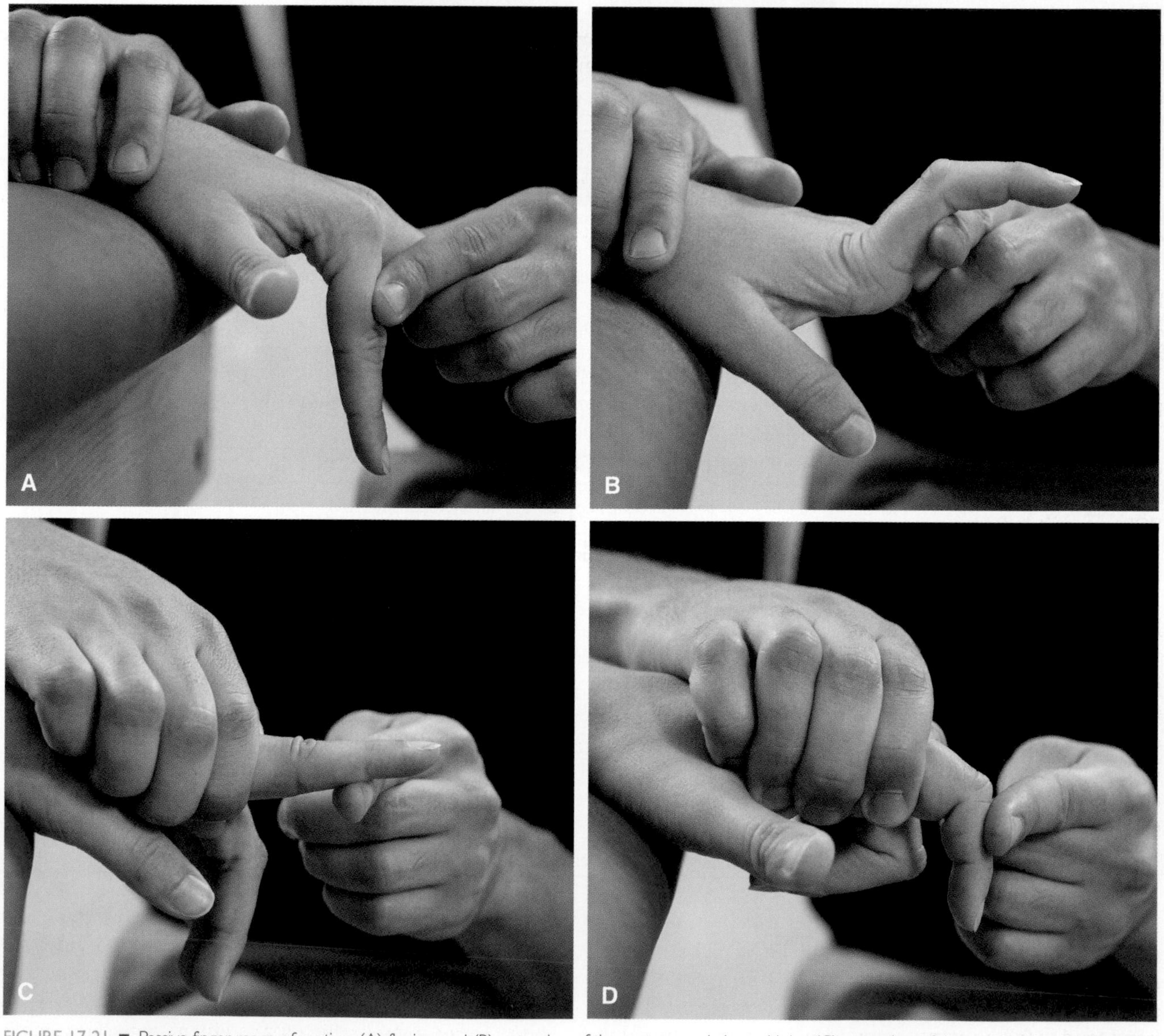

FIGURE 17-21 ■ Passive finger range of motion: (A) flexion and (B) extension of the metacarpophalangeal joint; (C) extension of the proximal interphalangeal joint; (D) flexion of the proximal interphalangeal joint.

Table 17-4 Ligaments Stressed During Wrist Passive Range of Motion

	Ligaments Stressed	
Passive Movement	Primary	Secondary
Extension	Palmar ulnocarpal Radial collateral	Palmar radiocarpal Ulnar collateral
Flexion	Dorsal radiocarpal	Radial collateral Ulnar collateral
Radial Deviation	Ulnar collateral	Palmar ulnocarpal
Ulnar Deviation	Radial collateral	Palmar radiocarpal

Stress Testing

Tests for collateral support of the wrist ligaments. The UCL provides lateral support against valgus forces (radial deviation), and the RCL checks varus forces (ulnar deviation). These two ligaments also function cooperatively to limit wrist flexion and extension. Although rarely injured in isolation, their involvement in pathology can be established through valgus and varus stress testing (Stress Test 17-1) and by assessing glide between the proximal carpal row and the radius (see Joint Play Assessment). These tests check the integrity of the collateral ligaments and may elicit signs of trauma to the triangular fibrocartilage.

Tests for collateral support of the interphalangeal joints. The integrity of the IP joints' collateral ligaments can be determined through stress testing the radial and ulnar ligaments (Stress Test 17-2).

Thumb ulnar collateral ligament stress test. The only MCP joint that is routinely stress tested is the thumb's UCL (Stress Test 17-3). Because of the alignment of the fingers, the only other MCP collateral ligaments commonly injured are the UCL of the MCP joint of the index finger and the RCL of the little finger.

Wrist and Hand Joint Play Assessment

Joint play of the many articulations of the wrist is performed using standard principles: stabilize one bone and glide the adjacent bone, noting any changes in mobility relative to the uninvolved side. Hypermobility may be associated with sprains and is common at the scapholunate articulation. Hypomobility frequently follows periods of immobilization. Radiocarpal and midcarpal joint play is presented in Joint Play 17-1; intercarpal joint play is presented in Joint Play 17-2.

Neurological Testing

Most commonly, nerves of the hand, wrist, and fingers are affected by pathology proximal to the forearm, but trauma in this region can lead to localized symptoms. Common sites for nerve entrapment resulting in symptoms in the hand tend to follow common patterns. Many of these radicular symptoms can originate along the nerve's path from the cervical spine. A complete upper-quarter screen may be indicated (see Neurological Screening 1-2).

- **Carpal tunnel:** Carpal tunnel syndrome (CTS), discussed later in this chapter, causes dysfunction in the distal median nerve distribution. The palmar surfaces of the thumb, index, middle, and half the ring finger are most commonly affected.
- **Guyon's canal:** Located between the hook of the hamate and the pisiform, this can compress the ulnar nerve, resulting in paresthesia in the little finger and ring fingers. Numbness or paresthesia on only the palmar side of the ulnar nerve distribution is indicative of ulnar nerve compression distal to Guyon's canal where the nerve diverges into palmar and dorsal branches.[24]
- **Cubital tunnel:** Entrapment of the ulnar nerve at the elbow can result in symptoms in the ring and little fingers.
- **Radial nerve:** Radial nerve entrapment can result in **drop-wrist syndrome**, the inability to actively extend the wrist and fingers, or it can cause paresthesia along the lateral dorsum of the hand.

Vascular Testing

Structural abnormalities that impede arterial and/or venous blood flow in the upper extremity often first present symptoms in the hand and fingers. Likewise, dislocation of the glenohumeral or elbow joints or fracture of the clavicle, humerus, radius, or ulna can compromise the neurovascular structures. Diseases such as cystic fibrosis or cardiovascular disorders may also reduce blood flow in the upper extremity.

Arterial blockage results in diminished radial and/or ulnar pulses and may produce cyanosis. Venous blockage causes swelling in the distal extremity.

Region-Specific Pathologies and Selective Tissue Tests

The potential for significant disability in both athletic participation and ADLs necessitates careful examination of any injury to the wrist, hand, and fingers. Although similar in nature, trauma to the thumb and trauma to the fingers are discussed in separate sections because of the potential differences in the functional outcomes.

Wrist Pathology

Trauma to the wrist can affect the distal portion of the radius and ulna; the collateral, palmar, and dorsal ligaments; the triangular fibrocartilage; or the neurovascular structures. Resulting hyper- or hypomobility at these small articulations changes the demands on proximal and distal structures. The mechanisms of injury for most of these conditions are similar, calling for careful inspection, palpation, and functional assessment of the involved structures.

Stress Test 17-1
Radial Collateral and Ulnar Collateral Ligament Stress Tests of the Wrist

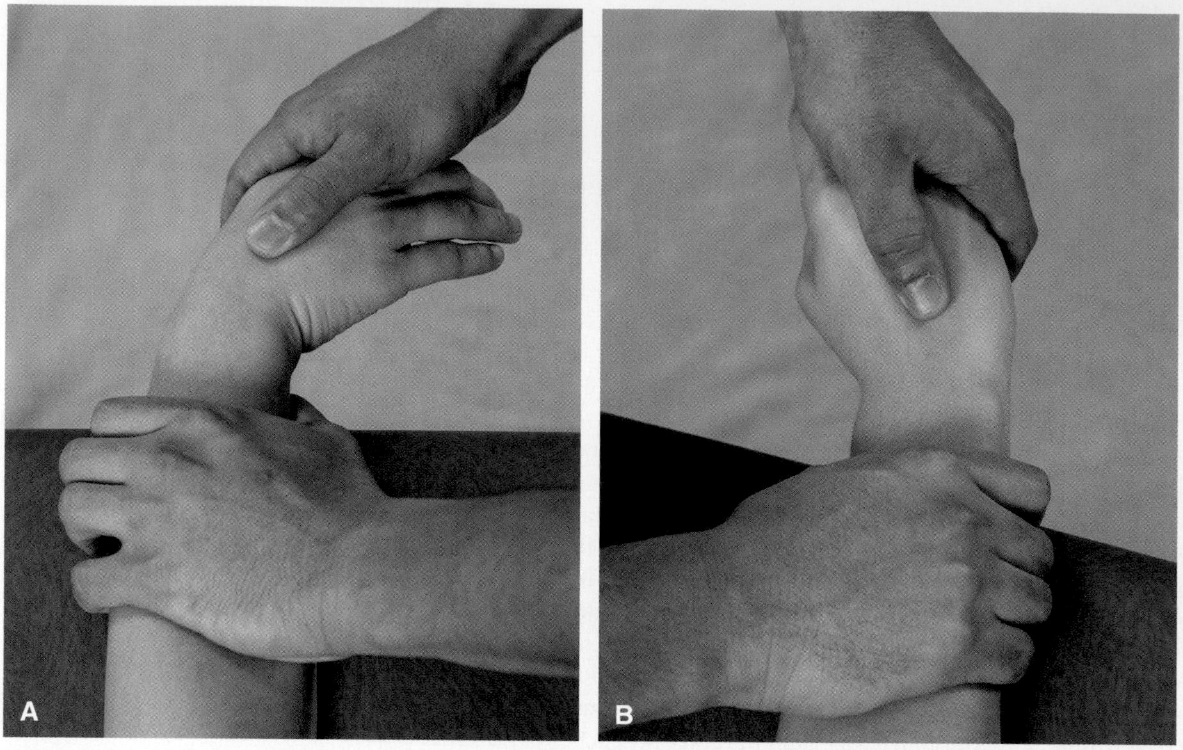

Although of limited clinical use, a passive ulnar deviation assesses the radial collateral ligament (A). Passive radial deviation stresses the ulnar collateral ligament of the wrist (B).

Patient Position	Sitting The elbow flexed to 90°, the forearm pronated, and the fingers assuming the relaxed position of flexion
Position of Examiner	Sitting or standing lateral to the wrist being tested One hand grips the distal forearm, and the other grasps the hand across the metacarpals.
Evaluative Procedure	UCL: A valgus stress is applied, radially deviating the wrist. RCL: A varus stress is applied, ulnarly deviating the wrist.
Positive Test	Pain or laxity (or both) compared with the same ligament on the opposite wrist
Implications	Sprain of the UCL or RCL
Comments	Pain may be elicited in the presence of trauma to the triangular fibrocartilage, scaphoid fractures, or the palmar or dorsal radiocarpal or ulnocarpal ligaments. These tests are rarely positive for hypermobility.
Evidence	Absent or inconclusive in the literature

RCL = radial collateral ligament; UCL = ulnar collateral ligament

Stress Test 17-2
Valgus and Varus Testing of the Interphalangeal Joints

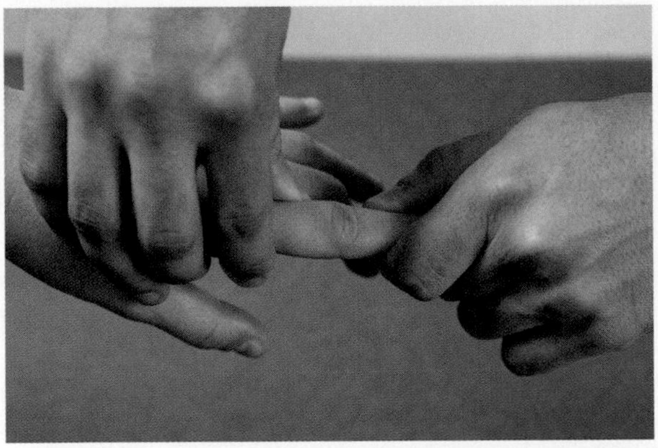

Stress test the ulnar collateral ligament of the PIP joint. This test should be repeated using varus stress for the radial collateral ligament.

Patient Position	Sitting or standing The joint being tested is in extension.
Position of Examiner	Standing in front of the patient, stabilizing the forearm, wrist, and phalanx proximal to the joint being tested
Evaluative Procedure	The examiner grasps the phalanx distal to the joint being tested and applies a valgus stress to the joint. A varus stress is then applied to the joint.
Positive Test	Increased gapping, compared with the same motion on the same finger of the opposite hand Pain
Implications	Collateral ligament sprain Avulsion fracture
Comments	Except in the case of a complete disruption of the ligament, the degree of injury to the ligament cannot be established. Avoid placing the stabilizing finger over the ligament being stressed.
Evidence	Absent or inconclusive in the literature

PIP = proximal interphalangeal

Stress Test 17-3
Test for Laxity of the Thumb MCP Collateral Ligaments

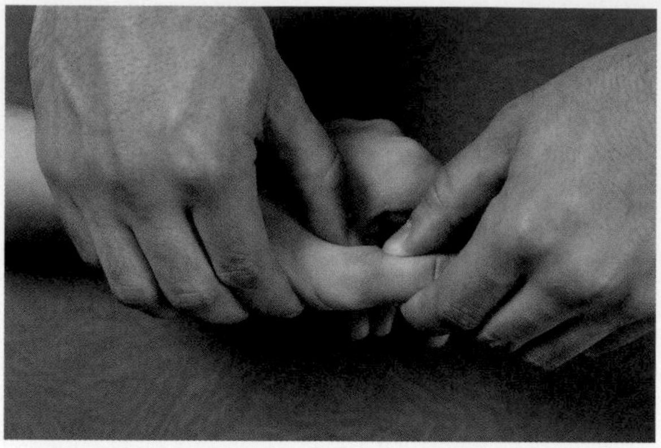

A valgus and varus stress is applied to the MCP joint to determine the integrity of the ulnar collateral and radial collateral ligaments.

Patient Position	Sitting or standing
Position of Examiner	Standing in front of the patient
Evaluative Procedure	The examiner stabilizes the 1st metacarpal with one hand and its proximal phalanx with the other. While stabilizing the 1st metacarpal with the thumb slightly abducted and extended, the examiner applies a valgus stress to the ulnar collateral ligament. In extension, the test stresses the accessory collateral ligament. In full flexion, the collateral ligament proper is stressed.
Positive Test	The ulnar or radial side of the first MCP joint gaps farther than the uninjured side or the patient describes pain (or both).
Implications	Sprain of the ulnar or radial collateral ligament Avulsion fracture
Comments	Avoid stabilizing over the ligament being stressed.
Evidence	Absent or inconclusive in the literature

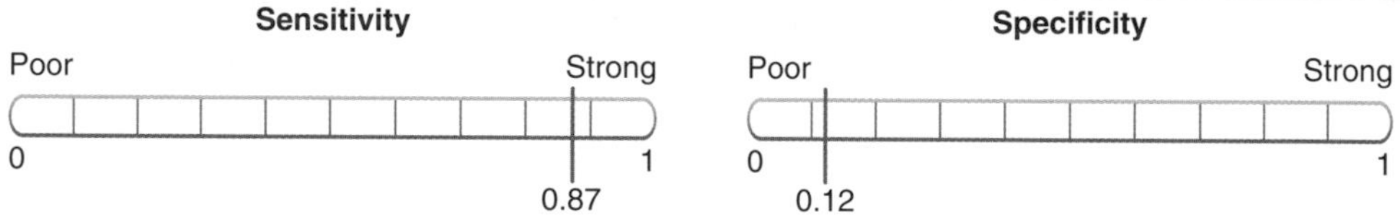

LR+: 0.99 **LR−: 1.08**

MCP = metacarpophalangeal

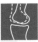

Joint Play 17-1
Radiocarpal and Midcarpal Joint Play

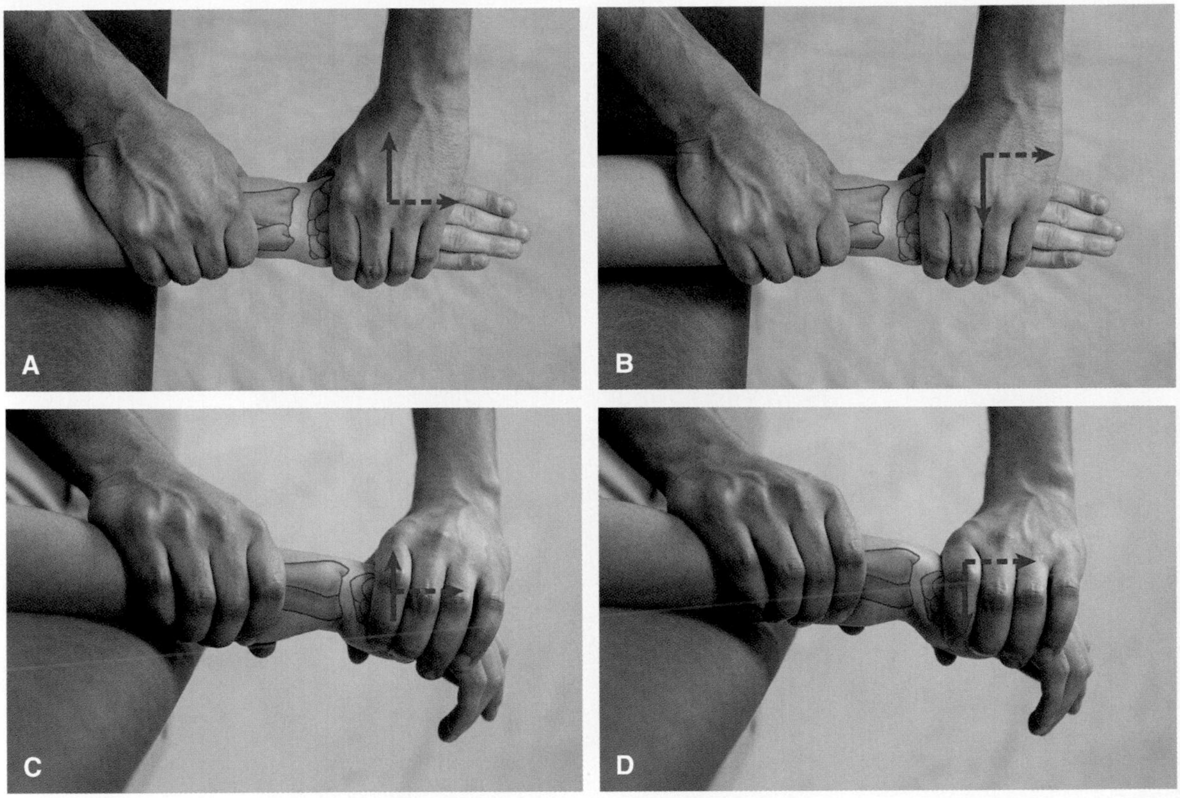

Joint play of the radiocarpal joint: (A) radial glide; (B) ulnar glide; (C) dorsal glide; and (D) palmar glide. Note that the hands are spread to allow visualization of the bones in the photographs. When performed clinically, the hands should almost be touching.

Patient Position	Sitting The elbow is flexed to 90°, the forearm pronated, and the fingers in a relaxed position.
Position of Examiner	Sitting or standing lateral to the wrist being tested Radiocarpal joint: One hand grips the distal radius, and the other hand grasps the proximal carpal row. Midcarpal joint: The proximal hand stabilizes the proximal carpal row, immediately distal to the radius. The other hand is immediately distal to the proximal row.
Evaluative Procedure	A shear force is applied to the wrist by gliding the distal segment in a radial and ulnar direction and then in a dorsal and palmar direction.
Positive Test	Pain or significant difference in glide compared with the opposite side
Implications	Sprain of the collateral or intercarpal ligaments or trauma to the triangular fibrocartilage. Decreased glide may indicate adhesions and capsular stiffness after injury or surgery.
Comment	Radial and ulnar glide stresses both collateral ligaments; the determination of which ligament is involved is based on the location of pain.
Evidence	Absent or inconclusive in the literature

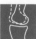

Joint Play 17-2
Intercarpal Joint Play

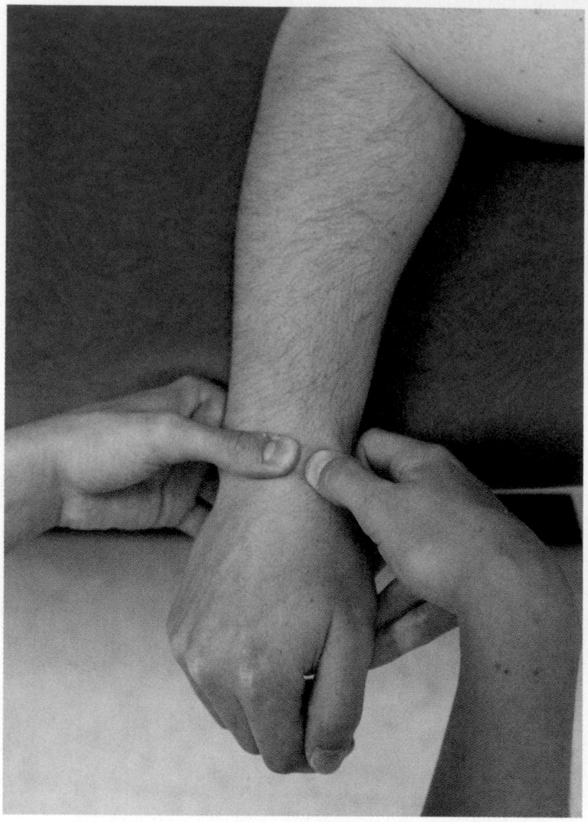

Joint play of the intercarpal articulations. Joint play of the scapholunate articulation is shown above.

Patient Position	Sitting The elbow is flexed to 90°, the forearm pronated, and the fingers in a relaxed position.
Position of Examiner	Sitting or standing lateral to the wrist being tested The thumb and index finger of one hand stabilize one carpal, with the thumb and index finger of the other hand stabilizing the other (or the radius).
Evaluative Procedure	A dorsal or palmar shear force is applied to one carpal while stabilizing the other.
Positive Test	Pain or significant change in glide compared with the opposite side
Implications	Sprain of the intercarpal ligaments. Decreased glide may indicate adhesions and capsular stiffness after injury or surgery.
Modification	Apply slight traction to the wrist during the test.
Comments	A systematic approach to testing each intercarpal articulation is required.
Evidence	

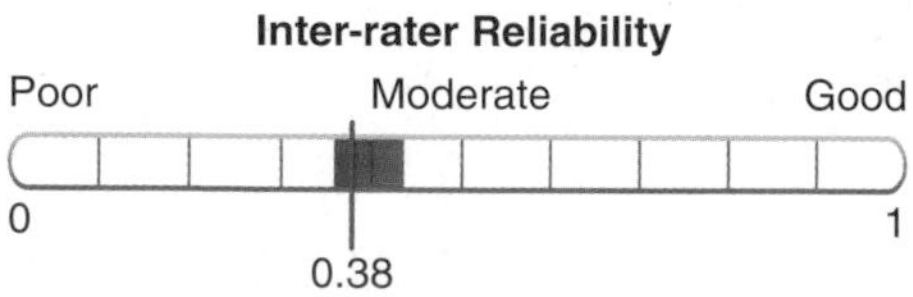

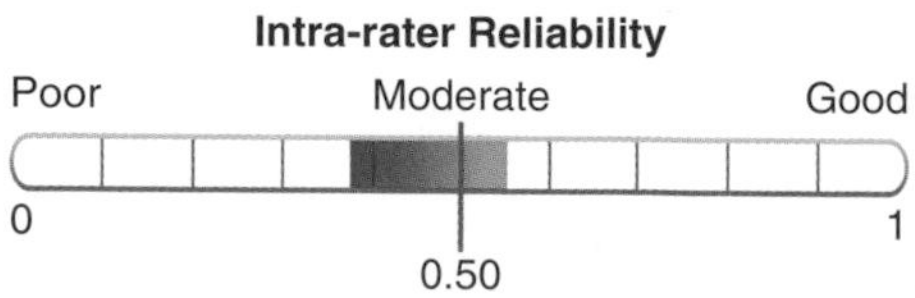

Distal Forearm Fractures

Fractures of the distal radius or ulna frequently occur secondary to landing on an outstretched arm. This region and its epiphyses are particularly vulnerable in the child and adolescent. The term "**Colles' fracture**" is often used to describe any fracture of the distal radius. However, a true Colles' fracture is a nonarticular fracture of the radius approximately 1.5 inches proximal to the radiocarpal joint, where the distal radius is displaced dorsally.[25] On a lateral radiographic view, the wrist appears as an upside-down fork (Fig. 17-22). Although not preferred nomenclature, the terms "**Smith's fracture**" and "**reverse Colles' fracture**" are used to describe a fracture in which the distal radius is displaced palmarly (Examination Findings 17-1).[26]

Forearm Fracture Intervention Strategies

As described in the On-Field Management section of this chapter, a splint should be applied and the patient referred for further evaluation. Distal forearm fractures are managed based on the extent of displacement, the patient's tolerance for a limitation in mobility, and whether or not the fracture line extends into the joint. Displaced fractures and fractures that extend into the joint often require surgical fixation for optimal outcomes.[27]

Scaphoid Fractures

The majority (over 80%) of all carpal fractures involve the scaphoid bone because of its function as a bony block limiting wrist extension.[28] Scaphoid fractures are most

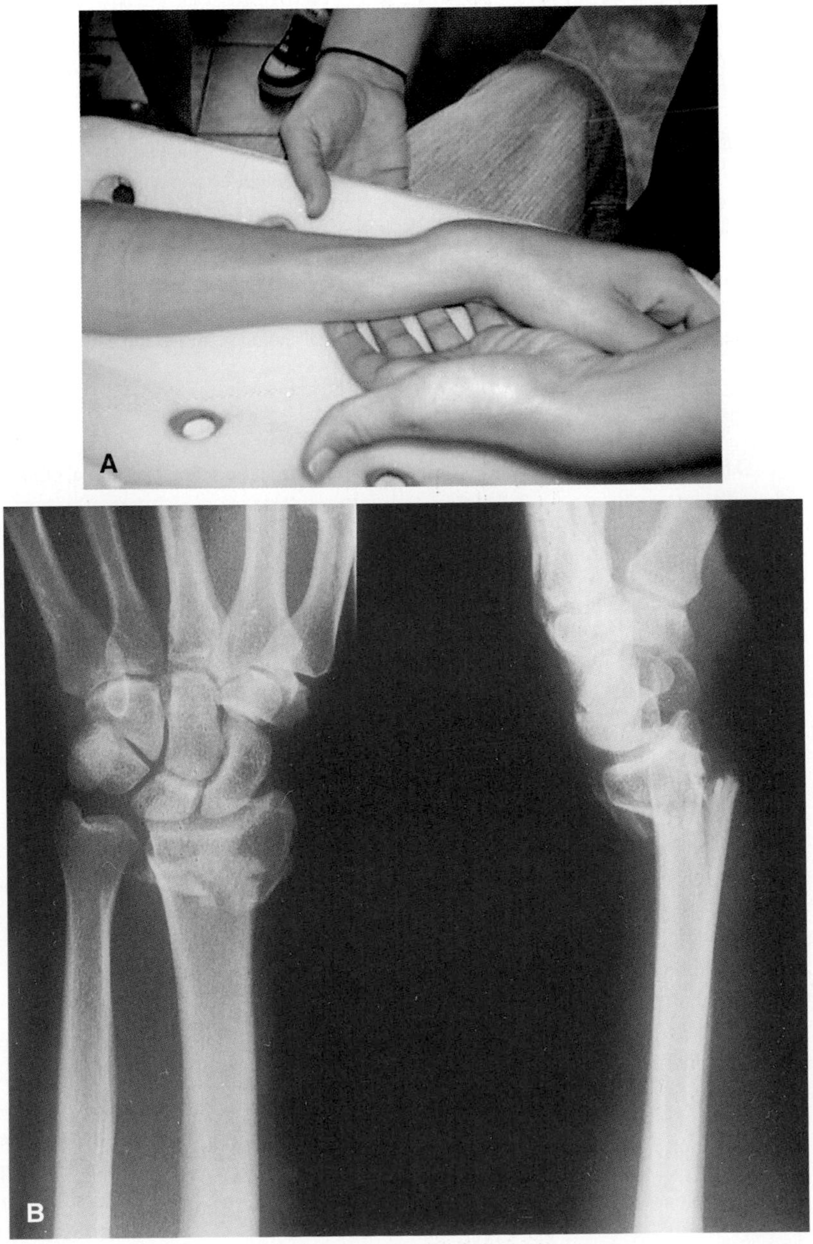

FIGURE 17-22 ■ Colles' fracture. (A) Obvious deformity. (B) Radiographic view.

Examination Findings 17-1
Distal Forearm Fractures

Examination Segment	Clinical Findings
History of Current Condition	*Onset:* Acute *Pain characteristics:* Immediate and sharp at distal forearm, proximal wrist *Other symptoms:* The patient may describe hearing and feeling a cracking sensation. *Mechanism:* A hyperextension mechanism, possibly combined with a rotatory component, placing tensile, compressive, or shear forces on the radius, ulna, or both (e.g., landing on an outstretched arm) *Risk factors:* Osteoporosis
Functional Assessment	None indicated
Inspection	Gross deformity of the radius and/or ulna possible; rapid onset of swelling Open fractures are readily apparent.
Palpation	Bony palpation may be omitted if gross deformity is present. Discontinuity of the long bones may be felt, and the area is tender to the touch.
Joint and Muscle Function Assessment	In the event of obvious gross deformity of the long bones, ROM testing and strength assessment is not conducted.
Joint Stability Tests	*Stress tests:* Should not be conducted if fracture is suspected *Joint play:* Should not be performed if fracture is suspected
Selective Tissue Tests	Not applicable
Neurological Screening	Assess distal neurological function in the radial, median, and ulnar nerve distributions.
Vascular Screening	Assess radial and ulnar pulses and check capillary refill to ensure an adequate blood supply to the hand and fingers.
Imaging Techniques	Radiographs
Differential Diagnosis	Distal radioulnar dislocation, radiocarpal dislocation, epiphyseal fracture
Comments	Suspected fractures should be appropriately splinted and the patient immediately referred to a physician. The patient should be monitored for shock.

AROM = active range of motion; MMT = manual muscle test; PROM = passive range of motion; ROM = range of motion

prevalent in the 15- to 40-year-old population.[29] In the very young and elderly populations, the scaphoid is spared at the expense of the weaker distal radius.[30] Receiving its blood supply from branches off the radial artery at the distal end, the proximal pole relies on a blood supply coming through the scaphoid. A fracture of the proximal pole compromises this blood supply and is a risk factor for nonunion secondary to avascular necrosis (Fig. 17-23).[19, 28] Unresolved fractures or chronically impaired circulation to the scaphoid may result in the development of **Preiser's disease**.

Preiser's disease Osteoporosis of the scaphoid, resulting from a fracture or repeated trauma

Practical Evidence

Scaphoid fractures are rare in patients older than the age of 50. The older the person, the more likely it is that the wrist will fracture at the distal radial metaphysis rather than at the scaphoid.[31]

An untreated fractured scaphoid can lead to instability of the proximal carpal row. The fracture fragment can displace dorsally or volarly. When the scaphoid becomes bipartite, the lunate rotates dorsally around the triquetrum while the proximal pole of the scaphoid rotates with the lunate. A **humpback** deformity results from the dorsal and radial angulation of the scaphoid fragments.[31]

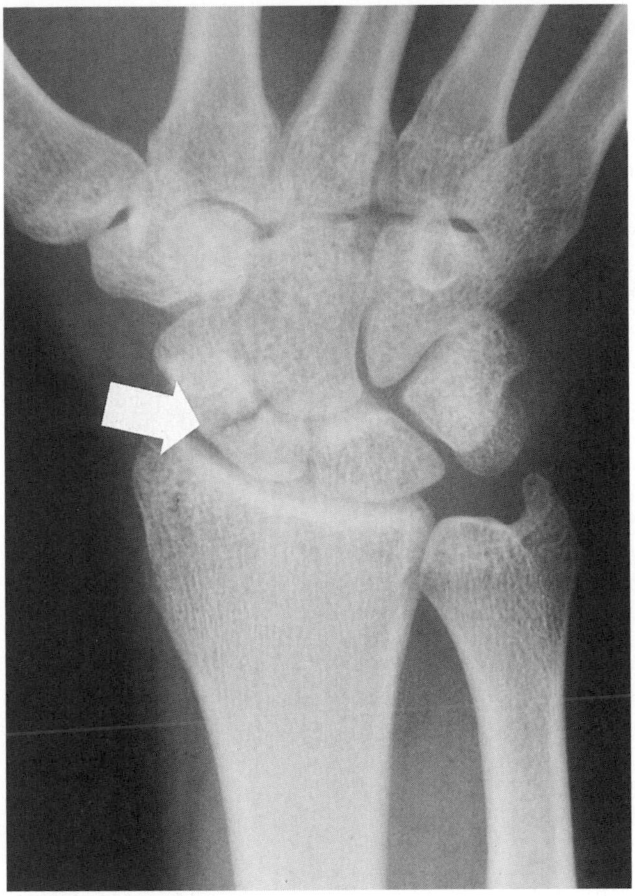

FIGURE 17-23 ■ Radiograph of a scaphoid fracture (palmar view).

Scaphoid fractures occur following a fall on an outstretched hand, a mechanism for many upper extremity injuries. The patient will describe pain in the area of the anatomic snuffbox, especially with ulnar deviation of the wrist.[32] Mild swelling and point tenderness at the anatomic snuffbox and scaphoid tubercle should also create a suspicion of a scaphoid fracture (see Fig. 17-19). To locate the scaphoid tubercle, palpate at the intersection of the distal wrist crease and the tendon of the flexor carpi radialis and ulnarly deviate the wrist.[33] The scaphoid is the prominent bump. Passive wrist extension and flexion may be painful at the end-range. Grip strength may be decreased on the involved side. The **scaphoid compression test,** in which an axial load is placed on the first metacarpal toward the scaphoid, may also produce pain (Examination Findings 17-2).[31] Absence of pain in the anatomic snuffbox is highly sensitive to the absence of a scaphoid fracture; however, point tenderness in the snuffbox demonstrates a low specificity, indicating that many false-positive results are associated with the test.[30,33]

*** Practical Evidence**

Sports-related injury in males, anatomic snuffbox pain with ulnar deviation of the wrist, and scaphoid tubercle tenderness 2 weeks postinjury are all independent predictors of scaphoid injury. When all four factors are present, the risk of scaphoid fracture is 91%.[32]

Patients with an injury that produces pain in the area of the anatomic snuffbox after a hyperextension mechanism, such as falling on an outstretched arm, must be treated as having a fracture of the scaphoid. Fracture lines are not always visible on the initial radiographic examination, and other imaging may be ordered.[28, 34] Computed tomography (CT) scans and magnetic resonance imaging (MRI) scans are both highly sensitive in ruling out scaphoid fractures, with MRI having a higher specificity in confirming scaphoid fractures.[34] Nonunion or malunion scaphoid fractures can lead to significant long-term disability. Most commonly associated with displaced fractures, fractures of the proximal pole, and in unrecognized fractures, decreased grip strength, reduced ROM, radiocarpal arthrosis, and pain significantly limit function.[29]

Scaphoid Fracture Intervention Strategies

Patients with suspected scaphoid fractures should be immobilized and referred for imaging and treatment. Many physicians will opt to treat patients with symptoms consistent with scaphoid fractures and equivocal or negative radiographs as having fractures. Immobilization options range from short-arm casts that may or may not include the thumb to above-the-elbow casts. No one type of immobilization has demonstrated effectiveness over the others.[35] Fractures of the distal pole and middle of the scaphoid that are well aligned with minimal gapping between the fragments respond well to immobilization. Fractures that are displaced and/or that occur in the proximal pole are more at risk for nonunion and are often treated with surgical fixation.[29] For some athletes, the treatment of choice regardless of the fracture location may also be to immediately surgically fixate the fracture, allowing for earlier return to activity.

Hamate Fractures

The hook of the hamate functions as a muscular attachment site for the flexor digiti minimi and the opponens digiti minimi and the point of attachment for the transverse carpal ligament and the pisohamate ligament. Hook of the hamate fractures occur following falls on an outstretched arm or, more commonly, as a result of trauma to the palm when playing racquet sports or baseball or golf.[36] The body of the hamate is fractured through an axial load applied to the fourth or fifth metacarpal and frequently occurs concurrently with a metacarpal fracture. The body may also be fractured secondary to a direct blow.

Acutely, the patient will describe sharp pain dorsally and/or volarly in the ulnar palmar and wrist region. Swelling in the hypothenar eminence may be present (Examination Findings 17-3). The patient may experience tenderness during firm palpation of the hamate. The multiple attachments to the hook of the hamate result in pain when the fifth finger is actively abducted or adducted or when flexion and abduction are resisted. Pain occurs during passive extension of the fifth finger.

The hook of the hamate pull test has been described as highly associated with hook of the hamate fractures. The

Examination Findings 17-2
Scaphoid Fractures

Examination Segment	Clinical Findings
History of Current Condition	*Onset:* Acute, although the patient may delay seeking assistance because of the initial "minor" nature of the injury *Pain characteristics:* Proximal portion of the lateral wrist in the anatomic snuffbox and at the scaphoid tubercle *Mechanism:* Forceful hyperextension of the wrist that compresses the scaphoid *Risk factors:* Younger than 40 years old; male; sports[32]
Functional Assessment	Reduced grip strength The patient may complain of pain and weakness with gripping actions and those that require ulnar deviation.
Inspection	Swelling possible in the anatomic snuffbox
Palpation	Palpation of the scaphoid as it sits in the anatomic snuffbox elicits pain and tenderness. Pain may also be produced during palpation of the distal tuberosity of the scaphoid on the palmar aspect of the hand.
Joint and Muscle Function Assessment	*AROM:* Pain is produced at the terminal wrist ROM, especially during extension and ulnar deviation.[32] *MMT:* Unremarkable. Some tests of the thumb muscles may be weak secondary to pain. *PROM:* Overpressure produces pain during extension and ulnar deviation. End-range of flexion may also be painful.
Joint Stability Tests	*Stress tests:* Stress of RCL increases lateral wrist pain due to compression. *Joint play:* The patient may have increased pain with radiocarpal joint play.
Selective Tissue Tests	Scaphoid compression test (compression of the 1st metacarpal toward the scaphoid)
Neurological Screening	Within normal limits
Vascular Screening	Within normal limits
Imaging Techniques	PA radiographs with the wrist in neutral and ulnarly deviated, lateral view, and 45° pronation and supination views are obtained. The sensitivity and specificity of plain film radiographs are low in the days immediately after the trauma.[31] MRI and CT are both sensitive in detecting scaphoid fractures; MRI is more specific than CT.[34] Up to 20% of scaphoid fractures are not detected using radiographs.[12]
Differential Diagnosis	Scapholunate sprain, fracture at the base of the 1st metacarpal (Bennett's fracture), trapezium fracture, distal radius fracture
Comments	Patients describing pain in the anatomic snuffbox after a mechanism involving forced hyperextension of the wrist should be managed as if they have a scaphoid fracture until it is ruled out by a physician. Scaphoid fractures may not appear on standard radiographs until several weeks after the injury. MRI or CT may be needed to confirm the diagnosis.

AROM = active range of motion; CT = computed tomography; MRI = magnetic resonance imaging; MMT = manual muscle test; PA = posterior-anterior; PROM = passive range of motion; RCL = radial collateral ligament; ROM = range of motion

patient's wrist is ulnarly deviated with resistance applied to finger flexion. This position creates a pull of the finger flexor tendons against the hook of the hamate and reproduces the sharp pain associated with the original injury.[36]

An unstable hamate can compress the ulnar nerve as it passes through Guyon's canal, leading to paresthesia of the fourth and fifth fingers. Decreased innervation of the fifth slip of the FDP can lead to its rupture.[37]

Hamate Fracture Intervention Strategies

Individuals with suspected hamate fractures should be immobilized with the wrist in slight flexion and the fourth and

Examination Findings 17-3
Hamate Fractures

Examination Segment	Clinical Findings
History of Current Condition	*Onset:* Acute *Pain characteristics:* Pain on the ulnar side of the hand, proximal to the 5th MC Over time, pain becomes diffuse in the wrist and hand. *Mechanism:* The hook of the hamate may be fractured secondary to a fall on the hand. The probability of a fracture is increased if the patient is gripping an object such as a bat, racquet, golf club, or hammer. An axial load applied to the 4th or 5th MC Direct blow to the hamate
Functional Assessment	Reduced grip strength, complaints of pain and secondary weakness when gripping objects
Inspection	Swelling may develop in the hypothenar eminence. A callus-like projection may develop over the hamate.
Palpation	Pain during palpation of the hamate; fractures of the hook result in pain in the palm of the hand.
Joint and Muscle Function Assessment	*AROM:* Pain during abduction and adduction of the 5th finger *MMT:* Pain during resisted flexion of the 4th and 5th fingers with the wrist in ulnar deviation; pain during resisted abduction of the 5th MCP *PROM:* Pain during passive extension of the wrist, 5th and possibly 4th, MCP
Joint Stability Tests	*Stress tests:* Within normal limits *Joint play:* Within normal limits
Selective Tissue Tests	None
Neurological Screening	Paresthesia may be present in the 4th and 5th fingers secondary to ulnar nerve trauma.
Vascular Screening	Within normal limits
Imaging Techniques	Radiographs are obtained using the carpal tunnel view and with the wrist supinated but may miss many hamate fractures.[19] CT scans are more specific for fractures of the hamate.[36]
Differential Diagnosis	CMC sprain, fracture of the 4th or 5th MC, intercarpal sprain, ulnar nerve palsy
Comments	Misdiagnosed or untreated hamate fractures may lead to a nonunion or malunion.

AROM = active range of motion; CT = computed tomography; CMC = carpometacarpal; MC = metacarpal; MCP = metacarpophalangeal; MMT = manual muscle test; PROM = passive range of motion

fifth MCP joints fully flexed.[19] Hook of the hamate fractures are often treated with surgical excision, which is associated with an excellent outcome.[36]

Perilunate and Lunate Dislocation

The biomechanics of the carpals cause the lunate to act as the keystone of the carpal group.[4] Perilunate and lunate dislocations fall on the same spectrum of injury and also involve the scaphoid and capitate.[38] Lunate dislocations occur when the lunate is disassociated from its contiguous carpals; perilunate dislocations involve the proximal carpal row being stripped from around the lunate.

High-energy forced hyperextension of the wrist and hand may disassociate the lunate from the rest of the carpals, resulting in its displacement either dorsally or palmarly. As the limits of the wrist and hand extension are exceeded, the scaphoid bone strikes the radius, rupturing the palmar interosseous ligaments connecting the scaphoid to the lunate. As the force continues, the distal carpal row is stripped away from the lunate, resulting in the lunate's resting dorsally relative to the other carpals—a perilunate dislocation. Further extension leads to rupture of the dorsal ligaments, relocating the carpals and rotating the lunate. Each of these types of dislocations may spontaneously reduce. Laxity of the interosseous ligaments alters the synchronous motion of the lunate, scaphoid, and triquetrum, called **dissociative carpal instability**.[4] As the scaphoid is bound to both the proximal and distal carpal rows, an associated scaphoid fracture and/or instability of the associated carpals must be considered.[4]

The chief complaint is pain along the radial side of the palmar or dorsal aspect of the wrist that limits ROM. A bulge may be visible on the palmar or dorsal aspect of the hand proximal to the third metacarpal (Examination Findings 17-4). The displacement of the lunate or swelling can cause paresthesia in the middle finger. With a lunate dislocation, the third knuckle is level with the other knuckles (it normally appears to be more distal).[39] A fracture of the scaphoid bone should be suspected with any lunate dislocation because of the similarity in their mechanisms of injury. However, patients with these injuries may present with no significant physical findings other than pain, so a definitive diagnosis of a lunate dislocation is made via radiographs or MRI.

Mobilization of the carpal joints can reproduce the patient's symptoms. A compressive force placed on the ulnar side of the triquetrum, compressing the proximal carpal row radially, and a palmar to dorsal force applied over the lunotriquetral joint stress the lunotriquetral ligament (Fig. 17-24).

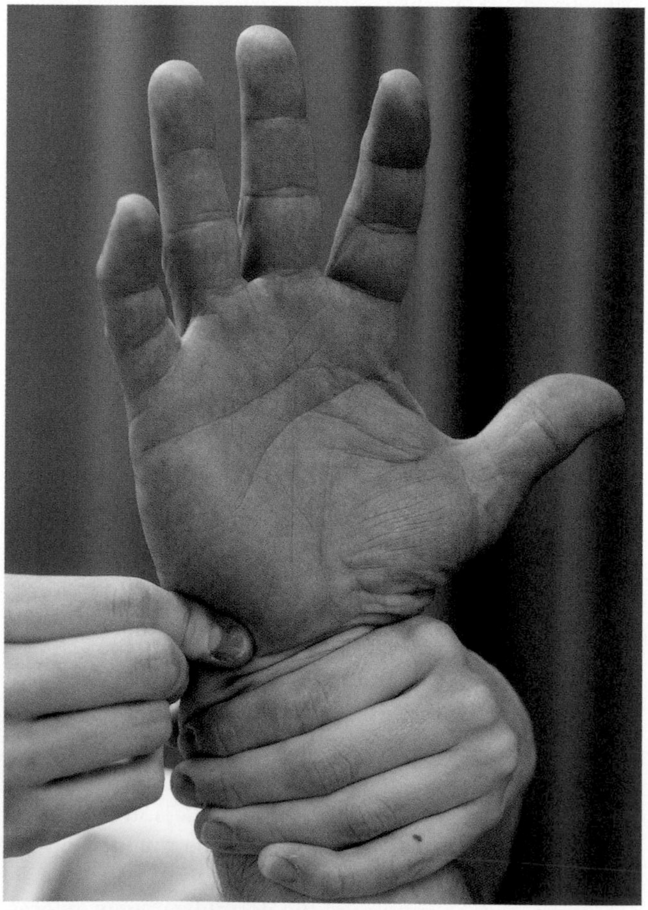

FIGURE 17-24 ■ A compressive force placed on the ulnar side of the triquetrum, compressing the proximal carpal row radially and a palmar to dorsal force applied over the lunotriquetral joint stress the lunotriquetral ligament.

Repeated trauma to the lunate may compromise its vascular supply, resulting in Kienböck's disease. Untreated, **Kienböck's disease** may result in a loss of ulnar deviation; tenderness, pain, and swelling over the lunate; decreased grip strength; and weakness during wrist extension. A characteristic finding of Kienböck's disease is pain during passive extension of the third finger.

Lunate Dislocation Intervention Strategies

Lunate dislocations that are seen early after the injury may be amenable to closed reduction. If reduction is successful, the wrist is then immobilized in flexion for 6 to 8 weeks. Frequent follow-up evaluations with radiographic examination are needed to make sure that the reduction is maintained. If the reduction is lost, percutaneous pinning of the lunate in the reduced position or open reduction may be needed.

Open surgical repair is the standard of care for perilunate dislocations. Even with good anatomic reduction, nonoperative management is associated with a worse functional outcome than operative management.[40]

Wrist Sprains

The diagnosis of wrist sprain is often based simply on pain or swelling around the wrist and an associated negative radiograph. This approach is apt to be overly broad and may preclude appropriate management.[41] Sprains of the UCL and RCL may be identified using the valgus and varus stress tests (see Stress Test 17-1). Based on the mechanism, these injuries rarely occur in isolation and require the examination of the related structures. The possibility of carpal fracture, triangular fibrocartilage tear, distal radioulnar joint pathology, and scapholunate ligament disruption must be considered for any wrist pain that does not subside within 2 weeks.[41]

*** Practical Evidence**

Because standard imaging techniques such as radiographs and MRI do not capture the dynamic instability associated with scapholunate dissociation, arthroscopy is considered the gold standard for diagnosis.[42]

Sprains of the scapholunate ligaments are the most common and outnumber sprains to the lunotriquetral joint by six to one.[20] Patients with acute scapholunate injury will present with pain and swelling at the dorsal scapholunate articulation, coupled with decreased range of motion (Examination Findings 17-5). The **Watson test** (scaphoid shift test) may be positive and is particularly meaningful if a clunk is accompanied by pain (Selective Tissue Test 17-2).[23,43,44] Radiographs, especially using a clenched-fist view, may show a gap between the scaphoid and lunate.[20] Some scapholunate ligament sprains result in the scaphoid assuming a static flexed position while

Kienböck's disease Osteochondritis or slow degeneration of the lunate bone

Examination Findings 17-4
Perilunate or Lunate Dislocation

Examination Segment	Clinical Findings
History of Current Condition	*Onset:* Acute *Pain characteristics:* Lateral (ulnar) wrist and hand *Other symptoms:* Paresthesia along the ulnar nerve distribution Descriptions of the wrist and hand giving way *Mechanism:* Forced hyperextension of the wrist and hand An ulnar deviation component may result in a perilunate dislocation. *Risk factors:* Participation in activities that require repetitive resisted wrist extension, such as weight lifting and football (offensive linemen)
Functional Assessment	Pain and decreased strength with gripping activities
Inspection	A bulge caused by the displacement of the lunate may be seen on the palmar or dorsal aspect of the hand. If the dislocation spontaneously reduces, this may not be present. The fingers may be postured in a semiflexed position.[4]
Palpation	The lunate can be prominent during palpation, especially if it is dorsally displaced. Ballottement of the triquetrum is indicative of lunotriquetral ligament tears.[5] Malalignment of the carpals may be noted. Point tenderness and crepitus are present over the lunate.
Joint and Muscle Function Assessment	ROM in all planes is limited secondary to pain. *AROM:* Limited wrist extension. Finger flexion may be painful. *MMT:* Pain and weakness with PIP and DIP flexion; possibly unremarkable *PROM:* Limited wrist extension; patient will be apprehensive at end-range. Passive extension of the fingers may produce pain.
Joint Stability Tests	*Stress tests:* Not applicable in the event of an obvious dislocation *Joint play:* Not applicable in the event of an obvious dislocation Radial translation of the proximal carpal row relative to the radius and ulna will produce pain.
Selective Tissue Tests	None
Neurological Screening	Median nerve may be impinged, resulting in paresthesia in its distribution.
Vascular Screening	Within normal limits
Imaging Techniques	Lateral, PA, and AP radiographs are required for diagnosis.[4]
Differential Diagnosis	Distal radioulnar joint subluxation, triangular fibrocartilage pathology, distal radius fracture, scaphoid fracture, hamate fracture, carpal instability, carpal tunnel syndrome, or other neuropathy
Comments	An associated scaphoid fracture must be suspected with both perilunate and lunate dislocations.

AP = anteroposterior; AROM = active range of motion; DIP = distal interphalangeal; MMT = manual muscle test; PA = posteroanterior; PIP = proximal interphalangeal; PROM = passive range of motion; ROM = range of motion

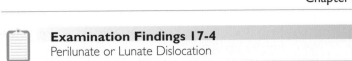

Examination Findings 17-5
Scapholunate Dissociation

Examination Segment	Clinical Findings
History of Current Condition	*Onset:* Acute; diagnosis may be made much later. *Pain characteristics:* Pain emanating from the palmar and dorsal aspects of the wrist near the joint line *Mechanism:* Tensile forces placed on the ligaments as the joint is forced past its normal ROM
Functional Assessment	Pain and weakness in gripping activities. Restricted range may further limit function.
Inspection	Acutely, swelling may be noted at the proximal wrist.
Palpation	Tenderness at the scapholunate joint; usually more diffuse over the wrist region than with other wrist injuries such as scaphoid fractures or tears of the triangular fibrocartilage
Joint and Muscle Function Assessment	*AROM:* Decreased wrist flexion and extension *MMT:* Unremarkable *PROM:* Limited wrist flexion and extension as the sprained tissues are placed on stretch
Joint Stability Tests	*Stress tests:* Possible associated hypermobility of the radiocarpal joint *Joint play:* Hypermobility at the scapholunate articulation
Selective Tissue Tests	Watson test
Neurological Screening	Within normal limits
Vascular Screening	Within normal limits
Imaging Techniques	MRI is more specific than CT. A clenched-fist AP view may reveal increased space between the scaphoid and lunate.
Differential Diagnosis	Scaphoid fracture, lunotriquetral sprain, midcarpal joint sprain, TFCC tear, radioulnar instability, lunate subluxation
Comments	Early recognition and management decreases long-term degenerative changes.

AP = anteroposterior; AROM = active range of motion; CT = computed tomography; MMT = manual muscle test; MRI = magnetic resonance imaging; PROM = passive range of motion; ROM = range of motion; TFCC = triangular fibrocartilage complex

the lunate and triquetrum are relatively extended; termed dorsal intercalated segmental instability (DISI). In other cases, the flexed position is assumed only during motion, a dynamic instability which can be detected using video fluoroscopy.[44] Arthroscopy is the gold standard for diagnosing ligamentous injuries to the wrist. MR and CT imaging are also used, but these are most helpful in detecting complete tears and are less effective in detecting partial disruption. Diagnostic ultrasound lacks the sensitivity (46.2%) to detect all of those with the pathology.[42]

Scapholunate Dissociation Intervention Strategies

Delayed management—even by a few weeks—can result in degenerative changes, so early detection is critical.[45] Conservative treatment of scapholunate dissociation is rarely effective, even if the condition is detected early. Surgical fixation of the unstable joint is associated with good outcomes and restoration of function.[44]

Triangular Fibrocartilage Complex Injury

Trauma or repeated insult to the TFCC and the UCL can result in permanent disability of the wrist if left unrecognized and untreated.[46] Athletes who compete in sports that place the upper extremity in a closed kinetic chain are at an increased risk of TFCC injury. A positive ulnar variance, where the ulna is unusually long compared with the radius, increases compressive forces on the TFCC and predisposes this structure to degeneration and injury (Fig. 17-25).[45]

When the TFCC is injured traumatically, forced hyperextension and ulnar deviation result in pain along the ulnar side of the wrist and are accompanied by decreased wrist motion secondary to pain. Acute injury can also occur by a force that distracts the ulnar aspect of the wrist.[47] Repeated loading, such as during gymnastic maneuvers and weight lifting, may cause degeneration of the TFCC, especially in those with positive ulnar variance. The TFCC may also be injured secondary to dorsally displaced fractures of the radius.[3]

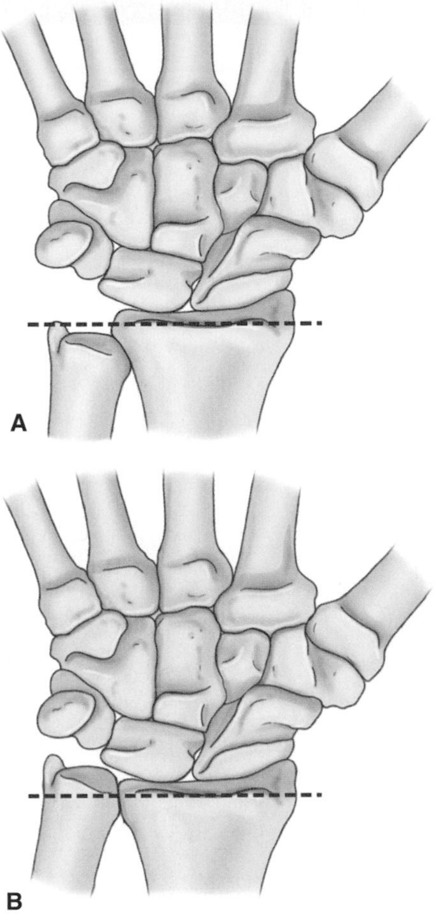

FIGURE 17-25 ■ Ulnar variance. The length relationship between the distal radius and ulna. (A) Negative ulnar variance: the ulna is shorter than the radius. (B) Positive ulnar variance: the ulna is longer than the radius.

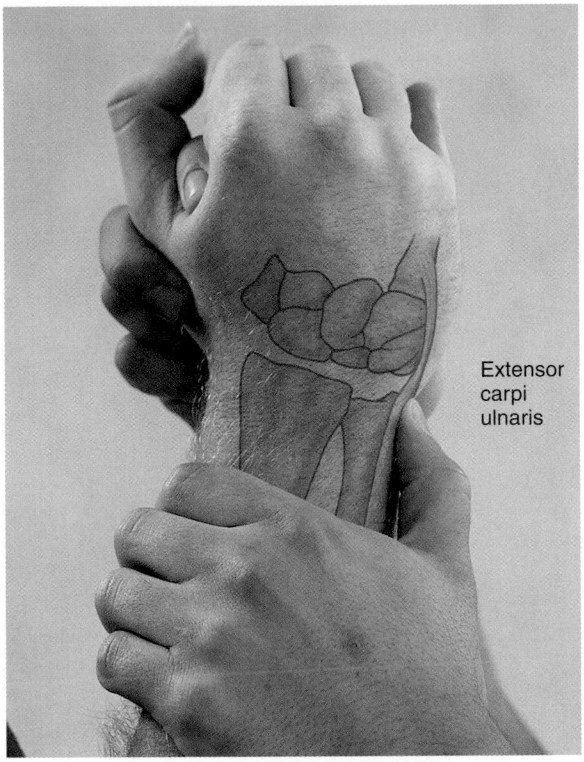

FIGURE 17-26 ■ Identifying TFCC lesions. Deep palpation over the ulnar joint line will yield pain in the presence of a TFCC tear.

*** Practical Evidence**

Approximately 48% of radiopalmar ganglion cysts that elicit pain during palpation combined with a positive ulnocarpal stress test have an associated TFCC tear.[48]

Functionally, the patient will describe pain when bearing weight on the arms, such as pushing up from a chair.[11] During palpation, pain over the TFCC is highly indicative of TFCC pathology (Fig. 17-26). Additionally, close attention must be devoted to the ulnar styloid process because it can be avulsed by the UCL concurrently with injury to the TFCC (Examination Findings 17-6). Any suspicion of injury to the TFCC warrants referral to a physician for further examination.

Triangular Fibrocartilage Complex Injury Intervention Strategies

Management of TFCC tears depends on the location of the tear and the underlying causes. Small, acute tears may be treated conservatively with short-arm casts or volar wrist splints. If conservative treatment is unsuccessful or if the tear is in a vascular zone or is unstable, surgical management is indicated. Tears to the avascular central articular disc, common in traumatic cases, respond well to debridement. Tears in the well-vascularized periphery can be repaired using open or arthroscopic procedures.[45] When a positive ulnar variance is the cause of degenerative changes, a procedure to shorten the ulna is required to prevent further damage and improve long-term outcomes.[45]

Carpal Tunnel Syndrome

CTS refers to the signs and symptoms caused by the compression of the median nerve as it passes through the carpal tunnel (see Fig. 17-11). Any pathology that decreases the size of the tunnel (e.g., carpal instability) or enlarges the structures inside it (e.g., wrist flexor tenosynovitis) can create the environment for compression of the nerve. Risk factors for CTS include diabetes, hypothyroidism, pregnancy, occupations or activities that require prolonged, repetitive wrist flexion and extension, and the use of equipment that vibrates (e.g., jackhammers).[50] The resulting symptoms of CTS can have detrimental effects on both athletic ability and ADLs.

Paresthesia and pain are described along the median nerve distribution (thumb, index, middle, and lateral half of the ring finger), with the symptoms often occurring at night and relieved with shaking.[50-53] In long-term cases, inspection of the hand may reveal atrophy of the thenar muscles, and grip strength is often decreased.[54] Manual muscle testing of the abductor pollicis brevis and the opponens pollicis reveals weakness on the involved side (Examination Findings 17-7).[55]

Selective Tissue Test 17-2
Watson Test for Scapholunate Instability

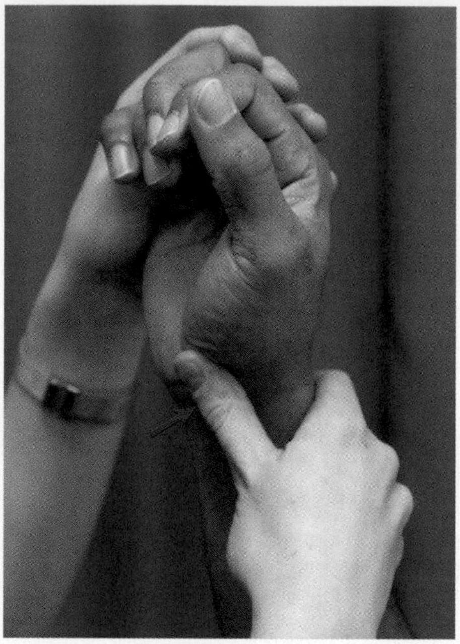

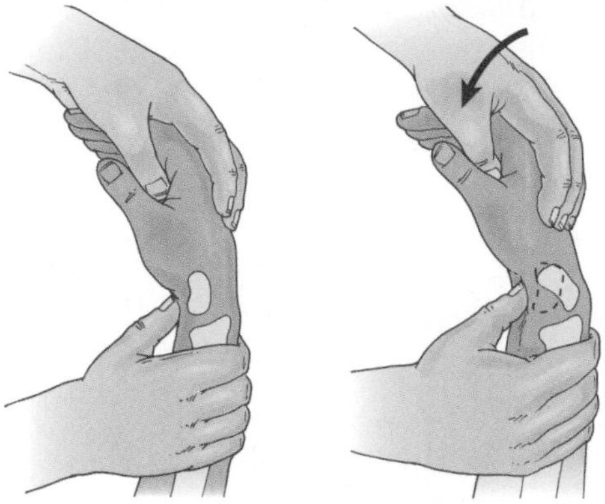

Application of a dorsally directed force attempts to shift the scaphoid from the lunate.

Patient Position	Seated with the elbow flexed and supported on the table and the forearm and hand pointing up, resembling the starting position for arm wrestling The wrist is in ulnar deviation.
Position of Examiner	In front of the patient
Evaluative Procedure	The examiner's thumb applies dorsal pressure to the distal pole of the scaphoid and then moves the patient's wrist from ulnar to radial deviation.
Positive Test	Reproduction of pain and a notable pop at the scapholunate articulation
Implications	Scapholunate dissociation
Comments	This test may be difficult to perform on the acutely injured patient. Bilateral comparison is important because many patients have nonpathological but positive findings.[20]
Evidence	

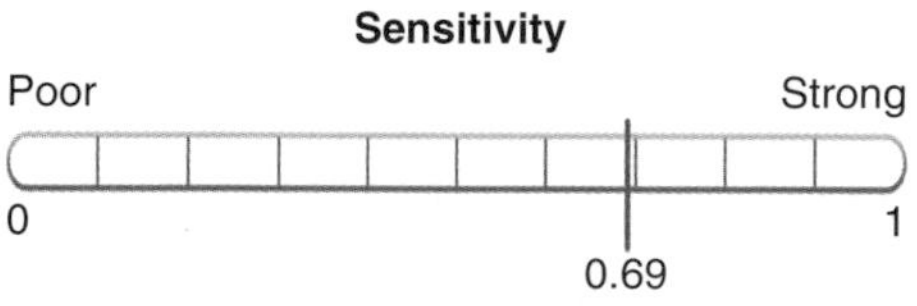

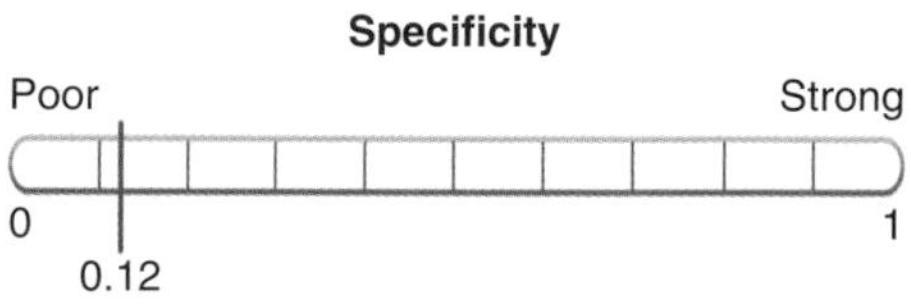

LR+: 2.03–2.88

LR−: 0.28–0.47

Examination Findings 17-6
Triangular Fibrocartilage Complex Injury

Examination Segment	Clinical Findings
History of Current Condition	*Onset:* Traumatic or degenerative Acute: The patient may not report the injury for some time after its onset. *Pain characteristics:* Distal to the ulna along the medial half of the wrist; the UCL of the wrist may also be tender. *Other symptoms:* The patient may complain of clicking on the ulnar side of the wrist with active motion. The click may be audible. *Mechanism:* Forced or repeated hyperextension of the wrist, compressing the triangular fibrocartilage, such as a fall Dorsally displaced radius fractures[3] *Risk factors:* Positive ulnar variance
Functional Assessment	Increased symptoms with weight-bearing activities on the arm (e.g., pushing off from table or chair, handstands) or activities that require repeated ulnar deviation and extension (e.g., hammering)
Inspection	Diffuse swelling around the wrist is possible, although, acutely, no swelling may be visible. Recurrent radiopalmar ganglion cysts may be associated with a TFCC tear.[48]
Palpation	Point tenderness distal to the ulna along the medial half of the wrist's joint line; the UCL may also be tender.
Joint and Muscle Function Assessment	*AROM:* Motion is limited secondary to pain, especially into extension and ulnar deviation. *MMT:* Unremarkable *PROM:* Motion is limited secondary to pain, especially at the end-ranges of extension and ulnar deviation. Ulnar deviation reproduces clicking symptoms.
Joint Stability Tests	*Stress tests:* Stressing the UCL elicits pain, although laxity may not be present. *Joint play:* Pain during lateral and/or medial radiocarpal glide
Selective Tissue Tests	None
Neurological Screening	Within normal limits
Vascular Screening	Within normal limits
Imaging Techniques	MRI, MRA TFCC abnormalities are frequently identified in asymptomatic patients, especially in individuals aged 50 or over.[49]
Differential Diagnosis	Lunotriquetral instability, extensor/flexor tendinopathy or subluxation, degeneration of distal radioulnar joint, wrist UCL sprain
Comments	Triangular fibrocartilage complex tears may be easily confused or occur in conjunction with a sprain of the wrist's UCL; persistence of symptoms should alert the examiner to injury beyond a simple wrist sprain and warrants referral to a physician for further evaluation.

AROM = active range of motion; MMT = manual muscle test; MRA = magnetic resonance arthrogram; MRI = magnetic resonance imaging; PROM = passive range of motion; TFCC = triangular fibrocartilaginous complex; UCL = ulnar collateral ligament

Examination Findings 17-7
Carpal Tunnel Syndrome

Examination Segment	Clinical Findings
History of Current Condition	*Onset:* Insidious *Pain characteristics:* Pain in the hand, wrist, and fingers, possibly radiating up the length of the arm and worsening during sleep secondary to a flexed posture of the elbow, wrist, and fingers *Other symptoms:* Paresthesia in the forearm, wrist, or hand (median nerve distribution) *Mechanism:* Repetitive wrist movement involving flexion and extension *Risk factors:* Occupations or activities that require repetitive and prolonged wrist flexion and extension and/or the use of equipment that vibrates; diabetes, rheumatoid arthritis, hypothyroidism, pregnancy, tenosynovitis[50]
Functional Assessment	Forward head, neck, and/or shoulder posture may be observed with activities of daily living. Shaking hands relieves symptoms.[51]
Inspection	Palmar aspect of the wrist possibly appearing thickened; atrophy of the thenar eminence after long duration of symptoms
Palpation	Possible tenderness on palpation or sustained pressure (carpal compression test) directly over the palmar aspect of the wrist
Joint and Muscle Function Assessment	*AROM:* The wrist motion may be slightly limited owing to stiffness, although AROM may be normal. *MMT:* In chronic cases, the strength of the abductor pollicis brevis, flexor pollicis brevis, or opponens pollicis may be decreased. *PROM:* Median nerve symptoms may increase as the wrist is fully extended or fully flexed.
Joint Stability Tests	*Stress tests:* Not applicable *Joint play:* Hypermobility or hypomobility of intercarpal or radiocarpal articulations may be an underlying cause of CTS.
Selective Tissue Tests	Tinel's sign; Phalen's test
Neurological Screening	Possible decreased sensation along the median nerve distribution of the hand (palmar aspect of the thumb, fingers II and III, and the lateral aspect of IV) Decreased 2-point discrimination tests within the median nerve distribution
Vascular Screening	Capillary refill and venous return are usually normal.
Imaging Techniques	Radiographs to rule out bony impingement within the tunnel MRI can be used to assist in identifying soft tissue compression of the tunnel.
Differential Diagnosis	Thoracic outlet syndrome, nerve root compression, proximal median nerve compressions (pronator syndrome, anterior interosseous nerve syndrome)
Comments	Nerve conduction studies are used to identify latency or slowed conduction of the median nerve.

AROM = active range of motion; CTS = carpal tunnel syndrome; MMT = manual muscle test; MRI = magnetic resonance imaging; PROM = passive range of motion

A positive **Tinel's sign** is elicited over the carpal tunnel, and **Phalen's test** is positive (Selective Tissue Test 17-3); although both of those examination techniques are associated with false negative results. Sustained pressure applied with both thumbs directly over the carpal tunnel (carpal tunnel test) will reproduce neurological symptoms.[52] An achy pain may be described in the palmar aspect of the forearm. The results of 2-point discrimination testing at less than 5 mm will be diminished.[56]

Replication of the functional demands that induce symptoms is important to determine the underlying cause of CTS. Although often reported as causative, use of a computer keyboard is not associated with the onset of CTS.[50] The postural examination may also reveal contributing factors, such as forward head and shoulders, that cause an increased demand and less-than-optimal biomechanics on the smaller distal joints and muscles.

The signs and symptoms of CTS closely resemble the peripheral symptoms associated with impingement of the C7 nerve root and proximal neuropathy of the median nerve. A careful differential evaluation must be made to identify the

Selective Tissue Test 17-3
Phalen's Test for Carpal Tunnel Syndrome

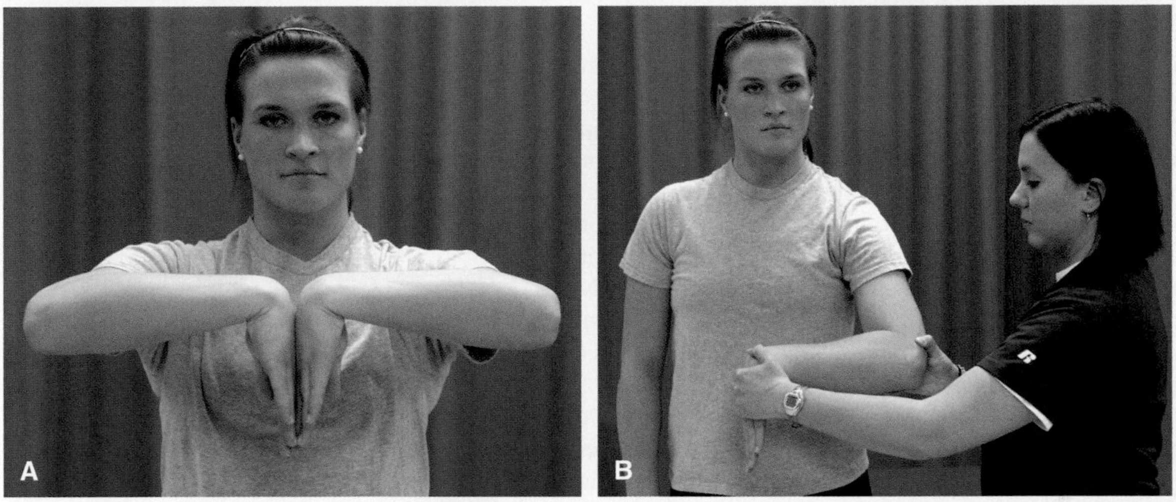

(A) Original test as described by Phalen. (B) Modification of Phalen's test (described below).

Patient Position	Standing
Position of Examiner	Standing in front of the patient
Evaluative Procedure	The examiner applies overpressure during passive wrist flexion and holds the position for 1 minute. Repeat this procedure for the opposite extremity.
Positive Test	Tingling develops or increases in the distribution of the median nerve distal to the carpal tunnel.
Implications	Median nerve compression
Modification	The traditional version of this test, in which the patient maximally flexes the wrists by pushing the dorsal aspects of the hands together, is not recommended because the patient may shrug the shoulders, causing compression of the medial branch of the brachial plexus as it passes through the thoracic outlet. **Reverse Phalen's test**, with the wrist positioned in maximum extension, is an alternate position to stress the median nerve, with approximately the same diagnostic value.[56,57]
Comments	Patients with numbness may not have an exacerbation of symptoms with this test, leading to a false-negative result.[56] This test is also frequently positive in those without CTS.
Evidence	

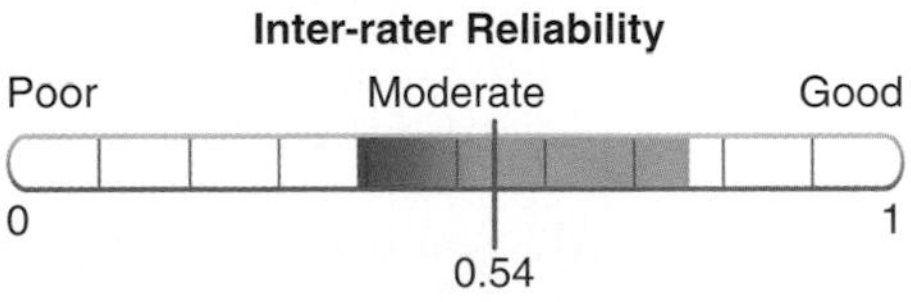

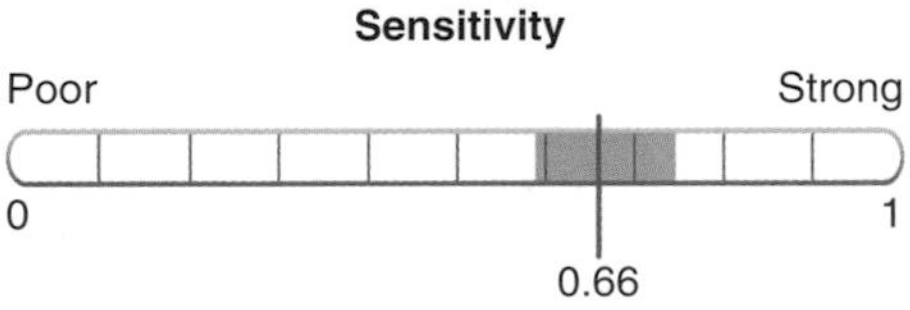

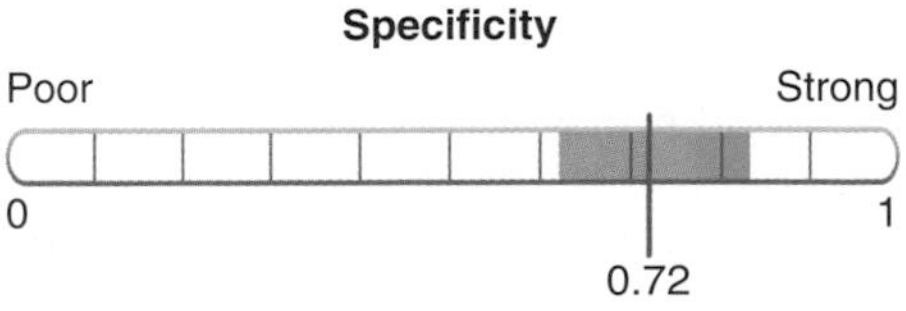

LR+: 2.06–3.39–4.71

LR−: 0.28–0.61–0.94

CTS = carpal tunnel syndrome

cause of the symptoms. An examination of the cervical spine and/or elbow is warranted if the patient reports a history of pain or injury in these regions.

Carpal Tunnel Syndrome Intervention Strategies

Because conservative management is successful for some people, initial management generally consists of the use of splints and/or corticosteroids.[58] Many other interventions have been described, including acupuncture, mobilization, ultrasound, and yoga, although the efficacy of these treatments has not been demonstrated.[53] Changes in the work or activity environment to incorporate rest breaks, modify the work pattern to minimize the duration of the repetitive activity, encourage good posture for efficient movement, and ensure that any equipment fits the individual are also important for treatment success.[50]

Surgical release of the carpal tunnel is associated with improved functional outcomes when compared with conservative treatment and is the treatment option for those with persistent symptoms following conservative treatment.[58]

Hand Pathology

The majority of injuries to the hand have an acute onset. Injury to the metacarpals and phalanges typically follows axial loading of the bone. Both groups of bones are also susceptible to crushing forces. Tendon ruptures or bony avulsions occur with eccentric stresses to the muscle–tendon unit.

Metacarpal Fractures

The metacarpals are typically fractured secondary to a compressive force along the bone's shaft, such as punching with a fist. In football players, the incidence of fractures involving metacarpals is evenly divided among the five digits. In basketball players, most fractures involve the fourth and fifth metacarpals.[20] It is common for the patient to hear the bone snapping as it fractures and describe immediate pain along one or more metacarpals. Gross deformity at the fracture site may be observed as one end of the bone rides over the other end, or the fracture site may be obscured by localized swelling along the dorsum of the hand (Fig. 17-27). Palpation reveals local tenderness over the fracture site. The actual bony fragments or crepitus may be palpated and the presence of a false joint established. The presence of a nondisplaced fracture may be confirmed through a variation of the long bone compression test (Fig. 17-28), although other symptoms usually make this unnecessary. The active range of motion (AROM) of the involved MCP is limited by pain.

In the absence of a metacarpal fracture, the fingers should point towards the scaphoid.[19] As the patient attempts to flex the hand, the fingers should remain parallel to one another. In the presence of a fracture, the patient is unable to make a fist (Examination Findings 17-8). With metacarpal fractures, the involved segment may rotate so that the finger flexes under or on top of the finger next to it.

Fractures of the fifth metacarpal are termed "**boxer's fractures**" because of their common incidence after an improperly thrown punch. This type of fracture is characterized by a depressed fifth MCP joint that, on radiographic examination, reveals an overlapping of the bone fragments.

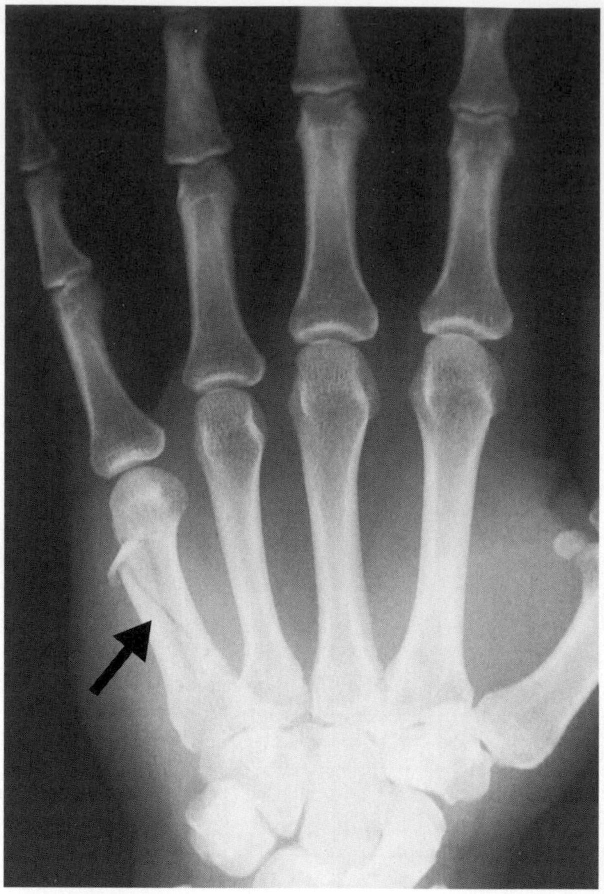

FIGURE 17-27 ■ Radiograph of a fractured 5th metacarpal, the so-called "boxer's fracture."

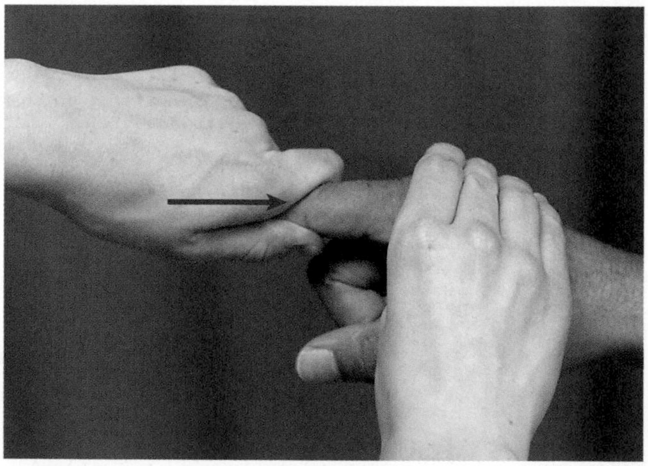

FIGURE 17-28 ■ Long bone compression test for phalanx fracture. For the middle and proximal phalanx and the metacarpals an axial load is applied to the ray.

Metacarpal Fracture Intervention Strategies

Treatment for metacarpal fractures depends on the presence of rotation and extent of angulation at the fracture site. Angulation less than 35 degrees is generally considered

Examination Findings 17-8
Metacarpal Fractures

Examination Segment	Clinical Findings
History of Current Condition	*Onset:* Acute *Pain characteristics:* Along the shaft of one or more metacarpals *Mechanism:* Longitudinal compression of the bone (direct contact), a crushing force (being stepped on), or a shear force (hyperextension of the finger)
Functional Assessment	Difficulty and pain when grasping objects
Inspection	Gross deformity of the bone may be visible. There is localized swelling over the involved metacarpal(s) and MCP joint(s), which may spread to the entire dorsum of the hand. Fractures of the 5th, and possibly 4th, metacarpals may result in a depression or shortening of the knuckles. The fingernail may be abnormally rotated when a fist is made.
Palpation	Palpation should not be performed if a fracture is evident. Severe tenderness is present over the fracture site. Bony fragments or crepitus may be present. A false joint may be evident.
Joint and Muscle Function Assessment	ROM testing is not performed if a fracture is evident.
Joint Stability Tests	*Stress tests:* Not applicable *Joint play:* Not applicable
Selective Tissue Tests	Long bone compression test Do not perform if a fracture is evident.
Neurological Screening	Within normal limits
Vascular Screening	Within normal limits
Imaging Techniques	Radiographs
Differential Diagnosis	MCP or CMC dislocation
Comments	If a fracture is evident, the hand should be appropriately splinted and the patient immediately referred to a physician.

CMC = carpometacarpal; MCP = metacarpophalangeal; ROM = range of motion

acceptable.[19,59] In the absence of rotation, a conservative approach of casting may be used. The presence of rotation at the fracture site that cannot be resolved with closed reduction necessitates open reduction with internal fixation to ensure favorable functional outcomes.[59,60] The amount of angulation deformity that can be tolerated while maintaining function differs among the metacarpals. At the fifth metacarpal, with its extensive mobility at its CMC, angulation of up to 70 degrees may be acceptable.[59,61] After adequate healing has taken place, AROM can be started and progressed to PROM, if needed, at about 8 weeks after the fracture. Strengthening of the wrist and hand is incorporated to counteract the effects of immobilization on the surrounding soft tissue.

Finger Pathology

Frequently, finger injuries go unreported or there is a significant lapse between the onset of the injury and its report. Often gross deformity is associated with these conditions, especially with joint dislocations. However, the patient may self-reduce a dislocation before seeking medical attention.

Collateral Ligament Injuries

Trauma to the collateral ligaments can range from simple sprains to complete dislocations caused by a unilateral stress being applied to an extended finger. Pain is experienced at the affected joint. Active motion and passive motion are limited secondary to pain and swelling. With the exception of a complete disruption of the ligament, valgus and varus stress testing does not accurately distinguish the severity of the injury.

Boutonnière Deformity

Boutonnière deformities can occur as occur as a result of a rupture of the central extensor tendon or secondary to the progression of osteoarthritis or rheumatoid arthritis.[62] A rupture of the central extensor tendon causes the lateral bands to slip palmarly on each side of the PIP joint, changing its line of pull on this joint from that of an extensor to one of a flexor. The resulting position of the finger is extension of the DIP and MCP joints and flexion of the PIP joint, called a boutonnière deformity (see Inspection Findings 17-2). The patient describes a longitudinal force on the finger, such as being struck with a ball. Pain occurs on the dorsal aspect of the PIP joint, and the boutonnière deformity is visible. In acute cases, the PIP joint cannot be actively extended, but the examiner can passively return the joint to its normal position. The signs and symptoms of a tendon rupture may not be recognized for some time after the injury.[63] In chronic cases, the remaining tendon becomes fibrotic, forming a mechanical block against even passive extension of the joint.

An injury to the volar plate can cause a flexion deformity of the PIP joint that resembles a boutonnière deformity—a **pseudoboutonnière deformity** (see Inspection Findings 17-2). Hyperextension of the finger causes the volar plate to split along the finger's long axis and slide dorsally past the joint's axis. The PIP joint cannot be extended either actively or passively.

Finger Fractures

Fractures of the **distal phalanx**, the most common fractures of the hand, occur most frequently in the thumb and middle finger. One reason for this high incidence of injury is the attachments of the flexor and extensor tendons. Avulsions of these tendons result in the inability to completely flex or extend the distal phalanx. The distal phalanx is also vulnerable to crushing mechanism (e.g., being stepped on) and longitudinal compression and rotation (e.g., a blow to the tip of the finger). The **middle phalanx** is the least frequently fractured phalanx and tends to fracture at the distal portion of the shaft. Injuries to the **proximal phalanx** usually have concurrent tendon and skin trauma. A direct blow to the finger often results in a transverse or comminuted fracture; a twisting or rotational force causes a spiral fracture (Fig. 17-29).

The signs and symptoms of phalanx fractures are similar to those of metacarpal fractures (see Examination Findings 17-8). An audible "snap" at the time of injury may be reported, especially when the proximal or middle phalanx is injured. Pain is centered over the fracture site, and gross deformity may be present. Soft tissue swelling and hematoma formation increase the amount of pain associated with the fracture. AROM is limited by pain or bony derangement. During finger flexion, a spiral or oblique fracture causes the portion of the finger distal to the fracture site to rotate so that the fingernails are not in line with each other (Fig. 17-30).

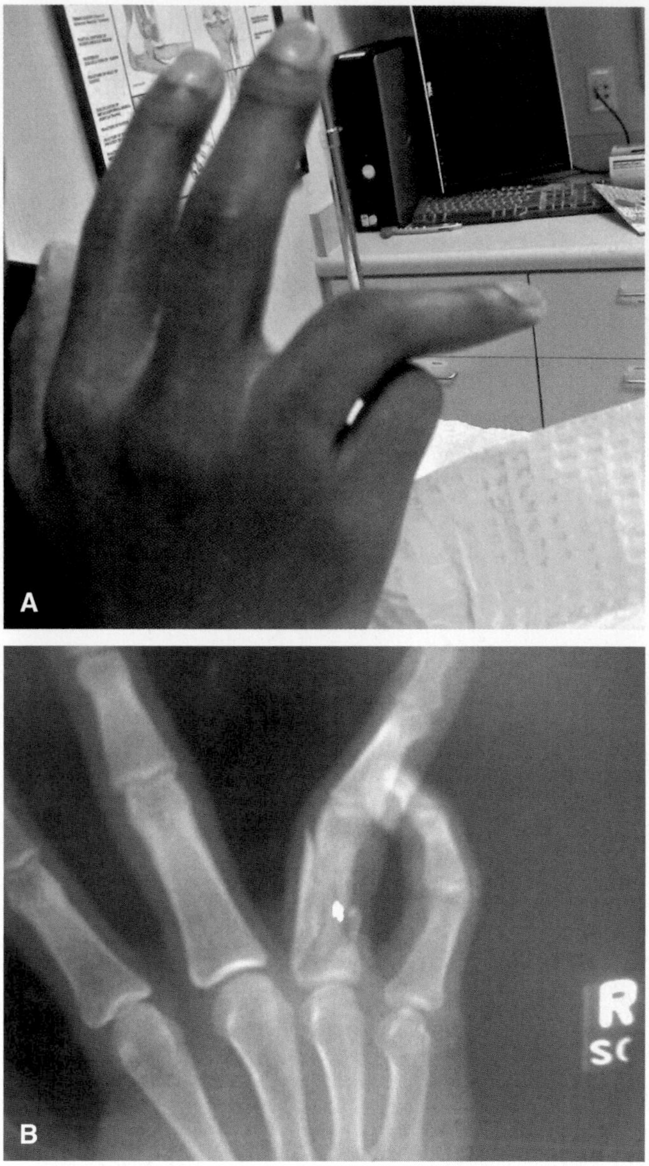

FIGURE 17-29 ■ Proximal phalanx fracture. (A) Note the ulnar displacement of the finger as the result of a displaced oblique fracture. (B) Radiographic view.

Radiographs obtained from the PA, lateral, and oblique views are used to diagnose phalangeal fractures.[19] Fractures that extended into the joint's articular surface can result in the long-term loss of ROM if not surgically realigned.

Finger Fracture Intervention Strategies

The acute management of suspected finger fractures is described in the on-field section of this chapter. Once radiographs have confirmed the fracture, further management

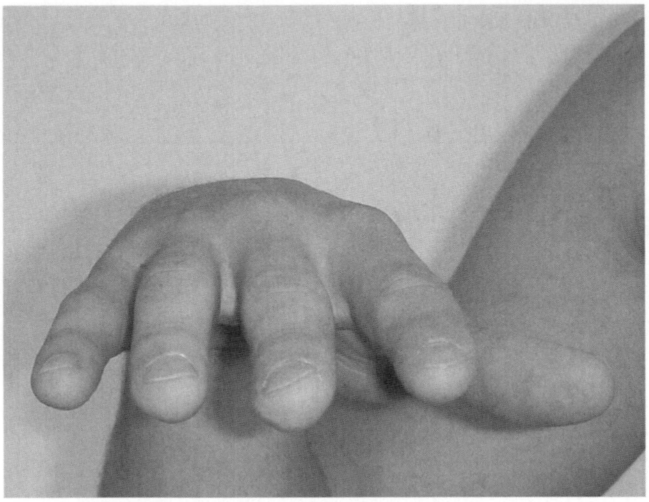

FIGURE 17-30 ■ Rotational malalignment associated with a spiral fracture of the phalanx or metacarpal. Note the rotational deformity of the third fingernail.

is determined by the extent of angulation and the location of the fracture. Surgery is usually indicated if the fracture crosses the joint surface in order to restore normal joint mechanics.[59]

Tendon Ruptures and Avulsion Fractures

Mallet finger occurs when an avulsion or rupture of an extensor tendon results in the inability to fully extend the distal phalanx (see Inspection Findings 17-2). This occurs when the DIP is forced into flexion, such as when the fingertip is struck with a ball. In addition to being unable to actively extend the finger, the patient will report pain at the distal phalanx, which rests at approximately 25 to 35 degrees of flexion. Active flexion is still present, and the phalanx can be passively moved into extension.

An avulsion of the FDP tendon off the palmar aspect of the DIP joint, **jersey finger**, results in the inability to flex the distal phalanx (see Inspection Findings 17-2). This commonly occurs when an athlete grasps another athlete's jersey, forcing the finger into extension as the finger is attempting to flex and hold onto the opponent. The jersey finger injury is described as being one of three types[64]:

- **First degree:** The bony attachment is left intact, and the ruptured tendon retracts to the PIP joint.
- **Second degree:** A portion of the bony attachment is avulsed, and the tendon retracts to the palm.
- **Third degree:** A fragment of bone is avulsed with the tendon's insertion and retracts to the PIP joint.

On casual inspection and functional testing, the involved finger appears to be normal. The finger is painful, but little swelling or disfiguration is noted. The fingers appear to flex and extend normally, with an increase in pain noted during flexion. The telltale sign occurs when the examiner stabilizes the PIP joint in extension and requests that the patient flex the DIP joint, but the patient is unable to do so.

Tendon Rupture and Avulsion Fracture Intervention Strategies

Acute management of suspected tendon ruptures involves splinting the involved finger in a position to shorten the involved tendon or in a position that is comfortable for the patient. For example, a suspected FDP tendon rupture should be splinted with the involved finger flexed. A mallet finger is splinted with the DIP in extension.

Following a definitive diagnosis, management might include a period of splinting or surgical management to repair the rupture tissue or restore bony congruency. Treatment of a mallet finger requires rigid patient compliance to maintain the DIP in extension for around 6 weeks.[65]

Thumb Pathology

The thumb is involved in most aspects of ADLs and athletics, and the position it assumes when gripping, catching, or in the "ready position" exposes it to potentially injurious forces in all planes. Unlike the other digits, the thumb is also susceptible to overuse conditions.

De Quervain's Syndrome

De Quervain's syndrome is a tenosynovitis of the extensor pollicis brevis and abductor pollicis longus tendons, which are encased by a fibrous sheath having a common synovial lining. De Quervain's syndrome is most common in women between the ages of 20 and 40.[66] Repetitive stress causes the compartment to become inflamed, with resulting thickening and narrowing of the tendon's sheath. A history of this condition reveals a mechanism of repetitive motions usually involving radial deviation.[67] Pain is located at the radial styloid process and dorsum of the thumb and radiates proximally into the forearm. Swelling may be located over the styloid process and thenar eminence. Radial and ulnar deviation of the wrist results in pain, as do flexion, extension, and abduction of the thumb (Examination Findings 17-9). Although not conclusive, **Finkelstein's test** may be used to support or refute the presence of de Quervain's syndrome (Selective Tissue Test 17-4).

De Quervain's Syndrome Intervention Strategies

Patients with de Quervain's syndrome are initially treated with corticosteroid injections.[15,68] The use of NSAIDs does not appreciably alter symptoms, but rest, ice, and splinting to limit ulnar deviation may be included in the treatment plan.[15] Surgery to release the sheaths surrounding the tendons has very high success rates with few complications.[15,69]

Thumb Ulnar Collateral Ligament Sprains

The UCL of the thumb's MCP joint is injured 10 times more often than its radial counterpart is.[70] This structure may be acutely sprained by hyperabduction or hyperextension of the MCP joint, or it may be traumatized secondary to a repetitive stress. In the case of acute trauma, an associated avulsion fracture may occur around the MCP joint. The term "gamekeeper's thumb" was coined to describe the stretching of this ligament suffered by individuals whose duty it was to

Examination Findings 17-9
De Quervain's Syndrome

Examination Segment	Clinical Findings
History of Current Condition	*Onset:* Insidious *Pain characteristics:* Over the length of the extensor pollicis brevis and abductor pollicis longus, the radial styloid process and thenar eminence, possibly extending into the distal forearm; complaints of pain increased during radial and ulnar deviation *Mechanism:* Repetitive stress often involving radial deviation *Risk factors:* Repetitive motion accompanied by poor biomechanics
Functional Assessment	Increased symptoms with activities requiring radial and ulnar deviation
Inspection	Swelling over the styloid process and in the involved tendons
Palpation	Pain felt over the styloid process, thenar eminence, and the length of the extensor pollicis brevis and abductor pollicis longus muscles
Joint and Muscle Function Assessment	*AROM:* Wrist: Pain with radial and ulnar deviation Thumb: Pain with flexion and adduction and extension and abduction *MMT:* Wrist: Pain with radial deviation Thumb: Pain with extension and abduction of CMC *PROM:* Wrist: Pain at the end-range of ulnar deviation Thumb: Pain with flexion and adduction of CMC
Joint Stability Tests	*Stress tests:* Not applicable *Joint play:* Not applicable
Selective Tissue Tests	Finkelstein's test
Neurological Screening	Within normal limits
Vascular Screening	Within normal limits
Imaging Techniques	Generally none used
Differential Diagnosis	Extensor carpi radialis brevis and/or extensor carpi radialis longus tendinopathy, ganglion, cervical radiculopathy, scaphoid fracture
Comments	Not applicable

AROM = active range of motion; CMC = carpometacarpal; MMT = manual muscle test; PROM = passive range of motion

snap the neck of small game that had just been captured during hunting. This injury is commonly seen in skiers, football players, and basketball players. UCL sprains limit opposition of the thumb and decrease grip strength.

The chief complaint is pain along the ulnar aspect of the MCP joint that hinders the ability to forcefully pinch or grasp smaller objects. Swelling, which can be extensive, is usually localized in the adductor compartment and thenar eminence. Ecchymosis may also be present. During palpation, tenderness is elicited over the UCL, with special attention paid to its proximal and distal attachments, noting for signs of an avulsion. Pain is produced, and a strength deficit is noted during opposition of the thumb and index finger (Examination Findings 17-10). Valgus stress testing of the UCL demonstrates an increase in the amount of gapping present as compared with the uninjured hand. Stress testing should be carried out with the first MCP joint extended and then again with the joint flexed to account for the geometry of the joint and to test the various bands of the UCL.[71]

Thumb Ulnar Collateral Ligament Sprains Intervention Strategies

The treatment of patients with sprains of the UCL of the first MCP joint is determined by the severity of the sprain.

Selective Tissue Test 17-4
Finkelstein's Test for de Quervain's Syndrome

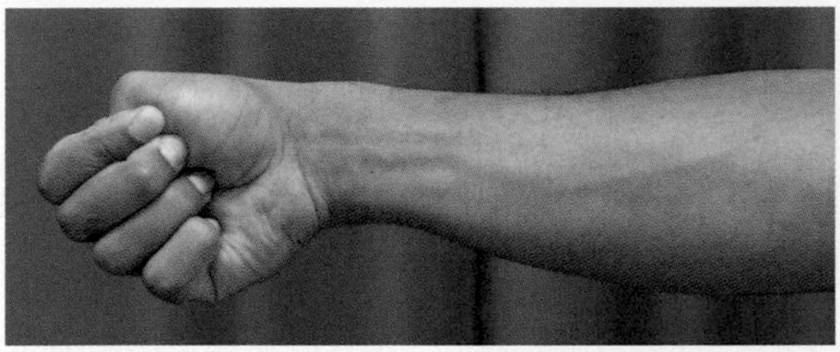

The patient ulnarly deviates the wrist while the thumb is clasped by the fingers.

Patient Position	Seated or standing
Position of Examiner	Standing in front of the patient
Evaluative Procedure	The patient tucks the thumb under the fingers by making a fist.
Positive Test	Increased pain in the area of the radial styloid process and along the length of the extensor pollicis brevis and abductor pollicis longus tendons
Implications	De Quervain's syndrome (tenosynovitis of the extensor pollicis brevis and abductor pollicis longus tendons)
Comments	This test often produces false-positive results, so the results must be correlated with other examination findings.
Evidence	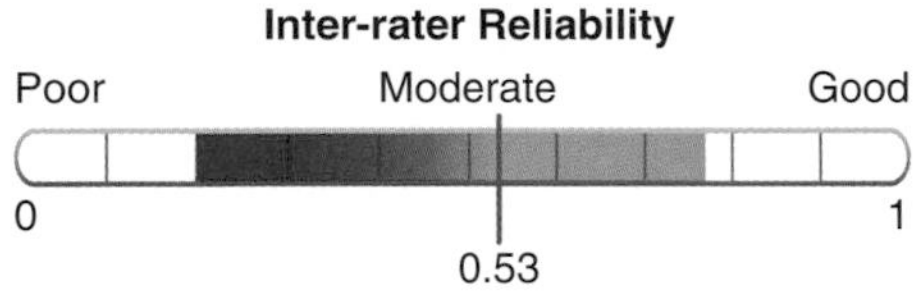

Instability of this joint will adversely affect ADLs as simple as gripping a soda can as well as more vigorous sports activities. Patients with incomplete tears with a firm endpoint and less than 30 degrees of opening compared with the opposite side during stress testing may be treated with a thumb spica splint for 4 to 6 weeks. Complete ruptures require early surgical repair to avoid long-term complications, but surgery can usually be attempted up to 3 weeks after the injury.[72] Periods longer than 3 weeks after the injury may require a reconstruction of the ligament with a graft versus a primary repair of the tissue. **Stener lesions**, in which the proximal end of the UCL dislocates from under the adductor aponeurosis, must be treated with surgery.[61]

Metacarpophalangeal Joint Dislocation
Dislocation of the MCP joint is most common in the thumb and occurs when the volar plate is avulsed from the head of the first metacarpal. The mechanism of injury is extension and abduction. A fracture of the proximal phalanx or first metacarpal joint may occur concurrently. The involved joint has obvious deformity and is unable to demonstrate AROM because of pain.

Thumb Fractures
Fractures of the first metacarpal are similar to the description given for metacarpal fractures of the hand. Fractures of the base of the first metacarpal that extend into the articular surface are termed **Bennett's fractures** (Fig. 17-31). Contracture of the abductor pollicus longus results in the metacarpal being displaced dorsally.[19]

Bennett's Fracture Intervention Strategies
Because of the thumb's potential loss of function secondary to instability at the CMC joint, patients with this type of fracture often require internal fixation to establish joint congruency.

On-Field Evaluation and Management of Wrist, Hand, and Finger Injuries

Most often, athletes with a wrist, hand, or finger injury leave the field on their own, cradling and protecting the injured extremity. The examiner must carry out a complete inspection of the injured area, a task that is somewhat simplified by the relatively superficial nature of the structures. With the exception of trauma to the carpal bones, deformity is usually obvious and may involve open or closed fractures or dislocation of the fingers.

Typically, the injured hand and wrist are not covered by equipment. In certain sports such as football, ice hockey,

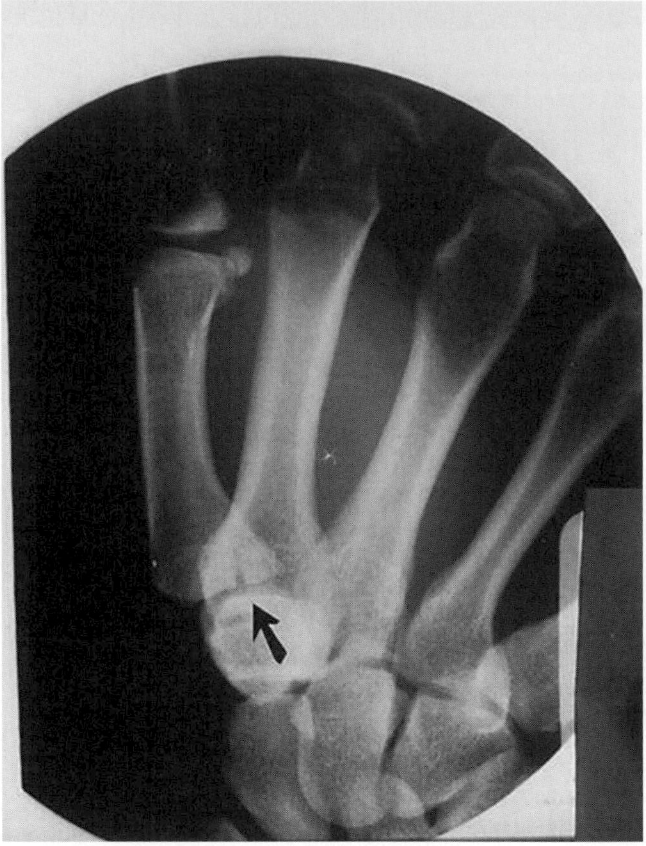

FIGURE 17-31 ■ Radiograph of a Bennett's fracture.

and lacrosse, the athlete may wear a glove. In these cases, the glove is removed most easily, and with the least amount of pain, by the athlete.

Wrist Fractures and Dislocations

Fractures of the radius or ulna as well as dislocations of the radiocarpal joint must be immobilized in the position in which they are found, using a vacuum or other type of splint (Fig. 17-32). Before splinting the area, the radial and ulnar arterial pulses must be evaluated. As with any fracture, the joint itself or the joint above and below the fracture site needs to be immobilized. Open fractures should be managed using universal precautions and with the fracture site covered before the splint is applied.

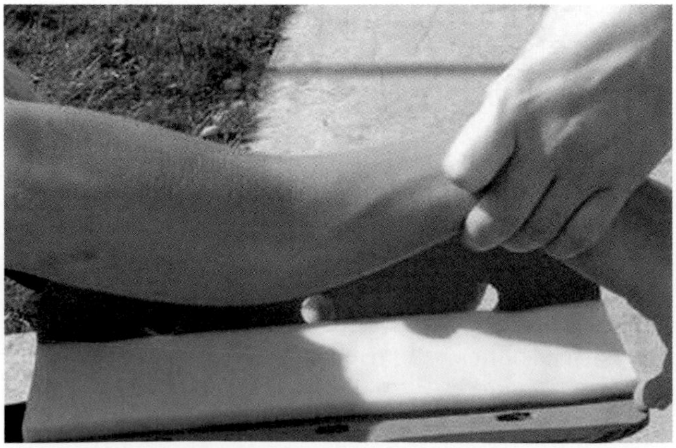

FIGURE 17-32 ■ Forearm fracture. Note the midshaft fracture of the radius and ulna.

Suspected fractures or dislocations of the carpal bones can be carefully supported and the athlete moved off the field for further evaluation. If a fracture is suspected, the wrist is immobilized as previously described.

Interphalangeal Joint Dislocations

Dislocation of an IP joint results in obvious deformity. In some instances, the athlete instinctively reduces the dislocation by applying traction to the finger. The on-field reduction of IP joint dislocations should be performed by trained personnel and followed by splinting, referral, and appropriate imaging (Box 17-2).

For unreduced dislocations, the palmar aspect of the injured finger must be splinted in the position in which it

Box 17-2
Reducing IP Joint Dislocations

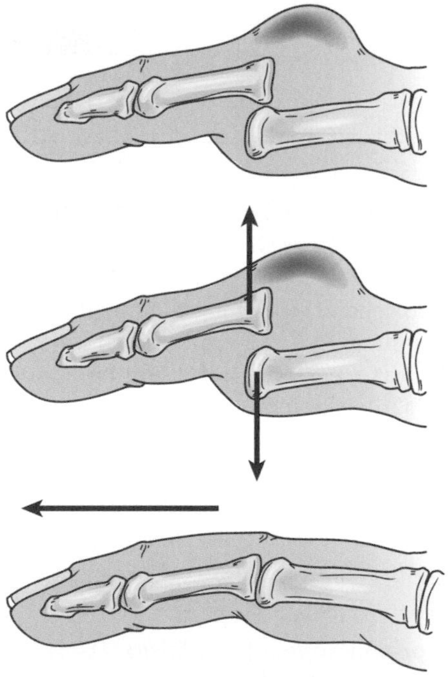

The potential for prolonged, severe pain coupled with the distressing visual deformity make prompt reduction of IP joint dislocations an appropriate intervention by qualified personnel. Reduction should not be attempted if a fracture is suspected or in the event of an open dislocation. Reduction is best achieved by stabilizing the phalanx proximal to the dislocation and applying a force to first increase the deformity (separating the bones) followed by distraction. Following reduction, AROM of the involved joint should be assessed, and the athlete should be referred for imaging and physician consultation.

Examination Findings 17-10
Ulnar Collateral Ligament Sprains

Examination Segment	Clinical Findings
History of Current Condition	*Onset:* Acute or chronic *Pain characteristics:* Along the ulnar aspect of the first MCP joint *Mechanism:* Acute: Hyperextension or hyperabduction (or both) of the first MCP joint Chronic: Repetitive flexion or adduction (or both) of the joint *Risk factors:* Repetitive motion that applies a valgus force to the MCP joint
Functional Assessment	Increased pain or weakness with any tasks requiring gripping
Inspection	Localized and possibly extensive swelling in the adductor compartment and thenar eminence Possible ecchymosis
Palpation	Pain is felt along the ulnar border of the MCP joint. The examiner should note for the presence of bony fragments indicating an avulsion of the ligament.
Joint and Muscle Function Assessment	*AROM:* Pain during extension, abduction, and opposition of the thumb *MMT:* Weakness experienced during MCP flexion and CMC adduction; pinch strength decreased (**Froment's sign**)[19] *PROM:* Pain at the end-range of thumb extension and abduction
Joint Stability Tests	*Stress tests:* Test for ulnar collateral ligament instability Valgus stress test for the MCP joint *Joint play:* Increased ulnar glide of MCP joint
Selective Tissue Tests	None
Neurological Screening	Within normal limits
Vascular Screening	Within normal limits
Imaging Techniques	Radiographs to rule out avulsion fracture
Differential Diagnosis	Metacarpal or proximal phalanx fracture, volar plate injury
Comments	UCL sprains should be referred to a physician for further evaluation to rule out an avulsion fracture.

AROM = active range of motion; CMC = carpometacarpal; MCP = metacarpophalangeal; MMT = manual muscle test; PROM = passive range of motion; UCL = ulnar collateral ligament

was found. An ice pack is applied to the dorsal side, and the athlete is referred to a physician.

Hand and Finger Fractures

When fractures of the hand are suspected, the hand is splinted so that the wrist and fingers are also immobilized. However, the fingernails must remain uncovered so that distal blood flow can be checked. Finger fractures are splinted in the position in which they are found using an aluminum splint that also immobilizes the MCP joint. Often a standard tongue depressor can be used to sufficiently splint the area. Table 17-5 describes the splinting position for other common finger injuries. Correct immediate management and

Table 17-5 Splinting of Common Finger Injuries

Deformity	Splinting Position
Jersey finger	DIP joint in flexion
Mallet finger	DIP joint in extension
Boutonnière deformity	PIP and DIP joints in extension
Phalanx fracture	Position found
Metacarpal fracture	Palmar surface of wrist and hand
Unreduced dislocations	Position found

DIP = distal interphalangeal; PIP = proximal interphalangeal proper immobilization techniques reduce the chance that the injury will require surgical correction.

Lacerations

Because of the relatively superficial location of the tendons and nerves in the wrist, hand, and fingers, they are vulnerable to damage from even shallow lacerations. As with any cut, the possibility of infection exists, especially when the laceration involves the joints. Any laceration involving the fascia below the cutaneous level requires referral to a physician to rule out the possibility of trauma to the underlying tendons and nerves and determine the possible need for suturing and prophylactic antibiotics.

REFERENCES

1. Austin, NM: The wrist and hand complex. In: Levangie, PK, and Norkin, CC (eds): *Joint Structure and Function: A Comprehensive Analysis* (ed 5). Philadelphia, PA: FA Davis, 2011, p 310.
2. Smith, TO, et al: Diagnostic accuracy of magnetic resonance imaging and magnetic resonance arthrography for triangular fibrocartilaginous complex injury. *J Bone Joint Surg Am*, 94:824, 2012.
3. Scheer, JH, and Adolfsson, LE: Patterns of triangular fibrocartilage complex (TFCC) injury associated with severely dorsally displaced extra-articular distal radius fractures. *Injury*, 43:926, 2012.
4. Kozin, SH: Perilunate injuries: diagnosis and treatment. *J Am Acad Orthop Surg*, 6:114, 1998.
5. Shin, AY, Battaglia, MJ, and Bishop, AT: Lunotriquestral instability: diagnosis and treatment. *J Am Acad Orthop Surg*, 8:170, 2000.
6. Newport, ML: Extensor tendon injuries in the hand. *J Am Acad Orthop Surg*, 5:59, 1997.
7. Strickland, JW: Flexor tendon injuries: I. foundations of treatment. *J Am Acad Orthop Surg*, 3:44, 1995.
8. McNamara, B: Clinical anatomy of the ulnar nerve. *ACNR*, 3:25, 2003.
9. McNamara, B: Clinical anatomy of the median nerve. *ACNR*, 2:18, 2003.
10. McNamara, B: Clinical anatomy of the radial nerve. *ACNR*, 3:28, 2003.
11. Nagle, DJ: Evaluation of chronic wrist pain. *J Am Acad Orthop Surg*, 8:45, 2000.
12. van Vugt, RM, et al: Chronic wrist pain: diagnosis and management: development and use of a new algorithm. *Ann Rheum Dis*, 58:665, 1999.
13. Forman, TA, Forman, SK, and Rose, NE: A clinical approach to diagnosing wrist pain. *Am Fam Phys*, 72:1753, 2005.
14. Saldana, MJ: Trigger digits: diagnosis and treatment. *J Am Acad Orthop Surg*, 9:246, 2001.
15. McAuliffe, JA: Tendon disorders of the hand and wrist. *J Hand Surg*, 35: 846, 2010.
16. Draeger, RW, and Bynum, DK: Flexor tendon sheath infections of the hand. *J Am Acad Ortho Surg*, 20:373, 2012.
17. Daluiski, A, Rahbar, B, and Meals, RA: Russell's sign: subtle hand changes in patients with bulimia nervosa. *Clin Orthop*, 343:107, 1997.
18. Hsu, SH, et al: Physical examination of the athlete's elbow. *Am J Sports Med*, 40:699, 2012.
19. Abraham, MK, and Scott, S: The emergent evaluation and treatment of hand and wrist injuries. *Emerg Med Clin N Am*, 28:789, 2010.
20. Rettig, AC: Athletic injuries of the wrist and hand. Part I: traumatic injuries of the wrist. *Am J Sports Med*, 31:1038, 2003.
21. Gunther, CM, et al: Grip strength in healthy Caucasian adults: reference values. *J Hand Surg Am*, 33:558, 2008.
22. Clarkson, HM: *Musculoskeletal Assessment. Joint Range of Motion and Manual Muscle Strength* (ed 2). Philadelphia, PA: Lippincott Williams & Wilkins, 2000.
23. Prosser, R, et al: Provocative wrist tests and MRI are of limited diagnostic value for suspected wrist ligament injuries: a cross-sectional study. *J Physiother*, 57:247, 2011.
24. Posner, MA: Compressive ulnar neuropathies at the elbow: I. etiology and diagnosis. *J Am Acad Orthop Surg*, 6:282, 1998.
25. Colles, A: On the fracture of the carpal extremity of the radius. *Edinb Med Surg J*, 10:182, 1814.
26. Thoms, FB: Reduction of Smith's fractures. *J Bone Joint Surg Br*, 39:463, 1959.
27. Black, WS, and Becker JA: Common forearm fractures in adults. *Am Fam Physician*, 80:1096, 2009.
28. Rhemrev, SJ, et al: Current methods of diagnosis and treatment of scaphoid fractures. *Int J Emerg Med*, 4:4, 2011.
29. Buijze, GA, Ochtman, L, and Ring, D: Management of scaphoid non-union. *J Hand Surg*, 37A:1095, 2012.
30. Phillips, TG, Reibach, AM, and Slomiany, WP: Diagnosis and management of scaphoid fractures. *Am Fam Physician*, 70:879, 2004.
31. Ring, B, Jupiter, JB, and Herndon, JH: Acute fractures of the scaphoid. *J Am Acad Orthop Surg*, 8:225, 2000.
32. Duckworth, AD, et al: Predictors of fracture following suspected injury to the scaphoid. *J Bone Joint Surg Br*, 94:961, 2012.
33. Schubert, HE: Scaphoid fracture. Review of diagnostic tests and treatment. *Can Fam Physician*, 46:1825, 2000.
34. Yin, Z, et al: Diagnosing suspected scaphoid fractures. *Clin Orthop Relat Res*, 468:723, 2010.
35. Doornberg, JN, et al: Nonoperative treatment for acute scaphoid fractures: a systematic review and meta-analysis of randomized controlled trials. *J Trauma*, 71:1073, 2011.
36. Wright, TW, Moser, MW, and Sahajpal, DT: Hook of the hamate pull test. *J Hand Surg*, 35:1887, 2010.
37. David, TS, Zemel, NP, and Mathews, PV: Symptomatic, partial union of the hook of the hamate fracture in athletes. *Am J Sports Med*, 31:106, 2003.
38. Green, DP, and O'Brien, ET: Classification and management of carpal dislocations. *Clin Orthop Relat Res*, 149:55, 1980.
39. Campbell, RD, Lance, EM, and Yeoh, CB: Lunate and perilunate dislocations. *J Bone Joint Surg Br*, 46:55, 1964.
40. Najarian, R, et al: Perilunate injuries. *Hand*, 6:1, 2011.
41. Bergh, TH, et al: A new definition of wrist sprain necessary after findings in a prospective MRI study. *Injury*, 43:1732, 2012.
42. Dao, KD, et al: The efficacy of ultrasound in the evaluation of dynamic scapholunate ligamentous instability. *J Bone Joint Surg Am*, 86-A:1473, 2004.
43. Park, MJ: Radiographic observation of the scaphoid shift test. *J Bone Joint Surg Br*, 85:358, 2003.
44. Rosati, M, et al: Treatment of acute scapholunate ligament injuries with bone anchors. *Musculoskel Surg*, 94:25, 2010.
45. Sachar, K: Ulnar-sided wrist pain: evaluation and treatment of triangular fibrocartilage complex tears, ulnocarpal impaction syndrome, and lunotriquetral ligament tears. *J Hand Surg Am*, 37:1489, 2012.
46. Nishikawa, S, and Satoshi, T: Anatomical study of the carpal attachment of the triangular fibrocartilage complex. *J Bone Joint Surg Br*, 84:1062, 2002.
47. Shih, J-T, Lee, H-M, and Tan, C-M: Early isolated triangular fibrocartilage complex tears: management by arthroscopic repair. *J Trauma*, 53:922, 2002.
48. Langer, I, et al: Ganglions of the wrist and associated triangular fibrocartilage lesions: a prospective study in arthroscopically treated patients. *J Hand Surg Am*, 37:1561, 2012.
49. Iordache, SD, et al: Prevalence of triangular fibrocartilage complex abnormalities on MRI scans of asymptomatic wrists. *J Hand Surg Am*, 37:98, 2012.
50. Palmar, KT: Carpal tunnel syndrome: the role of occupational factors. *Best Pract Res Clin Rheumatol*, 25:15, 2011.
51. Salerno, DF, et al: Reliability of physical examination of the upper extremity among keyboard operators. *Am J Ind Med*, 37:423, 2000.
52. Szabo, RM, et al: The value of diagnostic testing in carpal tunnel syndrome. *J Hand Surg Am*, 24:704, 1999.

53. Prime, MS, et al: Is there light at the end of the tunnel? controversies in the diagnosis and management of carpal tunnel syndrome. *Hand*, 5:354, 2010.
54. Bechtol, C: Grip test: the use of a dynamometer with adjustable handle spacings. *J Bone Joint Surg Am*, 36:L820, 1954.
55. Zimmerman, GR: Carpal tunnel syndrome. *J Athl Train*, 29:22, 1994.
56. MacDermid, JC, and Wessel, J: Clinical diagnosis of carpal tunnel syndrome: a systematic review. *J Hand Ther*, 17:309, 2004.
57. Aird, J, et al: The impact of wrist extension provocation on current perception thresholds in patients with carpal tunnel syndrome: a pilot study. *J Hand Ther*, 19:299, 2006.
58. Sui, Q, and MacDermid, JC: Is surgical intervention more effective than non-surgical treatment for carpal tunnel syndrome? a systematic review. *J Orthop Surg Res*, 6:17, 2011.
59. Haughton, DN, et al: Principles of hand fracture management. *Open Orthop J*, 6:43, 2012.
60. Capo, JT, and Hastings, H: Metacarpal and phalangeal fractures in athletes. *Clin Sports Med*, 17:491, 1998.
61. Leggit, JC, and Meko, CJ: Acute finger injuries: Part II: fractures, dislocations, and thumb injuries. *Am Fam Physician*, 73:827, 2006.
62. Williams, K, and Terrono, AL: Treatment of boutonniere finger deformity in rheumatoid arthritis. *J Hand Surg Am*, 36:1388, 2011.
63. Dawson, WJ: The spectrum of sports-related interphalangeal joint injuries. *Hand Clin*, 10:315, 1994.
64. Leddy, JP, and Packer, JW: Avulsion of the profundus tendon insertion in athletes. *J Hand Surg Am*, 2:66, 1977.
65. Andrade, A, and Hern, HG: Traumatic hand injuries: the emergency clinician's evidence-based approach. *Emerg Med Pract*, 13:1, 2011.
66. Rossi, C, et al: De Quervain disease in volleyball players. *Am J Sports Med*, 33:424, 2005.
67. Lipscomb, PR: Stenosing tenosynovitis at the radial styloid process. *Ann Surg*, 134:110, 1951.
68. Richie, CA 3rd, and Briner, WW Jr: Corticosteroid injection for treatment of de Quervain's tenosynovitis: a pooled quantitative literature evaluation. *J Am Board Fam Pract*, 16:102, 2003.
69. Crop, JA, and Bunt, CW: "Doctor my thumb hurts." *J Fam Practice*, 60:329, 2011.
70. Lane, LB: Acute grade III ulnar collateral ligament ruptures: a new surgical and rehabilitation protocol. *Am J Sports Med*, 19:234, 1991.
71. McCue, FC, Mayer, V, and Moran, DJ: Gamekeeper's thumb: ulnar collateral ligament rupture. *J Musculoskel Med*, 5:53, 1988.
72. Langford, SA, Whitaker, JH, and Toby, EB: Thumb injuries in the athlete. *Clin Sports Med*, 17:553, 1998.

SECTION 5

Examination of the Head

Unlike other body regions, many of the primary outcome measures used for the structures and systems located in the head are clinician rated. The head and face, including the eyes, ears, mouth, and nose, are the primary systems for the major senses of sight, hearing, taste, and smell (the fifth major sense, touch, is assessed using upper- and lower-quarter screens). Vision tests and hearing screens are among the most common functional assessments. These are discussed in Chapters 18 and 19.

The diagnosis and management of concussions rely on both patient-reported symptoms and clinician- and patient-rated function. Measures of balance, coordination, memory, and neurocognitive function used during the course of care are described in Chapter 20. Standardized assessments such as the Sport Concussion Assessment Tool provide scores for different subsections, allowing test–retest comparisons to gauge progress. Other scales can measure the impact of headaches, depressive symptoms, and mood states.[1] Broad health-related quality-of-life measures described in the Section I opener also provide helpful information regarding a patient's progress.

Headache Impact Test (HIT-6™)

The HIT-6™ assesses the effect of headaches on patient function and productivity.[2] Derived from a 54-item questionnaire, the HIT-6™ measures the level of headache-related dysfunction using a global score and four subscores: functional, psychological, social, and therapeutic. The resulting impact is then rated as "little to none," "moderate," "substantial," or "severe." [3]

Minimum Detectable Change: 2.5[4]
Minimum Clinically Important Difference: 1.5[4]

Beck Depression Inventory II (BDI II)

The BDI was developed to screen individuals for depression and has been used to monitor for depressive symptoms following concussion.[5] Because it assesses for the severity of depressive symptoms, the BDI II can also be used to monitor progress.[6] The BDI II list 21 symptoms such as sadness, potential for suicide, and changes in appetite. The patient selects an option relating to the severity of that symptom over the past 2 weeks. Scores are tallied, with a range from 0 to 63. Higher scores represent more severe symptoms and are interpreted as follows[7]:

Minimal range: 0–13
Mild depression: 14–19
Moderate depression: 20–28
Severe depression: 29–63

Profile of Mood States (POMS)

The POMS has a wide range of uses and is a common instrument in sports psychology. This instrument assesses the patient on six mood subscales: tension–anxiety, depression, anger–hostility, vigor, fatigue, and confusion. In the subscales of tension–anxiety, depression, anger–hostility, fatigue, and confusion, lower scores indicate a more positive mood state. In the subscale of vigor, a higher score is indicative of a positive mood state.[5]

Minimum Detectable Change: Variable based on the condition being monitored
Minimum Clinically Important Difference: Variable based on the condition being monitored

REFERENCES

1. Valovich McLeod, TC, and Register-Mihalik, JK: Clinical outcomes assessment for the management of sport-related concussion. *J Sport Rehabil*, 20:46, 2011.
2. Kosinski, M, et al: A six-item short-form survey for measuring headache impact: the HIT-6™. *Qual Life Res*, 12:963, 2003.
3. Nachit-Ouinekah, F, et al: Use of the headache impact test (HIT-6) in general practice: relationship with quality of life and severity. *Eur J Neurol*, 12:189, 2005.
4. Smelt, AFH, et al: What is a clinically relevant change on the HIT-6 questionnaire? An estimation in a primary-care population of migraine patients. *Cephalalgia*, July, 2013 34:29, 2014.
5. Strain, J, et al: Depressive symptoms and white matter dysfunction in retired NFL players with concussion history. *Neurology*, 81:25, 2013.
6. Smarr, KL, and Keefer, AL: Measures of depression and depressive symptoms: Beck Depression Inventory-II (BDI-II), Center for Epidemiologic Studies Depression Scale (CES-D), Geriatric Depression Scale (GDS), Hospital Anxiety and Depression Scale (HADS), and Patient Health Questionnaire-9 (PHQ-9). *Arthritis Care Res (Hoboken)*, 63(suppl 11):S454, 2011.
7. Beck, AT, Steer, RA, and Brown, GK: *Beck Depression Inventory: Second Edition Manual.* San Antonio, TX: The Psychological Corporation, 1996.
8. Yoshihara, K, et al: Profile of mood states and stress-related biochemical indices in long-term yoga practitioners. *Biopsychosoc Med*, 5:6, 2011.

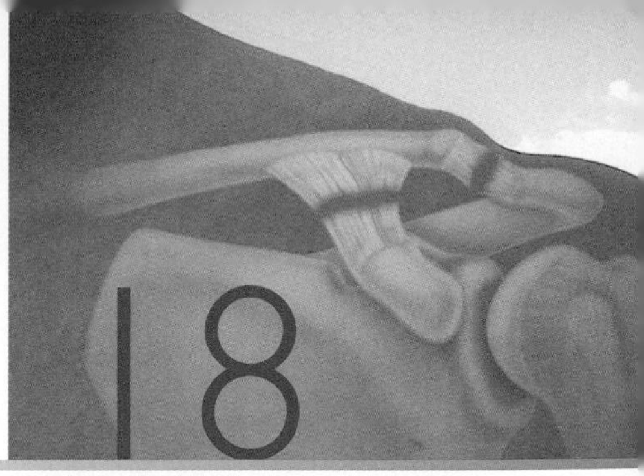

CHAPTER 18

Eye Pathologies

Resulting from a direct blow, impalement, or chemical invasion, trauma to the eye requires an accurate assessment so that proper management and further evaluation by an **ophthalmologist** can be initiated. Failure to recognize and properly manage eye trauma can result in permanent dysfunction, including blindness.

Racquet sports (in which the ball can reach speeds up to 140 mph), boxing, and golf are most often associated with catastrophic injury to the eye. However, traumatic injury to the eye can occur in all sports, with basketball being the most common.[1,2] An estimated 90% of all eye injuries can be prevented through the use of approved protective eye wear.

Clinical Anatomy

The eye, except for its anterior aspect, sits encased within the conical bony **orbit** (Fig. 18-1). In addition to protecting and stabilizing the eye, the orbit also serves as an attachment site for some of the extrinsic muscles acting on the eye. The **orbital margin** (periorbital region) is composed of the **frontal bone**, forming the supraorbital margin; the **zygomatic bone** and a portion of the frontal bone, forming the lateral margin; and the zygomatic bone and **maxillary bone**, forming the infraorbital margin.

The anterior portion of the orbit's roof is formed by the frontal bone. A portion of the **sphenoid bone** forms its posterior aspect. Medially, the orbit is formed by the thin **lacrimal**, **ethmoid**, **maxillary**, and **sphenoid bones**. The floor is formed by the maxillary, zygomatic, and **palatine bones**. Laterally, the orbit is composed of the zygomatic bone and the sphenoid bone. Here the orbit is the thickest. The **superior orbital fissure**, an opening between the lesser and greater wings of the sphenoid bone, is located between the lateral wall and the roof. This fissure allows the cranial nerves, arteries, and veins to communicate with the eye. The orbit's posterior aspect is marked by the **optic canal**, the foramen through which the optic nerve passes to reach the brain.

Eye Structures

The mass of the eye is a fibrous, fluid-filled structure collectively referred to as the **globe**. Its white layering, the **sclera**, encompasses the posterior five-sixths of the globe and becomes continuous with the sheath of the optic nerve as the nerve continues posteriorly and merges with the brain's fibrous lining. The dark central aperture of the eye, the **pupil**, is surrounded by pigmented contractile tissue, the **iris** (Fig. 18-2). The **conjunctiva**, a thin mucous membrane, covers the sclera and lines the inside of the eyelids. Anteriorly, the conjunctiva is continuous with the transparent **cornea**. The cornea is the main structure involved in focusing light rays entering the eye.

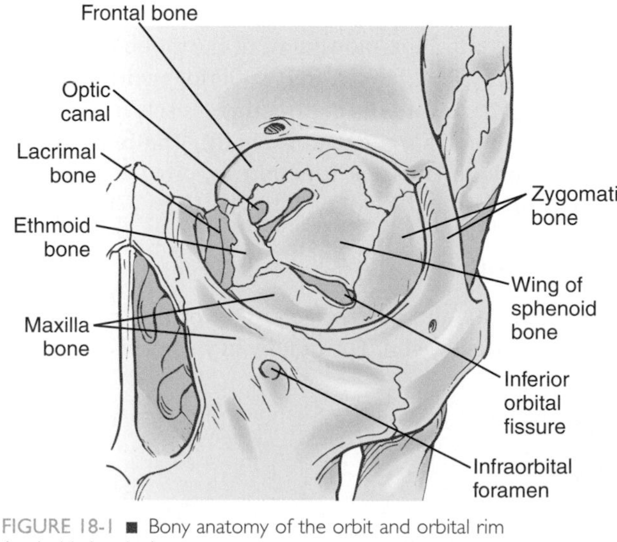

FIGURE 18-1 ■ Bony anatomy of the orbit and orbital rim (periorbital region).

Ophthalmologist A medical doctor specializing in injury, diseases, and abnormalities of the eye

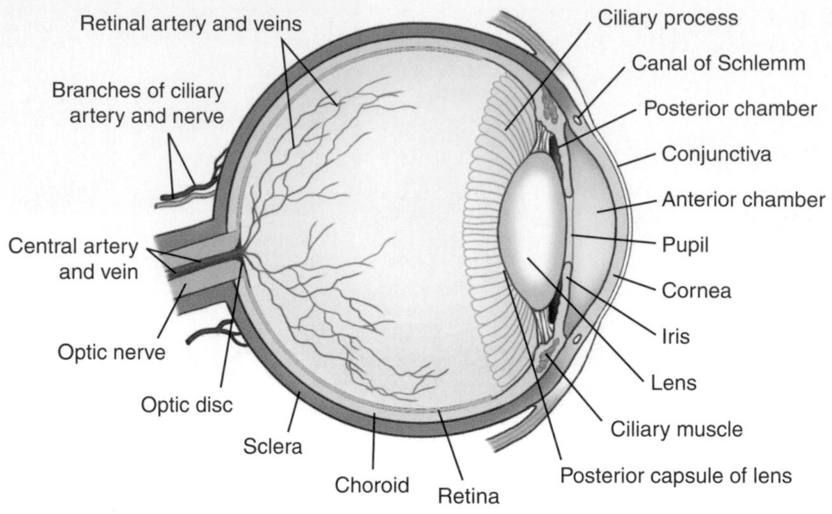

FIGURE 18-2 ■ Cross-sectional view of the anatomy of the globe of the eye.

Suspended by ligaments arising from the ciliary body, the lens is a clear elastic structure located behind the iris that serves to sharpen and focus visual rays on the globe's posterior surface, the retina. The area of the retina facing the center of the globe contains nervous tissues. The outer layer is composed of darkly pigmented vascular tissue, the choroid. Light rays strike the nervous tissues, stimulating the rods and cones, which are photoreceptors located on the globe's posterior surface. Each receptor passes its stimulus through a complex network of nerves until the impulses are collected and transmitted to the brain via the optic nerve. Rods and cones are absent at the optic nerve, thus causing a blind spot in the field of vision (Fig. 18-3).

Eyelids act as shutters to protect the eye from accidental direct contact by reflexively closing when an object comes close to the exposed globe and by preventing airborne dust and dirt from entering the eye. The conjunctiva of the globe is continuous with the inner surfaces of the eyelids. The **blink reflex** aids in lubricating the eye's ocular surface.

Muscular Anatomy

Six muscles control the movement of the globe (Fig. 18-4). The inferior, medial, lateral, and superior **rectus muscles** rotate the globe toward the contracting muscle (e.g., the inferior rectus rotates the eye downward). The **inferior** and **superior oblique muscles** function to provide a torsion (circular) motion to the globe (Table 18-1).

Visual Acuity

Proper anatomy and correct geometry of the lens are required for perfect vision. The quality of vision, visual acuity, can be assessed using a **Snellen chart** (Fig. 18-5). This method determines the person's ability to clearly see letters based on a normalized scale. **Emmetropia**, 20/20 vision, is the ability to read the letters on the 20-foot line of an eye chart when standing 20 feet from the chart, indicating that the light rays are focused precisely on the retina. **Myopia**, or nearsightedness, occurs when the light rays are focused in front of the retina, making only objects very close to the eyes distinguishable. **Hypermetropia** (hyperopia), or farsightedness, results when the light rays are focused at a point behind the retina. Diminished visual acuity may require further assessment to enhance performance and ensure safe participation in sports through corrective methods such as eyeglasses or contact lenses.

Clinical Examination of Eye Injuries

Blunt trauma to the eye can result in injury to the globe and its related structures, laceration of the periorbital skin, or a fracture of the bony orbit. Infections, diseases, allergies, and brain trauma can also lead to dysfunction of the eye. Because of the eye's delicate nature, all maladies involving the eye must be managed with the utmost care and urgency. The supplies necessary for the evaluation and management of eye injuries are presented in Table 18-2.

History

Past Medical History

- **Prior visual assessment:** Ask the patient about prior visual acuity, the need for corrective lenses (glasses or contact lenses), congenital pupillary changes,

FIGURE 18-3 ■ Determining the blind spot in the field of vision. Close one eye and focus on the "X." Move the page toward or away from you until the round spot disappears, indicating the blind area in your field of vision.

Table 18-1 Extrinsic Muscles Acting on the Eye

Muscle	Action	Origin	Insertion	Innervation	Root
Inferior Rectus	Downward rotation of the globe	From a tendinous ring on the posterior aspect of the orbit	Middle of the inferior aspect of the anterior globe	Oculomotor	CN III
Superior Rectus	Upward rotation of the globe	From a tendinous ring on the posterior aspect of the orbit	Middle of the superior aspect of the anterior globe	Oculomotor	CN III
Medial Rectus	Medial rotation of the globe	From a tendinous ring on the posterior aspect of the orbit	Middle of the medial aspect of the anterior globe	Oculomotor	CN III
Lateral Rectus	Lateral rotation of the globe	From a tendinous ring on the posterior aspect of the orbit	Middle of the lateral aspect of the anterior globe	Abducens	CN VI
Inferior Oblique	Adduction of the globe Elevation of the globe Rotation of the globe when abducted	From the periosteum of the maxilla	Inferolateral quadrant of the globe	Oculomotor	CN III
Superior Oblique	Abduction of the globe Depression of the globe Rotation of the globe when adducted	Greater wing of the sphenoid	Superolateral quadrant of the globe	Trochlear	CN IV

CN = cranial nerve

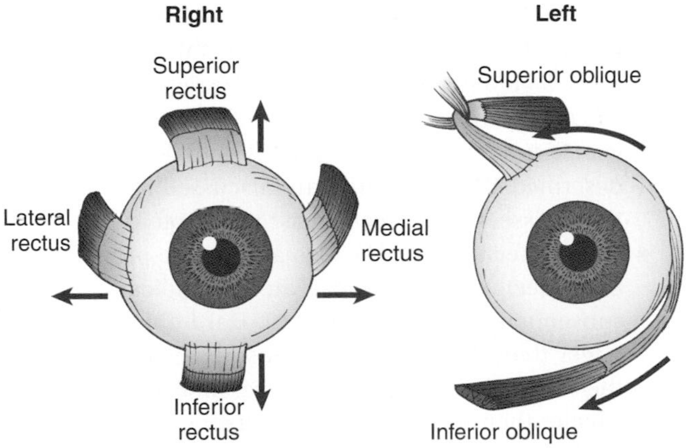

FIGURE 18-4 ■ Extrinsic muscles of the eye. The right eye is used to present the rectus muscles that move the globe in the cardinal planes. The left eye presents the oblique muscles that abduct and adduct the globe.

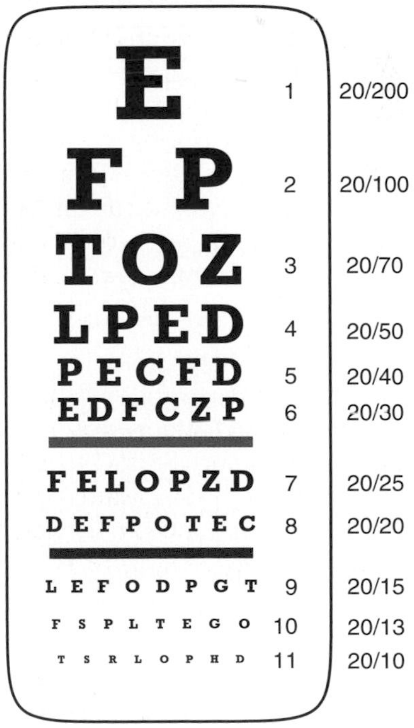

FIGURE 18-5 ■ Snellen-type chart. This device is commonly used to determine an individual's visual acuity.

Examination Map

HISTORY

Past Medical History
- Prior vision assessment
- Mental health status

History of the Present Condition
- General health status
- Location of pain
- Radicular symptoms
- Mechanism of injury
- Onset of condition

INSPECTION

Periorbital Area
- Discoloration
- Gross deformity

Inspection of the Globe
- General appearance
  - Eyelids
  - Cornea
  - Conjunctiva
  - Sclera
  - Iris
  - Pupil shape and size

PALPATION

Orbital Margin
Frontal Bone
Nasal Bone
Zygomatic Bone
Soft Tissue

FUNCTIONAL ASSESSMENT

Vision Assessment
Pupillary Reaction to Light

NEUROLOGICAL EXAMINATION

CN III, IV, VI

REGION-SPECIFIC PATHOLOGIES AND SELECTIVE TISSUE TESTS

Orbital Fractures
- Blowout fractures

Corneal Abrasion
Corneal Laceration
Traumatic Iritis
Hyphema
Retinal Detachment
Ruptured Globe
Conjunctivitis
Foreign Body Embedment

Table 18-2 Supplies Needed for the Evaluation and Management of Eye Injuries

Evaluation Supplies	Management Supplies
Snellen chart or similar	Eye shield
Occluder to cover the eye not being tested	Eye patch
Penlight	Tape
Cobalt blue light	Plunger for removing hard contact lenses
Small mirror	Sterile saline solution
Fluorescein strips	Sterile cotton swabs
	Sterile gauze
	Antibiotic eyedrops
	Contact lens case
	Steri-Strips™ or butterfly bandages
	Contact information of consulting ophthalmologist
	Contact information of hospital or poison control center

nystagmus (involuntary shaking of the eyes), other prior existing conditions, and any relevant history of previous eye injuries. This information should be noted in the medical file and be available for comparison with any subsequent examination findings.

- **General health:** Question the patient about any chronic illness. Certain conditions, such as diabetes, are associated with an increased risk of **retinopathy**.

History of the Present Condition

With the exception of dysfunction occurring secondary to infection, disease, or allergy, all eye injuries have an acute onset.

- **Location and description of the symptoms:** The patient may complain of **photophobia**. Complaints of scratchiness or "something in the eye" may be caused by a foreign body, displaced contact lens, seasonal allergies, or a **corneal abrasion**. Itching of the eye is usually associated with edema of the conjunctiva (**chemosis**) caused by an allergy or infection, such as conjunctivitis. Disruption of the normal visual field may also be described. These findings are discussed in the "Functional Assessment" section of this chapter.
- **Injury mechanism:** The size and elastic properties of the object striking the eye are key indicators of the subsequent injury (Table 18-3). Hard objects that are larger than the orbital rim transmit forces directly to the eye's bony margin. Elastic objects or objects smaller than the orbital margin may deliver forces directly to the eye. Elastic objects are of particular concern

Retinopathy A degenerative disease of the blood vessels supplying the retina, often associated with diabetes

Photophobia The eye's intolerance to light

Table 18-3 Blunt Eye Trauma and the Resulting Eye Pathology*

Size Relative to the Orbit	Elastic Property	Resulting Pathology
Larger	Hard	Orbital fracture, periorbital contusion
Larger	Elastic	Blowout fracture, ruptured globe, corneal abrasion, traumatic iritis, periorbital contusion
Smaller	Hard	Ruptured globe, corneal abrasion, corneal laceration, traumatic iritis
Smaller	Elastic	Ruptured globe, blowout fracture, corneal abrasion, traumatic iritis

*All of these mechanisms of injury can result in subconjunctival hemorrhage and retinal pathology

because the expansive force may be of a magnitude sufficient to rupture the globe.

Injury may also be caused by chemicals or other foreign substances entering the eye. In addition to dirt and sand, athletes commonly encounter substances such as field-marking agents, rubber granules from artificial turf, chlorine, and fertilizers and pesticides used for maintaining grass fields. If a foreign substance enters the eye, transport a sample of the substance to the hospital with the patient.

Inspection

Because all but the most anterior portion of the eye is hidden from view, trauma to its external structures, the eyelid and the eyebrow, may mask underlying pathology. A relatively normal outward appearance of the eye does not correlate well with the absence of internal damage. The presence of the findings listed in Table 18-4 indicates the need for immediate referral for further assessment by an ophthalmologist.

Inspection of the Periorbital Area

- **Discoloration:** A simple periorbital hematoma (or black eye) is common with blunt injuries and may have no consequence other than its abnormal appearance. However, external trauma to the eyelid, orbit, or conjunctiva may alter function and indicate trauma to the eye itself.
- **Gross deformity:** Gross bony deformity of the orbit, although rare, indicates a significant condition requiring immediate medical intervention. The loose skin surrounding the eye and eyelid is easily swollen after an injury, and the swelling is often less significant than it appears. Lacerations are common secondary to direct trauma and require management using the appropriate standard precautions.

Inspection of the Globe

- **General appearance:** The appearance of the globe is evaluated as it sits within the orbit relative to the uninvolved eye. Orbital fractures may cause the globe to be displaced medially, inferiorly, or posteriorly (**enophthalmos**) or to bulge anteriorly (**exophthalmos**) within the orbit.
- **Eyelids:** The eyelids are inspected for signs of acute injury, such as swelling, ecchymosis, or lacerations,

Table 18-4 Findings That Warrant Immediate Referral to an Ophthalmologist

History	Inspection	Palpation	Functional Tests	Neurological Tests
Loss of all or part of the visual field Persistent blurred vision Diplopia Photophobia Throbbing or penetrating pain around or within the eye Description of mechanism for a ruptured globe Air escaping from the eyelid or pain when blowing the nose	Foreign body protruding into the eye Laceration involving the margin of the eyelid Deep laceration of the lid Inability to open the eyelid because of swelling Protrusion of the globe (or other obvious displacement) **Injected** conjunctiva with a small pupil Loss of corneal clarity Hyphema Pupillary distortion Unilateral pupillary dilation or constriction	Crepitus and/or deformity of the orbital rim	Restricted eye movement Diplopia occurring with eye movement	Numbness or paresthesia over the lateral nose and cheek Abnormal pupillary reaction

Injected Congested with blood or other fluids forced into an area which may obscure serious underlying pathology of the globe (Fig. 18-6). A **stye**, an infection of a **ciliary gland** or **sebaceous gland**, is caused by bacteria. General eyelid edema, focal tenderness, and redness of the involved lid usually are noted.

- **Cornea:** Since the cornea is normally crystal clear, any discoloration indicates trauma warranting the immediate termination of the evaluation and subsequent referral to an ophthalmologist. Increased intraocular pressure may result in corneal cloudiness. **Hyphema**, the collection of blood within the anterior chamber of the eye, is caused by the rupture of a blood vessel supplying the iris (Fig. 18-7). See page 812 for further description of hyphema.

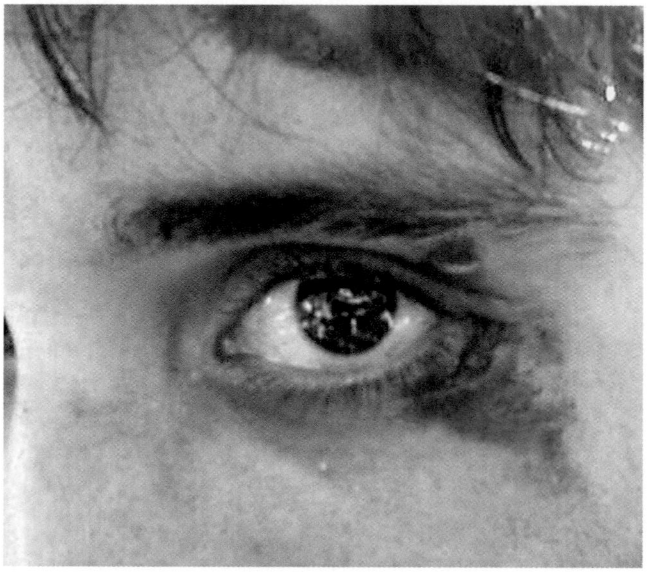

FIGURE 18-6 ■ Laceration of the eyelid. This injury may also conceal underlying eye trauma.

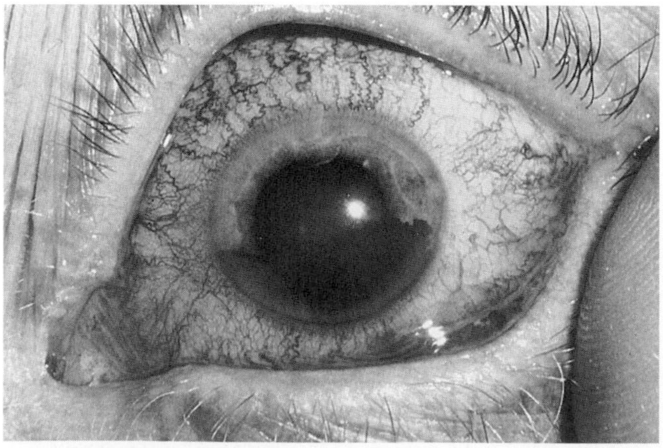

FIGURE 18-7 ■ Hyphema, a collection of blood within the anterior chamber of the eye.

Ciliary gland A form of sweat gland on the eyelid
Sebaceous gland Oil-secreting gland of the skin

- **Conjunctiva:** Normally, the conjunctiva appears transparent as it covers the white sclera anteriorly. To view the inferior portion of the conjunctiva, gently pull down on the eyelid as the patient looks upward. To view the upper conjunctiva, gently lift the upper eyelid while the patient looks downward. If a foreign body is suspected, the upper conjunctiva is viewed by gently inverting the upper eyelid using a cotton-tipped applicator. In some situations, the patient may be more comfortable doing this on his or her own (Fig. 18-8). Leakage of the superficial blood vessels, **subconjunctival hematoma**, is a common benign condition but is of concern because of its potential to conceal underlying pathology (Fig. 18-9).[3]
- **Sclera:** The appearance of a black object on the sclera must be viewed with concern because it may actually be the inner tissue of the eye that is bulging outward through a wound.
- **Iris:** Marked conjunctival injection adjacent to the cornea indicates the presence of inflammation, **iritis**.
- **Pupil shape and size:** The pupils are normally equal in size and shape, but **anisocoria** may be congenital or associated with brain trauma. Any irregularity in the pupil's shape is an ominous sign of a serious injury. An elliptical or **"teardrop" pupil** is of serious concern because of the possibility of a **corneal laceration** or **ruptured globe** (Fig. 18-10).

PALPATION

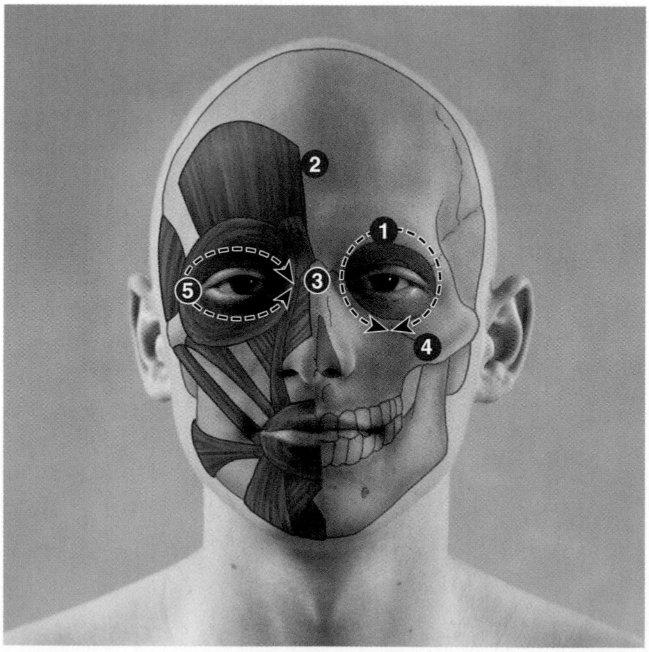

Anisocoria Unequal pupil sizes; possibly a benign congenital condition or secondary to brain trauma

Assessment of eye injuries should not include palpation or probing of the globe itself. However, the superficial bony structures and the soft tissue surrounding the eye may be safely palpated for signs of an injury. Palpation of the nose and other facial bones, often injured concurrently with the eye, is described in Chapter 19.

1 **Orbital margin:** Palpate the circumference of the **orbital rim** for signs of tenderness, deformity, or crepitus indicating the presence of an orbital fracture. The bony prominence of the orbit may become obscured secondary to swelling.

2–4 **Related areas:** Include a general palpation of the (2) **frontal**, (3) **nasal**, and (4) **zygomatic** bones to rule out concurrent injuries caused by blunt trauma.

5 **Soft tissue:** Palpate the **eyelid and skin** surrounding the eye, if appropriate. Keep in mind that injury to these areas is usually apparent during inspection.

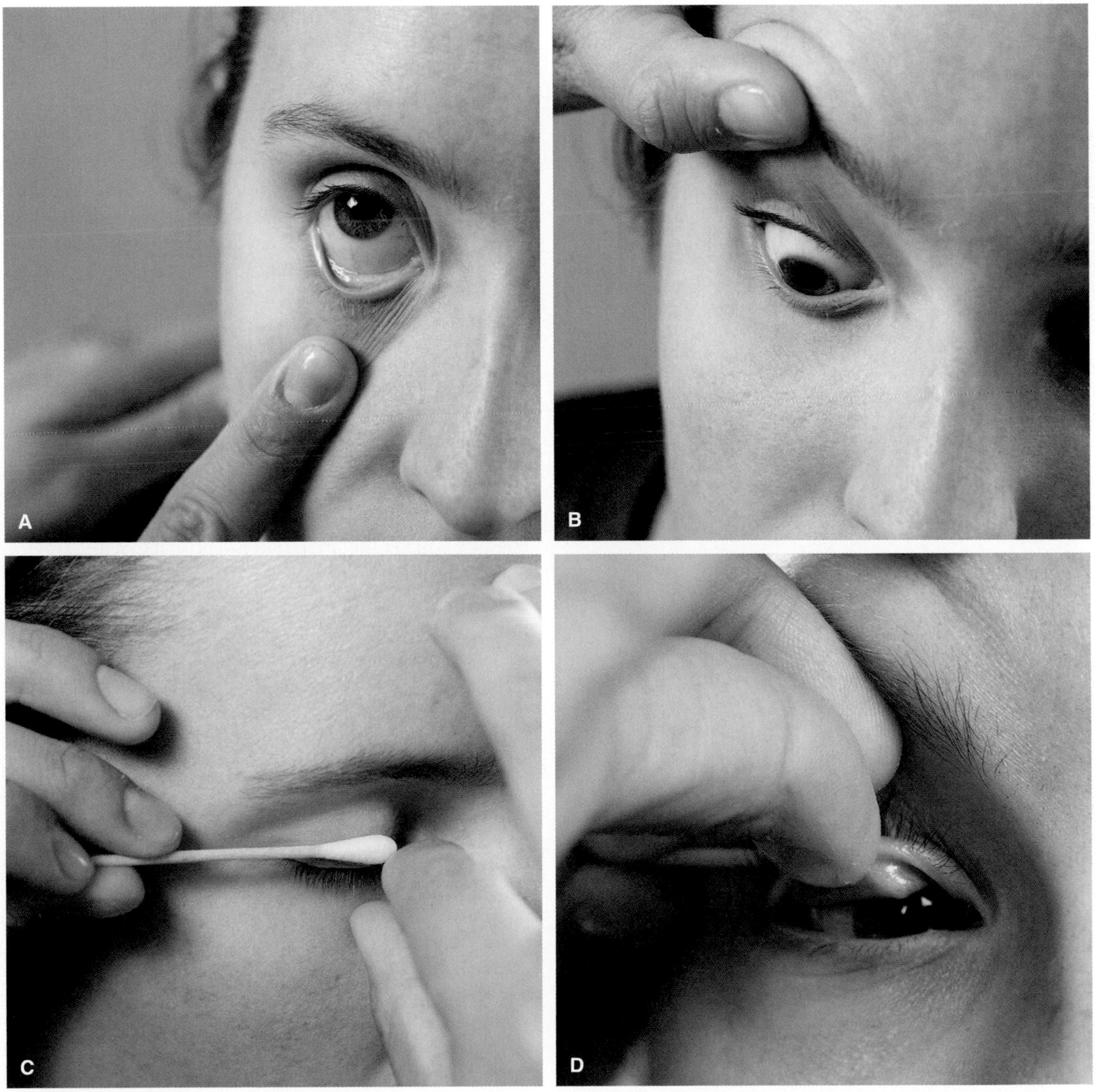

FIGURE 18-8 ■ Inspection of the upper surface of the eye. The upper eyelid is inverted around a cotton-tipped applicator to expose the upper portion of the sclera and conjunctiva.

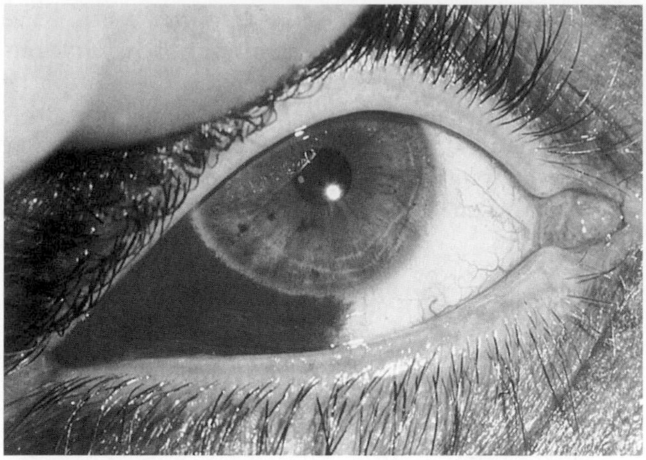

FIGURE 18-9 ■ Subconjunctival hemorrhage. This condition by itself is usually benign but may accompany underlying pathology.

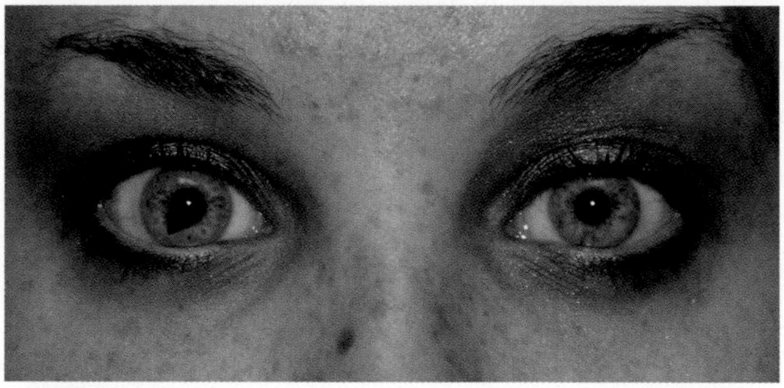

FIGURE 18-10 ■ Teardrop pupil. This condition, or any other deviation in the normally round shape of the pupil, indicates serious underlying pathology such as a corneal laceration or ruptured globe.

Functional Assessment

Vision Assessment

Vision can be assessed using the Snellen chart (see Fig. 18-5), a near-vision card, a newspaper, or a game program. Vision assessment is performed monocularly (one eye) and binocularly (both eyes). Individuals who require the use of glasses or contact lenses should be wearing these at the time of the vision assessment. A person younger than age 40 who has 20/20 vision should be able to read standard newspaper print held 16 inches from the eye. Individuals older than age 40 may have 20/20 distance vision but may have **presbyopia** and require the use of reading glasses.

If the patient is unable to read the chart, fingers may be used. When testing, the fingers are held at different distances, and vision is evaluated. The lack of normal visual acuity or the onset of **diplopia** after an injury to the eye requires a referral to an ophthalmologist for further evaluation. If these symptoms develop following a head injury, the patient should be examined for a concussion.

Presbyopia Loss of near vision as the result of aging
Diplopia Double vision

Blurred vision that clears on blinking the eye indicates the formation of mucus or other debris floating in the surface of the eye. This is not a significant finding. Blinking that clears the vision momentarily can indicate a corneal abrasion. Loss of portions of the visual field, typically described as resembling a shade or curtains being pulled over the eye, may indicate a detached retina. Diplopia may indicate an orbital fracture, brain trauma, damage to the optic or cranial nerves, or injury to the eye's extrinsic muscles.

Pupillary Reaction to Light

Pupillary dysfunction is also associated with significant head trauma and may include dilatation, diminished reactivity to light, or asymmetry (Selective Tissue Test 18-1). When a light is shined into one pupil, it should also result in constriction of the opposite pupil (cranial nerve III [CN III]).[4] The pupil not constricting when exposed to light suggests pathology to the optic nerve or retina.[4]

Eye Motility

The eyes' ability to perform a complete sweep of the range of motion (ROM) in a smooth, symmetrical manner through the eye's field of gaze is a key examination finding (Selective Tissue Test 18-2). Asymmetrical motion or movement that results in diplopia is considered significant.

Neurological Testing

The muscles of the eye are controlled sympathetically or parasympathetically by cranial nerves III, IV, and VI. A discussion of these nerves and their direct influence on the eyes is provided in Chapter 20. Numbness in the cheek and lateral nose corresponds to the distribution of the infraorbital nerve and may indicate an orbital floor fracture.

Region-Specific Pathologies and Selective Tissue Tests

Injury to the globe usually results in some degree of visual impairment, with or without outward signs of trauma. Periorbital injuries usually have no associated visual change. Following a recent history of head injury, associated brain pathology must be considered for those who complain of visual disturbances.

Orbital Fractures

A blow to the periorbital area from an object that is larger than the orbit itself may result in a fracture of the frontal, zygomatic, or maxillary bones of the orbital rim. A deformable or irregularly shaped object, such as a ball or an elbow, may also deliver force to the globe with a magnitude sufficient to cause the orbit to rupture at its weakest point, usually in the medial wall or the floor of the orbit (Fig. 18-11).[5,6] Fractures of the medial wall or floor are termed **blowout fractures**, and fractures of the orbital roof are termed **blowup fractures**.[6] In children, the elastic properties of growing bone can lead to another variant, a **trapdoor**

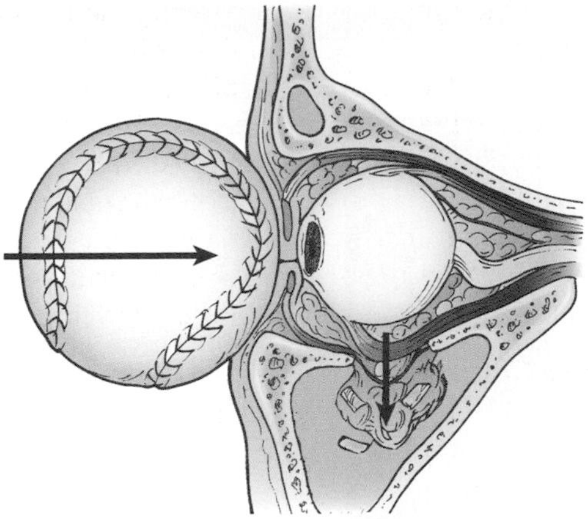

FIGURE 18-11 ■ Mechanism for an orbital floor "blow-out" fracture. The object striking the eye causes the globe to expand downward, rupturing the relatively thin floor.

blowout fracture. In this case, the fracture compresses intraorbital fat and muscle.[5]

After an orbital fracture, the globe may be sunken, medially displaced, or retracted (**enophthalmos**) in relation to the location and severity of the fracture (i.e., a fracture of the orbital floor would cause the globe to sit low within the orbit). Numbness may also be present in the infraorbital area. However, none of these symptoms may be present.[4,5] Pieces of the maxillary portion of the orbital floor may entrap the inferior rectus muscle, mechanically limiting the ability to look upward (Fig. 18-12). Entrapment of the inferior rectus muscle may lock the eye in a downward gaze. This finding, coupled with the absence of subconjunctival hemorrhage and other outward signs, is termed a **white-eyed blowout fracture,** a finding more common in children but potentially affecting individuals of all ages.[4,7]

✱ Practical Evidence

Plain radiographs are often inconclusive in diagnosing orbital floor fractures. Computed tomography (CT) imaging is the radiographic gold standard.[8]

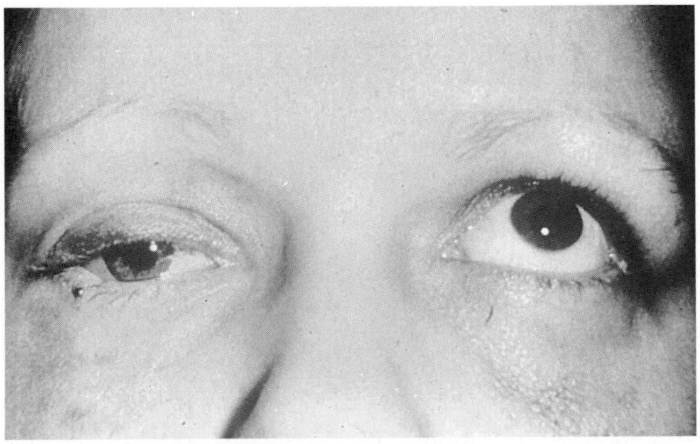

FIGURE 18-12 ■ Restriction of eye motion following a blow-out fracture of the orbital floor. The person's right eye is unable to gaze upward, indicating an entrapment of the inferior rectus muscle.

Initially, fractures of the medial wall of the orbit may be asymptomatic, remaining undiagnosed until the person attempts to blow his or her nose, at which time air escapes the nasal passage, enters the orbit, and exits from under the eyelids. A floor fracture or its subsequent swelling may cause infraorbital nerve entrapment, resulting in numbness in the lateral nose and cheek. Fracture of the lateral wall of the orbit can result in pain when the mouth is opened.[2]

Any deformity of the orbit, caused by bony fractures, entrapment of a muscle, or edema can disrupt the eye's alignment and result in diplopia.[6] Although not always associated with a blowout fracture, fractures of the orbital rim may produce focal tenderness and crepitus during palpation (Examination Findings 18-1). The definitive diagnosis of orbital fractures may require radiographic examination, CT scanning, or magnetic resonance imaging (MRI).

Orbital Fracture Intervention Strategies

Immediate management of a suspected orbital fracture is discussed in the on-field evaluation and management section. Many cases of orbital fractures are managed conservatively, especially when vision deficits are within acceptable limits. If participation in sports is permitted, the patient should be fitted with large protective goggles that would redirect forces away from the injured tissues. During the healing period, the patient may be instructed not to blow the nose.

Surgical decompression and release of entrapped muscles is indicated in cases where eye motility is restricted or in cases where there is pronounced diplopia.[5] The timing of surgery (early versus late) does not appear to affect outcomes.[6]

Corneal Abrasions

Because the cornea is so highly innervated, trauma to this part of the eye results in pain and photophobia.[9] Scratching of the cornea may be caused by an external force directly striking the eye or by a foreign object such as sand or dirt being caught between the cornea and the eyelid. Contact lenses may also create a corneal abrasion. Subsequent blinking of the eyelids results in pain and the sensation of a foreign body on the eye, which may or may not still be present.

The eye sympathetically tears in an attempt to wash any invading particles from the eye. Subsequent exposure of the corneal nerves may result in a sharp, stabbing pain. If the abrasion involves the central visual axis, the vision may be blurred (Examination Findings 18-2). Under normal conditions, the abrasion is not visible to the unaided eye. Definitive diagnosis is made using fluorescein strips and a cobalt blue light. A wet fluorescein strip is used to place dye in the eye. This dye is absorbed only by the cells exposed after a corneal laceration (Selective Tissue Test 18-3). When the examiner shines a cobalt blue light on the area, the abrasion becomes obvious.

Corneal Abrasion Intervention Strategies

An ophthalmologist will often prescribe a topical antibiotic and anesthetic eyedrops. If drying of the eye becomes

Selective Tissue Tests 18-1
Pupillary Reaction Assessment

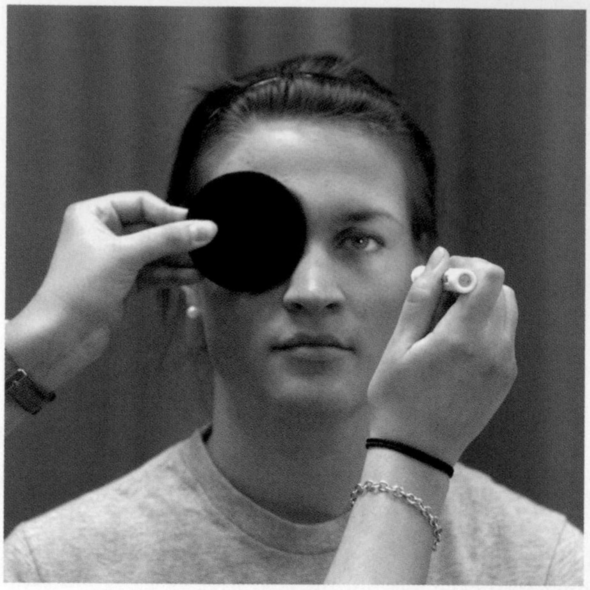

Checking for normal pupil reaction to light. If a penlight is not available, the eye tested can be covered and the pupil observed for constriction when the eye is exposed to light.

Patient Position	Sitting or standing
Position of Examiner	Standing in front of the patient
Evaluative Procedure	A card, an occluder, or the patient's hand is held in front of the eye not being tested. A penlight is used to shine light into the pupil for 1 second and then removed. The examiner observes for the pupil constricting when the light is applied and dilating when the light is removed. This process is repeated for the opposite eye.
Positive Test	A pupil that is unresponsive to light, reacts sluggishly compared with the opposite eye, or paradoxically dilates or constricts
Implications	*Afferent lesion (retina or optic nerve):* The involved pupil enlarges as the light is moved from the unaffected side to the affected side (paradoxical dilation). *Efferent lesion (CN III or pupillary muscle lesion):* The involved pupil does not react to light.[2]
Evidence	Absent or inconclusive in the literature

CN = cranial nerve

Selective Tissue Tests 18-2
Assessment of Eye Motility

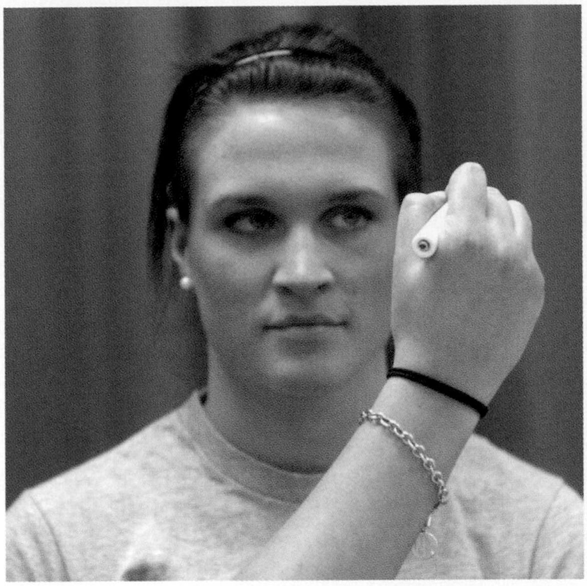

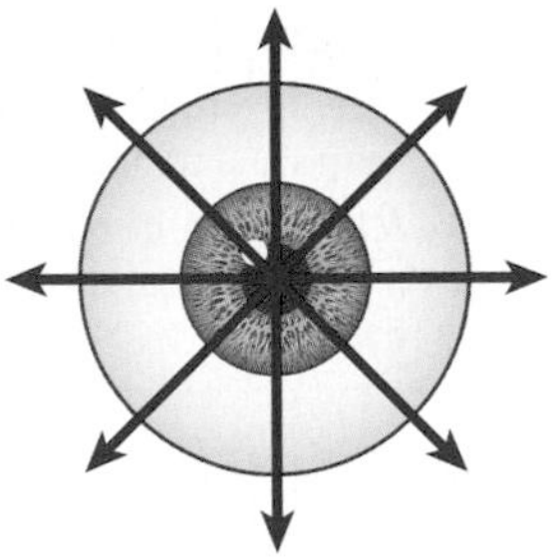

Checking the ROM (motility) of the eye. The eyes should track smoothly and travel an equal distance.

Patient Position	Sitting or standing
Position of Examiner	Standing in front of the patient, holding a finger approximately 2 feet from the patient's nose
Evaluative Procedure	The patient focuses on the examiner's finger and is instructed to report any double vision experienced during the test. The examiner moves the finger upward, downward, left, and right relative to the starting point. The patient follows this motion using only the eyes and is allowed to fix the gaze at the terminal end of each movement. The finger is then moved through the diagonal fields of gaze.
Positive Test	Asymmetrical tracking of the eyes or double vision produced at the end of the ROM
Implications	Decreased motility of the eyes as the result of neurological or muscular trauma or decreased vision
Evidence	Absent or inconclusive in the literature

ROM = range of motion

Examination Findings 18-1
Orbital Fracture

Examination Segment	Clinical Findings
History of Current Condition	*Onset:* Acute *Pain characteristics:* Orbital margin and possibly within the eye and orbit *Other symptoms:* Asymptomatic or possible complaints of air escaping from beneath the eyelid; nausea and vomiting *Mechanism:* A direct blow to the periorbital area or the globe itself A blowout fracture occurs when a blow increases the amount of pressure within the orbit, causing the orbital floor or medial wall to fracture.
Functional Assessment	*Vision:* Diplopia, especially on end-gaze, is caused by an alteration in the shape of the orbit or possibly secondary to the bony entrapment of the eye's intrinsic musculature or to edema; blurred vision may also be described. *Jaw function:* Fracture of the lateral orbital wall will produce pain when biting (trismus).[2]
Inspection	Ecchymosis and swelling may be present in the periorbital area. The eye may appear sunken inferiorly or posteriorly into the socket (enophthalmos), may bulge outward (exophthalmos), or may be medially displaced. An entrapped inferior rectus muscle may lock the eye in a downward gaze. A laceration of the periorbital area or eyelid may be associated with trauma.
Palpation	Possible tenderness in the periorbital area; however, there may be no tenderness elicited with a blowout fracture.
Joint and Muscle Function Assessment	*AROM:* Blowout fractures may result in the affected eye's inability to look upward or outward, although this is not a requisite symptom.
Joint Stability Tests	Not applicable
Selective Tissue Tests	Not applicable
Neurological Screening	Sensory testing of the cheek and lateral nose for infraorbital nerve involvement
Vascular Screening	Not applicable
Imaging Techniques	Radiography, CT scan, or MRI is used to view the orbit.
Differential Diagnosis	Hyphema, corneal or scleral abrasion, detached retina, infraorbital nerve entrapment
Comments	Individuals who are suspected of suffering from an orbital fracture should be referred to an ophthalmologist for further evaluation and be instructed to refrain from blowing their nose.

AROM = active range of motion; CT = computed tomography; MRI = magnetic resonance imaging

Examination Findings 18-2
Corneal Abrasions

Examination Segment	Clinical Findings
History of Current Condition	*Onset:* Acute *Pain characteristics:* Over the cornea and the surrounding conjunctiva, normally reported as "something in my eye;" pain possibly intense *Other symptoms:* Blurred vision, photophobia *Mechanism:* Direct contact to the cornea or a foreign object (e.g., sand) between the cornea and the eyelid, causing an abrasion
Functional Assessment	Vision possibly blurred secondary to increased watering of the eye or to scratching of the central cornea
Inspection	The patient's eyes may water. Conjunctival redness is present. A small foreign object may be present. The actual abrasion is not visible under normal conditions.
Palpation	Not applicable
Selective Tissue Tests	A corneal abrasion is definitively diagnosed through fluorescein strips and a cobalt blue light.
Neurological Screening	Not applicable
Vascular Screening	Not applicable
Imaging Techniques	Ocular CT scan; nonmetallic MRI studies
Differential Diagnosis	Laceration, orbital fracture, hyphema, retinal detachment
Comments	The visual symptoms of a corneal abrasion may momentarily clear when the surface is lubricated during blinking; however, the blurring of vision soon returns. Patients suspected of having a corneal abrasion should be immediately referred to an ophthalmologist, with the eye closed and patched.

CT = computed tomography; MRI = magnetic resonance imaging

problematic, "artificial tears" may be recommended.[9] A patch may or may not be used to cover the eye.[4] Contact lenses should not be worn during healing.

Corneal Lacerations

Direct trauma to the eye from a sharp object can result in partial- or full-thickness tears of the cornea.[3] Partial-thickness tears are similar in their signs and symptoms to corneal abrasions and do not penetrate into the anterior chamber (see Examination Findings 18-2). However, with these lacerations, the actual trauma to the cornea may be visible, especially if the laceration is large or irregularly shaped. Full-thickness tears penetrate into the anterior chamber. These tears are readily apparent by the disruption in the normal translucent appearance of the cornea, a shallow anterior chamber, or the obvious opening of the laceration and subsequent spilling of its contents. Air bubbles within the anterior chamber and an irregularly shaped (elliptical or teardrop) pupil are highly diagnostic of a corneal laceration.

Corneal Laceration Intervention Strategies

If the laceration was caused by a penetrating injury, the object should be left in place until it can be removed by an ophthalmologist. If no foreign object is embedded in the eye, an eye shield should be applied to protect the globe.

Partial thickness tears may be treated using topical antibiotics and anesthetics. Sutures or a fibrin glue are often used to correct full-thickness tears.[10]

Traumatic Iritis

Minor blunt trauma to the eye can activate an inflammatory reaction within the anterior chamber, resulting in the "red eye" appearance associated with iritis. Inflammation of the iris itself may occur without pain, but the sensation of pressure within the globe may be described along with marked sensitivity to light. On inspection, the involved pupil is constricted relative to the opposite side. In certain cases, however, the pupil appears dilated or normal. The inflammatory cells within the anterior chamber may cause

Selective Tissue Tests 18-3
Fluorescent Dye Test for Corneal Abrasions (Seidel Test)

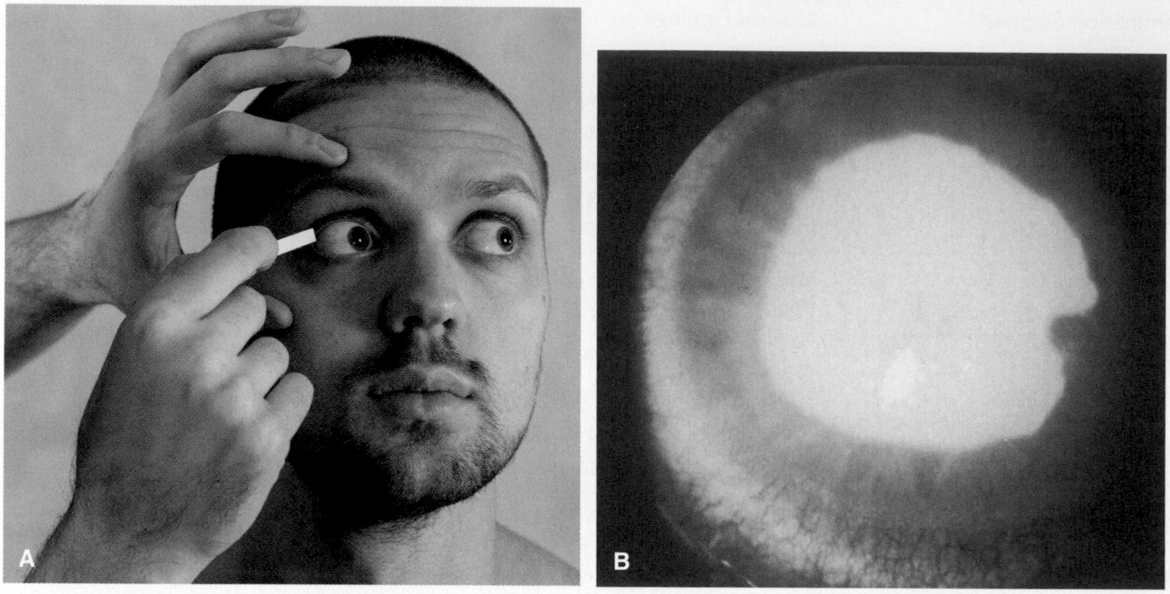

(A) A fluorescein strip is lightly touched to the conjunctiva. (B) A cobalt blue light is focused into the eye to highlight the abraded area.

Patient Position	Seated or supine
Position of Examiner	Standing in front of or beside the patient
Evaluative Procedure	Soak the fluorescein strip with sterile saline solution. Lightly touch the wet fluorescein strip to the conjunctiva of the lower eyelid for a few seconds. Avoid placing the strip directly on the cornea. Ask the patient to blink the eye a few times to spread the solution. Darken the room and use a cobalt blue light to illuminate the eye.
Positive Test	When viewed with the cobalt blue light, corneal abrasions appear as a bright yellow-green pattern on the eye.
Implications	A corneal abrasion
Evidence	Absent or inconclusive in the literature

blurred vision. Assessment of pupillary reaction, determined with a penlight, reveals that the pupil reacts sluggishly when compared with the pupil of the uninjured eye (Examination Findings 18-3).

Traumatic Iritis Intervention Strategies
In the absence of comorbid conditions, iritis is treated symptomatically. Corticosteroids may be prescribed in more complex conditions.

Hyphema

A hyphema, blood in the anterior chamber of the eye, can result from blunt eye trauma that causes a tear in the ciliary bodies. Less frequently, hyphemas occur spontaneously with no evidence of trauma. An increase in intraocular pressure is associated with hyphema approximately one-third of the time.[11] An individual presenting with a traumatic hyphema should be examined for other ocular and facial injuries.

* Practical Evidence

Nontraumatic hyphema or complications arising from explained hyphema in African Americans is suggestive of the presence of sickle cell trait.[12]

Hyphema Intervention Strategies
The management of a hyphema includes patching and shielding the eye with immediate referral to an emergency room. The patient should be placed in a semireclined position to encourage blood pooling in the inferior anterior chamber. Conservative treatment is generally effective; it includes relative rest and medications for pain to reduce the incidence of secondary hemorrhage or decrease

Examination Findings 18-3
Traumatic Iritis

Examination Segment	Clinical Findings
History of Current Condition	*Onset:* Acute *Pain characteristics:* Pain and burning in the eye *Other symptoms:* Photophobia *Mechanism:* A traumatic force to the eye that elicits an inflammatory response
Functional Assessment	The pupil is sluggishly reactive to light. Photophobia is usually described.
Inspection	The conjunctiva adjacent to the cornea may be **injected** (profused with blood). The involved pupil may be constricted. On occasion, the pupil may be dilated or normal.
Selective Tissue Tests	Not applicable
Neurological Screening	Pupillary reaction (CN III)
Vascular Screening	Not applicable
Imaging Techniques	Not applicable
Differential Diagnosis	Scleral or corneal abrasion
Comments	Blunt trauma can result in a tearing of the iris sphincter, leading to permanent pupillary deformity.

CN = cranial nerve

intraocular pressure. However, permanent visual impairment can result, particularly in the case of a total hyphema. Close monitoring is essential to ensure that the hyphema is resolving and that ocular pressure is decreasing. Hyphemas typically resolve in 5 to 7 days.

Retinal Detachment

A jarring force to the head can result in an interruption in the communication of the retina and the choroid. Although this mechanism can be delivered to the head, the jarring motion associated with sneezing may also be sufficient. Retinal detachments can also occur spontaneously, with no apparent mechanism. The actual detachment of the retina involves the interruption of the nerve pulses being relayed to the optic nerve, often occurring when the vitreous humor seeps between the retina and the choroid. Severely myopic, or nearsighted, individuals are more at risk for a retinal detachment.

The patient may complain of flashes of light (photopsia), halos, "floaters," and/or blind spots within the normal field of vision.[13] The patient may also describe a "curtain" or shape being pulled over the field of vision. Spontaneous retinal detachment may be indicative of Marfan's syndrome (see Chapter 14). The definitive diagnosis is made by an ophthalmologist.

Retinal Detachment Intervention Strategies

If a retinal detachment is suspected, protect the eye with a rigid shield that does not compress the globe and then transport the patient to an emergency room. Surgical correction is the standard course of care for symptomatic retinal detachment. Although some asymptomatic retinal detachments are managed conservatively, surgical correction for this condition is also recommended.[14]

Ruptured Globe

The most catastrophic injury to the eye is a ruptured globe. Severe blunt trauma delivered to the globe itself (i.e., little or no force being dissipated by the orbital rim) can result in a rupture of the cornea or sclera, subsequently causing it to spill its contents. Commonly, these tears occur behind the insertion of the eye's extrinsic muscles (where the sclera is the thinnest) and therefore may not be visible. However, black specks on the sclera indicate that the contents of the eye are spilling outward.

The primary complaints after a ruptured globe are pain and total or partial loss of vision. On inspection, the globe may appear disoriented in the orbit, and the anterior chamber may seem unusually deep. The conjunctiva has marked edema (**chemosis**), and the pupil may be elliptical or teardrop shaped. Hyphema or a dark, coffee ground–like substance also may be viewed within the anterior chamber (Examination Findings 18-4). However, many ruptured globes are often outwardly asymptomatic.

Ruptured Globe Intervention Strategies

Placement of an eye shield over the eye and immediate transport to the hospital are necessary for individuals suspected of suffering from a ruptured globe. Do not administer any type of eyedrops or touch the globe. Because of the possibility of the need for immediate surgery, advise the person not to eat or drink.

Conjunctivitis

Conjunctivitis is the result of a viral or bacterial infection of the conjunctiva. The first symptoms of conjunctivitis are usually experienced upon waking in the morning when the eyelids may stick together and the eye burns and itches. The involved eye typically is red and swollen. The nature of the discharge usually dictates the etiology. A watery discharge accompanied by redness of the conjunctiva indicates a viral infection (pink eye), while a yellow or green discharge indicates a bacterial infection. The affected eye may also be sensitive to light (Examination Findings 18-5). This condition may develop secondary to improper cleaning and care of contact lenses.

Conjunctivitis Intervention Strategies

Patients with conjunctivitis, a highly contagious condition, must be instructed not to touch the affected eye to avoid spreading the contamination to the uninvolved eye. Likewise, people diagnosed with this condition must be barred

Examination Findings 18-4
Ruptured Globe

Examination Segment	Clinical Findings
History of Current Condition	*Onset:* Acute *Pain characteristics:* Throughout the eye; asymptomatic cases have also been reported. *Mechanism:* Severe blunt trauma to the globe
Functional Assessment	Vision is lost or markedly decreased in the affected eye.
Inspection	The globe may be obviously deformed. The anterior chamber may appear deepened. Hyphema or a black, grainy substance may be visible within the anterior chamber. An elliptical or teardrop-shaped pupil may be observed. The contents of the globe may bulge outward through the sclera, appearing as a black "foreign object" on the eye.
Palpation	Not performed
Joint and Muscle Function Assessment	AROM is not assessed if a ruptured globe is suspected.
Selective Tissue Tests	Not applicable
Neurological Screening	Not applicable
Vascular Screening	Not applicable
Imaging Techniques	CT MR images may be obtained if there is no metal penetrating the orbit.[5]
Differential Diagnosis	Orbital fracture, hyphema, retinal detachment, laceration
Comments	Patients suspected of having a ruptured globe should immediately be transported to the hospital, with a shield covering the eye. Patches should not be used because direct pressure on the globe is to be avoided. No food or fluids should be permitted because immediate surgery may be required.

AROM = active range of motion; CT = computed tomography; MR = magnetic resonance

Examination Findings 18-5
Conjunctivitis

Examination Segment	Clinical Findings
History of Current Condition	*Onset:* Acute; symptoms normally appearing on awakening *Pain characteristics:* Itchy, burning sensation in the affected eye Photophobia also possible *Other symptoms:* Patient complains of the eyelids sticking together upon awakening. *Mechanism:* Viral or bacterial infection *Risk factor:* Improper cleaning and care of contact lenses
Functional Assessment	Vision may be hindered in the affected eye secondary to the inability to open the eye, swelling, and discharge.
Inspection	Reddening of the involved eye Eyelid swelling possibly present Discharge commonly seen; if a discharge is present, the color should be noted: • Clear or watery discharge: Viral infection • Yellow or green discharge: Bacterial infection
Palpation	Palpation is performed wearing gloves (and using all Universal Precautions) to prevent the infection from spreading to the examiner. The eyelids feel fluid filled and boggy.
Selective Tissue Tests	None
Neurological Screening	Not applicable
Vascular Screening	Not applicable
Imaging Techniques	Not applicable
Differential Diagnosis	Iritis, acute glaucoma, subconjunctival hemorrhage, allergic reaction
Comments	Conjunctivitis is highly contagious and will likely spread to the other eye. Individuals suffering from conjunctivitis should refrain from physical contact with other people or from entering a swimming pool. People suspected of suffering from conjunctivitis should be referred to a physician for further evaluation. The individual must refrain from wearing contact lenses. Patients with conjunctivitis should be advised to not share washcloths or makeup with others and to wash their hands frequently.

from contact sports or from entering a swimming pool to prevent transmission of the disease to other individuals.

Individuals suspected of suffering from conjunctivitis should be referred to a physician immediately. Bacterial conjunctivitis is easily treated with antibacterial eyedrops or ointment. Viral conjunctivitis may be treated with a topical antibiotic, topical antiviral, and/or topical steroid. For both types of conjunctivitis, an antihistamine may be prescribed to control itching.

Foreign Body Embedment

A foreign body in the eye is a troublesome but usually benign condition that clears after the object has been removed from the eye. On occasion, a foreign object can lead to corneal abrasions. Do not confuse foreign bodies with impalement of the eye by an object.

Foreign Body Embedment Intervention Strategies

An attempt to locate the material causing the discomfort, as described in the Inspection section of this chapter, is necessary. After the particle has been located, it may be flushed out of the eye using a saline solution or water. A moistened cotton applicator or the corner of a gauze pad may also be used to blot the contaminant from the eye. Dry cotton should not be used on the eye because the fibers will stick to it, possibly inducing a corneal abrasion. Instruct the person to refrain from rubbing the eye because this may worsen the problem. Discomfort may be reduced by having the person hold the upper eyelid outward, allowing the eye to tear, possibly washing the particle from the eye.

On-Field Examination and Management of Eye Injuries

The correct initial management of eye injuries greatly increases the chances of the long-term viability of the eye. Likewise, improper management can worsen the severity of the injury and increase the likelihood of permanent disability.

Contact Lens Removal

Trauma to the eye when swelling is imminent, such as with a periorbital contusion, requires that contact lenses be removed as soon as possible after the injury. Ideally, this is best performed by the athlete. However, in certain circumstances, athletes may require assistance, either because they are unable to do so or they cannot find the contact lens on the eye.

Hard contact lenses may be removed using a plunger-like device or may be manually manipulated from the eye in the following manner:

1. The patient opens the eyes as wide as possible.
2. The examiner laterally pulls the outer margin of the eyelids.
3. While holding a hand under the eye to catch the lens, the patient blinks, forcing the lens out of the eye.

Never pluck soft contact lenses directly from the eye, especially when they are resting on the cornea. Doing so may result in serious trauma to the eye. The following procedure is recommended for the removal of soft contact lenses (Fig. 18-13):

1. The patient is asked to look upward.
2. A clean finger is placed on the inferior edge of the contact lens.
3. The lens is manipulated inferiorly and laterally, to where it can be pinched between the fingers and safely removed from the eye.
4. If the contact lens is torn, it is important to remove all pieces from the eye.
5. Do not attempt to remove the contact lens if a ruptured globe is suspected because of the risk of further damaging the cornea or other structures.

Orbital Fractures

Fractures to the orbital rim that are asymptomatic (other than pain) may require no extraordinary treatment other than ice packs loosely applied to the periorbital area, avoiding direct pressure on the globe.[11] Fractures that cause pain during eye movement need to be shielded with a plastic or metal guard, again avoiding direct pressure on the globe. Because the eyes move in unison, the athlete is instructed to gaze straight ahead with the uninvolved eye, thus limiting voluntary eye movement.

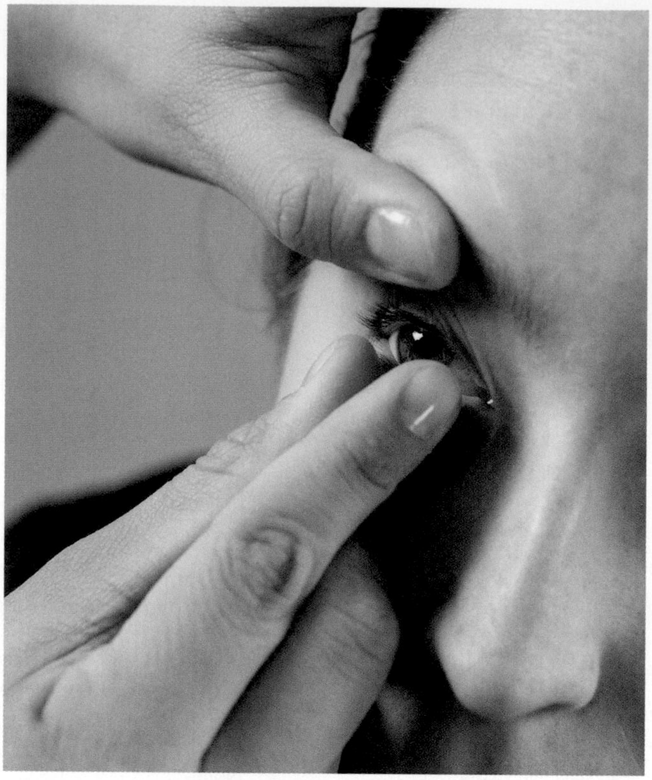

FIGURE 18-13 ■ Removing a soft contact lens. Care must be taken not to insult the cornea or conjunctiva during this procedure.

Penetrating Eye Injuries

Eye shields, as described previously, are used to manage corneal lacerations and ruptured globes. Do not attempt to remove an object that is impaling the eye and avoid applying direct pressure on the globe. If the object is protruding some distance outside of the eye, a foam, plastic, or paper cup may be used to cover and protect the eye. In this case, both eyes are covered to minimize movement. The patient must then be immediately transported to the hospital.

Chemical Burns

After a chemical burn, thoroughly irrigate the eye with large amounts of saline solution or water. Then patch the eye. The athlete, along with a sample of the invading substance, is immediately transported to a hospital.

REFERENCES

1. McGwin, G, et al: Consumer product-related eye injury in the United States, 1998–2002. *J Safety Res*, 37:501, 2006.
2. Rodriguez, JO, Lavina, AM, and Agarwal, A: Prevention and treatment of common eye injuries in sports. *Am Fam Physician*, 67:1481, 2003.
3. Boyd-Monk, H: Bringing common eye emergencies. *Nursing*, 35:46, 2005.
4. Pulalte, GGA: Eye injuries in sports. *Athl Ther Today*, 15:14, 2010.
5. Lane, K, Penne, RB, and Bilyk, JR: Evaluation and management of pediatric orbital fractures in a primary care setting. *Orbit*, 26:183, 2007.
6. Simon, GJB, et al: Early versus late repair of orbital blowout fractures. *Ophthalmic Surg Lasers Imaging*, 40:141, 2009.

7. Ethunandan, M, and Evans, BT: Linear trapdoor or "white-eye" blowout fracture of the orbit: not restricted to children. *Br J Oral Maxiofac Surg*, 49:142, 2011.
8. Ceallaigh, PÓ, et al: Diagnosis and management of common maxillofacial injuries in the emergency department. Part 4: orbital floor and midface fractures. *Emerg Med J*, 24:292, 2007.
9. Hua, L, and Doll, T: A series of three cases of corneal abrasions with multiple etiologies. *Optometry*, 81:83, 2010.
10. Kiire, C, Srinivasan, S, and Soddart, MG: A novel use of fibrin glue in the treatment of a partial thickness corneal laceration. *Br J Ophthalmol*, 94:810, 2010.
11. Walton, W, et al: Management of traumatic hyphema. *Surv Opthalmol*, 47:297, 2002.
12. John, N: A review of clinical profiles in sickle cell traits. *Oman Med J*, 25:3, 2010.
13. Kang, HK, and Luff, AJ: Management of retinal detachment: a guide for non-ophthalmologists. *BMJ*, 336:1235, 2008.
14. Ahmad, N, and West, J: Current opinion on treatment of asymptomatic retinal detachments. *Eye*, 21:1179, 2007.

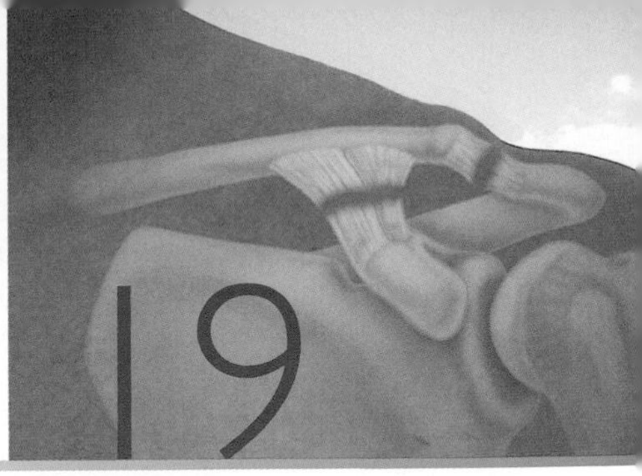

CHAPTER 19

Face and Related Structure Pathologies

Even when appropriate equipment is used, the face, nose, mouth, and ears are vulnerable to injury. However, rules requiring the use of face masks and mouthguards have reduced the number and severity of injuries to the maxillofacial area. For maximum protection, these devices must be properly fitted. The use of mouthguards during practices and games should be encouraged, even in low-risk sports in which their use is not mandated.

Injuries to the facial structures are significant because of their relationship to neurological function, the potential for permanent physical deformity and disability, and, in the case of throat injuries, the threat of a compromised airway. An accurate evaluation of injury to these areas is necessary to determine severity and initiate appropriate treatment and management immediately, lessening the probability of any long-term consequences.

Clinical Anatomy

The face is formed by the **frontal**, **maxillary**, **nasal**, and **zygomatic bones** (Fig. 19-1). Comprising a large portion of the anterior face, the maxilla forms a portion of the inferior orbit of the eye, nasal cavity, and oral cavity. The superior row of teeth is fixed within the **alveolar process** along the inferior border of the maxilla. The **zygoma** is fused to the maxilla anteriorly and the **temporal bones** posteriorly, forming the prominent **zygomatic arch** beneath the eyes. Providing the cheek with its surface structure, disruption of the zygomatic arch can drastically affect the face's physical appearance. The zygoma also plays an important role in ocular function by forming a portion of the lateral and inferior rim of the eye's orbit.

Anteriorly, the body of the **mandible** forms the chin. Diverging laterally from the point of the chin, the **ramus** of the mandible begins at the angle of the jaw and continues its course posteriorly and superiorly. The convex **mandibular condylar processes** are located at the end of the ramus, forming the inferior aspect of the **temporomandibular joint** (TMJ). Anterior to the mandibular condylar process is the site of attachment of the temporalis muscle, the **coronoid process**. Injury to the mandible can potentially involve the alveolar process and thus affect the **occlusion** of the teeth.

Temporomandibular Joint Anatomy

The TMJ is a synovial articulation located between the mandibular condylar process and the temporal bone.

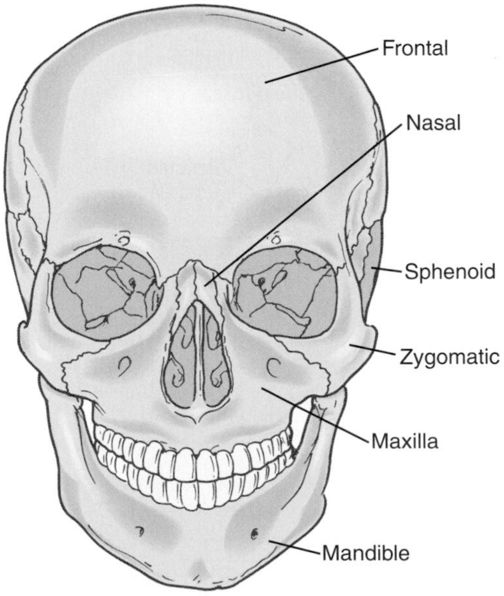

FIGURE 19-1 ■ Bony anatomy of the face and associated skull.

Occlusion The process of closing or being closed

Pathology to the TMJ can result in **malocclusion** of the teeth and is often cited as the cause of headaches, cervical muscle injury, and overall muscle weakness.[1,2] Correction of the malocclusion with specially formed mouthpieces has been suggested to solve these problems.

Movement at the TMJ is necessary for communication and the **mastication** of food. The superior temporal articulation, from anterior to posterior, consists of the **articular tubercle**, **articular eminence**, **glenoid fossa**, and **posterior glenoid spine** (Fig. 19-2). The actual articulating area for the mandibular condylar process is the convex articular eminence. The anterosuperior portion of the mandibular condylar process and the articular eminence are covered with the thickest area of fibrocartilaginous tissue, enabling these surfaces to withstand the stresses associated with joint movement.

The entire TMJ is encased in a synovial joint capsule. An **articular disc** is located between the two bones, dividing the joint into two separate cavities. The disc is concave on both its superior and inferior surfaces, allowing for a smooth articulation between two convex bones. The disc has sturdy attachments to the mandible, attaching anteriorly and posteriorly to the capsule and surrounding tissues, and divides the joint space into upper and lower compartments. Medially and laterally, there are no attachments to the joint capsule so that the disk can freely move in the anteroposterior direction as the mouth opens and closes.

To allow the mouth to open, the TMJ's mandibular condyles must roll and translate.[3] As the muscles of mastication (masseter, temporalis, medial pterygoid, and lateral pterygoid) relax, gravity causes the mandibular condyles to roll anteriorly on the articular disk as the disk rotates posteriorly until the midpoint of motion. At approximately the midpoint of the range of motion (ROM), the lateral pterygoid muscle contracts, translating the disk and condyle forward. Closing the mouth reverses this sequence of events. TMJ biomechanics tend to degrade with age as the articular disk begins to degenerate.[4]

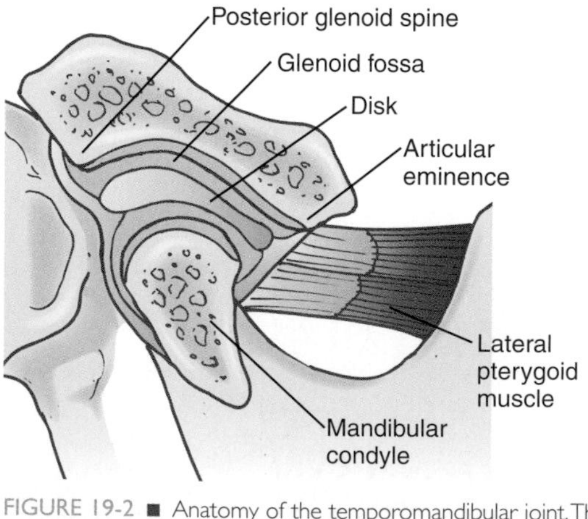

FIGURE 19-2 ■ Anatomy of the temporomandibular joint. The joint structure allows the mandibular condyle to glide forward as the mouth is opened. Trauma to the disk results in a locking or catching as the mouth is opened and closed.

Malocclusion A deviation in the normal alignment of two opposable tissues (e.g., the mandible and maxilla)

Mastication The chewing of food

The Ear

The ear is composed of three sections: the external ear, middle ear, and inner ear (Fig. 19-3). The design of the ear permits it to focus acoustical energy and convert it into an electrical signal that can be interpreted by the brain. The inner ear components also function to maintain balance.

The External Ear

The shape of the external ear is maintained by an accumulation of cartilaginous tissue, the **auricle (pinna)**. The shape of the external ear functions as a funnel, collecting and focusing sound waves into the **external auditory meatus** to be passed on to the middle ear. Although the auricle is sturdy enough to maintain the shape of the ear, the cartilage is capable of being deformed and quickly returning to its original shape, a mechanism that efficiently disperses many of the forces to which the external ear is exposed.

The Middle Ear

The **tympanic membrane**, or eardrum, is the outer barrier of the middle ear. With a function similar to a microphone picking up sound, sound waves strike the tympanic membrane, causing it to oscillate. Three small bones, the **auditory ossicles,** consisting of the **malleus**, **incus**, and **stapes**, are aligned in a chain. These bones transmit the vibrations of the tympanic membrane to the oval window of the inner ear.

The middle ear is connected to the nasal passages by the **eustachian tube**, which regulates the amount of pressure within the middle ear.

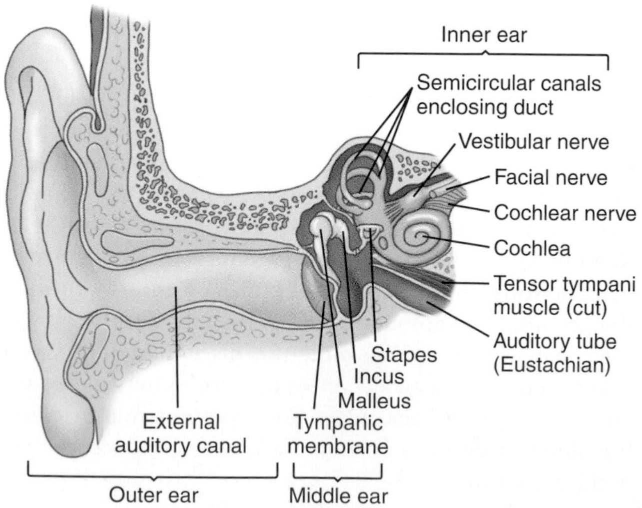

FIGURE 19-3 ■ Anatomy of the ear. The external and middle ear are separated by the tympanic membrane. The middle and inner ear are divided by the oval window.

The Inner Ear

Within the inner ear, the mechanical vibrations caused by sound waves are encoded into electrical impulses to be interpreted by the brain. The structures of the inner ear, the **cochlea** and the **semicircular canals**, sit within a bony, fluid-filled **labyrinth** formed inside the temporal bone (Fig. 19-4). Acoustic signals are passed along the cochlea, a bony structure that moves up and down in response to these signals. This movement is detected by fine hair cells and subsequently translated into electrical impulses by the **vestibulocochlear nerve**.

The semicircular canals are filled with fluid. As the head moves, the fluid in the canals shifts. The feedback from this movement is provided to the brain, assisting in maintaining balance and an upright posture of the head and body.

The Nose

The paired, wafer-thin **nasal bones** arise off the facial bones to meet with extensions of the **frontal bones** and **maxillary bones**, forming the **nasal bridge**. The **nasal septum**, formed on its posterior half by the **vomer bone** and the perpendicular plate of the **ethmoid bone**, meets with the **nasal cartilage** anteriorly to separate the nasal passage into two halves.[5] The floor of the nasal cavity is formed by the **hard palate** anteriorly and the **soft palate** posteriorly (Fig. 19-5).

The external nasal openings, the nostrils, allow air to flow into the nasal passages, through the inferior, middle, and superior **conchae** and into the **pharynx,** to be transmitted to the lungs via the trachea. The nasal passages are lined with **mucosal cells** that warm and humidify cool, dry air before inspiration into the lungs. These cells also produce mucus that acts in conjunction with the nasal hairs to trap foreign particles, preventing them from being passed along to the lungs.

Blood supply to the nasal passage is provided by the highly vascular **Kiesselbach's plexus**, a common source of **epistaxis**. Bleeding as the result of nasal fracture usually results from the **anterior ethmoid artery** (anterior bleeding) or the **sphenopalatine artery** (posterior bleeding).[5]

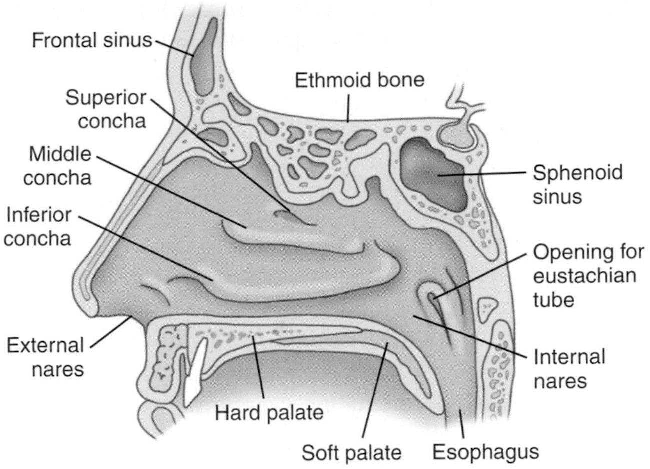

FIGURE 19-5 ■ Cross section of the nasal passage.

The Throat

Because the **larynx** is the most superficial and prominent structure of the throat, it is the area most susceptible to traumatic injury. Covered superiorly by the prominent **thyroid cartilage** (Adam's apple) and inferiorly by the **cricoid cartilage**, the larynx is well protected from all but the most severe blows. Inferior to the cricoid cartilage, the trachea's semicircular cartilage serves as its protective covering until it descends behind the sternum (Fig. 19-6).

The **hyoid bone**, located in the anterior neck between the mandible and the larynx, functions as the tongue's attachment site. This U-shaped bone is suspended by ligaments arising from the temporal bones. The hyoid bone, the only bone in the body that does not articulate with

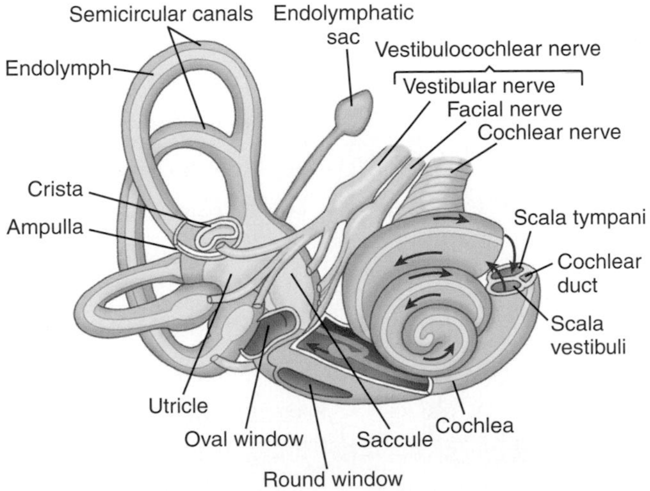

FIGURE 19-4 ■ Inner ear. Here mechanical sound waves are converted into nervous impulses that are sent along to the brain for processing.

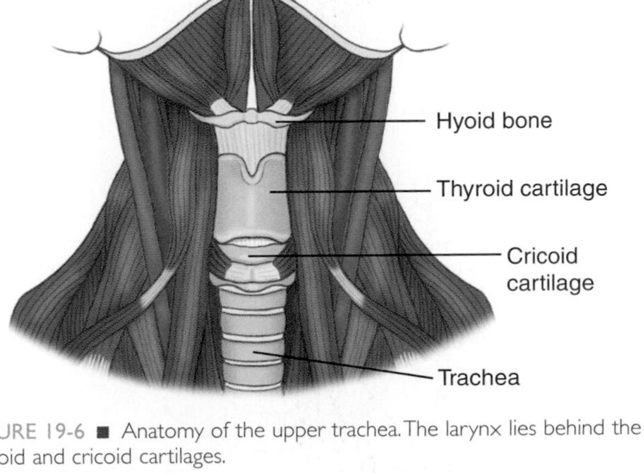

FIGURE 19-6 ■ Anatomy of the upper trachea. The larynx lies behind the thyroid and cricoid cartilages.

Epistaxis A nosebleed

another bone, consists of a central body with two pairs of laterally and posteriorly projecting structures, the greater and lesser **cornua**.

The Mouth

Formed by connective tissue and a thin covering of skin, the lips contain a small layer of transparent cells over a network of vascular capillaries. The lips meet the skin of the face at the **vermilion border**. The rest of the oral cavity is covered by a membrane that produces protective mucus throughout the digestive system. The mouth is divided into the **oral vestibule**, delineated as the area from the lips to the teeth, and the **oral cavity**, including everything past the teeth, leading to the trachea.

Lymphatic structures are located at the juncture between the oral cavity and throat. The **tonsils** and **adenoids** prevent bacteria and other germs from entering the respiratory and/or digestive system. Their function is more pronounced in the early years of life and decreases with time.

The tongue is a skeletal muscle covered by mucous membrane (Fig. 19-7). Its surface is covered with **papillae** and **taste buds**. The papillae are small, rough projections on the surface of the tongue that assist in the movement of food during chewing. The taste buds allow us to appreciate the flavor of whatever we are eating. The tongue is connected on its underside to the floor of the oral cavity by the **lingual frenulum**. This small piece of mucous membrane can be injured during trauma to the tongue or mouth.

The Teeth

Thirty-two permanent teeth, divided equally into upper and lower rows, are normally present. Each row is formed by four different types of teeth, each serving a different function (see Fig. 19-7; Table 19-1). Individually, each tooth has three major anatomical areas: the **root**, the **neck**, and the **crown**. The roots are anchored to the alveolar process by **cementum** and small **periodontal ligaments**. The **gums** cover the alveolar process and root to the base of the tooth's neck.

Each tooth is formed by **dentin**, a hard, calcified substance covered by an even harder substance, **enamel**. The tooth's core is formed by the **pulp chamber**, housing a strong connective tissue **(pulp)**, nerves, and blood vessels (Fig. 19-8). The nerves and blood vessels enter from the underlying bone through the apical foramen and course through the root canal up into the pulp cavity.

Muscular Anatomy

For the purposes of this chapter, the maxillofacial muscles are classified as being either the muscles of mastication or muscles of expression. Dysfunction of these muscles occurs secondary to lacerations, dislocations, fractures, or cranial nerve involvement. Additional facial muscles acting on the eye and eyelids are discussed in Chapter 18.

Muscles of Mastication

The primary muscle for flexing the jaw (closing the mouth) is the masseter, which spans the distance between the

Table 19-1 Classification and Function of the Teeth per Row

Type	Number	Function
Incisors	4	Cutting
Cuspids (Canines)	2	Tearing
Bicuspids (Premolars)	4	Crushing and grinding
Molars	6	Crushing and grinding

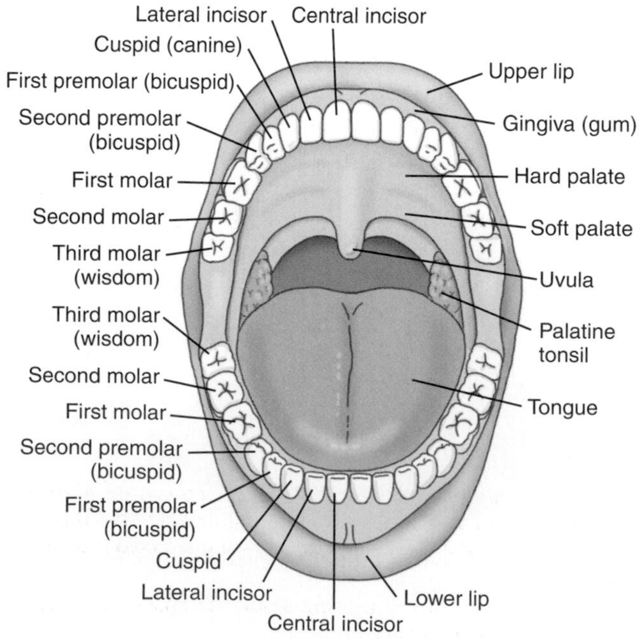

FIGURE 19-7 ■ Oral cavity.

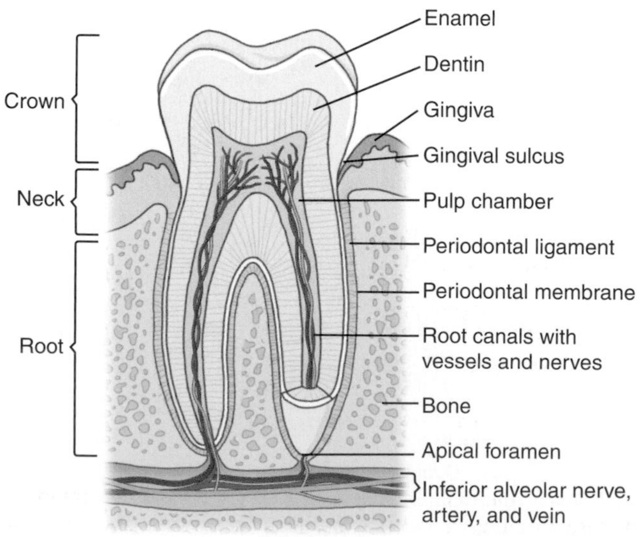

FIGURE 19-8 ■ Cross-sectional anatomy of a tooth.

mandibular angle and the inferior portion of the zygomatic arch. The mouth is opened by the contraction of the **digastric**, **mylohyoid**, **medial pterygoid**, and **lateral pterygoid** muscles.

Muscles of Expression

The muscles of expression—those that move the lips, cheeks, nose, eyebrows, and forehead—are presented in Table 19-2 and Figure 19-9. The lack of symmetrical movement or hypertonicity of the facial muscles indicates that there is trauma or disease to one or more cranial nerves, **Bell's palsy**, which may be caused by infection, disease, or stroke.

Clinical Examination of Facial Injuries

The evaluation of a specific segment of the face need not encompass all aspects of otherwise unrelated structures. However, a secondary screen of these areas should be conducted to rule out concurrent injury. For example, a direct blow to the face may fracture bones and damage teeth. In the event of direct blows to the head, the possibility of brain and cervical spine injury must be considered (see Chapter 20).

History

Despite the presence of an obvious injury to a particular structure, trauma to adjacent areas must also be ruled out. Injuries to the larynx may impede the ability to breathe and/or speak.

History Involving the Ear

- **Location of the pain:** Direct blows to the external ear result in pain in the affected area. Complaints of pressure within the middle or inner ear indicate an infection or a tympanic membrane rupture. Otitis externa, the infection of the external auditory meatus, causes intense, unremitting pain and itching.
- **Activity and injury mechanism:** Most ear injuries stem from a blunt trauma to the auricle, especially prevalent in sports in which headgear is not mandated. A tympanic membrane rupture can be caused by a slapping blow to the ear that produces pressure on the middle ear, thereby causing the membrane to rupture, an injury that is predisposed by infection of the middle ear. A physical puncture of the tympanic membrane may occur from an object entering the external auditory meatus. Infections to the middle ear are usually preceded by **upper respiratory infections**, resulting in inflamed mucous membranes that block the eustachian tubes. The tympanic membrane can also be injured secondary to external pressures during diving and airplane travel.
- **Other symptoms:** An infection of the inner ear, or labyrinth, can occasionally result from an upper respiratory infection (URI). In the acute stages, patients with labyrinthitis may complain of **vertigo**, nausea, and vomiting.[6] With infection, pressure changes within the middle or inner ear cause the ear to feel congested. This condition may be aggravated by pressure changes associated with airplane travel.

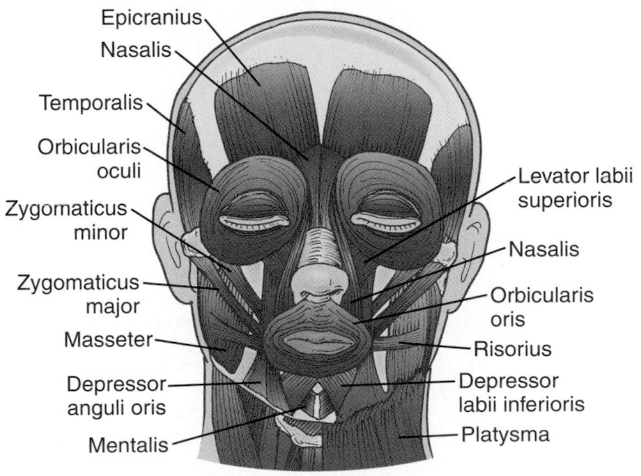

FIGURE 19-9 ■ The muscles of expression.

History Involving the Nose

- **Location of the pain:** Pain may be located over the nose but may also radiate throughout the eyes, face, and forehead.
- **Onset:** The onset of injury is often, if not always, acute. The insidious onset of nasal symptoms is suggestive of diseases such as **sinusitis** or URI.
- **Activity and injury mechanism:** The mechanism of injury is a direct blow to the nasal bone or nasal cartilage. Spontaneous epistaxis may occur as the result of a hot, dry environment drying out the highly vascularized nasal membrane.
- **Symptoms:** Pain and bleeding may be present. The patient requires evaluation for a possible concussion and orbital damage because the forces needed to fracture a nose may be sufficient to cause eye injury or closed head trauma (see Chapter 20).
- **Medical history:** Questioning the patient about a history of past nasal trauma is important. A prior nasal fracture may result in deformity that can be mistaken for an acute injury.

Bell's palsy Inhibition of the facial nerve secondary to trauma or disease, resulting in flaccidity of the facial muscles. In individuals suffering from Bell's palsy, the face on the involved side appears elongated.

Upper respiratory infection (URI) A categorical term encompassing a wide range of viral or bacterial infections of the nasal pathway, pharynx, and/or bronchi. The common cold is a form of URI.

Vertigo The sensation of moving around in space or of having objects move about the person

Sinusitis Inflammation of the nasal sinus

Table 19-2 Muscles of Expression (Partial List)

Muscle	Action	Origin	Insertion	Innervation	Root
Buccinator	Depresses the cheeks	Alveolar process of the maxilla and mandible	Angle of the mouth	Facial	CN VII
Depressor Anguli Oris	Draws the angle of the mouth downward (frowning)	Oblique line of the mandible	Angle of the mouth	Facial	CN VII
Depressor Labii Inferioris	Lowers the mouth	Oblique line of the mandible	Lower lip	Facial	CN VII
Digastric	Opens the mouth	Inferior border of the mandible	Superior aspect of the hyoid bone	Trigeminal	CN V
Geniohyoid	Opens the mouth	Median ridge of the mandible	Body of the hyoid bone	Ansa cervicalis	CN I, CN II
Levator Anguli Oris	Raises each side of the mouth (a bilateral muscle)	Just superior to the canine teeth	Angle of the mouth	Facial	CN VII
Masseter	Aids in biting	Superficial portion: Zygomatic process of maxilla; anterior two-thirds of the zygomatic arch Profundus portion: Posterior one-third of the zygomatic arch	Superficial portion: Inferior one-half of the lateral ramus of the mandible Profundus portion: Superior one-half of the ramus and coronoid process of the mandible	Trigeminal	CN V
Mentalis	Elevates the skin of the chin	Incisive fossa of the mandible	Point of the mandible	Facial	CN VII
Mylohyoid	Opens mouth	Inferior border of the mandible	Superior aspect of the hyoid bone	Trigeminal	CN V
Orbicularis Oris	"Puckers" lips	Originates off of the muscles surrounding the mouth	Skin surrounding the lips	Facial	CN VII
Procerus	Wrinkles the nose	Lower portion of the nasal bone Lateral nasal cartilage	Lower portion of the forehead between the eyebrows	Facial	CN VII
Temporalis	Aids in biting	Temporal fossa	Coronoid process and ramus of the mandible	Trigeminal	CN V
Zygomaticus Major	Used for smiling	Zygomatic bone	Angle of the mouth	Facial	CN VII

CN = cranial nerve

Examination Map

HISTORY

Location of Pain
Onset
Activity and Injury Mechanism
Symptoms

INSPECTION

Inspection of the Ear
- Auricle
- Tympanic membrane
- Periauricular area

Inspection of the Nose
- Alignment
- Epistaxis
- Septum and mucosa
- Eyes and face

Inspection of the Nose
- Respiration
- Thyroid and cricoid cartilage

Inspection of the Face and Jaw
- Bleeding
- Ecchymosis
- Symmetry
- Muscle tone

Inspection of the Oral Cavity
- Lips
- Teeth
- Tongue
- Lingual frenulum
- Gums

PALPATION

Palpation of the Anterior Structures
- Nasal bone
- Nasal cartilage
- Zygoma
- Maxilla
- Temporomandibular joint
- Periauricular area
- External ear
- Teeth
- Mandible
- Hyoid bone
- Cartilages

Palpation of the Lateral Structures
- Temporalis
- Masseter
- Buccinator

FUNCTIONAL ASSESSMENT

Ear
- Hearing
- Balance

Nose
- Smell

Temporomandibular Joint
- Range of motion
- Tracking

NEUROLOGICAL EXAMINATION

Cranial Nerve Assessment

REGION-SPECIFIC PATHOLOGIES AND SELECTIVE TISSUE TESTS

Ear Pathologies
- Auricular hematoma
- Tympanic membrane rupture
- Otitis externa
- Otitis media

Nasal Pathologies

Throat Pathologies

Facial Pathologies
- Mandibular fracture
- Zygoma fracture
- Maxillary fracture
- LeFort fracture

Dental Conditions
- Tooth fracture
- Tooth luxation
- Dental caries

Temporomandibular Joint Dysfunction

History Involving the Throat

- **Location of the pain:** Acute throat trauma causes pain in the anterior portion of the neck. Pain arising from illness (e.g., sore throat) is described as being deep within the neck.
- **Onset:** Throat injuries typically have acute onsets.
- **Activity and injury mechanism:** The throat is usually injured when it is struck with an object, such as a bat or ball, or by an opponent's elbow.
- **Symptoms:** A blow that crushes the larynx may result in the inability to speak. Respiratory distress may occur secondary to an obstruction of the airway and may result in the patient's speaking in a hoarse, raspy voice. This constitutes a medical emergency.

History Involving Maxillofacial Injuries

- **Location of the pain:** Normally, the exact site of pain can be located. Dental injuries usually can be pinpointed to one or more teeth. Oral pain may also be the result of neuralgia, TMJ conditions, sinusitis, migraine headaches, and myofascial inflammation.[7]
- **Onset:** Maxillofacial injuries are usually acute and the direct result of trauma. The exceptions are nonathletic dental problems (e.g., **dental caries**) and nerve conditions (e.g., Bell's palsy, **trigeminal neuralgia**).
- **Activity and injury mechanism:** The typical mechanism of injury is blunt trauma from an object or competitor. Balls, various forms of sticks and bats, and opponents all pose potential risks for inflicting maxillofacial injuries. Lacerating trauma to the lips or tongue can be accidentally self-inflicted by the patient's teeth.
- **Bruxing:** Bruxism (clenching or grinding of the teeth) may occur subconsciously or during sleep and can be habitual, the result of stress, or caused by TMJ dysfunction.[8] With time, bruxing can result in degeneration of the teeth's enamel and TMJ structures.
- **Other symptoms:** The facial bones are a large component of the eye orbit. The patient may report visual impairment and difficulty with eye movements. Initially,

---

Dental caries A destructive disease of the teeth; cavities

Trigeminal neuralgia A painful condition involving cranial nerve V, with possible motor involvement to one side of the mouth and paresthesia in the cheek

TMJ injuries may not be reported, but the patient may begin to notice pain or clicking in the TMJ while chewing. Difficulty chewing may indicate malocclusion of the teeth. Patients in the early stages of oral cancer may complain of **gingivitis**-like symptoms, and the tongue may feel thick and swollen (angioedema).

Inspection

Close inspection of the facial structures is vital for the accurate evaluation and management of injuries to this area. The primary inspection includes a check for obvious lacerations to the face and mouth because these injuries are usually found concurrently with other trauma. Because trauma to the face and mouth involves the respiratory system, the patency of the airway must also be immediately assessed. In cases of injury to the mouth, the oral cavity requires inspection for blockage by a mouthguard, displaced tooth, or other object that could become lodged in the airway.

Inspection of the Ear

- **The auricle:** Observe the outer ear for signs of a contusion or laceration. High-velocity impact of the auricle, as occurs when hit with a baseball, may cause a piece of the outer ear to be avulsed (Fig. 19-10). Formation of a hematoma within the auricle can result in the characteristic **pinna** or **auricular hematoma** (cauliflower ear) (Fig. 19-11). **Otitis externa** is evident as the external ear, including the external auditory meatus, is inflamed.

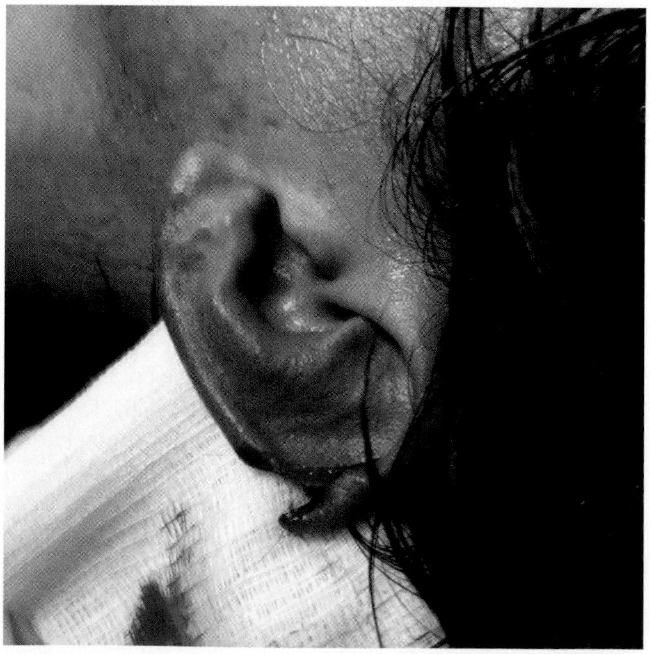

FIGURE 19-10 ■ Laceration of the external ear. This injury requires suturing to prevent permanent deformity of the ear.

Gingivitis Inflammation of the gums

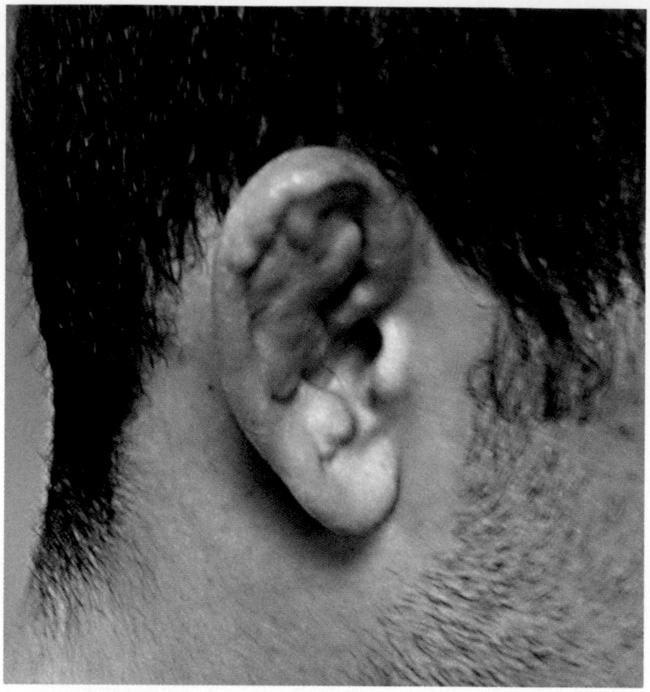

FIGURE 19-11 ■ Auricular hematoma, or "cauliflower ear." This condition is shown in its acute stage. If the hematoma is allowed to develop, the underlying cartilage is destroyed, resulting in permanent deformity of the external ear. Hearing acuity is affected secondary to the decreased ability to funnel sound waves into the middle ear.

- **The tympanic membrane:** Inspect the eardrum using an otoscope (Inspection Findings 19-1). The membrane normally appears shiny, convex, translucent, and smooth without any perforations. Suspected disruption of the tympanic membrane or fluid within the auditory canal requires immediate referral for further medical evaluation. Infection of the middle ear, otitis media, causes the membrane to appear distended secondary to the collection of fluids and pus. A collection of fluids may also be visible, otitis media with effusion. These substances may also occlude the membrane.
- **Periauricular area:** Carefully inspect the area surrounding the ear for signs of a basilar skull fracture, characterized by ecchymosis around the mastoid process, known as "**Battle sign**" (see Fig. 20-12, p 878).

Inspection of the Nose

- **Alignment:** Inspect the nose for proper alignment and symmetry on each side of the sagittal plane. Asymmetry may be caused by a fracture or swelling. Any question regarding the presence of a deformity can be resolved by asking the patient to view his or her nose in a mirror to see if it looks normal.
- **Epistaxis:** Bleeding from the nasal passage is common after trauma to the nasal bones and is usually the result of mucosal laceration. Light bleeding may indicate epistaxis from the anterior portion of the nose; moderate to heavy bleeding indicates posterior epistaxis.[9] Spontaneous or persistent epistaxis may be related to

Inspection Findings 19-1

Use of an Otoscope for Inspection of the Ear and Nose

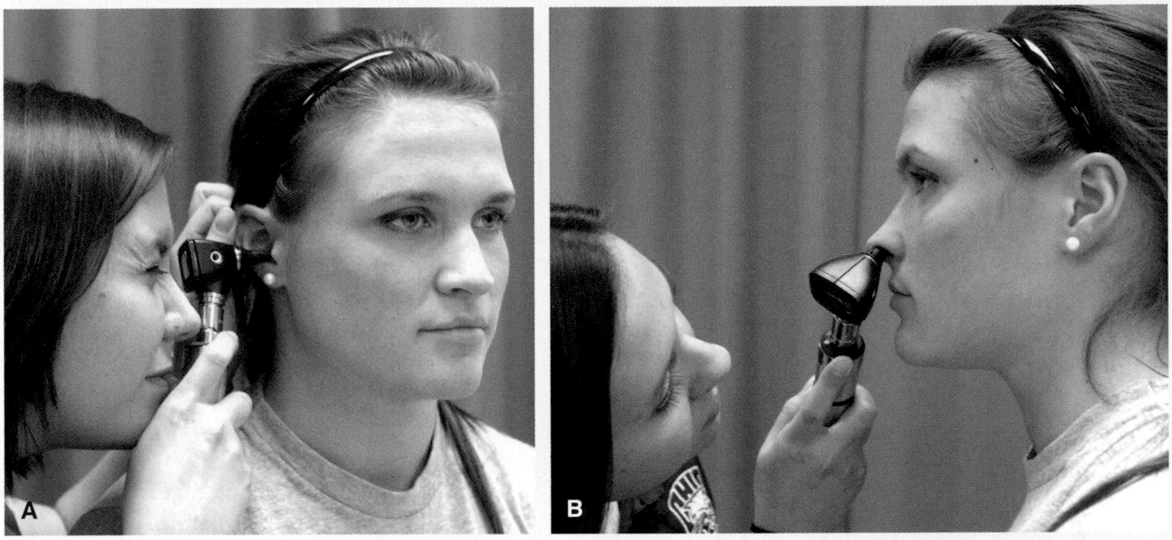

(A) An otoscope with a speculum that fits snugly within the ear canal without causing pain is used to inspect the tympanic membrane. The speculum needs to be placed only slightly into the ear canal to view the structures. Visualization is improved when the pinna is pulled upward and backward (some clinicians prefer to pull the earlobe downward). (B) The use of an otoscope to view the nasal passage.

Patient Position	Seated or standing
Position of Examiner	Positioned to easily access the patient's ear or nose
Evaluative Procedure	Select and fit a speculum on the otoscope that will fit snugly into the opening. When inspecting the ear, open the auditory canal by gently pulling upward and backward on the pinna or downward on the earlobe. Gently insert the speculum into the ear. Deep penetration is not necessary.
Positive Test	*Ear:* Reddened and/or bulging tympanic membrane; fluid buildup behind the tympanic membrane; fluid in the ear canal; ruptured tympanic membrane *Nose:* Deviation or deformity of the nasal passage(s)
Implications	*Ear:* A reddened and/or bulging tympanic membrane is indicative of middle ear infection (acute otitis media). Fluid behind the tympanic membrane (otitis media effusion) is not necessarily indicative of an infection. Fluid in the ear canal may represent otorrhea, or leakage of cerebrospinal fluid, and is associated with a skull fracture. A ruptured tympanic membrane may result from a blow to the ear. *Nose:* Fracture, deviated septum
Comments	Cerumen may obscure the tympanic membrane. To clear cerumen, gently flush the ear with hydrogen peroxide or warm water. Do not do this if a tympanic membrane rupture is suspected.
Evidence	Absent or inconclusive in the literature

high blood pressure.[10] Lacerations of the skin covering the nose are also common in patients with these injuries and may or may not have an associated fracture. Universal precautions are indicated.

- **Septum and mucosa:** View the nasal septum and its mucosal lining using an otoscope (see Inspection Findings 19-1) or penlight. On inspection, the septum appears symmetrical and straight; asymmetry or angulation of the nasal passage indicates a deviated septum. Bony fragments may also be seen within the nasal passage.
- **Eyes and face:** Inspect the area beneath the eyes for the presence of ecchymosis. After a nasal or skull fracture, blood follows the contour of the bone to rest beneath the eyes (periorbital ecchymosis), a clinical sign termed **raccoon eyes** (Fig. 19-12).

Inspection of the Throat

- **Respiration:** Observe the patient's breathing pattern for signs of respiratory distress (see Chapter 2). Even relatively minor blows to the throat can disrupt breathing, a medical emergency.
- **Thyroid and cricoid cartilage:** Inspect these cartilages for deformity. Swelling may appear rapidly and obliterate the borders of the thyroid cartilage. Any deformity in this structure must be treated as a medical emergency because of the potential jeopardy to the airway.[11]

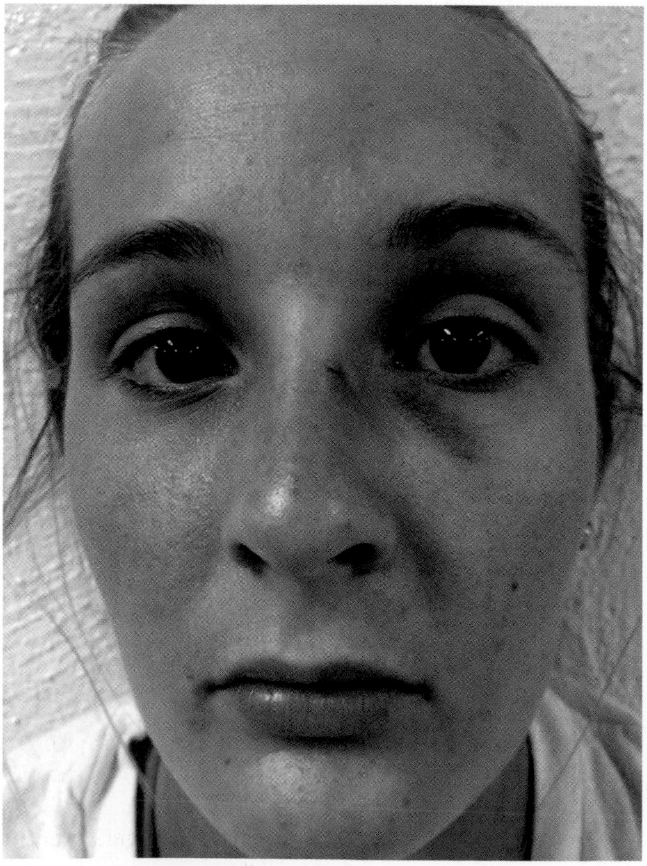

FIGURE 19-12 ■ Periorbital ecchymosis, or "Raccoon eyes". After a nasal fracture, hemorrhage follows the contour of the face and pools beneath the eyes. This condition can also result from a skull fracture.

*** Practical Evidence**

Acute hoarseness (85%) and dysphasia (52%) are the most common signs of laryngeal fractures.[11]

Inspection of the Face and Jaw

- **Bleeding:** Facial and tongue lacerations are often accompanied by profuse bleeding. Although controlling bleeding must be addressed, the possibility of underlying trauma must not be overlooked (see On-Field Management of Facial Lacerations).
- **Ecchymosis:** The presence of periorbital ecchymosis may be the result of fracture to the nasal bones, maxilla, or zygoma. In addition, it can occur without a fracture (e.g., black eye). Ecchymosis below the alveolar process and at the angle of the mandible is common after mandibular fracture.
- **Symmetry:** Inspection of the uninjured face usually reveals symmetry between the right and left halves. With facial pathology such as zygomatic fracture, TMJ injury, or mandibular fracture, this symmetry may be lost secondary to bony deformity or swelling. Inspection of the face also includes inspecting the patient's eye movements for equality. If the maxilla or zygoma is fractured, eye movement may be asymmetrical (see Chapter 18).
- **Muscle tone:** Watch the patient's mouth, eyebrows, and forehead for symmetrical motion while talking. A unilateral paralysis of the facial muscles, Bell's palsy, is the result of traumatic or organic inhibition of the facial nerves or can be associated with a stroke.

Inspection of the Oral Cavity

- **Lips:** Because of the high potential for infection and scarring, any laceration extending across the vermilion border onto the lips requires a referral to a physician for further evaluation.
- **Teeth:** Although most types of tooth fractures are readily apparent during gross inspection, chipped teeth and fractures involving the root are more subtle. Using a penlight and dental mirror, inspect both the inner and outer sides of the tooth's surfaces for chipped crowns and other defects. Although most acute dental trauma only involves one tooth, trauma to the surrounding teeth must also be ruled out (Fig. 19-13).[12]
- **Tongue:** The dorsal and ventral surfaces of the tongue are inspected for lacerations.
- **Lingual frenulum:** The integrity of the lingual frenulum is observed as the patient lifts the tongue (Fig. 19-14). This structure can become lacerated secondary to teeth fractures.
- **Gums:** The inner and outer border of the gums is inspected for lacerations, an abscess, or gingivitis. For conditions of insidious onset for patients with a history

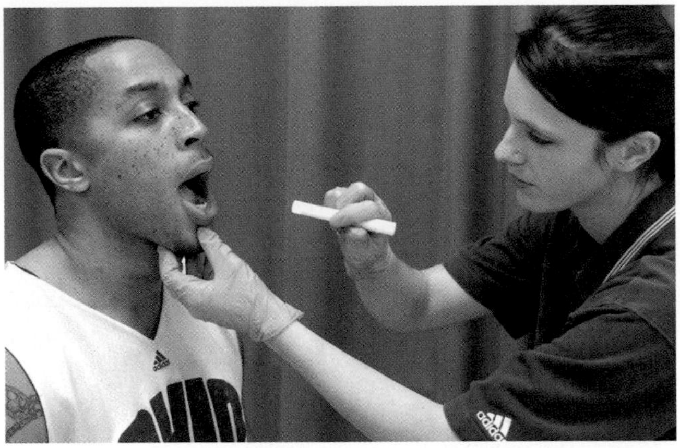
FIGURE 19-13 ■ Inspection of the oral cavity to rule out tooth fractures and to locate the source of bleeding.

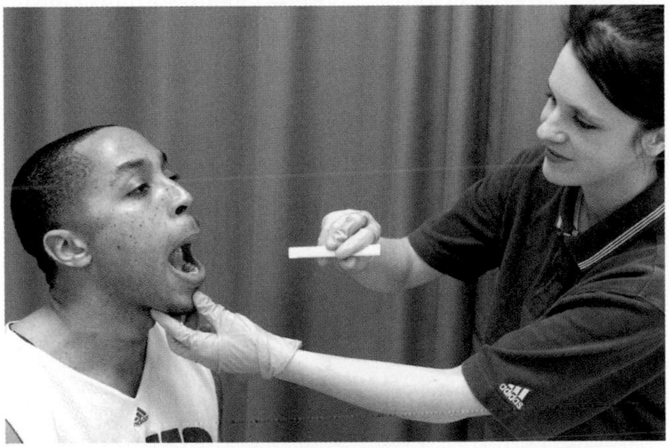
FIGURE 19-14 ■ Inspection of the lingual frenulum. The patient is asked to lift the tongue to the roof of the mouth.

of smoking or smokeless tobacco use, inspect the gums and tongue for white or red lesions and nonhealing open wounds. Leukoplakia, precancerous cells, often form in the area of contact with smokeless tobacco.

PALPATION

Because of the relatively subcutaneous location of the facial bones and mandible, these structures are easily palpated. Although the internal structures of the ears, nose, and throat cannot be palpated, the overlying and surrounding areas must be examined for tenderness and concurrent injury.

Palpation of the Anterior Structures

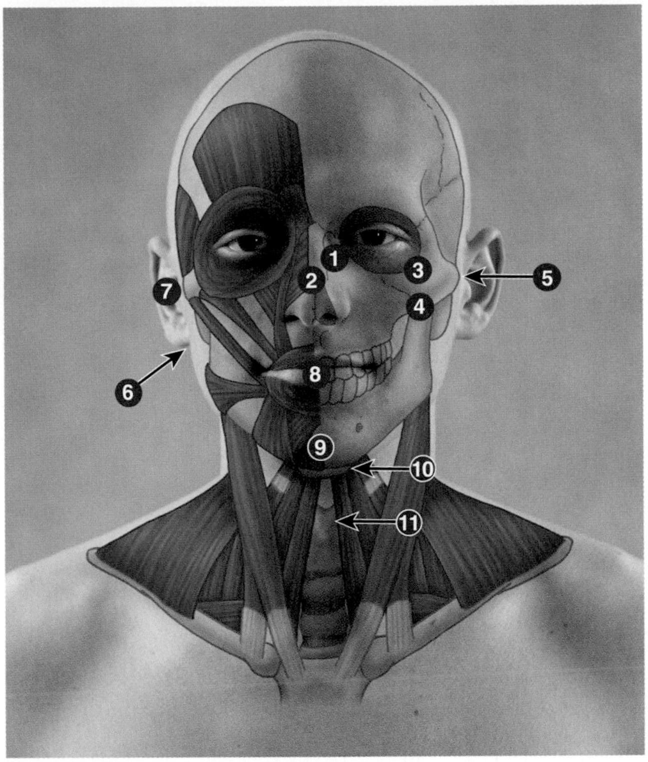

Palpation of the Anterior Structures

1 **Nasal bone:** Begin palpation of the **nasal bone** at the point that the zygomatic and maxillary bones merge beneath the medial portion of the orbit. Applying light yet firm pressure, continue to palpate medially to the base of the nasal bone and up to the bridge of the nose, noting painful areas or crepitus. Palpation of the nasal bone is not necessary if a fracture is visually apparent. From the upper boundaries of the nasal bone, proceed upward and laterally to palpate the frontal bone above the nose and eyes.

2 **Nasal cartilage:** From the bridge of the nose, continue palpating distal to the **nasal cartilage** at the tip of the nose. Normally, this structure should align with the center of the bridge.

3 **Zygoma:** Begin to palpate the face at the junction between the temporal and **zygomatic bones**, just anterior to the auditory canals and above the TMJ. Palpate anteriorly and medially along the zygomatic arches as they pass beneath the eyes and merge with the maxillary bones bilaterally.

4 **Maxilla:** From the crest of the zygomatic arch, palpate upward along the **maxilla**. The fused joint where the maxillary and nasal bones join is marked by a sudden slope. Palpation continues to the crest of the nasal bones. Palpate the remainder of the maxilla by moving inferiorly from the nose and outward along the upper margin of the teeth.

5 **TMJ:** Open the jaw to move the coronoid process from under the zygomatic arch. Although this structure is often not directly palpable, the area can be palpated for underlying tenderness.

Placing the tips of the index and middle fingers over the **TMJ**, note the presence of any clicking or crepitus as the mouth is opened and closed (Fig. 19-15). These conditions are pathological, indicating a disruption of the joint's normal

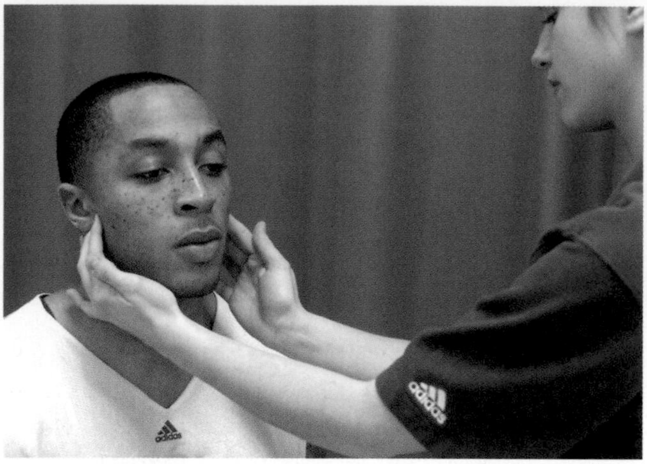

FIGURE 19-15 ■ External palpation of the external temporomandibular joint. The temporomandibular joint is palpated while the mouth is opened and closed. Asymmetry of movement and clicking or locking of the joint are noted.

biomechanics. As the mouth is opened wide, a small depression is normally felt within the joint as the mandibular head and neck slide forward. Swelling can fill this area.

Palpate the posterior aspect of the TMJ by placing the fifth finger in the opening of the external auditory meatus (Fig. 19-16). The bilateral movement of the TMJ normally is smooth and equal as the mouth is opened and closed. Any discrepancy in this motion may indicate TMJ dysfunction, a TMJ dislocation, or a mandibular fracture.

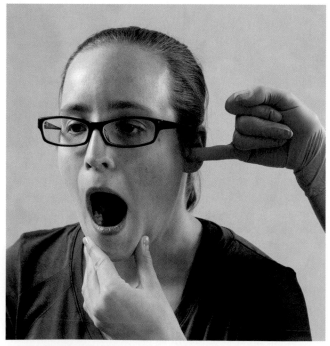

FIGURE 19-16 ■ Palpation of the internal temporomandibular joint. Wearing gloves, the examiner lightly places a finger in the outermost portion of the auditory canal to further palpate the mechanics of the temporomandibular joint as the mouth is opened and closed.

6 **Periauricular area:** To rule out the presence of a fracture, palpate the temporal bone surrounding the external ear and its mastoid process.

7 **External ear:** Palpate the auricle to determine tenderness and swelling. In cases of repeated trauma to the **external ear**, as commonly occurs in wrestlers, hard nodules may be felt within the auricle. Pain associated with a middle or inner ear infection is increased by tugging on the earlobe. Locate the lymph nodes just inferior and posterior to the ear. They can become enlarged secondary to infection.

8 **Teeth:** Wear gloves to palpate the **teeth** after an oral injury. Gentle pressure is sufficient to check the integrity of the tooth's attachment to the alveolar processes (Fig. 19-17). An alternative is to have the patient use the tongue to apply this pressure. Any suspicion of a loosened tooth warrants consultation with a dentist. The procedure for the management of an avulsed tooth is covered in the On-Field Management section.

9 **Mandible:** Begin the palpation of the chin at the mental protuberance (cleft of the chin). From here, progress posteriorly, palpating the lateral and posterior portion of the **mandible** and the lower alveolar processes. The mandibular ramus and the lateral border of the angle of the mandible become obscured by the masseter muscle.

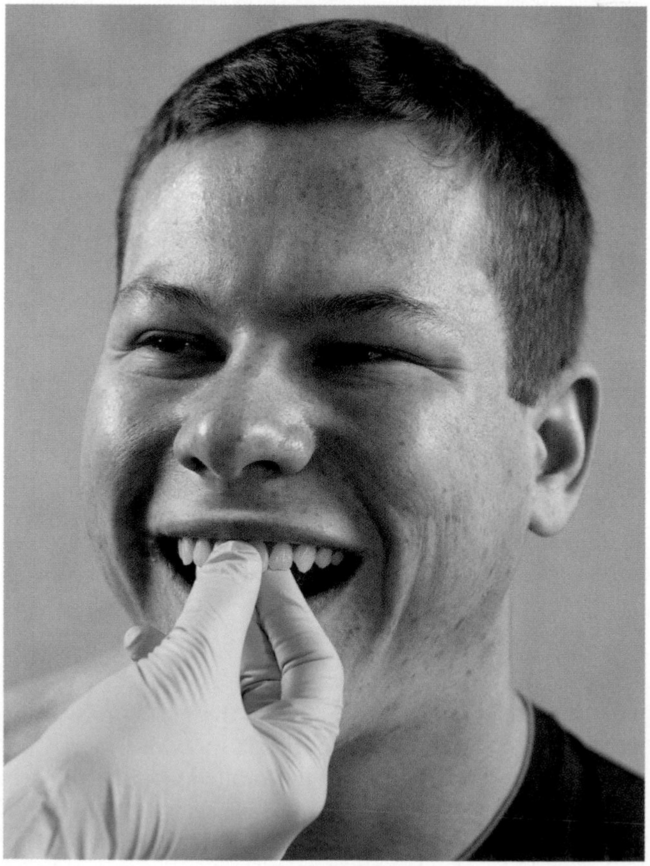

FIGURE 19-17 ■ Palpation of the teeth. Gloves must be worn during this process.

10 Hyoid: Palpate the **hyoid**, located approximately one finger breadth superior to the thyroid cartilage. The integrity of the hyoid can be determined by gently grasping it between the thumb and index fingers. The bone glides downward as the patient swallows.

11 Cartilages: Begin the palpation of the **cartilages** at the sternal notch. Continue upward to find the series of depressions and hardened bands of the tracheal cartilage. Then proceed upward to find the cricoid cartilage and the thick body of the thyroid cartilage.

Palpation of the Lateral Structures

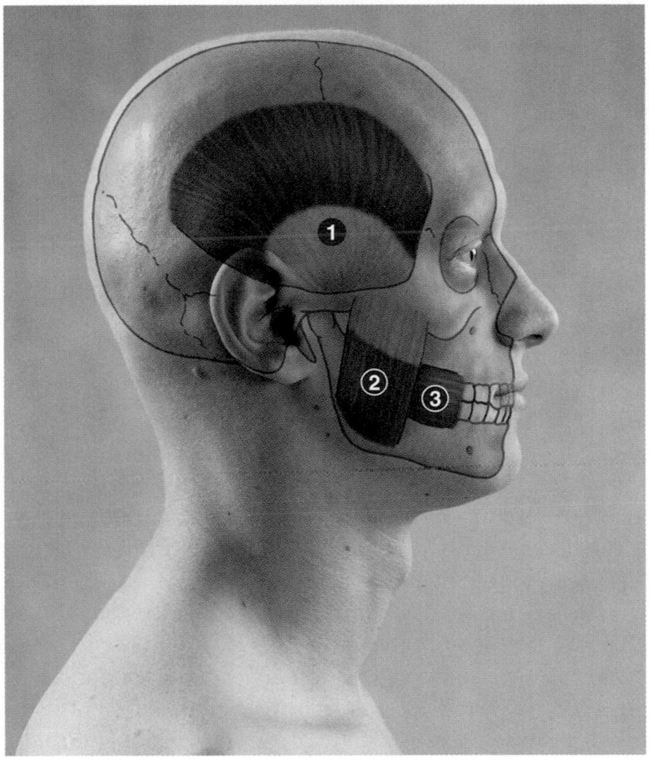

Palpation of the Lateral Structures

The four primary muscles of mastication are the temporalis, masseter, medial pterygoid, and lateral pterygoid.

1 Temporalis: Palpate the belly of the **temporalis** superior to the ears. To make the muscle more prominent, ask the patient to clench the teeth.

2 Masseter: The **masseter** is palpable superior to the mandible, near its angle. Clenching the teeth activates this muscle and makes it easily palpable. The medial and lateral pterygoid muscles lie beneath the masseter muscle.

3 Buccinator: Located in the space between the maxilla and mandible, the **buccinator** is a secondary muscle of mastication. The muscle is located just lateral to the mouth on both sides and becomes prominent with puffing the cheeks.

Functional Assessment

The functional tests for the ear, nose, and throat provide information about the pathology and impairment of hearing, balance, smell, and swallowing.

Tests for the Ear

- **Hearing:** Transitory hearing loss is to be expected immediately after a blow to the ear. Failure to regain normal hearing within 1 hour after injury is significant and warrants referral for further medical evaluation and visualization of the tympanic membrane.
- **Balance:** The patient is questioned regarding balance and dizziness, each of which may occur secondary to either ear or brain trauma. Neurological balance assessment is discussed in Chapter 20.

Tests for the Nose

- **Smell:** The olfactory senses may be obscured by epistaxis but should return after the bleeding has subsided. The loss of olfactory function is more commonly attributed to brain trauma than to trauma directly to the nose itself.

Tests for Temporomandibular Joint Involvement

Functional testing for TMJ pathology involves having the patient slowly open and close the mouth. Normally, the mouth can open wide enough to insert two knuckles (Selective Tissue Test 19-1).

To identify malocclusion, select a point, such as the junction between the two middle lower incisors, for use as a reference point (Fig. 19-18). Normally, the jaw moves smoothly and evenly with no interruption. After injury to the TMJ, mandible, or maxilla, opening and closing the jaw may demonstrate a lateral deviation, and the bite may be maloccluded.

Use the same reference point to evaluate the distance and quality of lateral excursion of the jaw. Then this can be compared with the point between the incisors of the upper jaw by asking the patient to move the jaw right and left. The distance that the lower reference point moves relative to the upper reference point is measured with a ruler and compared bilaterally. Normally, the movement is bilaterally equal and completed in a smooth and pain-free manner.

The point in the ROM where tracking deviations occur can be indicative of the nature of the pathology. Lateral deviations opposite of the involved side that occur early in the ROM are often the result of muscle spasm, deviations in the midpoint are associated with muscle spasm, and deviations at the end of the ROM are caused by posterior capsulitis.[13,14]

Neurological Testing

Loss of the associated special senses (hearing and smell) can indicate the presence of closed head trauma that has

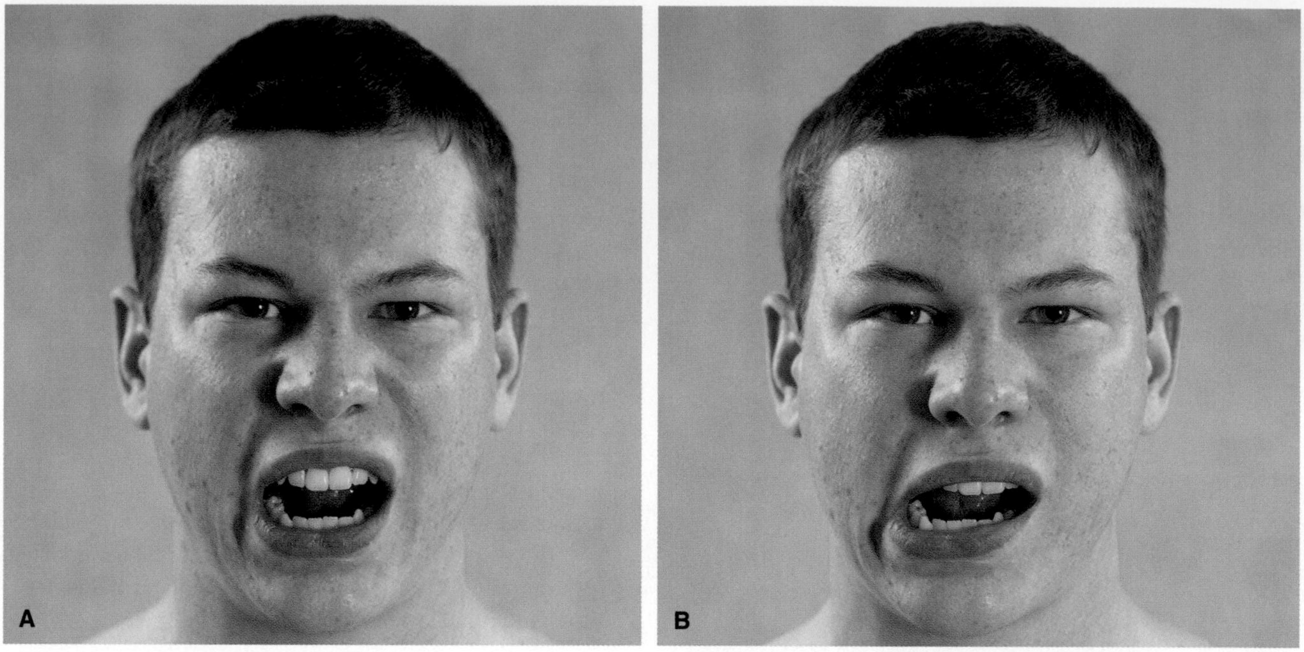

FIGURE 19-18 ■ Observation for malocclusion of the teeth. (A) Normally, the mandible travels in a straight line. (B) Trauma to the temporomandibular joint or a fracture of the mandible causes the jaw to track laterally and results in a malalignment of the teeth.

disrupted one or more cranial nerves. The evaluation of these conditions is described in Chapter 20. Decreased sensation in the upper cheek region may indicate involvement of the infraorbital nerve, such as entrapment associated with a blowout fracture (Chapter 18).

Region-Specific Pathologies and Selective Tissue Tests

Pathology to the ear, nose, and throat is relatively uncommon in athletes, largely because of the use of protective mouthguards and headgear. Also, rules have been implemented to decrease the possibility of injury by prohibiting blows to the face and head. Although limited in number, injuries to this area can involve major trauma with the potential for long-term complications of impaired hearing, smell, and speech and undesirable aesthetic changes. Laryngeal injury can be life threatening secondary to obstruction of the airway.

Ear Pathology

Most athletic-related ear injuries are the result of a single traumatic force or invading organisms and diseases. Because injuries do not always result in visible trauma, the decision to refer the patient to a physician is based on the complaints reported.

Auricular Hematoma

Repeated episodes of blunt trauma or shearing forces to the external ear can result in an auricular hematoma,[15] also termed "cauliflower ear." Swelling within the skin of the outer ear develops within hours of the injury. Pooling of blood between the skin and the cartilage separates the two, depriving the cartilage of its source of nutrition. With time, the hematoma can scar, causing a deformed appearance to the external ear (see Fig. 19-11).[16]

The chief complaint is pain in the external and middle ear, accompanied by ecchymosis and swelling of the auricle. The external ear is inspected for open wounds and drainage from the middle ear. Palpation reveals increased tenderness and, initially, the "boggy" feel of swelling. Untreated cases with scarring appear smooth but feel hardened on palpation (Examination Findings 19-1). The inner ear is also examined using an otoscope (see information on the tympanic membrane).

In cases caused by a blow to the head, brain trauma also must be ruled out. A concurrent basilar skull fracture may result in ecchymosis at the mastoid process (Battle sign). Patients suspected of having a concurrent skull fracture must be immediately referred to a physician for a definitive diagnosis.

Auricular Hematoma Intervention Strategies

Often, a small needle is used to aspirate the hematoma, decreasing the amount of separation between the skin and the cartilage. If the fluid accumulation is actually within the cartilage, a more extreme excision and drainage is needed to fully clear the hematoma.[15] Chronic cauliflower ear may require surgical correction.[16] After this procedure is performed, or as a method of initial management of a patient with this condition, the ear may be casted with pieces of plaster casting material or gauze and **flexible collodion** to prevent further fluid accumulation.[15] None of these treatments has

Flexible collodion A mixture of ether, alcohol, cellulose, and camphor that dries to form a firm, protective layer

Selective Tissue Tests 19-1
Temporomandibular Joint Range of Motion

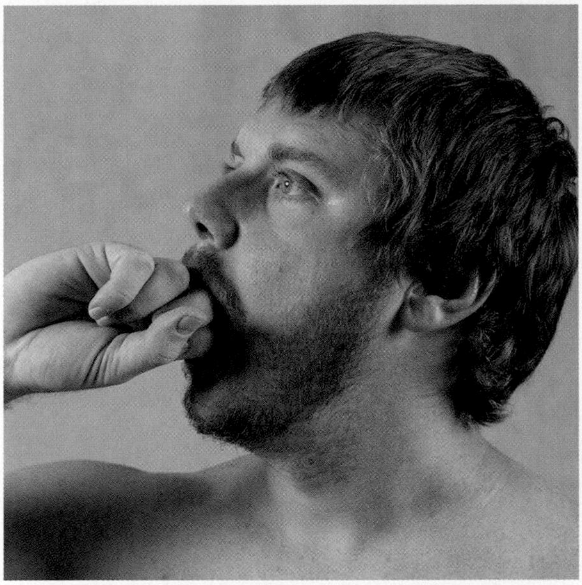

The TMJ should provide enough motion to allow two fingers to be inserted into the mouth.

Patient Position	Seated or standing
Position of Examiner	In front of the patient
Evaluative Procedure	The patient attempts to place as many flexed knuckles as possible between the upper and lower teeth.
Positive Test	The patient is unable to place a minimum of two knuckles within the mouth.
Implications	*Less than two fingers:* TMJ hypomobility *Three or more fingers:* TMJ hypermobility
Comments	Standardized measurement tools can also be used to quantify the amount of opening.
Evidence	Absent or inconclusive in the literature

TMJ = temporomandibular joint

been shown to be more effective than another.[18] Prophylactic antibiotics are used to reduce the chance of infection following drainage.[15]

Tympanic Membrane Rupture

The mechanism of injury for a tympanic membrane rupture is a sudden change of air pressure on the tympanic membrane caused by blunt trauma or by a decreased ability to regulate inner ear pressure secondary to an infection. The use of hyperbaric oxygen chambers may increase the risk of tympanic membrane ruptures secondary to the high atmospheric pressures used in this procedure.[19] The membrane may also be ruptured through direct trauma, such as sticking a sharp object in the ear (Examination Findings 19-2).

An otoscope is used to inspect the tympanic membrane. Reddish-brown **cerumen** may be seen as the speculum enters the ear canal, possibly obscuring the view of the tympanic membrane. Any fluids in the canal are unusual and minimally indicate a rupture to the tympanic membrane secondary to otitis media. In a worst-case scenario, this is caused by a skull fracture.

Tympanic Membrane Rupture Intervention Strategies

Disruption of the tympanic membrane warrants the referral for further examination by a physician. Pain medication

Cerumen A reddish-brown wax formed in the auditory meatus

Examination Findings 19-1
Auricular Hematoma

Examination Segment	Clinical Findings
History of Current Condition	*Onset:* Acute or chronic *Pain characteristics:* The external ear *Other symptoms:* Not applicable *Mechanism:* A single or repeated trauma to the external ear, resulting in a subcutaneous hematoma
Functional Assessment	Hearing and balance may be impaired.
Inspection	The ear and possibly the canal appear violently red. Swelling secondary to a hematoma is visible.
Palpation	Palpation of an acute injury produces pain and confirms the presence of a hematoma. Palpation of a chronic injury may reveal hardened nodules within the ear.
Joint and Muscle Function Assessment	Not applicable
Selective Tissue Tests	Not applicable
Neurological Screening	Impairment of cranial nerve VIII (acoustic nerve: hearing and balance)
Vascular Screening	Not applicable
Imaging Techniques	Not applicable
Differential Diagnosis	Not applicable
Comments	Auricular hematomas require referral to a physician.

and antibiotics may be prescribed. Instruct the patient to prevent water from entering the ear (e.g., during showering and swimming) while the rupture is healing.

The tympanic membrane's healing properties and process are different from those of other soft tissues. Although conservative management allows natural healing to occur, the defect must be closely monitored as it tends to heal without first closing, resulting in a permanent fissure in the tympanic membrane.[20,21] In some cases, a small graft may be placed over the wound.

Otitis Externa

Otitis externa is an infection of the external auditory meatus commonly termed "swimmer's ear" because of its prevalence in individuals who participate in water activities. The condition is usually caused by inadequate drying of the ear canal. The dark, damp environment encourages the growth of bacteria or fungus, resulting in the inflammation of the external auditory meatus. The presence of psoriasis, eczema, excessively oily skin, and open wounds within the ear can predispose an individual to otitis externa. Overcleaning of the external auditory canal may inadvertently remove a protective chemical layer, also predisposing a person to otitis externa. In addition, a narrow inner ear can predispose an individual to otitis externa by preventing adequate drying and encouraging the growth of bacteria.[22]

The chief complaint is one of constant pain and pressure, possibly accompanied by itching in the ear. The patient may complain of a hearing deficit and dizziness. The area is red, and a clear discharge from the middle ear may be present. The lymph nodes around the ear may be enlarged. In severe cases, the mastoid process may be enlarged and tender to the touch. Tugging on the earlobe usually increases pain.

Otitis Externa Intervention Strategies

A physician may prescribe acid-based drops mixed with antibiotics or corticosteroids (or both). A wick may be placed in the ear to maintain dryness. Patients, especially swimmers, should refrain from entering the water and keep their ears dry.

Otitis Media

Upper respiratory infections and bacterial or viral invasion can cause an inflammation of the ear's mucous membranes, blocking the eustachian tubes and increasing the pressure within the inner ear. URIs, airplane travel, and seasonal allergies may predispose an individual to acute otitis media,

Examination Findings 19-2
Tympanic Membrane Rupture

Examination Segment	Clinical Findings
History of Current Condition	*Onset:* Acute *Pain characteristics:* Pain, often excruciating, in the middle ear, radiating inward and outward *Other symptoms:* **Tinnitus** *Mechanism:* A mechanical pressure (e.g., a slap to the ear or a blocked sneeze) that causes the tympanic membrane to burst or a mechanical intrusion through the membrane (e.g., cleaning the ears with a ballpoint pen) A strong Valsalva maneuver that increases the inner ear pressure 5 to 14 psi can result in a tympanic membrane rupture.[20] *Risk factors:* URI, otitis media
Functional Assessment	There is a marked hearing loss in the involved ear. Valsalva maneuver may result in the audible escape of air from within the inner ear.
Inspection	Blood or fluids may be observed leaking from the ear. Inspection with an otoscope reveals redness, and the perforation will be visible.
Palpation	Not applicable
Selective Tissue Tests	Hearing assessment
Neurological Screening	Not applicable (in this case, hearing reduction is the result of a mechanical deficit)
Vascular Screening	Not applicable
Imaging Techniques	Not applicable
Differential Diagnosis	Not applicable
Comments	The resulting pain and inflammatory response may result in transient dizziness. The ear must be kept dry and the patient referred to a physician.

psi = pounds per square inch; URI = upper respiratory infection

and the condition is particularly prevalent in young children. Another condition, otitis media with effusion, occurs when fluid collects in the middle ear but no bacterial or viral infection is present.[23] In addition to having a history of upper respiratory problems, patients may also mention a feeling of the ear's being blocked and pressure and pain within the inner ear. Inspection with an otoscope reveals fluid buildup in the middle ear and an opaque, reddened, and bulging tympanic membrane. Otitis media may result in hearing loss in the affected ear. This hearing loss can be confirmed by striking a tuning fork and placing the stem on the center of the forehead (the **Weber test**); in the presence of otitis media, the patient hears the vibration louder in the affected ear. Otitis media may also lead to tympanic membrane rupture.

*** Practical Evidence**

A bulging tympanic membrane is highly suggestive of otitis media.

Tinnitus Ringing in the ears

Otitis Media Intervention Strategies

Oral antibiotics are usually prescribed for patients who are suffering from acute otitis media but are not warranted for otitis media with effusion. Antihistamine medications, commonly used to combat allergies, should not be used with acute otitis media or otitis media with effusion, as they may cause a longer duration of the middle ear effusion. Decongestants may help reduce nasal congestion, although neither antihistamines nor decongestants are associated with a shorter duration of acute otitis media.[23]

Nasal Injuries

The nasal bones are the most commonly fractured bones of the face and skull and the third most common of all fractures and most frequently occur from a direct blow.[24] Bleeding typically occurs immediately after the trauma but is usually easily controlled (see the section on on-field evaluation and management of nasal injuries). Athletes competing in contact or collision sports often have a history of nasal fractures. However, deformity of the nose should not be assumed to be preexisting.

Other than bleeding, the chief complaint is pain on and around the nose. On inspection, the nose may be visibly deformed, but the lack of a deformity does not conclusively rule out a nasal fracture. Swelling in and around the nose may obscure minor deformities. With time, ecchymosis develops and settles under the inferior aspect of the eyes ("raccoon eyes"). Palpation reveals tenderness at the fracture site and the surrounding areas. Crepitus may be identifiable at the fracture site as well (Examination Findings 19-3).

Using an otoscope or penlight, inspect the internal nose for deviation of the septum. The patient should attempt to breathe through one nostril while holding the opposite one closed. The nostril should close during inhalation, and breathing should be unobstructed. The exhalation should be easy and unencumbered. Inspection of the nasal cavity may reveal a deviated septum or septal hematoma. Although radiographs are often used to identify the presence of a nasal fracture, their use has low reliability as a diagnostic tool and is discouraged.[24,25] Computed tomography (CT) images are much more sensitive and specific in ruling in and ruling out nasal fractures.[26]

Nasal Fracture Intervention Strategies

Septal hematomas require immediate removal by a physician because of the associated risk of infection and subsequent necrosis of the articular cartilage, resulting in a saddle-nose deformity (Fig. 19-19).[24,25] If a nasal fracture, deviated septum, or septal hematoma is suspected, the patient requires a physician referral. Displaced nasal fractures or deviated septa require closed or open reduction for realignment. This procedure can be delayed to allow associated swelling to subside with no change in outcome.[25]

Throat Injury

Trauma to this area often results in respiratory distress and the inability to speak, leading to agitation of the patient.

Examination Findings 19-3
Nasal Fractures

Examination Segment	Clinical Findings
History of Current Condition	*Onset:* Acute *Pain characteristics:* The bridge of the nose and nasal cartilage, possibly radiating into the frontal and zygomatic bones *Other symptoms:* Bleeding normally accompanies nasal fractures. *Mechanism:* A direct blow to the nose
Functional Assessment	The sense of smell and breathing through the nose may be obstructed by bleeding or a deviated septum (or both).
Inspection	The nose may be visibly malaligned and/or swollen. Ecchymosis may accumulate beneath one or both eyes ("raccoon eyes"). The internal nose requires inspection with an otoscope or penlight for the presence of a deviated septum or septal hematoma. Swelling may mask any deviation.
Palpation	Palpation of the traumatized area elicits pain. Crepitus may be felt over the fracture site.
Selective Tissue Tests	Not applicable
Neurological Screening	Not applicable
Vascular Screening	Not applicable
Imaging Techniques	Radiographs may be obtained but are not accurate in identifying the presence of a nasal fracture, and their use is discouraged.[24] Optimal imaging is obtained from CT images, and pathology to the orbit or other facial structures can concurrently be assessed.[25]
Differential Diagnosis	Epistaxis resulting from URI, sinus conditions, or other general medical state; nasal cartilage pathology; septal hematoma
Comments	Patients who have suffered a nasal fracture should also be screened for injury to the eyes and head.

CT = computed tomography; URI = upper respiratory infection

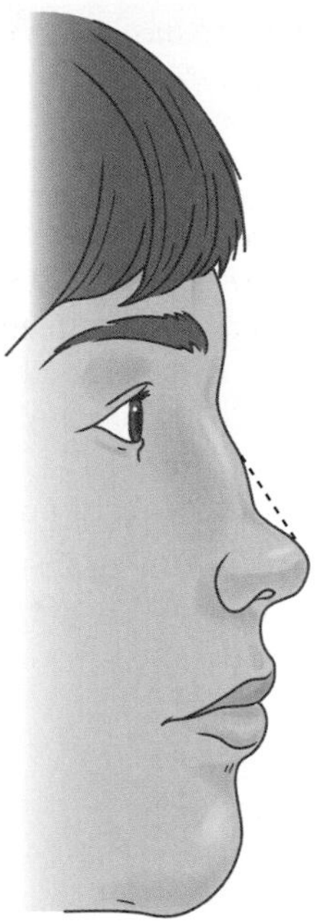

FIGURE 19-19 ■ Saddle-nose deformity. An untreated septal hematoma and its infection causing necrosis of the nasal cartilage can result in deformity of the nose.

The insulting blow to the anterior throat, if it includes the **carotid sinus**, can result in the loss of consciousness. Pain is increased during swallowing or while taking deep, gasping breaths of air. Bruising over and around the larynx is common, and the usual palpable definition of the larynx is lost because of deformity or swelling. There may be a noticeable change in the patient's voice.[11] The inside of the mouth is examined with the use of a penlight to detect the presence of bloody sputum, indicating an injury to the inside of the throat. Palpation may reveal a displaced cartilage and extreme tenderness or crepitus (Examination Findings 19-4).

Throat Injury Intervention Strategies

No attempt is made to correct any deviations because of the possibility of worsening the condition. Immediate referral to a physician or activation of the emergency action system is indicated because airway compromise may develop as swelling continues.

Facial Fractures

Protective facial equipment, such as a football helmet's face mask or a catcher's mask, is useful in deflecting many otherwise injurious forces. However, most equipment leaves at least a portion of the face exposed to potential injury. Also see Orbital Fractures, p. 806.

Mandibular Fractures

Mandibular fractures, the second most common type of facial fracture, ranking behind nasal fractures, are the result of a high-velocity impact to the jaw.[27] The chief complaint of a mandibular fracture is pain in the jaw that is increased by opening and closing the mouth. Difficulty with or discrepancies in jaw movement may also be noted by the patient (Fig. 19-20). Crepitus may be felt during palpation of the fracture site. Mandibular fractures typically result in a

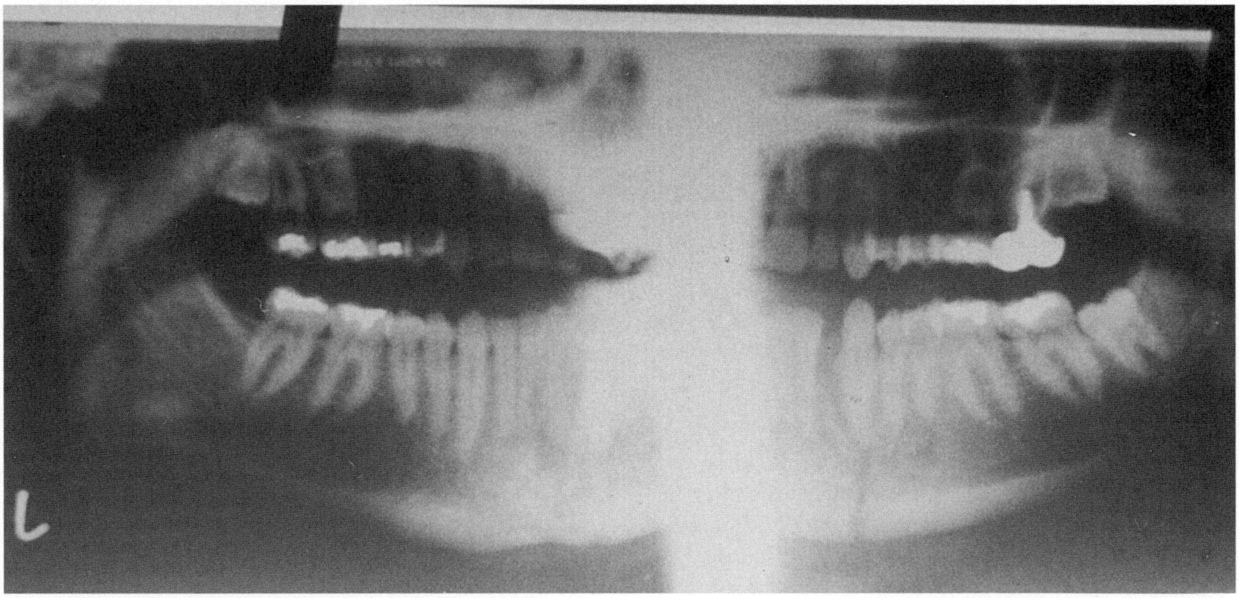

FIGURE 19-20 ■ Radiograph of a mandibular fracture.

Carotid sinus An area near the common carotid artery that, when stimulated, results in vasodilation and a lowering of the heart rate. When this happens suddenly, unconsciousness may occur.

Examination Findings 19-4
Throat Trauma

Examination Segment	Clinical Findings
History of Current Condition	*Onset:* Acute *Pain characteristics:* Anterior neck, possibly radiating into the chest secondary to an obstructed airway *Other symptoms:* Difficulty breathing *Mechanism:* A crushing force to the anterior neck
Functional Assessment	The patient has difficulty breathing. There is an inability to speak or difficulty speaking (aphasia).
Inspection	Bruising or other signs of trauma are present over the anterior throat. Swelling or deformity may be present. Bloody sputum may be visible in the mouth and throat. The patient may cough in an attempt to clear the airway. The patient's voice may be noticeably altered.
Palpation	Palpation produces tenderness. Crepitus is present. Displacement of the cartilage or fracture of the hyoid bone may be felt.
Selective Tissue Tests	Not applicable
Neurological Screening	Not applicable
Vascular Screening	Not applicable
Imaging Techniques	CT, MR, and ultrasonic images may be obtained.
Differential Diagnosis	Fractured larynx, contusion
Comments	Absence of breathing requires activation of the emergency action system. Immediate referral to a physician is indicated. Ice packs may be applied to control the swelling, but care must be taken not to compress the traumatized tissues. The vital signs require continuous monitoring.

CT = computed tomography, MR = magnetic resonance

malocclusion of the jaw and teeth, a finding that warrants referral to a physician (Examination Findings 19-5). The **tongue blade test** may be used to reinforce the suspicion of a mandibular fracture (Selective Tissue Test 19-2).

Zygoma Fractures

Direct blows to the cheek and inferior periorbital area may result in a fracture of the zygoma, especially at the arch. Examination findings reveal pain, discoloration, and possible depression of the zygomatic arch at the site of injury. Displaced fractures may result in malalignment of the eyes. Attempted eye movements may increase the pain or be performed with difficulty. Subconjunctival hematoma and periorbital swelling may be noted. Pain is elicited with palpation along the zygomatic arch and the lateral rim of the orbit. Occasionally, a step-off deformity is noted during palpation of the fracture site.[27] Definitive diagnosis of a zygomatic fracture is based on the findings of CT scans.

Maxillary Fractures

Fractures of the maxillae tend to occur concurrently with nasal fractures. Pain is described through the midportion of the face. Deformity found on inspection is rare, but ecchymosis and swelling along the alveolar processes are common. Crepitus may be elicited at the fracture site.

LeFort Fractures

The LeFort system is used to classify midface fractures. Because these fractures are normally the result of extremely high-impact forces (e.g., automobile accidents), their incidence in athletes is unusual. Figure 19-21 presents the LeFort classification system and identifies the bony segments

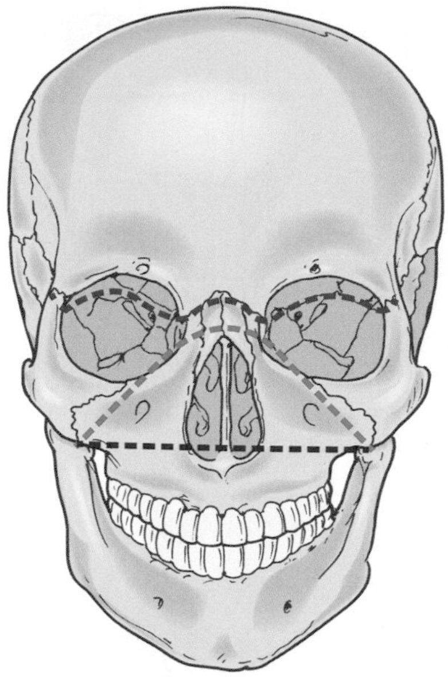

FIGURE 19-21 ■ Classification of LeFort fractures. Type I fractures involve only the maxillary bone; type II extend up into the nasal bone; type III cross the zygomatic bones and the orbit.

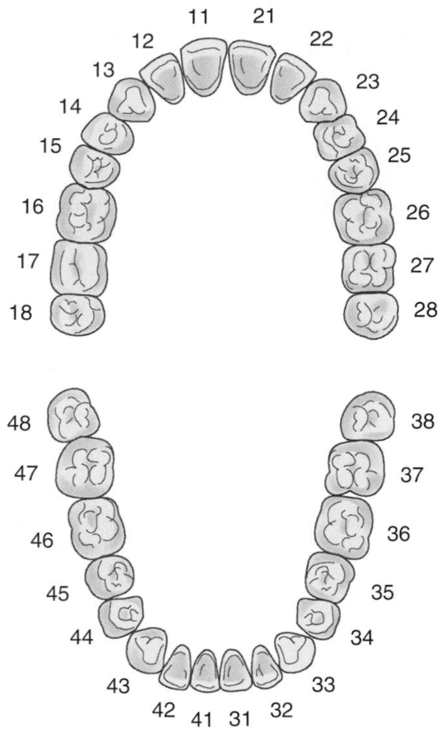

FIGURE 19-22 ■ Numbering system for referencing the teeth. The upper right teeth are numbered by 10s, the upper left by 20s, the lower left by 30s, and the lower right by 40s.

involved. This type of fracture is so extensive that, when the upper teeth are pulled forward, the fractured segment and the associated portion of the face are also displaced forward, roughly resembling the anterior drawer test in the knee. Sinus fluid may also be observed running from the nose. The tongue blade test may also be positive (see Selective Tissue Test 19-2).[29]

Facial Fracture Intervention Strategies

See On-Field Management of Facial Fractures.

Dental Conditions

Oral injury rates have been determined for both female and male intercollegiate athletes.[30,31] In female athletes, the injury rate ranges from 1.5% in softball players to 7.5% in basketball players; soccer, field hockey, and lacrosse players also have high rates. The highest oral injury rates for male athletes occur in basketball players, followed by ice hockey, lacrosse, football, soccer, baseball, and volleyball players.

The preparticipation physical examination questionnaire should ascertain the presence of dental appliances such as crowns, caps, or implants. This dental work must be evaluated for loosening, fracture, or luxation along with the natural dental structures. The numeric system used by dentists in referencing the teeth is presented in Figure 19-22. With all dental injuries, the examiner must establish the presence of a suitable airway, rule out the presence of head injury, and evaluate and manage concurrent lacerations.

Patients with oral injuries must be carefully evaluated to ensure prompt management to limit physical deformity and disability. The time and mechanism of injury define the risk of associated injuries and influence the treatment.[7]

Tooth Fractures

Tooth fractures, ranging from simple chips of the crown to full avulsions of the crown from its roots, are classified on a scale of I to IV (Fig. 19-23). Class I injuries, chip fractures, may be subtly noticed during eating, drinking, talking, or other activity in which the tongue is scraped across the teeth. These injuries may be self-evaluated when the patient looks in a mirror. Class II, III, and IV fractures are more easily recognized secondary to pain, sensitivity to extreme temperatures of food or drink, or obvious deformity. The degree of sensitivity depends on the extent of the fracture. Fractures into the enamel are usually minor irritations, but dental referral can be delayed.[7] Fractures involving the dentin and the pulp cavity are painful and sensitive to hot and cold temperatures. Fracture of the tooth's root generally requires radiographic identification.[7]

Tooth Luxations

A tooth luxation ranges from a tooth's being avulsed from the socket to its being driven into the bone (Fig. 19-24). A subtle tooth dislocation, one that is loosened in its socket, is not always visibly recognized. It may be discovered while the patient is chewing or applying pressure on it with the tongue. An **intruded tooth** is marked by its depression into the alveolar process relative to the contiguous teeth and to its match on the opposite side. An **extruded tooth** is partially withdrawn from the bone and may be tilted anteriorly

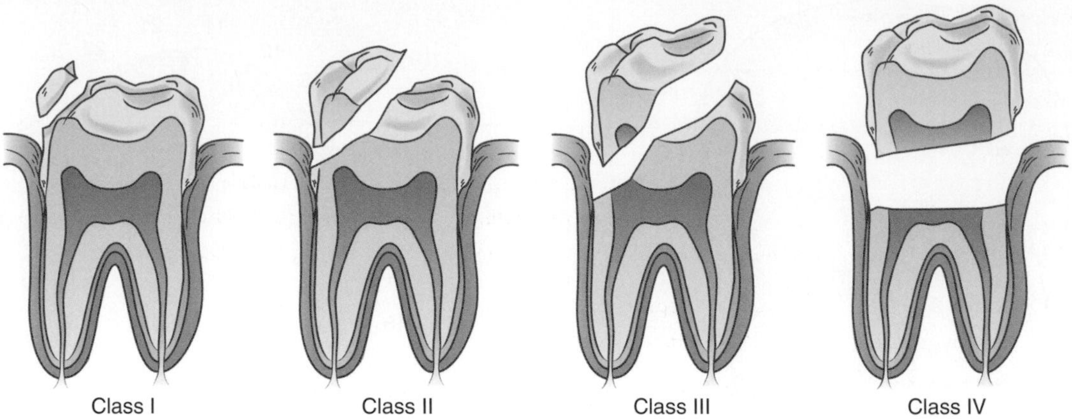

FIGURE 19-23 ■ Classification scheme for tooth fractures.

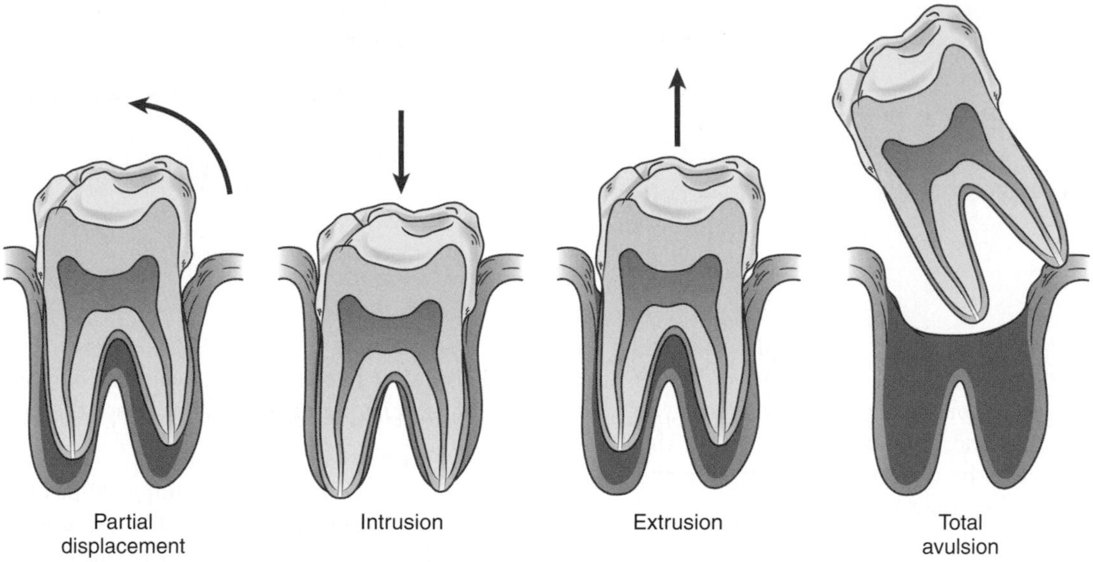

FIGURE 19-24 ■ Classification scheme for tooth luxations.

or posteriorly or may be twisted. A **tooth avulsion** is marked by the intact tooth's being displaced from the alveolar process and may represent a medical emergency.[7]

Fracture of the tooth's root can also result in luxation (Fig. 19-25). A fracture of the cervical third of the tooth may be repaired or permanently secured using dental hardware. Fractures to the middle third typically result in the loss of the tooth. The best prognosis occurs when the fracture occurs in the apical third (root) because the tooth is not greatly displaced in its socket.

The teeth can be evaluated for loosening through gentle palpation. If uncertainty exists as to whether a tooth has

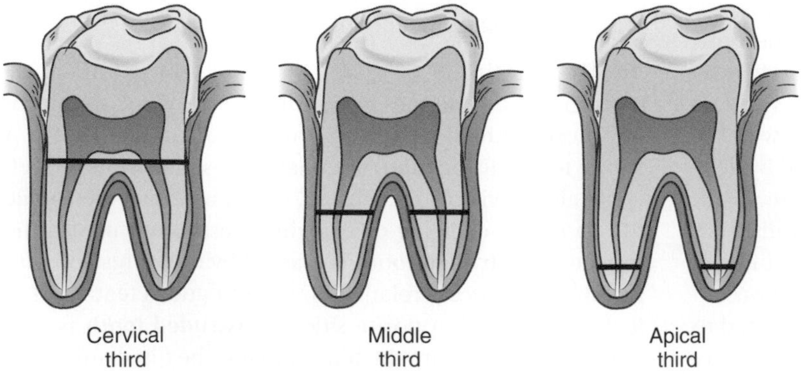

FIGURE 19-25 ■ Classification scheme for root fractures.

Examination Findings 19-5
Mandibular Fracture

Examination Segment	Clinical Findings
History of Current Condition	*Onset:* Acute *Pain characteristics:* Ramus or mental protuberance of mandible *Other symptoms:* Condylar fractures may cause headache, tinnitus, and/or balance disruptions.[28] *Mechanism:* Direct blow to the mandible on its anterior or lateral aspects
Functional Assessment	Difficulty opening and closing the mouth Chewing food is limited by pain.
Inspection	Swelling or gross deformity may be seen over the fracture site. A step deformity between the teeth may be noted on the involved side. Malocclusion of the teeth may be noted or described by the patient. Intraoral and extraoral ecchymosis may be noted.
Palpation	Tenderness, crepitus, or bony deformity is present over the fracture site.
Joint and Muscle Function Assessment	*AROM:* Pain is experienced when opening and closing the mouth, or this motion is prohibited secondary to pain. The mandible may track laterally or asymmetrically. *MMT:* See selective tissue tests. *PROM:* Not applicable
Joint Stability Tests	*Stress tests:* Not applicable *Joint play:* Not applicable
Selective Tissue Tests	Tongue blade test
Neurological Screening	Cranial nerves V or VII (or both) may be traumatized by the fracture (see Chapter 20).
Vascular Screening	Not applicable
Imaging Techniques	AP radiographs and/or CT scans are used to identify the presence and shape of fracture lines.
Differential Diagnosis	TMJ sprain, TMJ dislocation
Comments	Mandibular fractures may also be accompanied by a TMJ dislocation. Persons suspected of suffering a mandibular fracture or dislocation should be referred to a physician for further evaluation and treatment.

AP = anteroposterior; AROM = active range of motion; CT = computed tomography; MMT = manual muscle test; PROM = passive range of motion; TMJ = temporomandibular joint

Selective Tissue Tests 19-2
Tongue Blade Test

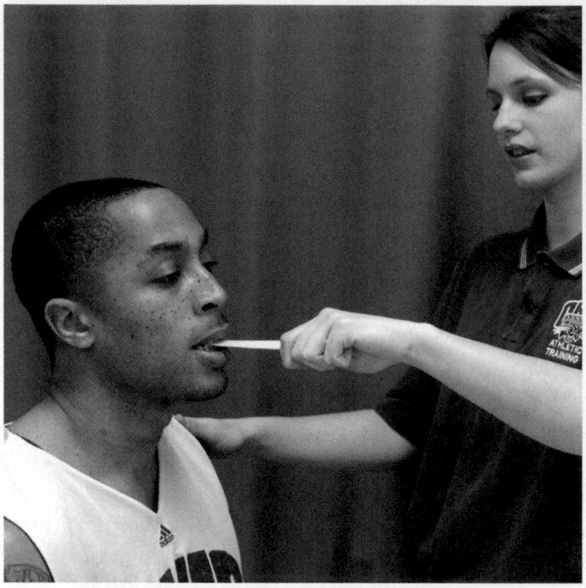

In the presence of a fractured mandible, the patient will not be able to bite down hard on the tongue depressor. This test should not be performed if a mandibular fracture is otherwise evident.

Patient Position	Seated
Position of Examiner	Standing in front of the patient
Evaluative Procedure	A tongue depressor is placed in the patient's mouth. As the patient attempts to hold the tongue blade in place, the examiner rotates (twists) the blade.
Positive Test	The patient is unable to maintain a firm bite or pain is elicited.
Implications	Possible mandibular fracture A positive test may also be indicative of a LeFort or maxillary sinus fracture.
Evidence	

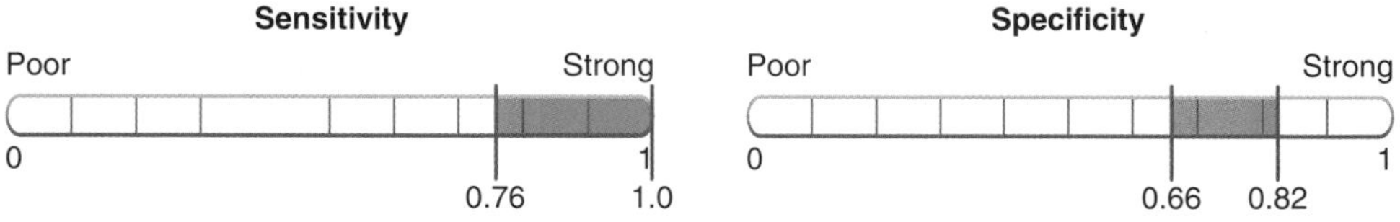

Sensitivity: Low = 759 High = 1.0

Specificity: Low 0.664 to High = 0.82

been partially dislodged, the patient may be given a mirror to conduct a self-assessment. A loose tooth should be left in place so that it can be properly managed by a dentist.

In the event of an avulsed tooth, the patient is keenly aware of the injury, and concomitant injuries, such as a mandible fracture, should be suspected. Other types of tooth luxations result in pain, bleeding from the socket, and temperature hypersensitivity. After the condition is recognized, the patient must be properly managed to maximize the potential of saving the tooth.

Dental Injury Intervention Strategies

Management of the luxated tooth is found in the "On-Field Evaluation and Management of Injuries to the Face and Related Areas" section of this chapter.

Temporomandibular Joint Dysfunction

Temporomandibular joint (TMJ) dysfunction is a broad term that encompasses pain, decreased range of motion, audible noises, and pain when opening and closing the mouth. Although TMJ dysfunction often has an insidious onset, a prior history of injury to the TMJ including sprains, cartilage tears, subluxations, or dislocations may be identified.

Acutely, the TMJ is usually injured when a blow is received on the point of the chin or across the jaw. The initial complaint is jaw pain and possibly clicking at the joint. Muscle guarding of either a physical or psychological nature increases tension in the lateral pterygoid muscle, pulling the articular disk posteriorly and stretching the joint capsule and its ligaments. TMJ derangements are classified as reducing or nonreducing.[3] Reducing derangements are characterized by "clicking" or "clunking" that represents the subluxation and reduction of the disk, usually at the midpoint of the ROM. Nonreducing derangements are characterized by the joint freezing and represent a torn portion of the disk presenting a mechanical block to motion. The nonreducing type often requires surgical correction. Intracapsular bleeding can result in joint ankylosis.[32]

On inspection, the mouth may open and close in an asymmetrical fashion, causing the lower jaw to deviate in one direction. The jaw may meet a mechanical block that limits the ROM. Palpation of the TMJ reveals localized tenderness and possibly crepitus or clicking at the joint. A stethoscope should be used to auscultate the TMJ during active ROM. Complaints of—or the presence of—audible crepitus alone are not indicative of TMJ dysfunction; these symptoms must be associated with other signs and symptoms of TMJ dysfunction (Examination Findings 19-6). Secondary symptoms including headache, earache, and dizziness may also be reported.[33]

Temporomandibular Joint Dysfunction Intervention Strategies

Interventions for TMJ dysfunction cover the spectrum from simple behavioral modifications, such as eating only soft food, to joint replacement.[34] Over-the-counter anti-inflammatory medications, moist heat, and focusing on normal biomechanics are common conservative clinical approaches to reduce the symptoms of TMJ dysfunction. Injected or oral corticosteroids may also be prescribed. Fluid around the joint may be aspirated (arthrocentesis). Mouthguard-type splints have proven to be useful in some cases.[35] Chronic or unrelenting cases may require surgical correction.[36]

Temporomandibular Joint Dislocation

Dislocations often result in an observable displacement of the mandible. However, subtle subluxations that spontaneously reduce may be less evident (Fig. 19-26). The mechanism of injury is a blow of sufficient force to move the mandible laterally, such as being punched. The rotation of the mandible causes the joint opposite the direction of displacement to anteriorly dislocate. The upper and lower teeth are malaligned, and movement of the jaw may be significantly impaired.

Blows to the point of the mandible, driving the bone toward the skull, may result in a fracture along the mandibular ramus or, on rare occasion, the temporal bone. Similar to TMJ dislocations, mandibular fractures result in malocclusion of the teeth, crepitus and deformity over the fracture site, and the inability to normally open and close the mouth.

Temporomandibular Joint Dislocation Intervention Strategies

See On-Field Management of Temporomandibular Joint Injuries.

On-Field Examination and Management of Injuries to the Face and Related Areas

The proximity of the maxillofacial area to the airway means that the presence of an unencumbered airway must be established. The athlete may concurrently sustain a laceration and injury to the maxillofacial structures. After establishing the presence of an airway, the responder must control bleeding before proceeding with a complete on-field examination.[37]

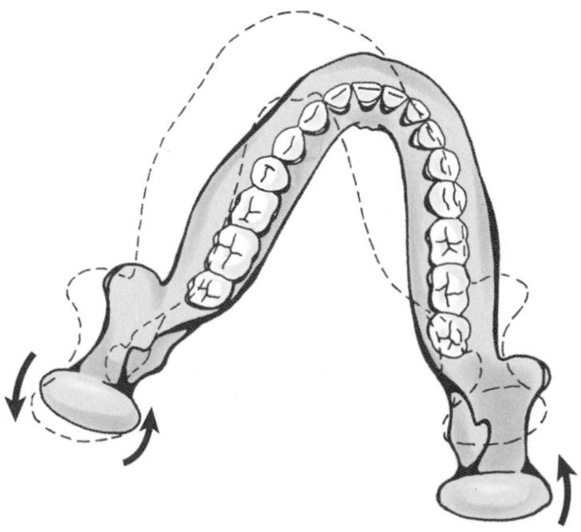

FIGURE 19-26 ■ Malocclusion of the jaw following a mandibular dislocation. Correlate this illustration with Figure 19-18B.

Examination Findings 19-6
Temporomandibular Joint Dysfunction

Examination Segment	Clinical Findings
History of Current Condition	*Onset:* Acute, insidious, or chronic *Pain characteristics:* Area of the TMJ *Other symptoms:* Clicking or locking of the joint Headache, earache, and dizziness may also be reported. *Mechanism:* Trauma to the mandible or progressive joint degeneration *Risk factors:* Laxity, disk degeneration, bruxing arthritis, missing or malaligned teeth, emotional stress
Functional Assessment	Observe the jaw for true inferior and superior movement as the mouth is opened or closed.
Inspection	Inspection of the joint may be unremarkable. Swelling may be located over the joint. Malocclusion of the jaw may be noted.
Palpation	Tenderness exists over the joint surfaces. Palpation of the external and internal structures may reveal clicking as the mouth is opened and closed.
Joint and Muscle Function Assessment	*AROM:* Active range of motion may be decreased secondary to pain or mechanical blockage of the TMJ. Any lateral deviation in the motion indicates joint pathology. *MMT:* Clenching the teeth may cause pain. *PROM:* Not applicable
Joint Stability Tests	*Stress tests:* Not applicable *Joint play:* Not applicable
Selective Tissue Tests	None
Neurological Screening	Not applicable; however, TMJ dysfunction has been implicated as a cause of headaches.
Vascular Screening	Within normal limits
Imaging Techniques	CT and MR images are obtained to identify joint structure and possible disk pathology.
Differential Diagnosis	Mandibular fracture
Comments	Individuals suffering from persistent TMJ pain should be referred to a physician or dentist for further evaluation. Instruct the patient not to eat hard foods (e.g., apples) that would cause pain during biting.

AROM = active range of motion; CT = computed tomography; MMT = manual muscle test; MR = magnetic resonance; PROM = passive range of motion; TMJ = temporomandibular joint

As with all open wounds, standard precautions for bloodborne pathogens must be implemented.

Lacerations

Lacerations may mask underlying injuries. After the bleeding is controlled, the area around the laceration is palpated for tenderness, with the examiner being careful to delineate between tenderness from the insulting blow that caused the injury and any fractures that may have occurred.

The presence of any foreign particles or objects within the laceration must be determined before beginning any subsequent treatment. An imbedded object must be left in place. The surrounding area can be cleaned and dressed until the object can be removed and the wound further managed by a physician.

Next, the extent of the wound must be determined. As a general rule, any facial laceration requires a referral to a physician for possible suturing or gluing to limit the extent and visibility of any scars. The sooner the referral occurs, the better it is, but the physician should see the patient within 24 hours after the injury.[27] If the bleeding can be controlled and the wound closed and dressed with a sterile bandage, the athlete may return to competition. The bandage covering the wound must be sufficient to protect other competitors from contact with the athlete's blood.

In the case of lacerations of the throat, the athlete is assessed for difficulty with breathing and transported by trained personnel who can aid the athlete on the way to the hospital. If the laceration avulses a piece of the ear, nose, or tongue, the avulsed tissue is cleaned with sterile water, wrapped in sterile gauze, put on ice, and transported with the athlete to the medical facility for possible reattachment. Microsurgical techniques may be able to salvage these parts, giving the athlete a better cosmetic repair and normal function.

Laryngeal Injuries

Laryngeal injuries present a difficult decision for the examiner because of their potential to become life threatening. Early signs of potentially catastrophic injury include progressive swelling (indicating bleeding), crepitation (indicating the presence of subcutaneous air), audible **stridor** (indicating a narrowing of the airway), and bleeding from the oral cavity.

The decision must be made to move the athlete to the sidelines before transport or to transport the athlete directly from the field. In cases in which the athlete has trouble breathing, it is prudent to stabilize and transport the athlete to a hospital using emergency medical personnel capable of managing an obstructed airway. The athlete may first be moved to the sidelines if no signs of breathing difficulty are noted. Ice may be applied to the anterior throat, but care must be taken not to compress the underlying structures. The pressure applied could be enough to displace the injured area, causing obstruction of the airway.

Stridor A harsh, high-pitched sound resembling blowing wind that is experienced during respiration

Facial Fractures

The forces required to fracture the facial bones (i.e., the zygoma, frontal, maxillary, and mandible bones) are usually of considerable magnitude. The athlete is not only "down" from the injury but may also be stunned or rendered unconscious by head injury from the incident. In this case, the examination and on-field management of the head injury take precedence (see Chapter 20).

LeFort fractures and other fractures around the nose and mouth can compromise the airway. In this case, maintaining an open airway is the highest treatment priority.[30] Athletes suffering stable facial fractures that do not jeopardize the airway can be carefully moved to the sidelines. If the athlete has an obvious fracture, movement of the athlete's head and neck is restricted. As long as it does not increase the athlete's discomfort, a Philadelphia collar can be used to stabilize the jaw and prevent unwanted motion while the athlete is transported to a medical facility (Fig. 19-27). Surgical correction involving open reduction and internal fixation techniques is commonly used.[38]

Temporomandibular Joint Injuries

A blow to the jaw may injure both the TMJ and the mandible. If a fracture of the mandible is unlikely, the athlete can be carefully assisted to the sidelines for a full assessment of the TMJ. Injuries that produce malocclusion warrant the immediate removal of the athlete from participation and referral

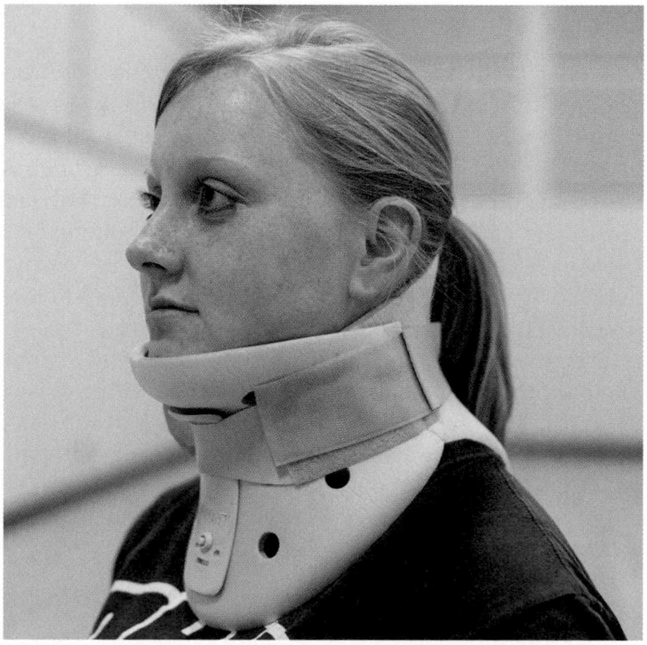

FIGURE 19-27 ■ Use of a Philadelphia collar for immobilizing a suspected mandibular fracture. Avoid applying too much pressure to the fracture site.

to a physician or dentist. If the TMJ is dislocated, the athlete can be immobilized with a Philadelphia collar as long as it does not create further pain. This athlete also requires a referral for immediate treatment.

Nasal Fracture and Epistaxis

Nasal fractures are usually accompanied by epistaxis, which must be controlled before further evaluation or management of the injury occurs. Palpate the nose, nasal cartilage, and adjacent maxillary, zygomatic, and frontal bones for tenderness and crepitus. If the nose is obviously deformed, the athlete is discouraged from viewing the injury in a mirror or physically touching the deformity because doing so may increase his or her anxiety or cause the onset of shock. Suspected nasal fractures may be packed with a small bag of ice to assist in controlling pain and limiting the amount of bleeding until the athlete can see a physician. Reduction of displaced fractures should be made 5 to 10 days after injury.[5]

Nasal Fracture and Epistaxis Intervention Strategies

Although squeezing the nostrils and tilting the head forward is an adequate form of management for nasal bleeding, this method may be prohibited secondary to pain arising from the fracture. Applying a cold pack to the nose and surrounding area also may stop the bleeding. The nose may be packed with rolled gauze or a tampon that has been cut into quarters. (These should be precut and kept in the medical kit.) Another technique to control bleeding involves placing a rolled cotton gauze pad between the anterior upper lip and gum. The pressure from the lip required to hold the gauze in place also applies pressure on the arteries that supply the anterior nasal mucosa, potentially stopping bleeding.

Dental Injuries

An athlete suffering tooth trauma usually reports to the sidelines for evaluation. Usually a fractured tooth is not a cause of immediate danger to the athlete unless the remaining portion is loose (Fig. 19-28). If no loosening has occurred and other concomitant injuries have been ruled out, the athlete can return to activity wearing a mouthguard. However, examination by a dentist must occur as soon as possible. The athlete should expect extreme discomfort, especially if the fracture penetrates the pulp cavity.

Every reasonable attempt must be made to find a tooth that has been luxated. The primary problem leading to failure of the tooth to survive involves the death of the periodontal ligament attached to the avulsed tooth. All treatment must focus on the survival of this ligament. To improve the tooth's chances of survival, the emergency procedures listed in Table 19-3 are recommended.[30,31]

*** Practical Evidence**

With proper care, the vast majority of all avulsed teeth can be permanently reimplanted.[30,31]

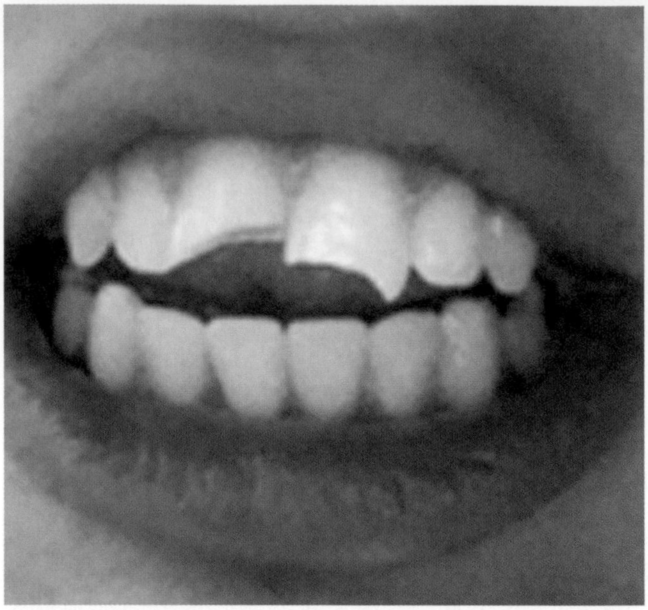

FIGURE 19-28 ■ A Class III fracture of the right central incisor and a Class II fracture of the left central incisor caused by direct impact from a blunt object.

Table 19-3 Emergency Management of Dental Injuries
• Before reimplanting an avulsed tooth, rinse it with water or saline solution. Allow the coherent athlete to hold the tooth in its socket by biting on gauze. Make sure that the tooth is reimplanted in its proper orientation.
• If the tooth is not reimplanted immediately, store it in a secure biocompatible storage environment such as an emergency tooth-preserving system or in fresh whole milk in a plastic container with a tightly fitting lid. Do not store it in water.[39]
• Do not attempt to clean, sterilize, or scrape the tooth in any way other than as noted above.
• Do not hold the tooth by the root.[30]
• A replanted or loose tooth can be immobilized using aluminium foil.[30]
• Transport the athlete and the tooth to a dentist as quickly as possible.

Current recommendations support the immediate reimplantation of an avulsed tooth.[39] If the tooth is visibly contaminated, wash it using cool tap water before reimplantation.

REFERENCES

1. Schiffman, E, et al: Diagnostic criteria for headache attributed to temporomandibular disorders. *Cephalalgia*, 32:683, 2012.
2. Walczyńska-Dragon, K, and Baron, S: The biomechanical and functional relationship between temporomandibular dysfunction and cervical spine pain. *Acta Bioeng Biomech*, 13:93, 2011.
3. Leader, JK, et al: Mandibular kinematics represented by a non-orthogonal floating axis coordinate system. *J Biomech*, 36:275, 2003.
4. Puzas, JE, et al: Degradative pathways in tissues of the temporomandibular joint: use of in vitro and in vivo models to characterize matrix metalloproteinase and cytokine activity. *Cells Tissues Organs*, 169:248, 2001.

5. Kucik, CJ, Clenney, T, and Phelan J: Management of acute nasal fractures. *Am Fam Physician*, 70:1315, 2004.
6. Labuguen, RH: Initial evaluation of vertigo. *Am Fam Physician*, 73:244, 2006.
7. Douglass, AB, and Douglass, JM: Common dental emergencies. *Am Fam Physician*, 67:511, 2003.
8. Guler, N, et al: Temporomandibular internal derangement: correlation of MRI findings with clinical symptoms of pain and joint sounds in patients with bruxing behavior. *Dentomaxillofac Radiol*, 32:304, 2003.
9. Supriya, M, et al: Epistaxis: prospective evaluation of bleeding site and its impact on patient outcome. *J Laryngol Otol*, 124:744, 2010.
10. Terakura, M, et al: Relationship between blood pressure and persistent epistaxis at the emergency department: a retrospective study. *J Am Soc Hypertens*, 6:291, 2012.
11. Juutilainen, M, et al: Laryngeal fractures: clinical findings and considerations on suboptimal outcome. *Acta Otolaryngol*, 128:213, 2008.
12. Beachy, G: Dental injuries in intermediate and high school athletes: a 15-year study at Punahou School. *J Athl Train*, 39:310, 2004.
13. Zhang, S, et al: Magnetic resonance imaging in the diagnosis of intra-articular adhesions of the temporomandibular joint. *Br J Oral Maxillofac Surg*, 47:389, 2009.
14. DePalma, AC: Clinical assessment of temporomandibular joint disorders. *J Pract Hyg*, 14:16, 2005.
15. Ghanem, T, Rasamny, JK, and Park, SS: Rethinking auricular trauma. *Laryngoscope*, 115:1251, 2005.
16. Roy S, Smith JP: A novel technique for treating auricular hematomas in mixed martial artists (ultimate fighters). *Am J Otolaryngol*, 31:21, 2010.
17. Yotsuyanagi, T, et al: Surgical correction of cauliflower ear. *Br J Plast Surg*, 55:380, 2002.
18. Jones, SEM, and Mahendran, S: Interventions for acute auricular haematoma. *Cochrane Database of Syst Rev*, 2:CD004166, 2004.
19. Plafki, C, et al: Complications and side effects of hyperbaric oxygen therapy. *Aviat Space Environ Med*, 71:119, 2000.
20. Baum, JD, et al: Clinical presentation and conservative management of tympanic membrane perforation during intrapartum Valsalva maneuver. *Case Report Med*, 2010:856045, 2010.
21. Gladstone, HB, Jackler, RK, and Varav, K: Tympanic membrane wound healing: an overview. *Otolarynol Clin North Am*, 28:913, 1995.
22. Wang, M, et al: Ear problems in swimmers. *J Chin Med Assoc*, 68:347, 2005.
23. Ramakrishnan, K, Sparks, RA, and Berryhill, WE: Diagnosis and treatment of otitis media. *Am Fam Physician*, 76:1650, 2007.
24. Mondin, V, Rinaldo, A, Ferlito, A: Management of nasal bone fractures. *Am J Otolaryngol*, 26:181, 2005.
25. Kucik, CJ, Clenney, T, and Phelan, J: Management of acute nasal fractures. *Am Fam Physician*, 70:1315, 2004.
26. Hwang, K, et al: Analysis of nasal bone fractures: a six-year study of 503 patients. *J Craniofac Surg*, 17:261, 2006.
27. Antoun, JS, and Lee, KH: Sports-related maxillofacial fractures over an 11-year period. *J Oral Maxillofac Surg*, 66:504, 2008.
28. Faralli, MM, et al: Correlations between posturographic findings and symptoms in subjects with fractures of the condylar head of the mandible. *Eur Arch Otorhinolaryngol*, 266:565, 2009.
29. Haydel, MJ, Meyers, R, and Mills, L: Use of the tongue-blade test to identify patients with mandible and maxillary sinus fractures. *Ann Emerg Med*, 46:S66, 2005.
30. Emerich, K, and Kaczmarek, J: First aid for dental trauma caused by sports activities: state of knowledge, treatment and prevention. *Sports Med*, 40:361, 2010.
31. American Academy of Pediatric Dentistry. Guideline on management of acute dental trauma. 2010. Retrieved from www.aapd.org/assets/1/7/G_Trauma.pdf#xml=http://pr-dtsearch001.americaneagle.com/service/search.asp?cmd=pdfhits&DocId=566&Index=F%3a%5cdtSearch%5caapd&HitCount=7&hits=267+268+269+26a+26b+26c+26d+&hc=42&req=%22Guideline+on+Management+of+Acute+Dental+Trauma%22. (Accessed February 4, 2013).
32. Muhtar_gullari, M, Demiralp, B, and Ertan, A: Non-surgical treatment of sports-related temporomandibular joint disorders in basketball players. *Dent Traumatol*, 20:338, 2004.
33. Schmitter, M, et al: Validity of temporomandibular disorder examination procedures for assessment of temporomandibular joint status. *Am J Orthod Dentofacial Orthop*, 133:796, 2008.
34. Brennan, PA, and Ilankovan, V: Arthrocentesis for temporomandibular joint pain dysfunction syndrome. *J Oral Maxillofac Surg*, 64:949, 2006.
35. Gahanem, WA: Arthrocentesis and stabilizing splint are the treatment of choice for acute intermittent closed lock in patients with bruxism. *J Craciomaxillofac Surg*, 39:256, 2011.
36. Güven, O: Management of chronic recurrent temporomandibular joint dislocations: a retrospective study. *J Craciomaxillofac Surg*, 37:24, 2008.
37. Mihalik, JP, et al: Maxillofacial fractures and dental trauma in a high school soccer goalkeeper: a case report. *J Athl Train*, 40:116, 2005.
38. Seemann, R, et al: Complication rates in the operative treatment of mandibular angle fractures: a 10-year retrospective. *J Oral Maxillofac Surg*, 68:647, 2010.
39. Flores, MT, et al: Guidelines for the management of traumatic dental injuries. II. avulsion of permanent teeth. *Dent Traumatol*, 23:130, 2007.

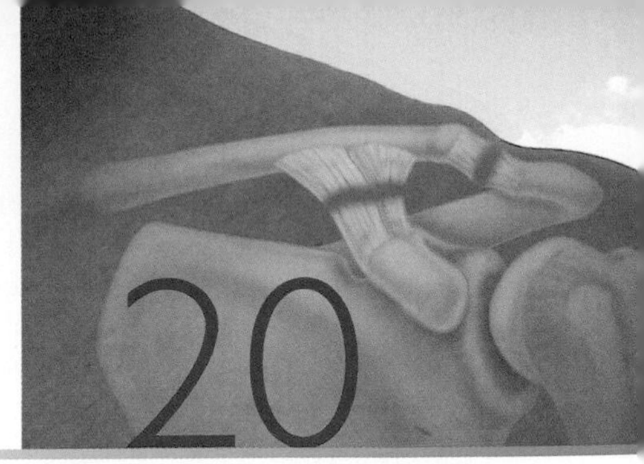

CHAPTER 20

Head and Acute Cervical Spine Pathologies

The potential for catastrophic head or cervical spine injuries and their life-ending or altering consequences necessitates development of a clear plan for evaluation and management. Fortunately, the overall rate of injury to these body areas is relatively low.[1] However, when it does occur, the outcomes can be fatal or result in long-term physical and/or mental deficits.[2]

Most often the result of direct contact with another player, head injuries occur more frequently in college athletics than in high school and tend to be more frequent in women's than in men's sports.[3] Sports in which blows to the head are commonplace—football, baseball, and ice hockey—have rules mandating the use of protective headgear. The use of helmets has greatly reduced the number and severity of head injuries in football, but various styles and brands have differing levels of effectiveness.[3–6]

Regular inspection of helmets is needed to ensure proper maintenance and continued protection. Athletes must be knowledgeable about the risks associated with participation in sports and be instructed in the proper techniques necessary to avoid serious head and cervical spine injuries.

This chapter focuses on the immediate and follow-up evaluation and management of athletes with head and cervical spine injuries. A well-organized procedure for the emergency management of head and cervical spine trauma is crucial to this process and must be rehearsed regularly by the medical staff to ensure appropriate care. Chapter 14 describes the anatomy of the cervical spine, examination of noncatastrophic cervical spine conditions, and injury to the brachial plexus.

Clinical Anatomy

With the exception the **foramen magnum**, a small opening on the skull's base through which the brainstem and spinal cord pass, the brain is almost fully encased in bone (Fig. 20-1). In adults, the cranial bones are rigidly fused by cranial sutures, making the skull a single structure. In infants and children, the sutures are more pliable because they are continually being remodeled during growth.

The skull's design allows for maximum protection of the brain. The density of the bone reduces the amount of physical shock transmitted inwardly. The rounded shape of the skull also has protective qualities. When an object strikes a rounded object, it tends to be deflected quickly. Consider, for example, two scenarios: dropping a brick on a tabletop and dropping a brick on a basketball. When the brick hits the tabletop, it stays there, transmitting its force into the table. When a brick is dropped onto a basketball, although some of the force is transmitted into the ball, the remaining force is dissipated as the brick deflects off the round surface. Suspended within cerebrospinal fluid, the brain floats within the cranium. The fluid suspension decreases the

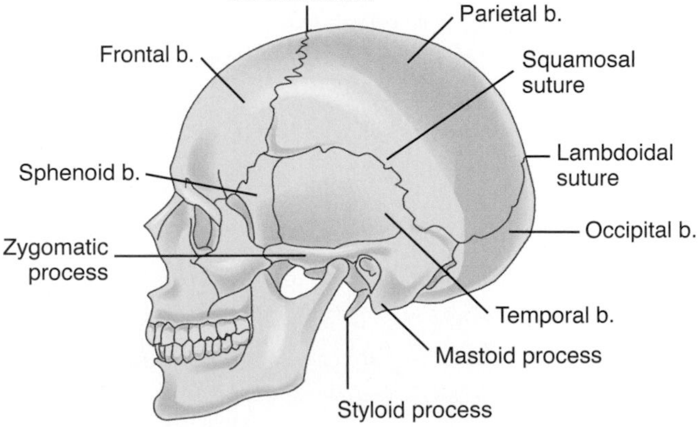

FIGURE 20-1 ■ Lateral view of the bones of the skull.

mechanical forces transmitted to the brain. Lastly, the skin covering the skull increases the cranium's ability to protect the brain by absorbing and redirecting forces from the skull. The skin greatly increases the skull's strength, increasing its breaking force from 40 pounds per square inch to 420 to 490 pounds per square inch.[7]

The Brain

The brain is the most complex and least understood part of the human body. Its anatomy and function are presented in this chapter only as they relate to athletic injuries. Table 20-1 presents an overview of the major brain areas and their primary functions.

The Cerebrum

The largest section of the brain, the cerebrum is composed of two **hemispheres** separated by the **longitudinal fissure**. Each hemisphere is divided into **frontal**, **parietal**, **temporal**, and occipital lobes, which are separated by sulci and fissures and are named for the overlying cranial bones (Fig. 20-2).

The cerebrum is responsible for controlling the body's primary **motor functions** and coordinates muscle contractions in a specific sequence. **Sensory information**, such as temperature, touch, pain, pressure, and proprioception, is processed in this region of the brain, along with the **special senses**: visual, auditory, olfactory, and taste. **Cognition**, including spatial relationships, behavior, memory, and association, also occurs in the cerebrum.

With a few exceptions, the cerebrum communicates contralaterally with the rest of the body. The right hemisphere controls the motor actions and interprets much of the sensory input of the body's left side, and vice versa. Clinically the same crossover occurs: motor impairment of the body's left side usually reflects damage to the brain's right hemisphere.

Table 20-1 Brain Function by Area

Area	Function
Cerebrum	Motor function Sensory information (e.g., touch, pain pressure, temperature) Special senses (vision, hearing, smell, taste) Cognition Memory
Cerebellum	Balance and coordination Smooth, synergistic muscle control
Diencephalon	**Thalamus** Routes afferent information to the appropriate cerebral areas Regulates consciousness, sleep, and alertness **Hypothalamus** Maintains the necessary water balance (via the posterior pituitary gland) Regulates the autonomic nervous system: Secretes neurohormones Regulates body temperature Regulates hunger, thirst, and sleep **Epithalamus** Secretes melatonin Regulates motor pathways Controls emotions (anger and fear)
Brainstem	Regulates heart rate Regulates respiratory rate Controls the amount of peripheral blood flow

The Cerebellum

Designed to allow the quick processing of both incoming and outgoing information, the cerebellum provides the functions necessary to maintain **balance and coordination**. Visual, tactile, auditory, and proprioceptive information from the cerebrum is routed to the cerebellum for immediate processing. The outgoing information is relayed to the muscles via the cerebrum and descending pathways to properly orchestrate the necessary movements.

Fluid, synergistic motions, whether performing a back flip in gymnastics or lifting a cup of coffee, are initiated and controlled by the cerebellum. Facilitative impulses are relayed from the cerebellum to the contracting muscles, and an inhibitory stimulus is sent to the antagonistic muscles. Individuals who have suffered trauma to the cerebellum are recognizable by their uncoordinated, segmental, robot-like movements. Cerebellar injuries are relatively rare in athletics. However, severe blows to the posterior aspect of the skull or acceleration and deceleration mechanisms that cause rotation of the brainstem can injure the cerebellum.

The Diencephalon

Formed by the **thalamus**, **hypothalamus**, and **epithalamus**, the **diencephalon** acts as a processing center for conscious and unconscious brain input. In its gatekeeping role, the thalamus monitors sensory information ascending the spinal cord, routing the specific types of information to the appropriate area of the brain. In addition to regulating some of the body's hormones, the hypothalamus is the center of the body's autonomic nervous system, regulating **sympathetic** and **parasympathetic nervous system** activity. Body temperature, water balance, gastrointestinal activity, hunger, and emotions are controlled by the hypothalamus.

The Brainstem

Formed by the **medulla oblongata** (medulla) and the pons, the brainstem serves to relay information to and from the central nervous system (CNS) and controls the involuntary systems. Literally translating as "bridge," the **pons** serves to

Sympathetic nervous system The part of the central nervous system that supplies the involuntary muscles

Parasympathetic nervous system A series of specific effects controlled by the brain regulating smooth muscle contractions, slowing the heart rate, and constricting the pupil

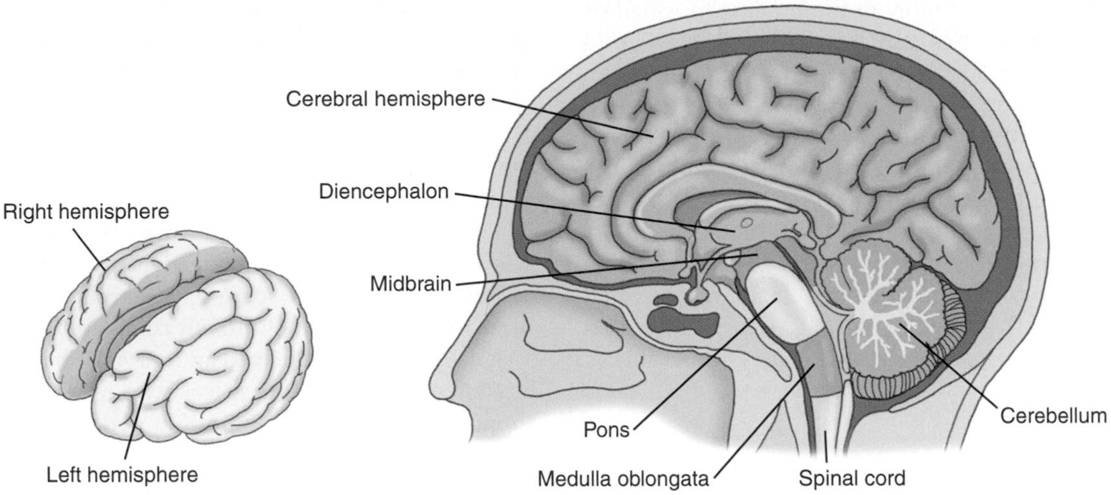

FIGURE 20-2 ■ Regions of the brain, with insert showing the cerebral hemispheres.

link the cerebellum to the brainstem and spinal cord, connecting the upper and lower portions of the CNS. In addition, receptors in the pons regulate the respiratory rate.

The medulla serves as the interface between the spinal cord and the rest of the brain. Involuntary functions of heart rate, respiration, blood vessel diameter (vasodilation and vasoconstriction), coughing, and vomiting are regulated by the **medullary centers**.

The Meninges

The brain and spinal cord are buffered from the bony surfaces of the cranium and spinal column by three meninges: the **dura mater**, **arachnoid mater**, and **pia mater**. The progressive densities of the meninges support and protect the brain and spinal cord. Arterial and venous blood supplies are provided through these structures, as are the production and introduction of the **cerebrospinal fluid** (CSF).

The Dura Mater

Literally translating as "hard mother," the dura mater is the outermost meningeal covering, also serving as the periosteum for the skull's inner layer. The **falx cerebri** is a fold in the dura mater in the longitudinal fissure between the two cerebral hemispheres. The void between the two cerebellar hemispheres is filled by another fold of the dura mater, the **falx cerebelli**.

Arteries in the dura mater, the **meningeal arteries**, primarily supply blood to the cranial bones. Blood supply to the dura mater is provided by fine branches from the meningeal arteries. At various points around the brain, the dura mater forms two layers. The space between these layers forms the **venous sinuses**, which serve as a drainage conduit to route deoxygenated blood into the internal jugular veins in the neck.

The Arachnoid Mater

The name "arachnoid" is gained from this structure's resemblance to a cobweb ("arachne" is the Greek word for "spider"). Similar to a cobweb, the fibers forming the arachnoid are thin yet relatively resilient to trauma. The arachnoid mater is separated from the dura mater by the narrow **subdural space**. Beneath the arachnoid is a wider separation, the **subarachnoid space**, containing the CSF.

The Pia Mater

The innermost meningeal membrane, the pia mater, envelops the brain, forming its outer "skin." This delicate membrane derives its name from the Latin word for "tender"; therefore, the pia mater is the "tender mother." The pia mater follows the brain's contour, intruding into its fissures and sulci.

Cerebrospinal Fluid

Originating from the **choroid plexuses** deep within the brain and secreted by cells surrounding the cerebrum's blood vessels, CSF slowly circulates around the brain and spinal cord within the subarachnoid space. From the lateral ventricles, CSF is forced into the third and fourth ventricles by a pressure gradient. After it is in the fourth ventricle, a small proportion of the CSF enters the central canal of the spinal cord. The remaining fluid flows down the spinal cord on its posterior surface and returns to the brain on the anterior portion of the subarachnoid space.

Because of the presence of the subarachnoid space and its watery content, the CNS floats within the body. This arrangement serves as another buffer against external forces being transmitted to the CNS. Although beneficial in dissipating the high-velocity impacts associated with collision sports, this protective configuration is most useful in buffering more repetitious forces, such as those seen when running.

Blood Circulation in the Brain

When the body is at rest, the brain demands 20% of the body's oxygen uptake. For each degree (centigrade) the body's core temperature increases, the brain's need for oxygen increases by 7%. Blood supply to the brain is provided by the two **vertebral arteries** and the two **common carotid arteries**. Each common carotid artery diverges to form an **internal carotid artery** and an **external carotid artery**. The external carotid arteries continue upward to supply blood to the head and neck, with the exception of the brain. The internal carotid arteries move toward the center of the cranium to assist in supplying the brain with blood.

The two internal carotid arteries and the two vertebral arteries converge to form a collateral circulation network, the **circle of Willis** (Fig. 20-3). If one of the cranial arteries is obstructed, the design of the circle of Willis permits at least a partial supply of blood to the affected area.

Examination Scenarios

Before discussing how to evaluate and manage athletes with head and cervical spine injuries, the possible scenarios under which an examination may have to be performed must be considered. The best-case scenario is one in which the athlete is conscious and responsive to stimuli. The worst-case scenario is that of a prone, unconscious athlete who is not breathing and has no pulse. In either case, the decisions made by the medical staff are critical in the optimal management of athletes with catastrophic conditions.

The basic premise of on-field management is: **All unconscious athletes must be managed as if a fracture or dislocation of the cervical spine exists until the presence of these injuries can be definitively ruled out.**

Ideally, athletes with head and cervical spine injuries are evaluated on the field by at least two responders. One responder must ensure stabilization and immobilization of the athlete's head and cervical spine by grasping the sides of the head or helmet and applying **in-line stabilization** on the cervical spine until significant pathology has been ruled out. A second responder performs the necessary palpation, sensory, and motor assessments (Fig. 20-4). One person

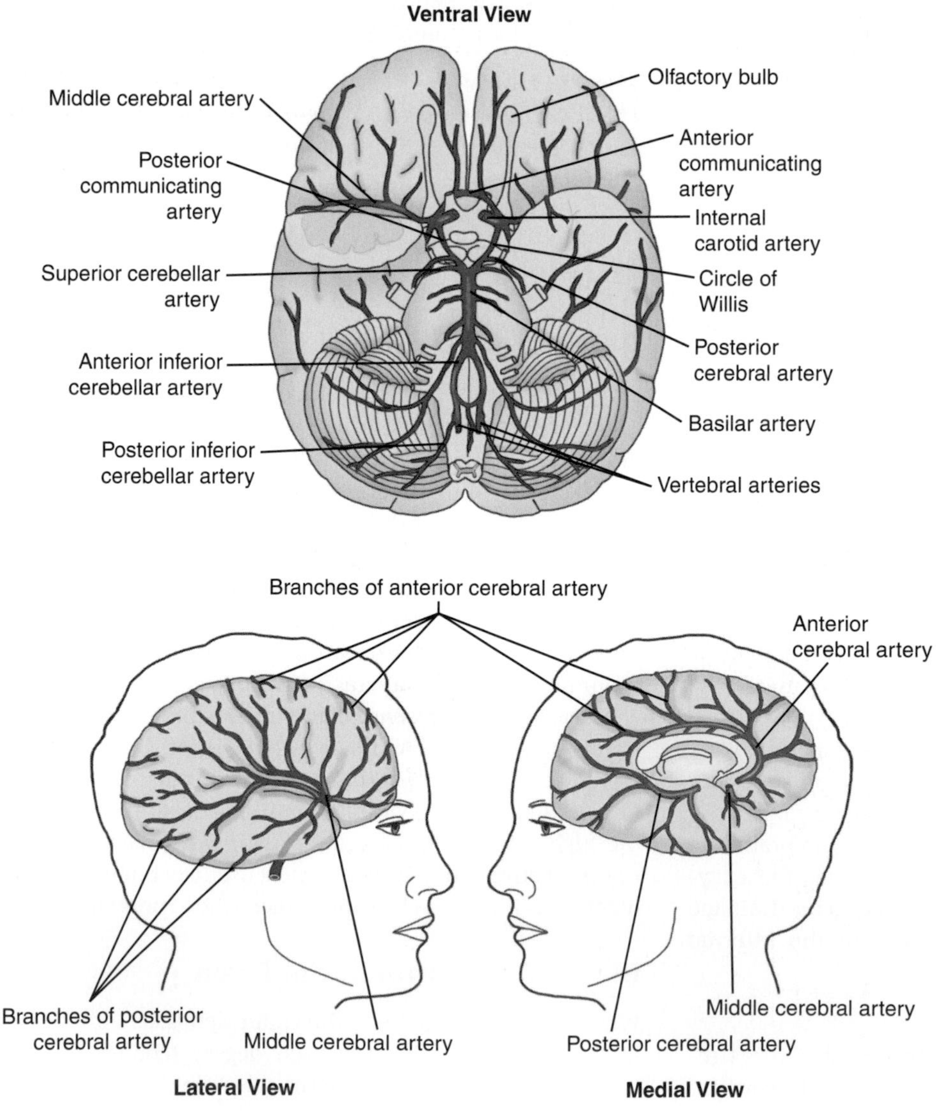

FIGURE 20-3 ■ Blood supply to the brain. The circle of Willis provides collateral circulation to the brain's regions.

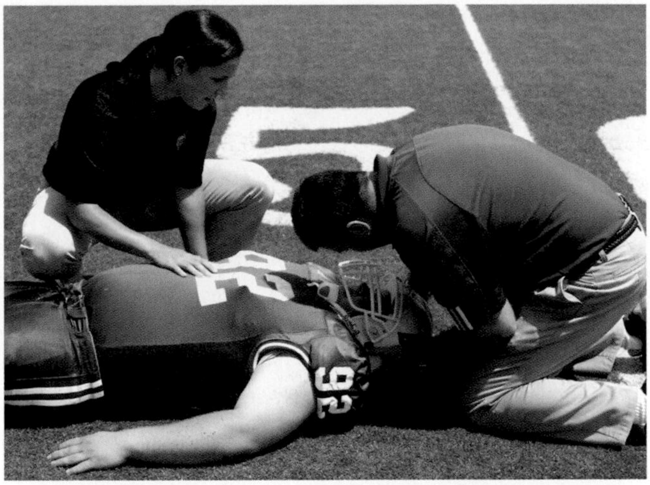

FIGURE 20-4 ■ Head and cervical spine trauma is best managed by two responders. One stabilizes the head while the second conducts the examination.

acts as the leader and directs the actions of all others at the injury scene. In situations in which only one responder is present, other on-site personnel may be directed to assist in the management of the athlete's condition. Prior discussion and practice are necessary to ensure orderly and precise action by the support staff.

Evaluation of the Athlete's Position

The initial assessment of an on-field head and cervical spine injury may be complicated further by the athlete's position. A supine athlete is in the optimal position for subsequent evaluation and management. When athletes are in the side-lying or prone position, the evaluation is more difficult.

If, as determined according to the assessments described in the next section, the athlete is conscious and vital signs are present, there is no need to move the athlete until a complete on-field evaluation is performed and the athlete's disposition is determined. However, when an athlete is prone or side-lying, the absence of vital signs takes precedence over the possibility of a spinal fracture. The athlete must be rolled into the supine position in the safest manner possible. These procedures are discussed in the On-Field Examination and Management of Head and Cervical Spine Injuries and the Unconscious Athlete section of this chapter.

Examination of Head Injuries

The ability to identify and properly manage patients with serious head and cervical spine injuries may affect whether the person lives, dies, or becomes permanently disabled. Although some signs and symptoms of brain trauma are blatantly obvious, such as unconsciousness, some potentially catastrophic head injuries initially have few, if any, outward

Examination Map

DETERMINATION OF CONSCIOUSNESS

Level of Consciousness
Primary Survey
Secondary Survey

HISTORY

Head pain
Mechanism of Injury
- **Coup**
- **Contrecoup**
- **Rotational**
- **Repeated subconcussive forces**

Loss of consciousness
History of concussion
Preexisting mood disorders
Emotional impairment
Weakness/fatigue
Cognitive impairment

INSPECTION

Inspection of the Bony Structures
- **Mastoid process**
- **Skull and scalp**

Inspection of the Eyes
- **General**
- **Nystagmus**
- **Pupil size**
- **Pupil reaction to light**

Inspection of the Nose and Ears
- **Fluid escaping**

PALPATION

Skull

FUNCTIONAL ASSESSMENT

Cranial Nerve Assessment

Neurocognitive Function
- **Behavior**
- **Analytical skills**
- **Information processing**
- **Memory**
- **SCAT3**

Balance and Coordination
- **Romberg test**
- **Tandem walking test**
- **Modified Balance Error Scoring System**

Vital Signs
- **Respiration**
- **Pulse**
- **Blood pressure**
- **Pulse pressure**

REGION-SPECIFIC PATHOLOGIES AND SELECTIVE TISSUE TESTS

Traumatic Brain Injury
- **Concussion**
- **Postconcussion Syndrome**
- **Diffuse Cerebral Swelling**
- **Intracranial Hemorrhage**
  - Epidural hematoma
  - Subdural hematoma

Skull Fractures
- Halo Test

signs or symptoms. This section describes the signs and symptoms of brain trauma. Acute cervical spine trauma and the on-field management of cervical spine-injured and unconscious athletes are covered in subsequent sections.

Determination of Consciousness

When an athlete is "down" on the field or court, the first priority is to establish the level of consciousness. A moving and speaking athlete demonstrates that the athlete's cardiovascular and respiratory systems are functioning. Even under these circumstances, a cervical fracture must be suspected, and the athlete's vital signs require regular monitoring.

- **Level of consciousness:** While moving toward the scene of the injury, note if the athlete is moving. At the scene, attempt to communicate with the athlete. If verbal communication fails, check the athlete's responsiveness to painful stimuli by applying pressure to the lumina of a fingernail or rubbing the sternum. Do not use ammonia inhalants because of the possibility of the athlete's jerking the head and cervical spine when awakening.
- **Primary survey:** If the athlete is unconscious or unable to communicate, check the athlete's cardiovascular and respiratory systems by looking, listening, and feeling for breathing (Fig. 20-5). The Emergency Action System should be activated if the athlete continues to remain unconscious. If the patient is not breathing, use a modified jaw thrust to open the airway. In the event that no carotid or radial pulse is found, initiate emergency cardiac procedures including automated external defibrillator (AED) use. The "On-Field Examination and Management of Head and Cervical Spine Injuries and the Unconscious Athlete" section of this chapter and Chapter 2 address further information on this topic.
- **Secondary survey:** Although the suspicion of cervical spine or brain trauma takes precedence, do not overlook the possibility of other trauma to the body. Inspect the extremities and torso for bleeding or indications of fractures or dislocations.

The examination of an individual with a head injury consists of assessing symptoms, a cognitive evaluation (including orientation, past and immediate memory, new learning and concentration), balance testing, and additional neurological examination.[8]

History

The history-taking process of an athlete with a head injury helps to identify the mechanism of injury, current symptoms, and underlying comorbidities that may impact the diagnostic and recovery process. Parts of this evaluation occur when the athlete is on the field and then are repeated at regular intervals. If the athlete loses consciousness, proceed to the inspection phase while continuing to monitor the vital signs. Throughout the examination, question the athlete and observe for the presence of subtle signs and symptoms indicating a head injury (see Graded Symptom Checklist, p. 866).

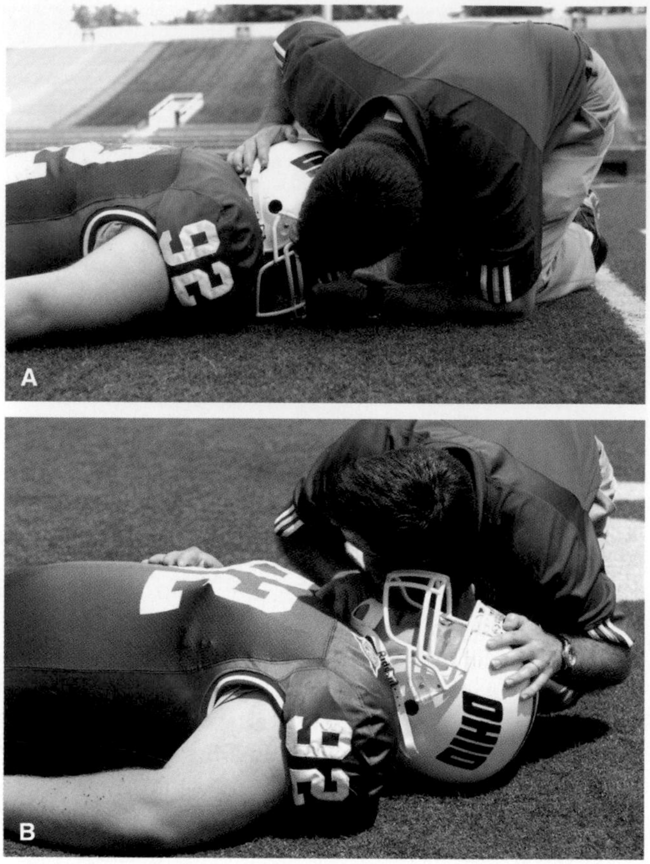

FIGURE 20-5 ■ Establishing the presence of consciousness. (A) If the athlete is unconscious and prone, (B) roll to the supine position and determine an open airway, breathing, and circulation.

- **Head pain:** Diffuse headaches are a common complaint after brain trauma. Localized pain can indicate a contusion, skull fracture, or intracranial hemorrhage.
- **Mechanism of head injuries:** The type of and severity of the injury inflicted to the head and cervical spine depends on the nature of the force delivered (Fig. 20-6). This information may be obtained from someone who witnessed the injury if the athlete is unconscious or groggy.
- **Coup:** A coup injury results when a relatively stationary skull is hit by an object traveling at a high velocity (e.g., being struck in the head with a baseball). This type of mechanism results in trauma on the side of the head that was struck.
- **Contrecoup:** A contrecoup injury occurs when the skull is moving at a relatively high velocity and is suddenly stopped, such as when falling and striking the head on the floor. The fluid within the skull fails to decrease the brain's momentum proportional to that of the skull, causing the brain to strike the skull on the

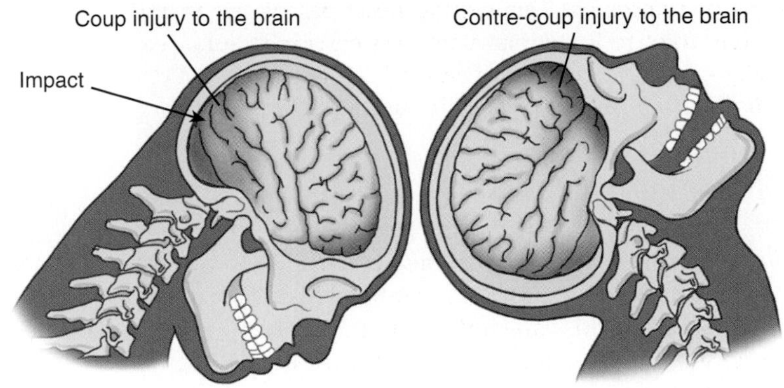

FIGURE 20-6 ■ Mechanisms of athletic head injuries. (A) Coup mechanism resulting in brain trauma on the side of the impact. (B) Contrecoup mechanism causing brain injury on the side opposite of the impact as it rebounds off the skull.

side opposite the impact. This mechanism includes forces that are transmitted up the length of the spinal column, such as when falling and landing on the buttocks.

- **Rotational or shear forces:** Sudden twisting forces or acceleration and deceleration can disrupt neural activity and result in cerebral concussion symptoms.
- **Repeated subconcussive forces:** Athletes receiving repeated nontraumatic blows to the head (e.g., in boxing or while heading a soccer ball) have a higher degree of degenerative changes within the CNS, including dementia.[9-11] A history of repeated concussions can result in cumulative neurological and cognitive deficits by disrupting electroencephalographic (EEG) activity.[10,12]

- **Loss of consciousness:** In the absence of a history of unconsciousness, question the athlete regarding a momentary loss of consciousness after the impact (e.g., "Did you black out?"). Record the responses given by the athlete immediately after the injury for future comparison. The athlete may also describe "seeing stars" at the time of the impact, which indicates transitory unconsciousness.

*** Practical Evidence**

Loss of consciousness was long thought to be the best predictor of the severity of the head injury and ensuing symptoms. Several studies suggest that loss of consciousness occurs in less than 10% of all concussions[8] and that the presence of amnesia is a more sensitive predictor of cognitive deficits and other symptoms.[13]

- **History of concussion:** A recent history of concussion increases the risk for subsequent concussions, increases the symptoms of the current condition, and delays recovery.[14,15] The history of concussions must be readily available from the athlete's medical file.
- **Preexisting mood disorders:** Identify if the patient has any preexisting mental health disorders, including learning disorders, attention deficit disorders, or a history of migraine headaches. Any of these conditions can complicate the diagnosis and management of head injury.[8]
- **Emotional impairment:** Irritability, sadness, and/or emotional instability are often signs of a concussion. These impairments and their duration are quantified using the Standardized Concussion Assessment Tool (SCAT3) or a graded symptom checklist.
- **Complaints of weakness:** A general malaise is to be expected after a cerebral concussion. Reports of muscular weakness in one or more extremities is a more serious finding, possibly indicating trauma to the brain, spinal cord, or one or more spinal nerve roots.
- **Fatigue:** Persistent fatigue may be present after a concussive event.
- **Cognitive impairment:** An inability to concentrate, confusion, and forgetfulness are symptoms associated with concussion.

Inspection

Individuals with head injuries may appear dazed. Many of traits associated with concussions are not directly observable.

- **Skull and scalp:** Inspect the athlete's skull and scalp for the presence of bleeding, swelling, or other deformities.

Inspection of the Eyes

- **General:** Note the general attitude of the athlete's eyes. A dazed, distant appearance may be attributed to mental confusion and disruption of cerebral function.
- **Nystagmus:** While observing both of the athlete's eyes simultaneously, look for the presence of involuntary shaking, or nystagmus. This clinical sign, although it may normally occur, may indicate pressure on the eyes' motor nerves or disruption of the inner ear.
- **Pupil size:** Observe the equality of the pupils. A unilaterally dilated pupil, anisocoria, can be indicative of an intracranial hemorrhage that is placing pressure on cranial nerve III (CN III), although some people may normally display unequal pupil sizes (Fig. 20-7). Although this condition may be benign, its presence should be detected during the preparticipation physical examination and recorded in the athlete's medical file to avoid confusion during the evaluation of a head injury.

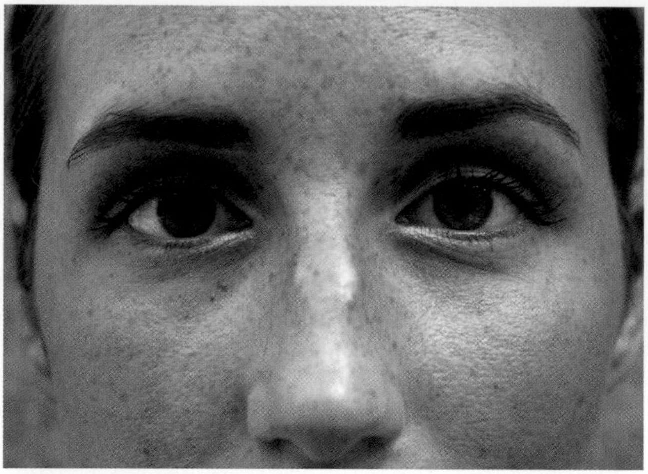

FIGURE 20-7 ■ Anisocoria, or unequal pupil size. Note the increased diameter of the patient's right pupil. This condition may result from pressure on the oculomotor nerve (cranial nerve III) or may be congenital.

- **Pupillary reaction to light:** Refer to Box 18.1 and see the "Neurological Testing" section of this chapter for the process and implications of negative pupillary reaction tests.

Inspection of the Nose and Ears

Bleeding from the ears, even in the absence of CSF in the fluid, may indicate a skull fracture. Bleeding from the nose could represent either a nasal fracture or a skull fracture. Ecchymosis under the eyes, "raccoon eyes," can indicate a skull fracture or nasal fracture. CSF may also leak from the ears and nose when a skull fracture is present and the dura is torn, opening the intracranial space to the nose or nasal tract.[16] The halo test is used to determine if CSF is present in fluids leaking from the nose or ears (see Selective Tissue Test 20-4).

Palpation

Palpate at the site of impact for any deformity. Because of the extensive blood supply in the scalp, swelling often has a rapid onset and can obscure any deformity. See Chapter 19 for details on palpation of the face and head.

Functional Assessment

Functional assessment involves the systematic review of the patient's memory, cognition, balance and coordination, and the integrity of the cranial nerves. Twelve pairs of cranial nerves (CNs), identified by Roman numerals (CN I to CN XII), arise from the brain and transmit both sensory and motor impulses (Table 20-2). The **ganglia** of the sensory component are located outside the CNS; the ganglia of the motor nerves are located within the CNS. Increased intracranial pressure results in impairment of the motor component of the cranial nerves involved but leaves their sensory component intact.

Practical Evidence

Unlike most musculoskeletal injuries, the diagnosis of concussions and return-to-play decisions are largely based on self-reported symptoms. Many athletes may be unaware that symptoms are present or may understate the magnitude of symptoms for fear of being withheld from competition.[13]

Cranial Nerve Function

An assessment of the cranial nerves must be conducted immediately after the injury and repeated at 15- to 20-minute intervals until intracranial bleeding has been ruled out as a potential diagnosis. Accumulation of blood within the cranium shifts the brain hemisphere, placing pressure on the cranial nerves, impairing their function. Information regarding the loss of many of these functions, such as vision, smell, and taste, is volunteered by the athlete. The following tests are ordered by the affected organ rather than by the cranial nerves themselves.

- **Eyes:** Vision (optic [CN II]) is assessed using a Snellen chart (see Fig. 18-5) or by reading an object of reasonable size for normal vision, such as the amount of time remaining on the scoreboard. With the use of a penlight, the **pupil's reaction to light** (oculomotor [CN III]) is determined by covering one of the athlete's eyes and briefly shining the light into the opposite pupil. Normally, the pupil should constrict when the light strikes it and dilate when the light is removed. Using a penlight, finger, or other object held approximately 2 feet from the athlete's nose, the equality of **eye movement** (cranial nerves: oculomotor [CN III], trochlear [CN IV], and abducens [CN VI]) is determined by moving the object up, down, left, right, and, finally, inward toward the athlete's nose.
- **Diplopia** experienced after the injury may indicate cerebral dysfunction resulting from pressure on CN III, IV, or VI, causing spasm of the eye's extrinsic muscles; or it may indicate a fracture of the eye's orbit. Diplopia that does not rapidly subside indicates the immediate need for advanced medical assistance.
- **Face:** Ask the athlete to raise the eyebrows and forehead, smile, and frown (facial [CN VII]); clench the jaw (trigeminal [CN V]), swallow (glossopharyngeal [CN IX] and vagus [CN X]); and stick out the tongue (hypoglossal [CN XII]).
- **Ears:** The functions of the vestibulocochlear nerve (CN VIII) include hearing, in which any disruption should be apparent. Tinnitus demonstrates possible malfunctions of CN VIII. Balance and equilibrium can be assessed through the Romberg test.
- **Shoulders and neck:** If the presence of a cervical injury has been ruled out, strength assessment of the cervical spine musculature should be performed (see

---

Ganglion (nerve) (pl. ganglia) A collection of nerve cell bodies housed in the central or peripheral nervous system

Table 20-2 Cranial Nerve Function

Number	Name	Type	Function
I	Olfactory	Sensory	Smell
II	Optic	Sensory	Vision
III	Oculomotor	Motor	Regulates pupillary reaction and size Elevation of upper eyelid Eye adduction and downward rolling
IV	Trochlear	Motor	Upward eye rolling
V	Trigeminal	Mixed	Motor: Muscles of mastication Sensation: Nose, forehead, temple, scalp, lips, tongue, and lower jaw
VI	Abducens	Motor	Lateral eye movement
VII	Facial	Mixed	Motor: Muscles of expression Sensory: Taste
VIII	Vestibulocochlear	Sensory	Equilibrium Hearing
IX	Glossopharyngeal	Mixed	Motor: Pharyngeal muscles Sensory: Taste
X	Vagus	Mixed	Motor: Muscles of pharynx and larynx Sensory: Gag reflex
XI	Accessory	Motor	Trapezius and sternocleidomastoid muscles
XII	Hypoglossal	Motor	Tongue movement

Clinical Application

Function	Cranial Nerves	How Tested
Eye Assessment	II, III, IV, VI	Visual acuity, pupillary reaction, and tracking
Balance	VIII	Romberg test, Balance Error Scoring System (BESS)
Speaking/Hearing	VIII, IX, X, XII	Speaking to the patient; the patient speaking
Facial Expression	V, VII, XII	Smile, frown, stick out tongue
Smelling	I	Based on self-reported symptoms (often a "bad smell")
Shoulder Shrug	XI	Resist shoulder girdle raise

Manual Muscle Tests 14-1 to 14-5). Resisted shoulder shrugs are used to determine the integrity of the accessory nerve (CN XI).

Neurocognitive Function

Trauma to the cerebrum can result in unusual communication between the patient and the examiner. This can manifest itself through inappropriate behavior, irrational thinking, and apparent mental disability or personality changes.

- **Behavior:** The individual's behavior, attitude, and demeanor may become altered after brain trauma. This may take the form of violent, irrational behavior; inappropriate behavior; and belligerence. After a head injury, the athlete may verbally or physically lash out at those attempting to assist.
- **Analytical skills:** The patient's analytical skills can be determined using **serial 7's**. The patient is asked to count backwards from 100 by 7 (e.g., 100, 93, 86, 79...).
- **Information processing:** The athlete's ability to process the information and assimilate facts should be noted. Confusion regarding relatively simple directions, such as "Sit on the bench," indicates profound cognitive dysfunction.

Memory

One of the most obvious dysfunctions after brain trauma is the loss of memory. The inability to recall events before the onset of the injury is termed **retrograde amnesia.** When the athlete cannot remember events after the onset of injury, it is termed **anterograde amnesia** or posttraumatic amnesia (Fig. 20-8). Although significant retrograde

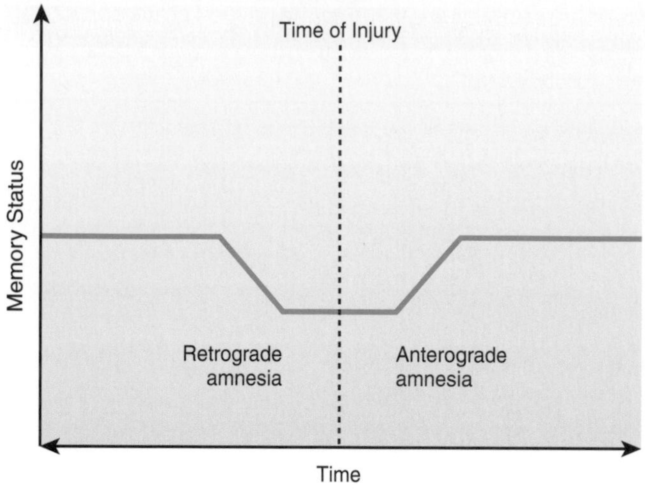

FIGURE 20-8 ■ Types of amnesia. Retrograde amnesia is the loss of memory from the onset of injury backward in time. Anterograde amnesia is the loss of memory after the onset of injury.

amnesia is a cause for concern, fading or fogging memory identifies a progressive deterioration of cerebral function. See the SCAT3 for determination of memory function (p. 867).

Neuropsychological Testing

Memory and cognitive testing provide a subjective assessment of the patient's mental abilities. The use of objective neuropsychological tests and objective balance tests (see the information on the Balance Error Scoring System [BESS] in the next section) objectively quantifies the amount of dysfunction demonstrated following the injury. These tests are more sensitive in identifying subtle cognitive impairment as compared with a clinical examination.[8,10,17–23]

Neuropsychological testing can identify attention deficits and delayed memory function in athletes suffering concussion.[10] Most cognitive deficits resolve within 7 to 10 days, although younger—high school aged—athletes tend to have a longer recovery time.[8] Neurocognitive symptoms may persist after physical symptoms have resolved,[24] and a history of multiple concussions further delays the recovery of neurological function.[25]

Several computer-based and smart phone–based programs such as ImPACT®, Axon®, and HeadMinder® are available for athletic neuropsychological testing. These systems measure variables such as memory, reaction time, and information processing speed, and the information obtained from them may be a valuable supplement to the return-to-play decision-making process.[14] Performance (scores) can be influenced by the patient's sex, sport(s) played, alertness at the time of testing, motivation, and other variables such as SAT scores.[26] Interestingly, a history of prior concussion does not appear to influence performance.[26]

Neuropsychological tests administered after the concussion are compared with the baseline scores and/or with other postconcussion tests (Box 20-1). However, many computer-based neuropsychological tests have low to moderate test–retest reliability.[27-29] In either case, these scores are only part of the return-to-play decision and must be considered alongside of other clinical examination findings.

Box 20-1

How Valuable (and Needed) Is Neuropsychological Baseline Testing?

The use of baseline neuropsychological tests has been recommended by several professional organizations, consensus/position statements, and researchers.[30,31] The baseline score is compared with scores obtained during the postconcussion recovery period to monitor the course of recovery. While improved scores are part of the overall clinical return-to-play decision, they are not the sole determinant of a person's ability to return to competition.

The usefulness of baseline neurological data has been called into question.[8,13,28,29,32–38] An inherent issue with most sport-specific neuropsychological tests is the lack of discrimination (range in scores) between otherwise-healthy people. Healthy individuals have varying levels of cognitive ability, memory, reaction time, and other measures. However, many neuropsychological tests—especially those addressing memory—are unable to differentiate among a general population, demonstrating a "ceiling effect," where perfect scores are common.[34,35,37] This lack of a representative baseline yields low sensitivity and poor reliability, making the identification of those with impaired cognitive function difficult.[28,29,36] Baseline neuropsychological testing will not be useful until the tests' psychometric properties improve.[29,36]

Balance and Coordination

After a head injury, the athlete's balance and coordination may be hindered secondary to trauma involving the cerebellum or the inner ear.[39] A profound loss of muscular coordination, ataxia, may be obvious as the athlete attempts to perform even simple tasks. The **Romberg test** (Selective Tissue Test 20-1) and **tandem walking test** (Selective Tissue Test 20-2) are used to determine cerebellar function by determining the level of balance and coordination.

After a head injury, an electronic balance system can be used to objectively determine the amount of balance disruption. In the absence of these devices and on the sidelines, a quantifiable clinical test should be used. The BESS, a clinical test that has been developed to evaluate impairment of balance and coordination, is more applicable and sensitive to the athletic population (Selective Tissue Test 20-3).[41,42] In this procedure, balance is first tested on a firm surface and then again with the patient standing on foam.

Baseline balance measurements should be obtained before the start of each season. During baseline testing, the patient should be well rested and free from any lower extremity musculoskeletal injury. After injury, the BESS can be administered on the sidelines or in the clinic with the results then compared with the baseline measures, but it should be performed under the same conditions as the baseline.[46] For example, if baseline measures were obtained in a quiet room, postinjury testing should also be performed in a quiet room. If baseline information is not available, the patient's BESS

Selective Tissue Tests 20-1
Romberg Test

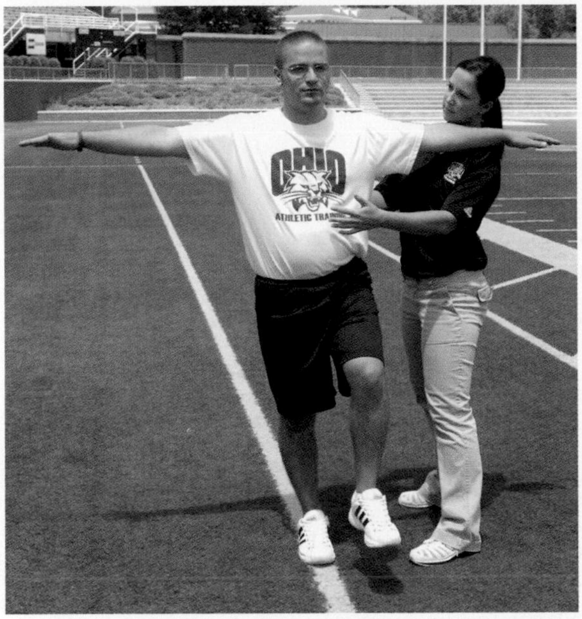

The Romberg test is used to determine the patient's balance and coordination.

Patient Position	Standing with the feet shoulder-width apart
Position of Examiner	Standing lateral or posterior to the patient, ready to support the patient as needed
Evaluative Procedure	The patient shuts the eyes and abducts the arms to 90° with the elbows extended. If this portion of the examination is adequately completed, the patient is asked to touch the index finger to the nose (with the eyes remaining closed).
Positive Test	The patient displays gross unsteadiness.
Implications	Lack of balance and/or coordination indicating cerebellar or cranial nerve VIII dysfunction
Comments	Changes in balance as measured by clinical balance equipment are commonly associated with concussions.[40] The modification of having the patient extending the neck is not recommended because of potential occlusion of the vertebral artery.
Evidence	Absent or inconclusive in the literature

Selective Tissue Tests 20-2
Tandem Walking Test

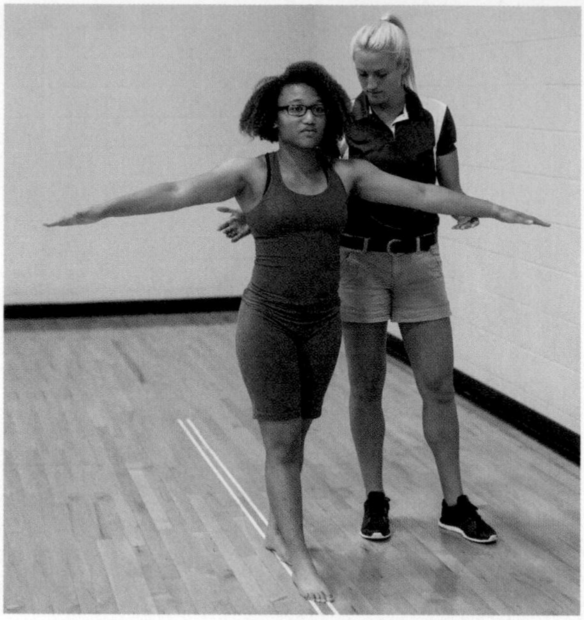

The tandem walking test determines the patient's balance.

Patient Position	Standing with the feet straddling a straight line (e.g., sideline or athletic tape) and 3 meters (9 feet, 10 in) long.
Position of Examiner	Beside the patient ready to provide support
Evaluative Procedure	The amount of time required for the patient to walk heel-to-toe along the length of the line, turn 180 degrees and return to the starting point is recorded. A total of four trials are performed, and the best time is used.
Positive Test	The test is failed if the patient's best time is more than 14 seconds, or if the patient steps off the line, grabs the examiner, or breaks the gait.
Implications	Cerebral or inner ear dysfunction that inhibits balance
Evidence	Absent or inconclusive in the literature

Selective Tissue Tests 20-3
Modified Balance Error Scoring System

Firm Surface Bout | **Soft Surface Bout**

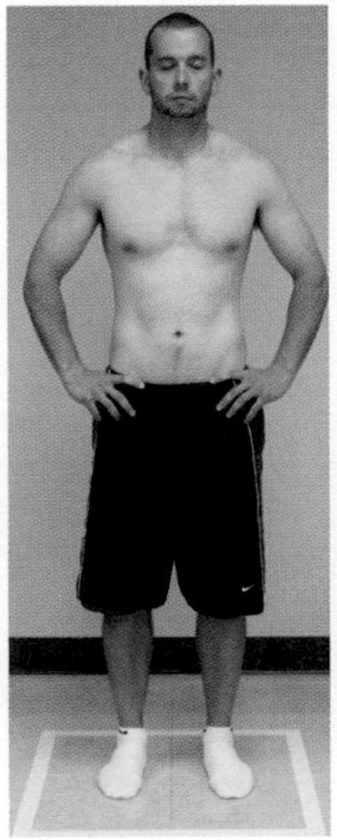
Double Leg Stance

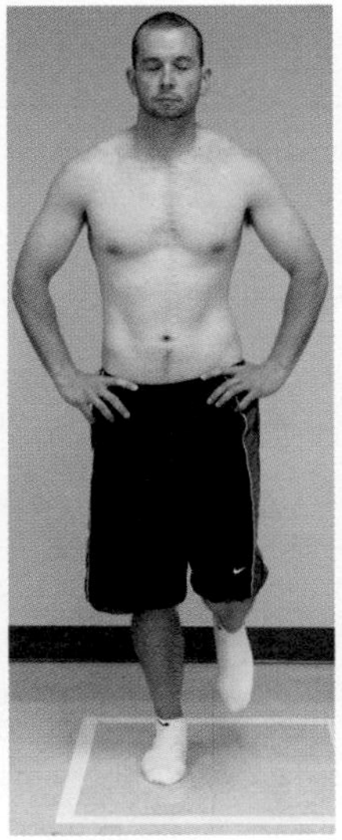
Single Leg Stance

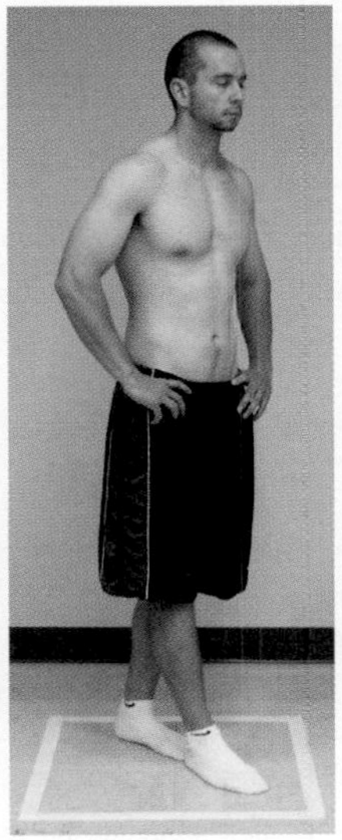
Tandem Stance

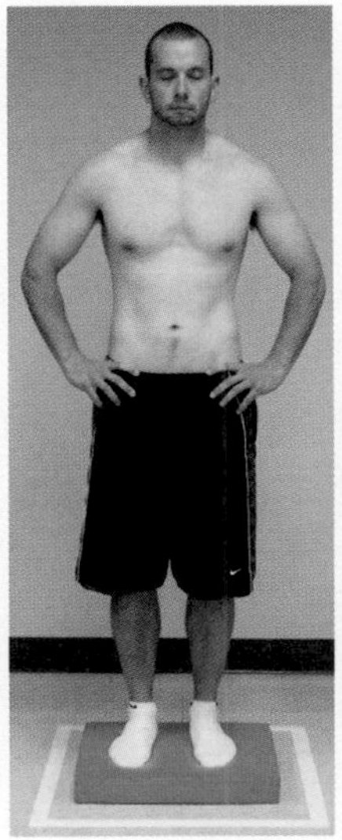
Double Leg Stance

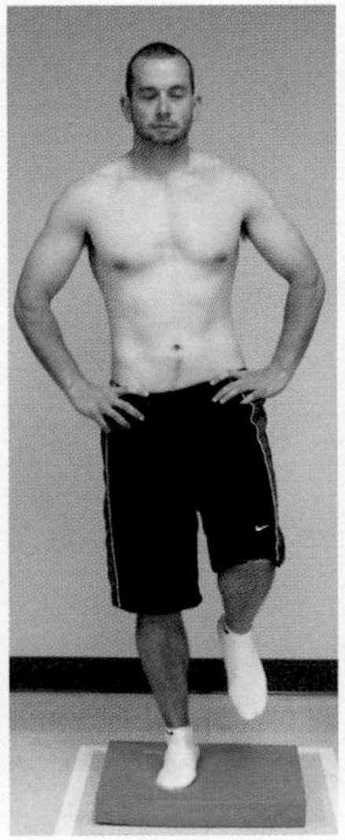
Single Leg Stance

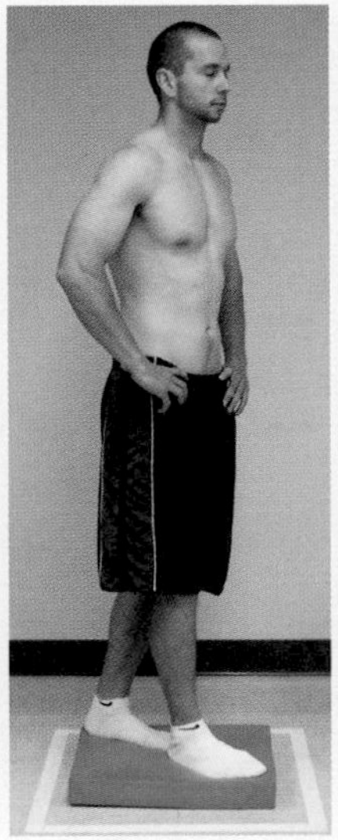
Tandem Stance

The BESS involves three different stances, each completed twice, once while standing on a firm surface and again while standing on a foam surface.

Patient Position	The patient is barefoot or wearing socks. The ankle must not be taped during the test. The patient assumes the following stances for each phase of the test. In each phase the patient's hands are placed on the hips, and the eyes are closed. **Phase 1:** Double leg stance. The patient attempts to remain stable standing with the weight evenly distributed between the two legs. **Phase 2:** Single leg stance. Standing on the dominant leg, the non–weight-bearing hip is flexed to 20=–30=, and the knee is flexed to 40=–50=. **Phase 3:** Tandem leg stance—The nondominant leg is placed behind the dominant leg, and the patient stands in a heel-to-toe manner.
Position of Examiner	The examiner stands in front of the athlete. A stopwatch is required to time the trials. A second clinician acts as a spotter.
Evaluative Procedure	The first battery of tests (Phases 1 through 3) is performed with the patient standing on a firm surface. The second battery of tests is performed with the patient standing on medium density foam (60 kg/m^3) that is 45 cm × 45 cm and 13 cm thick. Each bout consists of 20 seconds with the number of errors in each recorded. The trial is incomplete if the patient cannot hold the test position for a minimum of 5 seconds.

Continued

Selective Tissue Tests 20-3
Modified Balance Error Scoring System—cont'd

Scoring	One point is scored for each of the following errors: Lifting hands off the iliac crest Opening the eyes Stepping, stumbling, or falling Moving the hip into more than 30= of flexion or abduction Lifting the foot or heel Remaining out of the testing position for more than 5 seconds{boxul2: If more than one error occurs simultaneously, only one error is recorded. Patients who are unable to hold the test position for 5 seconds are assigned the score of 10.
Positive Test	Scores that are 25% above the patient's baseline or the norm[43] An increase in 3 BESS errors represents a clinically significant change (MCID). Performance on the BESS improves with repeated testing, a practice effect.[43,44]
Implications	Impaired cerebral function
Modification	As with repeated tests, patients learn how to take the BESS, thereby inflating scores. Using the mean score of three 20-second trials will reduce the learning effects and improve the test's reliability.[45]
Comments	To improve validity BESS pretests and postinjury tests should be administered in the same environmental conditions (e.g., athletic training facility, sideline).[46] BESS scores correlate well with scores acquired from more sophisticated balance equipment.[41]

BESS = balance error scoring system; MCID = minimal clinically important difference score can be compared with recovery curves for the normal population; however, because of wide individual variability, the sensitivity decreases if no baseline measurements are available.[8,20,41,42]

Vital Signs

Techniques for determining the vital signs are described in Chapter 1 (Review of Systems). The following are qualitative parameters that are relevant after a head or cervical spine injury.

- **Respiration:** In addition to the number of breaths per minute, the quality of the respirations is determined:

Type	Characteristics	Implications
Apneustic	Prolonged inspirations unrelieved by attempts to exhale	Trauma to the pons
Biot's	Periods of **apnea** followed by hyperapnea	Increased intracranial pressure
Cheyne-Stokes	Periods of **apnea** followed by breaths of increasing depth and frequency	Frontal lobe or brainstem trauma
Slow	Respiration consisting of fewer than 12 breaths per minute	CNS disruption
Thoracic	Respiration in which the diaphragm is inactive and breathing occurs only through expansion of the chest; normal abdominal movement is absent	Disruption of the phrenic nerve or its nerve roots

- **Pulse:** The pulse rate and quality must be monitored at regular intervals until the possibility of brain or spinal injury has been ruled out. Pulse abnormalities attributed to these conditions include:

Type	Characteristics	Implication
Accelerated	Pulse >150 beats per minute (bpm) (>170 bpm usually has fatal results)	Pressure on the base of the brain; shock
Bounding	Pulse that quickly reaches a higher intensity than normal, then quickly disappears	Ventricular systole and reduced peripheral pressure
Deficit	Pulse in which the number of beats counted at the radial pulse is less than that counted over the heart itself	Cardiac arrhythmia
High Tension	Pulse in which the force of the beat is increased; an increased amount of pressure is required to inhibit the radial pulse	Cerebral trauma
Low Tension	Short, fast, faint pulse having a rapid decline	Heart failure; shock

Apnea The temporary cessation of breathing

- **Blood pressure:** Blood pressure readings should be taken concurrently or immediately after each pulse measurement. These measurements are recorded and repeated at regular intervals. Blood pressure is normally high after physical exertion. Blood pressure that does not decrease over time or continues to increase may be a sign of severe intracranial hemorrhage.
- **Pulse pressure:** To calculate the pulse pressure, the diastolic pressure is subtracted from the systolic pressure. The normal pulse pressure is approximately 40 mm Hg. A pulse pressure of greater than 50 mm Hg may indicate increased intracranial bleeding.
- **Oxygenation:** Assess oxygenation using a pulse oximeter. Oxygenation levels under 95% suggests increased intracranial pressure and the need for supplemental oxygen.

Region-Specific Pathologies and Selective Tissue Tests

Although the death rate for organized football is relatively low, many fatalities are attributed to head or cervical spine trauma.[47] However, head and cervical spine trauma can—and does—occur in sports other than football. Therefore, emergency preparedness is not limited to the sport of football but, rather, should encompass all of an institution's or organization's athletic programs.

The ability to correctly identify and manage athletes with these conditions in a timely, safe, and efficient manner is a determining factor related to the outcome of a potentially catastrophic injury. More so than any other type of injury described in this text, a consistent standardized plan of action must be implemented immediately in the management of these conditions.[48]

Traumatic Brain Injury

The outcome of a single instance of brain injury can range from inconsequential to catastrophic. Recently, the potential long-term consequences of repeated mild brain injury have been identified. Multiple head injuries can result in organic changes within the structure—and therefore—the function of the brain (Box 20-2). Athletes with a history of multiple concussions can display the signs and symptoms of a current concussion in the absence of a recent history of head trauma.[25] In addition, a concussion may produce

Box 20-2
Chronic Traumatic Encephalopathy

Chronic traumatic encephalopathy (CTE) is the progressive degeneration of brain function caused by repeated mild traumatic brain injury.[8,49] Repeated trauma is thought to trigger a neurodegenerative disease associated with the tau protein that stabilizes microtubules in the CNS. Disruption of tau proteins is a characteristic finding in Alzheimer's disease. In postmortem studies of athletes' brains, 34 of 35 football players and 4 out of 5 professional ice hockey players demonstrated gross and/or microscopic signs of CTE during an autopsy.[49] Neurodegenerative-related causes of death such as Alzheimer's disease, Parkinson disease, and amyotrophic lateral sclerosis (ALS) is 3 to 4 times higher in former NFL players than in the general population.[12]

The onset of the signs and symptoms of CTE is progressive, with the characteristics of the prior stage carrying on into the next stages[49]:

Stage I Headache, decreased attention, impaired concentration

Stage II Depression, explosive behavior (impulse control), short-term memory loss

Stage III Disruption of higher brain function that regulates other brain processes (executive function), cognitive impairment

Stage IV Dementia, word-finding difficulty, aggression

Although CTE has been widely reported on—and speculated on—in the popular media, a definitive link between concussion and the development of CTE later in life has not been conclusively determined.[13] It should be noted that the early stages of CTE resemble the signs and symptoms of post-concussion syndrome.

lingering effects, be magnified by subsequent concussions, or mask underlying brain trauma.

Anyone who has sustained a head injury should be informed that symptoms can increase with time. For this reason, even athletes who are in apparently good health after a head injury need to be given information about signs and symptoms of worsening injury. These instructions should also be communicated to the athlete's parents, roommate, or spouse (see Home Instructions, p. 873).

Concussion

Concussion, a subset of mild traumatic brain injury, is defined by the 2012 **Zurich Guidelines** "a complex pathophysiological process affecting the brain, induced by biomechanical forces."[13] A concussion may be marked by direct or indirect trauma to the head followed by transient mental confusion, alteration of mental status, and amnesia.[13] Loss of consciousness may or may not occur.[1,13,14,30]

Some brain cells are destroyed as a direct result of the concussive force, and other cells are placed at risk of further trauma secondary to changes in cerebral blood flow, increased intracranial pressure, and apnea.[50] After the trauma, a paradoxical period occurs where there is an increased demand for glucose to fuel cell metabolism, but the blood flow that delivers the nutrients decreases.[50] Changes in the brain's metabolism may produce tell-tale metabolic changes (**biomarkers**) that potentially may assist in the diagnosis of concussion.[51] During this time of metabolic changes, the risk of further brain trauma may increase if the athlete is allowed to return to competition and suffers another head injury.[13,15,31]

Currently, no anatomic or physiological findings exist on which to base a diagnosis of a concussion although there is extensive on-going research in this area. In 2009 new guidelines fundamentally changed the procedures used to diagnose concussions and provided clear return-to-play guidelines.[13] One of the most significant changes proposed by these guidelines is eliminating the "grading" of concussions. A patient now either has a concussion or does not.

The diagnosis of a concussion is based on a battery of physical, behavioral, and cognitive findings.[14] Approximately 85% to 90% of concussions are not reported until after the practice or game, and up to 50% many go unrecognized or unreported.[8,20]

Symptoms associated with concussions include dizziness, tinnitus, nausea, memory loss, and motor impairment, with the symptoms occurring along a continuum ranging from no disruption to total disruption. Some cases may also result in loss of consciousness, convulsions, vomiting, and loss of bowel and bladder control (Examination Findings 20-1). Delayed symptoms may include personality changes, fatigue, sleep disturbances, lethargy, depression, and difficulty performing activities of daily living (ADLs).[50]

*** Practical Evidence**

The consensus guidelines state that the presence of at least one of the signs and symptoms (e.g., headache, dizziness, confusion, abnormal behavior) that emerges following a blow to the head is diagnostic of a concussion.[13]

Because concussion symptoms are multifaceted and vary from person to person, techniques that assess neurocognitive functioning, patient-described symptoms, and postural control should be used during the diagnostic process. Magnetic resonance imaging (MRI) may be used to identify other forms of traumatic brain injury, and computed tomography (CT) scans may be used to image intracranial bleeding or swelling, but neither technique is diagnostic for ruling in or ruling out concussions.[50]

A postconcussion symptom scale (or postconcussion checklist) should be used to monitor the patient following head injury (Table 20-3).[48] The presence or absence of these symptoms is a primary factor in determining return-to-play status.[52] When compared with baseline (preinjury) scores, these scales help to provide an objective assessment of changes in the patient's symptoms over time. Most

Examination Findings 20-1
Concussion

Examination Segment	Clinical Findings
History of Current Condition	*Onset:* Acute *Chief complaints:* Headache, ringing in the ears, blurred vision, dizziness, unconsciousness *Mechanism:* Blow to the skull or spinal column transmitting an injurious force to the brain; rapid acceleration/deceleration force to the head *Risk factors:* A recent history of a cerebral concussion or a past history of repeated subconcussive forces to the head
Functional Assessment	*Memory:* Transient retrograde amnesia of the events leading up to the injury is possible. An increased scope of memory loss may indicate more significant injury and an associated longer recovery. The presence of anterograde amnesia warrants immediate referral to a physician. *Cognitive function:* The patient may display confused, violent, or aggressive behavior and may have diminished analytical function. Balance and coordination: Romberg's test and heel-to-toe walk (balance and coordination) Instrumented assessment of balance may reveal abnormal balance as compared with baseline. *Eyes:* Blurred vision and unequal pupil size may be present. *Motor function:* Partial and transitory motor loss may occur secondary to trauma to the motor and premotor cortexes. *Vital signs:* Monitor pulse, blood pressure, blood oxygenation, and respiration for changes associated with intracranial bleeding.
Inspection	*Eyes:* Generally they may appear glazed or dazed. Pupil sizes should be equal; a unilaterally dilated pupil may indicate pressure on CN III. Nystagmus may indicate pressure on the CNs or inner ear dysfunction. *Nose and ears:* Any fluid draining from the nose and ears is checked for the presence of CSF, indicative of a skull fracture. *General:* Severe concussions may result in convulsions. The entire skull requires inspection for secondary bleeding or contusions. The area over the mastoid process and the area beneath the eyes are checked for ecchymosis, indicating a skull fracture.
Palpation	If the patient was not wearing a helmet at the time of injury, palpate the skull to determine areas of point tenderness, possibly indicating the presence of a skull fracture.
Neurological Screening	Retrograde amnesia test and anterograde amnesia test repeated at regular intervals Balance Error Scoring System Cerebral function tests (e.g., "What is 100 minus 7") Standardized Assessment of Concussion score Glasgow Coma Scale (used with profoundly head-injured patients) CN assessment Sensory testing Motor testing
Vascular Screening	Within normal limits
Imaging Techniques	MRI or CT scans are used to rule out intracranial hemorrhage or skull fractures, but these findings are not directly useful in diagnosing a concussion.
Differential Diagnosis	Intracranial hemorrhage, heat illness, drug overdose or interaction, skull fracture, hypoglycemia
Comments	The SCAT3 synthesizes many of these findings into a single instrument (see Box 20-3). The possibility of a cervical spine fracture must be assumed until such an injury can be ruled out. An athlete with a history of multiple head trauma or having symptoms after little or no physical trauma should always be referred for further assessment by a physician (see the Postconcussion Syndrome and the Diffuse Cerebral Swelling sections).

CN = cranial nerve; CSF = cerebrospinal fluid; CT = computed tomography; MRI = magnetic resonance imaging; SCAT = Sport Concussion Assessment Tool

Table 20-3 Graded Symptom Checklist

	Absent	Mild		Moderate		Severe		TOTAL
Headache	0	1	2	3	4	5	6	
Nausea	0	1	2	3	4	5	6	
Balance problems/ Dizziness	0	1	2	3	4	5	6	
Fatigue	0	1	2	3	4	5	6	
Drowsiness	0	1	2	3	4	5	6	
Feeling like "in a fog"	0	1	2	3	4	5	6	
Difficulty concentrating	0	1	2	3	4	5	6	
Difficulty remembering	0	1	2	3	4	5	6	
Sensitivity to light	0	1	2	3	4	5	6	
Sensitivity to noise	0	1	2	3	4	5	6	
Blurred vision	0	1	2	3	4	5	6	
Feeling slowed down	0	1	2	3	4	5	6	

Other symptoms evident since injury?

Adapted from Randolph, C, et al: Concussion symptom inventory: an empirically derived scale for monitoring resolution of symptoms following sport-related concussion. *Arch Clin Neuropsych*, 24:219, 2009.

standardized symptoms scales demonstrate moderate to good statistical reliability.[53,54]

✱ Practical Evidence

In contact sports such as football, an athlete who sustains a concussion has three to four times the risk of sustaining another concussion.[25,55]

Concussion Assessment Tools

Several different scales have been used to assist in the diagnosis of concussion. Quantifying concussion severity before all symptoms have cleared may provide inaccurate expectations of recovery.[56] The SCAT3 was based on the Zurich Guidelines and has been adopted by several medical and athletic organizations for assessing the presence of concussion in athletes aged 10 years and over.[13] The SCAT3 is a battery of clinical measurements that includes a graded symptom checklist, determination of loss of consciousness, the Glasgow Coma Scale, memory assessment, the **Standardized Assessment of Concussion** (SAC) instrument, and the assessment of balance and coordination (Box 20-3). Each section is awarded a point value based on the findings. These subscores are summed to yield a composite score. The compilation of scores from the various measurement systems improves the overall test properties and identifies variations in baseline scores based on sex, grade in school, and concussion history.[14] A modification of the SCAT3, the childSCAT3, is designed for use with children aged 5 to 12 years.[13]

✱ Practical Evidence

To reduce the effects of exertion and fatigue, wait at least 15 minutes following the trauma before administering neurocognitive and balance tests.[57]

The SAC has been developed specifically for athletes.[50,58] It consists of four scored sections that measure orientation, immediate memory, concentration, and delayed recall. The SAC protocol is included in the SCAT3 instrument.

The magnitude of severely brain-injured individuals can be quantified using the **Glasgow Coma Scale**. The normal score on this battery is 15. Patients scoring 11 or higher on this instrument have an excellent prognosis for recovery. Scores of 7 or less represent serious brain dysfunction.

Repeated measurements can be used to demonstrate an improvement or degradation of symptoms over time. The score itself is not used to clear a person to return to competition but is an element in the overall diagnostic process. The SCAT3 should be available during practices and games. The results of each test administered should be documented in the patient's medical file.

Concussion Intervention Strategies

Based on signs and symptoms, concussion management is individualized for each patient. Initially, those with concussion are removed from participation. Treatment of concussions may also require "cognitive rest" such as avoiding studying or attending classes and refraining from sensory

Box 20-3
Sport Concussion Assessment Tool 2 (SCAT3)

SCAT3™

FIFA® FEI

Sport Concussion Assessment Tool – 3rd Edition

For use by medical professionals only

Name

Date/Time of Injury:
Date of Assessment:

Examiner:

What is the SCAT3?[1]

The SCAT3 is a standardized tool for evaluating injured athletes for concussion and can be used in athletes aged from 13 years and older. It supersedes the original SCAT and the SCAT2 published in 2005 and 2009, respectively[2]. For younger persons, ages 12 and under, please use the Child SCAT3. The SCAT3 is designed for use by medical professionals. If you are not qualified, please use the Sport Concussion Recognition Tool[1]. Preseason baseline testing with the SCAT3 can be helpful for interpreting post-injury test scores.

Specific instructions for use of the SCAT3 are provided on page 3. If you are not familiar with the SCAT3, please read through these instructions carefully. This tool may be freely copied in its current form for distribution to individuals, teams, groups and organizations. Any revision or any reproduction in a digital form requires approval by the Concussion in Sport Group.

NOTE: The diagnosis of a concussion is a clinical judgment, ideally made by a medical professional. The SCAT3 should not be used solely to make, or exclude, the diagnosis of concussion in the absence of clinical judgement. An athlete may have a concussion even if their SCAT3 is "normal".

What is a concussion?

A concussion is a disturbance in brain function caused by a direct or indirect force to the head. It results in a variety of non-specific signs and/or symptoms (some examples listed below) and most often does not involve loss of consciousness. Concussion should be suspected in the presence of **any one or more** of the following:

- Symptoms (e.g., headache), or
- Physical signs (e.g., unsteadiness), or
- Impaired brain function (e.g. confusion) or
- Abnormal behaviour (e.g., change in personality).

SIDELINE ASSESSMENT

Indications for Emergency Management

NOTE: A hit to the head can sometimes be associated with a more serious brain injury. Any of the following warrants consideration of activating emergency procedures and urgent transportation to the nearest hospital:

- Glasgow Coma score less than 15
- Deteriorating mental status
- Potential spinal injury
- Progressive, worsening symptoms or new neurologic signs

Potential signs of concussion?

If any of the following signs are observed after a direct or indirect blow to the head, the athlete should stop participation, be evaluated by a medical professional and **should not be permitted to return to sport the same day** if a concussion is suspected.

Any loss of consciousness?	Y	N
"If so, how long?"		
Balance or motor incoordination (stumbles, slow/laboured movements, etc.)?	Y	N
Disorientation or confusion (inability to respond appropriately to questions)?	Y	N
Loss of memory:	Y	N
"If so, how long?"		
"Before or after the injury?"		
Blank or vacant look:	Y	N
Visible facial injury in combination with any of the above:	Y	N

1 Glasgow coma scale (GCS)

Best eye response (E)	
No eye opening	1
Eye opening in response to pain	2
Eye opening to speech	3
Eyes opening spontaneously	4
Best verbal response (V)	
No verbal response	1
Incomprehensible sounds	2
Inappropriate words	3
Confused	4
Oriented	5
Best motor response (M)	
No motor response	1
Extension to pain	2
Abnormal flexion to pain	3
Flexion/Withdrawal to pain	4
Localizes to pain	5
Obeys commands	6
Glasgow Coma score (E + V + M)	of 15

GCS should be recorded for all athletes in case of subsequent deterioration.

2 Maddocks Score[3]

"I am going to ask you a few questions, please listen carefully and give your best effort."

Modified Maddocks questions (1 point for each correct answer)

What venue are we at today?	0	1
Which half is it now?	0	1
Who scored last in this match?	0	1
What team did you play last week/game?	0	1
Did your team win the last game?	0	1
Maddocks score		of 5

Maddocks score is validated for sideline diagnosis of concussion only and is not used for serial testing.

Notes: Mechanism of Injury ("tell me what happened"?):

Any athlete with a suspected concussion should be REMOVED FROM PLAY, medically assessed, monitored for deterioration (i.e., should not be left alone) and should not drive a motor vehicle until cleared to do so by a medical professional. No athlete diagnosed with concussion should be returned to sports participation on the day of Injury.

Continued

BACKGROUND

Name: _____ Date: _____
Examiner: _____
Sport/team/school: _____ Date/time of injury: _____
Age: _____ Gender: ☐ M ☐ F
Years of education completed: _____
Dominant hand: ☐ right ☐ left ☐ neither
How many concussions do you think you have had in the past? _____
When was the most recent concussion? _____
How long was your recovery from the most recent concussion? _____
Have you ever been hospitalized or had medical imaging done for a head injury? ☐ Y ☐ N
Have you ever been diagnosed with headaches or migraines? ☐ Y ☐ N
Do you have a learning disability, dyslexia, ADD/ADHD? ☐ Y ☐ N
Have you ever been diagnosed with depression, anxiety or other psychiatric disorder? ☐ Y ☐ N
Has anyone in your family ever been diagnosed with any of these problems? ☐ Y ☐ N
Are you on any medications? If yes, please list: ☐ Y ☐ N

SCAT3 to be done in resting state. Best done 10 or more minutes post excercise.

SYMPTOM EVALUATION

3 How do you feel?
"You should score yourself on the following symptoms, based on how you feel now".

	none	mild		moderate		severe	
Headache	0	1	2	3	4	5	6
"Pressure in head"	0	1	2	3	4	5	6
Neck Pain	0	1	2	3	4	5	6
Nausea or vomiting	0	1	2	3	4	5	6
Dizziness	0	1	2	3	4	5	6
Blurred vision	0	1	2	3	4	5	6
Balance problems	0	1	2	3	4	5	6
Sensitivity to light	0	1	2	3	4	5	6
Sensitivity to noise	0	1	2	3	4	5	6
Feeling slowed down	0	1	2	3	4	5	6
Feeling like "in a fog"	0	1	2	3	4	5	6
"Don't feel right"	0	1	2	3	4	5	6
Difficulty concentrating	0	1	2	3	4	5	6
Difficulty remembering	0	1	2	3	4	5	6
Fatigue or low energy	0	1	2	3	4	5	6
Confusion	0	1	2	3	4	5	6
Drowsiness	0	1	2	3	4	5	6
Trouble falling asleep	0	1	2	3	4	5	6
More emotional	0	1	2	3	4	5	6
Irritability	0	1	2	3	4	5	6
Sadness	0	1	2	3	4	5	6
Nervous or Anxious	0	1	2	3	4	5	6

Total number of symptoms (Maximum possible 22) _____
Symptom severity score (Maximum possible 132) _____

Do the symptoms get worse with physical activity? ☐ Y ☐ N
Do the symptoms get worse with mental activity? ☐ Y ☐ N

☐ self rated ☐ self rated and clinician monitored
☐ clinician interview ☐ self rated with parent input

Overall rating: If you know the athlete well prior to the injury, how different is the athlete acting compared to his/her usual self?
Please circle one response:
| no different | very different | unsure | N/A |

Scoring on the SCAT3 should not be used as a stand-alone method to diagnose concussion, measure recovery or make decisions about an athlete's readiness to return to competition after concussion. Since signs and symptoms may evolve over time, it is important to consider repeat evaluation in the acute assessment of concussion.

COGNITIVE & PHYSICAL EVALUATION

4 Cognitive assessment
Standardized Assessment of Concussion (SAC)[4]

Orientation (1 point for each correct answer)
What month is it?	0	1
What is the date today?	0	1
What is the day of the week?	0	1
What year is it?	0	1
What time is it right now? (within 1 hour)	0	1
Orientation score		of 5

Immediate memory
List	Trial 1		Trial 2		Trial 3		Alternative word list		
elbow	0	1	0	1	0	1	candle	baby	finger
apple	0	1	0	1	0	1	paper	monkey	penny
carpet	0	1	0	1	0	1	sugar	perfume	blanket
saddle	0	1	0	1	0	1	sandwich	sunset	lemon
bubble	0	1	0	1	0	1	wagon	iron	insect
Total									

Immediate memory score total of 15

Concentration: Digits Backward
List	Trial 1		Alternative digit list		
4-9-3	0	1	6-2-9	5-2-6	4-1-5
3-8-1-4	0	1	3-2-7-9	1-7-9-5	4-9-6-8
6-2-9-7-1	0	1	1-5-2-8-6	3-8-5-2-7	6-1-8-4-3
7-1-8-4-6-2	0	1	5-3-9-1-4-8	8-3-1-9-6-4	7-2-4-8-5-6
Total of 4					

Concentration: Month in Reverse Order (1 pt. for entire sequence correct)
Dec-Nov-Oct-Sept-Aug-Jul-Jun-May-Apr-Mar-Feb-Jan	0	1

Concentration score of 5

5 Neck Examination:
Range of motion Tenderness Upper and lower limb sensation & strength
Findings: _____

6 Balance examination
Do one or both of the following tests.
Footwear (shoes, barefoot, braces, tape, etc.) _____

Modified Balance Error Scoring System (BESS) testing[5]
Which foot was tested (i.e. which is the **non-dominant** foot) ☐ Left ☐ Right
Testing surface (hard floor, field, etc.) _____
Condition
Double leg stance: _____ Errors
Single leg stance (non-dominant foot): _____ Errors
Tandem stance (non-dominant foot at back): _____ Errors
And/Or
Tandem gait[6,7]
Time (best of 4 trials): _____ seconds

7 Coordination examination
Upper limb coordination
Which arm was tested: ☐ Left ☐ Right
Coordination score of 1

8 SAC Delayed Recall[4]
Delayed recall score of 5

INSTRUCTIONS

Words in *Italics* throughout the SCAT3 are the instructions given to the athlete by the tester.

Symptom Scale

"You should score yourself on the following symptoms, based on how you feel now".

To be completed by the athlete. In situations where the symptom scale is being completed after exercise, it should still be done in a resting state, at least 10 minutes post exercise.

For total number of symptoms, maximum possible is 22.

For Symptom severity score, add all scores in table, maximum possible is 22 x 6 = 132.

SAC[4]

Immediate Memory

"I am going to test your memory. I will read you a list of words and when I am done, repeat back as many words as you can remember, in any order."

Trials 2 & 3:

"I am going to repeat the same list again. Repeat back as many words as you can remember in any order, even if you said the word before."

Complete all 3 trials regardless of score on trial 1 & 2. Read the words at a rate of one per second. **Score 1 pt. for each correct response.** Total score equals sum across all 3 trials. Do not inform the athlete that delayed recall will be tested.

Concentration

Digits backward

"I am going to read you a string of numbers and when I am done, you repeat them back to me backwards, in reverse order of how I read them to you. For example, if I say 7-1-9, you would say 9-1-7."

If correct, go to next string length. If incorrect, read trial 2. **One point possible for each string length.** Stop after incorrect on both trials. The digits should be read at the rate of one per second.

Months in reverse order

"Now tell me the months of the year in reverse order. Start with the last month and go backward. So you'll say December, November ... Go ahead"

1 pt. for entire sequence correct

Delayed Recall

The delayed recall should be performed after completion of the Balance and Coordination Examination.

"Do you remember that list of words I read a few times earlier? Tell me as many words from the list as you can remember in any order."

Score 1 pt. for each correct response

Balance Examination

Modified Balance Error Scoring System (BESS) testing[5]

This balance testing is based on a modified version of the Balance Error Scoring System (BESS)[5]. A stopwatch or watch with a second hand is required for this testing.

"I am now going to test your balance. Please take your shoes off, roll up your pant legs above ankle (if applicable), and remove any ankle taping (if applicable). This test will consist of three twenty second tests with different stances."

(a) Double leg stance:

"The first stance is standing with your feet together with your hands on your hips and with your eyes closed. You should try to maintain stability in that position for 20 seconds. I will be counting the number of times you move out of this position. I will start timing when you are set and have closed your eyes."

(b) Single leg stance:

"If you were to kick a ball, which foot would you use? [This will be the dominant foot] Now stand on your non-dominant foot. The dominant leg should be held in approximately 30 degrees of hip flexion and 45 degrees of knee flexion. Again, you should try to maintain stability for 20 seconds with your hands on your hips and your eyes closed. I will be counting the number of times you move out of this position. If you stumble out of this position, open your eyes and return to the start position and continue balancing. I will start timing when you are set and have closed your eyes."

(c) Tandem stance:

"Now stand heel-to-toe with your non-dominant foot in back. Your weight should be evenly distributed across both feet. Again, you should try to maintain stability for 20 seconds with your hands on your hips and your eyes closed. I will be counting the number of times you move out of this position. If you stumble out of this position, open your eyes and return to the start position and continue balancing. I will start timing when you are set and have closed your eyes."

Balance testing – types of errors

1. Hands lifted off iliac crest
2. Opening eyes
3. Step, stumble, or fall
4. Moving hip into > 30 degrees abduction
5. Lifting forefoot or heel
6. Remaining out of test position > 5 sec

Each of the 20-second trials is scored by counting the errors, or deviations from the proper stance, accumulated by the athlete. The examiner will begin counting errors only after the individual has assumed the proper start position. **The modified BESS is calculated by adding one error point for each error during the three 20-second tests. The maximum total number of errors for any single condition is 10.** If a athlete commits multiple errors simultaneously, only one error is recorded but the athlete should quickly return to the testing position, and counting should resume once subject is set. Subjects that are unable to maintain the testing procedure for a minimum of **five seconds** at the start are assigned the highest possible score, ten, for that testing condition.

OPTION: For further assessment, the same 3 stances can be performed on a surface of medium density foam (e.g., approximately 50 cm x 40 cm x 6 cm).

Tandem Gait[6,7]

Participants are instructed to stand with their feet together behind a starting line (the test is best done with footwear removed). Then, they walk in a forward direction as quickly and as accurately as possible along a 38mm wide (sports tape), 3 meter line with an alternate foot heel-to-toe gait ensuring that they approximate their heel and toe on each step. Once they cross the end of the 3m line, they turn 180 degrees and return to the starting point using the same gait. A total of 4 trials are done and the best time is retained. Athletes should complete the test in 14 seconds. Athletes fail the test if they step off the line, have a separation between their heel and toe, or if they touch or grab the examiner or an object. In this case, the time is not recorded and the trial repeated, if appropriate.

Coordination Examination

Upper limb coordination

Finger-to-nose (FTN) task:

"I am going to test your coordination now. Please sit comfortably on the chair with your eyes open and your arm (either right or left) outstretched (shoulder flexed to 90 degrees and elbow and fingers extended), pointing in front of you. When I give a start signal, I would like you to perform five successive finger to nose repetitions using your index finger to touch the tip of the nose, and then return to the starting position, as quickly and as accurately as possible."

Scoring: 5 correct repetitions in < 4 seconds = 1

Note for testers: Athletes fail the test if they do not touch their nose, do not fully extend their elbow or do not perform five repetitions. **Failure should be scored as 0.**

References & Footnotes

1. This tool has been developed by a group of international experts at the 4th International Consensus meeting on Concussion in Sport held in Zurich, Switzerland in November 2012. The full details of the conference outcomes and the authors of the tool are published in The BJSM Injury Prevention and Health Protection, 2013, Volume 47, Issue 5. The outcome paper will also be simultaneously co-published in other leading biomedical journals with the copyright held by the Concussion in Sport Group, to allow unrestricted distribution, providing no alterations are made.

2. McCrory P et al., Consensus Statement on Concussion in Sport – the 3rd International Conference on Concussion in Sport held in Zurich, November 2008. British Journal of Sports Medicine 2009; 43: i76-89.

3. Maddocks, DL; Dicker, GD; Saling, MM. The assessment of orientation following concussion in athletes. Clinical Journal of Sport Medicine. 1995; 5(1): 32–3.

4. McCrea M. Standardized mental status testing of acute concussion. Clinical Journal of Sport Medicine. 2001; 11: 176–181.

5. Guskiewicz KM. Assessment of postural stability following sport-related concussion. Current Sports Medicine Reports. 2003; 2: 24–30.

6. Schneiders, A.G., Sullivan, S.J., Gray, A., Hammond-Tooke, G. & McCrory, P. Normative values for 16-37 year old subjects for three clinical measures of motor performance used in the assessment of sports concussions. Journal of Science and Medicine in Sport. 2010; 13(2): 196–201.

7. Schneiders, A.G., Sullivan, S.J., Kvarnstrom. J.K., Olsson, M., Yden. T. & Marshall, S.W. The effect of footwear and sports-surface on dynamic neurological screening in sport-related concussion. Journal of Science and Medicine in Sport. 2010; 13(4): 382–386

Continued

ATHLETE INFORMATION

Any athlete suspected of having a concussion should be removed from play, and then seek medical evaluation.

Signs to watch for

Problems could arise over the first 24–48 hours. The athlete should not be left alone and must go to a hospital at once if they:

- Have a headache that gets worse
- Are very drowsy or can't be awakened
- Can't recognize people or places
- Have repeated vomiting
- Behave unusually or seem confused; are very irritable
- Have seizures (arms and legs jerk uncontrollably)
- Have weak or numb arms or legs
- Are unsteady on their feet; have slurred speech

Remember, it is better to be safe.
Consult your doctor after a suspected concussion.

Return to play

Athletes should not be returned to play the same day of injury.
When returning athletes to play, they should be **medically cleared and then follow a stepwise supervised program,** with stages of progression.

For example:

Rehabilitation stage	Functional exercise at each stage of rehabilitation	Objective of each stage
No activity	Physical and cognitive rest	Recovery
Light aerobic exercise	Walking, swimming or stationary cycling keeping intensity, 70% maximum predicted heart rate. No resistance training	Increase heart rate
Sport-specific exercise	Skating drills in ice hockey, running drills in soccer. No head impact activities	Add movement
Non-contact training drills	Progression to more complex training drills, eg passing drills in football and ice hockey. May start progressive resistance training	Exercise, coordination, and cognitive load
Full contact practice	Following medical clearance participate in normal training activities	Restore confidence and assess functional skills by coaching staff
Return to play	Normal game play	

There should be at least 24 hours (or longer) for each stage and if symptoms recur the athlete should rest until they resolve once again and then resume the program at the previous asymptomatic stage. Resistance training should only be added in the later stages.

If the athlete is symptomatic for more than 10 days, then consultation by a medical practitioner who is expert in the management of concussion, is recommended.

Medical clearance should be given before return to play.

Scoring Summary:

Test Domain	Score		
	Date:	Date:	Date:
Number of Symptoms of 22			
Symptom Severity Score of 132			
Orientation of 5			
Immediate Memory of 15			
Concentration of 5			
Delayed Recall of 5			
SAC Total			
BESS (total errors)			
Tandem Gait (seconds)			
Coordination of 1			

Notes:

CONCUSSION INJURY ADVICE

(To be given to the **person monitoring** the concussed athlete)

This patient has received an injury to the head. A careful medical examination has been carried out and no sign of any serious complications has been found. Recovery time is variable across individuals and the patient will need monitoring for a further period by a responsible adult. Your treating physician will provide guidance as to this timeframe.

If you notice any change in behaviour, vomiting, dizziness, worsening headache, double vision or excessive drowsiness, please contact your doctor or the nearest hospital emergency department immediately.

Other important points:

- Rest (physically and mentally), including training or playing sports until symptoms resolve and you are medically cleared
- No alcohol
- No prescription or non-prescription drugs without medical supervision. Specifically:
  - No sleeping tablets
  - Do not use aspirin, anti-inflammatory medication or sedating pain killers
- Do not drive until medically cleared
- Do not train or play sport until medically cleared

Clinic phone number

Patient's name

Treating physician /

Date/time of medical review

Treatingphysician

Contact details or stamp

stimuli such as playing video games or watching television.[59,60] Once symptoms subside, a graded return-to-play protocol is implemented.

The Zurich Guidelines recommend the following graduated return-to-play progression[13]:

Stage	Functional Exercise	Objective
1. No activity	Physical and cognitive rest based on symptoms	Recovery
2. Light aerobic activity	Low-intensity (< 70% maximum heart rate) exercise such as walking or stationary cycling. Avoid resistance training.	Increase heart rate
3. Sport-specific exercise	Gradual progression in sport-specific motion patterns and activities. Avoid activities that involve —or may involve—head impact.	Functional movement
4. Noncontact training drills	Advanced sport/skill progression relative to Stage 3. Begin resistance training exercise.	Exercise, coordination, cognitive load
5. Full-contact practice	Medical clearance to participate in normal training activities	Restore confidence. Allow coaching staff to assess functional ability.
6. Return to play	Normal game play	

Adapted from: McCrory, P, et al: Consensus statement on concussion in sport: the 4th international conference on concussion in sport held in Zurich, November 2012. *Br J Sports Med*, 47:250, 2013.

Once a patient is asymptomatic in one stage, the progression to the next stage is made. A minimum of 24 hours is recommended between each stage. If the patient's symptoms reoccur, the progression reverts to the prior stage (e.g., if symptoms reoccur in Stage 5, start the next session at Stage 4).[13] Student-athletes who are recovering from a concussion may require adjunctive accommodations such as extended test taking time, use of a note taker, and a tutor during their recovery.[59]

✱ Practical Evidence

A general theme among concussion guidelines is that an athlete who displays the signs and symptoms of concussion or other brain injury must not return to competition that day.[31] Likewise, an individual should not return to activity while any of the signs and/or symptoms of a concussion are present.[61]

Postconcussion Syndrome

Athletes suffering a cerebral concussion may describe a number of cognitive impairments for some time after the injury as the result of altered neurotransmitter function.[62–64] Although this syndrome is widely reported, its definition is not standardized.[65]

✱ Practical Evidence

Adolescents who sustained a blow to the head, have a headache, and are admitted to the hospital[66] and those with a history of migraine headaches[67] are at increased risk of postconcussion syndrome.

In general, postconcussion syndrome is characterized by decreased attention span, trouble concentrating, impaired memory, and irritability over both the short and long term.[68] Exercise may cause headaches, dizziness, and premature fatigue.[63] Long-term consequences of postconcussion syndrome are balance disruptions, decreased cognitive performance, and emotional depression.[14,69] With time, social interaction, academic performance, and job performance are significantly impaired.[14]

Many of the clinical measures used to diagnose a concussion are also used to identify postconcussion syndrome. Findings such as decreased concentration, memory dysfunction, balance disturbance, and a graded symptom checklist can reveal postconcussive symptoms. The cranial nerves, especially those that control tracking (IV and VI) should be assessed since postconcussion syndrome can affect extraocular movement. The cervical spine should also be assessed since some postconcussive symptoms such as headache and dizziness may originate from the spinal nerves.[67]

Postconcussion Syndrome Intervention Strategies

Postconcussion syndrome is managed similarly to a concussion.[67] As with concussion management, cognitive rest, possibly including reduced (or no) schoolwork or screen time and no exertion during ADLs, is often indicated.[56,60] The athlete should not be returned to competition until postconcussion syndrome symptoms have resolved, and the athlete can progress through a progressive exertional protocol. CT scans and neuropsychological tests must show normal or baseline findings.

Diffuse Cerebral Swelling (Second impact syndrome)

Second impact syndrome (SIS), sustaining a second concussion while the individual is still symptomatic from an earlier concussion, has been proposed as a major risk factor for head injury–related deaths. Recent research suggests that SIS does not exist—or has been overdiagnosed—as it has been historically described.[28,33] Of those individuals who have died as the result of head injuries other than intracranial hemorrhage such as an epidural hematoma, the majority did not have a history of prior head injury.[33]

Deaths that were originally associated with SIS may actually be the result of **diffuse cerebral swelling** (diffuse cerebral edema), an abnormality of the brain's autoregulation following trauma that causes vasodilation and engorgement of the intracranial vasculature.[8,33,70] As a result, cerebrovascular congestion and brain edema occurs, leading to increased intracranial pressure.[14] The increased blood flow and vascular expanse increase the intracranial pressure and quickly disrupt the normal function of the brainstem.

Initially, the athlete may display the signs and symptoms of a concussion but quickly collapses in a semicomatose state. Pressure on the cranial nerves results in rapidly dilating pupils that are unresponsive to light and the loss of eye motion.[63] As the pressure continues to build, the athlete displays signs of respiratory distress secondary to disruption of phrenic nerve activity.

Diffuse Cerebral Swelling Intervention Strategies

Intervention must be swift and concise. The physician, paramedic, or other qualified personnel should intubate the athlete and may induce hyperventilation to facilitate vasoconstriction secondary to decreased carbon dioxide in the bloodstream. Even in the best-case scenarios, diffuse cerebral swelling has a 50% mortality rate. This severity emphasizes the importance of preventing this occurrence by prohibiting athletes from returning to athletic competition until all symptoms of a cerebral concussion have subsided and a physician has cleared the athlete's return to activity.

Intracranial Hemorrhage

Rupture of the blood vessels supplying the brain results in an intracranial hematoma, named relative to the meninges (Fig. 20-9). Intracranial hematoma may also develop after disruption of the sinus separating the two brain hemispheres. Subsequent hematoma formation within the enclosed space (the cranium) places pressure on the brain and may have catastrophic results (see Table 20-2). The length of time until the onset of symptoms varies, depending on the type of bleeding involved (arterial or venous) and the location relative to the dura mater (above or below it).

Epidural Hematoma

Arterial bleeding between the dura mater and the skull results in the rapid formation of an epidural hematoma, with the onset of symptoms occurring within hours after the initial injury. The mechanism of this injury is that of a concussion, a blow to the head that jars the brain. Because of the concussive mechanism, the athlete may be briefly unconscious and may show the signs and symptoms of mild concussion, although these are not prerequisite symptoms. These symptoms quickly subside, and the athlete progresses through a very **lucid** period (Table 20-4).

As the size of the hematoma increases, the athlete's condition deteriorates at a rate proportional to the amount of intracranial bleeding. The individual becomes disoriented, displays abnormal behavior, and complains of or displays drowsiness. A headache of increasing intensity may be reported, indicating pressure on the periosteum of the skull or an insult to the dura mater. Continued expansion of the hematoma results in outward symptoms via the cranial nerves; a unilaterally dilated pupil is the most common sign.

Subdural Hematoma

Hematoma formation between the brain and dura mater usually involves venous bleeding. This type of injury accounts for the majority of deaths resulting from athletic-related head trauma.[28] Because venous bleeding occurs at a lower pressure than arterial bleeding and because the blood collects within the fissures and sulci, the symptoms occur hours, days, or even weeks after the initial trauma. Whereas acute subdural hematomas become symptomatic within 48 hours, chronic hematomas may not manifest symptoms until 30 days after the trauma.[71]

Subdural hematomas are classified as simple or complex. No direct cerebral damage is associated with a simple

Evidence for Concussion Testing and Diagnosis

Throughout this text, we have presented the available diagnostic evidence for various orthopedic tests. The evidence surrounding the diagnosis and management of concussion is well summarized and clinically applied in widely available clinical guidelines such as the Zurich Consensus Statement. We encourage you to remain current on the ever-changing evidence and best practices in concussion diagnosis and return-to-play guidelines by reviewing the current literature.

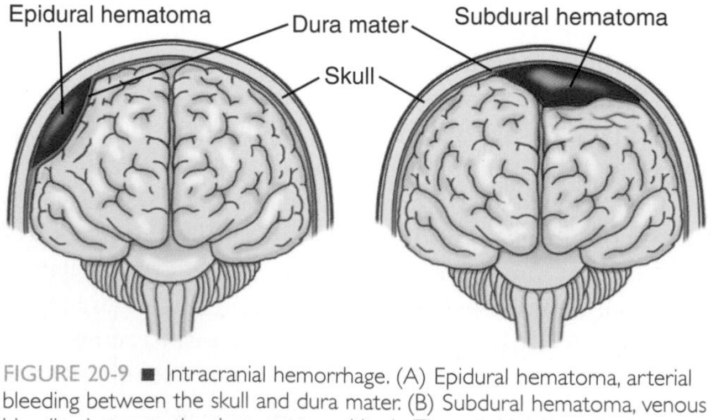

FIGURE 20-9 ■ Intracranial hemorrhage. (A) Epidural hematoma, arterial bleeding between the skull and dura mater. (B) Subdural hematoma, venous bleeding between the dura mater and brain. The meningeal spaces have been enlarged for clarity.

Table 20-4 Progression of Symptoms Associated With an Epidural Hematoma

The patient is unconscious or has other signs of a concussion (these are not prerequisite findings).
The patient has a period of very lucid consciousness, perhaps eliminating the suspicion of a serious concussion.
The patient appears to become disoriented, confused, and drowsy.
The patient complains of a headache that increases in intensity with time.
The patient develops signs and symptoms of cranial nerve disruption.
The patient slips into a coma.
If untreated, death or permanent brain damage occurs.

Lucid Mentally clear

subdural hematoma. Complex subdural hematomas are characterized by contusions of the brain's surface and associated cerebral swelling.

Initially after the injury, the individual is very lucid, even to the point of not displaying any of the signs or symptoms of a cerebral concussion. However, as blood accumulates within the brain, the patient begins to develop headaches, accompanied by a clouding of consciousness.[72] Further hematoma formation results in the impairment of cognitive, behavioral, and motor ability, and signs of cranial nerve dysfunction may be observed. The potentially long duration between the trauma and the onset of symptoms illustrates the need for home instructions identifying the latent signs and symptoms of head injuries.

Intracranial Hemorrhage Intervention Strategies

The management of intracranial hemorrhage requires diagnostic imaging and, if indicated, medical intervention including hospitalization and possible surgery to reduce intracranial pressure.

Home Instructions

Because of the delayed onset of symptoms associated with intracranial hemorrhage, there is always the potential for a more serious condition to develop. In some cases, the attending physician may elect to admit the patient to the hospital for observation. In other cases, the patient is allowed to return home.

Educate the patient's parents, roommates, and coaches of the consequences of concussion and the possibility of delayed progression of the signs and symptoms of possible intracranial injury and alert them to the appropriate course of action. A good method of doing this is by using a business card-sized instruction booklet. A list of emergency numbers (e.g., athletic trainer, physician, emergency room) is printed on the front cover. The card then opens to display a list of signs and symptoms to alert the individual to a deteriorating condition (Fig. 20-10).

Behavioral changes, forgetfulness, confusion, anger, aggression, and malaise are the most outward signs. In addition, the patient may describe nausea, vomiting, a headache with increasing severity, and a loss of appetite. Although these symptoms may be caused by other conditions, their presence after a head injury is cause for concern.

The use of medications should be judicious. Some medications such as aspirin inhibit the clotting mechanism, potentially increasing the rate of intracranial bleeding.

Prohibiting sleep after a concussion is largely founded in fiction rather than fact. Although it is necessary to keep the athlete conscious immediately after the injury, sleep should—and must—be permitted as needed. The patient's parents or roommate can be asked to check on the athlete at regular intervals. If enough doubt surrounds the athlete's condition to prohibit sleep, the physician will admit the athlete to the hospital for observation. The medical staff or emergency room personnel should be contacted immediately if any of the latent signs or symptoms of intracranial hemorrhage are manifested.

Skull Fractures

The prevalence of skull fractures is much higher in athletes who are not wearing headgear than in those who are. However, skull fractures can still occur in a head that is protected, especially in the bones around the helmet's periphery. Skull fractures are typically classified as **linear, comminuted,** or **depressed** (Fig. 20-11).

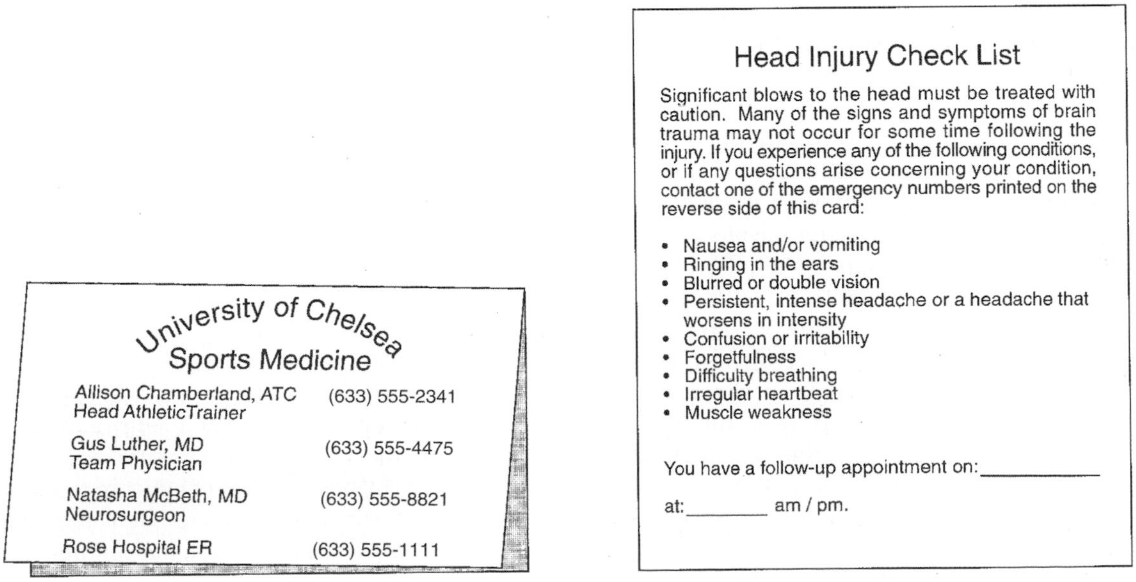
University of Chelsea
Sports Medicine

Allison Chamberland, ATC Head AthleticTrainer	(633) 555-2341
Gus Luther, MD Team Physician	(633) 555-4475
Natasha McBeth, MD Neurosurgeon	(633) 555-8821
Rose Hospital ER	(633) 555-1111

Head Injury Check List

Significant blows to the head must be treated with caution. Many of the signs and symptoms of brain trauma may not occur for some time following the injury. If you experience any of the following conditions, or if any questions arise concerning your condition, contact one of the emergency numbers printed on the reverse side of this card:

- Nausea and/or vomiting
- Ringing in the ears
- Blurred or double vision
- Persistent, intense headache or a headache that worsens in intensity
- Confusion or irritability
- Forgetfulness
- Difficulty breathing
- Irregular heartbeat
- Muscle weakness

You have a follow-up appointment on:__________

at:________ am / pm.

FIGURE 20-10 ■ Business card method of communicating home instructions to a head-injured athlete.

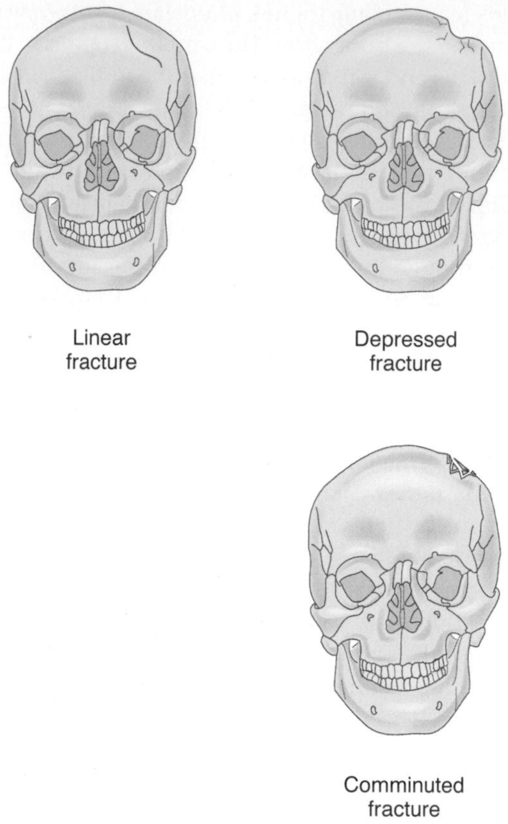

FIGURE 20-11 ■ Types of skull fractures: linear, depressed, and comminuted.

Linear fractures, referred to as hairline fractures in long bones, are caused by a blunt impact to the cranium. The subsequent swelling causes the loss of the skull's rounded contour in the traumatized area. Comminuted skull fractures result in fragmentation of the skull. A slight depression is felt during gentle palpation of the fractured area. If the blunt force is of enough intensity or fails to become deflected by the round shape of the skull, a depressed fracture can occur. The skull's indentation is obvious on gross inspection. Additional concern is focused around the possibility of the fractured pieces of bone lacerating the meninges and brain.

Although depressed skull fractures are often obvious during inspection, linear and comminuted fractures are less evident. The traumatic impact often results in a laceration of the overlying skin. Although the bleeding must be controlled, no material or object should be inserted into the laceration or possible fracture site. Fractures of the ethmoid or temporal bones may result in the leakage of CSF from the nose or ears or in bleeding from the ears (Selective Tissue Test 20-4). With time, ecchymosis may accumulate beneath the eyes and over the mastoid process (Fig. 20-12) (Examination Findings 20-2). In addition to these symptoms, the patient may also describe the signs and symptoms of a concussion caused by the blow to the skull.

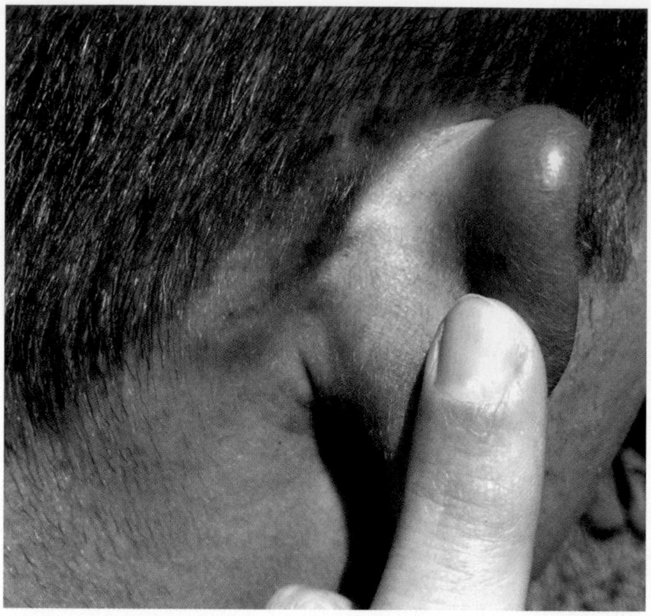

FIGURE 20-12 ■ Ecchymosis over the mastoid process, Battle's sign, may suggest a skull fracture.

*** Practical Evidence**

After a blow to the head and one or more episodes of vomiting, the probability of a skull fracture triples in adults and more than doubles in children.[73]

Examination of Acute Cervical Spine Injuries

Injuries to the cervical spine range from nagging to catastrophic. This section focuses on examination and management of potentially serious neck pathology. Noncatastrophic injuries including brachial plexus pathology are described in Chapter 14.

History

- **Location of symptoms:** Question the athlete about the location and type of pain or other symptoms experienced after the injury.
    - **Cervical pain:** The most significant finding during this portion of the examination is cervical pain or muscle spasm. The significance of this finding is magnified when it is accompanied by pain, numbness, or burning, which may or may not radiate into the extremities (Box 20-4).
- **Mechanism of cervical spine injuries:** Most of the forces directed toward the cervical spine are capable of being dissipated by the energy-absorbing properties of the cervical musculature and intervertebral discs.[75] The mechanisms of injury to the cervical spine involve flexion, extension, or lateral bending and may be accompanied by a rotational component.

Selective Tissue Tests 20-4
Halo Test

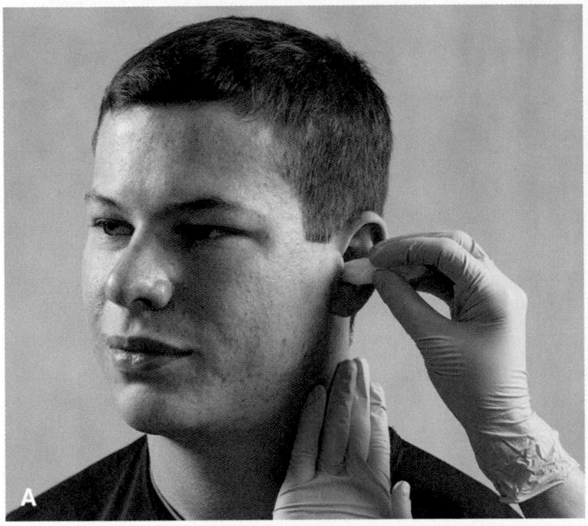

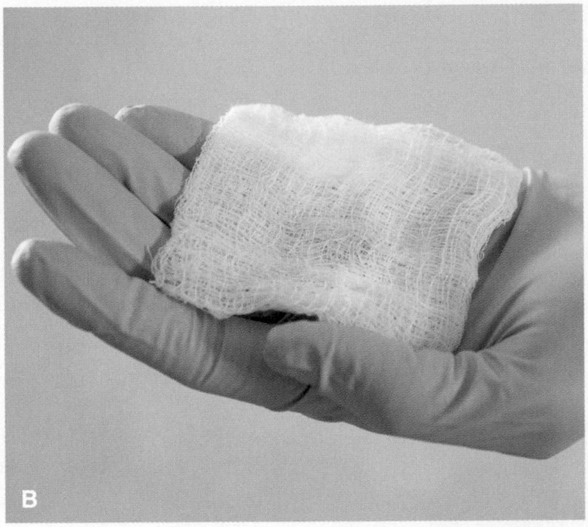

The halo test determines the presence of cerebrospinal fluid (CSF) in any fluid escaping from the ears or nose.

Patient Position	Lying or sitting
Position of Examiner	Lateral to the patient's ear
Evaluative Procedure	Fold a piece of sterile gauze into a triangle. Using the point of the gauze, collect a sample of the fluid leaking from the ear or nose and allow it to be absorbed by the gauze.
Positive Test	A pale yellow "halo" will form around the sample on the gauze.
Implications	CSF leakage, indicative of a skull fracture. The frontal bone and ethmoid bone are most commonly involved.[16]
Comments	CSF leakage from the intracranial space to the nose significantly increases the risk of infection.[16]
Evidence	Absent or inconclusive in the literature

Examination Map: Cervical Spine

HISTORY

Location of Symptoms
Cervical pain
Mechanism of Injury
- Flexion/axial loading
- Extension
- Lateral bending/rotation

Weakness

INSPECTION

Inspection of the Bony Structures
Position of the head
Cervical vertebrae
Mastoid process

FUNCTIONAL ASSESSMENT

Assess ability to move distal extremities (e.g., fingers, toes).

PALPATION

Palpation of the Bony Structures
Spinous processes
Transverse processes
Skull

Palpation of Soft Tissue
Musculature
Throat

NEUROLOGICAL EXAMINATION

Spinal Nerve Root Evaluation
Upper quarter screen
Lower quarter screen

REGION-SPECIFIC PATHOLOGIES AND SELECTIVE TISSUE TESTS

Cervical Fracture/Dislocation
Transient Quadriplegia

Examination Findings 20-2
Skull Fractures

Examination Segment	Clinical Findings
History of Current Condition	*Onset:* Acute *Pain characteristics:* Pain over the point of impact; a headache may be described secondary to the trauma. *Other symptoms:* Possible vomiting[73] *Mechanism:* Blunt trauma to the head; either the skull's being struck by a moving object or the skull's striking a stationary object
Functional Assessment	General unwillingness to move
Inspection	Bleeding may occur secondary to the blow. Ecchymosis under the eyes ("raccoon eyes") and over the mastoid process (Battle's sign) may be noted. The rounded contour of the skull over the impacted area may be lost.
Palpation	Crepitus may be felt over the fracture site. Palpation should not be performed over areas of obvious fracture.
Selective Tissue Tests	Halo test
Neurological Screening	Same as for evaluation of a cerebral concussion: cranial nerve assessment, sensory testing, and motor testing
Vascular Screening	Within normal limits, unless there are associated shock symptoms
Imaging Techniques	Computed tomography
Differential Diagnosis	Traumatic brain injury
Comments	The presence of a cervical fracture or dislocation must be ruled out. No object should be inserted into the site of a skull laceration (e.g., cleaning the wound, removing deeply impaled objects). Athletes suspected of suffering from a skull fracture should be immediately referred to a physician.

Box 20-4
Cervical Spine Clinical Decision Rules

The Canadian C-spine Rules are used to determine the need for radiography in conscious patients who have sustained traumatic cervical spine injury.[74]

Radiographs are needed if:

1. A high-risk factor is present:
   - Patient age of 65 or older
   - A history of a "dangerous mechanism" such as fall from a height, axial loading of the cervical spine, bicycle accident
   - Paraesthesia in the extremities
2. If none of the above risk factors is present, the next step is to determine if assessing range of motion (ROM) is safe. The ability to assess ROM is indicated by the ABSENCE of the following checks. If the response to any is "No," then radiographs are warranted:
   - Simple rear-end motor vehicle accident (if applicable)
   - Seated position
   - Ambulatory at any time
   - Delayed onset of neck pain
   - Absence of midline cervical spine pain
3. If any of the low-risk factors are present, then assess the patient's ability to rotate the cervical spine.
   - If the patient cannot actively rotate 45 degrees to the left AND right, then radiographs are warranted.

Flexion of the cervical spine combined with an axial load applied to the crown of the head is the mechanism most likely to produce catastrophic injury.[76,77] As the crown of the head makes contact, the cervical spine and skull flexes. As soon as the cervical spine is flexed to approximately 30 degrees, its lordotic curve is lost (Fig. 20-13). In this position, the effectiveness of the cervical spine's energy-dissipating mechanism is rendered ineffective, thus transmitting forces to the cervical vertebrae, creating an axial load through the vertical axis of the segmented columns (Fig. 20-14).

Inspection

If the athlete is wearing protective headgear at the onset of the inspection process, a decision must be made regarding whether and when to remove it. In general, football helmets should not be removed if there is any lingering suspicion of a cervical spine fracture or dislocation. In an unconscious athlete, if the helmet is loosely fitting and/or the airway cannot be accessed, then the helmet should be removed. For properly fitting helmets, the face mask can be removed to access the airway. Much of the inspection and palpation process can be performed with the helmet still in place.

Inspection of the Bony Structures

- **Position of the head:** Observe the way in which the head is positioned. Normally, the head should be upright in all planes. A laterally flexed and rotated skull that is accompanied by muscle spasm on the side opposite that of the tilt may indicate a dislocation of a cervical vertebra.
- **Cervical vertebrae:** If possible, view the athlete from behind and observe the alignment of the spinous processes. A vertebra that is obviously malaligned (i.e., rotated or displaced anteriorly or posteriorly) can signify a vertebral dislocation.
- **Mastoid process:** Note any ecchymosis over the mastoid process, Battle's sign, which may indicate a basilar skull fracture. This finding would emerge several hours following the injury.

PALPATION

Palpation should not be performed over areas of obvious deformity or suspected fracture, especially in the cervical spine and skull. Placing too much pressure on these structures may cause the bony fragment to displace, possibly resulting in catastrophic consequences. Refer to Chapter 14 for a detailed description of the palpation of the cervical spine and Chapter 19 for the description of palpating the skull and face.

Palpation of the Bony Structures

- **Spinous processes:** Keeping the athlete in the position found, palpate the **spinous processes** of the cervical and upper thoracic spine, noting any pain or deformity. If the athlete walks off the field and complains of neck pain, position the patient sitting. Standing behind the athlete, palpate the spinous processes of C7, C6, and C5 (Fig. 20-15). At approximately the C5 level, the spinous processes become less defined. Continue to palpate the area over the spinous processes of C4 and C3, noting for tenderness or crepitus.
- **Transverse processes:** Although the transverse processes of C1 are the only ones that are directly

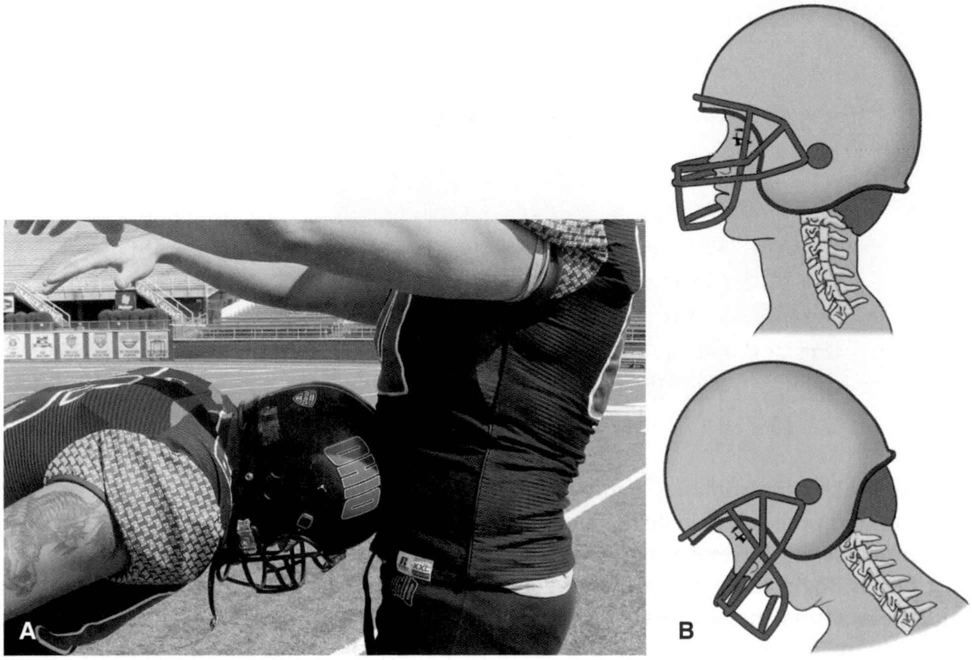

FIGURE 20-13 ■ Making Contact With the Crown of the Helmet Results in Axial Loading

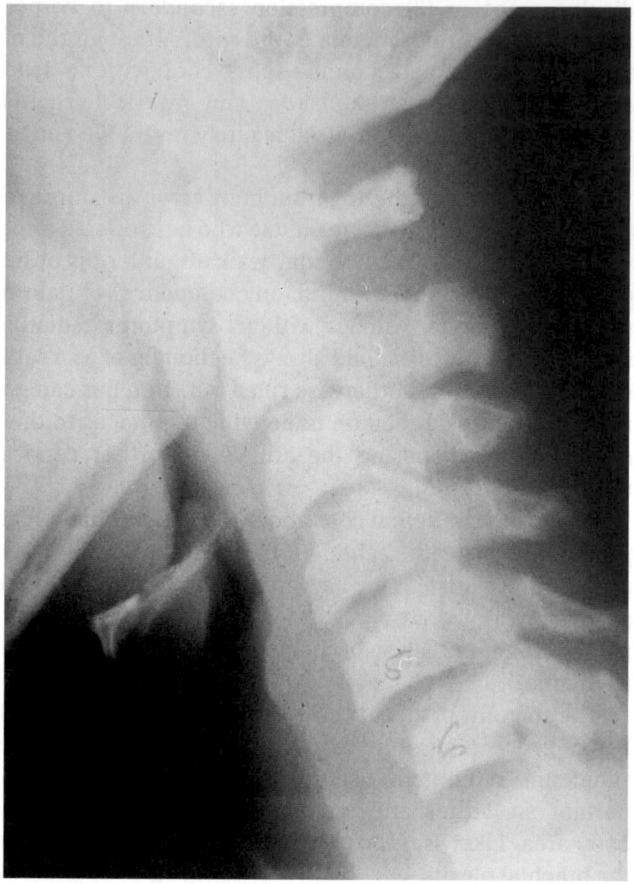

FIGURE 20-16 ■ Fracture–dislocation of the C6 vertebra. Note the posterior displacement of the vertebral body relative to C5 and the fracture of the C6 spinous process.

secondary to vertebral fractures results when a bony fragment lacerates the cord; swelling compresses the cord; ischemia affects the cord's cells; or the vertebra shifts, narrowing the spinal canal.

Cervical dislocations represent a much more serious direct threat to the spinal cord. Most often affecting the lower cervical vertebrae (C4–C6) when the cervical spine is forced into flexion and rotation, the superior articular facet passes over the inferior facet. The resulting dislocation decreases the diameter of the spinal canal, often compressing the cord.

The signs and symptoms of a stretch or pinch of the brachial plexus can mimic many of those of a spinal cord injury. The primary differences are found in the relatively rapid fading of symptoms associated with brachial plexus trauma and the fact that the symptoms most often occur unilaterally.

Trauma to the cervical spine itself is identified by pain along its posterior and lateral structures and possible spasm of the surrounding muscles. If there is associated damage to the spinal cord or if displaced bone or swelling is compressing the cord, symptoms are referred to the involved nerve distributions and in those nerves located distal to the site of the insult. Typically, these symptoms involve pain, burning, or numbness radiating into the extremities (Examination Findings 20-3). Fractures of the vertebral body may produce little or no symptoms unless the cervical spine and head are positioned in a manner that places a load on the involved body.

Other than the actual physical trauma, the spinal cord tissue is further damaged by ischemia. Pharmacologically, the use of ganglioside (GM-1), methylprednisolone, and other medications has shown promise in limiting spinal cord trauma.[81,82] The strategy of medically increasing the patient's mean arterial blood pressure above 85 mm Hg has also been demonstrated to assist in reducing the long-term effects of spinal cord trauma.[83]

Cervical Spine Fracture or Dislocation Intervention Strategies

Bony cervical spine injury that does not involve the cervical spine requires judicious, supervised return to activity. Surgical intervention to repair damaged tissue such as vertebral fusion, cervical instability, residual neurological deficit, spinal stenosis, or permanent malalignment usually contraindicates further participation in contact sports.[84] Patients who are medically cleared for competition should demonstrate appropriate strength and ROM.

Transient Quadriplegia

Blows to the head that force the cervical spine into hyperextension, hyperflexion, or create an axial load may result in transient quadriplegia (quadriparesis), a body-wide state of decreased or absent sensory and motor function.[79,85,86] This results from neurapraxia of the cervical spinal cord and is predisposed by stenosis of the spinal foramen (especially at the C3–C4 level), congenital fusion of the cervical canal, abnormalities of the posterior arch, or cervical instability.[79] The risk of transient quadriplegia is increased when the ratio between the diameter of the spinal canal and the diameter of the vertebral body is 0.80 or less.[79,86] The narrowing of the spinal canal predisposes the spinal cord to compressive and contusive forces, a condition referred to as spear tackler's spine.[84]

Initially, the signs and symptoms of transient quadriplegia resemble those of a catastrophic cervical injury. Symptoms range from sensory dysfunction to burning pain, numbness, or paresthesia in the upper and lower extremities. Likewise, upper and lower extremity motor function is inhibited, ranging from muscular weakness to complete paralysis. However, these symptoms clear within 15 minutes to 48 hours. Pain within the cervical spine is limited to burning paresthesia.[79]

The definitive diagnosis of transient quadriplegia is made through imaging and electrophysiological testing. Radiographic examination is used to rule out fractures or congenital abnormalities of the cervical spine, and CT scans are used to gain a better definition of the cervical bony anatomy. The integrity of the spinal cord and its roots is determined by using MRI scans, **electromyelograms**, and nerve conduction velocity testing.

Electromyelogram The recording of the electrical activity within a muscle

Examination Findings 20-3
Cervical Spine Fracture or Dislocation

Examination Segment	Clinical Findings
History of Current Condition	*Onset:* Acute *Pain characteristics:* Pain in the cervical spine Chest pain *Other symptoms:* Numbness, weakness, or paresthesia radiating into the extremities Cervical muscle spasm Loss of bladder or bowel control *Mechanism:* Fractures most commonly secondary to an axial load placed on the cervical vertebrae Dislocations most commonly resulting from hyperflexion or hyperextension and rotation of the cervical spine *Risk factors:* Increased risk of cervical fracture if the normal lordotic curve of the cervical spine is decreased[79]
Functional Assessment	Determine if patient can move fingers and toes.
Inspection	Malalignment of the cervical spine spinous processes may be observed. The head may be abnormally tilted and rotated. Unilateral cervical dislocations result in the head's tilting toward the site of the dislocation. The muscles on the side opposite the dislocation (tilt) are in spasm. Those muscles on the side of the dislocation are flaccid.
Palpation	Tenderness, crepitus, or swelling may be present over the cervical spine. Unilateral or bilateral muscle spasm may be present.
Joint and Muscle Function Assessment	ROM testing should only be performed if warranted by the Canadian C-Spine Rules (see Box 20-4).
Joint Stability Tests	*Stress tests:* Not performed acutely *Joint play:* Not performed acutely
Selective Tissue Tests	Not applicable in acute conditions in which a fracture or dislocation is suspected
Neurological Screening	Upper quarter and lower quarter neurological screens
Vascular Screening	Within normal limits
Imaging Techniques	Radiographs, MRI, CT scans[80]
Differential Diagnosis	Brachial plexus neuropathy, intervertebral disc injury, cervical vertebra sprain, injury of the cervical musculature
Comments	Athletes suspected of suffering a spinal cord injury should be immediately stabilized and transported. Trauma to the brainstem or phrenic nerve may result in cardiac arrest.

CT = computed tomography; MRI = magnetic resonance imaging; ROM = range of motion

Transient Quadriplegia Intervention Strategies

Athletes must not be returned to competition while neurological symptoms including pain, motor weakness, paresthesia, or numbness are present. The athlete's cervical region must have a preinjury level of strength and ROM. Clinical and radiographic examination should reveal no evidence of spinal stenosis, disc injury, or vertebral instability, and the cervical spine should have its normal lordotic curvature. Athletes who experience more than one episode of transient quadriplegia should be disqualified from contact sports.[79]

On-Field Examination and Management of Cervical Spine Injuries and the Unconscious Athlete

The decisions made during a crisis situation are key to the proper management of head and cervical spine trauma. It is the medical staff's responsibility to have a planned course of action that has been discussed and approved by the athletic training staff, physician, emergency medical service (EMS), and administration (see Chapter 2). Before the start of each season, these procedures must be reviewed by the involved parties, with each understanding not only his or her own roles but also those of the others. Further, the techniques discussed in this text must be reviewed and rehearsed until each member is comfortable performing them. The procedures described in this section assume that more than one responder knowledgeable of the plan is present.

Because of the importance of not unnecessarily moving an athlete with a spinal injury and the potentially catastrophic ramifications of doing so, athletic trainers should conduct meetings with each team, instructing the athletes not to help injured players to their feet. In too many instances, these well-intentioned actions have resulted in an athlete's death or permanent paralysis.

This section assumes that the responder has a minimum of emergency cardiac care (ECC) certification which includes cardiopulmonary resuscitation (CPR) and use of an AED. The procedures discussed in this section are not intended to supersede formal ECC training. Refer to Chapter 2 for more information on emergency preparedness.

Equipment Considerations

When, where, and how to remove a helmet after a spinal injury is a debatable issue.[87] Central to the decision of removing equipment is whether or not the cervical spine can be maintained in a neutral position.[88] The consensus opinion is the football helmet should not be removed during the prehospital care of a patient with a spinal injury except in three circumstances:

1. The helmet is does not fit properly, thereby allowing of movement of the head within the helmet, or
2. The equipment prevents neutral alignment of the cervical spine, or
3. The equipment prevents airway or chest access.[87]

Football helmets are radiographic translucent (Fig. 20-17). In most cases, a definitive diagnosis can be made before removal.[80]

The strongest argument in support of removing the helmet and shoulder pads involves the necessity, or the potential necessity, of **defibrillating** the athlete's heart.[87] Proper protocol for the use of an AED requires that the athlete's chest be completely exposed and dry to place the electrodes over the apex of the heart and inferior to the right clavicle.

This section first discusses making the airway and chest accessible for CPR or the physical examination of these areas. Regardless of the athlete's condition, the helmet or shoulder pads must be removed at some point, whether on the field or in the hospital, and safely doing so is not an easy task. These techniques must be practiced and rehearsed before actually performing them on stricken athletes requiring assistance. Often it is necessary to assist hospital personnel with this procedure because they may be unfamiliar with the sport's equipment.

Face Mask Removal

An alternative to removing the athlete's helmet is to remove the face mask, which is commonly held in place by four plastic clips (Fig. 20-18).[89] The face mask should be completely removed if spinal cord injury is suspected, if there is any possibility that rescue breathing or CPR will be administered, or if the patient will be transported on a spine board.[88] The fastest method of face mask removal that imposes the least amount of movement is a cordless electric screwdriver. Because the screwdriver is not 100% reliable in removing screws, an alternative tool to cut the clips should always be available (Fig. 20-19).[88,90–92]

*** Practical Evidence**

Many "quick release" face mask attachment systems allow faster access to the airway and result in less cervical spine motion than traditional "loop and strap" attachment devices.[93]

Regardless of the method used to remove the face mask, this procedure requires two people. In-line stabilization of the head and cervical spine must be maintained, and the cervical spine must be guarded against any movement that may occur during this process, especially avoiding hyperflexion of the cervical spine.

Chest Exposure

Auscultation of heart sounds, external cardiac compression during CPR, and use of an AED require that the athlete's sternum be exposed. First the athlete's shirt is cut to expose the shoulder pads, and, if the shirt is particularly tight fitting, it is cut along the anterior portion of the sleeves. Next, the clinician cuts or unfastens the rib straps on the sternal

Defibrillation (defibrillating) The process of restoring a normal heartbeat

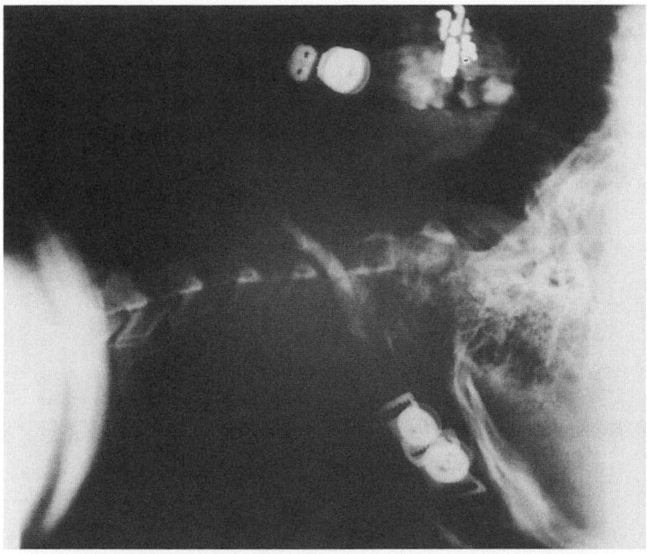

FIGURE 20-17 ■ Radiograph of the cervical spine through a helmet. Note the metal snaps for the chin strap.

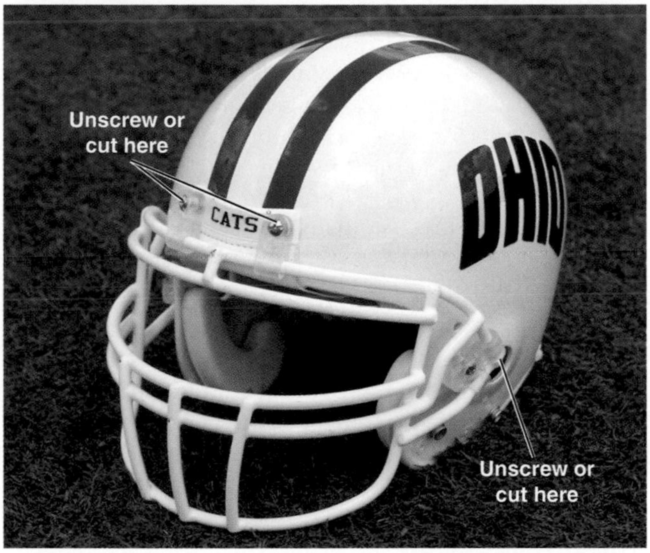

FIGURE 20-18 ■ Clips attaching the face mask to the helmet.

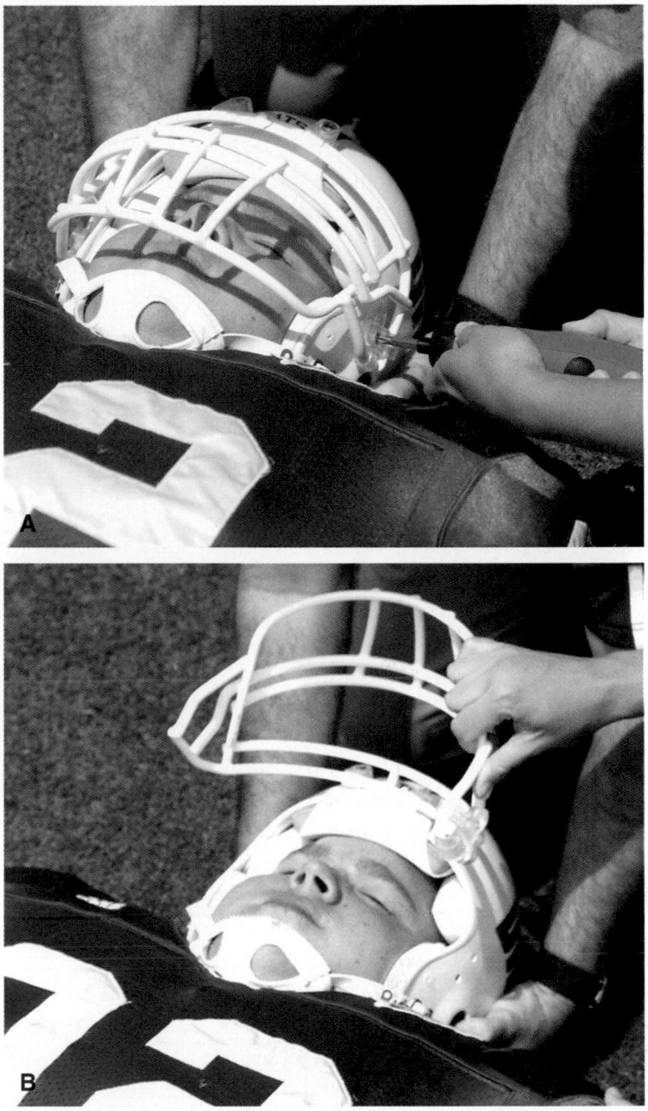

FIGURE 20-19 ■ Using an electric screwdriver to remove the screws attaching the face mask to the helmet and exposing the athlete's airway. Because of the possibility of damage or rusting of the screw or bolt, a cutting-type face mask removal tool should always be available.

portion of the pads and cuts the laces holding together the anterior portion of the pad. The halves are spread to expose the sternum (Fig. 20-20). At this point, an AED can be applied (Fig. 20-21).

Helmet Removal

In cases necessitating the removal of the helmet (e.g., improperly fitting helmet, inability to secure the head to the spine board with the helmet on), two people are necessary to perform the process in a manner that minimizes the amount of cervical spine motion (Fig. 20-22). A semirigid collar can be fitted to the cervical spine before removing the helmet if the relationship of the helmet, shoulder pads, and surface provides sufficient room to do this with a minimum of movement; this may also require removing the shoulder pads (see Using a Spine Board, p. 889).

While maintaining in-line stabilization, the other responder cuts the chin strap or straps. A flat instrument, such as the handle of a pair of scissors, is slid between the cheek pad and the helmet. A twist of this instrument causes the pad to unsnap and separate from the helmet. The pad is removed, and the procedure is repeated on the opposite side. The person who has been applying the in-line stabilization now slips a finger in each ear hole and spreads the helmet. As the helmet is slowly slid off the head, the second responder reaches behind the neck to support the cervical spine and provide a firm grip on the head.

Shoulder Pad Removal

When a serious cervical spine injury is suspected, the shoulder pads are removed only when the athlete's life is—or will be—in jeopardy.[88] This decision warrants that the

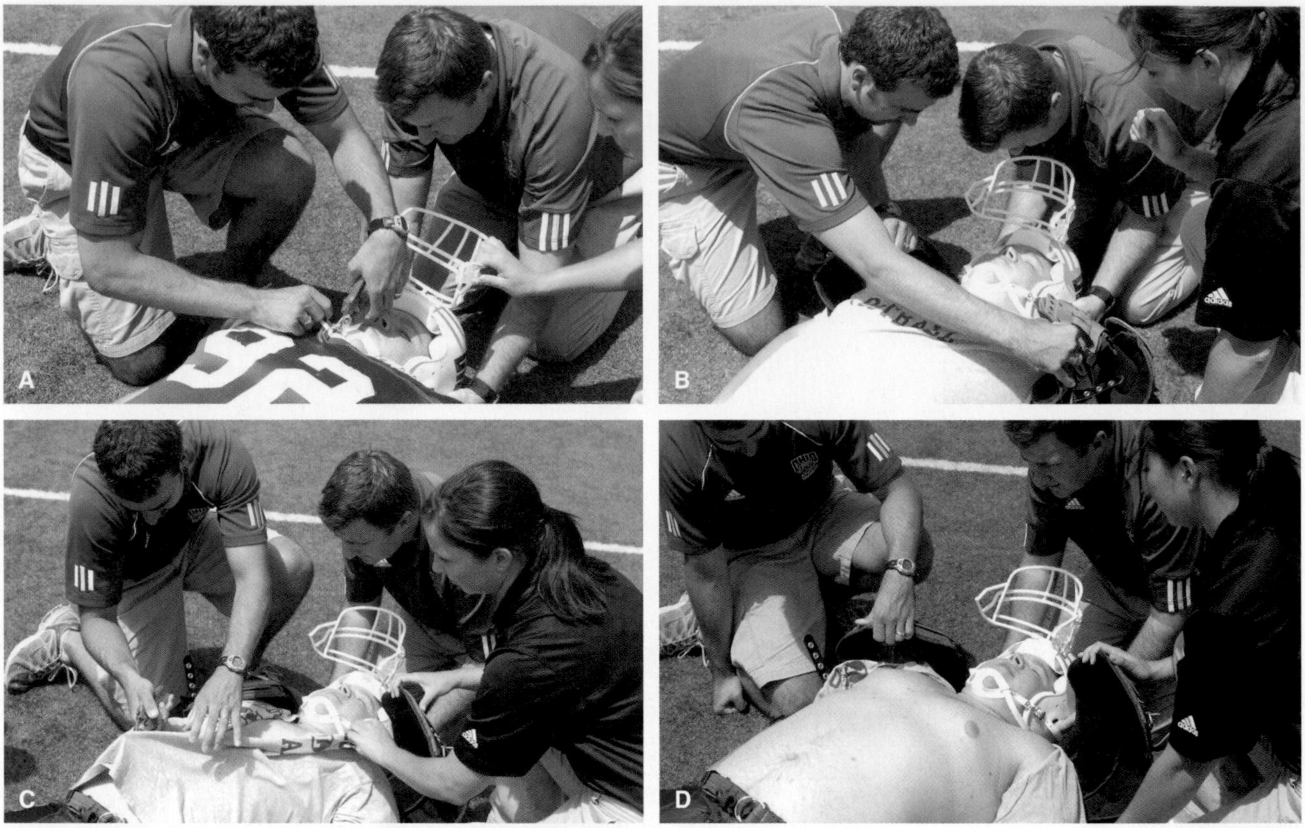

FIGURE 20-20 ■ Exposing the athlete's sternum so that cardiopulmonary resuscitation can be performed. (A) The jersey is cut. (B) The laces holding the shoulder pads together are cut and the halves of the shoulder pads are spread. (C) The underlying t-shirt is cut. (D) The shoulder pads and shirts are moved back to expose the athlete's chest. See also Figure 20.21 for the placement of AED electrodes. Note that in the event of cervical spine injury the facemask should be completely removed.

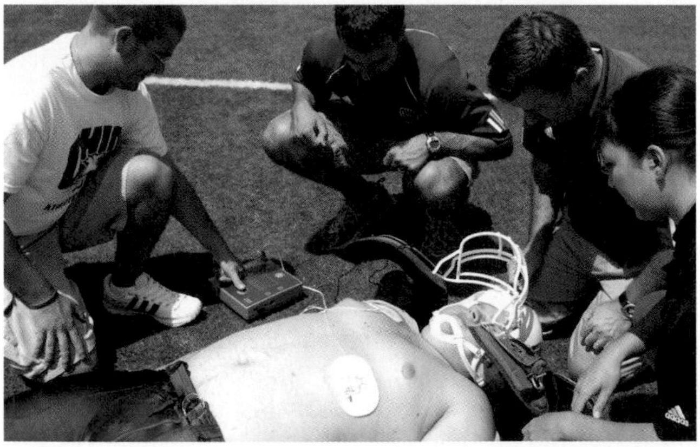

FIGURE 20-21 ■ Preparing the patient for AED application.

immediate threat to the athlete's life outweighs the possibility of spinal cord injury that may result from moving the athlete. This decision should be made by a physician, if one is present. Otherwise, the decision is made by the attending athletic trainer, emergency medical technician, or paramedic.

This procedure is most safely performed after the cervical spine has been stabilized by a hard or firm collar and the helmet removed. The responder begins this procedure by performing the steps described in the section on exposing the chest. After the anterior and axillary shoulder straps have been cut, the two halves of the shoulder pads may be widened. While one person continues to support the athlete's head, the shoulder pads are slid off the shoulders and over the head (Fig. 20-23).

Initial Inspection

The initial inspection encompasses contingencies that must be noted on arrival at the accident scene. These factors provide clues to the severity of the injury and insight regarding the proper on-field management of the patient.

- **Encumbering circumstances:** Encumbering circumstances are factors that make the worst-case scenarios even more difficult to handle. Examples of these include a diver who is still in the water, a football player who is lying on top of another player, a gymnast in a soft landing pit, or a hockey player whose head and neck are still against the boards.
- **Movement:** Any movement by the athlete must be noted. Unconscious athletes may be lying perfectly still or may have a seizure. Likewise, conscious athletes may lie still out of fear or grogginess.
- **Position:** Ideally, the athlete should be supine. Athletes who are side-lying or prone eventually must be

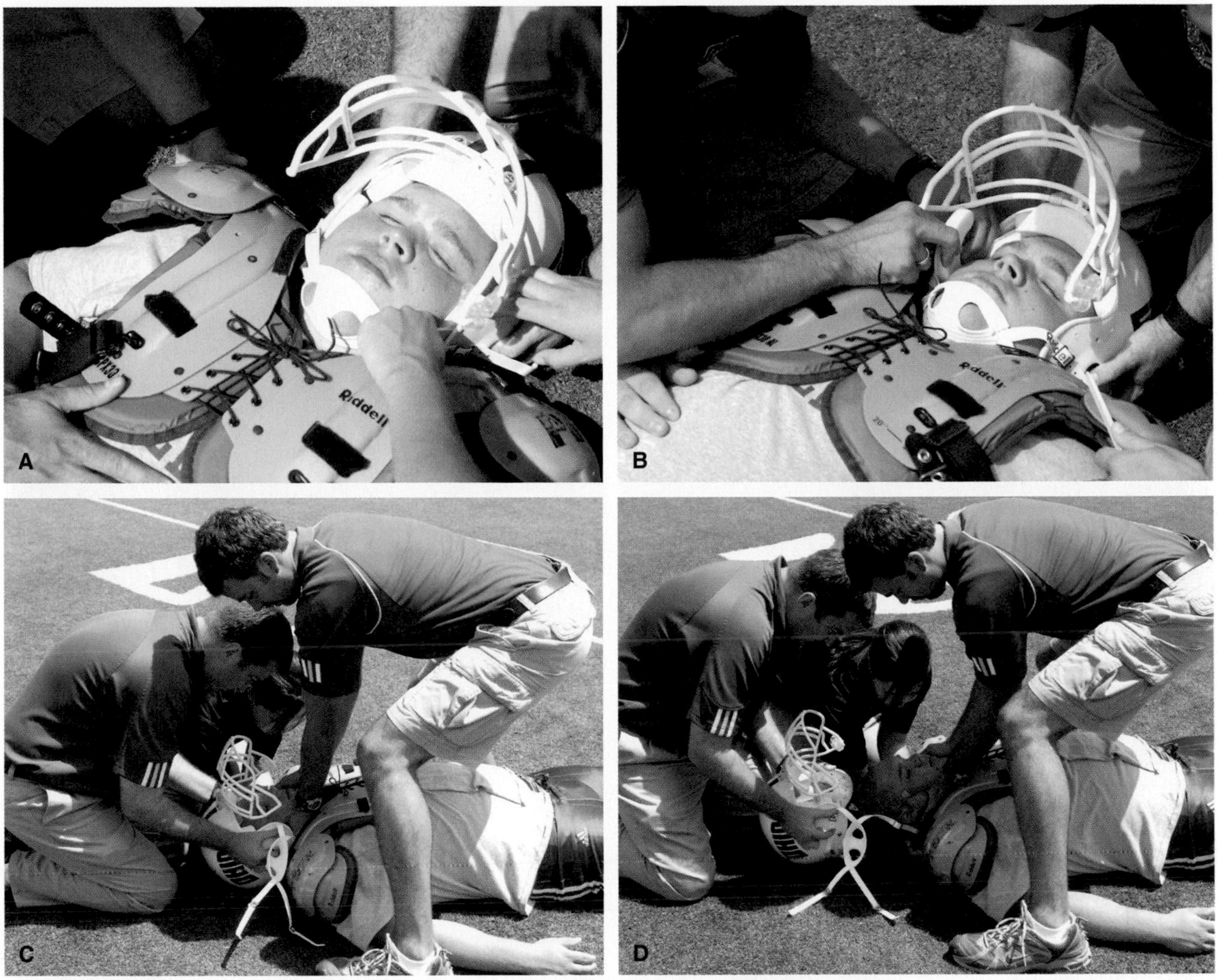

FIGURE 20-22 ■ Removing a football helmet. (A) In-line stabilization is maintained while a cheek pad is removed using a blunt object. (B) The opposite cheek guards is removed. (C) The chin strap is uncut or unsnapped. (D) Secondary stabilization is applied to the cervical spine as the helmet is spread and slid off the athlete's head.

rolled, but these initial assessments must be made before the decision to move the athlete is made.

- **Posture:** The alignment of the athlete's arms, legs, and cervical spine relative to the trunk is noted (Inspection Findings 20-1). Splayed extremities must be aligned with the rest of the body if spine boarding or rolling the athlete is required. Male athletes who are suffering from a lesion of the spinal cord at the thoracic or cervical level may also demonstrate **priapism**.

Initial Action

After arriving at the scene, the responder's actions within the first 3 or 4 minutes strongly determine whether the athlete lives, dies, or becomes permanently disabled. Despite this urgency, the responder must not rush through these processes but must perform each with care and diligence.

Priapism Spontaneous penile erection

- **Stabilize the cervical spine:** One responder must immediately assume control of the head by applying in-line stabilization. If the athlete is wearing a helmet, in-line stabilization is achieved by firmly grasping the sides of the helmet in the area of the ear holes and applying firm stabilization along the vertical axis of the cervical spine (Fig. 20-24). If the athlete is not wearing a helmet, stabilization is applied by grasping the skull beneath the occipital bone and mandible on each side, maintaining in-line stabilization.

From t[hcb8]his point until the situation resolves, either by the determination that no cervical spine injury exists or by the athlete's placement on a spine board, the person at the head maintains the in-line stabilization and directs the other individuals providing assistance. Movement of the spinal column may result in a fragmented or displaced piece of bone lacerating the spinal cord and causing death or permanent disability.

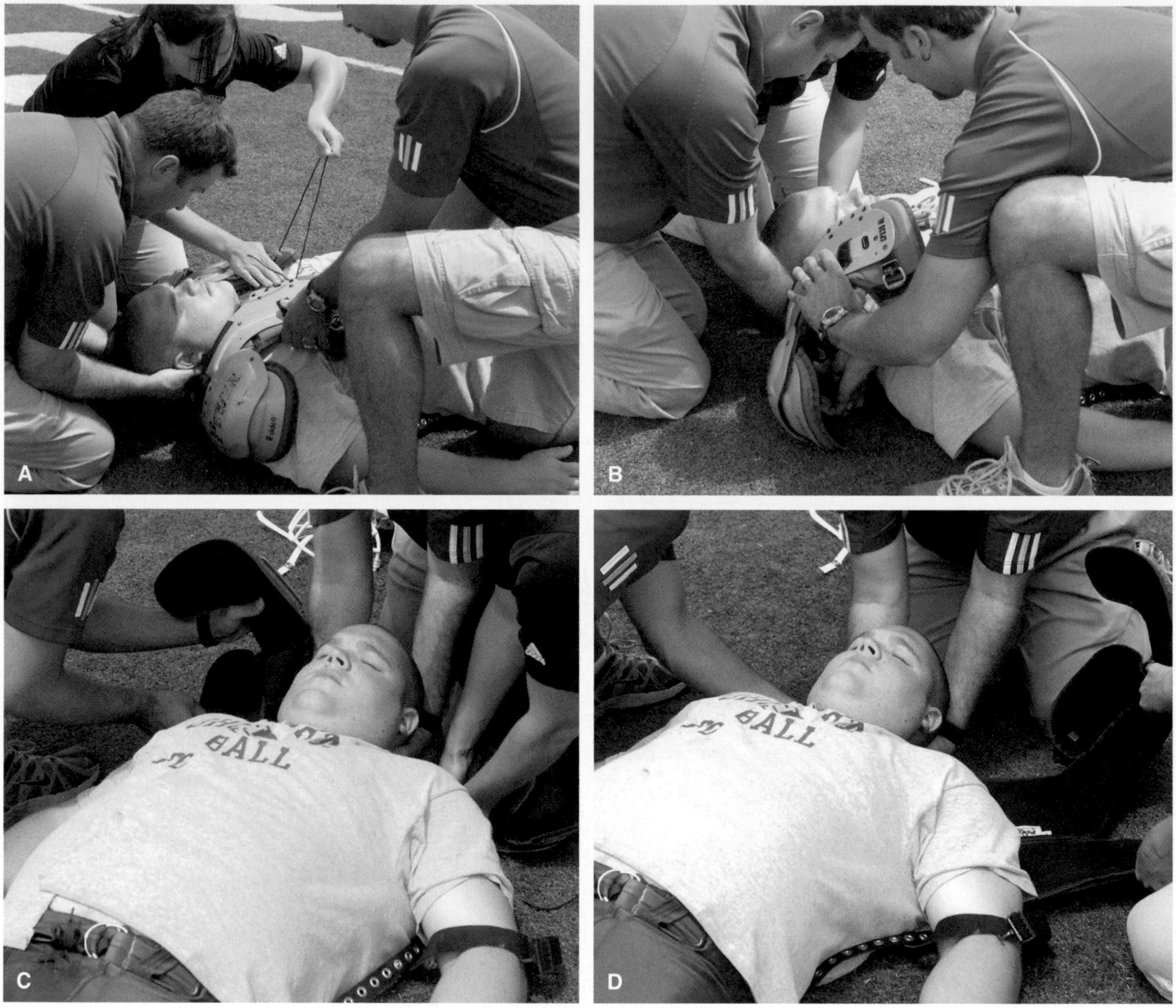

FIGURE 20-23 ■ Removing the shoulder pads. After removing the athlete's jersey and unsnapping or cutting the axial straps: (A) The sternal laces holding the pads together are cut or untied. (B) The shoulder pad is spread. (C) The one half of the shoulder pads are slid from under the athlete. (D) The shoulder pads are pulled from under the athlete. Note that in-line cervical stabilization is maintained throughout this procedure.

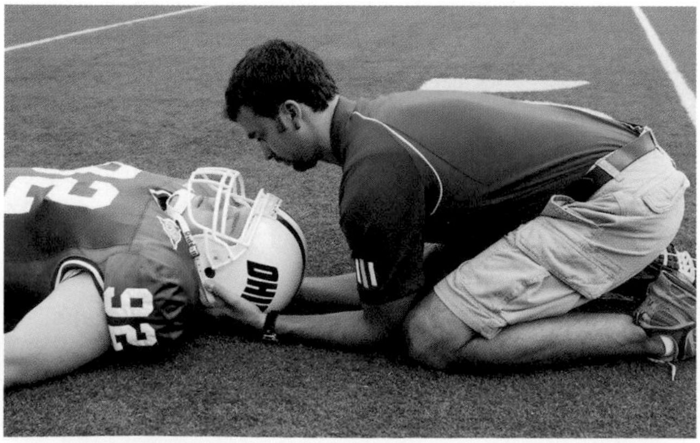

FIGURE 20-24 ■ Applying in-line stabilization to the cervical spine.

- **Clear airway:** Remove the athlete's mouthpiece. In addition, inspect the mouth for other objects that may become lodged in the athlete's airway.
- **Determine the level of consciousness:** In cases in which the athlete is not obviously responsive, the level of consciousness can be determined by calling the athlete's name and asking, "CAN YOU HEAR ME?" If this verbal stimulus fails to evoke a motor response, the athlete's response to a painful stimulus can be determined by applying pressure to the bed of a fingernail (see Fig. 20-5). Failure to evoke a response through either of these methods indicates that the athlete is unconscious. At this time, reevaluate the athlete's cardiovascular and respiratory status.

Inspection Findings 20-1
Postures Assumed After Spinal Cord Injury

Decerebrate Posture

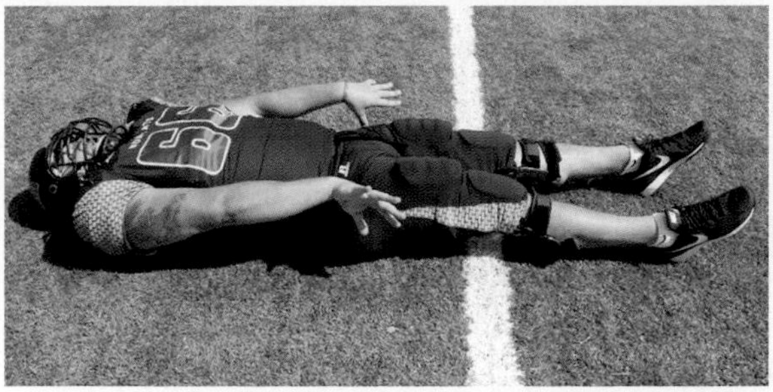

Description Extension of the extremities and retraction of the head
Pathology Lesion of the brainstem; also possible secondary to heat stroke

Decorticate Posture

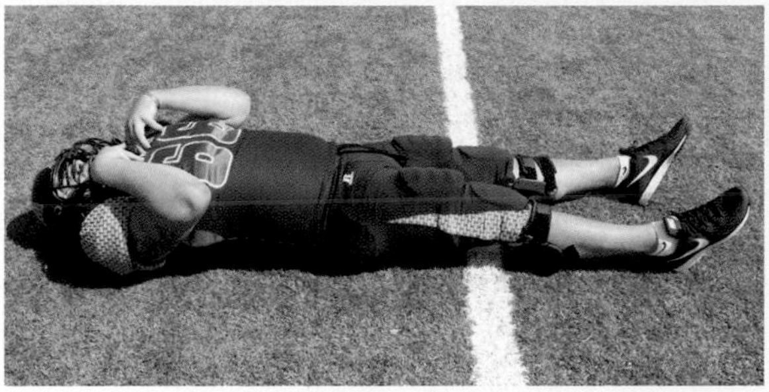

Description Flexion of the elbows and wrists, clenched fists, and extension of the lower extremity
Pathology Lesion above the brainstem

Flexion Contracture

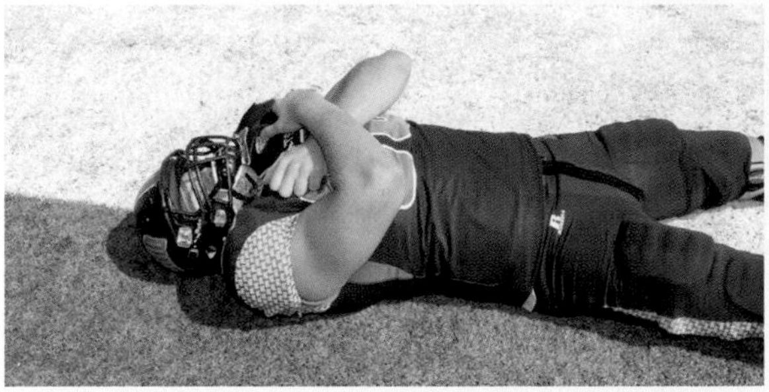

Description Arms flexed across the chest
Pathology Spinal cord lesion at the C5–C6 level

- **Secondary screen:** The torso and extremities are observed for any signs of additional trauma such as a fracture, joint dislocation, or bleeding. Of these pathologies, controlling bleeding takes the highest priority because of the need to preserve the athlete's blood pressure.

Management of the Unconscious Athlete

Unconsciousness that is more than transient warrants the activation of the emergency medical system. If the athlete regains consciousness, follow the procedures described in the "Management of the Conscious Athlete" section. The athlete's cervical spine continues to be stabilized using in-line stabilization during these procedures.

Patient Positioning: Following activation of the emergency plan and while maintaining in-line cervical spine stabilization, if the athlete is prone or side-lying, reposition to the supine position. Bystanders must be recruited to quickly roll the athlete to the supine position, foregoing the immediate use of a spine board. Once the patient is in the supine position, assess for breathing and circulation. As this is happening, another provider should be working to remove the face mask to access the patient's airway. Adjunctive airways (nasopharyngeal or oropharyngeal) must be available for use as indicated.

Immediately follow the current Emergency Cardiac Care Guidelines (Note: Because these guidelines change, they are not included in this text).

Management of the Unconscious but Breathing Athlete

This section assumes that the athlete has an open airway and the cardiopulmonary system is functioning normally. Although these findings initially appear to be normal, they require continuous monitoring because the worst-case scenario involves the athlete's progressing to cardiac arrest. Lesions in the C1 region of the spinal cord alter brainstem function and result in almost immediate cardiac arrest. C2 to C4 lesions or subsequent hemorrhage and hematoma formation at these levels can interrupt the phrenic nerve, possibly resulting in a delayed onset of respiratory arrest.

- **Cervical spine evaluation:** Gently palpate the cervical spine for signs of gross bony deformity or swelling. The absence of these signs, however, does not rule out the possibility of cervical spine injury.
- **Blood pressure:** The athlete's blood pressure is monitored and recorded so that any change over time may be identified. If a blood pressure cuff is not immediately available, the athlete's blood pressure can be estimated based on where the pulses can be palpated[94]:

Palpable Pulse	Minimum Systolic Blood Pressure, mm Hg
Carotid artery	60
Femoral artery	70
Radial artery	90

- **Pupil responsiveness:** The athlete's eyelids are opened to observe for pupillary response. The act of opening the eyelids alone should cause the pupils to constrict. The absence of pupillary response indicates that the brain is not receiving oxygen or that substantial brain trauma has occurred.
- **Continuation of monitoring:** The athlete's respirations, blood pressure, pupillary reflex, and pulse are monitored and recorded every 5 minutes. Decreased respiration, increased blood pressure, and decreased heart rate are signs of an expanding intracranial lesion.

Management of the Conscious Athlete

The on-field management described in this section assumes that the athlete has been determined to be conscious, in-line stabilization has been applied to the athlete's cervical spine, the athlete's mouthpiece has been removed, and the presence of an open airway has been established.

As long as the athlete displays stable vital signs, no attempts should be made to move the athlete until the possibility of a spinal fracture has been ruled out or the athlete is stabilized with a spine board and cervical collar. The athlete may express the desire to move or may attempt to do so. Either through verbal commands or gentle restraint, the athlete should not be allowed to move until the possibility of a fracture has been ruled out.

History

Question the athlete regarding any loss of consciousness, the mechanism of the injury, and any areas of pain or paresthesia in the cervical spine or radiating into the extremities. Any significant findings of pain or numbness radiating into the extremities or cervical pain warrant the immediate spine boarding of the athlete and transport to the hospital.

- **Loss of consciousness:** Determine if the athlete lost consciousness, even for a brief period of time. A transitory loss of consciousness may be described as "blacking out" or "seeing stars."
- **Mechanism of injury:** Identify how the injurious force was delivered. A direct blow to the head can result in either brain or cervical spine trauma. If this mechanism forces the cervical spine into flexion or extension, cervical spine trauma should be suspected. If the athlete cannot recall the onset of injury, bystanders or witnesses may be able to describe it.
- **Symptoms:** Question the athlete regarding the symptoms that indicate spinal pathology. Positive findings for any of the following support the assumption that a spinal cord or cervical vertebral injury is present:
  - Pain in the cervical spine
  - Numbness, tingling, or burning pain radiating through the upper or lower extremities
  - Sensation of weakness in the cervical spine, upper extremities, or lower extremities
  - Burning or aching in the chest secondary to cardiac pathology

Inspection

This inspection process supplements the information gained during the observations made on the way to the scene and may be conducted concurrently with the previously described segments of the examination. If the athlete is supine, the inspection of the posterior cervical structures can be delayed until the athlete is moved to the sidelines or omitted if the athlete is being transported to the hospital.

- **Cervical vertebrae:** Observe the cervical vertebrae spinous processes, if visible. They should display a normal alignment.
- **Cervical musculature:** Observe for the presence of muscle spasm indicating a cervical fracture, a dislocation, or a strain of the cervical muscles.

PALPATION

Palpation is conducted to confirm any visual findings of malalignment and identify underlying pathology. Too much pressure during palpation must be avoided to prevent the possible displacement of a bony fragment. If the athlete is supine, palpation can be performed by reaching beneath the athlete. Certain pieces of equipment, such as cervical collars, can prohibit palpation while the athlete is either prone or supine.

- **Cervical spine:** Palpate the area over the spinous and transverse processes for signs of vertebral malalignment, crepitus, or tenderness. Any of these signs signifies the possibility of a **cervical spine** fracture or dislocation.
- **Cervical musculature:** Palpate the **cervical musculature** for signs of spasm in the upper portion of the trapezius, levator scapulae, scalenes, or sternocleidomastoid muscles. Unilateral spasm is an indication of a cervical vertebral dislocation, especially when the skull is rotated and tilted toward the opposite side.

Neurological Testing

- **Sensory testing:** Although formal dermatome testing may be conducted while the athlete is on the field, the essential finding is that of normal and bilaterally equal sensation in the upper and lower extremities. Sensation is assessed by comparing bilateral perception of touch along the following body areas:

Upper Extremity		Lower Extremity	
Area	**Dermatome**	**Area**	**Dermatomes**
Superior shoulder	C4	Lateral thigh	L1, L2, L3
Lateral humerus	C5	Lateral lower leg and foot	L5, S1
Lateral forearm	C6	Medial lower leg and foot	L4
Middle finger	C7		
Medial forearm	C8		
Medial humerus	T1		

- **Active motion:** Active movements are first performed on the small joints because motion of the large joints (e.g., knees and hips) may result in a significant shift of the body. Begin by asking the athlete to wiggle the toes and fingers, progressing to movement of the ankles, wrists, knees, elbows, hips, and shoulders. Each of these motions should be performed smoothly and appear bilaterally equal.
- **Motor testing:** If no other signs and symptoms of cervical vertebral involvement exist and active motion is available, the athlete's ability to resist movements of the upper extremity may be assessed.

Removing the Athlete From the Field

Each on-field incident ends with the decision of how to remove the athlete from the field. The extremes of the possible scenarios range from the athlete walking off the field without assistance to rolling and placing the athlete on a spine board. Cases that lie between these extremes require that the medical staff make a decision about the best method to safely remove the athlete.

Any suspected cervical spine trauma mandates that the athlete be placed on a spine board and transported to a hospital via an ambulance. The use of stretchers without a spine board is to be avoided in these cases. In addition, if any doubt exists, the most conservative form of management should be chosen.

Walking the Athlete off the Field

Removing athletes from the field under their own power is not as straightforward as standing the athlete up and having him or her walk off the field. After a head injury, the sudden change from a lying to a standing position may make the blood pressure drop suddenly, causing the athlete to faint or become unsteady.

The athlete's body should be allowed to gradually adjust to the change in positions, using a three-step process. First, the athlete is brought to a sitting position with the knees bent. The athletic trainer is positioned behind the athlete, providing support and being ready to assist the athlete if dizziness occurs. This position is maintained until the athlete feels comfortable with the position. The athlete then kneels forward on one knee and again waits, to ensure that dizziness does not occur. Finally, the athlete is brought to the standing position, with assistance being provided on either side. If the symptoms increase in any of these positions, the athlete should be transported in a supine or sitting position.

Using a Spine Board

In-line stabilization is maintained throughout these procedures until the athlete's head is securely affixed to the spine board. These procedures should be discussed and practiced with the emergency medical squad.

Cervical spine stabilization. If possible, the cervical spine should be stabilized using a semirigid collar, such as a Philadelphia collar, prior to spine boarding (Fig. 19-27). These devices are most easily applied when the athlete is not wearing shoulder pads or a helmet. Other types of collars, such as a vacuum splint cervical immobilizer, can be used for stabilization when the helmet and shoulder pads are still in place.[95]

After the two halves of the collar are separated, the posterior shell is compressed and slid behind the cervical spine, taking care to prevent spinal movement. This section should fit snugly beneath the athlete's occipital and mastoid processes. The anterior shell is fitted so that it envelops the chin. Most models have an opening on the sternal pad that allows access to the trachea in case a **tracheotomy** must be performed.

The supine athlete. When spine boarding spinal injury, the six-plus person lift is recommended.[96] In this case, one person applies in-line stabilization (referred to as the leader) as an appropriate number of people control the athlete's torso and legs, while another person manipulates the spine board (Fig. 20-25). The leader maintains in-line stabilization throughout the lift and subsequent stabilization of the athlete on the spine board and is responsible for instructing and guiding the remaining personnel in the sequence to be performed.

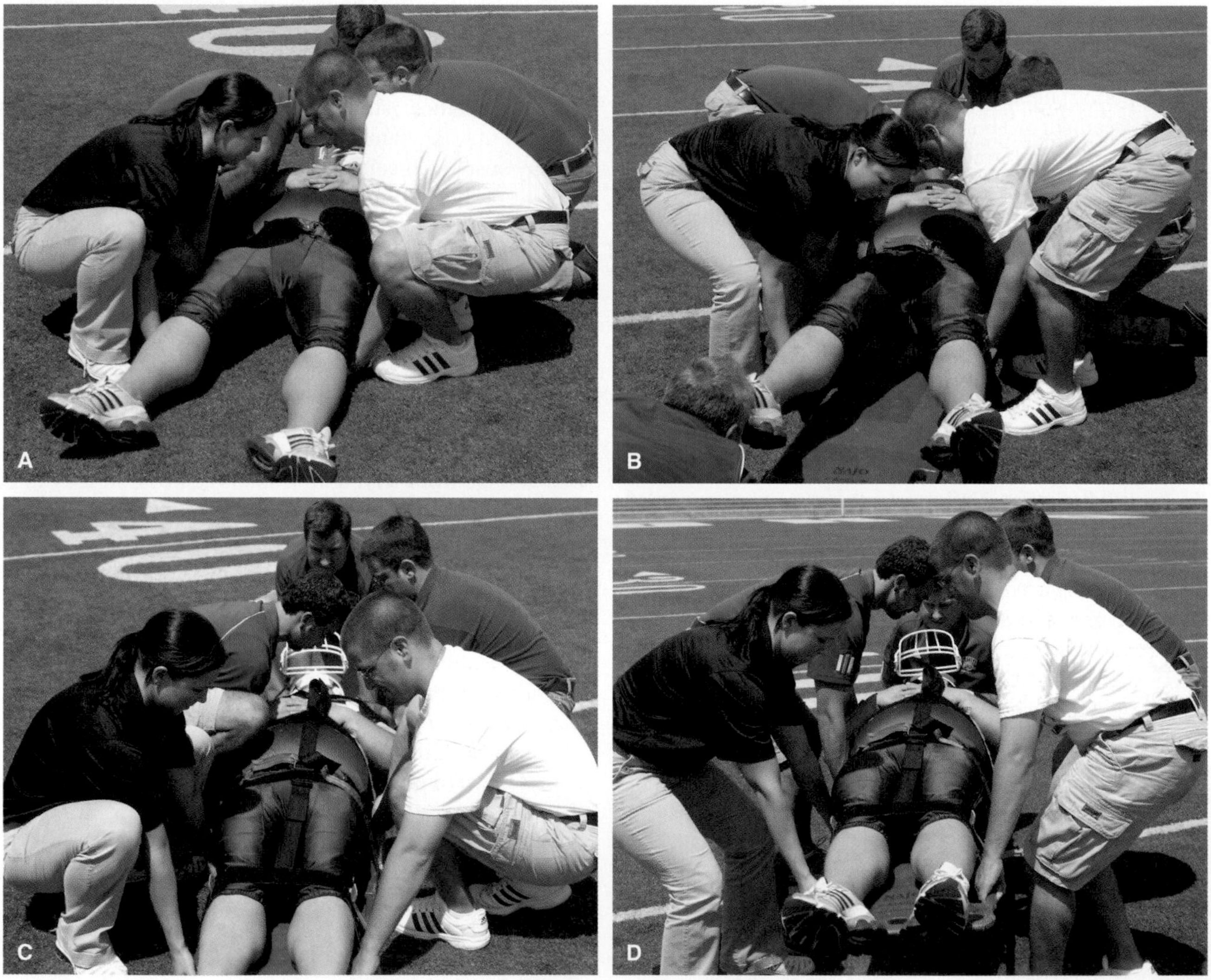

FIGURE 20-25 ■ The six-person lift for spine boarding a supine athlete; see text for details.

Tracheotomy A method of delivering air to the lungs by incising the skin and trachea and inserting a tube to form an airway; an emergency technique used only when the person's life is threatened by an immovable obstruction to the upper airway. Training is required to perform this technique properly.

The process of using a spine board for an athlete who is supine involves lifting the athlete, sliding the board under the person, and then placing the athlete on the board.

1. **Align the athlete:** Before the athlete is placed on the board, the extremities must be aligned with the body. If possible, cross the athlete's arms across the chest.
2. **Position the personnel:** Depending on the height and weight of the athlete, at least one person should be positioned on each side of the chest, pelvis, and legs. Larger athletes will require more rescuers.
3. **Lift the athlete:** On the leader's command, the athlete is lifted 4 to 6 inches. The following command is used: "On the count of three, we will lift the athlete until I say 'stop.' Start and stop on my command. Ready? One, two, three, lift." The personnel positioned at the torso and legs are responsible for maintaining axial alignment of the spinal column by staying with the leader's pace.
4. **Slide the spine board:** With the board on the ground, slide the spine board from the athlete's feet toward the head. The final position should place the board under the athlete so that the top of the spine board is matched with the athlete's head.
5. **Return the athlete:** After the leader is satisfied with the board's position relative to the athlete, he or she gives the command, "On the count of three, we lower the athlete to the board. Start and stop on my command. Ready? One, two, three, lower." Again, it is the torso personnel who are responsible for meeting the pace of the leader. Minor adjustments may be needed after the athlete is positioned on the board.
6. **Secure the athlete:** After the athlete is properly positioned on the spine board, the torso is secured, using the strapping techniques applicable to the equipment being used. The cervical spine must be secured, using the equipment supplied by the ambulance squad or using commercially available equipment (Fig. 20-26). If the helmet is left on, the head may be secured to the board by tape.

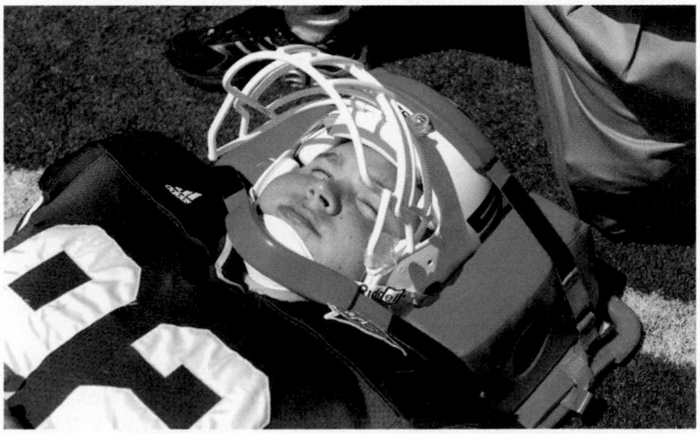

FIGURE 20-26 ■ The spine boarding process is completed by immobilizing the patient's head.

The prone athlete. Athletes in the prone position who are breathing but unconscious may be rolled onto the spine board in a safer and more orderly manner than that described in the section on the on-field management of an unconscious athlete who is not breathing. The basic procedures are the same as those described for spine boarding an athlete in the supine position, but the athlete must be rolled 180 degrees (Fig. 20-27). The person who is providing in-line stabilization to the cervical spine is again the operation's leader. A minimum of three additional people is necessary for this procedure to be safely performed. A fourth additional person is recommended to manipulate the spine board.

*** Practical Evidence**

The efficacy and safety of the use of a full-length spine board and the log-rolling technique have been questioned. Research has suggested that there is an "unacceptable" amount of cervical spine motion associated with spine boarding using the log roll method.[97–99]

1. **Align the athlete:** Before the athlete is placed on the board, the extremities are aligned with the body. The arm on the side toward which the athlete is to be rolled is abducted to 180 degrees. In Figure 20-27, the right arm is fully abducted prior to rolling.
2. **Position the personnel:** When the minimum of three personnel is used at the torso, one is positioned at the shoulders, one at the hips, and one along the legs. The hands should be spaced along the athlete, gripping underneath the athlete. Tall, heavy, or large individuals may require more personnel in order to be moved safely.
3. **Roll to the side:** On the leader's instructions, the athlete is rolled 90 degrees. The command is given: "On the count of three, we will roll the athlete to his side. Start and stop on my command. Ready? One, two, three, roll." The personnel used at the torso are responsible for maintaining axial alignment of the spinal column by staying with the leader's pace.
4. **Slide the spine board:** If a single person is given the responsibility of manipulating the spine board, it should be slid so that it is resting against the athlete. The board is positioned longitudinally so that its head is matched with the athlete's head.
5. **Placement:** After the leader is satisfied with the board's position relative to the athlete, he or she gives the command: "On the count of three, we will roll the athlete on the board. Start and stop on my command. Ready? One, two, three, roll." The torso personnel are responsible for meeting the pace of the leader. Minor adjustments may be needed after the athlete is positioned on the board.
6. **Secure the athlete:** The athlete is secured on the spine board as described in the previous section.

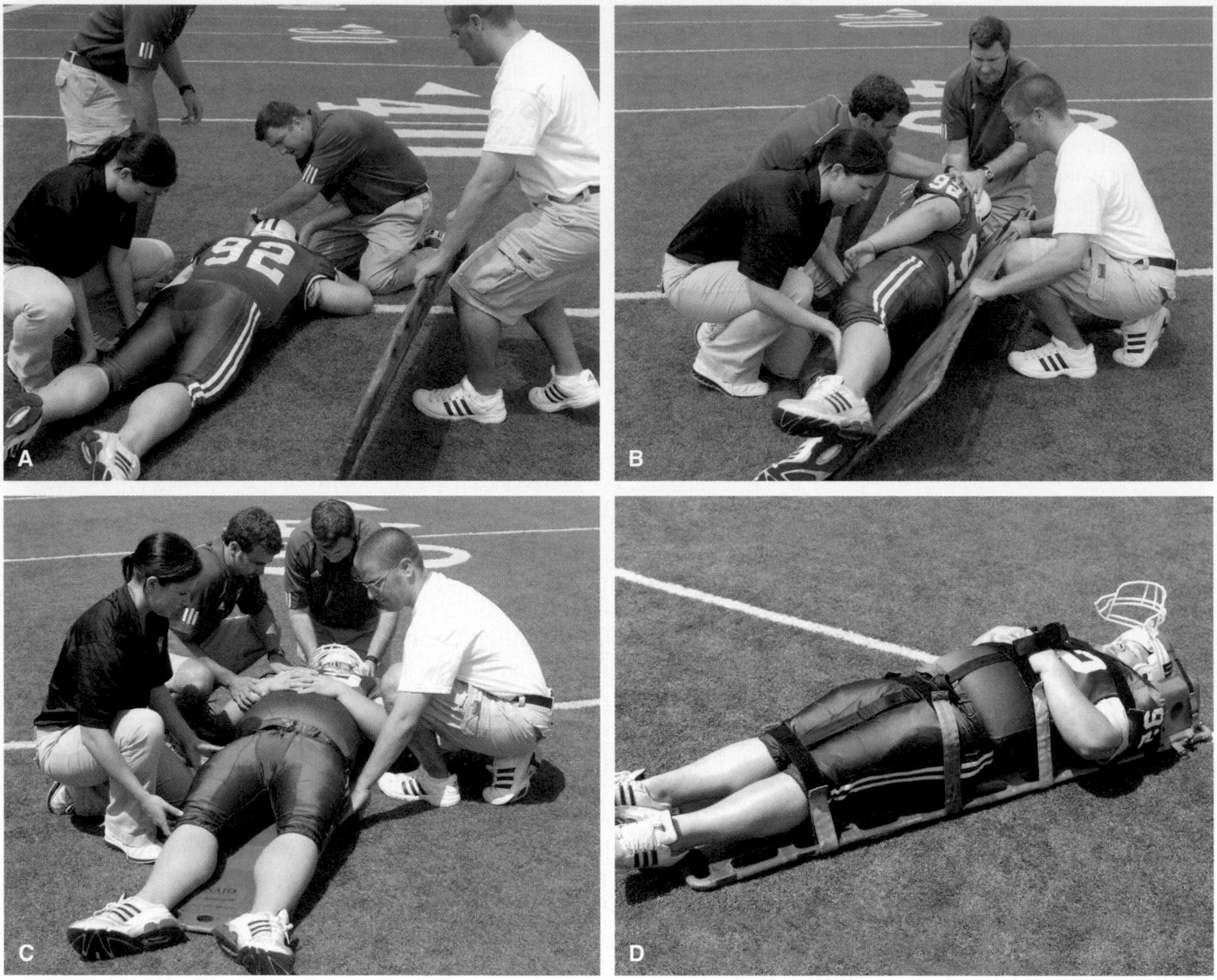

FIGURE 20-27 ■ Spine boarding a prone athlete; see text for details. Note the cross-armed position of the leader applying in-line stabilization.

REFERENCES

1. Tommasone, BA, Valovich McLeod, TC: Contact sport concussion incidence. *J Athl Train*, 41:470, 2006.
2. Boden, BP, et al: Catastrophic head injuries in high school and college football players. *Am J Sports Med*, 35:1075, 2007.
3. Gessel, LM, et al: Concussions among United States high school and college athletes. *J Athl Train*, 42:495, 2007.
4. Duhaime, AC, et al: Spectrum of acute clinical characteristics of diagnosed concussions in college athletes wearing instrument helmets: clinical article. *J Neurosurg*, 117:1092, 2012.
5. Bartsch, A, et al: Impact test comparisons of 20th- and 21st-century American football helmets. *J Neurosurg*, 116:222, 2012.
6. Heck, JF, et al: National Athletic Trainers' Association position statement: head-down contact and spearing in tackle football. *J Athl Train*, 39:101, 2004.
7. Nelson, WE: Athletic head injuries. *J Athl Train*, 19:95, 1984.
8. Harmon, KG, et al: American Medical Society for sports medicine position statement: concussion in sport. *Br J Sports Med*, 47:15, 2013.
9. Tysvaer, AT, and Lochen, EA: Soccer injuries to the brain: a neuropsychologic study of former soccer players. *Am J Sports Med*, 19:56, 1991.
10. Killam, C, et al: Assessing the enduring residual neuropsychological effects of head trauma in college athletes who participate in contact sports. *Arch Clin Neuropsych*, 20:599, 2005.
11. Gavett, BE, et al: Chronic traumatic encephalopathy: a potential late effect of sport-related concussive and subconcussive head trauma. *Clin Sports Med*, 30:179, 2011.
12. Lehman, EJ, et al: Neurodegenerative causes of death among retired National Football League players. *Neurology*, 79:1970, 2012.
13. McCrory, P, et al: Consensus statement on concussion in sport: the 4th International conference on concussion in sport held in Zurich, November 2012. *Br J Sports Med*, 47:250, 2013.
14. Theye, F, and Mueller, KA: "Heads up": concussions in high school sports. *Clin Med Res*, 2:165, 2004.
15. Guskiewicz, KM, et al: Epidemiology of concussions in collegiate and high school football players. *Am J Sports Med*, 28:643, 2000.
16. Abuabara, A: Cerebrospinal fluid rhinorrhea: diagnosis and management. *Med Oral Patol Oral Cir Bucal*, 12:E397, 2007.
17. Miller, JR, et al: Comparison of preseason, midseason, and postseason neurocognitive scores in uninjured collegiate football players. *Am J Sports Med*, 35:1284, 2007.

18. Oliaro, SM, et al: Establishment of normative data on cognitive tests for comparison with athletes sustaining mild head injury. *J Athl Train*, 33:36, 1998.
19. Onate, JA, et al: A comparison of sideline versus clinical cognitive test performance in collegiate athletes. *J Athl Train*, 35:155, 2000.
20. Guskiewicz, KM: Concussion in sport: the grading system dilemma. *Athl Ther Today*, 6:18, 2001.
21. Bohnen, N, et al: Performance in the Stroop color word test in relationship to the persistence of symptoms following mild head injury. *Acta Neurol Scand*, 85:116, 1992.
22. Hinton-Bayre, AD, et al: Mild head injury and speed of information processing: a prospective study of professional rugby league players. *J Clin Exp Neuropsychol*, 19:275, 1997.
23. Iverson, G, et al: Normative comparisons for the controlled oral word association test following acute traumatic brain injury. *J Clin Exp Neuropsychol*, 13:437, 1999.
24. Broglio, SP, et al: Neurocognitive performance of concussed athletes when symptom free. *J Athl Train*, 42:504, 2007.
25. Guskiewicz, KM, et al: Cumulative effects associated with recurrent concussion in collegiate football players: the NCAA concussion study. *JAMA*, 290:2549, 2003.
26. Brown, CN, et al: Athlete characteristics and outcome scores for computerized neuropsychological assessment: a preliminary analysis. *J Athl Train*, 42:515, 2007.
27. Broglio, SP, et al: Test–retest reliability of computerized concussion assessment programs. *J Athl Train*, 42:509, 2007.
28. Randolph, C: Baseline neuropsychological testing in managing sport-related concussion: does it modify risk? *Curr Sports Med Rep*, 10:21, 2011.
29. Mayers, LB, and Redick, TS: Clinical utility of ImPACT assessment for postconcussion return-to-play counseling: psychometric issues. *J Clin Exp Neuropsychol*, 34:235, 2012.
30. McLeod, TCV, et al: Representative baseline values on the Sport Concussion Assessment Tool 2 (SCAT2) in adolescent athletes vary by gender, grade, and concussion history. *Am J Sports Med*, 40:927, 2012.
31. Herring, SA, et al: Concussion (mild traumatic brain injury) and the team physician: a consensus statement—2011 update. *Med Sci Sports Exerc*, 43:2412, 2011.
32. Randolph, C, et al: Is neuropsychological testing useful in the management of sport-related concussion? *J Athl Train*, 40:139, 2005.
33. McCrory, P: Does second impact syndrome exist? *Clin J Sport Med*, 11:144, 2001.
34. Ragan, B, et al: Psychometric evaluation of the standardized assessment of concussion: evaluation of baseline score validity using item analysis. *Athl Train Sports Health Care*, 1:180, 2009.
35. Echemendia, RJ, and Julian, LJ: Mild traumatic brain injury in sports: neuropsychology's contribution to a developing field. *Neuropsychol Rev*, 11:69, 2001.
36. Kirkwood, MW, et al: Returning pediatric athletes to play after concussion: the evidence (or lack thereof) behind neuropsychological testing. *Acta Paediatr*, 98:1409, 2009.
37. Ragan, BG, and Kang, M: Measurement issues in concussion testing. *Athl Ther Today*, 12:2, 2007.
38. Jinquji, TM, et al: Sport assessment tool-2: baseline values for high school athletes. *Br J Sports Med*, 46:365, 2012.
39. Register-Mihalik, JK: Balance deficits after sports-related concussion in individuals reporting posttraumatic headache. *Neurosurgery*, 63:76, 2008.
40. Broglio, SP, et al: Sensitivity of the concussion assessment battery. *Neurosurgery*, 60:1050, 2007.
41. Riemann, BL, and Guskiewicz, KM: Effects of mild head injury on postural stability as measured through clinical balance testing. *J Athl Train*, 35:19, 2000.
42. University of North Carolina. *Balance Error Scoring System (BESS) User's Manual.* Chapel Hill, NC: University of North Carolina Sports Medicine Research Laboratory.
43. Valovich, TCV, et al: Psychometric and measurement properties of concussion assessment tools in youth sports. *J Athl Train*, 41:399, 2006.
44. Valovich, TC, et al: Repeat administration elicits practice effect with the Balance Error Scoring System but not with the Standardized Assessment of Concussion in high school athletes. *J Athl Train*, 38:51, 2003.
45. Broglio, SP, et al: Generalizability theory analysis of balance error scoring system reliability in healthy young adults. *J Athl Train*, 44:497, 2009.
46. Onate, JA, et al: On-field testing environment and Balance Error Scoring System Performance during preseason screening of healthy collegiate baseball players. *J Athl Train*, 42:446, 2007.
47. Mueller, FO, and Colgates, B: Annual survey of catastrophic football injuries 1997–2011: National Center for Catastrophic Sport Injury Research. Retrieved from www.unc.edu/depts/nccsi/FBCATReport2011.pdf . (Accessed March 9, 2013).
48. Oliaro, S, et al: Management of cerebral concussion in sports: the athletic trainer's perspective. *J Athl Train*, 36:257, 2001.
49. McKee, AC, et al: The spectrum of disease in chronic traumatic encephalopathy. *Brain*, 136:43, 2013.
50. Wojtys, EM, et al: Current concepts: concussion in sports. *Am J Sports Med*, 27:676, 1999.
51. Jeter, CB, et al: Biomarkers for the diagnosis and prognosis of mild traumatic brain injury/concussion. *J Neurotrauma*, 30:657, 2013.
52. Randolph, C, et al: Concussion symptom inventory: an empirically derived scale for monitoring resolution of symptoms following sport-related concussion. *Arch Clin Neuropsych*, 24:219, 2009.
53. Lovell, MR, et al: Measurement of symptoms following sports-related concussion: reliability and normative data for the postconcussion scale. *Appl Neuropsych*, 13:166, 2006.
54. Piland, SG, et al: Structural validity of self-report concussion-related symptom scale. *Med Sci Sport Exerc*, 38:27, 2006.
55. Gerberich, SG, et al: Concussion incidences and severity in secondary school varsity football players. *Am J Public Health*, 73:1370, 1983.
56. McCrory, P, et al: Summary and agreement statement of the 2nd International Conference on Concussion in Sport, Prague 2004. *Clin J Sport Med*, 15:48, 2005.
57. Guskiewicz, KM, et al: Evidence-based approach to revising the SCAT2: introducing the SCAT3. *Br J Sports Med*, 47:289, 2013.
58. McCrea, M, et al: Standardized assessment of concussion in football players. *Neurology*, 48:586, 1997.
59. McGrath, N: Supporting the student-athlete's return to the classroom after a sport-related concussion. *J Athl Train*, 45:492, 2010.
60. McLeod, TCV, and Gioia, GA: Cognitive rest: the often neglected aspect of concussion management. *Athl Ther Today*, 15:1, 2010.
61. American Academy of Neurology: Position statement: sports concussion (AAN Policy 2010-36). 2010. Retrieved from www.aan.com/globals/axon/assets/7913.pdf. (Accessed March 9, 2013).
62. Cantu, RC: Criteria for return to competition after a closed head injury. In: Torg, JS (ed): *Athletic Injuries to the Head, Neck, and Face* (ed 2). St Louis, MO: Mosby-Year Book, 1991, p 326.
63. Cantu, RC: Head and spine injuries in youth sports: the young athlete. *Clin Sports Med*, 14:517, 1995.
64. Bigler, ED: Neuropsychology and clinical neuroscience of persistent post-concussive syndrome. *J Int Neuropsychol Soc*, 14:1, 2008.
65. Boake, C, et al: Diagnostic criteria for postconcussion syndrome after mild to moderate traumatic brain injury. *J Neuropsychiatry Clin Neurosci*, 17:350, 2005.

66. Babcock, L, et al: Predicting postconcussion syndrome after mild traumatic brain injury in children and adolescents who present to the emergency department. *JAMA Pediatr*, 167:156, 2013.
67. Leddy, JJ, et al: Rehabilitation of concussion and post-concussion syndrome. *Sports Health*, 4:147, 2012.
68. Erlanger, DM, et al: Neuropsychology of sports-related head injury: dementia pugilistica to post-concussion syndrome. *Clin Neuropsychol*, 13:193, 1999.
69. Geurts, AC, et al: Is postural control associated with mental functioning in the persistent postconcussion syndrome? *Arch Phys Med Rehabil*, 80:144, 1999.
70. Sanders, RI, and Harbaugh, RE: The second impact in catastrophic contact: sports head trauma. *JAMA*, 252:538, 1984.
71. White, RJ: Subarachnoid hemorrhage: the lethal intracranial explosion. *Emerg Med Clin North Am*, 74, May 1994.
72. Logan, SM, et al: Acute subdural hematoma in a high school football player after 2 unreported episodes of head trauma: a case report. *J Athl Train*, 36:433, 2001.
73. Nee, PA, et al: Significance of vomiting after head injury. *J Neurol Neurosurg Psychiatry*, 66:470, 1999.
74. Stiell, IG, et al: Canadian C-spine rule study for alert and stable trauma patients: I. background and rationale. *CJEM*, 4:84, 2002.
75. Ivanic, PC: Head-first impact with head protrusion causes noncontiguous injuries of the cadaveric cervical spine. *Clin J Sport Med*, 22:390, 2012.
76. Heck, JF: The incidence of spearing by high school football carriers and their tacklers. *J Athl Train*, 27:120, 1992.
77. Ivancic, PC: Biomechanics of sports-induced axial-compression injuries of the neck. *J Athl Train*, 47:489, 2012.
78. Torg, JS: Criteria for return to collision activities after cervical spine injury. *Oper Techn Sports Med*, 1:236, 1993.
79. Torg, JS, et al: Spear tackler's spine: an entity precluding participation in tackle football and collision activities that expose the cervical spine to axial energy inputs. *Am J Sports Med*, 21:640, 1993.
80. Waninger, KN: Management of the helmeted athlete with suspected cervical spine injury. *Am J Sports Med*, 32:1331, 2004.
81. Chikuda, H, et al: Mortality and morbidity after high-dose methylprednisolone treatment in patients with acute cervical spinal cord injury: a propensity-matched analysis using a nationwide administrative database. *Emerg Med J*, e-pub, 2013.
82. Robins-Steele, S, et al: The delayed post-injury administration of soluble fas receptor attenuates post-traumatic neural degeneration and enhances functional recovery after traumatic cervical spinal cord injury. *J Neurotrauma*, 29:1586, 2012.
83. Vale, FL, et al: Combined medical and surgical treatment after acute spinal cord injury: results of a prospective pilot study to assess the merits of aggressive medical resuscitation and blood pressure management. *J Neurosurg*, 87:239, 1997.
84. Kepler, CK, and Vaccaro, AR: Injuries and abnormalities of the cervical spine and return to play criteria. *Clin Sports Med*, 31:499, 2012.
85. Concannon, LG, et al: Radiating upper limb pain in the contact sport athlete: an update on transient quadriparesis and stingers. *Curr Sports Med Rep*, 11:28, 2012.
86. Davis, G, et al: Clinics in neurology and neurosurgery of sport: asymptomatic cervical canal stenosis and transient quadriparesis. *Br J Sports Med*, 43:1154, 2009.
87. Casa, DJ, et al: National Athletic Trainers' Association position statement: preventing sudden death in sports. *J Athl Train*, 47:96, 2012.
88. Waninger, KN, and Swartz, EE: Cervical spine injury management in the helmeted athlete. *Curr Sports Med Rep*, 10:45, 2011.
89. Gale, SD, et al: The combined tool approach for face mask removal during on-field conditions. *J Athl Train*, 43:14, 2008.
90. Decoster, LC, et al: Football face-mask removal with a cordless screwdriver on helmets used for at least one season of play. *J Athl Train*, 40:169, 2005.
91. Swartz, EE, et al: The influence of various factors on high school football helmet face mask removal: a retrospective, cross-sectional analysis. *J Athl Train*, 42:11, 2007.
92. Swartz, EE, et al: Football equipment design affects face mask removal efficiency. *Am J Sports Med*, 33:1, 2005.
93. Swartz, EE, et al: Emergency face-mask removal effectiveness: a comparison of traditional and nontraditional football helmet face-mask attachment systems. *J Athl Train*, 45:560, 2010.
94. Caroline, N, et al: *Emergency Care in the Streets* (ed 7). Burlington, MA: Jones & Bartlett Learning, 2013.
95. Ransone, J, et al: The efficacy of rapid form cervical vacuum immobilizer in the cervical spine immobilization of the equipped football player. *J Athl Train*, 35:65, 2000.
96. Kleiner, DM, et al: *Prehospital Care of the Spine-Injured Athlete: A Document from the Interassociation Task Force for Appropriate Care of the Spine-Injured Athlete*. Dallas, TX: National Athletic Trainers' Association, 2001.
97. Del Rossi, G, et al: Are scoop stretchers suitable for use on spine-injured patients? *Am J Emerg Med*, 28:751, 2010.
98. Del Rossi, G, et al: Spine-board transfer techniques and the unstable cervical spine. *Spine*, 29:E134, 2004.
99. Horodyski, M, et al: Removing a patient from the spine board: is the lift and slide safer than the log roll? *J Trauma*, 70:1282, 2011.

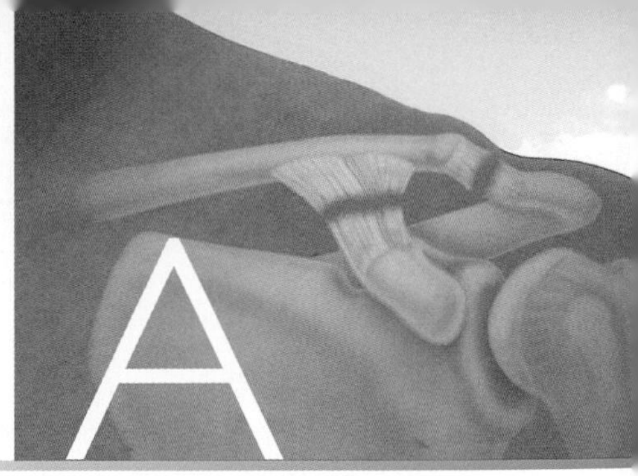

APPENDIX A

Diagnostic Evidence References

The following is a list of references used to calculate the scores of diagnostic accuracy (inter- and intrarater reliability, sensitivity, specificity, and positive and negative likelihood ratios). We calculated the confidence interval for those procedures having 12 or more data points to yield the mean, low- and high values. For those procedures having 5 to 11 data points we calculated the interquartile range. For those tests having two to four data points, the low value, high value, and median value were reported.

Chapter 1

Procedure	Reference(s)
Abdominal Percussion	304
Ankle Girth Measurement	24, 84, 184, 220, 237, 271, 305
Blood Pressure Assessment	69
Lung Auscultation	25
"Clean Catch" Dipstick Urinalysis	256

Chapter 6

Procedure	Reference(s)
Measured Block Method of Detecting Leg-Length Discrepancies	103, 129, 225, 272
Tape Measure Method of Detecting Leg-Length Discrepancies	12, 203, 238, 272
Muscle Length – Gastrocnemius	223, 225
Muscle Length – Hamstrings	225
Muscle Length – Rectus Femoris	225

Chapter 8

Procedure	Reference(s)
Arch Angle	109, 129, 245
Dorsiflexion – Eversion Test	146
Forefoot Valgus/Varus Inspection	27, 261, 285
Goniometry Rearfoot Inversion/Eversion	72
Joint Play – Tarsometatarsal Joint	93
Mulder Sign	48
Navicular Drop Test	166, 222, 223, 252, 290
Subtalar Joint Neutral	222
Windlass Test	59

Chapter 9

Procedure	Reference(s)
Anterior Drawer Test	32, 230, 283, 284
External Rotation Test	3, 58, 215
Goniometry – Plantarflexion/Dorsiflexion	72, 129, 305
Squeeze Test	3, 58
Talar Tilt Test	88, 286
Thompson Test	177

Chapter 10

Procedure	Reference(s)
Anterior Drawer Test	15, 20, 23, 65, 105, 106, 123, 126, 131, 137, 145, 149, 161, 169, 195, 212, 242, 249, 278, 301
Apley's Compression/Distraction Test	71, 82, 132, 149, 154, 190, 249
Ballotable Patella Test	85, 95, 135
Dynamic Posterior Shift Test	242
External Rotation Recurvatum	40, 242
Flexion Reduction Drawer	208
Girth Measurement	260
Godfrey's Test	83, 242
Goniometry – Knee Flexion/Extension	26, 44, 56, 86, 94, 108, 162, 240, 297, 301
Lachman's Test	15, 20, 23, 51, 61, 65, 105, 126, 131, 137, 161, 169, 195, 242, 249, 265, 278
McMurray Test	5, 11, 54, 61, 74, 82, 109, 126, 132, 154, 190, 207

Pivot Shift Test	15, 20, 65, 105, 126, 137, 173, 242, 249, 265
Posterior Drawer Test	47, 106, 123, 172, 196, 242
Quadriceps Active Test	55, 57, 242
Reverse Lachman's Test	242
Reverse Pivot Shift	242
Sweep Test	86, 95
Thessally Test	107, 132
Valgus Stress	89, 106, 134, 186, 301
Varus Stress Test	106, 301

Chapter 11

Procedure	Reference(s)
Apprehension Test	101, 205, 206, 244
Joint Play – Medial Lateral Glide	202, 270
Joint Play – Patellar Tilt	77, 166, 223, 276, 298
Q-Angle (Standing)	45, 99, 251
Q-Angle (Supine)	96, 97, 99, 112, 223, 251, 276

Chapter 12

Procedure	Reference(s)
Acetabular Impingement	14, 31, 138, 167, 181, 257, 279
Angle of Torsion	166, 194, 223, 255
Goniometry – Abduction/ Adduction	42, 118, 147, 228
Goniometry – Flexion/Extension	42, 118, 147, 228
Goniometry – Internal/ External Rotation	42, 118, 147, 228
Hip Scouring	43, 183, 269
Ober's Test	42, 223, 232
Thomas Test	42, 166, 185, 201, 267, 300
Trendelenburg Test	19, 42, 163, 302, 306

Chapter 13

Procedure	Reference(s)
Active Straight-Leg Raise	241
Adams Forward Bend Test	53, 303
Extension Endurance	160
Fabere Test	7, 42, 66, 150, 181, 183, 213, 236, 269, 279
Femoral Nerve Traction Test	227, 268
Gaenslen's Test	66, 79, 150, 158, 213
Inclinometer – Flexion/Extension	28, 64, 189, 204, 221, 234
Prone Instability Test	87, 115, 248
Sacral Thrust Test	66, 158
Sacroiliac Compression Test	79, 150, 157, 158, 213, 214, 236, 267
Sacroiliac Distraction Test	79, 150, 157, 158, 213, 267
Single-Leg Stance Test	182, 274
Slump Test	179, 214, 280
Sorensen Test	60
Spring Test (Joint Play)	1, 18, 66, 85, 121, 178, 214, 248
Straight-Leg Raise Test	2, 36, 39, 63, 100, 102, 116, 124, 130, 140, 148, 151, 152, 179, 214, 239, 262, 267, 268, 287, 291
Thigh Thrust Test	66, 158, 282
Valsalva Test	37, 293
Well Straight-Leg Raise Test	63, 102, 130, 140, 148, 152, 262, 268

Chapter 14

Procedure	Reference(s)
Adson's Test	226
Babinski Test	49, 50, 73, 192
Brachial Plexus Neuropathy	289
Cervical Compression Test	231, 289
Cervical Distraction Test	17, 49, 180, 288, 289, 292, 294
Inclinometer – Flexion/Extension	33, 46, 117, 122, 224, 292
Inclinometer – Lateral Bending	33, 46, 117, 122, 224, 292
Inclinometer – Rotation	33, 117, 122, 224
Joint Play	78, 111
Roos Test	92
Shoulder Abduction Test	180, 231, 288, 289, 292
Spurling Test	17, 49, 180, 246, 254, 277, 289, 292
Upper Limb Tension Test	231, 246, 292, 293, 294
Vertebral Artery Test	235

Chapter 15

Procedure	Reference(s)
Acromioclavicular Joint Compression Test	296
Active Compression Test (SLAP Lesions)	29, 34, 41, 62, 68, 81, 98, 127, 141, 143, 187, 188, 197, 199, 200, 210, 211, 216, 217, 247, 266, 281, 295, 296
Anterior Release ("Surprise!" Test)	171, 174, 281
Anterior Slide Test	91, 127, 141, 142, 143, 187, 200, 211, 217, 247
Apprehension Test	52, 75, 81, 98, 127, 143, 171, 174, 200, 263
Compression Rotation Test	62, 98, 143, 170, 187, 199, 200, 211, 217, 259
Drop Arm Test	4, 34, 35, 127, 193, 198, 219
Empty Can Test	119, 125, 139, 191, 219
Gerber Lift-Off Test	113, 125, 127, 188, 193
Hawkins Test (Impingement)	4, 10, 13, 34, 35, 80, 81, 91, 110, 127, 128, 139, 165, 176, 191, 219
Hawkins Test (SLAP lesions)	81, 127, 143, 200, 217
Jerk Test	144, 164, 200, 253
Neer Test (Impingement)	10, 35, 109, 139, 165, 176, 188, 191, 219
Neer Test (SLAP lesions)	127, 143, 200, 217
Posterior Apprehension Test	127, 263
Posterior Jerk Test	200
Relocation Test (Anterior Instability)	75, 98, 170, 171, 174, 281

Relocation Test (SLAP lesions)	98, 143, 197, 200, 211, 217
Speed's Test (Biceps tendon involvement)	8, 16, 21, 35, 91, 119, 127, 141, 165, 188, 211, 219
Speed's Test (SLAP lesion)	68, 98, 110, 127, 141, 143, 144, 197, 200, 217, 218
Sulcus Sign	174, 200, 281
Yeargson's Test (Long Head of Biceps Involvement)	35, 98, 119, 141, 143
Yeargson's Test (SLAP Lesion)	98, 141, 143, 200, 217

Chapter 16

Procedure	Reference(s)
Goniometry – Flexion/Extension	9, 38, 240,
Goniometry – Pronation/Supination	9, 133
Moving Valgus Stress Test	209
Posterolateral Rotatory Instability (Pivot Shift) Test	233
Valgus Stress Test	209, 275

Chapter 17

Procedure	Reference(s)
Finklestein's Test	258
Goniometry – Flexion/Extension	120
Goniometry – Radial/Ulnar Deviation	120
Grip Dynamometry	168, 250
Joint Play – Intercarpal Joints	264
Phalen's Test	6, 22, 30, 67, 70, 76, 90, 104, 136, 153, 155, 156, 175, 243, 258, 273, 293, 299
Thumb Valgus Stress Test	114
Watson Test	159, 229

REFERENCES

1. Abbott, JH: Lumbar segmental instability: a criterion-related validity study of manual therapy assessment. *BMC Musculoskelet Disord*, 6:56, 2005.
2. Albeck, MJ: A critical assessment of clinical diagnosis of disc herniation in patients with monoradicular sciatica. *Acta Neurochir*, 138:40, 1996.
3. Alonso, A, Khoury, L, and Adams, R: Clinical tests for ankle syndesmosis injury: reliability and prediction of return to function. *J Orthop Sports Phys Ther*, 27:276, 1998.
4. Alqunaee, M, Galvin, R, and Fahey, T: Diagnostic accuracy of clinical tests for subacromial impingement syndrome: a systematic review and meta-analysis. *Arch Phys Med Rehabil*, 93:229, 2012.
5. Anderson, AF, and Lipscom, AB: Clinical diagnosis of meniscal tears: description of a new manipulative test. *Am J Sports Med*, 14:291, 1986.
6. Ann, DS: Hand elevation: a new test for carpal tunnel syndrome. *Ann Plast Surg*, 46:120, 2001.
7. Arab, AM, et al: Inter- and intra-examiner reliability of single and composites of selected motion palpation and pain provocation tests for sacroiliac joint. *Man Ther*, 14:213, 2009.
8. Ardic, F, et al: Shoulder impingement syndrome: relationships between clinical, functional, and radiologic findings. *Am J Phys Med Rehabil*, 85:53, 2006.
9. Armstrong AD, et al: Reliability of range-of-motion measurements in the elbow. *J Elbow Shoulder Surg*, 7:573, 1998.
10. Bak, K, and Fauno, P: Clinical findings in competitive swimmers with shoulder pain. *Am J Sports Med*, 25:254, 1997.
11. Barry, OC, et al: Clinical assessment of suspected meniscal tears. *Ir J Med Sci*, 24:164, 1996.
12. Beattie, P, et al: Validity of derived measurements of leg-length differences obtained by use of a tape measure. *Phys Ther*, 70:150, 1990.
13. Beaudreuil, J, et al: Contribution of clinical tests to the diagnosis of rotator cuff disease: a systematic literature review. *Joint Bone Spine*, 76:15, 2009.
14. Beaulé, PE, et al: Three-dimensional computed tomography of the hip in the assessment of femoroacetabular impingement. *J Orthop Res*, 23:1286, 2005.
15. Benjaminse, A, Gokeler A, and van der Schans, CP: Clinical diagnosis of an anterior cruciate ligament rupture: a meta-analysis. *J Orthop Sports Phys Ther*, 36:267, 2006.
16. Bennett, WF: Specificity of the Speed's test: arthroscopic technique for evaluating the biceps tendon at the level of the bicipital groove. *Arthroscopy*, 14:789, 1998.
17. Bertilson, BC, et al: Reliability of clinical tests in the assessment of patients with neck/shoulder problems: impact of history. *Spine*, 28:2222, 2003.
18. Binkley, J, Stratford, PW, and Gill, C: Interrater reliability of lumbar accessory motion mobility testing. *Phys Ther*, 75:786, 1995.
19. Bird, PA, et al: Prospective evaluation of magnetic resonance imaging and physical examination findings in patients with greater trochanteric pain syndrome. *Arthritis Rheum*, 44:2138, 2001.
20. Boeree, NR, and Ackroyd, CE: Assessment of the menisci and cruciate ligaments: an audit of clinical practice. *Injury*, 22:291, 1991.
21. Boileau, P, Ahrens, PM, and Hatzidakis, AM: Entrapment of the long head of the biceps tendon: the hourglass biceps—a cause of pain and locking in the shoulder. *J Shoulder Elbow Surg*, 13:249, 2004.
22. Boland, RA, and Kieman, MC: Assessing the accuracy of a combination of clinical tests for identifying carpal tunnel syndrome. *J Clin Neurosci*, 16:929, 2009.
23. Braunstein, EM: Anterior cruciate ligament injuries: a comparison of arthographic and physical diagnosis. *AJR Am J Roentgenol*, 168:423, 1982.
24. Brodovicz, KG, et al: Reliability and feasibility of methods to quantitatively assess peripheral edema. *CMR*, 7:21, 2009.
25. Brooks, D, and Thomas, J: Interrater reliability of auscultation of breath sounds among physical therapists. *Phys Ther*, 75:1082, 1995.
26. Brosseau, L, et al: Intratester and intertester reliability and criterion validity of the parallelogram and universal goniometers for active knee flexion in healthy subjects. *Physiother Res Int*, 2:150, 1997.
27. Buchanan, KR, and Davis, I: The relationship between forefoot, midfoot, and rearfoot static alignment in pain-free individuals. *J Orthop Sports Phys Ther*, 35:559, 2005.
28. Burdett, RG, et al: Reliability and validity of four instruments for measuring lumbar spine and pelvic positions. *Phys Ther*, 66:677, 1986.
29. Burkart, S, Morgan, CD, and Kibler, WB: Shoulder injuries in overhead athletes: the "dead arm" revisited. *Clin Sports Med*, 19:125, 2000.
30. Burke, DT, et al: Subjective swelling: a new sign for carpal tunnel syndrome. *Am J Phys Med Rehabil*, 78:504, 1999.
31. Burnett, R, et al: Clinical presentation of patients with tears of the acetabular labrum. *J Bone Joint Surg Am*, 88:1448, 2006.
32. Burns, S: Anterior drawer of the ankle: technique. Retrieved August 27, 2013 from www.physio-pedia.com/index.php?title=Anterior_Drawer_of_the_Ankle.
33. Bush, KW, et al: Validity and intertester reliability of cervical range of motion using inclinometer measurements. *J Man Manip Ther*, 8:52, 2000.
34. Cadogan, A, et al: Interexaminer reliability of orthopaedic special tests used in the assessment of shoulder pain. *Man Ther*, 16:131, 2011.
35. Calis, M, et al: Diagnostic values of clinical diagnostic tests in subacromial impingement syndrome. *Ann Rheum Dis*, 59:44, 2000.

36. Capra, F, et al: Validity of the straight-leg raise test for patients with sciatic pain with or without lumbar pain using magnetic resonance imaging results as a reference standard. *J Manipulative Physiol Ther*, 34:231, 2011.
37. Cecin, HA: Cecin's sign ("X" sign): improving the diagnosis of radicular compression by herniated lumbar discs. *Bras J Rheumatol*, 50:44, 2010.
38. Chapleau, J, et al: Validity of goniometric elbow measurements: comparative study with a radiographic method. *Clin Orthop Relat Res*, 469:3134, 2011.
39. Charnley, J: Orthopaedic signs in the diagnosis of disc protrusion: with special reference to the straight-leg-raising test. *Lancet*, 1:186, 1951.
40. Chen, FS, Rokito, AS, and Pitman, MI: Acute and chronic posterolateral rotatory instability of the knee. *J Am Acad Orthop Surg*, 8:97, 2000.
41. Chronopoulos, E, et al: Diagnostic value of physical tests for isolated chronic acromioclavicular lesions. *Am J Sports Med*, 32:655, 2004.
42. Cibere, J, et al: Reliability of the hip examination in osteoarthritis: effect of standardization. *Arthritis Rheum*, 59:373, 2008.
43. Cilborne, AV, et al: Clinical hip tests and a functional squat test in patients with knee osteoarthritis: reliability, prevalence of positive test findings, and short-term response to hip mobilization. *J Orthop Sports Phys Ther*, 34:676, 2004.
44. Clapper, MP, and Wolf, SL: Comparison of the reliability of the Orthoranger and the standard goniometer for assessing active lower extremity range of motion. *Phys Ther*, 68:214, 1998.
45. Clark, J, and Stechschulte, DJ: The interface between bone and tendon at insertion site: a study of the quadriceps tendon insertion. *J Anat*, 192:605, 1998.
46. Cleland, JA, et al: Interrater reliability of the history and physical examination in patients with mechanical neck pain. *Arch Phys Med Rehabil*, 87:1388, 2006.
47. Clendenin, MB, DeLee, JC, and Heckman, JD: Interstitial tears of the posterior cruciate ligament of the knee. *Orthopedics*, 3:764, 1980.
48. Cloke, DJ, and Greiss, ME: The digital nerve stress test: a sensitive indicator of Morton's neuroma and neuritis. *Foot Ankle Surg*, 12:201, 2006.
49. Cook, C, et al: Clustered clinical findings for diagnosis of cervical spine myelopathy. *J Man Manip Ther*, 18:175, 2010.
50. Cook, C, et al: Reliability and diagnostic accuracy of clinical special tests for myelopathy in patients' need for cervical dysfunction. *J Orthop Sports Phys Ther*, 39:172, 2009.
51. Cooperman, JM, Riddle, DL, and Rothstein, JM: Reliability and validity of judgments of the integrity of the anterior cruciate ligament of the knee using the Lachman's test. *Phys Ther*, 70:225, 1990.
52. Cordasco, FA, et al: Arthroscopic treatment of glenoid labral tears. *Am J Sports Med*, 21:425, 1993.
53. Côté, P, et al: A study of the diagnostic accuracy and reliability of the Scoliometer and Adam's forward bend test. *Spine*, 23:796, 1998.
54. Couture, J, et al: Joint line fullness and meniscal pathology. *Sports Health*, 4:47, 2012.
55. Cross, MJ, Schmidt, DR, and Mackie, IG: A no-touch test for the anterior cruciate ligament. *J Bone Joint Surg Br*, 69:300, 1987.
56. Currier, LL, et al: Development of a clinical prediction rule to identify patients with knee pain and clinical evidence of knee osteoarthritis who demonstrate a favorable short-term response to hip mobilization. *Phys Ther*, 87:1106, 2007.
57. Daniel, DM, et al: Use of the quadriceps active test to diagnose posterior cruciate ligament disruption and measure posterior laxity of the knee. *J Bone Joint Surg Am*, 70:386, 1988.
58. de César, PC, Avila, EM, and de Abreu, MR: Comparison of magnetic resonance imaging to physical examination for syndesmotic injury after lateral ankle sprain. *Foot Ankle Int*, 32:1110, 2011.
59. De Garceau, D, et al: The association between diagnosis of plantar fasciitis and windlass test. *Foot Ankle Int*, 24:251, 2003.
60. De Paula Lima, PO, et al: Reproducibility of the pressure biofeedback unit in measuring transversus abdominis muscle activity in patients with chronic nonspecific low back pain. *J Bodyw Mov Ther*, 16:251, 2012.
61. Dervin, GF, et al: Physicians' accuracy and interrator reliability for the diagnosis of unstable meniscal tears in patients having osteoarthritis of the knee. *Can J Surg*, 44:267, 2001.
62. Dessaur, WA, and Magarey, ME: Diagnostic accuracy of clinical tests for superior labral anterior posterior lesions: a systematic review. *J Orthop Sports Phys Ther*, 38:341, 2008.
63. Devillé, WLJM, et al: The test of Lasegue: Systematic review of the accuracy in diagnosing herniated discs. *Spine*, 25:9, 2000.
64. Dillard, J, et al: Motion of the lumbar spine: reliability of two measurement techniques. *Spine*, 16:321, 1991.
65. Donaldson, WF, Warren RF, and Wickiewicz, T: A comparison of acute anterior cruciate ligament examinations: initial versus examination under anesthesia. *Am J Sports Med*, 15:5, 1985.
66. Dreyfuss, P, et al: The value of medical history and physical examination in diagnosing sacroiliac joint pain. *Spine*, 21:2594, 1996.
67. Durkan, JA: A new diagnostic test for carpal tunnel syndrome. *J Bone Joint Surg Am*, 73:535, 1991.
68. Ebinger, N, et al: A new SLAP test: the supine flexion resistance test. *Arthroscopy*, 24:500, 2008.
69. Edmonds, ZV, et al: The reliability of vital sign measurements. *Ann Emerg Med*, 39:233, 2002.
70. El Miedany, Y, et al: Clinical diagnosis of carpal tunnel syndrome: old tests—new concepts. *Joint Bone Spine*, 75:451, 2008.
71. Ellis, MR, Griffin, KW, and Meadows, S: For knee pain, how predictive is physical examination for meniscal injury? *J Fam Pract*, 53:918, 2004.
72. Elveru, RA, Rothstein, JM, and Lamb, RL: Goniometric reliability in a clinical setting. *Phys Ther*, 68:672, 1988.
73. Estanol, B, et al: Babinski's sign: statistical validity of a classic sign in medicine. *Neurologica*, 10:307, 1995.
74. Evans, PJ, Bell, GD, and Frank, C: Prospective evaluation of the McMurray test. *Am J Sports Med*, 21:604, 1993.
75. Farber, AJ, et al: Clinical assessment of three common tests for traumatic anterior shoulder instability. *J Bone Joint Surg Am*, 88:1467, 2006.
76. Fertl, E, Wober, C, and Zeitlhofer, J: The serial use of two provocative tests in the clinical diagnosis of carpal tunnel syndrome. *Acta Neurol Scand*, 98:328, 1998.
77. Fitzgerald, GK, and McClure, PW: Reliability of measurements obtained with four tests for patellofemoral alignment. *Phys Ther*, 75:84, 1995.
78. Fjelhner, A, et al: Interexaminer reliability in physical examination of the cervical spine. *J Manipulative Physiol Ther*, 22:511, 1999.
79. Flynn, T, et al: A clinical prediction rule for classifying patients with low back pain who demonstrate short-term improvement with spinal manipulation. *Spine*, 27:2835, 2002.
80. Fodor, D, et al: Shoulder impingment syndrome: correlations between clinical tests and ultrasonographic findings. *Orthop Traumatol Rehabil*, 11:120, 2009.
81. Fowler, EM, et al: Clinical and arthroscopic findings in recreationally active patients. *Sports Med Arthrosc Rehabil Ther Technol*, 2:2, 2010.
82. Fowler, PJ, and Lubliner, JA: The predictive value of five clinical signs in the evaluation of meniscal pathology. *Arthroscopy*, 5:184, 1989.
83. Fowler, PJ, and Messieh, SS: Isolated posterior cruciate ligament injuries in athletes. *Am J Sports Med*, 15:553, 1987.
84. Friends, J, Augustine, E, and Danoff, J: A comparison of different assessment techniques for measuring foot and ankle volume in healthy adults. *J Am Podiatr Med Assoc*, 98:85, 2008.
85. Fritz, JM, et al: Accuracy of the clinical examination to predict radiographic instability of the lumbar spine. *Eur Spine J*, 14:743, 2005.

86. Fritz, JM, Delitto, A, Erhard, RE, and Roman, M: An examination of the selective tissue tension scheme, with evidence for the concept of a capsular pattern of the knee. *Phys Ther*, 78:1046, 1998.
87. Fritz, JM, et al: An examination of the reliability of a classification algorithm for subgrouping patients with low back pain. *Spine*, 31:77, 2006.
88. Gaebler, C, et al: Diagnosis of lateral ankle injuries. *Acta Orthop Scand*, 68:286, 1997.
89. Garvin, GJ, Munk, PL, and Vellet, AD: Tears of the medial collateral ligament: magnetic resonance imaging findings and associated injuries. *Can Assoc Radiol J*, 44:199, 1993.
90. Gellman, H, et al: Carpal tunnel syndrome: an evaluation of the provocative diagnostic tests. *J Bone Joint Surg Am*, 68:735, 1986.
91. Gill, HS, et al: Physical examination for partial tears of the biceps tendon. *Am J Sports Med*, 35:1334, 2007.
92. Gillard, J, et al: Diagnosing thoracic outlet syndrome: contribution of provocative tests, ultrasonography, electrophysiology, and helical computer tomography in 48 patients. *Joint Bone Spine*, 68:416, 2001.
93. Glascoe, WM, et al: Criterion-related validity of a clinical measure of dorsal first ray mobility. *J Orthop Sports Phys Ther*, 35:589, 2005.
94. Gogia, PP, et al: Reliability and validity of goniometric measurements at the knee. *Phys Ther*, 67:192, 1987.
95. Gogus, F, et al, for the American College of Rheumatology, 2008 Scientific Meeting: Reliability of physical knee examination for effusion: verification by musculoskeletal ultrasound (abstract). Retrieved August 25, 2013 from https://acr.confex.com/acr/2008/webprogram/Paper2759.html.
96. Greene, CC: Reliability of the quadriceps angle measurement. *Am J Knee Surg*, 14:97, 2001.
97. Greslsamer, RP: Men and women have similar Q-angles: a clinical and trigometric evaluation. *J Bone Joint Surg Am*, 87:1498, 2005.
98. Guanche, CA, and Jones, DC: Clinical testing for tears of the glenoid labrum. *Arthroscopy*, 19:517, 2003.
99. Guerra, JP, et al: Q-angle: effects of isometric quadriceps contraction and body position. *J Orthop Sports Phys Ther*, 19:200, 1994.
100. Gurdjian, ES, et al: Herniated lumbar intervertebral discs: an analysis of 1,176 operated cases. *J Trauma*, 1:158, 1961.
101. Haim, A, et al: Patellofemoral pain syndrome: validity of clinical and radiological features. *Clin Orthop Rel Res*, 451:69, 2006.
102. Hakelius, A, and Hindmarsh, J: The significance of neurological signs and myelographic findings in the diagnosis of lumbar root compression. *Acta Orthop Scand*, 43:239, 1972.
103. Hanada, E, et al: Measuring leg-length discrepancy by the "iliac crest palpation and book correction" method: reliability and validity. *Arch Phys Med Rehabil*, 82:938, 2001.
104. Hansen, PA, Micklesen, P, and Robinson, LR: Clinical utility of the flick maneuver in diagnosing carpal tunnel syndrome. *Am J Phys Med Rehabil*, 83:363, 2004.
105. Hardaker, WT, Garrett, WE, and Bassett FH: Evaluation of acute traumatic hemarthrosis of the knee joint. *South Med J*, 83:640, 1990.
106. Harilainen, A: Evaluation of knee instability in acute ligamentous injuries. *Ann Chir Gynaecol*, 76:269, 1987.
107. Harrison, BK, Abell, BE, and Gibson, TW: The Thessaly test for detection of meniscal tears: validation of a new physical examination technique for primary care medicine. *Clin J Sport Med*, 19:9, 2009.
108. Hayes, KW, Petersen, C, and Falconer, J: An examination of Cyriax's passive motion tests with patients having osteoarthritis of the knee. *Phys Ther*, 74:697, 1994.
109. Hegedus, EJ, et al: Measures of arch height and their relationship to pain and dysfunction in people with lower limb impairments. *Physiother Res Int*, 15:160, 2010.
110. Hegedus, EJ, et al: Physical examination tests of the shoulder: a systematic review with meta-analysis of individual tests. *Br J Sports Med*, 42:80, 2008 (update 2012).
111. Heiderscheit, B, and Boissonnault, W: Reliability of joint mobility and pain assessment of the thoracic spine and rib cage in asymptomatic individuals. *J Man Manip Ther*, 16:210, 2008.
112. Herrington, L, and Nester, C: Q-angle undervalued? the relationship between Q-angle and medio-lateral position of the patella. *Clin Biomech*, 19:1070, 2004.
113. Hertel, R, et al: Lag signs in the diagnosis of rotator cuff rupture. *J Shoulder Elbow Surg*, 5:307, 1996.
114. Heyman, P, et al: Injuries of the ulnar collateral ligament of the thumb metacarpophalangeal joint: biomechanical and prospective clinical studies on the usefulness of valgus stress testing. *Clin Orthop Relat Res*, Jul:165, 1993.
115. Hicks, GE, et al: The reliability of clinical examination measures used for patients with suspected lumbar instability. *Arch Phys Med Rehabil*, 84:1858, 2003.
116. Hirsch, C, and Nachemson, A: The reliability of lumbar disc surgery. *Clin Orthop*, 29:189, 1963.
117. Hole, DE, et al: Reliability and concurrent validity of two instruments for measuring cervical range of motion: effects of age and gender. *Man Ther*, 1:36, 1995.
118. Holm, I, et al: Reliability of goniometric measurements and visual estimates of hip ROM in patients with osteoarthritis. *Physiother Res Int*, 5:241, 2000.
119. Holtby, R, and Razmjou, H: Accuracy of the Speed's test and Yergason's test in detecting biceps pathology and SLAP lesions: comparison with arthroscopic findings. *Arthroscopy*, 20:231, 2004.
120. Horger, MM: The reliability of goniometric measurements of active and passive wrist motions. *Am J Occup Ther*, 44:342, 1990.
121. Horneij, E, et al: Clinical tests on impairment level related to low back pain: a study of test reliability. *J Rehabil Med*, 34:176, 2002.
122. Hoving, JL, et al: Reproducibility of cervical range of motion in patients with neck pain. *BMC Musculoskelet Disord*, 6:59, 2005.
123. Hughston, JC, et al: Classification of knee ligament instabilities. I. the medial compartment and cruciate ligaments. *J Bone Joint Surg Am*, 58:159, 1976.
124. Hunt, DG, et al: Reliability of the lumbar flexion, lumbar extension, and passive straight-leg raise test in normal populations embedded within a complete physical examination. *Spine*, 26:2714, 2001.
125. Itoi, E, et al: Which is more useful, the "full can test" or the "empty can test" in detecting the torn supraspinatus tendon? *Am J Sports Med*, 27:65-68, 1999.
126. Jackson, JL, O'Malley, PG, and Kroenke, K: Evaluation of acute knee pain in primary care. *Ann Intern Med*, 139:575, 2003.
127. Jai, X, et al: Examination of the shoulder: the past, the present, and the future. *J Bone Joint Surg Am*, 91(Suppl 6):10, 2009.
128. Johansson, K, and Ivarson, S: Intra- and interexaminer reliability of four manual shoulder maneuvers used to identify subacromial pain. *Man Ther*, 14:231, 2009.
129. Jonson, SR, and Gross, MT: Intraexaminer reliability, interexaminer reliability, and mean values for nine lower extremity skeletal measures in healthy naval shipmen. *J Orthop Sports Phys Ther*, 25:253, 1997.
130. Jonsson, B, and Stromqvist, B: The straight-leg raising test and the severity of symptoms in lumbar disc herniation: a preoperative evaluation. *Spine*, 20:27, 1995.
131. Jonsson, T, et al: Clinical diagnosis of ruptures of the anterior cruciate ligament: a comparative study of the Lachman test and the anterior drawer sign. *Am J Sports Med*, 10:100, 1982.

132. Karachalios, T, et al: Diagnostic accuracy of a new clinical test (the Thessaly test) for early detection of meniscal tears. *J Bone Joint Surg Am*, 87:955, 2005.
133. Karagiannopoulos, C, et al: Reliability of two functional goniometric methods for measuring forearm pronation and supination active range of motion. *J Orthop Sports Phys Ther*, 33:523, 2003.
134. Kastelein, M, et al: Assessing medial collateral ligament knee lesions in general practice. *Am J Med*, 121:982, 2008.
135. Kastelein, M, et al: Diagnostic value of history taking and physical examination to assess effusion of the knee in traumatic knee patients in general practice. *Arch Phys Med Rehabil*, 90:82, 2009.
136. Katz, JN, et al: The carpal tunnel syndrome: diagnostic utility of the history and physical examination findings. *Ann Intern Med*, 112:321, 1990.
137. Katz, JG, and Fingeroth, RJ: The diagnostic accuracy of ruptures of the anterior cruciate ligament comparing the Lachman test, the anterior drawer sign, and the pivot shift test in acute and chronic knee injuries. *Am J Sports Med*, 14:88, 1986.
138. Keeney, JA, et al: Magnetic resonance arthrography versus arthroscopy in the evaluation of articular hip pathology. *Clin Orthop Relat Res*, 6:163, 2004.
139. Kelly, SM, Brittle, K, and Allen, GM: The value of physical tests for subacromial impingement syndrome: a study of diagnostic accuracy. *Clin Rehabil*, 24:149, 2010.
140. Kerr, RS, et al: The value of accurate clinical assessment in the surgical management of the lumbar disc protrusion. *J Neurol Neurosurg Psychiatry*, 51:169, 1988.
141. Kibler, WB, et al: Clinical utility of traditional and new tests in the diagnosis of biceps tendon injuries and superior labrum anterior and posterior lesions in the shoulder. *Am J Sports Med*, 37:1840, 2009.
142. Kibler, WB: Specificity and sensitivity of the anterior slide test in throwing athletes with superior glenoid labral tears. *Arthroscopy*, 11:296, 1995.
143. Kim, TK, et al: Clinical features of the different types of SLAP lesions: an analysis of 139 cases. *J Bone Joint Surg Am*, 85:66, 2003.
144. Kim, SH, Ha, KI, and Han, KY: Biceps load test: a clinical test for superior labrum anterior and posterior lesions in shoulders with recurrent anterior dislocations. *Am J Sports Med*, 27:300, 1999.
145. Kim, SJ, and Kim, HK: Reliability of the anterior drawer test, the pivot shift test, and the Lachman test. *Clin Orthop*, 317:237, 1995.
146. Kinoshita, M, et al: The dorsiflexion-eversion test for diagnosis of tarsal tunnel syndrome. *J Bone Joint Surg Am*, 83:1835, 2001.
147. Klassbo, M, et al: Examination of passive ROM and capsular patterns in the hip. *Physiother Res Int*, 5:241, 2003.
148. Knutsson, B: Comparative value of electromyographic, myelographic, and clinical-neurological examination in diagnosis of lumbar root compression syndrome. *Acta Orthop Scand*, 49(S):1, 1961.
149. Kocabey, Y, et al: The value of clinical examination versus magnetic resonance imaging in the diagnosis of meniscal tears and anterior cruciate ligament rupture. *Arthroscopy*, 20:696, 2004.
150. Kokmeyer, DJ, et al: The reliability of multitest regimens with sacroiliac pain provocation tests. *J Manipulative Physiol Ther*, 25:42, 2002.
151. Kosteljanetz, M, et al: Predictive value of clinical and surgical findings in patients with lumbago-sciatica: a prospective study. *Acta Neurochir*, 73:67, 1984.
152. Kosteljanetz, M, et al: The clinical significance of straight-leg raising (Lasegue's sign) in the diagnosis of prolapsed lumbar disc: interobserver variation and correlation with surgical finding. *Spine*, 13:393, 1988.
153. Kuhlman, KA, and Hennessey, WJ: Sensitivity and specificity of carpal tunnel syndrome signs. *Am J Phys Med Rehabil*, 76:451, 1997.
154. Kurosaka, M, et al: Efficacy of the axially loaded pivot shift test for the diagnosis of a meniscal tear. *Int Orthop*, 23:271, 1999.
155. Kuschner, SH, et al: Tinel's sign and Phalen's test in carpal tunnel syndrome. *Orthopedics*, 15:1297, 1992.
156. LaJoie, AS, et al: Determining the sensitivity and specificity of common diagnostic tests for carpal tunnel syndrome using latent class analysis. *Plast Reconstr Surg*, 116:502, 2005.
157. Laslett, M, and Williams, M: The reliability of selected pain provocation tests for sacroiliac joint pathology. *Spine*, 19:1243, 1994.
158. Laslett, M, et al: Diagnosis of sacroiliac joint pain: validity of individual provocation tests and composites of tests. *Man Ther*, 10:207, 2005.
159. LaStayo, P, and Howell, J: Clinical provocative tests used in evaluating wrist pain: a descriptive study. *J Hand Ther*, 8:10, 1995.
160. Latimer, J, et al: The reliability and validity of the Biering-Sorensen test in asymptomatic subjects and subjects reporting current or previous nonspecific low back pain. *Spine*, 24:2085, 1999.
161. Lee, JK, et al: Anterior cruciate ligament tears: MR imaging compared with arthroscopy and clinical tests. *Radiology*, 166:861, 1988.
162. Lenssen, AF, et al: Reproducibility of goniometric measurement of the knee in the in-hospital phase following total knee arthroplasty. *BMC Musculoskelet Disord*, 8:83, 2007.
163. Lequesne, M, et al: Gluteal tendinopathy in refractory greater trochanter pain syndrome: diagnostic value of two clinical tests. *Arthritis Rheum*, 59:241, 2008.
164. Lerat, JL, et al: Dynamic anterior jerk of the shoulder: a new clinical test for shoulder instability: preliminary study. *Rev Chir Orthop Reparatrice Appar Mot*, 80:461, 1994.
165. Leroux, JL, et al: Diagnostic value of clinical tests for shoulder impingement syndrome. *Rev Rheum Engl Ed*, 62:423, 1995.
166. Lesher, JD, et al: Development of a clinical prediction rule for classifying patients with patellofemoral pain syndrome who respond to patellar taping. *J Orthop Sports Phys Ther*, 36:854, 2006.
167. Leunig, M, et al: Evaluation of the acetabular labrum by MR arthrography. *J Bone Joint Surg Br*, 79:230, 1997.
168. Lindstrom-Hazel, D, et al: Interrater reliability of students using hand and pinch dynamometers. *Am J Occup Ther*, 63:193, 2009.
169. Liu, SH, et al: The diagnosis of acute complete tears of the anterior cruciate ligament: comparison of MRI, arthrometry and clinical examination. *J Bone Joint Surg Br*, 77:586, 1995.
170. Liu, SH, Henry, MH, and Nuccion, SL. A prospective evaluation of a new physical examination in predicting glenoid labral tears. *Am J Sports Med*, 24:721, 1996.
171. Lo, IK, et al: An evaluation of the apprehension, relocation, and surprise tests for anterior shoulder instability. *Am J Sports Med*, 32:301, 2004.
172. Loos, WC, et al: Acute posterior cruciate ligament injuries. *Am J Sports Med*, 9:86, 1981.
173. Lucie, RS, Wiedel, JD, and Messner, DG: The acute pivot shift: clinical correlation. *Am J Sports Med*, 12:189, 1984.
174. Luime, JJ, et al: Does this patient have an instability of the shoulder or a labrum lesion? *JAMA*, 292:1989, 2004.
175. MacDermid, JC, and Wessel, J: Clinical diagnosis of carpal tunnel syndrome: a systematic review. *J Hand Ther*, 17:309, 2004.
176. MacDonald, PB, Clark, P, and Sutherland, K: An analysis of the diagnostic accuracy of the Hawkins and Neer subacromial impingement signs. *J Shoulder Elbow Surg*, 9:299, 2000.
177. Maffulli, N: The clinical diagnosis of subcutaneous tear of the Achilles tendon: a prospective study in 174 patients. *Am J Sports Med*, 26:266, 1998.
178. Maher, C, and Adams, R: Reliability of pain and stiffness assessments in clinical manual lumbar spine examination. *Phys Ther*, 7:801, 1999.
179. Majlesi, J, et al: The sensitivity and specificity of the slump and straight-leg raising tests in patients with lumbar disc herniation. *J Clin Rheumatol*, 14:87, 2008.
180. Malanga, GA, Landes, P, and Nadler, SF: Provocative tests in cervical spine examination: historical basis and scientific analysis. *Pain Physician*, 6:199, 2003.

181. Martin, RL, and Sekiya, JK: The interrater reliability of four clinical tests used to assess individuals with musculoskeletal hip pain. *J Orthop Sports Phys Ther*, 38:71, 2008.
182. Masci, L, et al: Use of the one-legged hyperextension test and magnetic resonance imaging in the diagnosis of active spondylolysis. *Br J Sports Med*, 40:940, 2006.
183. Maslowski, E, et al: The diagnostic validity of hip provocation maneuvers to detect intra-articular hip pathology. *PMR*, 2:174, 2010.
184. Mawdsley, RH, Hoy, DK, and Erwin, PM: Criterion-related validity of the figure-8 method of measuring ankle edema. *J Orthop Sports Phys Ther*, 30:149, 2000.
185. McCarthy, J, and Busconi, B: The role of hip arthroscopy in the diagnosis and treatment of hip disease. *Can J Surg*, 38(Suppl 1):S13, 1995.
186. McClure, PW, Rothstein, JM, and Riddle, DL: Intertester reliability of clinical judgments of medial knee ligament integrity. *Phys Ther*, 69:268, 1989.
187. McFarland, EG, Kim, TK, and Savino, RM: Clinical assessment of three common tests for superior labral anterior posterior lesions. *Am J Sports Med*, 30:810, 2002.
188. McFarland, EG: *Examination of the Shoulder: The Complete Guide*. New York: Thieme Medical Publishers, Inc., 2006. Data from the Johns Hopkins University Shoulder Database.
189. Mellin, G: Measurement of thoracolumbar posture and mobility with a Myrin inclinometer. *Spine*, 11:759, 1986.
190. Meserve, BB, Cleland, JA, and Boucher, TR: A meta-analysis examining clinical test utilities for assessing meniscal injury. *Clin Rehabil*, 22:143, 2008.
191. Michener, LA, et al: Reliability and diagnostic accuracy of five physical examination tests and combination of tests for subacromial impingement. *Arch Phys Med Rehabil*, 90:1898, 2009.
192. Miller, TM, and Johnston, SC: Should the Babinski sign be part of the routine neurologic examination? *Neurology*, 25:1165, 2005.
193. Miller, CA, Gorrester, GA, and Lewis, JS: The validity of the lag signs in diagnosing full-thickness tears of the rotator cuff: a preliminary investigation. *Arch Phys Med Rehabil*, 89:1162, 2008.
194. Mitchell, B, et al: Hip joint pathology: clinical presentation and correlation between magnetic resonance arthrography, ultrasound, and arthroscopic findings in 25 consecutive cases. *Clin J Sports Med*, 13:152, 2003.
195. Mitsou, A, and Vallianatos, P: Clinical diagnosis of ruptures of the anterior cruciate ligament: a comparison between the Lachman test and the anterior drawer sign. *Injury*, 19:247, 1988.
196. Moore, JA, and Larson, RL: Posterior cruciate ligament injuries: results of early surgical repair. *Am J Sports Med*, 8:86, 1980.
197. Morgan, CD, et al: Type II SLAP lesions: three subtypes and their relationships to superior instability and rotator cuff tears. *Arthroscopy*, 14:553, 1998.
198. Murrell, GA, and Walton, JR: Diagnosis of rotator cuff tears. *Lancet*, 357:769, 2001.
199. Myers, TH, Zemanovic, JR, and Andrews, JR: The resisted supination external rotation test: a new test for the diagnosis of superior labral anterior posterior lesions. *Am J Sports Med*, 3:1315, 2005.
200. Nakagawa, S, et al: Forced shoulder abduction and elbow flexion test: a new simple clinical test to detect superior labral injury in the throwing athlete. *Arthroscopy*, 22:1290, 2005.
201. Narvani, AA, et al: A preliminary report on prevalence of acetabular labrum tears in sports patients with groin pain. *Knee Surg Sports Traumatol Arthrosc*, 11:403, 2003.
202. Nashlund J, et al: Comparison of symptoms and clinical findings in subgroups of individuals with patellofemoral pain. *Physiother Theory Pract*, 22:105, 2006.
203. Neelly, K, Wallmann, HW, and Backus, CJ: Validity of measuring leg length with a tape measure compared to a computed tomography scan. *Physiother Theory Pract*, 29:487, 2013.
204. Ng, KG, et al: Range of motion and lordosis of the lumbar spine: reliability of measurement and normative values. *Spine*, 26:53, 2001.
205. Nijs, J, et al: Diagnostic value of five clinical tests in patellofemoral pain syndrome. *Man Ther*, 11:69, 2006.
206. Niskanen, RO, et al: Poor correlation of clinical signs with patellar cartilaginous changes. *Arthroscopy*, 17:307, 2010.
207. Noble, J, and Erat, K: In defence of the meniscus: a prospective study of 200 menisecectomy patients. *J Bone Joint Surg Br*, 62:B7, 1980.
208. Noyes, F, et al: Arthroscopy in acute traumatic hemarthrosis of the knee. *J Bone Joint Surg Am*, 62:687, 1980.
209. O'Driscoll, SWM, Lawton, RL, and Smith, AM: The "moving valgus stress test" for medial collateral ligament tears of the elbow. *Am J Sports Med*, 33:231, 2005.
210. O'Brien, SJ, et al: The active compression test: a new and effective test for diagnosing labral tears and acromioclavicular joint abnormality. *Am J Sports Med*, 26:610, 1983.
211. Oh, JH, et al: The evaluation of various physical examinations for the diagnosis of type II superior labrum anterior and posterior lesion. *Am J Sports Med*, 36:353, 2008.
212. Ostrowski, JA: Accuracy of three diagnostic tests for anterior cruciate ligament tears. *J Athl Train*, 41:120, 2006.
213. Ozgocmen, S, et al: The value of sacroiliac pain provocation tests in early active sacroiliitis. *Clin Rheumatol*, 10:1275, 2008.
214. Paatelma, M, et al: Clinical perspective: how do clinical test results differentiate between chronic and subacute pain patients from "nonpatients"? *J Man Manip Ther*, 17:11, 2009.
215. Pakarinen, H, et al: Intraoperative assessment of the stability of the distal tibiofibular joint in supination-external rotation injuries of the ankle sensitivity, specificity, and reliability of two clinical tests. *J Bone Joint Surg Am*, 93:2057, 2011.
216. Parentis, MA, Mohr, KJ, and El Attrache, NS: Disorders of the superior labrum: review and treatment guidelines. *Clin Orthop Relat Res*, 77, July 2002.
217. Parentis, MA, et al: An evaluation of the provocative tests for superior labral anterior posterior lesions. *Am J Sports Med*, 34:265, 2006.
218. Parentis, MA, Mohr, KJ, and El Attrache, NS: Disorders of the superior labrum: review and treatment guidelines. *Clin Orthop Relat Res*, 77, July 2002.
219. Park, HB, et al: Diagnostic accuracy of clinical tests for the different degrees of subacromial impingement syndrome. *J Bone Joint Surg Am*, 87:1446, 2005.
220. Petersen, EJ, et al: Reliability of water volumetry and the figure of eight method on subjects with ankle joint swelling. *J Orthop Sports Phys Ther*, 29:609, 1999.
221. Petra, M, et al: Lumbar range of motion: reliability and validity of the inclinometer technique in the clinical measurement of trunk flexibility. *Spine*, 21:1332, 1996.
222. Picciano, AM, Rowlands, MS, and Worrell, T: Reliability of open and closed kinetic chain subtalar joint neutral positions and navicular drop test. *J Orthop Sport Phys Ther*, 18:553, 1993.
223. Piva, SR, et al: Reliability of measures of impairments associated with patellofemoral pain syndrome. *BMC Musculoskelet Disord*, 7:33, 2006.
224. Piva, SR, et al: Intertester reliability of passive intervertebral and active movements of the cervical spine. *Man Ther*, 11:321, 2006.
225. Piva, SR, Goodnite, EA, and Childs, JD: Strength around the hip and flexibility of soft tissues in individuals with and without patellofemoral pain syndrome. *J Orthop Sports Phys Ther*, 35:793, 2005.
226. Plewa, MC, and Delinger, M: The false-positive rate of thoracic outlet syndrome shoulder maneuvers in healthy subjects. *Acad Emerg Med*, 5:337, 1998.
227. Porchet, F, et al: Extreme lateral lumbar disc herniation: clinical presentation in 178 patients. *Acta Neurochir*, 127:203, 1994.

228. Prather, H, et al: Hip range of motion and provocative physical examination tests reliability and agreement in asymptomatic volunteers. *PMR*, 2:888, 2010.

229. Prosser, R, et al: Provocative wrist tests and MRI are of limited diagnostic value for suspected wrist ligament injuries: a cross-sectional study. *J Physiother*, 57:247, 2011.

230. Raatikainen, T, et al: Arthrography, clinical examination, and stress radiograph in the diagnosis of acute injury to the lateral ligaments of the ankle. *Am J Sports Med*, 20:2, 1992.

231. Raney, NH, et al: Development of a clinical prediction rule to identify patients with neck pain likely to benefit from cervical traction and exercise. *Eur Spine J*, 3:382, 2009.

232. Reese, NB, and Bandy, WD: Use of an inclinometer to measure flexibility of the iliotibial band using the Ober test and modified Ober test: differences in the magnitude and reliability of measurements. *J Orthop Sports Phys Ther*, 33:326, 2003.

233. Regan, W, and Lapner PC: Prospective evaluation of two diagnostic apprehension tests for posterolateral instability of the elbow. *J Elbow Surg*, 15:344, 2006.

234. Reynolds, PMG: Measurement of spinal mobility: a comparison of three methods. *Rheumatol Rehabil*, 14:180, 1975.

235. Richter, RR, and Reinking, MF: How does evidence on the diagnostic accuracy of the vertebral artery test influence teaching of the test in a professional physical therapist education program? *Phys Ther*, 85:589, 2005.

236. Robinson, HS, et al: The reliability of selected motion- and pain-provocation tests for the sacroiliac joint. *Man Ther*, 12:72, 2007.

237. Rohner-Spengler, M, Mannion, AF, and Babst, R: Reliability and minimal detectable change for the figure-of-eight-20 method of measurement of ankle edema. *J Ortho Sports Phys Ther*, 37:199, 2007.

238. Rondon, CA, et al: Observer agreement in the measurement of leg length. *Rev Invest Clin*, 44:85, 1992.

239. Rose, MJ: The statistical analysis of the intraobserver repeatability of four clinical measurement techniques. *Physiotherapy*, 77:89, 1991.

240. Rothstein, JM, Miller, PJ, and Roettger, RF: Goniometeric reliability in a clinical setting: elbow and knee measurements. *Phys Ther*, 63:1611, 1983.

241. Roussel, NA, et al: Low back pain: clinimetric properties of the Trendelenburg test, active straight-leg raise test, and breathing pattern during active straight-leg raising. *J Manipulative Physiol Ther*, 30:270, 2007.

242. Rubinstein, RA, et al: The accuracy of the clinical examination in the setting of posterior cruciate ligament injuries. *Am J Sports Med*, 22:550, 1994.

243. Salerno, DF, et al: Reliability of physical examination of the upper extremity among keyboard operators. *Am J Ind Med*, 37:423, 2000.

244. Sallay, PI, et al: Acute dislocation of the patella: a correlative pathoanatomic study. *Am J Sports Med*, 24:52, 1996.

245. Saltzman, CL, Nawoczenski, DA, and Talbot, KD: Measurement of the medial longitudinal arch. *Arch Phys Med Rehabil*, 76:45, 1995.

246. Sandmark, H, and Nisell, R: Validity of five common manual neck pain provoking tests. *Scand J Rehabil Med*, 27:131, 1995.

247. Schlechter, JA, Summa, S, and Rubin, BD: The passive distraction test: a new diagnostic aid for clinically significant superior labral pathology. *Arthroscopy*, 25:1374, 2009.

248. Schneider, M, et al: Spinal palpation for lumbar segmental mobility and pain provocation: an interexaminer reliability study. *J Manipulative Physiol Ther*, 31:465, 2008.

249. Scholten, RJPM, et al: Accuracy of physical diagnostic tests for assessing ruptures of the anterior cruciate ligament: a meta-analysis. *J Fam Pract*, 52:689, 2003.

250. Schreuders, TAR, et al: Measurement error in grip and pinch force measurements in patients with hand injuries. *Phys Ther*, 83:806, 2003.

251. Schultz S, et al: Intratester and intertester reliability of clinical measures of lower extremity anatomic characteristics: implications for multi-center studies. *Clin J Sport Med*, 16:155, 2006.

252. Sell, KE, et al: Two measurement techniques for assessing subtalar joint position: a reliability study. *J Orthop Sports Phys Ther*, 19:162, 1994.

253. Seung-Ho, K, et al: The Kim test: a novel test for posteroinferior labral lesion of the shoulder—a comparison to the jerk test. *Am J Sports Med*, 33:1188, 2005.

254. Shah, KC, and Rajshekhar, V: Reliability of diagnosis of soft tissue disc prolapse using Spurling's test. *Br J Neurosurg*, 18:480, 2004.

255. Shultz, SJ, et al: Intratester and intertester reliability of clinical measures of lower extremity anatomic characteristics: implications for multicenter studies. *Clin J Sport Med*, 16:155, 2006.

256. Simerville, JA, Maxted, WC, and Pahira, JJ: Urinalysis: a comprehensive review. *Am Fam Physician*, 71:1153, 2005.

257. Sink, EL, et al: Clinical presentation of femoroacetabular impingement in adolescents. *J Pediatr Orthop*, 28:806, 2008.

258. Smith, CK, et al: Interrater reliability of physical examinations in a prospective study of upper extremity musculoskeletal disorders. *J Occup Environ Med*, 52:1014, 2010.

259. Snyder, SJ, et al: SLAP lesions of the shoulder. *Arthroscopy*, 6:274, 1990.

260. Soderberg, GL, Ballantyne, BT, and Kestel, LL: Reliability of lower extremity girth measurements after anterior cruciate ligament reconstruction. *Physiother Res Int*, 1:7, 1996.

261. Somers, DL, et al: The influence of experience on the reliability of goniometric and visual measurements of forefoot position. *J Orthop Sports Phys Ther*, 25:192, 1997.

262. Spangfort, EV: The lumbar disc herniation: a computer-aided analysis of 2,504 operations. *Acta Orthop Scand*, 142:5, 1972.

263. Speer, KP, et al: An evaluation of the shoulder relocation test. *Am J Sports Med*, 22:177, 1994.

264. Staes, FF, et al: Reliability of accessory motion testing at the carpal joints. *Man Ther*, 14:292, 2009.

265. Steiner, ME, et al: Measurement of anterior–posterior displacement of the knee. *J Bone Joint Surg Am*, 72:1307, 1990.

266. Stetson, WB, and Templin, K: The crank test, the O'Brien test, and routine magnetic resonance imaging scans in the diagnosis of labral tears. *Am J Sports Med*, 30:806, 2002.

267. Strender, L, et al: Interexaminer reliability in physical examination of patients with low back pain. *Spine*, 22:814, 1997.

268. Suri, P, et al: The accuracy of the physical examination for the diagnosis of midlumbar and low lumbar nerve root impingement. *Spine*, 36:63, 2011.

269. Sutlive, TG, et al: Development of a clinical prediction rule for diagnosing hip osteoarthritis in individuals with unilateral hip pain. *J Orthop Sports Phys Ther*, 38:542, 2008.

270. Sweitzer, BA, et al: The interrater reliability and diagnostic accuracy of patellar mobility tests in patients with anterior knee pain. *Phys Sportsmed*, 38:90, 2010.

271. Tatro-Adams, D, McGann, SF, and Carbone, W: Reliability of the figure-of-eight method of ankle measurement. *J Orthop Sports Phys Ther*, 22:161, 1995.

272. Terry, MA, et al: Measurement variance in limb length discrepancy: clinical and radiographic assessment of interobserver and intraobserver variability. *J Pediatr Orthop*, 25:197, 2005.

273. Tetro, AM, et al: A new provocative test for carpal tunnel syndrome: assessment of wrist flexion and nerve compression. *J Bone Joint Surg Br*, 80:493, 1998.

274. Tidstrand, J, and Homeij, E: Interrater reliability of three standardized functional tests in patients with low back pain. *BMC Musculoskelet Disord*, 2:10, 2009.

275. Timmerman, LA, et al: Preoperative evaluation of the ulnar collateral ligament by magnetic resonance imaging and computed tomography arthrography. *Am J Sports Med*, 22:26, 1994.
276. Tomsich, DA, et al: Patellofemoral alignment: reliability. *J Orthop Sports Phys Ther*, 23:200, 1996.
277. Tong, HC, et al: The Spurling test and cervical radiculopathy. *Spine*, 27:156, 2002.
278. Torg, JS, Conrad, W, and Kalen, V: Clinical diagnosis of anterior cruciate ligament instability in the athlete. *Am J Sports Med*, 4:84, 1976.
279. Troelsen, A, et al: What is the role of clinical tests and ultrasound in acetabular labral tear diagnostics? *Acta Orthopaedica*, 80:314, 2009.
280. Tucker, N, et al: Reliability and measurement error of active knee extension range of motion in a modified slump test position: a pilot study. *J Man Manip Ther*, 15:E85, 2007.
281. Tzannes, A, and Murrell, GAC: Clinical examination of the unstable shoulder. *Sports Med*, 32:447, 2002.
282. van der Wurff, P, et al: Clinical tests of the sacroiliac joint: a systematic methodological review. 1: reliability. *Man Ther*, 5:30, 2000.
283. van Dijk, CN, et al: Diagnosis of ligament rupture of the ankle joint. physical examination, arthrography, stress radiography and sonography compared in 160 patients after inversion trauma. *Acta Orthop Scand*, 67:566, 1996.
284. van Dijk, CN, et al: Physical examination is sufficient for the diagnosis of sprained ankles. *J Bone Joint Surg Br*, 78:958, 1996.
285. Van Gheluwe, B: Reliability and accuracy of biomechanical measurements of the lower extremities. *J Am Podiatr Med Assoc*, 92:317, 2002.
286. Vela, L, Tourville, TW, and Hertel, J: Physical examination of acutely injured ankles: an evidence-based approach. *Athl Ther Today*, 8:13, 2003.
287. Viikari-Juntura, E, et al: Standardized physical examination protocol for low back disorders: feasibility of use and validity of symptoms and signs. *J Clin Epidemiol*, 51:245, 1998.
288. Viikari-Juntura, E, et al: Validity of clinical tests in the diagnosis of root compression in cervical disease. *Spine*, 14:253, 1989.
289. Viikari-Juntura, E: Interexaminer reliability of observations in physical examinations of the neck. *Phys Ther*, 67:1526, 1987.
290. Vinicombe, A, Raspovic, A, and Menz, HB: Reliability of navicular displacement measurement as a clinical indicator of foot posture. *J Am Podiatr Med Assoc*, 91:262, 2001.
291. Vroomen, PC, et al: Consistency of history taking and physical examination in patients with suspected lumbar nerve root involvement. *Spine*, 25:91, 2000.
292. Wainner, RS, et al: Reliability and diagnostic accuracy of the clinical examination and patient self-report measures for cervical radiculopathy. *Spine*, 28:52, 2003.
293. Wainner, RS, et al: Development of a clinical prediction rule for the diagnosis of carpal tunnel syndrome. *Arch Phys Med Rehabil*, 86:609, 2005.
294. Wainner, RS, and Gill H: Diagnosis and nonoperative management of cervical radiculpathy. *J Orthop Sports Phys Ther*, 30:728, 2000.
295. Walsworth, MK, et al: Reliability and diagnostic accuracy of history and physical examination for diagnosing glenoid labral tears. *Am J Sports Med*, 36:162, 2007.
296. Walton, J, et al: Diagnostic values of tests for acromioclavicular joint pain. *J Bone Joint Surg Am*, 86:801, 2004.
297. Watkins, MS, et al: Reliability of goniometric measurements and visual estimates of knee range of motions obtained in a clinical setting. *Phys Ther*, 71: 90, 1991.
298. Watson, CJ, et al: Reliability of McConnell's classification of patellar orientation in symptomatic and asymptomatic subjects. *J Orthop Sports Phys Ther*, 29:378, 1999.
299. Williams, TM, et al: Verification of the pressure provocative test in carpal tunnel syndrome. *Ann Plast Surg*, 29:8, 1992.
300. Winters, MV, et al: Passive versus active stretching of hip flexor muscles in subjects with limited hip extension: a randomized clinical trial. *Phys Ther*, 84:800, 2004.
301. Wood, L, et al: A study of noninstrumented physical examination of the knee found high observer variability. *J Clin Epidemiol*, 59:512, 2006.
302. Woodley, SJ, et al: Lateral hip pain: findings from magnetic resonance imaging and clinical examination. *J Orthop Sports Phys Ther*, 38:313, 2008.
303. Yawn BP, et al: A population-based study of school scoliosis screening. *JAMA*, 282:1427, 1999.
304. Yen, K, et al: Interexaminer reliability in physical examination of pediatric patients with abdominal pain. *Arch Pediatr Adolesc Med*, 159:373, 2005.
305. Youdas, JW, et al: Reliability of goniometric measurements and visual estimates of ankle joint range of motion obtained in a clinical setting. *Arch Phys Med Rehabil*, 74:1113, 1993.
306. Youdas, JW, Madson, TJ, and Hollman, JH: Usefulness of the Trendelenburg test for identification of patients with hip joint osteoarthritis. *Physiother Theory Pract*, 26:184, 2010.

Index

Note: The letter b indicates content appears in a box on the cited page. The letter f indicates a figure and the letter t indicates a table.

D

M

N

O

P

S

T

U